Childhood asthma and other wheezing disorders

Childhood asthma and other wheezing disorders

Second edition

Edited by

Michael Silverman
Professor and Head
Department of Child Health and
Institute for Lung Health
University of Leicester
Leicester, UK

ARNOLD

A member of the Hodder Headline Group
LONDON

First published in Great Britain in 2002 by
Arnold, a member of the Hodder Headline Group,
338 Euston Road, London NW1 3BH

http://www.arnoldpublishers.com

Co-published in the United States of America by
Oxford University Press Inc.,
198 Madison Avenue, New York, NY10016
Oxford is a registered trademark of Oxford University Press

Whilst the advice and information in this book are believed to be
true and accurate at the date of going to press, neither the
author[s] nor the publisher can accept any legal responsibility
or liability for any errors or omissions that may be made.
In particular (but without limiting the generality of the preceding
disclaimer) every effort has been made to check drug dosages;
however it is still possible that errors have been missed.
Furthermore, dosage schedules are constantly being revised and
new side-effects recognized. For these reasons the reader is
strongly urged to consult the drug companies' printed
instructions before administering any of the drugs recommended
in this book.

British Library Cataloguing in Publication Data
A catalogue record for this book is available from the
British Library

Library of Congress Cataloging-in-Publication Data
A catalog record for this book is available from the
Library of Congress

ISBN 0 340 76318 3 (hb)

1 2 3 4 5 6 7 8 9 10

Commissioning Editor: Joanna Koster
Production Editor: James Rabson
Production Controller: Bryan Eccleshall
Cover Designer: Terry Griffiths

Typeset in 10/12 Minion by Charon Tec Pvt Ltd., Chennai, India
Printed and bound in Great Britain by The Bath Press

What do you think about this book? Or any other Arnold title?
Please send your comments to feedback.arnold@hodder.co.uk

Contents

List of contributors

John Alexander
Paediatric Intensive Care Unit, North Staffordshire Hospital, Stoke on Trent, Staffordshire, UK

Ian Balfour-Lynn
Consultant in Paediatric Respiratory Medicine, Royal Brompton & Harefield NHS Trust, London, UK

Hans Bisgaard
National University Hospital, Rigshospitalet, Copenhagen, Denmark

Isobel M Brookes
Department of Child Health, University of Leicester, Leicester Royal Infirmary, Leicester, UK

KN Chan
Specialist in Paediatrics, St Paul's Hospital, Hong Kong

Jonathan M Couriel
Consultant in Paediatric, The Respiratory Unit, Royal Liverpool Children's Hospital, Alder Hey, Liverpool, UK

Isi Dab
Kinderpneumologie, Academisch Ziekenhuis, Free University of Brussels, Brussels, Belgium

Robert Dinwiddie
Consultant Paediatrician, Respiratory Medicine Unit, Great Ormond Street Hospital, London, UK

Felicity S Flack
Division of Clinical Sciences, Institute for Child Health Research, Princess Margaret Hospital for Children, West Perth, Western Australia

Jonathan Grigg
Department of Child Health, University of Leicester, Leicester Royal Infirmary, Leicester, UK

Per A Gustafsson
Division of Child and Adolescent Psychiatry, Linkoping University Hospital, Linkoping, Sweden

Alison A Hislop
Department of Cardiology, Institute of Child Health, London, UK

Patrick G Holt
Head, Division of Cell Biology, Institute for Child Health Research, Princess Margaret Hospital for Children, Perth, Western Australia

Yoji Ikura
Department of Paediatrics, Showa University School of Medicine, Shinagawa-ku, Tokyo, Japan

Peter K Jeffery
Lung Pathology Unit (Department of Gene Therapy), ICSM at Royal Brompton Hospital, London, UK

Kevin Jones
Senior Lecturer, Department of Primary Health Care, School of Health Sciences, The Medical School, Newcastle-upon-Tyne, UK

Michael Kabesch
Respiratory Sciences Center, College of Medicine, Tucson, Arizona, USA

Jennifer M Knight-Madden
Sickle Cell Unit, University of West Indies, Mona, Kingston, Jamaica

Carlos D Kofman
Respiratory Center, Ricardo Gutiérrez Children's Hospital, Buenos Aires, Argentina

Bryan Lask
Department of Psychiatry, St George's Hospital Medical School, London, UK

Warren Lenney
Academic Department of Child Health, North Staffordshire Hospital, Stoke on Trent, Staffordshire, UK

Anne Malfroot
Kinderpneumologie, Academisch Ziekenhuis, Free University of Brussels, Brussels, Belgium

Fernando D Martinez
Respiratory Sciences Center, College of Medicine, Tucson, Arizona, USA

Sheila McKenzie
Queen Elizabeth Children's Services, Royal London Hospital, London, UK

Anne Milner
Professor of Clinical Respiratory Physiology, Department of Child Health, King's College Hospital, London, UK

Anthony D Milner
Professor of Neonatology, Department of Paediatrics, St Thomas' Hospital, London, UK

Erica von Mutius
University Children's Hospital, Munchen, Germany

S Noel Narayanan
Professor and Head, Department of Paediatrics, Paediatric Pulmonologist, SAT Hospital Medical College, Trivandrum, Kerala, India

Christopher L O'Callaghan
Professor of Paediatrics, Department of Child Health and Institute for Lung Health, University of Leicester, Leicester, UK

Peter JM Openshaw
Professor of Experimental Medicine and Honorary Consultant, National Heart & Lung Institute, Imperial College School of Medicine, London, UK

Liesl M Osman
Senior Research Fellow, Chest Clinic, Aberdeen Royal Infirmary, Aberdeen, UK

Mustafa Osman
Department of Child Health, Medical School, Aberdeen, UK

Hitesh C Pandya
Department of Child Health, University of Leicester, Leicester Royal Infirmary, Leicester, UK

James Y Paton
Senior Lecturer in Paediatric Respiratory Disease, and Consultant Paediatrician, Department of Child Health, Royal Hospital for Sick Children, Glasgow, UK

Søren Pedersen
Department of Paediatrics, Kolding Hospital, Kolding, Denmark

John F Price
Department of Child Health, King's College Hospital, London, UK

William R Roche
Department of Pathology, Southampton General Hospital, Southampton, UK

George Russell
Consultant Paediatrician, Department of Medical Paediatrics, Royal Aberdeen Children's Hospital, Aberdeen, UK

Susan M Sawyer
Deputy Director, Centre for Adolescent Health, Royal Children's Hospital, Melbourne, Australia

Michael Silverman
Professor and Head, Department of Child Health and Institute for Lung Health, University of Leicester, Leicester, UK

Peter D Sly
Head, Division of Clinical Sciences, Institute for Child Health Research, Princess Margaret Hospital for Children, West Perth, Western Australia

Peter N le Souëf
Professor of Paediatrics, University of Western Australia, Children's Hospital Medical Centre, Perth, Western Australia

Alejandro M Teper
Respiratory Center, Ricardo Gutiérrez Children's Hospital, Buenos Aires, Argentina

Ezekiel M Wafula
Chairman, Department of Paediatrics & Child Health, University of Nairobi, Kenyatta National Hospital, Nairobi, Kenya

Jill A Warner
Senior Lecturer in Allergy & Immunology, Allergy & Inflammation Sciences, School of Medicine, University of Southampton, Southampton, UK

John O Warner
Professor of Child Health & Director of Allergy & Inflammation Sciences, School of Medicine, University of Southampton, Southampton, UK

Trisha Weller
Head of Quality Assurance, National Respiratory Training Centre, Warwick, UK

Karen E Willet
Division of Clinical Sciences, Institute for Child Health Research, Princess Margaret Hospital for Children, Perth, Western Australia

Nicola M Wilson
Department of Paediatrics, Royal Brompton Hospital, London, UK

Foreword

Wheezing, as a sign and/or symptom, and asthma, as a clinical diagnosis, are extremely common in childhood and are increasing in prevalence. As many as a third of all children may wheeze in the first three years of life and nearly 50 per cent may wheeze by the age of six years. Infants and young children wheeze because of smaller airways, increased compliance of airways and the chest wall, decreased lung recoil, increased airway reactivity, more mucous glands and poor cough clearance, as well as, perhaps, other anatomic and physiologic factors. Since so many young children wheeze, it is possible that it is the non-wheezing infant/child who is 'abnormal' and deserves study! Why don't these children wheeze? The prevalence rates for asthma vary around the world but as many as 10 to 20 per cent of children receive this diagnosis. Clearly, not all children who wheeze are asthmatic.

Recent studies have described different wheezing syndromes and their predisposing factors, associated characteristics, prognosis, and therapeutic implications. These studies have shown that a high percentage (as much as 60 per cent) of wheezing that occurs in the first three years of life is transient and disappears by the age of three. Recognizing which wheezing infant will continue to wheeze and subsequently be diagnosed as asthmatic (loosely defined as a genetic disorder related to chronic airway inflammation usually associated with atopy and increased airway reactivity) remains difficult at the present time. In the future, the outcomes from genetic and immunologic studies may serve as predictive factors for those infants and children who are destined to develop asthma. Since the first edition of this book, additional investigations have begun to elucidate mechanisms (e.g., hygiene hypothesis) which help to explain the increasing rates of asthma and atopy worldwide. What all of these studies have shown is that wheezing illnesses are a complex group of heterogeneic disorders.

The morbidity and, perhaps, mortality from childhood asthma continue to rise. The total impact – medical, social, psychological, and economic – of these illnesses is immense. In order to reduce the morbidity from these illnesses and to avoid over-treatment and inappropriate treatment of wheezing infants and children who do not have asthma, or under-treatment of wheezing children who do have asthma, it is incumbent upon physicians and other health care providers involved with the care of children to understand the causes of wheezing in childhood, the pathophysiologic processes involved, diagnostic considerations, the clinical significance and prognosis for the various causes of wheezing, approaches to treatment, and primary and secondary prevention strategies. The second edition of this outstanding textbook provides a most comprehensive review of all aspects of these disorders in erudite, concise, and clearly written chapters. The chapters are very current and provide an insight into the new discoveries that surely will come in the next few years and will allow us to understand these disorders better. The new chapters added to this second edition markedly enhance an already excellent book.

The authors of the individual chapters are world leaders in their respective fields, making this an international book of relevance and importance to anyone, anywhere, caring for children. The authors are clinicians with extensive experience with wheezing children as well as investigators who have personally studied the subjects about which they are writing.

Congratulations to Professor Silverman and the contributing authors for what I consider *the* reference source on childhood asthma and other wheezing disorders.

Lynn M Taussig, MD
President and CEO
The Carole and Albert Angel Family
Presidential Chair
National Jewish Medical and Research Center
Professor of Pediatrics
University of Colorado Health Sciences Center
Denver, Colorado, USA

Preface

Surely the era of the textbook is over! Are we not on the threshold of an entirely paperless world of computer-based information access? It seems not. Like others, health professionals do not simply follow the dictates of logic, but enjoy the traditional values embodied in books. Predictions suggest that their conservatism is likely to persist for many years to come, possibly until a generation is produced whose learning has been largely conducted via electronic media.

This particular book came to be published for several reasons. The first was the need for a comprehensive international textbook dealing with childhood asthma. It is surprising that paediatricians should have been so badly served with information about the condition which provides their bread and butter. Most of the many textbooks and monographs which deal with asthma in general or with the genetics, immunopharmacology, or molecular biology of asthma fail to consider those aspects which are relevant to childhood. Obvious examples range from the mundane, such as the range of problems encountered in the management and clinical assessment of wheezy infants on the one hand and teenagers on the other, to the arcane, such as fetal and neonatal allergen handling and its relationship to the origins of asthma. These important themes, clinical asthma in the developing child and the early life origins of asthma, permeate this book.

The methodology and many of the results of research in adults into the epidemiology, clinical aspects, and inflammatory processes of asthma clearly apply to older children. It is not the aim of this book to replicate all of this information, but to complement it.

The Second Edition not only brings up to date the many advances in knowledge in existing chapters, but incorporates significant topics which have emerged recently. New chapters deal with the Natural History of Asthma, Impact of Asthma and Asthma Around the World. The chapters on Epidemiology, Viral Infection, Passive Smoking, Asthma in Young People, Psychological Factors, Growth, Primary Care, and Education have been completely rewritten, often by new authors.

The book has been written for all those health professionals who deal with wheezy children and for those whose patients may have begun their illness in childhood. While general paediatricians, those in training, and paediatric respiratory physicians (or pulmonologists) may find relevant information throughout the book; others will wish to delve selectively.

The timely completion of a multiauthor book depends almost entirely on the enthusiasm of the team of contributors. Their professionalism and personal commitment as clinical scientists is evident from their writing. I thank them all.

Finally, thanks to my wife, who demonstrated the patience of Penelope each time I vanished into 'hibernation' in order to indulge in the selfish pleasures of writing and editing.

Michael Silverman
Children's Asthma Centre
Institute for Lung Health
Leicester, UK

Abbreviations

AHR	airway hyper-reactivity	EPX	eosinophil protein X
AM	alveolar macrophage	Ers	elastance of respiratory system
AMP	adenosine monophosphate	ETS	environmental tobacco smoke
APC	antigen-presenting cell	Ew	elastance of chest wall
ASM	airway smooth muscle	Fas L	fas ligand
ATP	adenosine triphosphate	FBM	fetal breathing movements
ATPS	ambient temperature and pressure saturated	FEV_t	forced expiratory volume (in t seconds)
BAL(F)	broncho-alveolar lavage (fluid)	FEFx	forced expiratory flow (after exhalation of x% of VC)
BALT	bronchus-associated lymphoid tissue	FGF(R)	fibroblast growth factor (receptor)
BCG	bacille Calmette-Guérin	FOT	forced oscillation technique
BDP	beclomethasone dipropionate	FRC	functional residual capacity (end-expiratory lung volume)
BDR	bronchodilator responsiveness		
BHR	bronchial hyper-responsiveness	FVC	forced vital capacity
BMD	bone mineral density	GCS	gluco-corticosteroid
BPD	bronchopulmonary dysplasia	GINA	Global Initiative for Asthma
BR	bronchial responsiveness	GM-CSF	granulocyte-macrophage colony stimulating factor
BTPS	body temperature and pressure saturated		
BUD	budesonide	GMP	guanosine monophosphate
CC	clara cell	GOR	gastro-oesophageal reflux
CDH	congenital diaphragmatic hernia	GR	glucocorticoid receptor
CF	cystic fibrosis	GSD	geometric standard deviation
CLD	chronic lung disease (of prematurity)	GTP	guanosine triphosphate
CMI	cell mediated immunity	HFA	hydrofluoroalkane
CRS	cough receptor sensitivity	HNF	hepatocyte nuclear factor
Crs	compliance of the respiratory system	Irs	inertance of respiratory system
CT	computerised tomography	ICAM	intercellular adhesion molecule
CTMC	connective tissue mast cell	ICS	inhaled corticosteroid
DC	dendritic cell	IEL	intra-epithelial lymphocyte
DPI	dry power inhaler	IFNαIg	interferon (α, etc)
DZ	dizygotic	Ig	immunoglobulin (A, E, G, M)
EBM	evidence-based medicine	IGF	insulin-like growth factor
ECM	extracellular matrix	IL-1	interleukin (1, etc)
ECP	eosinophil cationic protein	IMCI	Integrated Management of Childhood Illness (WHO)
EDT	eosinophil derived toxin		
EEV	elastic equilibrium volume	IRV	inspiratory reserve volume
EGF	epithelial growth factor	ISAAC	International Study of Allergies and Asthma in Children
El	lung elastance		
EIA (or B)	exercise induced asthma (or bronchoconstriction)	LABA	long acting beta-agonist
		LPS	lipopolysaccharide (bacterial endotoxin)
ELF	epithelial lining fluid	LRI	lower respiratory tract illness
eNO	exhaled nitric oxide	LTRA	leukotrene receptor antagonist
EpDRF (or EDRF)	epithelium-derived relaxing factor	MAB	monoclonal antibody
		MBP	major basic protein
EPO	eosinophil peroxidase	MC	mast cell

M-CSF	macrophage colony stimulating factor	RCT	randomised controlled trial
MEFV	macrophage expiratory flow volume (manoeuvre or curve)	RDS	respiratory distress syndrome
MEFx	maximum expiratory flow (at x% of VC)	Rint	interrupter resistance
MHC	major histocompatibility complex	Rrs	resistance of respiratory system
MMAD	mass median aerodynamic diameter	RSV	respiratory syncitial virus
MMC	mucosal mast cell	RTC	rapid thoracic compression
MMD	mass median diameter	Tri	lung tissue resistance
MPC	mononuclear phagocytic cell	RTK	receptor with intrinsic tyrosine kinase
MPO	myeloperloxidase	RV	residual volume
Mrna	messenger RNA	RVRTC	raised volume rapid thoracic compression
MZ	monozygotic	SABA	short acting beta-agonist
NAC	(UK) National Asthma Campaign	SCG	sodium cromoglycate
NANC	non-adrenergic, non-cholinergic inhibitory (nerve)	SDS	standard deviation score
		SHH	sonic hedgehog
NF	nuclear factor	SIDS	sudden infant death syndrome
NHS	(UK) National Health Service	SM	smooth muscle
NIEV	neonatal intensive care unit	SM-MHC	smooth muscle myosin heavy chain
NK	natural killer (cell)	SPARC	secreted protein, acid rich in cysteine (osteonectin)
NO	nitric oxide		
NRT	nictotine replacement therapy	τrs	time constant of respiratory system
P_A	alveolar pressure	TGF	transforming growth factor
P_a	arterial pressure (or partial pressure)	TGV	thoracic gas volume
PAF	platelet activating factor	TH (or Th)	helper T-lymphocyte
PCx	provocative concentration (causing x% response)	TLC	total lung capacity
		TNFα	tumour necrosis factor (α, etc)
PGDF	platelet-derived growth factor	TOF	tracheo-oesophageal fistula
PDx	provocative dose (causing x% response)	TTF	thyroid transcription factor
Pel	elastic recoil pressure	V'	flow (of gas)
PEF	peak expiratory flow	V''	acceleration (of gas)
PEFV	partial expiratory flow volume (or peak expiratory flow variability)	V'_{max}	maximum flow
		V'_{max}FRC	maximum expiratory flow at FRC (by RTC)
PG	prostaglandin (D, F_{2a} etc)	VC	vital capacity
PHA	phytohemagalutinin	VCAM	vascular cell adhesion molecule
PICU	paediatric intensive care unit	VCD	vocal cord dysfunction
pMDI	pressurised metered dose inhaler	VEGF	vascular endothelial growth factor
PMN	polymorphonuclear leukocyte	VIP	vasoactive intestinal peptide
Ptp	transpulmonary pressure	VLBW	very low birth weight
QOL	quality of life	Vt	tidal volume
RAST	radio-allergo-sorbent test	Vtg	volume of thoracic gas
Raw	airway resistance	V/Q	ventilation-perfusion (balance)
		z-Score	standard deviation score

1

Introduction

MICHAEL SILVERMAN

ASTHMA AND OTHER WHEEZING DISORDERS

The type-form and its phenotypes

A steady but important change has been taking place over recent years, quite as important as the explosions of genetic and immunological knowledge, in our understanding of the nature of childhood asthma. The title of this volume with its suffix 'and other wheezing disorders', implies that we are not facing a single disorder, but a number of 'asthmas'. This represents a 'paradigm shift' over the last 20 years from the era in which it was expedient to lump all the non-specific childhood wheezing illnesses under the diagnosis of asthma. One of the major themes running through this volume is the awareness that, especially in the youngest children (but also at all other ages – including the elderly), 'other wheezing disorders', some of them ill-defined, are emerging as distinct disorders under the umbrella term 'asthma'.

From a clinical perspective, the time is not ripe for us to cast aside the term asthma, but we should be more ready to qualify it, in order to more clearly describe to each other and our patients, its different forms, often referred to as phenotypes.[1] This brings us to the heart of the problem: defining asthma.[2]

The term asthma, although initially based simply on the physiological criterion of variable or reversible airway obstruction,[3] has been all but usurped by allergists and clinical immunologists to imply variable or reversible airway obstruction on a basis of (allergic, IgE-mediated) inflammation. Thus almost all recent work on mechanisms has focused on the single nosological entity of atopic asthma.[4] This is the most frequent severe form of reversible airway disease to occur in the young adult population, an age group in which volunteers are readily available for invasive investigations such as bronchoscopy, bronchial biopsy and bronchoalveolar lavage. This is an acceptable approach, as long as its limitations are realized by clinicians and epidemiologists. Atopic asthma in this age group has *de facto* become the type-form.

Similar arguments are used to define asthma for epidemiological purposes: wheeze + allergy + bronchial hyperresponsiveness = asthma.[5] As well as creating problems when applied to the very young, for whom we do not yet have the tools to measure bronchial hyperresponsiveness (BHR), or even allergy, definitions such as these create statistical difficulties. Both allergy and BHR are continuously distributed in the population. Where is the line to be drawn between normal and abnormal? (Chapter 6c).

There have been attempts to squeeze all of asthma (or physician-diagnosed asthma, a vague and confusing term) in adult life[6] and in middle childhood[7] into this IgE inflammatory mould, despite the obvious problems posed by chronic obstructive lung disease in later life.[8] But the main criticism of the physician-centred approach is that it ignores population-based data which suggest that in the community there is a huge and dimly recognized group of people with perhaps only occasional wheezing with colds, who do not easily fit the diagnosis of asthma and who rarely if ever attend a hospital (Figure 1.1). Whether the gradation of symptoms recorded in Figure 1.1 coincides with the population distribution of IgE levels or of bronchial responsiveness is unknown. I would suggest that in the mild, intermittent, virus-associated wheeze of adult life, we are seeing the cooling remnants of the

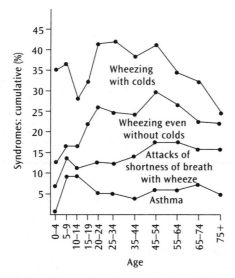

Figure 1.1 *Prevalence of asthma and asthma-like symptoms in a general population (from ref. 9 with permission).*

Big Bang – that enormous explosion of non-atopic airway disease of infancy and early childhood.[10,11]

It has become popular to label some of these variants as 'phenotypes'. Is this a useful term, or simply a passing fashion? Where a cluster of features associate to form a distinct entity of clinical significance (as for example, Type 1 and Type 2 diabetes), then phenotypic labels are important. This is clearly the case for distinct forms of asthma characterized by, for example, (a) episodes of non-atopic viral wheezing of early childhood, or (b) chronic variable wheeze with multiple triggers in atopic children.[10,11] But it would be wrong to label every individual variant of each aetiological mechanism (high or low eosinophil levels, for example) or therapeutic response (good or poor responders to inhaled corticosteroids) as a new phenotype: this threatens to create a new Tower of Babel, rendering the complex more opaque rather than more transparent.

The evidence for distinct clinical varieties of wheezing disease in childhood comes from several sources[12] and will be reviewed in depth at appropriate points in this book (Chapters 2, 3 and 9).

We await techniques which will permit us to explore the structural and cellular basis for some of these phenotypes of asthma. In particular, the role of patterns of inflammation is becoming clearer, as different invasive techniques (biopsy or lavage) find an ethical place in clinical research in children.[13]

The value of splitting asthma into several wheezing disorders in childhood will be realized when:

- it is possible to focus therapeutic trials more precisely on specific clinical problems;
- we have a better understanding of cause before setting up programs of prevention;
- more accurate information on response to treatment and prognosis are acquired.

The building blocks

Science and the practice of clinical medicine have one important feature in common: uncertainty. Scientific facts and clinical statements are provisional hypotheses, coconuts awaiting the next accurate blow to send them toppling. It should be no surprise to find that even our most cherished assumptions are tottering and may be about to fall. Wheeze is the cardinal feature of asthma, but what is it? (Chapter 6a). Peak flow measurement is the basis for diagnosis and monitoring – or is it? (Chapter 4b). Allergy explains much of the recent asthma epidemic – or does it?[14,15,16] Even the concept that the eosinophil is king has come under renewed scrutiny recently,[15] while the star of the mast cell is once again in the ascendant.[17] NO may not always be the aggressor.[18]

New views incorporate the results of better science. But part of the problem is that in the past, we have portrayed asthma as a simple model of cause and effect: Trigger + BHR = Airway obstruction. It is, of course, far more complex.

COMPLEXITY

A complex system

Life used to be simple. We could convey the story of asthma in a few simple diagrams in which A → B→ C and responded to therapy with drug D. To some extent this works. Simple protocols, such as those embodied in the WHO Guidelines, help health professionals in developing countries cope effectively with respiratory illness in real situations – except that they tend to ignore asthma!

Attempts to find 'the gene' or 'the cytokine' or 'the inflammatory cell'… for asthma are doomed to fail, because asthma is at the heart of a system, influenced by genes on one hand and human behaviour on the other, in a series of interacting processes of staggering complexity (Figure 1.2). This is not to say that scientific endeavour will not elucidate cause and effect (quite the contrary), but that the results will be uncertain and often unexpected. Weather forecasting works and is improving – despite the mythological effect of the butterfly flapping in the Amazon rainforest on our weather. But El Nino still surprises us. By analogy sudden death in a child with asthma is devastating and baffling. It differs from 'usual' severe asthma. It sometimes seems as if something has flipped into an irretrievable positive feedback spiral – an El Nino event in asthma?

On a more mundane level, the unpredictability of asthma, embodied in daily symptom or PEF charts which has the features of complexity, monitored at smaller scales (minute to minute as airway resistance fluctuates) and larger (year to year as asthma waxes and wanes) is

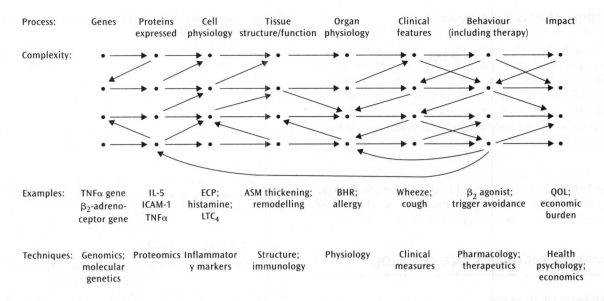

Process:	Genes	Proteins expressed	Cell physiology	Tissue structure/function	Organ physiology	Clinical features	Behaviour (including therapy)	Impact
Complexity:								
Examples:	TNFα gene β₂-adreno-ceptor gene	IL-5 ICAM-1 TNFα	ECP; histamine; LTC₄	ASM thickening; remodelling	BHR; allergy	Wheeze; cough	β₂ agonist; trigger avoidance	QOL; economic burden
Techniques:	Genomics; molecular genetics	Proteomics	Inflammatory markers	Structure; immunology	Physiology	Clinical measures	Pharmacology; therapeutics	Health psychology; economics

Figure 1.2 *Asthma as a complex system. Although a linear process (gene protein cell physiology, etc.) is often assumed, the interactions between one level and another are extremely complex.*

reminiscent of the fractal pattern which describes a complex system.

The important features of the complex illustration in Figure 1.2 are as follows:

1 For each process, there are several independent components (there may, for instance, be many hundreds of relevant genes).
2 The interactions operate forward and backward, and may skip adjacent processes, so that, for instance, change in behaviour (sleep) may alter any physiology or change in therapy (corticosteroid) may directly alter gene transcription.
3 Individual components may have opposite effects under different circumstances: NO, eosinophils and PGE₂ for example may have negatively damaging or positively adaptive effects.
4 The techniques which we use to measure asthma (or markers of asthma) are often context dependent;[19]
5 The weakest link is at the clinical level, where the features are most poorly characterized (Chapter 6a);
6 We intervene to alter any one of these processes at our peril, since the more distant the process from the clinical level, the more unpredictable the clinical outcome.

Evolution

In the final analysis, asthma and allergy need to be understood on an evolutionary timescale. Modern man evolved in (rural) Africa, and emerged in relatively small numbers to populate the rest of the world. Our immune systems, both adaptive and innate, have had insufficient time to adapt to the modern world. This could be a clue to

the 'epidemic' of allergic disease,[20,21] in which vigorous immune responses more appropriate to host defence against parasitic infection, are directed at trivial environmental allergens. An alternative explanation for the discrepancy between the prevalence of asthma inside and outside Africa is a founder effect: the emigrants who populated the rest of the world bore the relevant genes. Could Adam and Eve have had asthma?

DEVELOPMENT AND DISEASE

Age and development affect clinical asthma

Asthma provides excellent examples of the way in which development during fetal life and childhood, and chronic disease may interact. The developmental theme runs throughout this book, as befits a paediatric text. The terms infant (under 12 months in the UK, but up to 24 months in many reports from N. America), preschool child (1 or 2 to 5 years), schoolchild (6 years to adolescence) and 'young person' (post-pubertal teenager) have more than terminological simplicity. They may match:

• clinical features, such as bronchiolitis and episodic viral wheeze which predominate in infancy;
• the clinical approach to children and families;
• possibilities for physiological measurement, which are being rapidly extended to the former Dark Ages of the preschool child;
• immune mechanisms and expression of allergy;
• therapeutic techniques, especially aerosol therapy and devices;
• prognosis in the growing child.

Asthma affects development

Conversely, there are ways in which asthma and its therapy alter childhood growth and development. Stunting is a feature of chronic severe and poorly controlled asthma. This is thankfully a thing of the past, with modern therapy (Chapter 15). More insidious, and as yet unquantified, is the possibility that high-dose inhaled corticosteroid therapy given to infants with asthma, could impair lung development at a time of rapid alveolization (Chapter 4a). We lack the tools to measure alveolar development and cannot therefore assess the risk/benefit balance for young infants.

Psychological development too may be affected by chronic disease, an issue which is addressed in Chapter 13c.

PATTERN, DIAGNOSIS AND CONTROL

Patterns of disease

The variability of asthma seems to be far greater in children than in adults. Changes are apparent in pattern and severity between children and over the passage of time within individuals. This variability is at the same time both problematic, if one tries too vigorously to apply adult-based management protocols to children, and illuminating, since analysing its causes can help to improve management at all ages.

For example, paediatricians have been aware for many years that troublesome acute episodes of wheeze are especially common in young children, usually in association with viral respiratory tract infections. The prevention and management of such episodes is a major task, since they constitute the severest aspects of asthma, cause much discomfort, lead to about 25% of all hospital admissions in childhood in the UK and are occasionally fatal. There is good reason to believe that standard management protocols do not work very well in young children with episodic asthma (Chapter 9).[22] This is not simply because the majority of troublesome attacks occur in children too young to use peak flow meters (in any case, lower respiratory tract symptoms are more sensitive than peak flow measurements in guiding self-management in children).[23] The protocols work well for relatively stable adults whose

asthma varies gradually but are inadequate for childhood asthma with its sudden changes.

It is useful to consider the *pattern of asthma* at any age as being composed of three component parts (Figure 1.3):

acute episodes of airway obstruction, usually provoked by viral respiratory tract infection, but sometimes by antigen exposure or other environmental factors, which cause a sudden decline in PEF or worsening of symptoms, usually lasting for a few days and with a variable degree of reversibility during the episodes;

day-to-day (interval) symptoms which include nocturnal cough or wheeze, antigen-, exercise- or laughter-induced wheeze, wheeze triggered in a variety of situations or early morning symptoms; reversibility is a feature; acute viral episodes may also occur;

suboptimal function, even in the steady state, which represents adaptation to a functionally inadequate level as a result of persistent airway obstruction; in the absence of symptoms, only physiological measurement will pick up the problem; this is often referred to as the irreversible element of asthma, since by definition, there is a poor response to usual therapy, even a trial of oral corticosteroids.

Recognition of the pattern of symptoms in an individual has major implications for management, whether by altering lifestyle or by drug therapy. Patterns change with time, from year to year. They also change with age, particularly in the preschool period and around puberty. The reversible element may change quite rapidly over hours or days in an acute episode, from poorly responsive to bronchodilators early in an attack to highly responsive later.

The empirical approach to asthma which is embodied in consensus management protocols makes few assumptions about the underlying mechanisms or pathophysiology of these patterns of airway obstruction. The 'science' of medicine has yet to make an impact here.

Severity

An aspect of self-management terminology which often confuses is the difference between severity and control. An excellent set of definitions has been provided in conjunction with one International Consensus Management

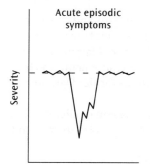

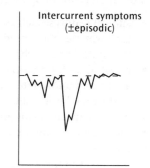

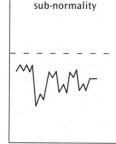

Figure 1.3 *Disease patterns in childhood. There are three components to the pattern of asthma, whether measured by symptom score or lung function: acute episodes; intercurrent reversible features; chronic unremitting features (which are rare in children).*

statement.[24] Severity during treatment is defined by the level of treatment required to maintain control. Thus, in the hierarchy of severity, the use of high-dose topical corticosteroids indicates more severe asthma than do low-dose steroids or intermittent bronchodilators. Unfortunately, this system is of little value in young children. How can a single term describe the level of management of the three largely independent features of asthma illustrated in Figure 1.3? If it is necessary to define severity for epidemiological purposes or for therapeutic trials, then a new classification is needed, describing separately the three features: steady state – reversible element; steady state – irreversible element; episodic element.

Diagnosis

Diagnosis may seem to be impossible if asthma is both difficult to define and split into several phenotypes. The topic is discussed at several points in this book, in relation to symptoms, lung function, inflammatory markers, and clinical management. The diagnosis can be considered as an empirical process (Figure 1.4). This is simply a description of good clinical practice! At the heart of the process is the question 'Is it asthma?' This implies a questioning approach at all stages in the process. The final step is the response to a treatment plan. Failure to respond triggers a re-iteration of some of the steps. In practice, this sort of algorithm defines asthma as a disease which responds to anti-asthma therapy!

Control

The adequacy of control is defined by the degree to which symptoms (or lung function or inflammation) deviate from normality during treatment. Again, the term is unsatisfactory unless the various components of asthma

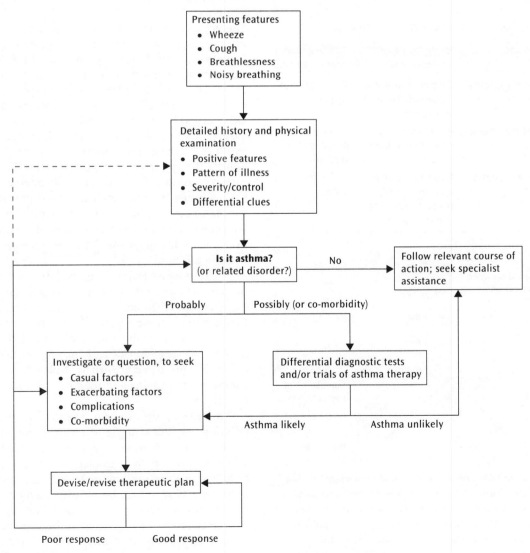

Figure 1.4 *A diagnostic algorithm for asthma. At its heart is the key question 'Is it asthma?'*

are all considered. In young children, steady-state (interval) symptoms may be easy to abolish with preventer therapy, but acute severe episodes are often difficult to control. Since self-management plans depend on symptom (or PEF) based steps, definitions of good or poor control and consequent action should cover the three components in Figure 1.3 separately and explicitly.

As professionals, it is important to remember that controlling asthma has different implications from the perspective of the child or parents (Table 1.1). Understanding what motivates our patients and ourselves is an important prerequisite to good practice, and therefore to better control and better outcomes!

Outcome measurement

One of the key themes of this book relates to clinical assessment and measurement (Chapters 6a–e and 7a–e). These are essential tools to monitor the outcome of our interventions in individual patients, i.e. clinical trials or in populations.[25] Many of the techniques have been described in greater detail elsewhere.[26]

No investigation should be performed in clinical practice, without a clear aim. The same stricture applies to the measurement of outcome. It is not just a matter of performing the technique properly, but of choosing the appropriate measure. The choice will depend on the age of the child, the complexity of the outcome variable and the interval over which outcome is to be monitored (Figure 1.5). For instance, measuring the response to a bronchodilator in a schoolchild requires spirometry and takes 15 minutes. Measuring the impact of allergen avoidance in infancy on the prevalence of atopic asthma may require a large population to be studied over 5–10 years by clinical, immunological and physiological methods.

PROFESSIONAL PERSPECTIVES

Clinical practice

The advances in clinical practice have been significant since the first edition of this book appeared in 1995. The first new class of *drugs* to be introduced for thirty years (discounting long-acting β_2 agonists as variations on a theme), the (cysteinyl) leukotriene receptor antagonists (LTRA), are finding their place in clinical care (Chapter 8a). Other agents have had their places properly evaluated for the first time by systematic review conducted in a thorough and transparent manner. Some 20 reviews of childhood asthma therapy have been published by the Cochrane Airways Group and many more will emerge, providing both a secure base for evidence-based practice and an agenda for further research to fill the gaps.[27] These reviews and others dealing with issues such as allergen avoidance, from the backbone of the advice on management provided in this book.

Evidence-based practice has its detractors. It is clear that subjectivity creeps into the process at several points. The selection of studies for systematic review, the degree to which the results are generalizable and the uniqueness of each clinical consultation, all require individual judgement. Even when the evidence is incontrovertible, effecting change in clinical practice can be challenging. It demands commitment, training and resources to break the habits of many years.[28]

Advances in some areas of practice have been disappointing. We still struggle to measure *lung function* in children under 5 years, although advances have been achieved using both spirometry and the interrupter technique in older preschool children (Chapters 6b and 9). In the next few years, non-invasive methods to monitor *airway inflammation* will change clinical practice for wheezy children of all ages, and at the same time lead to greater understanding of mechanisms and targeting of therapy.

Table 1.1 *Perspectives on control of asthma*

Patients and parents	Personal health professionals	Public health professionals
Relief of symptoms	Demonstration of personal skill and sensitivity	Prevention of disease
Safety of treatment	Application of evidence-based practice	Early diagnosis by screening
Good symptomatic outcome	Good functional outcome (lung function, BHR or inflammation)	Value for money

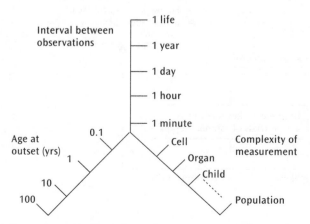

Figure 1.5 *The dimensions of outcome measurement. The appropriate measure of outcome depends not only on the type of intervention (environmental change, short-term or long-term drug therapy) but on the age of the patient, the duration of outcome and the complexity of the measurement target.*

The *public health* impact of childhood asthma has received relatively little attention. This is surprising, since the cost of wheezing disorders in the under-5s, a group which places great demands on primary care and inpatient services, must be substantial. Similarly preventive programmes await development, the fruits of research into the hygiene hypothesis (Chapter 2).

RESEARCH

There has been an explosion of research in all aspects of asthma genetics, cell and organ physiology, clinical measurement and pharmacology over the recent years. New ideas continue to emerge from epidemiology, to be tested in clinical populations or to provide clues for geneticists. The hygiene hypothesis, the effect of diet, ethnicity and migration and air pollution (including passive smoking) have all provided important clues. Research into the early life origins of allergy and asthma, reinforced by the work of Barker,[29] will lead to strategies to divert the developing immune system over the next decade (Chapters 4c and 14).

A number of important issues remain to be resolved. The contribution and control of viral infections in wheezing disorders has barely been explored, despite their personal and public cost. Fetal lung growth and its contribution to lifelong respiratory health is being investigated in only a handful of laboratories world-wide. Translation of new immunopharmacological information into new therapies takes many years of developmental work. Even so, the benefits only reach a tiny proportion of the world's asthmatic children. It is also in the Developing World that the political fight continues to reduce children's exposure to tobacco smoke.

One of the greatest challenges is to be able to measure chronic inflammation and remodelling in the airways of young children,[13] and to demonstrate that early intervention can modulate these processes, thereby altering the natural history of asthma lifelong.[30] This is the Holy Grail.

THE SCOPE OF THIS BOOK

The purpose of this book is to educate and enthuse the reader, but above all to provoke thought and to encourage change. Better management of childhood asthma and ultimately prevention of asthma at all ages are the goals.

The emphasis is on clinical science and its application to the management of children. With a plethora of textbooks and reviews on the basic mechanisms and pharmacology of asthma, we have not attempted to complete, but rather sought to complement existing literature. Each chapter forms a comprehensive review of its subject, presenting the scientific background which informs clinical management.

REFERENCES

1. Silverman M, Wilson NM. Asthma time for a change of name? *Arch Dis Child* 1997;**77**:62–4.
2. Burrows B, Taussig LM. As the twig is bent, the tree inclines. *Am Rev Respir Dis* 1980;**122**:813–16.
3. Clarke TJH, Godfrey S, Lee TH, Thomson NC. *Asthma*, 4th edn. Arnold, London, 2001.
4. Djukanovic R, Roche WR, Wilson JW *et al*. Mucosal inflammation in asthma. *Am Rev Respir Dis* 1990;**142**:434–57.
5. Peat JK, Toelle BG, Marks GB, Mellis CM. Continuing the debate about measuring asthma in population studies. *Thorax* 2001;**56**:406–11.
6. Burrows B, Martinez FD, Halonen M, Barbee RA, Cline MG. Association of asthma with serum IgE levels and skin-test reactivity to allergens. *New Engl J Med* 1989;**320**:271–7.
7. Burrows B, Sears MR, Flannery EM, Herbison GP, Holdaway MD. Relationship of bronchial responsiveness assessed by methacholine challenge to serum IgE, lung function, symptoms and diagnosis in 11 year old New Zealand children. *J All Clin Immunol* 1992;**90**:376–85.
8. Calverley P, Pride NB. *Chronic Obstructive Pulmonary Disease*. Chapman and Hall, London, 1994.
9. Dodge RR, Burrows B. The prevalence and incidence of asthma and asthma-like symptoms in a general population sample. *Am Rev Respir Dis* 1980;**122**:567–75.
10. Martinez F, Wright AL, Toussing LM, Holberg CJ, Halonen M, Morgon WJ. Asthma and wheezing in the first six years of life. The Group Health Medical Associates. *New Engl J Med* 1995;**332**:181–2.
11. Stein RT, Holberg CJ, Morgan WJ, Wright AL, Lombardi E, Taussig L, Martinez FD. Peak flow variability, methacholine responsiveness and atopy as markers for detecting different wheezing phenotypes in childhood. *Thorax* 1997;**52**:946–52.
12. Silverman M. Out of the mouths of babes and sucklings – lessons from early childhood asthma. *Thorax* 1993;**48**:1200–4.
13. Silverman M, Grigg J, Pedersen S. Measurement of airway inflammation in young children. *Am J Respir Crit Care Med* 2001;**162**:Part 2.
14. Pearce N, Pekkanen J, Beasley R. How much asthma is really attributable to atopy? *Thorax* 999;**54**:268–72.
15. Chu HW, Martin RJ. Are eosinophils still important in asthma? *Clin Exp All* 2001;**31**:525–8.
16. Kuehni CE, Davis A, Brooke AM, Silverman M. Are all wheezing disorders in very young (preschool) children increasing in prevalence? *Lancet* 2001;**357**:1821–5.
17. Brightling CE, Bradding P, Symon FA, Holgate ST, Wardlaw AJ, Pavord ID. Mastcell infiltration of airway smooth muscle in asthma. *New Engl J Med* 2002;**346**:1699–705.

18. Baraldi E, Zanconato S. The labyrinth of asthma phenotypes and exhaled NO. *Thorax* 2001;**56**:333–5.
19. Martinez FD. Context dependency of markers of disease. *Am J Respir Crit Care Med* 2000;**162**:S56–7.
20. Le Souef PN, Goldblatt J, Lynch NR. Evolutionary adaptation of inflammatory immune responses in human beings. *Lancet* 2000;**356**:242–4.
21. Holt PG. Parasites, atopy and the hygiene hypothesis: resolution of a paradox? *Lancet* 2000;**356**:1699–1701.
22. Stevens CA, Wesseldine LJ, Couriel JM, Dyer AJ, Osman LM, Silverman M. Parental education and guided self-management of asthma and wheezing in the pre-school child: a randomised controlled trial. *Thorax* 2002;**57**:39–44.
23. Wensley D, Silverman M. Routine peak flow measurements in guided self management of childhood asthma: are they useful? *Thorax* 2002 (in press).
24. International Asthma Management Project. International consensus report on the diagnosis and management of asthma. *Clin Exp All* 1992;**22**:Suppl 1.
25. Silverman M, Pedersen S. Outcome measures in early childhood asthma and other wheezing disorders. *Eur Respir J* 1996;**9**:Suppl 21.
26. Silverman M, O'Callaghan CLP (Editors). *Practical Paediatric Respiratory Medicine*. Arnold, London, 2001.
27. The Cochrane Library. Update Publications, Oxford. http://www.update-software.com/default.htm
28. Powell CVE, Maskell GR, Marks MK, South M, Robertson CF. Successful implementation of spacer treatment guideline for acute asthma. *Arch Dis Child* 2001;**84**:142–6.
29. Barker DJP. A new model for the origins of chronic disease. *Med Health Care Philos* 2001;**4**:31–4.
30. Silverman M, Martinez FD, Pedersen S. Early intervention in childhood asthma. *Eur Respir J* 1998;**12**:Suppl 27.

2

Epidemiology and public health

MICHAEL KABESCH AND ERIKA VON MUTIUS

INTRODUCTION

Epidemiology is defined as 'the study of the distribution and determinants of disease frequency in human populations' under the assumption that through systematic investigation of different populations or subgroups of individuals within a population in different places or at different times, causal and preventable factors of human disease can be identified. Thus, the first task in epidemiology is to quantify the *occurrence* of illness, i.e. its frequency and distribution within populations. The goal is then to evaluate hypotheses about the *causation* of disease by measuring the effects of people's characteristics and their environment on the occurrence of illness. Thirdly, epidemiology has great potential to improve the understanding of *disease mechanisms* by longitudinally observing and meticulously describing different phenotypes of chronic diseases and their natural course from infancy, through childhood and adolescence into adulthood. The advent of modern genetic and statistical tools has created the new field of genetic epidemiology, which attempts to tackle the role of a subject's genetic make-up in the development of chronic, multifactorial disease. These techniques may in the future help to overcome one major drawback of epidemiological studies, relating population data to individual subjects. Since most epidemiological studies describe group characteristics, a prediction for an individual patient on the basis of findings from epidemiological studies is often difficult, if not impossible. Eventually, by combining individual information on a subject's genetic background with knowledge about that subject's exposure to environmental determinants, epidemiological findings may be made more relevant to clinical practice and to preventative programmes.

This chapter summarizes the contribution of epidemiology to the understanding of childhood asthma and wheezing. Although limitations exist, epidemiology has proven to be a valuable tool in documenting the increase of wheezing disorders in childhood over the last decades and pointing out the differences in disease prevalence between populations. Furthermore, epidemiological studies have identified risk factors for the development of childhood asthma and wheezing illnesses thereby influencing the formulation of a disease hypothesis. Last, but not least, epidemiology has provided insight into the natural history of wheezing illnesses and their prognosis.

DISEASE DEFINITION

A major problem in studying asthma is the lack of a gold standard for the definition of the disease. In clinical practice asthma is often defined as bronchial hyperresponsiveness (BHR), the excessive response of the airways to a variety of stimuli leading to a reversible airway obstruction, in an IgE-mediated disease. Wheezing is a common symptom associated with airway obstruction due to asthma. However, wheezing also occurs with other airway diseases such as viral infections, bronchopulmonary dysplasia and cystic fibrosis. Furthermore, a wide range in the clinical expression and severity of asthma symptoms exists. Wheezing, chest tightness, nocturnal cough and exercise-induced shortness of breath are all regarded as typical asthma symptoms but they might not share the same underlying disease mechanisms. The individual expression of asthma symptoms depends on numerous environmental as well as genetic factors. It is not possible to relate specific symptoms to certain bio-chemical, immunological and structural changes in the lungs.

In epidemiological studies a number of different disease definitions have been used to characterize asthma.[1,2] In children, assessment of disease status often relies on parental questionnaire-derived data. *Life-time prevalence* of asthma can be ascertained either as physician-diagnosed asthma or as wheezing symptoms, ever based on parental recall. Both definitions are subjected to parental recall bias. While the term *physician-diagnosed asthma* reflects a more specific disease definition it also tends to focus on a more severe form of the disease. Conversely, parental reports of lifetime prevalence of wheeze are more inclusive but less specific, reflecting milder forms of asthma. Another common variable used in cross-sectional studies of asthma is '*current wheeze*' which is defined as wheezing during the 12 months prior to the survey. This also relies on recall by the parent or child. To distinguish current wheezing due to asthma from other respiratory diseases further criteria may be included. Thus, current wheeze in children with a prior diagnosis of asthma by a physician may be labelled *current asthma*. Some authors have suggested incorporating measurements of bronchial challenge testing, so that the definition of current asthma *includes BHR* as well as recent wheeze.[1,2] However, BHR is not equivalent to asthma and cannot be used as a single disease marker. BHR alone is sometimes referred to as an 'intermediate' or 'partial' phenotype. Overall, disease definitions of childhood asthma in cross-sectional studies should be based on a number of *intermediate phenotypes* and different methods of assessment. These definitions represent a rather broad view of the disease. In longitudinal studies early onset, late onset, transient and persistent wheezing can be distinguished which may better reflect the natural history of asthma, and its phenotypic variation, during childhood[3] (see Figure 2.1 and Chapter 3).

None of these epidemiological disease definitions relates directly to the causes of asthma. In particular, only rarely is distinction made between wheezing phenotypes caused by viral infections alone and those caused by other agents too, in addition to viral infections.[4] This may be a task for future prospective studies of childhood asthma. Due to the lack of a global disease definition for asthma, it is the hypothesis to be answered, that must determine the formulation of the disease definition for each epidemiological study. A number of tools are available for phenotype characterization in study subjects and the most important ones are discussed here.

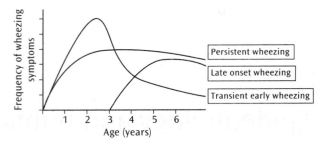

Figure 2.1 *Schematic depiction of putative development of wheezing during childhood. Difference in prognosis and natural history of symptoms in three distinct groups of wheezing children. (Data extracted from ref. 3.)*

Questionnaires

For epidemiological studies of childhood asthma, a pragmatic disease definition is often required with the danger of oversimplification. Questionnaires are widely used to assess asthma in population-based studies. Physician-diagnosed asthma is a key variable in most of these questionnaires. There is, however, substantial variation between doctors in labelling a wheezing disease as asthma. Furthermore, if information about a certain diagnosis is based only on parental reports, their response may be influenced by access to medical care resources, recall bias and language problems. Although efforts to standardize these questionnaires have been made[5,6] and translations as well as video questionnaires exist, cultural differences may still influence the response. One has to further keep in mind that by solely using a physician's diagnosis of asthma, subjects with more severe disease may be selected. Conversely, relying only on parental reports of wheezing may result in an overestimation of asthma prevalence because of misinterpretation of other respiratory noises as wheeze (Chapter 6a), and because some wheezing episodes may be attributable to other conditions. Therefore, it seems reasonable to seek additional information on the frequency and pattern of wheezing and on other symptoms such as cough and shortness of breath. Such an inclusive approach may help to evaluate the overall burden of respiratory disease.

Bronchial hyperresponsiveness (BHR)

It is well known that asthma is strongly associated with BHR and allergy. By measuring these indirect markers, a further characterization of asthma by more objective techniques is possible. While the assessment of pulmonary function and bronchial hyperresponsiveness in infants and toddlers is technically difficult and therefore not well established in epidemiological studies, these techniques have been successfully applied in surveys of school-children. In a clinical setting BHR can be measured in several different ways (Chapter 6c), using 'indirect' challenge with cold dry air, nebulized hypertonic saline, exercise or 'direct' challenge with increasing doses of pharmacological bronchoconstrictors such as histamine or methacholine. However, due to the equipment involved, the time-consuming procedures and the potential for side effects, bronchial challenges are difficult to implement outside a clinical setting, and thus rarely performed on a wide scale.

Although BHR is highly associated with asthma in childhood, it is not synonymous with asthma. In some individuals BHR can be shown in the absence of symptoms. Conversely, BHR is a condition which varies over time and therefore can be missed by a single assessment in epidemiological studies, even among asthmatic subjects. Thus, measurements of BHR are not an objective 'gold standard' for asthma diagnosis in epidemiological studies, but can help in determining the nature of different lower respiratory tract illnesses among participants of field studies. Therefore, measures of airway responsiveness should be included in field studies whenever possible.

Assessment of atopy

Asthma, allergic rhinitis and atopic dermatitis (eczema) are atopic diseases which share numerous characteristics such as elevated total serum IgE levels, specific sensitization to ubiquitous allergens, eosinophilic inflammation and alterations in T-cell dependent immune responses. As many of these features are easily accessible to objective measurements they are frequently included in epidemiological studies of childhood asthma. Total serum IgE can be determined by simple laboratory tests while atopic sensitization to one or more allergens can be assessed by skin-prick tests or with blood-based detection systems. These measurements can be used as an indicator for the presence and degree of atopic sensitization and may therefore be used to further characterize childhood asthma as atopic or non-atopic. As with BHR, measurements of atopy are not synonymous with asthma (Figure 2.2). Although most school-children with asthma are atopic (increased production of total and specific IgE), not all atopics are asthmatic. This fact is obvious, as the prevalence rates for atopy in any given population are generally significantly higher than the prevalence of asthma itself. At this point it is not entirely clear why some children develop atopy alone while others suffer from asthma.

PREVALENCE OF CHILDHOOD ASTHMA

Although many reports of asthma prevalence in childhood have existed for different populations and for different age

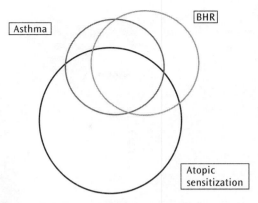

Figure 2.2 *Schematic depiction of the relationship between asthma, bronchial hyperresponsiveness (BHR) and atopic sensitization in school-children. While most school-aged children with asthma also display signs of BHR and atopic sensitization the majority of children labelled atopic do not suffer from respiratory symptoms.*

groups, the lack of standardization in disease definition and methodology makes it difficult to compare these data. Only recently have efforts been successful to standardize questionnaires and other methods, thereby providing the opportunity to compare the prevalence of the disease between different countries all around the world.[7,8] While comparing disease prevalence and their changes over time within a country has immediate benefits for healthcare planners, comparisons between countries are important in generating hypotheses concerning the development of childhood asthma. The wide range of genetic and environmental differences between countries and populations allow for a better analysis of putative disease related factors. Only when differences between lifestyle or environmental factors are significantly different between populations, as is the case between Western European countries and those in Eastern Europe, can the effect of these factors on disease development be studied adequately.

World-wide variation in childhood asthma and allergy

In general, asthma rates are higher in affluent, western countries with a high degree of industrialization than in developing countries with a large rural population. In the large scale International Study of Asthma and Allergy in Childhood (ISAAC) the world-wide prevalence of allergic diseases was assessed in the 1990s.[8] More than 450 000 school-aged children from 56 countries participated in this survey. Identical methods in all study centres were used in an effort to draw a picture of present-day asthma prevalence around the globe (Figure 2.3). A 20-fold difference between study centres was found for childhood

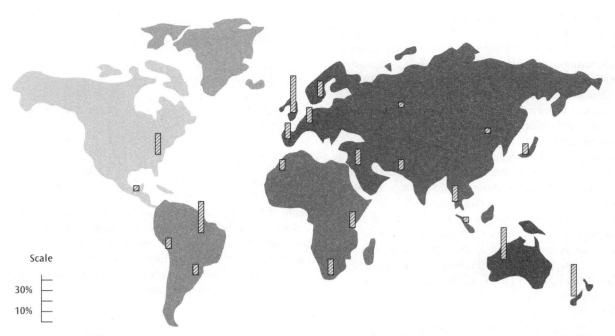

Figure 2.3 *World-wide variation in asthma prevalence. Schematic depiction of asthma prevalence (in %) in arbitrarily selected countries around the world. (From ref. 8.)*

asthma, while the variation for other allergic diseases was between 20 and 60-fold. The highest prevalence of current asthma symptoms (assessed by questionnaire as 'Wheezing in the last 12 months') was found in the UK, New Zealand and Australia while most developing countries had comparatively low prevalence rates. In general, centres with low asthma rates also showed low levels of other atopic diseases. However, countries with the highest prevalence for atopic rhinitis and atopic eczema were not necessarily identical to those with the highest asthma rates, indicating either differences in aetiology and risk factors for these disorders or problems in disease definition and recognition.

Furthermore, within European countries a west-east gradient in the prevalence of childhood asthma is apparent. German re-unification in 1992 opened a window of opportunity to study a genetically homogeneous population that had lived under very different economic and environmental circumstances for 40 years. At that time, allergic rhinitis and atopic sensitization was significantly higher in West Germany than in the East.[9] Likewise, in a study from the Baltic area of northern Europe, Swedish children had a higher prevalence of atopic sensitization and asthma than did those from Poland and Estonia.[10,11] When a cross-sectional survey was repeated in 1996, atopic sensitization measured by skin-prick tests had increased significantly in East German children though not as much as to attain prevalence rates of atopy previously observed among school-children in Munich.[12] The children from East Germany participating in this repeated survey were born 3 years before the downfall of

communism and were therefore only exposed to Western living conditions after their third birthday. This may indicate that factors early in life are particularly important for the development of asthma, while environmental factors beyond infancy may influence the development of other allergic disorders. Thus it could be shown that the prevalence of hay fever more than doubled in children from East Germany within 4 years after exposure to Western lifestyle coming closer to prevalence rates found in the West. It remains to be seen whether the prevalence of asthma will increase in the countries of the former communist Eastern Europe, once children are born and raised in a more 'western' lifestyle.

Migration

Migration studies may be helpful to determine the relative effects of genetic compared to environmental factors in the world-wide variation of childhood asthma and atopy. However, as the interactions between these two factors are very complex, it seems difficult to predict the effect immigration may have on the development of these diseases. Migration from countries with lower to countries with higher prevalence of asthma and atopy may either result in increased[13,14] or decreased[15,16] disease prevalence in immigrants compared with the indigenous population of their adopted country. Moreover, children of immigrants may have a lower prevalence of asthma and atopy than those still living in the country of origin.[15] In Turkish children living in Germany, the prevalence of atopy depended on the degree of adaptation to a western lifestyle.[17] Adoption studies from Sweden further investigated the relationship between age of arrival in a new country and the development of atopic diseases.[18] Adopted children who came to Sweden before the age of 2 years suffered from asthma, hay fever and eczema significantly more often than those who came to Sweden between 2 and 6 years of age. Moreover, differences existed in the prevalence of hay fever and eczema between children of different ethnic origins. These findings would suggest that both genetic and environmental factors, operating early in life, have a profound influence on the development of atopic disorders.

Urbanization

In some developing and developed countries a lower prevalence of childhood asthma in rural compared with urban areas has been reported, but the evidence is not conclusive. Airway challenges performed in urban and rural areas of Africa suggested that bronchial hyperresponsiveness was almost non-existent in rural areas in the late 1980s and early 1990s.[19,20] In turn, among the more affluent urban populations of South Africa and Zimbabwe BHR reached a prevalence of 3.2% and 5.9%, respectively. Similar results have been reported from other studies in Africa. However, over the last decade BHR seems to have increased also in rural Africa.[21]

Differences in childhood asthma between rural and urban populations in Western countries are less pronounced. In a large British study only marginal differences in the prevalence of childhood asthma between rural and urban areas were observed.[22] However, children from rural Scotland tended to show a lower prevalence of severe asthma symptoms.[23] Data from Sweden indicated a higher prevalence of atopic sensitization to aeroallergens

in children from urban centres compared with rural areas, but no information was available for childhood asthma.[10] The increased risk for children to develop an atopic disease in an urban environment was largely attributed to increased levels of air pollution, particularly related to heavy car traffic exposure. However, recent findings from Switzerland,[24] Austria[25] and Southern Germany[26] provide evidence that lower prevalences of atopic diseases in rural populations may rather be attributable to the presence of protective factors in a farm environment than to the absence of urban risk factors.

TIME TRENDS IN ASTHMA PREVALENCE

Numerous studies have investigated the trends in the occurrence of childhood asthma over time.[27] Data collected over the last 40 years in industrialized countries indicate a significant increase in asthma prevalence. A wide array of survey methods, disease definitions, sample populations and age groups have been used by different investigators, making direct comparisons between studies difficult. However, many reports have used identical questionnaires in similar population samples at different time points and are therefore relatively reliable indicators of changes in prevalence (Table 2.1). Unfortunately, most studies lack the assessment of more objective measurements related to asthma such as BHR or atopic sensitization. Studies relying only on parental questionnaires may be subject to potential bias, as the perception of childhood asthma may have changed considerably over recent years due to increased public awareness.

In some studies but not in others, the prevalence of diagnosed asthma increased much more rapidly than the prevalence of wheezing,[28] suggesting either that a loosening of the definition of asthma has occurred, or

Table 2.1 *Changes in prevalence of asthma and wheezing symptoms in children and adolescents*

Prevalence (%)						
Country	Reference	Age (yr)	Period	Outcome variable	1st study	2nd study
Australia	Peat[33]	8–10	1982–1992	Asthma diagnosis	11.0	31.8
Canada	Manfreda[147]	5–14	1983–1988	Asthma diagnosis	1.9	4.2
England	Whincup[148]	6–7.5	1966–1990	Lifetime wheezing	18.3	21.8
England	Anderson[35]	7–8	1978–1991	Current wheezing	8.8	11.6
England	Kuehni[38]	1–5	1990–1998	Current wheezing	12.4	23.7
New Zealand	Shaw[34]	12.4–18.9	1975–1989	Asthma diagnosis	7.9	13.3
Norway	Nystad[149]	6–16	1981–1994	Asthma diagnosis	3.4	9.3
Scotland	Ninan[36]	8–13	1964–1989	Asthma diagnosis	4.1	10.2
Scotland	Omran[37]	11–13	1989–1994	Asthma diagnosis	10.2	19.6
Taiwan	Hsieh & Shen[150]	7–14	1974–1985	Asthma diagnosis	1.3	5.1
USA	Gergen[151]	6–11	1974–1980	Asthma diagnosis or current wheezing	4.8	7.6
USA	Weitzman[44]	0–17	1981–1988	Current asthma	3.1	4.3
Wales	Burr[29]	12	1973–1988	Asthma diagnosis	5.5	12.0

that former under-diagnosis has been corrected. Another possibility is an increase in the severity of asthma symptoms over time, leading to a more easily recognisable disease pattern. This was observed in a survey of Welsh school-children,[29] where exercise-induced BHR was assessed alongside questionnaire-derived information over a time period of 15 years. An increase in the prevalence and severity of exercise induced symptoms, which matched the increase of asthma as reported by the parents, was reported. Other surveys have, however, failed to document an increase in the severity of asthma symptoms as assessed by speech limiting attacks, school absenteeism and activity restriction.[30] Interestingly, over the same time period a declining trend in the prevalence of bronchitis was found,[31,32] suggesting that at last some of the increase in the prevalence of asthma may have been due to diagnostic transfer.

A well documented study from Australia, applying a histamine challenge, skin-prick tests and questionnaires, showed that the prevalence of BHR had almost doubled between 1982 and 1992.[33] In this study the increase in the prevalence of BHR was mainly observed among atopic children, while the total prevalence of atopy remained unchanged. Furthermore, during the same period of time the prevalence of current wheeze (assessed as wheezing in the last 12 months) also doubled in this study population of 8 to 10-year-old school-children. Another study from New Zealand investigated trends of asthma prevalence in adolescents in 1975 and 1989.[34] The prevalence of self-reported asthma or wheeze increased significantly in children from European origin as well as in those from Maori families.

Though using different methods and definitions of asthma, these studies from countries all over the developed world suggest an overall increase in the prevalence of asthma and concurrent wheezing symptoms between 1960 and 1990. This is not the case for other respiratory diseases such as bronchitis. While Anderson et al. suggested that the prevalence of wheezing illnesses and childhood asthma may have reached a plateau in the mid-1980s,[35] studies from Scotland indicated a continuous rise of self-reported asthma and asthma related symptoms from 1964 well into the 1990s.[36,37] In fact, between 1989 and 1994 the prevalence of diagnosed asthma increased from 10.2% to 19.6% in this study, while the prevalence of hay fever stayed almost the same. The prevalence of both viral wheeze and of wheeze due to multiple triggers has increased over the 1990s in preschool children.[38] The increase in prevalence may be even greater for non-atopic than for atopic wheeze and asthma.[39] Therefore, it cannot be determined with certainty if the peak in asthma prevalence has yet been reached.

Another study from Scotland investigated the changes in prevalence of different types of wheezing over two generations.[40] In this study, children from individuals originally studied as children in the 1960s were selected as probands. Children of probands classified as having wheezy bronchitis (wheezing with viral infections alone) in the 1960s had a lower prevalence of current wheezing symptoms than those children whose parents had been diagnosed with asthma during their childhood. Thus it can be speculated that virus induced wheezing (wheezy bronchitis) and multiple cause wheezing (childhood asthma) differ in their heritability. However, it has been shown in the same study population, that atopic asthma increased significantly within one generation. This is occurring in children from families with no pre-existing history of asthma or atopy, previously considered to be of low risk of developing asthma.[41]

Trends in hospital admission rates for childhood asthma

The increase in prevalence of childhood asthma during the last decades was accompanied by an increase in hospital admissions during the same time period. The association between these two observations is not necessarily straightforward. When interpreting hospitalization data additional factors have to be taken into consideration.

A striking increase in hospital admissions for asthma has been reported in children between 0 and 14 years of age since the 1960s in many parts of the world (Table 2.2; Figure 2.4). Hospital admission data in the form of the international classification of disease (ICD-9) was available in all these countries for analysis except for the US, where disease data was obtained at the discharge from the hospital. In this international comparison hospital admission showed a 10-fold increase in New Zealand between the mid-1960s and the early 1980s, while rates in England and Wales rose by six-fold. In the US a three-fold increase was observed and in Australia the increase varied between three and eight-fold dependent on the study region. This increase was strongest in the 0 to 4-year-olds but rates in the 5 to 14-year-olds have more than doubled since the early 1970s. There are indications, however, that the increasing trend in hospitalization has stopped in the late 1980s and even a small decrease in hospital admission has been reported from some countries in the 1990s.[42]

In many countries the rate of hospitalization has risen much faster than the prevalence of asthma. There is, however, little evidence to suggest that asthma requiring hospital admission has increased in severity. Changes in coding of respiratory conditions might have contributed to the increasing trends observed, since the diagnosis of bronchitis seems to overlap with that of asthma in some cases. While a US study suggested a sudden 40% shift from a diagnosis of bronchitis to asthma as a consequence of changes in the ICD coding that occurred in 1979, no such trends were found in studies from New Zealand, England and Wales or Australia. However, in

Table 2.2 *Changes in admission rates for asthma and wheezing in children and adolescents*

Country	Reference	Age (yr)	Period	Admission rate (per 1000 children per year)	
				1st timepoint	2nd timepoint
Australia	Carman[43]	0–17	1971–1987	3.25	10
Netherlands	Wever-Hess[154]	0–4	1980–1994	1.02	2.1
New Zealand	Jackson[157]	0–14	1966–1981	0.6	6.29
New Zealand	Horwood[158]	0–13	1974–1989	1.4	6
Norway	Jonasson[159]	0–14	1980–1995	0.8[a]	2.9[a]
Norway	Jonasson[159]	0–14	1980–1995	0.7[b]	0.4[b]
Spain	Benito[153]	2–14	1987–1992	2.98	4.05
Sweden	Wennergren[152]	2–18	1985–1993	350*	200*
USA, CA	Von Behren[42]	0–15	1983–1996	2.17	1.90
USA, NH	Goodman[155]	0–17	1985–1994	1.4	1.03
USA, NY	Goodman[155]	0–17	1985–1994	3.55	4.77
USA, Maine	Goodman[155]	0–17	1985–1994	1.74	1.33
USA, Vermont	Goodman[155]	0–17	1985–1994	1.98	1.09
USA, national	Gergen[156]	0–17	1979–1987	1.73	2.57

* Total admissions per year.
[a] First admissions.
[b] Re-admissions.

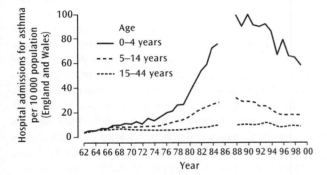

Figure 2.4 *Trends in the rate of hospital admissions for asthma by age group for England and Wales. (From ref. 160.)*

a Western Australian study a significant shift from the diagnosis of bronchitis to asthma was observed over a 17-year time period and this at least partly contributed to the increase in hospital admissions attributed to asthma over recent decades.[43] In the United States, the prevalence of childhood asthma and respiratory symptoms was assessed in 1981 and 1988[44] showing a significant increase of asthma symptoms without evidence for an increase of disease severity or hospitalization due to asthma.

Apart from changes in disease coding other factors may also have contributed to the increasing rate of hospitalization for asthma between the 1960s and 1980s. Changes in the accessibility of hospital care compared with primary care may play a role. Indeed, a five-fold increase of self-referrals for asthma attacks in children was observed in a British study.[42] This reflects the increasing tendency of parents to take their children directly to emergency departments in the event of an asthma attack instead of consulting their primary care

physician first.[45,46] A lack of accessible primary care facilities may also be a reason why children of minority backgrounds such as African–American children in the US or Polynesian children in New Zealand show much higher admission rates for asthma than their Caucasian peers. The availability of appropriate healthcare for children is clearly linked to the economic status of families. Thus, when controlling for family income, black and white children of comparable poverty levels showed nearly identical rates of hospitalization for asthma in a US study.[47]

Asthma treatment in primary care settings may also be expected to influence the rate of hospital admissions. A Swedish study demonstrated a drastic reduction in the total number of hospital days as well as hospital admissions for childhood asthma between 1985 and 1993, which coincided with the introduction of inhaled steroids for anti-inflammatory treatment of asthma in this age group in Sweden. These findings were confirmed by a second study from Sweden, which correlated the decrease in numbers of childhood asthma hospitalization days with increased regional sales of inhaled corticosteroids.[48] An alternative explanation for the decrease in hospitalization rates observed lately in some US surveys was suggested by a very recent study from Rochester.[49] Investigating the severity of asthma by measuring oxygen saturation levels within the first 24 hours of admission, a three-fold increase in severe asthma admissions was observed between 1991 and 1995 while the overall hospitalization rate remained almost constant. This might indicate that the threshold for asthma admissions has increased during the 1990s to keep hospitalization rates low.

Many hospital admissions for asthma are re-admissions. There is evidence that re-admission rates are falling, especially in preschool children, and that this could be hiding a continued rise in first admissions.[158]

Trends in childhood asthma mortality

Asthma is a rare cause of death during childhood, and mortality rates due to asthma have remained fairly low for the second half of the 20th century in most developed countries. However, there appeared to be two major epidemics of asthma deaths in children and young adults; one in the 1960s and a second in the late 1970s. Both epidemics were linked to the overuse of certain high-dose bronchodilators but the evidence was not fully conclusive. However, when these drugs were removed from the market, the death rate fell accordingly.[50]

Trends in death rates differ greatly between countries. An increase in asthma related deaths in childhood between the mid-1970s and mid-1980s was observed in the UK,[51] Australia and Germany.[52] In the US, the mortality rate for childhood asthma almost doubled between 1978 and 1987.[53] Furthermore, asthma mortality in non-Caucasian Americans was found to be three times as high as in white children. Other countries like Japan, Switzerland and France showed little variation in mortality rates over the same period of time.[52] However, more recent studies from the UK showed a decrease in asthma mortality beginning in the late 1980s.[54] Thereafter death rates remained stable in the 1990s, approximately below 1 per 100 000 in the 15 to 24-year-olds and below 3 per 100 000 in the age group 0–14 years.[55] For the US a further increase in asthma mortality was reported until as recently as 1994[56] at which point death rates for asthma among children and young adults were similar to those reported from England. This increase was observed despite growing sales and use of anti-inflammatory drugs during this period.

Data on asthma mortality in developing countries are sparse. However, a survey from Mauritius reported an overall dramatic decline of asthma deaths in children.[57] Between 1982 and 1991 asthma mortality steadily dropped from 20 to 5 per 100 000 in 0 to 4-year-old children while numbers dropped from 2.6 to 1.0 per 100 000 in the 5 to 34-year age group. This probably reflects improvements in general healthcare and better availability of treatment. At the beginning of the 1990s, there was no significant difference in childhood asthma mortality between Mauritius and other more industrialized countries.

RISK FACTORS FOR CHILDHOOD ASTHMA AND WHEEZING

Risk factors are characteristics present more frequently in people that have or develop a disease than in those that do not. However, not all risk factors are causally involved in the development of a given disease and some risk factors can be associated indirectly. So it can be argued that drinking alcohol is a risk factor for lung cancer as it is found more frequently in people with the disease than without it. However, it has been shown that people who drink also smoke cigarettes more frequently. Thus, although drinking alcohol is associated with lung cancer and therefore is a risk factor, a causal relationship exists only between smoking and the occurrence of the disease. Conversely, all causes are also risk factors. However, in chronic diseases such as asthma causal factors and expression of the disease will generally be separated by a period of time thus making it more difficult to establish causal relationships. Therefore, even if risk factors assessed by epidemiological studies are not causally related to the disease, they may be a necessary first step towards the identification of causal factors.

Risk factors for the development of childhood asthma may not be identical to risk factors for the exacerbation of symptoms or triggers for asthma attacks. Furthermore, risk factors may vary between different subtypes of asthma such as viral induced wheezing and atopic asthma. Some risk factors will also play a role in determining the prognosis of the disease as well as the severity of symptoms over time.

Which risk factors are necessary and what is sufficient to lead to the expression of childhood asthma? Without a necessary factor disease expression is not possible while sufficiency indicates a threshold of factors that permits disease expression. As for many other chronic disorders, childhood asthma is likely to be determined by multiple factors, some of which constitute host characteristics such as gender, race and genetic background while others consist of extrinsic, environmental influences. These factors interact on several different levels. In addition, certain windows of opportunity for different exposures may exist and differ between types of wheezing and atopic conditions. Therefore, the timing of exposure may play a crucial role for a certain factor to affect either the onset or the progression of illness.

Most studies of risk factors have used cross-sectional study designs, which are less suitable to allow different wheezing phenotypes to be identified. Studies performed in infants and preschool children are therefore likely to identify different risk factors than surveys of school-children or adolescents. Unless wheezing phenotypes are carefully characterized in a longitudinal study, a substantial misclassification bias is likely to significantly hamper the understanding of factors determining the onset and persistence of childhood asthma and wheezing illnesses (Chapter 3).

Potential gene by environment interactions must become a focus of attention since complex diseases such as asthma and allergic conditions are likely to result from interactions between multiple major and minor genes and important environmental factors. The search for genes and for environmental determinants relies on increasing knowledge about the mutual cofactors.

Genetic factors

Convincing evidence exists for a strong genetic component in asthma and other atopic disorders. Twin studies estimated the genetic contribution to preschool and childhood asthma as high as 75%.[58,59] Segregation analysis has suggested that in large family pedigrees the patterns of asthma occurrence match best with models of either polygenetic or oligogenetic inheritance.[60,61] This would indicate that multiple genes are involved in determining the susceptibility for childhood asthma, which may thereby contribute to the variability in the phenotypic expression of the disease. Purely genetic models were rejected in theses studies stressing the importance of environmental cofactors for the development of childhood asthma.

Our knowledge about the genetic mechanisms involved in the development of asthma is beginning to evolve as more candidate genes are identified and screened for polymorphisms. Since numerous genes are likely to be involved in these putative gene-by-environment interactions, a great effort is needed to fully understand the impact of genetics in childhood asthma (Chapter 4d).

Environmental tobacco smoke

Tobacco smoke has been identified as a main source of indoor air pollution. The effects of exposure to environmental tobacco smoke (ETS) on children have been extensively studied and numerous surveys have reported an association between ETS exposure and respiratory diseases. Strong evidence exists that passive smoking increases the risk of lower respiratory tract illnesses such as bronchitis, wheezy bronchitis and pneumonia in infants and young children. Maternal smoking during pregnancy and early childhood has been shown to be strongly associated with impaired lung growth and diminished lung function[62,63] which in turn may predispose infants to develop transient early wheezing. In children with asthma parental smoking is independently associated with increases symptoms and frequency of asthma attacks.

A series of epidemiological studies has been performed to determine the effect of ETS exposure on the inception, prevalence and severity of asthma and other wheezing illnesses during childhood. In most cross-sectional studies ETS exposure appears to be an important risk factor for the development of childhood asthma. Furthermore, in the longitudinal Tucson Cohort Study maternal smoking was related to both transient early wheezing and persistent wheezing.[3] A recent meta-analysis of 51 publications investigating the effect of ETS exposure on the development of asthma estimated a 37% increased risk for acquiring asthma up to the age of 6 and a 13% increased risk after the age of 6 if the parents smoked.[64] The effects of ETS exposure on the development of childhood asthma and atopic diseases are further discussed in Chapter 7e.

Nutrition

The rise in childhood asthma prevalence over the last 30 years in industrialized countries has coincided with a substantial change in dietary habits. Therefore, the hypothesis was proposed that dietary change may be a contributory factor for the development of atopic diseases. In general, the intake of fresh fruit and vegetables, milk, and fish has been replaced by the consumption of highly processed foods in western societies and increasingly in many developing countries.

Furthermore, *breast-feeding* rates declined in most affluent countries over the last decades as feeding formulas became more popular. Breast-feeding has shown a transient protective effect towards the development of eczema, food allergy and wheezing during the first 3 years of life in some studies but not in others. These studies are confounded by the frequency with which transient viral wheeze (as distinct from atopic asthma) occurs in the first 2–3 years of life (Chapter 3). Recently, prospective cohort studies from Australia investigating the association between infant nutrition and asthma have shown protective effects of breast-feeding in 3 to 5-year-olds[65] and 6-year-olds.[66] In contrast, recent data from the Tucson cohort suggested that the effects of breast-feeding may differ between children at high and low risk of asthma.[67] Among children of non-asthmatic mothers, breast-feeding was associated with a lower prevalence of recurrent wheezing during the first two years of life (transient wheeze) and was unrelated to the occurrence of wheezing after the age of 6 years (late or persistent wheeze). Conversely, in children of asthmatic mothers breast-feeding was associated with a higher risk of developing wheezing after the age of 6 years. A meta-analysis of published evidence suggests an overall protective effect from breast-feeding.[68] Based on current knowledge it seems impossible to predict the effects of breast-feeding on the development of asthma and atopic diseases in an individual child. Breast milk has been shown to contain various fatty acids and immunomodulatory agents which may influence a child's susceptibility to develop asthma and wheezing illnesses.

Intervention studies in a cohort of high-risk children (determined by a strong familial background of asthma and atopy) showed a benefit when a combination of maternal allergen avoidance during pregnancy and hydrolysed formulas was applied.[69] However, the effects were only transient, resulting in a reduction of early wheeze, eczema and gastrointestinal food allergy. No protective effect on the development of asthma later in childhood was found. Obesity in children is an increasing problem. The Tucson Cohort study has shown a 7-fold increase in the incidence of new asthma symptoms as well as BHR in girls who become obese in middle-childhood.[70]

In the late 1980s it was first suggested that high levels of *sodium intake* may contribute to the development of asthma.[71] This was based on the ecological observation that asthma mortality was highest in those regions of England and Wales, with the highest levels of salt intake. In subsequent studies, an association between sodium intake and BHR was reported,[72] although population-based studies did not confirm a relation between asthma and salt intake.[73]

Magnesium is involved in a wide range of biological pathways. In adults aged 18 to 70, low levels of magnesium intake were related to a decrease in lung function, the occurrence of airway hyperreactivity and self-reported wheezing within the past 12 months.[74] However, data on the effect of magnesium in childhood are sparse. A study from Saudi Arabia indicated that low levels of magnesium, together with a low intake of milk, vegetables, and fibre may be associated with wheezing illnesses in children.[75]

Furthermore, the balance between *unsaturated and saturated fatty acids* may have shifted towards a higher consumption of unsaturated oils and *trans*-fatty acids over recent decades. While meat and margarine have high levels of unsaturated arachidonic acid, deep-sea fish like tuna, salmon and herring provide high levels of unsaturated eicosapentanoic acid.[76] In population based studies subjects who regularly consumed fresh oily fish showed a lower prevalence of asthma and BHR as well as better baseline levels of lung function.[77–79] Among asthmatic children interventional studies failed to document a positive effect of oily fish consumption on the severity of symptoms.[80] In preschool children, a diet high in polyunsaturated fats significantly increased the risk of recent asthma.[65]

Finally, low levels of intake of the *antioxidant* vitamin C have been associated with the increasing prevalence of childhood asthma in Western societies. An ecological study found evidence that fresh fruit intake was associated with reduced allergic sensitization.[81] Epidemiological studies have reported lower levels of lung function in individuals with a low intake of vitamin C.[82,83] In a large British study of young adults the frequency and severity of asthma attacks was negatively associated with the intake of fresh fruit and positively associated with smoking.[84] Furthermore, it was reported that the intake of fresh fruit during winter was inversely correlated with the presence of asthma symptoms in more than 4000 Italian children.[85] The results suggested that the consumption of fruit rich in vitamin C, even at a low levels, may reduce wheezing symptoms in childhood, especially among already susceptible individuals. To date, however, the majority of supplementation studies have provided only inconclusive evidence for the effects of short-term vitamin C administration in adults. No intervention data are available in childhood asthma.

In summary,[86] based on the current knowledge from epidemiological studies some evidence exists that a diet low in sodium and rich in fish and vitamin C has a positive effect on the course of asthma symptoms. However, intervention studies in childhood are needed to test the hypothesis that nutrition may be involved in the development of childhood asthma. After all it seems unlikely that changes in nutrition alone are responsible for the increase in asthma prevalence in Western societies over the last decades. Nevertheless, changes in diet may have contributed to other disease patterns observed today in industrial societies.

Air pollution

Air pollution is perceived by the public as a major health problem all around the world. What would be more obvious than to suspect that it may also play a role in the development of respiratory diseases and especially asthma? Thus numerous studies have been performed to investigate if an association between ambient air pollution and childhood asthma exists. However, based on evidence derived from many epidemiological surveys, it seems very unlikely that air pollution significantly contributes to the development (inception) of childhood asthma.[87] Nevertheless, findings from a number of studies suggested that air pollution is a trigger of symptoms in individuals who already suffer from asthma.[88,89]

Prior to re-unification in 1990, differences between East and West Germany were not limited to political and economical systems but differences also existed in the amount and quality of environmental pollution. Areas of heavy industry in the East reached excessively high levels of classic air pollutants such as sulphur dioxide and smoke particles. Conversely, West German cities showed considerably higher levels of pollution with nitrogen dioxide reflecting the higher density of vehicular traffic. Surveys in the now reunited Germany[90,91] have consistently shown that the prevalence of childhood asthma, BHR and atopy were significantly lower in East than in West Germany. Confirmation of these observations has been obtained in other parts of Eastern Europe.[10,11]

As the comparisons between East and West Europe indicated, a higher prevalence of childhood asthma was observed in Western cities.[90] Hence, it was argued that other components of air pollution other than sulphur dioxide and smoke particles are associated with childhood asthma. Pollutants characteristic for Western cities are traffic related and therefore some interest in the potential effects of *automobile exhausts* on the development of asthma arose. Diesel exhaust is the single most important component of particulate matter in most urban areas in cities world-wide.[92] Diesel particles are ultrafine (<1 micron) and therefore small enough to penetrate deep into the peripheral airways.[93] In addition, they can act as carriers for ubiquitous airborne allergens thus facilitating their deposition in the lung. Several experimental studies have established that the exposure to diesel exhaust increases levels of IgE and allergy-specific cytokines in previously sensitized subjects.[94] These results suggest that diesel particles are capable of aggravating pre-existing allergic symptoms but do not necessarily imply that exposure to diesel fumes also induces the development of new cases of atopy. In fact, epidemiological studies suggested no major role for the exposure to car and truck traffic, which are the main sources of diesel particles, on the inception of asthma and atopy.[95,96]

A potential role for *ozone* was implied by the observation that a single high-dose ozone exposure can evoke respiratory obstruction, cough and chest pain. In addition ozone can induce neutrophilic inflammation of the airway submucosa and increase airway reactivity in sensitive subjects.[97] These effects are, however, at least in part reversible after continuous exposure indicating adaptation of subjects exposed for more than two days in experimental studies. Epidemiological data on the effects of ozone on childhood asthma are sparse. While the prevalence of childhood asthma was shown to increase according to the level of long-term ozone exposure in an American study,[98] no such relation was observed in a Swiss survey.[99] However, neither of these two studies included objective measures of atopy or BHR. Likewise, results in adults are inconclusive.

Socio-economic status and housing

A higher prevalence of asthma has been found in affluent Western societies compared to developing countries. Thus it has been suggested that the *socio-economic status* of countries and individual families may influence the development of childhood asthma. Low prevalence rates of asthma in rural and poor areas of Africa seem to support this hypothesis, as children from more affluent centres in these countries showed a higher prevalence of asthma symptoms.[20] Results from British studies indicated an increased risk for atopic diseases in children from high social class families compared to those from lower classes.[100] However, asthma rates were less affected by socio-economic status. Moreover, the association between socio-economic status and an increased prevalence of asthma is inverted in urban areas of the USA.[101] Here, poverty and living in run-down inner city districts were shown to be strong predictors for the development of childhood asthma in a number of studies.

These results, which seem contradictory at first sight, may indicate that socio-economic status may be a surrogate for living conditions and lifestyle, rather than a risk factor for asthma in itself. Factors influenced by social status include availability of and access to healthcare, nutrition and physical exercise, housing conditions, exposure to allergens and family size.

The quality of *housing*, which is strongly related to family income, has been suspected to influence the prevalence of asthma diagnosis, asthma symptoms and asthma severity. Indoor dampness[99] and exposure to certain fungal spores[102] have repeatedly been shown to be associated with a higher risk of asthma and respiratory symptoms in children, independent of parental socio-economic status. Furthermore, an American case control study, which quantified the asthma symptoms and the severity of dampness at home in more than 200 adults, reported a dose–response relation between the extent of dampness and the presence of asthma and asthma like symptoms.[103] In children with asthma, exposure to dampness at home may be a significant risk factor for the persistence of BHR and respiratory symptoms.[104]

Allergen exposure

There is increasing evidence to suggest that the level of allergen exposure is a risk factor for the development of *atopic sensitization* in children.[105–107] In the German Multicentre Atopy Study,[108] a large birth cohort following newborn children up to the age of 7 years, house-dust mite and cat allergen concentrations in domestic carpet dust were strongly related to the development of atopic sensitization to that specific allergen in the first three years of life and up to the age of 7 years. A clear dose-response relationship was found as well as a strong effect modification by the family background. In children with a positive family history of atopy, mite allergen concentrations below 750 ng/mg dust resulted in a sensitization rate of 3%, whereas in the group of children with a negative family history an exposure up to 25 000 ng/mg dust (over 30-fold higher) was necessary to achieve the same sensitization rate. These findings indicate that no general exposure threshold can be proposed and that in fact children with a genetic risk are susceptible to even very low levels of exposure. The relevance of allergen concentration for the inception of atopic sensitization extends beyond infancy, since similar findings have been reported for new-onset house-dust mite allergy in school age children.[106] These observations question the effectiveness of primary prevention procedures to reduce dust mite sensitization in infancy, especially in those at greatest risk.

Whether environmental allergen exposure affects the *inception of asthma* in similar ways as the development of atopic sensitization remains doubtful. In a prospective, longitudinal study of infants born to atopic parents, Sporik and colleagues[109] showed a strong correlation between wheezing and sensitization to mites at the age of 11. Exposure to house-dust mites in infancy was weakly associated with sensitization at age 11 ($p = 0.062$). There was considerable overlap in the degree of exposure in infancy and no difference in mean exposures between asymptomatic and wheezing school-children was found. However, a significantly increased risk of current asthma was apparent if a subject had in infancy been exposed to an arbitrary value of more than 10 µg per gram dust of Der p I, a major mite allergen.

If the level of exposure to mites in early infancy is indeed crucial for the expression of asthma, children brought up in a mite-free environment at high altitude or in a desert zone should have a significantly lower prevalence of asthma and wheeze than children from humid, mite-infested areas.

The results of two studies performed in the Alps and in New Mexico failed, however, to document a significant effect of a mite-free environment on the occurrence of asthma.[110,111] Furthermore, in desert areas such as Tucson, Arizona, US or inland Australia, where mites are rarely detected, asthma is just as common as elsewhere.[112,113] A recent report from the German Multicentre Study has pointed out that while allergen levels strongly predict specific sensitization the incidence of asthma up to the age of 7 years remains unaffected.[108] Thus, in contrast to the immunological processes involved in the production of specific IgE antibodies, the mechanisms inducing asthma might not be susceptible to changes in allergen exposure levels. The characteristic feature of an asthmatic subject may rather lie in that person's capacity to mount particularly strong IgE responses towards perennial, but not seasonal allergens, the strength of response being dependent on the level of exposure to that respective allergen.

Family size

Strachan first reported that sibship size is inversely related to the prevalence of childhood atopic diseases.[114] This observation has since been confirmed by numerous studies,[115–119] in relation to hay fever, atopic eczema and positive skin-prick tests and levels of allergen-specific IgE. In the majority of large studies the protective effect of having older siblings was stronger than having younger ones.

However, a number of earlier studies did not see a protective effect of a large family size for the development of asthma and BHR.[120]

Several hypotheses have been examined in an effort to explain the intriguing association between sibling numbers and the occurrence of atopic diseases. The effect of a larger family size is independent of parental socioeconomic status. Furthermore, maternal age at birth is not responsible for the protective effects of having older siblings, since a lower prevalence of atopic diseases was still observed after adjustment for maternal age. Some studies have even linked increasing maternal age to an increase in the prevalence of atopy.[115] Having more older siblings increases exposure to more viral infections thereby possibly directing the development of the immune system in a non-atopic direction (Chapter 4d). However, it is also conceivable that multiple pregnancies alter the immune status of the mother in a way that protects a child from developing atopic diseases. What causes the strong protective effect for asthma observed in children from large families still remains a topic of investigation.

Infections

The role of infection in the development of atopy and childhood asthma is still a matter of heated debate. Until some years ago it was commonly assumed that respiratory infections during infancy increased a child's risk of subsequently developing asthma. Conversely, recent epidemiological data have suggested a more complex and potentially protective effect of infections.

Viral infections of the upper as well as the lower respiratory tract are very common during infancy and early childhood, and most children do not suffer any aftermath.[121] There is, however, still an ongoing debate about a potential causal role of non-specific virus infections such as *respiratory syncytial virus* (RSV), for the subsequent development of childhood wheezing illness, asthma and atopy. Two major hypotheses have been proposed to explain the association between respiratory tract infections and subsequent respiratory abnormalities. One hypothesis states that viral infections early in life damage the growing lung or alter the host immune regulation. The second hypothesis holds that respiratory infections are more severe in infants and children with an underlying predisposition to wheeze, such as lower pre-morbid airway calibre.[126] In the latter case, the symptomatic viral infection is merely an indicator of an otherwise silent predisposition, whereas if the former hypothesis holds true, viral infections were causal risk factors. These two arguments are not mutually exclusive. It is conceivable that severe viral lower respiratory tract infections occur primarily in infants and children with an inherent predisposition, and that both the infection and the predisposition contribute to the development of wheezing illness or other long-term respiratory abnormality.

RSV infection is very common in the first year of life. According to Long and colleagues[121] 80% or more of all infants are infected with RSV by their first birthday, but only approximately 1% of all infants are hospitalized for RSV disease, and 0.1% require intensive care. Thus, most children undergo an inapparent RSV infection (causing only cold symptoms) in the first year of life suggesting that there is at least one host factor which determines the development of bronchiolitis after RSV infection.

Several investigators have followed children with proven RSV bronchiolitis for several years. Most authors reported reductions in lung function and increased prevalence of symptoms and airway hyperresponsiveness in the early years, compared with controls. These results are, however, also consistent with the notion of an underlying premorbid respiratory abnormality rather than a subsequent damage of the airways through the RSV infection. Pullen and co-workers[122] followed 130 infants with proven RSV bronchiolitis admitted to hospital at a mean age of 14 weeks and compared them with matched controls. Of the RSV group 6.2% were wheezing at the age of 10 years as compared with 4.5% of the control group. A slightly increased prevalence of repeated mild episodes of wheeze was found during the first 4 years of age (38% vs 15%), but no increased rate of atopic sensitization was seen in the cases as compared with the controls. A recent report from the longitudinal Tucson Birth Cohort Study corroborated the previous observations in a general population sample devoid of potential selection bias through follow-up of a selected hospital population. In the Tucson study, RSV lower respiratory tract illness was associated with a diminishing risk of recurrent wheezing with increasing age, with a 4-fold increased risk at age 6 years falling to no additional risk at age 13.[123] The occurrence of RSV lower respiratory tract illnesses was unrelated to the development of atopic sensitization. Other forms of virus-associated wheezing may be less related to atopy and BHR and have a better prognosis than atopic asthma.[124] The evidence for an inverse relationship between asthma and the overall burden of respiratory viral infections is reviewed in Chapter 7b.

A recent report from Southern Italy showed that military recruits who were sero-positive for hepatitis A, *Toxoplasma gondii* or *Helicobacter pylori* had a significantly lower prevalence of atopic sensitization to common aeroallergens and a lower prevalence of allergic asthma than their peers who did not have antibodies.[125] A dose–response relationship was observed: the more oro–fecal, the lower was the prevalence of allergic asthma.

In a recent study from East Germany the development of asthma at the age of 5–14 years was reduced in children from small families entering *day nursery* between 6–11 months of age compared with those entering day care after the first year of life.[126] These findings have recently been confirmed by a report from the Tucson Children's Respiratory Study showing that children in day care in the first 6 months of life were at significantly reduced risk of wheezing at school age and adolescence.[127] Likewise, frequent episodes of runny nose in the first year of life were inversely associated with the incidence of asthma and BHR up to the age of 7 years in the German multicentre study.[128]

The potential protective effect of *parasitic infections* in the developing world has not yet been explored adequately. The link between nematode infection and the host adaptive response[129,130] may hold the clue to the difference in prevalence of asthma between children in rural Africa and those in the industrialized world.[131]

Microbial stimulation, both from normal commensals and pathogens in the gut may be another route of exposure, which may have altered the normal intestinal colonization pattern in infancy. Thereby, the induction and maintenance of oral tolerance of innocuous antigens, such as food proteins and inhaled allergens may substantially be hampered.[132,133] These hypotheses, though intriguing, have to date not been supported by epidemiological evidence since significant methodological difficulties arise when attempting to measure the microbial pattern of the intestinal flora.

A 'human model' which may prove interesting in this context is the recent observation reported by several authors that growing up on a *traditional farm* confers significant protection against the development of asthma and atopy.[24–26,134,135] This protective effect was not seen in children growing up in a rural environment in non-farming households. Living conditions on farms differ in many respects from those of other families: more pets, larger family size, heating with wood and coal, less maternal smoking, more dampness and different dietary habits. None of these factors could sufficiently explain the strong inverse association between atopy, asthma and growing up on a farm. Therefore, it was suggested that the exposure to certain immune modulating agents specific for farm life may prevent the occurrence of these conditions. Frequent contact with livestock seems to explain the protective effect of farm life. A dose–response relationship between exposure to farm animals and the prevalence of atopic disease was reported among farmers' children in Bavaria.[26] This protective effect was not limited to children growing up on a farm. Frequent contact with farm animals by children who did not live on a farm, but had exposure through their peers, was reported to confer significant protection against the development of atopic sensitization.[25]

These findings suggest that factors prevalent in animal houses and presumably thereby also in the homes of farming families, confer the protection which is associated with a farming lifestyle. A potential candidate among other factors is exposure to bacterial products such as the endotoxin lipopolysaccharide (LPS) which may through binding with the CD14 receptor result in increased production of IL-12 and thereby activation of the Th1 pathway[136,137] (Chapter 4c). Polymorphisms in the CD14 gene have recently been identified[138] which may be of importance for a subject's response to the environmental exposure to bacterial products. Increased or altered microbial exposure may also arise through the consumption of unpasteurized milk. Further investigations including measurements of microbial contamination, a child's immune response and his/her genetic background in farming households are needed.

These findings have prompted investigators to speculate about a potential harmful effect of *vaccinations* and antibiotic use. This discussion was further fuelled by a report that, amongst BCG immunized Japanese schoolchildren, asthmatic symptoms and several indices of atopy were significantly less likely in positive tuberculin responders compared with negative responders, and that remission of atopic symptoms between the ages of 7 and 12 years was much more likely in positive tuberculin responders.[139] The interpretation of these findings has been debated intensively. The inverse association between allergic status and tuberculin reactivity may simply reflect the imbalance of Th1/Th2 responsiveness characteristic of atopic individuals who have been shown to express smaller delayed type hypersensitivity skin reactions to recall antigens than non-atopic subjects.[140] This imbalance may relate to genetic or other constitutional factors rather than to exposure to Mycobacteria. Such an interpretation is supported by findings of a Swedish group showing that a single immunization for BCG after birth does not affect the prevalence of atopic diseases at school age.[141]

Likewise, the role of vaccination for measles has been questioned. The generalization to western populations of the findings from Guinea-Bissau, West-Africa, that measles infection (in contrast to vaccination) reduced the risk of atopic sensitization,[142] must be called in question. Several studies have been unable to detect an adverse effect of childhood immunization on the development of allergic diseases.[143,144] Moreover, there is no evidence to date to suggest that the use of antibiotics may causally be related to the inception of childhood asthma or allergies. A recent retrospective study by Farooqi and Hopkin[145] showing a positive association between antibiotic use and asthma must be interpreted with great caution since there is potential severe bias by reverse causation: children with pre-existing symptoms of asthma may receive more antibiotics because of their respiratory symptoms. This study also pointed towards a potential risk associated with pertussis immunization, as seen in another investigation from New Zealand.[146] In the latter study, no recorded asthma episodes or consultations for asthma or other allergic illness before age 10 years were seen in the 23 children who received no diphtheria/pertussis/tetanus (DPT) and polio immunizations. These numbers are, however, quite small and other studies have failed to show significant associations with immunization status.[143,144]

THE FUTURE OF ASTHMA EPIDEMIOLOGY

There are several ways in which we can improve our understanding of causal factors in epidemiological studies of childhood asthma. Firstly, *informative study populations* must be identified. These may include populations over a broad range of exposure to a suspected risk factor, where after adjustment for confounding factors a potential dose-response effect can be investigated. Alternatively, populations with significant differences in the prevalence of asthma can be sought. Ideally, such populations should not differ in many exposures, which should furthermore not be strongly interrelated, otherwise the specific effect of an individual factor is almost impossible to identify. A comparison of envir-onmental influences in ethnically similar groups with presumably similar genetic background may prove particularly interesting.

Genetic epidemiology will open new avenues for research into the causes of asthma. Recent developments suggest that no single gene will be identified as explaining the clinical manifestations of asthma. Rather, a complex interplay of different genes will form a subject's genetic predisposition to disease. Such predisposition will, however, only result in illness in the context of exposure to certain environmental stimuli. The future challenge may thus consist in the identification of the relevant environmental exposures for a given subject's genetic make-up. These approaches may lead away from group data, which lumps subjects with very different susceptibilities in exposure groups, thereby increasing the ability to individually predict disease. When considering childhood asthma such gene-by-environment interactions will need to take one other element into consideration: the timing of the exposure. There is accumulating evidence to suggest that it is the very early years of life (including fetal life) which confer a risk for the inception of asthma whereas later exposures do not significantly affect the risk of disease, except in special circumstances, such as occupational exposures.

REFERENCES

1. Toelle BG, Peat JK, Salome CM, Mellis CM, Woolcock AJ. Toward a definition of asthma for epidemiology. *Am Rev Respir Dis* 1992;**146**:633–7.
2. Peat JK, Toelle BG, Marks GB, Mellis CM. Continuing the debate about measuring asthma in population studies. *Thorax* 2001;**56**:406–11.
3. Martinez FD, Wright AL, Taussig LM, Holberg CJ, Halonen M, Morgan WJ. Asthma and wheezing in the first six years of life. The Group Health Medical Associates. *N Engl J Med* 1995;**332**:133–8.
4. Wilson NM. Wheezy bronchitis revisited. *Arch Dis Child* 1989;**64**:1194–9.
5. de Marco R, Zanolin ME, Accordini S, Signorelli D, Marinoni A, Bugiani M, Lo Cascio V, Woods R, Burney P. A new questionnaire for the repeat of the first stage of the European Community Respiratory Health Survey: a pilot study. *Eur Respir J* 1999;**14**:1044–8.
6. Manual for the International Study of Asthma and Allergies in Childhood (ISAAC). Bochum and Auckland; 1992.
7. Burney PG, Luczynska C, Chinn S, Jarvis D. The European Community Respiratory Health Survey. *Eur Respir J* 1994;**7**:954–60.
8. Worldwide variation in prevalence of symptoms of asthma, allergic rhinoconjunctivitis, and atopic eczema: ISAAC. The International Study of Asthma and Allergies in Childhood (ISAAC) Steering Committee. *Lancet* 1998;**351**:1225–32.
9. von Mutius E, Fritzsch C, Weiland SK, Roll G, Magnussen H. Prevalence of asthma and allergic disorders among children in united Germany: a descriptive comparison. *BMJ* 1992;**30**:1395–9.
10. Bråbäck L, Breborowicz A, Dreborg S, Knutsson A, Pieklik H, Björksten B. Atopic sensitization and

respiratory symptoms among Polish and Swedish school children. *Clin Exp Allergy* 1994;**24**:826–35.

11. Bråbäck L, Breborowicz A, Julge K, Knutsson A, Riikjarv MA, Vasar M, Björksten B. Risk factors for respiratory symptoms and atopic sensitization in the Baltic area. *Arch Dis Child* 1995;**72**:487–93.

12. von Mutius E, Weiland SK, Fritzsch C, Duhme H, Keil U. Increasing prevalence of hay fever and atopy among children in Leipzig, East Germany. *Lancet* 1998;**351**:862–6.

13. Pattemore PK, Asher MI, Harrison AC, Mitchell EA, Rea HH, Stewart AW. Ethnic differences in prevalence of asthma symptoms and bronchial hyperresponsiveness in New Zealand schoolchildren. *Thorax* 1989;**44**:168–76.

14. Beckett WS, Belanger K, Gent JF, Holford TR, Leaderer BP. Asthma among Puerto Rican Hispanics: a multi-ethnic comparison study of risk factors. *Am J Respir Crit Care Med* 1996;**154**:894–9.

15. Kabesch M, Schaal W, Nicolai T, von Mutius E. Lower prevalence of asthma and atopy in Turkish children living in Germany. *Eur Respir J* 1999;**13**:577–82.

16. Leung RC, Carlin JB, Burdon JG, Czarny D. Asthma, allergy and atopy in Asian immigrants in Melbourne. *Med J Aust* 1994;**161**:418–25.

17. Grueger C, Plieth A, Taner C, Schmidt D, Sommerfeld C, Wahn U. Less allergic sensitization, wheezing, and itching eczema in Turkish children than in German children raised in Berlin, Germany. *J Allergy Clin Immunol* 2000;**105**:S32.

18. Hjern A, Rasmussen F, Hedlin G. Age at adoption, ethnicity and atopic disorder: a study of internationally adopted young men in Sweden. *Pediatr Allergy Immunol* 1999;**10**:101–6.

19. Van Niekerk CH, Weinberg EG, Shore SC, Heese HV, Van Schalkwyk J. Prevalence of asthma: a comparative study of urban and rural Xhosa children. *Clin Allergy* 1979;**9**:319–24.

20. Keeley DJ, Neill P, Gallivan S. Comparison of the prevalence of reversible airways obstruction in rural and urban Zimbabwean children. *Thorax* 1991;**46**:549–53.

21. Ng'ang'a LW, Odhiambo JA, Mungai MW, Gicheha CM, Nderitu P, Maingi B, Macklem PT, Becklake MR. Prevalence of exercise induced bronchospasm in Kenyan school children: an urban-rural comparison. *Thorax* 1998;**53**:919–26.

22. Strachan DP, Anderson HR, Limb ES, O'Neill A, Wells N. A national survey of asthma prevalence, severity, and treatment in Great Britain. *Arch Dis Child* 1994;**70**:174–8.

23. Strachan DP, Golding J, Anderson HR. Regional variations in wheezing illness in British children: effect of migration during early childhood. *J Epidemiol Community Health* 1990;**44**:231–6.

24. Braun-Fahrlander C, Gassner M, Grize L, Neu U, Sennhauser FH, Varonier HS, Vuille JC, Wuthrich B. Prevalence of hay fever and allergic sensitization in farmer's children and their peers living in the same rural community. SCARPOL team. Swiss Study on Childhood Allergy and Respiratory Symptoms with Respect to Air Pollution. *Clin Exp Allergy* 1999;**29**:28–34.

25. Riedler J, Eder W, Oberfeld G, Schreuer M. Austrian children living on a farm have less hay fever, asthma and allergic sensitization. *Clin Exp Allergy* 2000;**30**:194–200.

26. Von Ehrenstein OS, Von Mutius E, Illi S, Baumann L, Bohm O, von Kries R. Reduced risk of hay fever and asthma among children of farmers. *Clin Exp Allergy* 2000;**30**:187–93.

27. von Mutius E. In: Naspitz CK *et al.* Environmental factors and rising time trends in prevalence and severity. *The Textbook of Pediatric Asthma: An International Perspective*. Martin Dunitz, London, 1999.

28. Hill R, Williams J, Tattersfield A, Britton J. Change in use of asthma as a diagnostic label for wheezing illness in schoolchildren. *BMJ* 1989;**299**:898.

29. Burr ML, Butland BK, King S, Vaughan Williams E. Changes in asthma prevalence: two surveys 15 years apart. *Arch Dis Child* 1989;**64**:1452–6.

30. Anderson HR, Butland BK, Strachan DP. Trends in prevalence and severity of childhood asthma. *BMJ* 1994;**308**:1600–4.

31. Burney PG, Chinn S, Rona RJ. Has the prevalence of asthma increased in children? Evidence from the national study of health and growth 1973–86. *BMJ* 1990;**300**:1306–10.

32. Rona RJ, Chinn S, Burney PG. Trends in the prevalence of asthma in Scottish and English primary school children 1982–92. *Thorax* 1995;**50**:992–3.

33. Peat JK, van den Berg RH, Green WF, Mellis CM, Leeder SR, Woolcock AJ. Changing prevalence of asthma in Australian children. *BMJ* 1994;**308**:1591–6.

34. Shaw RA, Crane J, O'Donnell TV, Porteous LE, Coleman ED. Increasing asthma prevalence in a rural New Zealand adolescent population: 1975–89. *Arch Dis Child* 1990;**65**:1319–23.

35. Anderson HR. Is asthma really increasing? *Paediat Respir Med* 1993;**2**:6–10.

36. Ninan TK, Russell G. Respiratory symptoms and atopy in Aberdeen schoolchildren: evidence from two surveys 25 years apart. *BMJ* 1992;**304**:873–5.

37. Omran M, Russell G. Continuing increase in respiratory symptoms and atopy in Aberdeen schoolchildren. *BMJ* 1996;**312**:34.

38. Kuehni CE, Davis A, Brooke AM, Silverman M. Are all wheezing disorders in very young (preschool) children increasing in prevalence? *Lancet* 2001;**357**:1821–5.

39. Downs SH. Continued increase in the prevalence of asthma and atopy. *Arch Dis Child* 2001;**84**: 20–23.

40. Christie GL, Helms PJ, Ross SJ, Godden DJ, Friend JA, Legge JS, Haites NE, Douglas JG. Outcome of children of parents with atopic asthma and transient childhood wheezy bronchitis. *Thorax* 1997;**52**:953–7.

41. Christie GL, Helms PJ, Godden DJ, Ross SJ, Friend JA, Legge JS, Haites NE, Douglas JG. Asthma, wheezy bronchitis, and atopy across two generations. *Am J Respir Crit Care Med* 1999;**159**:125–9.

42. Von Behren J, Kreutzer R, Smith D. Asthma hospitalization trends in California, 1983–1996. *J Asthma* 1999;**36**:575–82.

43. Carman PG, Landau LI. Increased paediatric admissions with asthma in Western Australia – a problem of diagnosis? *Med J Aust* 1990;**152**:23–6.

44. Weitzman M, Gortmaker SL, Sobol AM, Perrin JM. Recent trends in the prevalence and severity of childhood asthma. *JAMA* 1992;**268**:2673–7.

45. Anderson HR. Increase in hospital admissions for childhood asthma: trends in referral, severity, and readmissions from 1970 to 1985 in a health region of the United Kingdom. *Thorax* 1989;**44**:614–19.

46. Strachan DP, Anderson HR. Trends in hospital admission rates for asthma in children. *BMJ* 1992;**304**:819–20.

47. Wissow LS, Warshow M, Box J, Baker D. Case management and quality assurance to improve care of inner-city children with asthma. *Am J Dis Child* 1988;**142**:748–52.

48. Gerdtham UG, Hertzman P, Jonsson B, Boman G. Impact of inhaled corticosteroids on acute asthma hospitalization in Sweden 1978 to 1991. *Med Care* 1996;**34**:1188–98.

49. Russo MJ, McConnochie KM, McBride JT, Szilagyi PG, Brooks AM, Roghmann KJ. Increase in admission threshold explains stable asthma hospitalization rates. *Pediatrics* 1999;**104**:454–62.

50. Pearce N, Beasley R, Crane J, Burgess C, Jackson R. End of the New Zealand asthma mortality epidemic. *Lancet* 1995;**345**:41–4.

51. Burney PG. Asthma mortality in England and Wales: evidence for a further increase, 1974–84. *Lancet* 1986;**2**:323–6.

52. Jackson R, Sears MR, Beaglehole R, Rea HH. International trends in asthma mortality: 1970 to 1985. *Chest* 1988;**94**:914–18.

53. Weiss KB, Wagener DK. Changing patterns of asthma mortality. Identifying target populations at high risk. *JAMA* 1990;**264**:1683–7.

54. Campbell MJ, Cogman GR, Holgate ST, Johnston SL. Age specific trends in asthma mortality in England and Wales, 1983–95: results of an observational study. *BMJ* 1997;**314**:1439–41.

55. Anderson HR, Strachan DP. Asthma mortality in England and Wales, 1979–89. *Lancet* 1991;**337**:1357.

56. Johnson CA, Mannino DM, Ashizawa A. Trends in asthma mortality. Asthma mortality in United States has risen but is similar to that in England and Wales. *BMJ* 1997;**315**:1012–13.

57. Fakim N, Subratty AH, Manraj M, Surrun SK, Hoolooman K. Asthma mortality in Mauritius: 1982–1991. *Ann Allergy Asthma Immunol* 1997;**79**:423–6.

58. Harris JR, Magnus P, Samuelsen SO, Tambs K. No evidence for effects of family environment on asthma. A retrospective study of Norwegian twins. *Am J Respir Crit Care Med* 1997;**156**:43–9.

59. Koeppen-Schomerus G, Stevenson J, Plomin R. Genes and environment in asthma: a study of 4 year old twins. *Arch Dis Child* 2001;**85**:398–400.

60. Sampogna F, Demenais F, Hochez J, Oryszczyn MP, Maccario J, Kauffmann F, Feingold J, Dizier MH. Segregation analysis of IgE levels in 335 French families (EGEA) using different strategies to correct for the ascertainment through a correlated trait (asthma). *Genet Epidemiol* 2000;**18**:128–42.

61. Martinez FD, Holberg CJ. Segregation analysis of physician-diagnosed asthma in Hispanic and non-Hispanic white families. *Clin Exp Allergy* 1995;**25**(Suppl 2):68–70; discussion 95–6.

62. Tager IB, Hanrahan JP, Tosteson TD, Castile RG, Brown RW, Weiss ST, Speizer FE. Lung function, pre- and post-natal smoke exposure, and wheezing in the first year of life. *Am Rev Respir Dis* 1993;**147**:811–17.

63. Hanrahan JP, Tager IB, Segal MR, Tosteson TD, Castile RG, Van Vunakis H, Weiss ST, Speizer FE. The effect of maternal smoking during pregnancy on early infant lung function. *Am Rev Respir Dis* 1992;**145**:1129–35.

64. Strachan DP, Cook DG. Health effects of passive smoking. 6. Parental smoking and childhood asthma: longitudinal and case–control studies. *Thorax* 1998;**53**:204–12.

65. Haby MM, Peat JK, Marks GB, Woolcock AJ, Leeder SR. Asthma in preschool children: prevalence and risk factors. *Thorax* 2001;**56**:589–95.

66. Oddy WH, Holt PG, Sly PD, Read AW, Landau LI, Stanley FJ, Kendall GE, Burton PR. Association between breast feeding and asthma in 6 year old children: findings of a prospective birth cohort study. *BMJ* 1999;**319**:815–19.

67. Wright AL, Holberg CJ, Toussing M, Martinez FD. Factors influencing the relation of infant feeding to asthma and recurrent wheeze in childhood. *Thorax* 2001;**56**:192–7.

68. Gdalevich M, Mimouni D, Mimouni M. Breast-feeding and the risk of bronchial asthma in childhood: a systematic review with meta-analysis of prospective studies. *J Pediatr* 2000;**139**:261–6.

69. Zeiger RS, Heller S. The development and prediction of atopy in high-risk children: follow-up at age seven years in a prospective randomized study of combined maternal and infant food allergen avoidance. *J Allergy Clin Immunol* 1995;**95**:1179–90.

70. Castro-Rodriguez JA, Holberg CJ, Morgan WJ, Wrist AL, Martinez FD. Increased incidence of asthma-like symptoms in girls who become overweight or obese during the school years. *Am J Resp Crit Care Med* 2001;**163**:1344–9.

71. Burney PG. The causes of asthma – does salt potentiate bronchial activity? Discussion paper. *J R Soc Med* 1987;**80**:364–7.

72. Burney PG, Britton JR, Chinn S, Tattersfield AE, Platt HS, Papacosta AO, Kelson MC. Response to inhaled histamine and 24 hour sodium excretion. *BMJ (Clin Res Ed)* 1986;**292**:1483–6.

73. Pistelli R, Forastiere F, Corbo GM, Dell'Orco V, Brancato G, Agabiti N, Pizzabiocca A, Perucci CA. Respiratory symptoms and bronchial responsiveness are related to dietary salt intake and urinary potassium excretion in male children. *Eur Respir J* 1993;**6**:517–22.

74. Britton J, Pavord I, Richards K, Wisniewski A, Knox A, Lewis S, Tattersfield A, Weiss S. Dietary magnesium, lung function, wheezing, and airway hyperreactivity in a random adult population sample. *Lancet* 1994;**344**:357–62.

75. Hijazi N, Abalkhail B, Seaton A. Diet and childhood asthma in a society in transition: a study in urban and rural Saudi Arabia. *Thorax* 2000;**55**:775–9.

76. Greene LS. Asthma, oxidant stress, and diet. *Nutrition* 1999;**15**:899–907.

77. Weiland SK, von Mutius E, Husing A, Asher MI. Intake of trans fatty acids and prevalence of childhood asthma and allergies in Europe. ISAAC Steering Committee. *Lancet* 1999;**353**:2040–1.

78. Hodge L, Salome CM, Peat JK, Haby MM, Xuan W, Woolcock AJ. Consumption of oily fish and childhood asthma risk. *Med J Aust* 1996;**164**:137–40.

79. Schwartz J, Weiss ST. The relationship of dietary fish intake to level of pulmonary function in the first National Health and Nutrition Survey (NHANES I). *Eur Respir J* 1994;**7**:1821–4.

80. Hodge L, Salome CM, Hughes JM, Liu-Brennan D, Rimmer J, Allman M, Pang D, Armour C, Woolcock AJ. Effect of dietary intake of omega-3 and omega-6 fatty acids on severity of asthma in children. *Eur Respir J* 1998;**11**:361–5.

81. Heinrich J, Hölscher B, Bolte G, Winkler G. Allergic sensitization and diet: ecological analysis in selected European cities. *Eur Resp J* 2001;**17**:395–402.

82. Britton JR, Pavord ID, Richards KA, Knox AJ, Wisniewski AF, Lewis SA, Tattersfield AE, Weiss ST. Dietary antioxidant vitamin intake and lung function in the general population. *Am J Respir Crit Care Med* 1995;**151**:1383–7.

83. Cook DG, Carey IM, Whincup PH, Papacosta O, Chirico S, Bruckdorfer KR, Walker M. Effect of fresh fruit consumption on lung function and wheeze in children. *Thorax* 1997;**52**:628–33.

84. Butland BK, Strachan DP, Anderson HR. Fresh fruit intake and asthma symptoms in young British adults: confounding or effect modification by smoking? *Eur Respir J* 1999;**13**:744–50.

85. Forastiere F, Pistelli R, Sestini P, Fortes C, Renzoni E, Rusconi F, Dell'Orco V, Ciccone G, Bisanti L. Consumption of fresh fruit rich in vitamin C and wheezing symptoms in children. SIDRIA Collaborative Group, Italy (Italian Studies on Respiratory Disorders in Children and the Environment). *Thorax* 2000;**55**:283–8.

86. Fogarty A, Britton J. The role of diet in the aetiology of asthma. *Clin Exp All* 2000;**30**:615–27.

87. von Mutius E. The environmental predictors of allergic disease. *J Allergy Clin Immunol* 2000;**105**:9–19.

88. Bascom R, Bromberg PA, Costa DA. State of the art: health effects of outdoor air pollution; part I. *Am J Respir Crit Care Med* 1996;**153**:3–53.

89. Bascom R, Bromberg PA, Costa DA. State of the art: health effects of outdoor air pollution; part II. *Am J Respir Crit Care Med* 1996;**153**:477–98.

90. von Mutius E, Martinez FD, Fritzsch C, Nicolai T, Roell G, Thiemann HH. Prevalence of asthma and atopy in two areas of West and East Germany. *Am J Respir Crit Care Med* 1994;**149**:358–64.

91. Nowak D, Heinrich J, Jorres R, Wassmer G, Berger J, Beck E, Boczor S, Claussen M, Wichmann HE, Magnussen H. Prevalence of respiratory symptoms, bronchial hyperresponsiveness and atopy among adults: west and east Germany. *Eur Respir J* 1996;**9**:2541–52.

92. Salvi SS, Frew A, Holgate S. Is diesel exhaust a cause for increasing allergies? *Clin Exp Allergy* 1999;**29**:4–8.

93. Bunn H, Dinsdale D, Smith T, Grigg J. Ultra fine particles in alveolar macrophages from normal children. *Thorax* 2002;**56**:932–4.

94. Salvi S, Holgate ST. Mechanisms of particulate matter toxicity. *Clin Exp Allergy* 1999;**29**:1187–94.

95. Wjst M, Reitmeir P, Dold S, Wulff A, Nicolai T, von Loeffelholz Colberg EF, von Mutius E. Road traffic and adverse effects on respiratory health in children. *BMJ* 1993;**307**:596–600.

96. Oosterlee A, Drijver M, Lebret E, Brunekreef B. Chronic respiratory symptoms in children and adults living along streets with high traffic density. *Occup Environ Med* 1996;**53**:241–7.

97. Koenig JQ, Pierson WE, Covert DS, Marshall SG, Morgan MS, van Belle G. The effects of ozone and nitrogen dioxide on lung function in healthy and asthmatic adolescents. *Res Rep Health Eff Inst* 1988;**14**:5–24.

98. Dockery DW, Speizer FE, Stram DO, Ware JH, Spengler JD, Ferris BG, Jr. Effects of inhalable

particles on respiratory health of children. *Am Rev Respir Dis* 1989;**139**:587–94.

99. Braun Fahrlander C, Kunzli N, Domenighetti G, Carell CF, Ackermann Liebrich U. Acute effects of ambient ozone on respiratory function of Swiss schoolchildren after a 10-minute heavy exercise. *Pediatr Pulmonol* 1994;**17**:169–77.

100. Lewis SA, Britton JR. Consistent effects of high socioeconomic status and low birth order, and the modifying effect of maternal smoking on the risk of allergic disease during childhood. *Respir Med* 1998;**92**:1237–44.

101. McConnochie KM, Russo MJ, McBride JT, Szilagyi PG, Brooks AM, Roghmann KJ. Socioeconomic variation in asthma hospitalization: excess utilization or greater need? *Pediatrics* 1999;**105**:1171.

102. Garrett MH, Rayment PR, Hooper MA, Abramson MJ, Hooper BM. Indoor airborne fungal spores, house dampness and associations with environmental factors and respiratory health in children. *Clin Exp Allergy* 1998;**28**:459–67.

103. Williamson IJ, Martin CJ, McGill G, Monie RD, Fennerty AG. Damp housing and asthma: a case-control study. *Thorax* 1997;**52**:229–34.

104. Nicolai T, Illi S, von Mutius E. Effect of dampness at home in childhood on bronchial hyperreactivity in adolescence. *Thorax* 1998;**53**:1035–40.

105. Lau S, Falkenhorst G, Weber A, Werthmann I, Lind P, Buettner Goetz P, Wahn U. High mite-allergen exposure increases the risk of sensitization in atopic children and young adults. *J Allergy Clin Immunol* 1989;**84**:718–25.

106. Kuehr J, Frischer T, Meinert R, Barth R, Forster J, Schraub S, Urbanek R, Karmaus W. Mite allergen exposure is a risk for the incidence of specific sensitization. *J Allergy Clin Immunol* 1994;**94**:44–52.

107. Wahn U, Lau S, Bergmann R, Kulig M, Forster J, Bergmann K, Bauer CP, Guggenmoos-Holzmann I. Indoor allergen exposure is a risk factor for sensitization during the first three years of life. *J Allergy Clin Immunol* 1997;**99**:763–9.

108. Lau S, Illi S, Sommerfeld C, Niggemann B, Bergmann R, von Mutius E, Wahn U, Multicentre Allergy Study Group. Early exposure to house dust mite and cat allergens and the development of childhood asthma: a cohort study. *Lancet* 2000;**356**:1392–7.

109. Sporik R, Holgate ST, Platts Mills TA, Cogswell JJ. Exposure to house-dust mite allergen (Der p I) and the development of asthma in childhood. A prospective study. *N Engl J Med* 1990; **323**:502–7.

110. Charpin D, Birnbaum J, Haddi E, Genard G, Lanteaume A, Toumi M, Faraj F, Van der Brempt X, Vervloet D. Altitude and allergy to house-dust mites.

A paradigm of the influence of environmental exposure on allergic sensitization. *Am Rev Respir Dis* 1991;**143**:983–6.

111. Sporik R, Ingram JM, Price W, Sussman JH, Honsinger RW, Platts Mills TA. Association of asthma with serum IgE and skin test reactivity to allergens among children living at high altitude. Tickling the dragon's breath. *Am J Respir Crit Care Med* 1995;**151**:1388–92.

112. Halonen M, Stern DA, Wright AL, Taussig LM, Martinez FD. Alternaria as a major allergen for asthma in children raised in a desert environment. *Am J Respir Crit Care Med* 1997;**155**:1356–61.

113. Peat JK, Woolcock AJ. Sensitivity to common allergens: relation to respiratory symptoms and bronchial hyper-responsiveness in children from three different climatic areas of Australia. *Clin Exp Allergy* 1991;**21**:573–81.

114. Strachan DP. Hay fever, hygiene, and household size. *BMJ* 1989;**299**:1259–60.

115. Strachan DP, Taylor EM, Carpenter RG. Family structure, neonatal infection, and hay fever in adolescence. *Arch Dis Child* 1996;**74**:422–6.

116. Wickens KL, Crane J, Kemp TJ, *et al.* Family size, infections, and asthma prevalence in New Zealand children. *Epidemiology* 1999;**10**(6):699–705.

117. Ponsonby AL, Couper D, Dwyer T, Carmichael A, Kemp A. Relationship between early life respiratory illness, family size over time, and the development of asthma and hay fever: a seven year follow up study. *Thorax* 1999;**54**:664–9.

118. Ball TM, Castro-Rodriguez JA, Griffith KA, Holberg CJ, Martinez FD, Wright AL. Siblings, day-care attendance, and the risk of asthma and wheezing during childhood. *N Engl J Med* 2000;**343**:538–43.

119. Rona RJ, Duran-Tauleria E, Chinn S. Family size, atopic disorders in parents, asthma in children, and ethnicity. *J Allergy Clin Immunol* 1997;**99**: 454–60.

120. Rona RJ, Hughes JM, Chinn S. Association between asthma and family size between 1977 and 1994. *J Epidemiol Community Health* 1999;**53**:15–19.

121. Long CE, McBride JT, Hall CB. Sequelae of respiratory syncytial virus infections. A role for intervention studies. *Am J Respir Crit Care Med* 1995;**151**:1678–80.

121a. Turner SW, Young S, Landau LI, LeSouef PN. Reduced lung function both before bronchiolitis and at eleven years. *Arch Dis Child* 2002 (in press).

122. Pullen CR, Hey EN. Wheezing, asthma and pulmonary dysfunction 10 years after infection with respiratory syncytial virus in infancy. *Br Med J* 1982;**284**:1665–9.

123. Stein RT, Sherrill D, Morgan WJ, Holberg CJ, Halonen M, Taussig LM, Wright AL, Martinez FD. Respiratory syncytial virus in early life and risk of wheeze and allergy by age 13 years. *Lancet* 1999;**354**:541–5.

124. von Mutius E, Illi S, Hirsch T, Leupold W, Keil U, Weiland SK. Frequency of infections and risk of asthma, atopy and airway hyperresponsiveness in children. *Eur Respir J* 1999;**14**:4–11.

125. Matricardi PM, Rosmini F, Riondino S, Fortini M, Ferrigno L, Rapicetta M, Bonini S. Exposure to foodborne and orofecal microbes versus airborne viruses in relation to atopy and allergic asthma: epidemiological study. *BMJ* 2000;**320**:412–17.

126. Kramer U, Heinrich J, Wjst M, Wichmann HE. Age of entry to day nursery and allergy in later childhood. *Lancet* 1999;**353**:450–4.

127. Ball TM, Castro-Rodriguez JA, Griffith KA, Holberg CJ, Martinez FD, Wright AL. Siblings, day-care attendance, and the risk of asthma and wheezing during childhood. *N Engl J Med* 2000;**343**:538–43.

128. Illi S, von Mutius E, Bergmann R, Lau S, Niggeman B, Wahn U, group tMS. Upper respiratory tract infections in the first year of life and asthma in children up to the age of 7 years. *BMJ* 2000 (in press).

129. Scrivener S, Britton J. Immunoglobulin E and allergic disease in Africa. *Clin Exp All* 2000;**30**:304–7.

130. Scrivener S, Yemaneberhan H, Zebenigus M, *et al.* Independent effects of intestinal parasite infection and domestic allergen exposure on risk of wheeze in Ethiopia: a nested case-control study. *Lancet* 2001;**358**:1493–9.

131. Le Souëf PN, Goldblatt J, Lynch NR. Evolutionary adaptation of inflammatory immune responses in human beings. *Lancet* 2000;**356**:24244–6.

132. Wold AE. The hygiene hypothesis revised: is the rising frequency of allergy due to changes in the intestinal flora? *Allergy* 1998;**53**:20–5.

133. Holt PG. Mucosal immunity in relation to the development of oral tolerance/sensitization. *Allergy* 1998;**53**:16–19.

134. Ernst P, Cormier Y. Relative scarcity of asthma and atopy among rural adolescents raised on a farm. *Am J Respir Crit Care Med* 2000;**161**:1563–6.

135. Kilpelainen M, Terho EO, Helenius H, Koskenvuo M. Farm environment in childhood prevents the development of allergies. *Clin Exp Allergy* 2000;**30**:201–8.

136. Holt PG, Sly PD, Bjorksten B. Atopic versus infectious diseases in childhood: a question of balance? *Pediatr Allergy Immunol* 1997;**8**:53–8.

137. Martinez FD. Maturation of immune responses at the beginning of asthma. *J Allergy Clin Immunol* 1999;**103**:355–61.

138. Baldini M, Lohman IC, Halonen M, Erickson RP, Holt PG, Martinez FD. A polymorphism in the 5′ flanking region of the CD14 gene is associated with circulating soluble CD14 levels and with total serum immunoglobulin E. *Am J Respir Cell Mol Biol* 1999;**20**:976–83.

139. Shirakawa T, Enomoto T, Shimazu S, Hopkin JM. The inverse association between tuberculin responses and atopic disorder. *Science* 1997;**275**:77–9.

140. Strannegård IL, Larsson LO, Wennergren G, Strannegård O. Prevalence of allergy in children in relation to prior BCG vaccination and infection with atypical mycobacteria. *Allergy* 1998;**53**: 249–54.

141. Alm JS, Lilja G, Pershagen G, Scheynius A. Early BCG vaccination and development of atopy. *Lancet* 1997;**350**:400–3.

142. Shaheen SO, Aaby P, Hall AJ, Barker DJ, Heyes CB, Shiell AW, Goudiaby A. Measles and atopy in Guinea-Bissau. *Lancet* 1996;**347**:1792–6.

143. Henderson J, North K, Griffiths M, Harvey I, Golding J. Pertussis vaccination and wheezing illnesses in young children: prospective cohort study. The Longitudinal Study of Pregnancy and Childhood Team. *BMJ* 1999;**318**:1173–6.

144. Nilsson L, Kjellman NI, Bjorksten B. A randomized controlled trial of the effect of pertussis vaccines on atopic disease. *Arch Pediatr Adolesc Med* 1998;**152**:734–8.

145. Farooqi IS, Hopkin JM. Early childhood infection and atopic disorder. *Thorax* 1998;**53**:927–32.

146. Kemp T, Pearce N, Fitzharris P, Crane J, Fergusson D, St. George I, Wickens K, Beasley R. Is infant immunization a risk factor for childhood asthma or allergy? *Epidemiology* 1997;**8**:678–80.

147. Manfreda J, Becker AB, Wang PZ, Roos LL, Anthonisen NR. Trends in physician-diagnosed asthma prevalence in Manitoba between 1980 and 1990. *Chest* 1993;**103**:151–7.

148. Whincup PH, Cook DG, Strachan DP, Papacosta O. Time trends in respiratory symptoms in childhood over a 24 year period. *Arch Dis Child* 1993;**68**:729–34.

149. Nystad W, Magnus P, Gulsvik A, Skarpaas IJ, Carlsen KH. Changing prevalence of asthma in school children: evidence for diagnostic changes in asthma in two surveys 13 years apart. *Eur Respir J* 1997;**10**:1046–51.

150. Hsieh KH, Shen JJ. Prevalence of childhood asthma in Taipei, Taiwan, and other Asian Pacific countries. *J Asthma* 1988;**25**:73–82.

151. Gergen PJ, Mullally DI, Evans RD. National survey of prevalence of asthma among children in the United States, 1976 to 1980. *Pediatrics* 1988;**81**:1–7.

152. Wennergren G, Kristjansson S, Strannegard IL. Decrease in hospitalization for treatment of childhood asthma with increased use of antiinflammatory treatment, despite an increase in prevalence of asthma. *J Allergy Clin Immunol* 1996;**97**:742–8.

153. Benito J, Bayon JL, Montiano J, Sanchez J, Mintegui S, Vazquez C. Time trends in acute childhood asthma in Basque Country, Spain. *Pediatr Pulmonol* 1995;**20**:184–8.

154. Wever-Hess J, Wever AM. Asthma statistics in The Netherlands 1980–94. *Respir Med* 1997;**91**:417–22.

155. Goodman DC, Stukel TA, Chang CH. Trends in pediatric asthma hospitalization rates: regional and socioeconomic differences. *Pediatrics* 1998;**101**:208–13.

156. Gergen PJ, Weiss KB. Changing patterns of asthma hospitalization among children: 1979 to 1987. *JAMA* 1990;**264**:1688–92.

157. Jackson RT, Mitchell EA. Trends in hospital admission rates and drug treatment of asthma in New Zealand. *N Z Med J* 1983;**96**:728–30.

158. Horwood LJ, Dawson KP, Mogridge N. Admission patterns for childhood acute asthma: Christchurch 1974–89. *N Z Med J* 1991;**104**:277–9.

159. Jonasson G, Lodrup Carlsen KC, Leegaard J, Carlsen K-H, Mowinckel P, Halvorsen KS. Trends in hospital admissions for childhood asthma in Oslo, Norway, 1980–95. *Allergy* 2000;**55**:232–9.

160. National Asthma Campaign. Out in the open – a true picture of asthma in the United Kingdom today. *Asthma J* 2001;**6**(Special Suppl 3):9.

3

The natural history of asthma during childhood

FERNANDO D MARTINEZ

CHILDHOOD ASTHMA AS A HETEROGENEOUS DISEASE

There is renewed interest in the patterns of expression of different forms of asthma-like symptoms during childhood. The main reason for this interest is the understanding that at least some forms of asthma (often referred to as 'asthma phenotypes') begin during the early years of life and later become lifelong conditions associated with significant morbidity, need for chronic therapy and frequent use of healthcare resources. For years, clinical experience indicated that these forms of more severe, persistent disease, co-exist with other forms of asthma, characterized by intermittent and less predictable symptomatology. It was not known, however, if this diversity was the expression of a spectrum of severity within a single disease caused by the same underlying pathogenetic mechanism or if asthma was heterogeneous in nature. Perhaps the most important advance in our understanding of childhood asthma in the last 30 years is the realization that asthma is not a single condition and that the same clinical manifestations may be the expression of different disease mechanisms.

In describing the natural history of childhood asthma, therefore, we will subdivide the disease into three main clinical expressions. We caution the reader, however, that in classifying childhood asthma we are faced with problems similar to those rheumatologists have to deal with in classifying the wide spectrum of autoimmune diseases. Although we believe that there is strong evidence indicating that the three basic conditions described below do exist as separate entities, there is wide overlap between them and they no doubt share common risk factors. No single risk factor has a one-to-one relation to any of the three main forms of childhood asthma. Therefore, it is often difficult to unmistakably classify every single patient into one group or the other. The fact that the prevalence of each group predominates during specific age periods no doubt helps, but at no age is there only one form of asthma.

It could be argued that distinguishing different forms of childhood asthma in order to describe the natural history of the disease may be artificial. It is true that, from a therapeutic point of view, it may be presently of little benefit to accurately classify any single patient as having a specific form of asthma. None of the treatment currently available has been unequivocally shown to be more effective in the control of asthma symptoms for one form or the other. However, this speaks more about the limitations of current asthma treatment, than against the existence of different forms of the disease in children. None of the treatments currently available for asthma truly address the underlying 'cause' of the disease because there is simply no way to know what that cause may be for each individual patient. Therefore, available treatments are either broadly 'anti-inflammatory' or symptomatic. It is thus not surprising that they are used in all forms of childhood asthma, with different (and often unpredictable) degrees of effectiveness. As well as potential therapeutic differences, there are other good reasons to differentiate different forms of asthma (Table 3.1).

There is little doubt that this situation will change in the near future. Studies of the genetics, immunology and

Table 3.1 *Clinically important reasons for differentiating between types of asthma (phenotypes)*

- Responses to treatment
- Causes (therefore preventive programmes)
- Natural history (prognosis)
- Genetic basis

cellular biology of asthma will help us to identify forms of the disease in which certain underlying disease mechanisms are predominant. The final goal of these studies is not only to identify therapies that will control symptoms, but to identify interventions to prevent lung damage or restore normality.

TRANSIENT WHEEZING OF INFANCY

The fact that infants and very young children are more likely to wheeze during viral infections has been known for many decades.[1] Although there has been controversy on the right nomenclature, for many years this condition was usually called 'bronchiolitis', and it was widely recognized that it was 'for the most part an acute, usually non-recurrent infection occurring in infancy and very early childhood'.[1] Recent longitudinal studies have indeed demonstrated that the majority of infants and young children who develop airway obstruction during acute viral infections will only have one or at most a few such episodes confined to the first 2–3 years of life.[2,3] We have proposed to call this condition transient early wheezing (see also Chapter 9).

The cumulative *incidence* of all episodes of bronchial obstruction associated with viral infection during the first years of life varies depending on the methods used to ascertain such episodes. However, the results of studies that have used prospective methodologies in general population samples suggest that no less than 30% of all children have at least one attack of bronchial obstruction during the first three years of life.[4] Peak incidence rates occur between the ages of 3 and 6 months,[5] and the frequency of new cases decreases markedly after the end of the first year. Epidemiologic studies have suggested that over two-thirds of all incident cases are due to respiratory syncytial virus (RSV), with parainfluenza and other viruses accounting for only a minority of such events.[6] In developed countries, no less than 60% of all infants and young children who have one or more episodes of wheezing during the first three years of life will have stopped wheezing by the early school years.[3] Thus up to 20% of all children will have transient early wheezing.

For the most part, transient early wheezers have mild symptoms that seldom occur away from concurrent upper respiratory illnesses. *Longitudinal studies* have demonstrated that infants who will stop wheezing are less likely to be hospitalized for this condition, and usually have

fewer and shorter episodes of bronchial obstruction than those who will have wheezing episodes that persist beyond the early years.[3] When compared with children who do not wheeze, these children are not more likely to have eczema, rhinitis apart from colds, or a maternal history of asthma.

The factors that determine this transient form of airway obstruction have been difficult to study, because there is no reliable way to distinguish these infants from those who will go on to have more persistent forms of asthma. Most of the data thus come from a small number of longitudinal studies.[7,8] The two main risk factors for transient early wheezing that have been quite conclusively identified are maternal smoking during pregnancy[9–11] and lower levels of lung function measured usually during the very first weeks of life and before any lower respiratory tract illness (LRI) developed.[4,11,12] Interestingly, young children whose mothers smoked during pregnancy have been consistently reported to have lower values for different parameters of lung function.[13] This has suggested the possibility that exposure to tobacco smoke products during pregnancy may alter the development of the lung *in utero*, thus predisposing to airway obstruction during LRIs. However, the relation between lower levels of lung function and transient early wheezing is also observed in children not exposed to tobacco smoke, so that factors other than maternal smoking must influence lung function in early life. Among these factors, it is important to consider the role of genetic predisposition. Several studies of familial aggregation have shown that levels of spirometric lung function are significantly correlated between siblings and between parents and offspring.[14,15] Many genes may determine lung size and airway size and tone, and it is thus unlikely that a single inherited factor may be responsible for the types of abnormality observed in transient early wheezers.

The nature of the alteration(s) in *lung function* in transient early wheezers is not well understood. A more detailed analysis of the characteristics of children who wheezed at different times during the first two years of life has been recently reported.[4] These studies show that children who started wheezing during the first year of life but were not wheezing during the second year of life, those who started wheezing during the second year of life, and those who wheezed both during the first and second year of life had significantly diminished levels of VmaxFRC (maximal flows obtained by the chest compression technique) before any LRIs occurred.[4] However, for those children who only wheezed during the first year of life, the neonatal lung function deficits had resolved by 12 months of age. On the contrary, among children who started wheezing during the second year of life or whose wheezing persisted into the second year of life lung function differences remained throughout the first year of life. The authors also found that children who wheezed only during the first year of life had significantly *increased* compliance of the respiratory system when measured shortly after birth and before any LRI. Conversely, children who wheezed during the first and second year of life had significantly *decreased* compliance of their respiratory system measured shortly after birth. Although these studies did not assess persistence of wheezing beyond the first two years of life, the results clearly suggest that different mechanisms may lead to transient infant wheezing, but all of them seem to point towards a final common pathway of reduced airway calibre predisposing to airway obstruction in this age group. In children with increased respiratory system compliance shortly after birth, this reduced airway calibre may spontaneously resolve with lung maturation during the first year of life, while in those with reduced compliance of the respiratory system shortly after birth the abnormalities appear to be more persistent and associated with recurrent wheezing during the first years of life.

It goes without saying that any of the abnormalities described above, especially those that persist beyond the first year of life, may predispose to forms of childhood asthma other than transient infant wheezing, especially if they are associated with risk factors that are more specific for these other forms of asthma. However, in the absence of such risk factors, it appears that the alterations in airway function that are responsible for transient infant wheezing reverse spontaneously with age. Since this reversion occurs concomitantly with remission of respiratory systems, it seems plausible to surmise a causal relation between pre-existing airway abnormalities and the likelihood of transient early wheezing.

PERSISTENT WHEEZING AFTER RSV INFECTION

Observations made in the 1980s first suggested that children who were infected with RSV and developed airway obstruction were more likely to have continued wheezing episodes years after the original RSV infection than those who did not.[16] This has been recently confirmed by the results of several long-term longitudinal studies.[17,18] The factors that determine this association have been the matter of intense controversy. One proposed explanation has been that RSV could cause damage to the airways and lungs, thus predisposing to subsequent recurrent obstructive illnesses. This contention was not devoid of empirical support. It has been known for years that some infants with severe acute adenoviral infection develop obliterative bronchiolitis, with persistent airflow limitation and marked abnormalities in lung function years after the initial episode. A consistent observation among children with a history of LRIs due to RSV in early life has been the presence of abnormalities in lung function many years after the original episode.[16,18,19] It was thus plausible to surmise that, as in the case of adenovirus, RSV could also cause lung and airway damage in susceptible children. As explained earlier, longitudinal studies have demonstrated that, in children who were destined to become transient early wheezers, lower levels of lung function were consistently found during the first months of life, before any sign of airway obstruction had occurred. However, among children with confirmed acute RSV infections whose wheezing episodes persisted up to age 6 and beyond (called 'persistent wheezers') lung function measured shortly after birth was only slightly (and not significantly) lower than that of children who never wheezed during the first years of life. When mean lung function in these same children was again assessed at age 6 it was found to be significantly lower than that of children who never wheezed before that age.[3,20] It was thus apparent that there was indeed a group of children who had RSV–LRIs and who showed progressive deficits in (pre-bronchodilator) airway function.

We also showed that children with a predisposition to allergic disease (eczema, parental history of asthma and allergies, high total serum IgE levels, among others) were more likely to become persistent wheezers than those who did not have such predisposition (see below: Atopic Asthma). Nevertheless, for the purpose of this discussion, it became relevant to assess if the association between RSV infection, low lung function, and subsequent asthma-like symptoms could be explained by the development of an acute, IgE-mediated response to RSV. This idea was first suggested by Welliver *et al.*,[21] who reported RSV-specific IgE in nasal secretions of a high proportion of infants who wheezed during RSV infection and subsequently developed recurrent wheezing episodes. Studies done by other groups could not confirm this.[22] Following those studies it was suggested that RSV infection could activate a Th2-type immune response not only against the virus itself but also facilitate the development of IgE responses against local aeroallergens.[23] We could not confirm this hypothesis. We found that children with confirmed RSV–LRI during the first 3 years of life were no more likely to have at least one positive skin test against aeroallergens at ages 6 or 11 than those with no such a history. Children with confirmed RSV–LRI were 4–5 times more likely to have wheezing episodes at age 6 than their peers, but this risk diminished significantly with age up to age 13[18] (Figure 3.1).

These results apparently contradict a recent report in a Swedish study by Sigurs *et al.*[17,24] These authors followed 47 infants hospitalized with RSV bronchiolitis and 89 controls up to age 7 years. They found that the RSV group had a 23% prevalence of current asthma at age 7 compared with only 2% among control subjects. Allergic sensitization was reported in 41% of the RSV children and 22% of controls. The authors suggest that their data support the contention that RSV increases the mechanisms involved in the development of both asthma and allergies in children. The population under study, however, was different to that in our study in Tucson: whereas all their subjects were hospitalized with severe bronchiolitis, over 95% of the children with RSV–LRI in our study were seen and diagnosed as outpatients. It is possible that a pre-existing predisposition to allergies may make it more likely that subjects with RSV infection develop severe airway obstruction needing hospitalization.

But in addition, their controls had a very low prevalence of current wheezing episodes (<5%) at age 7, compared with other reports from Sweden suggesting 2–3 times higher prevalence of current wheezing in school-age children.[25] It is thus possible that Sigurs *et al.*[24] may have used controls that were inadvertently biased towards less asthma and atopy than the general population.

An inherited or acquired predisposition for atopy does not seem therefore to explain the association between RSV–LRI and subsequent persistent wheezing. Support for this contention comes from our own observation (and that of others) of changes with age in the risk of subsequent wheezing after RSV–LRI.[18] We observed that, after adjusting for several known risk factors for asthma, children with confirmed RSV–LRI were 3–4 times more likely to have either infrequent (≤3) or frequent (>3) episodes of wheezing during the previous year at age 6. However, this risk decreased significantly with age and was barely significant by age 13 (Figure 3.1). Conversely, the association between asthma symptoms and sensitization to local aeroallergens increased significantly with age: 60% of children with current wheezing were skin test positive at age 6, compared with over 90% at age 11–13. The pattern of the association between current wheezing during childhood and RSV infection during infancy was thus exactly opposite to that between current wheezing and sensitization to local aeroallergens.

All of the factors that explain the association between RSV–LRI and subsequent wheezing/LRI have not been clearly identified. An important clue may come from our own observation (also reported by others) that, as a group, children with a history of RSV–LRI have lower levels of lung function and increased airway hyperresponsiveness when compared with those without such a history.[26] We observed, for example, that the abnormalities in FEV_1 after RSV–LRI could be entirely reversed by the administration of a single dose of albuterol (salbutamol). It is not clear whether the increased airway responsiveness precedes the development of the first episode of LRI or is a consequence of some direct and persistent effect of the virus on the regulation of airway tone. It is possible that both mechanisms may exist, in different children.[27]

Recent observations also suggest that, in some children, persistence of wheezing after RSV may be the consequence of alterations in the nature of the immune response to the virus. Bont and co-workers[28] studied cytokine responses of peripheral blood mononuclear cells to non-specific stimuli (LPS/IFN-γ and PHA) during the acute and convalescent phase of RSV infections requiring hospitalization. They then compared these responses in children who did or did not have episodes of wheezing during the subsequent year. They found that subsequent wheezing was unrelated to IL-12 or IFN-γ/IL-4 responses during the acute or convalescent phase of the infection. However, children who had continued wheezing episodes had significantly higher IL-10 responses during the convalescent phase of the acute illness than those who did not have subsequent wheezing episodes. Moreover, there was a strong positive correlation between the number of wheezing episodes during the subsequent year and the intensity of the IL-10 response (Figure 3.2).

The mechanisms by which IL-10 responses could predispose to persistent wheezing after RSV remain unresolved. Bont *et al.* did not specifically determine the cells responsible for the production of IL-10 in their studies, but speculated that most likely these were antigen presenting cells, since the results were obtained after stimulation with lipopolysaccharide and IFN-γ. IL-10 is a potent down-regulator of both Th1 and Th2 responses

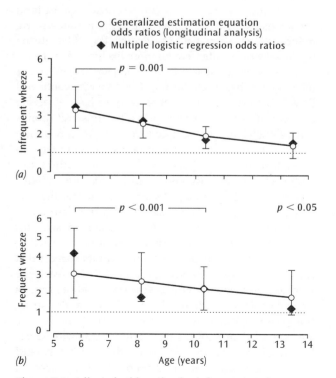

(a)

(b)

Figure 3.1 *Adjusted odds ratios for infrequent and frequent wheeze associated with RSV lower respiratory infections before age 3. (From ref. 18.)*

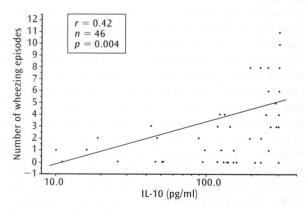

Figure 3.2 *Relation between IL-10 production and number of wheezing episodes during a 1-year follow-up period. (From ref. 28.)*

in humans.[29] It is thus possible that individuals with strong IL-10 responses may foster the activity of an invasive virus such as RSV by excessive down-regulation of the immune response to the infectious agent. However, an alternative explanation is also possible. Recent studies in animal models suggest that IL-10 may have a direct effect in airway smooth muscle and in the regulation of airway tone.[30] Mice sensitized to certain allergens developed increased responsiveness of their airways and of isolated smooth muscle. However, when the same experiments were performed in animals in which the IL-10 gene had been rendered dysfunctional and which were unable to produce IL-10, no such bronchial responsiveness developed. These results suggest that IL-10 not only has direct activity on immune cells, but may also have a direct role in the regulation of airway tone. The mechanisms involved are not well understood but open a new field in our understanding of the potential role of cytokines that, until recently, were not known to be able to exert their function in cells other than those of the immune system.

The finding of a potential role of interleukins such as IL-10 on airway function/responsiveness independent of the Th1/Th2 paradigm may offer a new basis for our understanding of those forms of recurrent wheezing during childhood that are not associated with increased risk of allergic sensitization.

ATOPY-ASSOCIATED ASTHMA

The most persistent and usually the most severe form of recurrent airway obstruction is almost invariably associated with evidence of IgE-mediated immune responses to local aeroallergens. Both prospective and retrospective studies have shown that most cases of atopy-related asthma have their first asthma-like symptoms during early life.[31,32] Recently the pattern of initiation of symptoms has become clearer from the analysis of results of longitudinal studies started at birth. Based on data from the Tucson Children's Respiratory Study, Halonen and co-workers [33] divided a population of children who had recurrent wheezing episodes during the early school years into two groups: one group was sensitized against *Alternaria*, the main local aeroallergen associated with asthma, whereas a second group was not sensitized against this particular antigen. They observed that symptoms had started preferentially during the second and third years of life for the group sensitized against *Alternaria*, while in the group that was not sensitized against *Alternaria*, symptoms had usually started during the first year of life. Moreover, children who were sensitized against *Alternaria* were much more likely to have continued symptoms by the age of 11 years. This type of analysis probably addresses the same issues discussed above in relation to the long-term consequences of RSV–LRIs, because wheezing episodes that start during the first year of life are

usually associated with virus (often RSV) infection and have a better prognosis than those that start during the second or third years of life, which are more likely to be associated with an atopic predisposition.

Results of a similar longitudinal study undertaken in Perth, Australia, point in the same direction. Young *et al.*[4] reported that approximately 50% of 160 infants wheezed during the first two years of life. Of these, 28 wheezed during the first year of life only, 21 during the second year of life only, and 32 in both the first and second years of life. Although all groups of children who wheezed had lower levels of lung function measured during the first months of life and before any lower respiratory illness had occurred, abnormalities were more persistent among those who wheezed during the first and second years of life. Moreover, bronchial hyperresponsiveness (BHR), which was measured by use of histamine during the first month of life, was significantly increased mainly in children who wheezed during the second year of life.[4]

A subsequent re-analysis of this same data set,[27] in conjunction with data at the age of 6 years, enhanced the understanding of the natural history of asthma in early life. BHR measured during the first month of life was strongly associated with the likelihood of having physician-diagnosed asthma and wheezing, both with and without colds, at the age of 6 years. Of great interest was the observation that bronchial responsiveness to histamine at 1 month was unrelated to lung function at that same age, and was also unrelated to BHR to histamine at the age of 6 years. However, bronchial responsiveness at the age of 1 month was strongly correlated with the level of lung function observed at the age of 6 years. There was also a strong correlation between BHR at 6 years and wheezing and asthma at that same age.

Taken together, these results suggest that level of lung function and response to bronchoconstrictors measured shortly after birth measure different properties of the airways. The former seems to be strongly associated with the likelihood of wheezing very early in life, but in the absence of other risk factors, the effect tends to rapidly subside with age. The effect of 'congenital' BHR, on the other hand, is not readily observed during the first year of life, perhaps because it is masked by the strong role of 'congenital' lung function on early wheezing. The effect of 'congenital' BHR is first observed during the second year of life and persists up to age of 6 years.

Of particular importance in the Australian data set is the observation that 'congenital' BHR and BHR observed at the age of 6 years are not correlated with each other and have independent effects on the likelihood of wheezing at the age of 6.[27] Studies from our Tucson group suggest that one of the most important determinants of BHR at the age of 6 is the development of allergic sensitization.[34] The data thus suggest the existence of two separate, independent determinants of BHR: 'congenital' BHR is unrelated to allergic markers[27] whereas BHR measured at age 6 seems to be an acquired characteristic of the lung, most probably associated with allergic sensitization. Both forms of BHR are strong determinants of the level of lung function observed at the age of 6.

The observations made both by the Tucson study and the Perth study, therefore, provide new insights as to the factors that determine persistence of BHR and, therefore, persistence of asthma symptoms beyond the preschool years. This is an important observation, because in developed countries, most children with persistent asthma during the school years show evidence of sensitization against local aeroallergens. The evidence clearly suggests that, in these children, BHR is the consequence of the process that leads, on the one hand, towards allergic sensitization, and on the other hand, towards the development of BHR.

The nature of the relation between allergic sensitization and the development of atopy-related asthma is not well understood. For years it was believed that atopic asthma was the direct consequence of exposure to aeroallergens and that it was this exposure, in susceptible individuals, that triggered the disease mechanisms responsible for the disease.[35,36] The fact that children who develop asthma and live in different environments become sensitized to different allergens, however, suggests that the association between sensitization to aeroallergens and asthma is not simply one of cause–effect. More likely, atopic asthmatics have a defect in immune development that determines, on the one hand, an increased likelihood of becoming sensitized to local aeroallergens and, on the other hand, an increased likelihood of developing asthma-like symptoms.

Studies of the development of IFN-γ responses during the first year of life strongly suggested that this could indeed be the case. Both in environments where the predominant aeroallergen is *Dermatophagoides pteronyssinus*[37,38] and in an environment where *Alternaria* is the main asthma-related allergen,[39] subjects who became sensitized to these allergens were more likely to show impaired development of IFN-γ responses by peripheral blood mononuclear cells during the first year of life. Interestingly, this impairment was not usually observed or was much less pronounced at birth, as assessed by studies of cord blood. However, in both locales, IFN-γ responses were markedly impaired during the first year of life in subjects who would go on to become sensitized to asthma-related allergens, and 'caught up' with those of non-atopic children between the ages of 3–6 years.[40] These results clearly suggest that atopy-associated asthma may be the result of a delay in the maturation of normal, IFN-γ mediated responses in the immune system. Clearly, genetic factors may be important,[41] but environmental influences also seem to be significant.

Of clear relevance are the recent observations that, in environments where exposure to microbial burden in early life is quite significant, both allergic sensitization and asthma tend to be much less prevalent in school-age children.[42,43] Several studies have suggested that exposure to endotoxin, a component of the cell wall of Gram-negative bacteria, may be an important consequence of the level of microbial burden during the first years of life. Studies by Gereda and co-workers showed that subjects exposed to higher levels of endotoxin in the dust present in their homes during the first year of life were less likely to become sensitized to aeroallergens during these first years.[44] These same subjects were more likely to show enhanced IFN-γ responses to non-specific stimuli by peripheral blood mononuclear cells. It has been suggested that decreased microbial burden during the last 50 years may have delayed the normal maturation process of the immune system thus explaining, at least in part, the recently observed increases in the prevalence of asthma.

The factors that determine the persistence of asthma symptoms in children who are sensitized against local allergens has been the matter of considerable debate. Large studies performed in the United States suggest that, among subjects who are sensitized against local allergens, exposure to these allergens is an important risk factor for the persistence and severity of symptoms.[45] Unfortunately, few controlled studies are available to support the hypothesis that decreased exposure to allergens would decrease asthma symptoms in sensitized subjects. Nevertheless, it is unlikely that exposure to aeroallergens is a cause of the development of asthma, as clearly shown recently by a carefully performed study in Germany,[46] in which exposure to house-dust mites was measured in the homes of a large number of children. The likelihood of becoming sensitized to house-dust mite increased with increased exposure, but the likelihood of developing asthma during the early school years was similar in children with very high and very low exposure to house-dust mites in their homes. These results clearly suggest that the thresholds for sensitization to house-dust mites among subjects who are destined to become asthmatics are extremely low. Moreover, most asthmatic children by the age of 7 are pluri-sensitized[47] and therefore, their basic abnormality is not their susceptibility to becoming sensitized to one aeroallergen in particular. For this reason, strategies to prevent asthma by preventing sensitization to single allergens are very likely to fail.

CONCLUSIONS

Recently longitudinal studies have uncovered the complexity of the phenotypic presentations of childhood asthma. Recurrent airway obstruction with wheezing is the final common pathway for many different disease mechanisms. All these disease mechanisms can be summarized in two main potential alterations: a structurally narrow airway or an airway that is narrowed functionally by either, smooth muscle contraction, oedema, or mucus secretion. Naturally these mechanisms may co-exist and overlap, determining different degrees of severity and persistence of symptoms. Wheezing in infancy and during the toddler years is determined by a combination of 'congenital' BHR, congenitally narrow airways, and potential sequels of abnormal immune responses to RSV and other viruses. Atopy-associated asthma, on the other hand, also starts during the toddler years, but only becomes the most frequent expression of asthma during the school years. This form of asthma appears to be determined by a combination of genetic and environmental factors that predispose to a delay in the maturation of the immune system during the first years of life. The main consequences of this delayed maturation are the development of early allergic sensitization, increased BHR, and losses in lung function that persist until adult life.

REFERENCES

1. Nelson W. Comment. In: S Gellis, ed. *The Year Book of Pediatrics*, 1960, p. 131.
2. Holberg CJ, Wright AL, Martinez FD, Ray CG, Taussig LM, Lebowitz MD. Risk factors for respiratory syncytial virus-associated lower respiratory illnesses in the first year of life. *Am J Epidemiol* 1991;**133**:1135–51.
3. Martinez FD, Wright AL, Taussig LM, Holberg CJ, Halonen M, Morgan WJ, The Group Health Medical Associates. Asthma and wheezing in the first six years of life. *New Engl J Med* 1995;**332**:133–8.
4. Young S, Arnott J, O'Keeffe PT, Le Souef PN, Landau LI. The association between early life lung function and wheezing during the first 2 years of life. *Eur Respir J* 2000;**15**:151–7.
5. Martinez FD. Sudden infant death syndrome and small airway occlusion: facts and hypothesis. *Pediatrics* 1991;**87**:190–8.
6. Wright AL, Taussig LM, Ray CG, Harrison HR, Holberg CJ. The Tucson Children's Respiratory Study. II. Lower respiratory tract illness in the first year of life. *Am J Epidemiol* 1989;**129**:1232–46.
7. Taussig LM, Wright AL, Morgan WJ, Harrison HR, Ray CG. The Tucson Children's Respiratory Study. I. Design and implementation of a prospective study of acute and chronic respiratory illness in children. *Am J Epidemiol* 1989;**129**:1219–31.
8. Le Souef P, Turner S, Rye P, *et al.* Pulmonary function at four weeks correlates with pulmonary function at 6 and 12 years. *Am J Respir Crit Care Med* 2001;**163**:A541.
9. Stein RT, Holberg CJ, Sherrill D, Wright AL, Morgan WJ, Taussig LM, Martinez FD. The influence of parental smoking on respiratory symptoms in the first decade of life: the Tucson Children's Respiratory Study. *Am J Epidemiol* 1999;**149**:1030–7.
10. Tager IB, Ngo L, Hanrahan JP. Maternal smoking during pregnancy. Effects on lung function during the first 18 months of life. *Am J Respir Crit Care Med* 1995;**152**:977–83.
11. Tager IB, Hanrahan JP, Tosteson TD, Castile RG, Brown RW, Weiss ST, Speizer FE. Lung function, pre- and post-natal smoke exposure, and wheezing in the first year of life. *Am Rev Respir Dis* 1993;**147**:811–17.
12. Morgan WJ, Martinez FD. Risk factors for developing wheezing and asthma in childhood. *Pediatr Clin N Am* 1992;**39**:1185–1203.
13. Dezateux C, Stocks J, Dundas I, Fletcher ME. Impaired airway function and wheezing in infancy: the influence of maternal smoking and a genetic predisposition to asthma. *Am J Respir Crit Care Med* 1999;**159**:403–10.
14. Holberg CJ, Morgan WJ, Wright AL, Martinez FD. Differences in familial segregation of FEV1 between asthmatic and nonasthmatic families. Role of a maternal component. *Am J Respir Crit Care Med* 1998;**158**:162–9.
15. Chen Y, Horne SL, Rennie DC, Dosman JA. Segregation analysis of two lung function indices in a random sample of young families: the Humboldt Family Study. *Genet Epidemiol* 1996;**13**:35–47.
16. Pullen C, Hey E. Wheezing, asthma, and pulmonary dysfunction 10 years after infection with respiratory syncytial virus in infancy. *BMJ* 1982;**5**:1665–9.
17. Sigurs N, Bjarnason R, Sigurbergsson F, Kjellman B, Bjorksten B. Asthma and immunoglobulin E antibodies after respiratory syncytial virus bronchiolitis: a prospective cohort study with matched controls. *Pediatrics* 1995;**95**:500–5.
18. Stein RT, Sherrill D, Morgan WJ, Holberg CJ, Halonen M, Taussig LM, Wright AL, Martinez FD. Respiratory syncytial virus in early life and risk of wheeze and allergy by age 13 years. *Lancet* 1999;**353**:541–5.
19. Mok JY, Simpson H. Symptoms, atopy, and bronchial reactivity after lower respiratory infection in infancy. *Arch Dis Child* 1984;**59**:299–305.
20. Martinez FD, Morgan WJ, Wright AL, Holberg CJ, Taussig LM. Diminished lung function as a predisposing factor for wheezing respiratory illness in infants. *New Engl J Med* 1988;**319**:1112–17.
21. Welliver RC, Wong DT, Sun M, Middleton E, Jr., Vaughan RS, Ogra PL. The development of respiratory syncytial virus-specific IgE and the release of histamine in nasopharyngeal secretions after infection. *New Engl J Med* 1981;**305**:841–6.
22. De Alarcon A, Walsh EE, Carper HT, La Russa JB, Evans BA, Rakes GP, Platts-Mills TA, Heymann PW. Detection of IgA and IgG but not IgE antibody to respiratory syncytial virus in nasal washes and sera from infants with wheezing. *J Pediatr* 2001;**138**:311–17.
23. Welliver RC, Sun M, Rinaldo D, Ogra PL. Predictive value of respiratory syncytial virus-specific IgE

responses for recurrent wheezing following bronchiolitis. *J Pediatr* 1986;**109**:776–80.

24. Sigurs N, Bjarnason R, Sigurbergsson F, Kjellman B. Respiratory syncytial virus bronchiolitis in infancy is an important risk factor for asthma and allergy at age 7. *Am J Respir Crit Care Med* 2000;**161**:1501–7.

25. Bjorksten B, Dumitrascu D, Foucard T, *et al.* Prevalence of childhood asthma, rhinitis and eczema in Scandinavia and Eastern Europe. *Eur Respir J* 1998;**12**:432–7.

26. Kattan M. Epidemiologic evidence of increased airway reactivity in children with a history of bronchiolitis. *J Pediatr* 1999;**135**:8–13.

27. Palmer LJ, Rye PJ, Gibson NA, Burton PR, Landau LI, Lesouef PN. Airway responsiveness in early infancy predicts asthma, lung function, and respiratory symptoms by school age. *Am J Respir Crit Care Med* 2001;**163**:37–42.

28. Bont L, Heijnen CJ, Kavelaars A, van Aalderen WM, Brus F, Draaisma JT, Geelen SM, Kimpen J. Monocyte IL-10 production during respiratory syncytial virus bronchiolitis is associated with recurrent wheezing in a one-year follow-up study. *Am J Respir Crit Care Med* 2000;**161**:1518–23.

29. Rennick D, Berg D, Holland G. Interleukin 10: an overview. *Prog Growth Factor Res* 1992;**4**:207–27.

30. Makela MJ, Kanehiro A, Borish L, *et al.* IL-10 is necessary for the expression of airway hyperresponsiveness but not pulmonary inflammation after allergic sensitization. *Proc Natl Acad Sci USA* 2000;**97**:6007–12.

31. Yunginger J, Reed CE, O'Connell EJ, Melton LJ, O'Fallon WM, Silverstein MD. A community-based study of the epidemiology of asthma. Incidence rates, 1964–1983. *Am Rev Respir Dis* 1992;**146**:888–94.

32. Barbee RA, Dodge R, Lebowitz ML, Burrows B. The epidemiology of asthma. *Chest* 1985;**87**(Suppl):21S–5S.

33. Halonen M, Stern DA, Lohman C, Wright AL, Brown MA, Martinez FD. Two subphenotypes of childhood asthma that differ in maternal and paternal influences on asthma risk. *Am J Respir Crit Care Med* 1999;**160**:564–70.

34. Lombardi E, Morgan WJ, Wright AL, Stein RT, Holberg CJ, Martinez FD. Cold air challenge at age 6 and subsequent incidence of asthma. A longitudinal study. *Am J Respir Crit Care Med* 1997;**156**:1863–9.

35. Peat JK, Tovey E, Toelle BG, Haby MM, Gray EJ, Mahmic A, Woolcock AJ. House dust mite allergens. A major risk factor for childhood asthma in Australia. *Am J Respir Crit Care Med* 1996;**153**:141–6.

36. Platts-Mills TAE, Weck ALD. Dust mite allergens and asthma – a worldwide problem. *J Allergy Clin Immunol* 1989;**83**:416–27.

37. Prescott SL, Macaubes C, Yabuhara A, Venaille TJ, Holt BJ, Habre W, Loh R, Sly PD, Holt PG. Developing patterns of T cell memory to environmental allergens in the first two years of life. *Internat Arch Allergy Immunol* 1997;**113**:75–9.

38. Prescott SL, Macaubas C, Smallacombe T, Holt BJ, Sly PD, Holt PG. Development of allergen-specific T-cell memory in atopic and normal children. *Lancet* 1999;**353**:196–200.

39. Halonen M, Stern DA, Wright AL, Taussig LM, Martinez FD. *Alternaria* as a major allergen for asthma in children raised in a desert environment. *Am J Respir Crit Care Med* 1997;**155**:1356–61.

40. Holt PG, Rudin A, Macaubas C, Holt BJ, Rowe J, Loh R, Sly PD. Development of immunologic memory against tetanus toxoid and pertactin antigens from the diphtheria–tetanus–pertussis vaccine in atopic versus nonatopic children. *J Allergy Clinical Immunol* 2000;**105**:1117–22.

41. Martinez FD, Stern DA, Wright AL, Holberg CJ, Taussig LM, Halonen M. Association of interleukin-2 and interferon-gamma production by blood mononuclear cells in infancy with parental allergy skin tests and with subsequent development of atopy. *J Allergy Clin Immunol* 1995;**96**:652–60.

42. Riedler J, Eder W, Oberfeld G, Schreuer M. Austrian children living on a farm have less hay fever, asthma and allergic sensitization. *Clin Exp Allergy* 2000;**30**:194–200.

43. Von Mutius E, Braun-Fahrlander C, Schierl R, Riedler J, Ehlermann S, Maisch S, Waser M, Nowak D. Exposure to endotoxin or other bacterial components might protect against the development of atopy. *Clin Exp Allergy* 2000;**30**:1230–4.

44. Gereda JE, Leung DYM, Thatayatikon A, Streib JE, Price MR, Klinnert MD, Liu AH. Relation between house-dust endotoxin exposure, type 1 T-cell development, and allergen sensitization in infants at high risk of asthma. *Lancet* 2000;**355**:1680–3.

45. Rosenstreich DL, Eggleston P, Kattan M, *et al.* The role of cockroach allergy and exposure to cockroach allergen in causing morbidity among inner-city children with asthma [see comments]. *New Engl J Med* 1997;**336**:1356–63.

46. Lau S, Illi S, Sommerfeld C, Niggemann B, Bergmann R, von Mutius E, Wahn U. Early exposure to house-dust mite and cat allergens and development of childhood asthma: a cohort study. *Lancet* 2000;**356**:1392–7.

47. Sears MR, Herbison GP, Holdaway MD, Hewitt CJ, Flannery EM, Silva PA. The relative risks of sensitivity to grass pollen, house dust mite and cat dander in the development of childhood asthma. *Clin Exp Allergy* 1989;**19**:419–24.

Structural development

ALISON A HISLOP AND HITESH C PANDYA

INTRODUCTION

It is important to understand normal lung development when considering childhood disease and its treatment since the lung's response to either will differ depending on the stage of development.

The lung at birth is not a miniature version of the adult lung. Each of the structural components of the lung has it own timetable of development and at any one time each will be at a different stage of maturity. External factors such as air pollution or infection will affect immature or small lungs differently from those of older subjects. Any change in normal development is likely to have a long-term effect. A small lung at birth tends to remain small during growth: so-called tracking. Also, the 'Barker hypothesis' suggests a link between early morphogenesis and long-term outcome in adulthood.[1]

Much lung development occurs during fetal life and the lung is unique in growing while failing to fulfil its main postnatal function, suggesting that the pattern of fetal lung growth is genetically determined. By term the lung has grown sufficiently to support the respiratory needs of the infant and is able to adapt rapidly to its new function. During infancy and childhood as the body surface increases, the lung grows in size, increasing the size of airways and the surface area for gas exchange in the alveolar region with a concomitant increase in the size of blood vessels and number of capillaries. The structure of these components also matures.

Although the development of the conducting airways is of primary interest in relation to asthma, other structures are important in the pathophysiology of the disease including the respiratory acinus.[2] The airways regulate and direct the flow of air and they also act as a barrier to prevent harmful substances reaching the alveolar region.

The branching system is an efficient method of increasing surface area within a given volume. The alveoli, which make up the greatest volume of the lung, have evolved to produce the largest possible gas exchange area: thin walls interdigitating into the air space. A single balloon would give little gas exchange area for the volume of gas involved. The conducting airways are supplied with oxygenated blood (epithelial cells probably get their oxygen directly from the airway) via the bronchial arteries, which originate from the aorta and are at a high internal pressure. The low pressure pulmonary arteries carry deoxygenated blood to the alveoli. Both systems are drained via pulmonary veins. The blood supply to the alveoli must pass through the capillary bed at a linear velocity that will allow gas exchange to take place and at a bulk flow which matches ventilation. All these structures and their functions are controlled by the nervous system, by circulating humoral factors and by local homeostatic mechanisms.

The growth of all these structures is complex and though each follows its own timetable, they are not independent of each other. In humans, by birth all the major components of the lung have developed but during childhood they mature in structure and grow in size and in the case of peripheral structures, in number.

NORMAL LUNG DEVELOPMENT

Fetal development

The classic descriptions of lung growth have divided fetal development into four major stages based on the appearance of the lung tissue: embryonic, pseudoglandular, canalicular and alveolar; the last is sometimes divided into an earlier saccular or terminal sac phase and

Table 4a.1 *Phases of lung development*

Embryonic	0–7 weeks gestation	Lung buds form Blood vessels connect to heart
Pseudoglandular	6–17 weeks gestation	Preacinar airways and blood vessels develop
Canalicular	16–27 weeks gestation	Respiratory (intra-acinar) region develops. Thinning of peripheral epithelium and mesenchyme. Type I and II pneumonocytes
Alveolar (or terminal sac or saccular)	27 weeks to term	Development of saccules and then alveoli
Postnatal	Up to 18 months Up to adulthood	Alveoli and small blood vessels multiply All structures increase in size

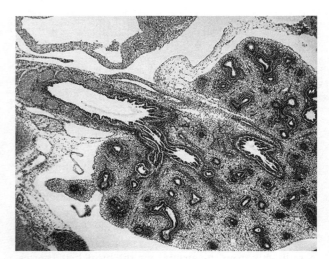

Figure 4a.1 *Photomicrograph of a longitudinal section through the left lung of a fetus at nine weeks of gestation. The lung is in the glandular phase of development with a large number of airway branches within the matrix. The main bronchus has cartilage plates in the wall and pulmonary arteries can be seen running alongside proximal airways (×64).*

a later alveolar stage[3] (Table 4a.1). The alveolar stage continues after birth and in some species is entirely postnatal; the time span varying between different species. There is also considerable individual variation and one stage gradually merges into the next.

During the *embryonic period* the lung appears as a ventral diverticulum from the endodermal foregut in the fourth week after ovulation. The complete lining epithelium of the lung is derived from the endoderm. A first division produces the left and right bronchi by 26–28 days of age. Further dichotomous division of airways into the surrounding mesenchyme continues until the end of the *pseudoglandular stage* (17 weeks) by which time all preacinar airways to the level of the terminal bronchiolus are present. The majority of divisions occur during the 10–14th weeks of gestation[4] (Figures 4a.1 and 4a.2).

As successive airways form, their walls first develop smooth muscle closely followed by cartilage, submucosal glands and connective tissue. Epithelial differentiation

also begins during this period. These structural elements of the airway wall appear from the hilum towards the periphery from 6 weeks of age, and by 24 weeks of gestation the airways have the same structure as they do in the adult.[4,5] Smooth muscle cells are present in human trachea and lobar bronchi by 8–10 weeks of gestation (Figure 4a.3).[6–8] As in adult lungs, fetal airway smooth muscle expresses contractile smooth muscle specific myofilaments such as smooth muscle α-actin and smooth muscle myosin heavy chains (SM-MHCs). However the relative content of SM-MHC in immature and mature smooth muscle is different.[9] Fetal smooth muscle cells are smaller than adult cells and express a wider repertoire of potassium ion channels, the proteins that control their resting membrane potential.[10] *In vitro* studies of first trimester human tracheal ASM[7] and peripheral lung explants of first trimester human lung have shown that 'fetal' airway smooth muscle cells have a fluctuating resting membrane potential which is associated with the spontaneous development of tone and peristalsis-like contractions of the compliant airway. These contractions cause active movement of intraluminal fluid and rhythmic distension of more peripheral airways, at least *in vitro*, and may stimulate 'strain-induced' growth of airway cells especially in epithelial tubes lacking airway smooth muscle.[6] Blocking spontaneous contractions leads to lung hypolasia *in vitro*.[11] The smooth muscle contractions are not blocked by agents which abolish neural transmission, indicating their myogenic nature, but are sensitive to acetylcholine and isoproterenol suggesting that neuro-humoral factors could modulate smooth muscle activity.[6,7] Airway smooth muscle activity during lung development *in utero* may therefore contribute to airway wall growth in a number of ways. 'Synthetic' airway smooth muscle activity such as cell proliferation, hypertrophy and elaboration of extracellular matrix will thicken the airway wall. In addition, smooth muscle contractile activity will promote growth and development of cells in more distal parts of the lung.

Viewed microscopically during the pseudoglandular stage the lung has numerous airways lined by columnar epithelium separated from each other by a meshwork of mesenchyme containing capillaries (Figure 4a.3). Throughout this period, new capillaries appear around

Fetal stage

Lung structure

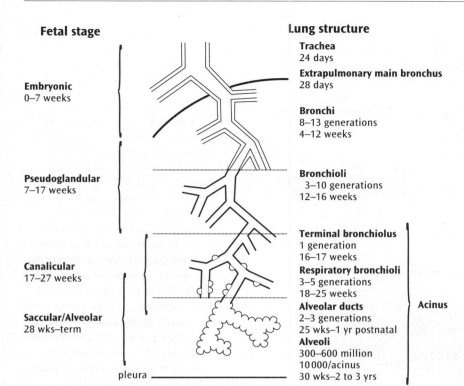

Embryonic
0–7 weeks

Pseudoglandular
7–17 weeks

Canalicular
17–27 weeks

Saccular/Alveolar
28 wks–term

Trachea
24 days

Extrapulmonary main bronchus
28 days

Bronchi
8–13 generations
4–12 weeks

Bronchioli
3–10 generations
12–16 weeks

Terminal bronchiolus
1 generation
16–17 weeks

Respiratory bronchioli
3–5 generations
18–25 weeks

Alveolar ducts
2–3 generations
25 wks–1 yr postnatal

Alveoli
300–600 million
10 000/acinus
30 wks–2 to 3 yrs

Acinus

pleura

Figure 4a.2 *The number of airway generations in the human lung and the stage and gestational age at which they appear.*

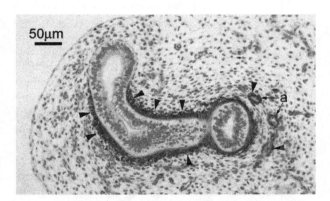

50μm

Figure 4a.3 *Photomicrograph of a peripheral airway in an 8-week-old fetus. Section immunostained for α-smooth muscle actin. Muscle cells (arrowheads) are seen around the airway epithelium except in the final branch. Smooth muscle cells also surround the pulmonary arteries (a) lined up alongside the airways.*

the end of the lung bud. These coalesce to form the pulmonary arteries, which line up alongside the airways, as are seen in the adult lung.[8] During fetal life the arteries and airways develop together and all preacinar arteries, including supernumerary arteries which will eventually supply the alveoli, are present by the end of the pseudoglandular period.[12] The pulmonary veins grow at the same time as the arteries. They do not accompany the airways but lie in the inter-segmental planes.[8a] However, the number of veins is similar to the number of arteries.[13]

During the *canalicular period* (16–27 weeks), the peripheral airways continue to divide to form the prospective respiratory bronchioli (2–3 generations in humans) and beyond these the prospective alveolar ducts, alongside which arteries and veins also develop. The preacinar airways increase in diameter and length. The mesenchymal region between the airways thins and capillaries come to lie beneath the epithelium of the peripheral airways apparently causing the epithelium to become thinner.

The larger (prospective bronchi) airways are lined by columnar epithelium (Figure 4a.4) but the distal bronchioli are lined by cuboidal cells. At the level of the prospective respiratory bronchioli part of the wall is lined by flattened cells, as are the prospective alveolar ducts which at this stage are sac-shaped (saccules). By 20–22 weeks of gestation type I and type II alveolar epithelial cells can be identified lining all saccular air spaces. The type I cells are flat and elongated and cover the majority of the surface. The type II cells maintain a cuboidal shape and develop lamellar bodies around 24 weeks of gestation which is 4–5 weeks before surfactant can be detected in the amniotic fluid. By the end of the canalicular stage the air to blood barrier is thin enough to support gas exchange (about 0.6 μm) but the gas exchange units are the large thin walled saccules.

At the beginning of the *alveolar stage* the saccules have discrete bundles of elastin at intervals around their luminal edge forming small crests which are subdividing the saccules (Figure 4a.5).[14] Between 28 and 32 weeks of gestation these crests elongate sufficiently to form primitive alveoli.[14,15] The walls of these alveoli are still quite thick, having a double capillary supply and mesenchymal tissue between the epithelial cells. With age the crests increase in length, become thinner and have only a single capillary

Preacinar airway

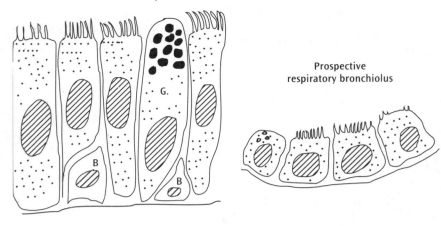

Prospective
respiratory bronchiolus

Prospective alveolar duct

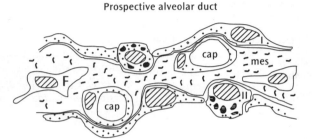

Figure 4a.4 *The cell types lining the airways during the canalicular phase. The preacinar airways are lined by columnar epithelium mainly of ciliated cells. The most peripheral airways, which are destined to become the respiratory bronchioli are lined by cuboidal cells. In the region of canalization – the prospective alveolar ducts – the capillaries (cap) lie under thinned epithelial cells, the type I pneumonocytes (I). The type II (cuboidal) pneumonocytes contain lamellated bodies (II). There is still considerable mesenchymal tissue (mes) between adjacent air spaces. B: basal cell; G: goblet cell; F: fibroblast.*

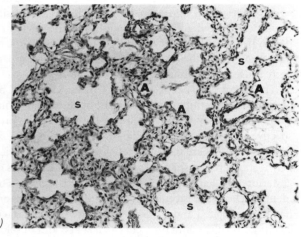

(a)

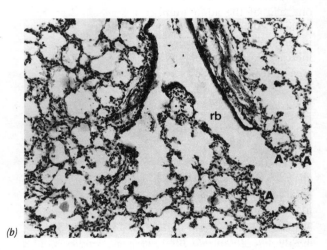

(b)

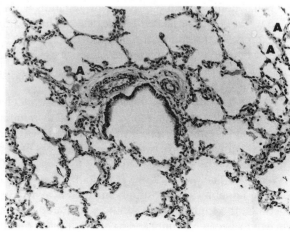

(c)

Figure 4a.5 *Alveolar development illustrated by photomicrographs of lung. (a) At 28 weeks' gestation, saccules (s), many with shallow thick walled alveoli (A), are separated by relatively thick interstitial tissue. (b) At 34 weeks' gestation, a respiratory bronchiolus (rb) leads into an alveolar duct lined by alveoli. Saccules are present at the edge of the acinus. (c) At term, alveoli are mature in shape and thin walled (from ref. 14 with permission) (×187).*

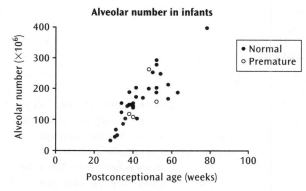

Figure 4a.6 *The number of alveoli in the developing lung related to postconceptional age in weeks.* ●: *control lungs;* ○: *prematurely born infants not artificially ventilated; their number is not different from normal.*

network.[16] The formation of these alveolar walls has been described in detail in the rat where the alveoli develop from the saccules in the postnatal period.[17,18] Eventually mature cup-shaped alveoli line the elongated saccules, now called alveolar ducts, and they are also found lining part of the walls of the respiratory bronchioli.

Counts of the alveoli (Figure 4a.6) show an increase with gestational age and by term between one third and one half of the adult number is present, around 150 million[14,15] (adult number 300–600 million[19]). The increase in lung volume seen during this stage is due mainly to the increase in number of the alveoli. The alveolar surface area increases and shows a linear relationship to age and body weight.

The lung at birth

At birth the lung has the adult number of airways with an airway wall consisting of the components found in the adult lung. Within the respiratory portion of the lung the majority of respiratory airways are present and there are up to half the adult number of alveoli present. The alveoli, though smaller than in the adult, have a blood–gas barrier of mature thickness. The blood supply to the lung is complete save for the blood vessels that will supply the enlarging alveolar region.

During fetal life the lung is filled with liquid but immediately after birth fluid is removed, triggered by a large rise in the fetal adrenaline (epinephrine) level which leads to the opening of sodium channels and hence salt and water reabsorption. In fetal lambs absorption rates of up to 50 ml/h have been recorded.[20] The presence of adrenaline also triggers the release of surfactant by the lamellar bodies of type II pneumonocytes. Surfactant synthesis which begins at the start of the second trimester of pregnancy and normally accelerates as partuition approaches can be pharmacologically accelerated by stressor hormones, especially glucocorticoids.[21]

During fetal life blood flow is directed away from the lung due to high pulmonary artery resistance. The pulmonary arterial lumen is small with a relatively thick wall. Immediately after birth, pulmonary vascular resistance falls, there is a decrease in the wall thickness of the small muscular arteries in the first few days. In the larger vessels the low adult level is reached by three months of age.[22–24] Studies on neonatal pigs have shown that the rapid thinning at the periphery is due to reorganization of the shape and orientation of both pulmonary vascular smooth muscle and endothelial cells.[24,25] The rapid dilation of the pulmonary vasculature is stimulated by the rise in arterial oxygen partial pressure that occurs with air-breathing and is mediated, in part, by the release of prostacyclin and bradykinin.[26] Endothelial-derived relaxation factor or nitric oxide[27,28] also plays an important role in vascular dilatation. Studies suggest that nitric oxide is produced during fetal life, blocking its production increases pulmonary vascular resistance.[29] The enzyme nitric oxide synthase which is present in the endothelial cells at birth, increases in amount at 2–3 days of age, suggesting a role in the adaptation process,[30] and shows a rapid increase in activity immediately after birth.[31] Nitric oxide is used successfully in treatment of infants with persistent pulmonary hypertension of the newborn.

Postnatal development

AIRWAY DEVELOPMENT

Increase in airway size in the perinatal period is linear and continuous with antenatal growth. Premature delivery does not alter this rate of growth. After the first year of life there is a slowing in the growth, there being an approximately two-fold increase between 22 weeks of gestation and eight months postnatal age and a two- to three-fold increase between birth and adulthood.[32] A previous study measuring airway length and diameter for all generations along main and lateral pathways in children from birth to adulthood showed symmetrical growth throughout the lung.[33] During infancy and early childhood the airways are large relative to total volume. Girls have wider and or shorter airways than boys during early childhood and this may explain their lesser tendency to wheeze, but by adulthood males have relatively large airways.[34] The enhanced growth in males at puberty may be a factor in the relative decline in reversible obstructive airways disease in teenage boys.

AIRWAY WALL STRUCTURE

In the newborn, airway wall structure is similar to that of the adult, containing cartilage, submucosal glands, smooth muscle, connective tissue; with bronchial arteries and veins the amount of each component for a given sized airway is generally less than in the adult (Figure 4a.7).[32,35] During the first year of life there is a rapid increase in

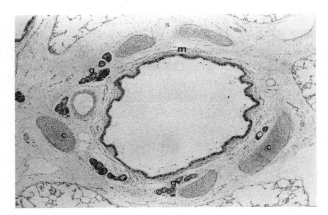

Figure 4a.7 *Transverse section through a bronchus from an 8-month-old infant stained with periodic acid Schiff stain. c: cartilage; m: bronchial smooth muscle; g: submucosal gland. The goblet cells can be seen in the epithelium (×50).*

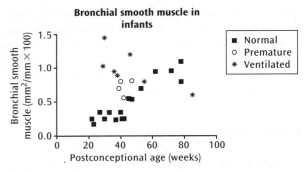

Figure 4a.8 *The area of bronchial smooth muscle per mm of airway perimeter in cross-section small bronchi related to postconceptional age. ▪: normal fetus and infant; ○: premature infant; ∗: ventilated premature infant.*

submucosal gland and bronchial smooth muscle mass relative to airway size with cartilage mass only increasing at the same rate as the increase in size of the airways. After infancy the airway wall increases in proportion to airway diameter. The increase in airway smooth muscle is particularly rapid in the first few weeks after birth. The relative amount of airway smooth muscle in the bronchioli is close to the adult level by 8 months of age whereas there is still a considerable increase in muscle mass in the bronchi after this time.[32] In children there is therefore a greater proportion of airway smooth muscle in the smaller non-cartilaginous airways than in the bronchi. This rapid increase is probably related to the change to air breathing since it occurs at a similar postnatal age and therefore an earlier gestational age in babies that are born prematurely (Figure 4a.8). Airway smooth muscle mass increases above normal in artificially ventilated babies[32] and in children and adults with asthma where airway wall thickness is also increased by connective tissue.[36] An increased airway smooth muscle mass, whether absolute or due to premature development, may predispose to airflow obstruction by a number of mechanisms including

increased force generation for a given amount of smooth muscle cell shortening.

Human airway smooth muscle responds to acetylcholine and isoproterenol as early as the glandular stage of fetal development.[6] Postnatally there is reactivity to methacholine and subsequent bronchodilation after addition of metaproterenol in healthy infants less than 15 months of age.[37] The drop in the bronchoconstrictor response with age is controversial (Chapter 9), but if true could be related to changes in muscle cell myofilament, ion channel or receptor expression or to the relative amount of muscle mass at different stages of lung growth. Alterations in the nerve supply of airway smooth muscle could also account for the differences in bronchodilator response with age although structural studies have shown that the distribution and density of nerves at birth is similar to that seen in the adult.[38]

The submucosal glands are responsible for producing most of the mucus found in the airways. They are located in the submucosa between the cartilage and the surface epithelium and are made up of acinar regions of mucous and serous cells which lead to the surface via a ciliated duct which is continuous with the airway epithelium. They appear in the trachea of the human at ten weeks of gestation and gradually extend towards the periphery of the lung. During childhood there is relatively more submucosal gland mass than in the adult,[35,39] but it is only at 13 years of age that the glands have the adult appearance. They continue to grow in size in normal subjects until 28 years of age.

The airways are supplied with oxygenated blood via the bronchial arteries which originate from the aorta or intercostal arteries and there are commonly two to each lung entering at the hilum. They divide to form a subepithelial plexus and an adventitial plexus on either side of the bronchial smooth muscle layer. True bronchial veins drain the trachea and upper bronchi and return blood to the right atrium while the veins in the more peripheral airways drain via the pulmonary veins to the left atrium.[40] The bronchial supply appears at the end of the first trimester and extends down the airway wall as the bronchial smooth muscle, cartilage and glands differentiate.

AIRWAY EPITHELIUM

The epithelium is the first line of defence in the lung and also responds to environmental stimuli. The epithelial cells develop by differentiation and maturation of the primitive endodermal cells. In the adult human, four cell types predominate in the surface epithelium of the conducting airways. Ciliated cells are found from the trachea to the respiratory bronchioli and at all levels are the most numerous cells. Mucous-secreting or goblet cells are found from the trachea to the end of the bronchioli. Basal cells are found in the larger airways and in addition, indeterminate cells can also be found. During development neuroendocrine cells are identified. In the terminal bronchioli a further cell type, the Clara cell is found in addition to ciliated cells.

Maturation begins in the proximal airways and progresses distally. In the early pseudoglandular stage all airways are lined by elongated cells overlying basally situated cells over a basement membrane. The elongated cells have a prominent nucleus and a cytoplasm containing a large amount of glycogen.

Ciliated cells first appear at 11 weeks of gestation.[41] Cilia develop from centrioles which are formed by division of the pre-existing single centriole or by aggregations in the Golgi region to form a generative complex of precentrioles. By the time cilia reach one third of their final length the internal microfilaments have formed first as single strands and then as doublets. Cilia can be motile before they achieve mature length and from this time they can develop a coordinated beat. There are 200–300 cilia per cell in the adult.[42] The ciliated cells do not divide but originate from basal or secretory cells.

The presence of intracellular mucus has been demonstrated in the human fetal lung at 13 weeks of gestation but at this age the *goblet cells* are sparse. There is extension of goblet cells from the bronchi into the bronchioli but at birth there is still a relatively low number of goblet cells, less than 10% of the total number of epithelial cells. After birth there is a rapid increase in the number of goblet cells, reaching up to 40% of the total in the bronchi by three months of age.[32] The goblet cells are predominantly mucous in type and they produce mainly acidic mucus.[43] The mucous cells increase in airway disease such as chronic bronchitis and with inhalation of sulphur dioxide, cigarette smoke and ozone. They also increase in asthma relative to ciliated cells.[44]

Basal cells can be identified from 12–14 weeks of gestation and have been considered to be the stem cell in the tracheobronchial epithelium. Cells from basal cell colonies grown from rabbit trachea have been able to establish a columnar, pseudostratified epithelium when inoculated onto denuded tracheal grafts. This epithelium had basal, ciliated and goblet cells.[45] It is not known whether basal cells form ciliated cells directly or whether they form via goblet cells. Basal cells also aid the adherence of columnar cells to the basal lamina since they are firmly attached via hemidesmosomes to both the basal lamina and the columnar cells.

Clara cells are thought to develop in the second half of gestation from glycogen-containing, non-ciliated cells in the terminal bronchioli.[42] The Clara cell 10-kDa protein (CC10) has been shown to have immunomodulatory and anti-inflammatory activity and may play a role in controlling airway inflammation. Lower serum levels than normal have been found in asthmatics.[46] They are also the source of some surfactant apoprotein, under β-adrenergic control. Clara cells are progenitors for the ciliated cells in peripheral airways.[47]

Neuroendocrine (dense-core granulated) cells are the first types of cell to differentiate within the primitive airway epithelium. They are peptide-producing and are often innervated and probably derive from the neural crest. They are distributed singly or in pairs by eight weeks of gestation when they are weakly argyrophilic and show immunoreactivity for serotonin and neurone-specific enolase. It has been suggested that they play an important part in cell differentiation[48] since they are not found in such large numbers in the adult and they increase in number in babies with chronic lung disease of prematurity.[49]

The epithelium, as well as producing the fluid and mucus for the ciliary escalator to remove particles from inside the lung, also produces a number of factors that can modulate the function of airway smooth muscle.[50] Removal of the airway epithelium results in an increase in the contractile response to histamine and muscarinic agonists in human airways. The nature of the epithelium-derived inhibitory factor is unknown. The increase in sensitivity of smooth muscle strips to these agonists persists in the presence of prostanoid and nitric oxide synthesis inhibitors.[51] Although these observations indicate that airway epithelium is a source of smooth muscle inhibitory factor(s), it can also generate endothelin which is a contractile agonist as well as a smooth muscle cell mitogen.

Airway epithelial injury and denudation is a characteristic feature of atopic asthma and airway epithelial cells are an important source of locally acting mediators. Some of these mediators may modulate airway smooth muscle force generation. Others may promote the thickened basement membrane and the increased fibrosis and airway smooth muscle characteristic of chronic asthma (Chapter 5).

However, the role of the epithelium in wheezing diseases of infancy and early childhood is unclear.

ALVEOLAR DEVELOPMENT

After birth the alveolar region of the lung grows rapidly. There is proportionately much less growth in the airways than in the alveolar region in the first years after birth. Up to half of the alveoli are present by birth[14] and it is likely that the adult number is almost complete by 18 months of age.[15,16,52] During this postnatal period blunt crests with elastic bundles at their tips can be seen dividing the air spaces (similar to those seen in the alveolar stage of fetal development) and then lengthening and thinning by loss of interstitial matrix and loss of the double capillary bed.

The formation of alveoli is dependent upon the deposition of elastin. Mice lacking elastin have impaired peripheral airway development.[53] The elastin is thought to be produced by smooth muscle cells that have migrated from terminal bronchioli since failure of alveogenesis is coupled to lack of distal spreading of alveolar smooth muscle cell progenitors during lung development in PDGF-A-deficient mice.[54] At first elastin is seen only at the tips of alveolar crests, that is, at the mouth of the alveolus. With age the amount increases but at 5 years of age is still only at the luminal edge. By 12 years of age it extends around the alveolar walls and by 18 years there are many fibres throughout the walls.[3] The relative lack of elastin in the young lung allows the growth in size of the alveoli. Babies ventilated after birth have abnormal deposition of elastin and this may lead to the failure of normal shaped alveoli to develop so that the total number may be reduced.[55]

Males generally have a greater number of alveoli[56] than females at all ages over one year, independent of size as well as age. In the first 18 months the increase in lung volume is brought about by an increase in size of air spaces as well as their multiplication while the relative amount of tissue decreases[52] due to a loss of interstitial cells while the endothelial and epithelial cells continue to grow. After 18 months all lung compartments of the gas exchanging region increase equally relative to body mass, so by this time the lung is a miniature version of the adult lung. Lung volumes (as measured by the vital capacity) continues to increase until the early twenties in normal adults.

DYSANAPTIC GROWTH

Many authors have concluded that airways and lung parenchyma develop disproportionately in size, that is, there is dysanaptic growth, during the first few years of life.[34,57] The conducting airways are complete in number at birth and increase only in size,[33] whereas alveoli increase both in size and in number. After about 2 years of age, parenchymal growth is mainly due to alveolar enlargement. It is therefore likely that airways and air spaces grow isotropically (i.e. in proportion to each other) thereafter throughout childhood. A recent longitudinal study suggested that airways and air spaces continue to grow isotropically in boys during adolescence, whereas in girls airway growth lags behind that of the parenchyma at this stage.[58]

PULMONARY VASCULATURE

During childhood as new alveoli form and enlarge, new pulmonary blood vessels develop at the periphery of the lung. The majority of these new vessels develop in the first 18 months of life.[23] After the newborn period the ratio of pulmonary arteries and veins to alveoli remains similar, there always being more veins than arteries. The small pulmonary arteries reach adult wall thickness within the first few days of life while the larger vessels take up to three months.[22,23] Beyond this period there is an increase in lumen diameter and capacity as arteries and veins increase in size along with the increase in lung volume.

Neural development

The nerves of the lung develop from neural crest cells which migrate via the vagus to the future trachea and lung before it separates from the gut. There is progressive extension and increase in complexity of the nerve supply as the structures of the lung develop.[59,60] By four months of gestation the trachea has a nerve supply to smooth muscle, submucosal glands and epithelium and there are nerves present in all but the smallest bronchi and the arteries and veins. By term and in the neonate the distribution and density of nerves is similar to that seen in the adult with parasympathetic nerve fibres forming a meshwork within the airway wall (Figure 4a.9).[38] Sensory nerves are also found in the epithelium. There are few nerves within the air spaces of the alveolar region of the lung.

The efferent innervation to airways consists of parasympathetic (cholinergic) excitatory nerves and inhibitory non-adrenergic, non-cholinergic (NANCi) nerves. Release of acetylcholine by cholinergic nerves stimulates airway

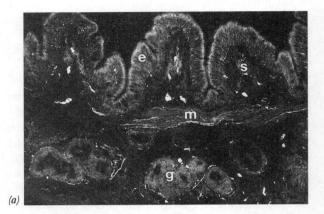

(a)

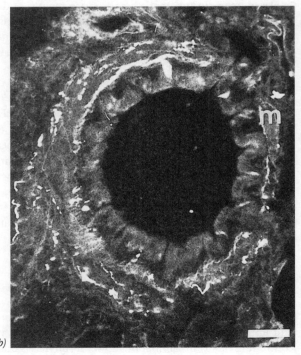

(b)

Figure 4a.9 *Photomicrographs of a section of (a) bronchus and (b) bronchiolus from a newborn infant immunostained for the general neuronal marker PGP 9.5. Nerve fibres supply epithelium (e), submucosal gland (g), bronchial smooth muscle (m) and submucosal region (s). Bar = 50 μ (from ref. 38 with permission).*

smooth muscle contraction and an increase in submucosal gland mucous production. NANCi nerves provide inhibitory signals via vasoactive intestinal peptide (VIP) and perhaps, as recent evidence would suggest, through generation of nitric oxide which stimulates cyclic-GMP production in airway smooth muscle cells. The effect of NANCi innervation is greatest in the trachea and decreases towards the periphery.[61] β-receptor-induced bronchodilation is mediated by circulating epinephrine (adrenaline) since there are no functional adrenergic nerves to airway smooth muscle. Circulating epinephrine also contributes to the regulation of mucus production and bronchial and pulmonary blood flow. β-receptors on the epithelium probably induce production of an epDRF, that affects the airway smooth muscle.[50]

We have little information on the development of receptors, although functional studies by Tepper[37] suggest that they are present in the first year of life. Current data suggest that the number of β$_2$-receptors on airway smooth muscle may remain relatively consistent through life. However, the level of sensitivity appears to peak in early adult life with a progressive increase throughout the early childhood years and a decline in responsiveness with increasing age in patients over 40 years of age.[62]

REGULATION OF LUNG GROWTH

Factors associated with early lung growth

The development of the human lung is regulated by a number of mechanisms which, although poorly defined at present, interact at many levels including the molecular and cellular. The complexity of this regulation is highlighted by the fact that the interplay between the various mechanisms alters with the phase of lung growth and that their outcomes depend and build upon the growth sustained in preceding stages. The normal development of the lung can be altered *in utero* and postnatally (Figure 4a.10). During early intrauterine life, adverse factors will influence airway growth while factors having their effect in later weeks of gestation and infancy will affect alveolar development. Abnormalities in airway branching cannot be corrected once the period of airway multiplication is complete. Thus airflow is likely to be abnormal in these subjects throughout life. Indeed it is now recognized that major adverse events occurring during the period of rapid growth and development in early life may have long-term and irreversible effects.[63–65] This leaves the probability that many subtle changes in lung development could contribute to the risk of subsequent wheezing disease.

GENES AND TRANSCRIPTION FACTORS

Early studies showed the importance of the interaction of endoderm and mesenchyme in lung morphogenesis. Recent studies at the molecular level have extended our knowledge on the control of lung growth but the mechanisms are still not fully understood. Approaches used to define the molecular control of lung development have hitherto largely relied on loss- or gain-of-function phenotypes of candidate genes or gene families in fruit flies (*Drosophila*) and mice. These studies indicate that despite the vast phenotype divide between various species there

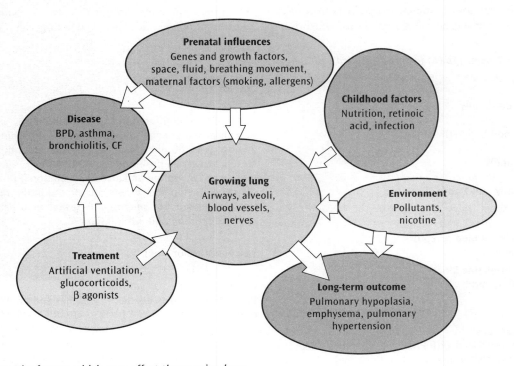

Figure 4a.10 *The factors which may affect the growing lung.*

is a marked degree of conservation of gene function so that homologues of genes are found across species including humans.[66,67] The studies have also shown that early lung development is largely controlled by transcription factors but at present, many of the target genes of the transcription factors so far implicated in lung development are unknown.

The earliest event in lung morphogenesis, the development of foregut endoderm cells committed to the formation of the lung bud, appears to be critically dependent on the transcription factor, *hepatocyte nuclear factor-3β* (*HNF-3β*). Foregut endoderm morphogenesis from an apparently normal endoderm is severely affected in *HNF-3β*$^{-/-}$ knockout mice.[68] The next stage of lung development clearly associated with a specific transcription factor is cleavage of the tracheal tube from the primitive foregut and branching morphogenesis. *Thyroid transcription factor* (*TTF-1*) also known as Nkx2.1 and thyroid enhancer-binding protein (T/ebp) is expressed in the endoderm of the foregut, the thyroid gland and the developing edge of the lung bud and in addition in specific respiratory epithelial cell lineages later in lung development. It is not expressed by lung mesenchyme. *TTF-1* null mutant mice have a common tracheo-oesophageal tube which fails to branch significantly. Inhibition of *TTF-1* mRNA with anti-sense oligonucleotides results in restricted branching morphogenesis and a hyperplastic, poorly differentiated respiratory epithelium in fetal mouse lung explants.[69,70]

Gli proteins form yet another group of transcription factors controlling lung development. *Gli* proteins are implicated in the mesenchymal–epithelial cell interactions that characterize much of lung branching morphogenesis. In developing mouse lungs, *Gli* proteins are activated in pulmonary mesenchymal cells in response to the product of a gene called *smoothened* which is also associated with segmentation in early embryonic development. Smoothened is released by the binding of the morphogenetic protein *sonic hedgehog* (*SHH*), which is produced by the respiratory epithelium, to the *patched* gene receptor on pulmonary mesenchyme. Abrogation of any of the factors in this signalling pathway has similar effects on mouse lung development, namely right lung hypoplasia, left lung agenesis and a tracheo-oesophageal fistula.[71,72] In man, mutation of one member of the *Gli* protein family (*Gli3*) is linked with three dominant genetic disorders associated with polydactyly. One of these disorders, Pallister–Hall syndrome, is also associated with foregut abnormalities including lung lobulation defects, tracheal stenosis and tracheo-oesophageal fistula in some patients.[73] The linkage of transcription factors to non-lethal human lung disorders serves to indicate that their effects on lung development may range from the subtle to the catastrophic.

GROWTH FACTORS

A wide variety of biochemical factors have been linked with lung cell proliferation and growth. Most belong to a super-family of polypeptide ligands, which bind to cognate, membrane-spanning receptors with intrinsic tyrosine kinase (RTKs) activity (kinase = phosphorylation). Lung cell growth mediators which are not part of the RTK super-family form a heterogeneous group. Some 'non-RTK' growth factors mediate their intracellular effects through membrane-spanning receptors coupled to guanine triphosphate (GTP) binding proteins (G-proteins).

The potential role of some growth factors in lung development is listed in Table 4a.2. Two of these deserve further mention. Fibroblast growth factors (FGFs) are a key group of polypeptides involved in lung cell proliferation,

Table 4a.2 *Some growth factors associated with lung development*

Factor	Role in lung development
RTK super-family	
EGF	Epithelial cell proliferation and differentiation
Acidic- and basic-FGF family	Branching morphogenesis, epithelial cell differentiation, angiogenesis, fibroblast and endothelial cell proliferation
PDGF family	Mesenchymal cell proliferation (PDGF-BB), airway smooth muscle cell migration and alveolar septation (PDGF-AA)
IGF family (IGF-1 and -2)	Airway epithelial and smooth muscle cell proliferation
VEGF	Vascular (fibroblasts, smooth muscle and endothelium) cell proliferation and differentiation
G-protein coupled receptors	
Endothelin-1	Vascular development
Serine-threonine kinases	
TGF-β (I, II and III)	Promotion of matrix synthesis. Inhibition of matrix degrading enzymes and branching morphogenesis
Miscellaneous	
Factors associated with PNEC cells (bombesin-like peptides, calcitonin gene related peptide)	Lung cell proliferation

differentiation and branching morphogenesis. All FGF receptors are expressed in the lung although their expression is regulated in time and in space. Acidic FGF (FGF-1) is linked with epithelial cell branching whereas paradoxically FGF-7 (keratinocyte growth factor), which binds to the same receptor subtype as FGF-1 (FGFR-2IIIb), induces epithelial cell differentiation. FGF-10 also appears to be critical to branching morphogenesis. It is expressed by distal lung mesenchyme and may act as a guidance signal for distal epithelial cells. Fetal mouse lung cultures treated with FGF-10-coated beads show increased amounts of airway branching at the site of a bead. In contrast, FGF-10 null mutant mice show no lung formation distal to the carina. The integration of the FGF-10 signal in the lung appears to be modulated or controlled by *SHH*. In *SHH* null mutant mice, FGF-10 is broadly expressed in distal mesenchyme whereas in wild-type mice FGF-10 expression is localized to areas of the lung where *SHH* is lacking. Thus, *SHH* produced by developing epithelium appears to control epithelial tube branching by spatially restricting the expression of FGF10.[74–77]

The platelet-derived growth factor (PDGF) family of mitogens is another important group of growth factors linked to lung development. Three biologically active forms of PDGF are recognized. Studies of mouse lung explants exposed to PDGF-AA and -BB anti-sense oligonucleotides suggest that the PDGF-AA is important for branching morphogenesis whereas PDGF-BB stimulates lung cell proliferation. PDGF-AA probably also plays an important role in alveolar development since PDGF-AA null mutant mice show absence of alveolar septation linked to a failure of ASM migration from terminal airways.[54] Disorganized airway wall smooth muscle migration could explain the increased alveolar smooth muscle and reduced alveolar septation associated with chronic lung disease of prematurity and bronchopulmonary dysplasia.[78]

EPITHELIAL MESENCHYMAL INTERACTIONS

Airway branching requires the presence of both the endodermal tube lined by epithelial cells and the surrounding mesenchyme. An airway tube will continue to grow in length but will not branch if its mesenchyme is stripped away[79,80] whereas mesenchyme transplanted from an area of active branching will stimulate an otherwise dormant epithelial tube to divide. Bifurcation may be initiated by local contraction of filaments within the cytoplasm of the epithelial cells causing a cleft or alternatively by some cells migrating while others remain stationary and thus forming a cleft. The process is partly dependent upon interactions between cell adhesion molecules and matrix proteins.[81]

CELL ADHESION

It has become evident over the last few years that cell adhesion is crucial to the proper progression of lung development. Lung cells adhere to each other and the various extracellular matrix (ECM) proteins through a large family of transmembrane receptors called integrins which recognize, as ligands, components of the extracellular matrix or cell surface counter-receptors of the cadherin and immunoglobulin families. Evidence for the role of cell adhesion comes from studies of SPARC (secreted protein acidic rich in cysteine, or osteonectin), a secreted glycoprotein that inhibits cell adhesion. SPARC is widely distributed expressed in airways during the pseudoglandular stage of lung development and the mesenchyme around airways during the canalicular and saccular stage of lung development. Addition of anti-SPARC antisera or synthetic SPARC antisera or synthetic SPARC-like peptide to rat lung explant cultures reduced epithelial bud formation and altered bud morphology but did not affect cell proliferation during branching morphogenesis.[82]

INTEGRATION OF LUNG GROWTH REGULATORY SIGNALS

Initiation of lung development from the embryonic foregut requires transcriptional factors. Subsequent airway branching events and pulmonary vasculogenesis involve reciprocal epithelial-mesenchymal interactions mediated by growth factors and their receptors as well extracellular matrix and proteins and their cognate receptors on cells. In general, receptor tyrosine kinases and their ligands (bFGF, PDGF-AA and EGF) positively modulate lung growth and branching morphogenesis while transforming growth factor-beta (TGF-β) family members have an inhibitory effect on branching morphogenesis. An interplay may also occur between soluble negative and positive growth factors and physical stimuli such as spontaneous airway contractions and fetal breathing movements. For the present, much of the integration of positive and negative signalling pathways is unknown.[83]

GENDER, ETHNICITY AND LUNG GROWTH

Gender and ethnicity also affect lung growth. Tracheal size does not differ between the sexes during early life[84] but adult males have a larger trachea than females.[34] Although lung volume and alveolar number are greater in boys than girls,[56] girls have larger expiratory flows than boys in infancy[85] and the narrower peripheral airways of boys may predispose them to wheeze.[63,86,87] This is not just a growth effect, since dexamethasone given to infants leads to a better outcome in females,[88] and studies in sheep using lung function tests to study the growth and function of the lung after prenatal treatment support this finding.[89]

Marked ethnic differences in infant mortality and respiratory morbidity have been reported.[90] Prematurely delivered Afro-Caribbean infants are less likely to develop respiratory distress syndrome (RDS) than white infants of similar gestational age, which suggests that the respiratory system is either more mature or that airway function is enhanced in black preterm infants.[91] Some of these differences may be attributed to their lower nasal resistance.[92]

PHYSICAL FACTORS AND LUNG GROWTH

Lung growth *in utero* is also influenced by a number of biophysical factors, including the space available in the chest cavity, fluid in the lungs and the amniotic sac, pressures within the chest cavity and fetal breathing movements all of which interact to contribute to overall lung growth.

The *space available* within the thoracic cavity has considerable impact on growth of the lung. Infants with congenital diaphragmatic hernia (CDH) have lungs with reduced airway number and size suggesting that the effects of space restriction begin before airway branching is complete.[93] Indeed, the diaphragm normally separates the thoracic cavity between weeks 8 and 9 of human gestation, well before the completion of branching morphogenesis. Increase in space available as seen after pneumonectomy leads to an increase in lung volume. Experimental studies show that the increase is both by increase in alveolar number during development and in size after multiplication is complete.[94] There is evidence of similar factors in human lung expansion after correction of hypoplastic lungs.[95,96]

Sufficient quantities of *lung fluid* are needed for normal lung development: babies with oligohydramnios as a result of renal anomalies have small lungs and in these the airways are reduced in number.[97] Premature rupture of membranes reduces the number and size of alveoli. Even removal of amniotic fluid as in amniocentesis affects alveolar and airway growth.[98] Increased fluid in fetal lungs as seen in laryngeal atresia accelerated lung growth[99] and experimental studies on lambs in which the lung is overdistended by plugging the trachea promotes lung growth[100] and has been used to overcome the effects of CDH.[101–103]

The role of *fetal breathing* in lung development has been reviewed recently.[104] Intermittent lung expansion stimulates lung growth[105] whereas ablation of the phrenic nerves leads to lung hypoplasia in fetal rabbits[106] and diminished alveolar growth and maturation in lambs.[105] Studies on fetal lung explants have shown that repetitive stretch results in cell proliferation.[107] Fetal breathing movements are diminished by exposure to hypoxia, nicotine and various drugs.

The association between disorders of lung growth and wheezing disorders is discussed in Chapter 4b.

NUTRITION

Recent epidemiological evidence showing a relationship between adult airway function and birth weight suggests that intrauterine nutrition in humans may be more important than recognized previously.[108] Malnutrition will affect lung growth both pre and postnatally and will have the greatest affect at the time of rapid alveolar development.[109,110] This suggests that in humans the most important time for nutrition is during late fetal life and up to 2 years of age. However, a study on rats found that re-feeding resulted in catch up growth of both lung volume and gas exchange area.[111] In children with cystic fibrosis (CF), nutritionally reduced body weight is associated with reduced lung function parameters although wheezing in CF has other causes.[112] Asthma may itself lead to poor weight gain.[113] In addition to calorie intake, Vitamin A (retinoic acid) has been shown to be essential for normal alveolar development[114]; deficiency decreases alveolar septal development. More importantly Vitamin A supplementation led to redevelopment of alveoli in rats with elastase-induced emphysema[115] and retinoic acid treatment given to young rats with dexamethasone induced failure of alveolar development induced new septal formation. This may be an important finding in improving alveolar growth in prematurely born infants (see below).[116] It is worth noting that Vitamin A transcriptionally regulates the expression of a number of genes including some cytokines.[117,118]

INFECTION AND MATERNAL TOBACCO SMOKING

Intrauterine infection may affect lung growth. Low-grade amniotic infection and chorioamnionitis is associated with an increased risk of bronchopulmonary dysplasia.[119–121] Experimental administration of endotoxin *in utero* also affects the development of alveoli.[122]

Maternal smoking during pregnancy leads to an increased risk of low birth weight, preterm delivery, and sudden death in infancy.[123–125] The risk of lower respiratory illness, wheezing and asthma is also increased among young children whose mothers smoke[126–128] (Chapter 7e). However, cessation of smoking during pregnancy has been associated with improved morbidity.[129] A marked reduction in fetal movements lasts for at least an hour after the mother has smoked a cigarette.[130] Animal studies have shown maternal exposure to cigarette smoke results in offspring with small lungs and decreased air spaces,[114] reduces elastin production,[131] produces up-regulation of nicotinic receptors in the lung[132] and leads to an increase in collagen around airways.[132] Decreased coupling between parenchyma and airways in guinea pigs exposed to passive smoking *in utero* may explain their increased airway responsiveness.[133] These findings may explain results from functional studies in human infants shortly after birth, which show changes in the pattern of breathing and diminished airflows in those whose mothers smoked during pregnancy.[126] Recent measurements in preterm infants have shown that these changes are evident at least seven weeks before an infant is due to be born.[134] The mechanisms associated with tobacco smoke-induced airflow obstruction in humans may involve abnormal airway modelling as in animals. An increased airway wall thickness and smooth muscle mass have been reported at postmortem in SIDS infants whose mothers smoked during pregnancy.[135]

Factors associated with abnormal lung growth in infancy and later childhood

Many prenatal factors will continue to have an effect after birth. The most common factor is preterm birth. Preterm birth on its own does not seem to affect normal alveolar development (Figure 4a.6).[55] However the airways are small for postnatal age and have an increase in smooth muscle mass and mucus secreting cells (Figure 4a.8).[32] These structural changes are accentuated by ventilator therapy.[55] Babies who go on to get bronchopulmonary dysplasia (BPD) have a reduced number of alveoli beyond the age when normal alveolar development is complete.[136] Experimental studies on baboons show that extreme prematurity can lead to impaired alveolar development.[137]

Early respiratory disease and subsequent airway function

Childhood respiratory problems such as inhalation of foreign or toxic material and infectious or non-infectious respiratory disease may interfere with the normal development of the respiratory tract and lung parenchyma.

There is a well-established association between *viral bronchiolitis* in infancy and recurrent wheezing in later childhood (Chapters 3 and 7b). However, the role of viruses such as respiratory syncitial virus (RSV) in the initiation of asthma is controversial.[138] Some viruses, in particular adenovirus, may cause permanent airway and parenchymal lung damage in infants although such cases are the exception rather than the rule. Virus-induced wheeze in rats is modulated by age (neonatal vs weanling vs adult) and the strain of rat suggesting the importance of host susceptibility factors.[139] The mechanisms associated with viral infections and recurrent wheezing in humans or in experimental rats have yet to be elucidated although in rats viruses have been shown to impair both alveolar and airway development.[140]

Pulmonary *bacterial infections* appear to affect preterm neonates more than term infants. Neonatal bacterial infection is synergistic with high oxygen levels in producing abnormal alveolar development in baboons,[141] and is a risk factor in the development of BPD and chronic lung disease of prematurity (CLD).[142] However, BPD and CLD are multifactorial diseases with lung immaturity, hyperoxia, barotrauma, inflammation as well as chronic pulmonary infection being major factors in their pathogenesis.[143,144] Wheezing occurs more frequently in adolescents and young adults who had BPD in infancy than in age-matched controls of similar or normal birth weight (Chapter 13b).[145,146]

Chronic airway inflammation in *asthma* might be expected to interfere with lung development. However, despite intensive investigation, this remains a very controversial area. While reduced expiratory flows prior to bronchodilator therapy have been documented in several studies of asthmatic or ex-asthmatic subjects, these do not necessarily reflect disturbed airway growth providing such abnormalities are reversible by adequate bronchodilator and anti-inflammatory treatment.[147] The issue of airway remodelling, which is affected by many of the same factors that control airway growth, is dealt with in Chapter 5.

Effects of treatment

Abnormal lung development has been linked to management strategies associated with the treatment of bronchopulmonary disease (BPD) and chronic lung disease (CLD). There are also major concerns regarding the effects of glucocorticoids and bronchodilators on long-term lung development and function.

ARTIFICIAL VENTILATION

Experimental evidence suggests that normal oxygen tensions are necessary for normal alveolar development. In preterm baboons, ventilation with appropriate oxygen levels allowed alveoli to develop normally while high oxygen tensions led to reduced alveolar septation.[148] In neonatal rats hyperoxia also prevented alveolar multiplication and led to enlarged alveoli in adulthood.[149] Animal studies have shown that hyperoxia is associated with fibroblast hyperplasia and up-regulation of growth factors,[150,151] alveolar damage and reduced septation,[148,149,152] parenchymal thickening[153] and increased airway responsiveness.[154]

High-volume ventilation (previously referred to as barotrauma) may also be associated with airway and alveolar mal-development. In a study on piglets where high oxygen and volutrauma were used together or independently Davis *et al.*[152] found that high oxygen tensions had a much greater effect on alveolar appearance than barotrauma. The independent effect of these factors are much more difficult to determine in human infants who are usually exposed to both insults simultaneously.[143,144]

THERAPEUTIC AGENTS

Glucocorticoids are administered before birth to accelerate maturation and prevent surfactant deficiency syndrome. In the airways of asthmatics, glucocorticoids reduce inflammation, restore the airway epithelium as manifested by a return of the normal proportions of ciliated and mucus epithelial cells[155] and partially reverse basement membrane thickening.[44] Cell culture studies show that production of matrix is altered by dexamethasone.[156] Similarly, in cultured adult human airway smooth muscle cells, glucocorticoids reduce mitogen-stimulated thymidine incorporation, an indirect marker of cell proliferation.[157–159] All of these processes will tend to reduce both airway obstruction and bronchial responsiveness. The use of glucocorticoids in children may affect total lung growth, especially since lung morphogenesis is regulated by glucocorticoid-affecting growth factors.[160,161]

Structural studies in sheep and rats[162–164] treated with prenatal and postnatal dexamethasone have shown accelerated alveolar wall thinning and maturation, at the expense of subsequent normal alveolar development.[165] Glucocorticoids have been shown to reduce elastin, decrease procollagen mRNA and reduce cross-linking, all of which may alter the stability of the alveoli and the calibre of the peripheral airways, possibly leading to enhanced 'small airways disease' in the long term.

The mechanism by which glucocorticoids affect alveolar formation is unclear.

New interalveolar walls (septae) are formed by pleating up of part of the wall[166] producing a double capillary system. This is reduced to a single layer by an apoptosis-dependent process which leads to thinning of the interalveolar septa and loss of interstitial tissue. Glucocorticoids induce thinning of the septal wall probably by promoting the fusion of the microvasculature. If this occurs before the alveolar development is complete it will truncate the period of development of new alveolar walls.[165] Too few alveolar septae will eventually lead to alveoli that are too large and more smoothly contoured, an apparent emphysematous appearance.[167] In addition to causing abnormal gas-exchange physiology, reduced septal growth will decrease the 'load' placed on the airways and airway smooth during normal tidal breathing and thus increase the risk of airway collapse and excessive smooth muscle shortening. The clinical effects of such events may not become apparent until the ageing process is well established and may be similar to those found in patients with chronic obstructive pulmonary disease. Recent experimental studies have shown that the failure of alveolar growth can be overcome by the use of transretinoic acid.[116]

The largely experimental data in relation to glucocorticoids shows that therapeutic intervention at critical stages of development may have unwanted or unexpected sequelae. Even brief treatment at low doses may have a profound effect even at a later stage in development.

Little is known about the effect of *β₂-adrenoreceptor agonists* on growth, but glucocorticoids given during fetal life increase the number of β-receptors. Inhaled terbutaline exerted no effect on epithelial appearance[168] but β-agonists do appear to inhibit proliferation of adult human airway smooth muscle cells[169] and long-term use of bronchodilators may lead to abnormally small amounts of muscle in the airway walls. Improvement in lung function as a result of use of anticholinergics has been reported, but nothing is known of the effect on the airway smooth muscle cells of the developing lung.[170]

Lung growth and asthma

In recent times a number of researchers have re-emphasized the fact that processes active during lung development can impact on lung function in later life. The quest now is to identify the biological mechanisms underlying their observations so that their effects can be ameliorated.

It is not difficult to imagine that processes acting during lung morphogenesis could contribute to the development of asthma, its severity and/or the responsiveness of individuals to treatment. Sparrow and colleagues have suggested that phasic, myogenic airway contractions during the pseudoglandular phase of lung development may be important in airway wall and lung development.[171] The airway contractions are dependent on the activity of fetal airway smooth muscle which like adult airway smooth muscle is influenced by a number of contractile agonists. Nicotine could interfere with the phenotype and/or the contractile and synthetic functions of airway smooth muscle either directly or indirectly by its effect on the developing autonomic nervous system or the airway epithelium.

Major advances have been made over the past decade using candidate gene approaches in determining the function of several important molecules such as HNF-3β and TTF-1 in lung morphogenesis. Over the next decade the role of many more genes and their products in human lung development are likely to be determined as a direct result of powerful molecular biology techniques such as DNA 'chip' technology and rt-PCR.[83] In relation to asthma diagnosis, some of the products of these genes may be markers of lung disease or alternatively may be thought of as risk factors and used to identify children at high-risk of developing asthma. Moreover, these genes and their products are also likely to be amenable to therapeutic intervention in such a way that their downstream effects on lung structure and function can be manipulated.

The last decade has seen a shift towards earlier use of corticosteroids in children with atopic asthma/recurrent wheezing, based on the premise that early treatment with corticosteroids will suppress inflammation-mediated airway modelling. However, the majority of children with recurrent wheezing have a good prognosis and only a minority is at risk of impaired growth of lung function during childhood due to their disease.[172] For the majority, the risks of early steroids on lung growth may be greater than the clinical benefits. Using inhaled corticosteroids and bronchodilators at an early age also raises questions relating to drug delivery. The importance of particle size for lung deposition and clinical effect has been determined for adult patients. The optimal particle size for infants and children is not known but it may be smaller (because of their smaller calibre airways) than delivered by currently available aerosol devices.

Thus, future research will need to focus on methodologies to measure lung development in fetal or early postnatal life and to relate alterations in function to subsequent clinical outcomes and continue to assess lung growth into adulthood.

REFERENCES

1. Shaheen SO, Barker DJP. Early lung growth and chronic airflow obstruction. *Thorax* 1994;**49**:533–6.
2. Verbanck S, Schuermans D, Noppen M, Van Mulem A, Paiva M, Vincken W. Evidence of acinar airway involvement in asthma. *Am J Respir Crit Care Med* 1998;**159**:1545–50.
3. Loosli CG, Potter EL. Pre and postnatal development of the respiratory portion of the human lung. *Am Rev Resp Dis* 1959;**80**:5–20.
4. Bucher U, Reid L. Development of the intrasegmental bronchial tree: the pattern of branching and development of cartilage at various stages of intra-uterine life. *Thorax* 1961;**16**:207–18.
5. Bucher U, Reid L. Development of the mucus-secreting elements in human lung. *Thorax* 1961;**16**:219–25.
6. McCray PB. Spontaneous contractility of human foetal airway smooth muscle. *Am J Resp Cell Mol Biol* 1993;**8**:573–80.
7. Richards IS, Kulkarni A, Brooks SM. Human foetal tracheal smooth muscle produce spontaneous electromechanical oscillations that are calcium dependent and cholinergically potentiated. *Dev Pharmacol Ther* 1991;**16**:22–8.
8. Hall SM, Hislop AA, Pierce C, Haworth SG. Prenatal origins of human intrapulmonary arteries: formation and maturation. *Am J Respir Cell Mol Biol* 2000;**23**:194–203.
8a. Hall SM, Hislop AA, Haworth SG. Origin, differentiation and maturation of human pulmonary veins. *Am J Respir Cell Mol Biol* 2002;**26**:330–40.
9. Mohammad MA, Sparrow MP. The distribution of heavy-chain isoform of myosin in airways from adult and neonate humans. *Biochem J* 1989;**260**:421–6.
10. Snetkov VA, Pandya HC, Hirst SJ, Ward JPT. Potassium channels in human foetal airway smooth muscle cells. *Pediatr Res* 1998;**43**:548–54.
11. Roman, J. Effects of calcium channel blockade on mammalian lung branching morphogenesis. *Exp Lung Res* 1995;**21**:489–502.
12. Hislop A, Reid L. Intrapulmonary arterial development during foetal life – branching pattern and structure. *J Anat* 1972;**113**:35–48.
13. Hislop A, Reid L. Foetal and childhood development of the intrapulmonary veins in man – branching pattern and structure. *Thorax* 1973;**28**:313–19.
14. Hislop A, Wigglesworth JS, Desai R. Alveolar development in the human foetus and infant. *Early Hum Dev* 1986;**13**:1–11.
15. Langston C, Kida C, Reed M, Thurlbeck WM. Human lung growth in late gestation and in the neonate. *Am Rev Resp Dis* 1984;**129**:607–13.
16. Zeltner TB, Caduff JH, Gehr P, Pfenninger J, Burri PH. The postnatal development and growth of the human lung. I. Morphometry. *Respir Physiol* 1986;**67**:247–67.
17. Burri PH, Dbaly J, Weibel ER. The postnatal growth of the rat lung. I. Morphometry. *Anat Rec* 1974;**178**:711–30.
18. Burri PH. The postnatal growth of the rat lung. III. Morphology. *Anat Rec* 1974;**180**:77–98.
19. Angus GE, Thurlbeck WM. Number of alveoli in the human lung. *J Appl Physiol* 1972;**32**:483–5.
20. Strang LB. Foetal lung liquid: secretion and reabsorption. *Physiol Rev* 1991;**71**:991–1016.
21. Robertso B, Van Golde LMG, Batenburg JJ. *Pulmonary Surfactant from Molecular Biology to Clinical Practice.* Elsevier Science, Amsterdam, 1992.
22. Haworth SG, Hislop AA. Normal structural and functional adaptation to extra-uterine life. *J Pediatr* 1981;**98**:915–18.
23. Hislop A, Reid L. Pulmonary arterial development during childhood: branching pattern and structure. *Thorax* 1973;**28**:129–35.
24. Allen K, Haworth SG. Human postnatal pulmonary arterial remodelling: ultrastructural studies of smooth muscle cell and connective tissue maturation. *Lab Invest* 1988;**59**:702–9.
25. Haworth SG. Pulmonary vascular remodeling in neonatal pulmonary hypertension. State of the art. *Chest* 1988;**93**:133S–8S.
26. Glasgow RE, Heymann MA. Endothelium-derived relaxing factor as a mediator of bradykinin-induced perinatal pulmonary vasodilatation. *Clin Res* 1990;**38**:211A.
27. Abman SH, Chatfield BA, Rodman DM, Hall SL, McMurtry IV. Maturational changes in endothelium-derived relaxing factor activity of ovine pulmonary arteries in vitro. *Am J Physiol* 1991;**260**:L280–5.
28. Kinsella JP, Ivy DD, Abman SH. Ontogeny of NO activity and response to inhaled NO in the developing ovine pulmonary circulation. *Am J Physiol* 1994;**267**:H1955–61.
29. Abman SH, Chatfield BA, Hall, SL, McMurtry IF. Role of endothelium-derived relaxing factor during transition of pulmonary circulation at birth. *Am J Physiol* 1990;**259**:H1921–7.
30. Hislop AA, Springall DR ,Buttery LDK, Pollock JS, Haworth SG. Abundance of endothelial nitric oxide synthase in newborn intrapulmonary arteries. *Arch Dis Child* 1995;**12**:F17–21.
31. Arrigoni FI, Hislop AA, Pollock J, Haworth SG, Mitchell JA. Changes in nitric oxide synthase activity in the porcine lung. *Am J Respir Crit Care Med* 1999;**159**(3), A898 (abstract).
32. Hislop AA, Haworth SG. Airway size and structure in the normal foetal and infant lung and the effect

of premature delivery and artificial ventilation. *Am Rev Respir Dis* 1989;**140**:1717–26.

33. Hislop A, Muir DCF, Jacobsen M, Simon G, Reid L. Postnatal growth and function of the pre-acinar airways. *Thorax* 1972;**27**:265–74.

34. Martin TR, Castile RG, Fredberg JJ, Wohl B, Mead J. Airway size is related to sex but not lung size in normal adults. *J Appl Physiol* 1987;**63**:2042–7.

35. Matsuba K, Thurlbeck WM. A morphometric study of bronchial and bronchiolar walls in children. *Am Rev Resp Dis* 1972;**105**:908–13.

36. James AL, Pare PD, Hogg JC. The mechanics of airway narrowing in asthma. *Am Rev Respir Dis* 1989; **139**:242–6.

37. Tepper RS. Airway reactivity in infants: a positive response to metacholine and metaproterenol. *J Appl Physiol* 1987;**62**:1155–9.

38. Hislop AA, Wharton J, Allen KM, Polak J, Haworth SG. Immunohistochemical localisation of peptide-containing nerves in the airways of normal young children. *Am J Respir Cell Mol Biol* 1990;**3**:191–8.

39. Field WEH. Mucous gland hypertrophy in babies and children aged 15 years or less. *Br J Dis Chest* 1968;**62**:11–18.

40. Baile EM. The anatomy and physiology of the bronchial circulation. *J Aerosol Med* 1996;**9**:1–6.

41. Jeffery PK, Reid L. The ultrastructure of the airway lining and its development. In: A Hodson, ed. *The Development of the Lung*. Marcel Dekker, New York, 1977, pp. 87–134.

42. Harkema JR, Mariassy A, St George J, Hyde DM, Plopper CG. Epithelial cells of the conducting airways: a species comparison. In: SP Farmer, DW Day, eds. *The Airway Epithelium. Physiology, Pathophysiology and Pharmacology*. Marcel Dekker, New York, 1991, pp. 3–40.

43. Lamb D, Reid L. Histochemical types of acid glycoprotein produced by mucous cells of the tracheobronchial glands in man. *J Pathol* 1969;**98**:213–28.

44. Laitinen A, Laitinen LA. Airway morphology: epithelium/basement membrane. *Am J Respir Crit Care Med* 1994;**150**:S14–17.

45. Jetten AM. Growth and differentiation factors in tracheobronchial epithelium. *Am J Physiol* 1991;**260**: L361–73.

46. Shijubo N, Itoh Y, Yamaguchi T, Imada A, Hirasawa M, Yamada T, Kawai T, Abe S. Clara cell protein-positive epithelial cells are reduced in small airways of asthmatics. *Am J Respir Crit Care Med* 1999; **160**(3):930–3.

47. Hermans C, Bernard A. Lung epithelium-specific proteins – characteristics and potential applications as markers. *Am J of Respir Crit Care Medicine* 1999; **159**:646–78.

48. Cutz E. Neuroendocrine cells of the lung. An overview of morphologic characteristics and development. *Exp Lung Res* 1982;**3**:185–208.

49. Johnson DE. Pulmonary neuroendocrine cells. In: SG Farmer, DWP Hay, eds. *The Airway Epithelium: Physiology, Pathophysiology and Pharmacology*. Marcel Dekker, New York, 1991, pp. 335–97.

50. Spina D. Epithelium smooth muscle regulation and interactions. *Am J Respir Crit Care Med* 1998; **158**:S141–5.

51. Tamaoki J, Tagaya E, Isono K, Kondo M, Konno K. Role of Ca^{2+}-activated K^+ channel in epithelium-dependant relaxation of human bronchial smooth muscle. *Br J Pharmacol* 1997;**121**:794–8.

52. Zeltner TB, Burri PH. The postnatal development and growth of the human lung. II. Morphology. *Respir Physiol* 1986;**67**:269–82.

53. Wendel DP, Taylor DG, Albertine KH, Keating MT, Li DY. Impaired distal airway development in mice lacking elastin. *Am J Respir Cell Mol Biol* 2000; **23**:320–6.

54. Lindahl P, Karlsson L, Hellstrom M, Gebre-Medhin S, Willetts K, Heath JK, Betsholtz C. Alveogenesis failure in PDGF-A-deficient mice is coupled to lack of distal spreading of alveolar smooth muscle cell progenitors during lung development. *Development* 1997; **124**:3943–53.

55. Hislop A, Wigglesworth JS, Desai R, Aber V. The effects of preterm delivery and mechanical ventilation on human lung growth. *Early Hum Dev* 1987; **15**:147–64.

56. Thurlbeck WM. Postnatal growth and development of the lung. *Am Rev Respir Dis* 1975;**3**:803–44.

57. Lanteri CJ, Sly PD. Changes in respiratory mechanics with age. *J Appl Physiol* 1993;**74**:369–78.

58. Merkus PJFM, Borsboom GJJM, Van Pelt W, Schrader PC, Van Houwelingen HC. Growth of airways and air spaces in teenagers is related to sex but not to symptoms. *J Appl Physiol* 1993;**75**:2045–53.

59. Loosli CG, Hung KS. Development of pulmonary innervation. In: WA Hodson, ed. *Development of the Lung*. Marcel Dekker, New York, 1977, p. 269.

60. Sparrow MP, Weichselbaum M, McCray PB. Development of the innervation and airway smooth muscle in human foetal lung. *Am J Resp Cell Mol Biol* 1999;**20**:550–60.

61. Ward JK, Belvisi MG, Fox AJ, Miura M, Tadjkarimi S, Yacoub MH, Barnes PJ. Modulation of cholinergic neural bronchoconstriction by endogenous nitric oxide and vasoactive intestinal peptide in human airways in vitro. *J Clin Invest* 1993;**92**:736–42.

62. Ullah MI, Newman GB, Saunders KB. Influence of age on response to ipratropium and salbutamol in asthma. *Thorax* 1981;**36**:523–9.

63. Dezateux CA, Stocks J. Lung development and early origins of childhood respiratory illness. *Br Med Bull* 1997;**53**:40–57.

64. Shaheen SO, Barker DJP, Shiell AW, Crocker FJ, Wield GA, Holgate ST. The relationship between pneumonia in early childhood and impaired lung

function in late adult life. *Am J Respir Crit Care Med* 1994;**149**:616–19.

65. Martinez FD, Wright AL, Taussig LM, Holberg CJ, Halonen M, Morgan WJ. Asthma and wheezing in the first six years of life. *N Eng J Med* 1995; **332**:133–8.

66. Sutherland DC, Samkovlis C, Drasnow MA. Branchless encodes a Drosophila FGF homolog that controls tracheal cell migration and patterning of branching. *Cell* 1996;**87**:1091–101.

67. Hogan BLM, Yingling JM. Epithelial/mesenchymal interactions and branching morphogenesis of the lung. *Curr Opin Genet Dev* 1998;**8**:481–6.

68. Ang S-L, Rossan J. HNF-3b is essential for node and notochord development in mouse development. *Cell* 1994;**78**:561–74.

69. Bruno MD, Bohinski RJ, Huelsman KM, Whitsett JA, Korfhagen TR. Lung cell specific expression of the murine surfactant A gene is mediated by interactions between the SP-A promoter and thyroid transcription factor. *J Biol Chem* 1995;**270**:6531–6.

70. Minoo P, Hamdan H, Bu D, Warburton D, Stepanik P, deLemos R. TTF-1 regulates lung epithelial morphogenesis. *Dev Biol* 1995;**172**:694–8.

71. Motoyoma J, Liu J, Mo R, Ding Q, Post M, Hui CC. Essential function of Gli2 and Gli3 in the formation of the lung, trachea and esophagus. *Nat Genet* 1998;**20**:54–7.

72. Whitsett J. A lungful of transcription factors. *Nat Genet* 1998;**20**:7–8.

73. Kang S, Graham Jr JM, Olney AH, Biesecker LG. Gli3 frameshift mutations cause autosomal dominant Pallister–Hall syndrome. *Nature Genet* 1997; **17**:259–60.

74. Bellusci S, Grindley H, Emoto H, Itoh N, Hogan BL. Fibroblast growth factor 10 (FGF-10) and branching morphogenesis in embryonic mouse lung. *Development* 1997;**124**:4867–78.

75. Cardoso WV, Itoh A, Nogawa H, Mason I, Brody JS. FGF-1 and FGF-7 induce distinct patterns of growth and differentiation in embryonic lung epithelium. *Dev Dyn* 1997;**298**:398–405.

76. Park WY, Miranda B, Lebeche D, Hashimoto G, Cadoso WV. FGF-10 is a chemotactic factor for distal lung epithelium buds during development. *Dev Biol* 1998;**15**:125–34.

77. Pepicelli CV, Lewis PM, McMahon AP. Sonic hedgehog regulates branching morphogenesis in the mammalian lung. *Dev Biol* 1998;**8**:1083–6.

78. Bostrom H, Willets K, Pekny M, *et al.* PDGF-a signalling is a critical event in lung myofibroblast development and alveogenesis. *Cell* 1996;**85**:863–73.

79. Masters JRW. Epithelial-mesenchymal interaction during lung development: the effect of mesenchymal mass. *Develop Biol* 1976;**51**:98–108.

80. Minoo P, Ring RJ. Epithelial-mesenchymal interactions in lung development. *Ann Rev Physiol* 1994;**56**:13–45.

81. McGowan SE. Extracellular matrix and the regulation of lung development and repair. *FASEB J* 1992; **6**:2895–904.

82. Strandjord TP, Sage EH, Clark JG. SPARC participates in the branching morphogenesis of developing foetal rat lung. *Am J Respir Cell Mol Biol* 1995;**13**:279–87.

83. Warburton D, Zhao J, Berberich MA, Bernfield M. Molecular embryology of the lung: then, now and in the future. *Am J Physiol* 1999;**276**:L697.

84. Griscom NT, Wohl MEB, Fenton T. Dimensions of the trachea to age 6 years related to height. *Pediatr Pulmonol* 1989;**6**:186–90.

85. Stocks, J, Henschen M, Hoo A-F, Costeloe K, Dezateux CA. The influence of ethnicity and gender on airway function in preterm infants. *Am J Respir Crit Care Med* 1997;**156**:1855–62.

86. Taussig LM, Cota K, Kaltenborn W. Different mechanical properties of the lung in boys and girls. *Am Rev Respir Dis* 1981;**123**:640–3.

87. Gold DR, Wypij D, Wang XZ, Speizer FE, Pugh M, Ware JH. Gender and race-specific effects of asthma and wheeze on level and growth of lung function in children in six US cities. *Am J Respir Crit Care Med* 1994;**149**:1198–208.

88. Collaborative Study Group on Antenatal Steroid Therapy. Effect of antenatal dexamethasone administration on the prevention of respiratory distress syndrome. *Am J Obstet Gynecol* 1981;**141**: 276–87.

89. Willet KE, Jobe AH, Ikegami M, Polk DH, Newnham J, Kohan R, Gurrin L, Sly PD. Postnatal lung function after prenatal steroid treatment in sheep: effect of gender. *Pediatric Res* 1997;**42**:885–92.

90. Greenberg DN, Yoder BA, Clark RH, Butzin CA, Null DM. Effect of maternal race on outcome of preterm infants in the military. *Pediatrics* 1993; **91**:572–7.

91. Stocks J, Gappa M, Rabbette PS, Hoo A-F, Mukhtar Z, Costeloe KL. A comparison of respiratory function in Afro-Caribbean and Caucasian infants. *Eur Respir J* 1994;**7**:11–16.

92. Stocks J, Godfrey S. Nasal resistance during infancy. *Respir Physiol* 1978;**34**:233–46.

93. Kitagawa, M, Hislop A, Boyden EA, Reid L. Lung hypoplasia in congenital diaphragmatic hernia. A quantitative study of airway, artery and alveolar development. *Br J Surg* 1971;**58**:342–6.

94. Holmes CWM, Thurlbeck WM. Normal lung growth and response after pneumonectomy in the rat at various ages. *Am Rev Respir Dis* 1979;**120**:1125–36.

95. Hislop A, Reid L. Persistent hypoplasia of the lung after repair of congenital diaphragmatic hernia. *Thorax* 1976;**31**:450–5.

96. Ijsselstijn H, Tibboel D, Hop WJC, Molenaar JC, de Jongste JC. Long-term pulmonary sequelae in children with congenital diaphragmatic hernia. *Am J Respir Crit Care Med* 1997;**155**:174–80.

97. Hislop A, Hey E, Reid L. The lungs in congenital bilateral renal agenesis and dysplasia. *Arch Dis Child* 1979;**54**:32–8.

98. Hislop A, Fairweather DVI, Blackwell RJ, Howard S. The effect of amniocentesis and drainage of amniotic fluid on lung development in *Macaca fascicularis*. *Br J Obstet Gynecol* 1984;**91**:835–42.

99. Wigglesworth JS, Hislop A, Desai R. Foetal lung growth in congenital laryngeal atresia. *Ped Pathol* 1987;**7**:515–25.

100. Alcorn D, Adamson TM, Lambert TF, Maloney JE, Ritchie BC, Robinson PM. Morphological effects of chronic tracheal ligation and drainage in the foetal lamb lung. *J Anat* 1977;**123**:649–60.

101. Hooper SB, Harding R. Foetal lung liquid: a major determinant of the growth and functional development of the foetal lung. *Clin Exp Pharmacol Physiol* 1995;**22**:235–47.

102. Hedrick MH, Estes JM, Sullivan KM, Bealer JF, Kitterman JA, Flake AK, Adzick NS, Harrison MR. Plug the lung until it grows (PLUG): a new method to treat congenital diaphragmatic hernia in utero. *J Ped Surg*1994;**29**:612–17.

103. Harrison MR, Adzick NS, Flake AW, *et al.* Correction of congenital diaphragmatic hernia in utero: VI. Hard-earned lessons. *J Ped Surg* 1993; **28**:1411–17.

104. Harding R. Foetal breathing: relation to postnatal breathing and lung development. In: MA Hanson, JAD Spencer, CH Rodeck, D Walters, eds. *Foetus and Neonate: Physiology and Clinical Applications.* Cambridge University Press, Cambridge, 1994, pp. 63–84.

105. Liggins GC, Vilos GA, Campos GA, Kitterman JA, Lee CH. The effect of bilateral thoracoplasty on lung development in foetal sheep. *J Develop Physiol* 1981;**3**:275–82.

106. Wiggleswort JS, Desai R. Is foetal respiratory function a major determinant of perinatal survival? *Lancet* 1982;**1**:264–7.

107. Liu M, Skinner SJMXJ, Han RNN, Transwell AK, Post M. Stimulation of foetal rat lung cell proliferation in vitro by mechanical stretch. *Am J Physiol* 1992;**263**:L376–83.

108. Barker DJP. The intrauterine environment and adult cardiovascular disease. In: G Bock, J Whelan, eds. *The Childhood Environment and Adult Disease.* John Wiley, Chichester, 1991, pp. 3–15.

109. Gaultier C. Malnutrition and lung growth. *Pediatr Pulmon* 1991;**10**:278–86.

110. Sekhon HS, Thurlbeck WM. Lung cytokinetics after exposure to hypobaria and/or hypoxia and undernutrition in growing rats. *J Appl Physiol* 1995;**79**:1299–309.

111. Kalenga M, Tschanz SA, Burri PH. Protein deficiency and the growing rat lung. II. Morphometric analysis and morphology. *Pediatr Res* 1995;**37**:789–95.

112. Thomson MA, Quirk P, Swanson CE, Thomas BJ, Holt TL, Francis PJ, Shepherd RW. Nutritional growth retardation is associated with defective lung growth in cystic fibrosis: a preventable determinant of progressive pulmonary dysfunction. *Nutrition* 1995;**11**:350–4.

113. Neville RG, McCowan C, Thomas G, Crombie IK. Asthma and growth – cause for concern? Asthma and growth in Tayside children. *Ann Hum Biol* 1996;**23**:323–31.

114. Massaro GD, Massaro D. Formation of pulmonary alveoli and gas exchange surface area: quantitation and regulation. *Ann Rev Physiol* 1996;**58**:73–92.

115. Massaro GD, Massaro D. Retinoic acid treatment abrogates elastase-induced pulmonary emphysema in rats. *Nat Med* 1997;**3**:675–7.

116. Massaro GD, Massaro D. Retinoic acid treatment partially rescues failed septation in rats and in mice. *Am J Physiol* 2000;**278**:L955–60.

117. Noy N. Retinoid-binding proteins: mediators of retinoid action. *Biochem J* 2000;**348**:481–95.

118. McGowan S, Jackson SK, Jenkins-Moore M, Dai HH, Chambon P, Snyder JM. Mice bearing deletions of retinoic acid receptors demonstrate reduced lung elastin and alveolar numbers. *Am J Respir Cell Mol Biol* 2000;**23**:162–7.

119. Watts DH, Krohn MA, Hillier SL, Echenbach DA. The association of occult amniotic fluid infection with gestational age and neonatal outcome among women in preterm labor. *Obs Gynecol* 1992; **79**:351–7.

120. Watterberg KL, Demers LM, Scott SM, Murphy S. Chorioamnionitis and early lung inflammation in infants in whom bronchopulmonary dysplasia develops. *Pediatrics* 1996;**97**:210–15.

121. Yoon BH, Romero R, Jun JK, Park KH, Park JD, Ghezzi F, Kim BI. Amniotic fluid cytokines (interleukin-6, tumor necrosis factor-alpha, interleukin-1 beta and interleukin-8) and the risk for the development of bronchopulmonary dysplasia. *Am J Obstet Gynecol* 1997;**177**:825–30.

122. Jobe AH, Newnham JP, Willet KE, Sly P, Ervin MG, Bachurski C, Possmayer F, Hallman M, Ikegami M. Effects of antenatal endotoxin and glucocorticoids on the lungs of preterm lambs. *Am J Obstet Gynecol* 2000;**182**:401–8.

123. Haglund B, Cnattingius S. Cigarette smoking as a risk factor for Sudden Infant Death Syndrome: a population based study. *Am J Public Health* 1990;**80**:29–32.

124. Blair PS, Fleming PJ, Bensley D. Smoking and the sudden infant death syndrome: results from 1993–5 case–control study for confidential inquiry into stillbirths and deaths in infancy. *Br Med J* 1996;**313**:195–8.

125. Cook DG, Strachan DP. Summary of effects of parental smoking on the respiratory health of

children and implications for research. *Thorax* 1999;**54**:357–66.

126. Dezateux C, Stocks J, Dundas I, Fletcher ME. Impaired airway function and wheezing in infancy. *Am J Respir Crit Care Med* 1999;**159**:403–10.

127. Tager IB, Hanrahan JP, Tostesan TD. Lung function, pre and postnatal smoke exposure and wheezing in the first year of life. *Am Rev Respir Dis* 1993; **147**:811–17.

128. Young S, O'Keeffe PT, Arnott J, Landau LI. Lung function, airway responsiveness and respiratory symptoms before and after bronchiolitis. *Arch Dis Child* 1995;**72**:16–24.

129. Ahlsten G, Cnattingius S, Lindmark G. Cessation of smoking during pregnancy improves foetal growth and reduces infant morbidity in the neonatal period. A population-based prospective study. *Acta Paediatr* 1993;**82**:177–81.

130. Thaler I, Goodman JDS, Dawes GS. Effects of maternal cigarette smoking on foetal breathing and foetal movements. *Am J Obstet Gynecol* 1980; **138**:282–7.

131. Maritz GS, Woolward K. Effect of maternal nicotine exposure on neonatal lung elastic tissue and possible consequences. *S Afr Med J* 1992;**81**:517–19.

132. Sekhon HS, Jia Y, Raab R, Kuryatov A, Pankow JF, Whitsett JA. Prenatal nicotine increases pulmonary a7 nicotine receptor expression and alters foetal lung development in monkeys. *J Clin Invest* 1999; **103**:637–47.

133. Elliot J, Carroll N, Bosco M, McCrohan M, Robinson P. Increased airway responsiveness and decreased alveolar attachment points following in utero smoke exposure in the guinea pig. *Am J Resp Crit Care Med* 2001;**163**:140–4.

134. Hoo AF, Henschen M, Dezateux C, Costeloe K, Stocks J. Respiratory function among preterm infants whose mothers smoked during pregnancy. *Am J Respir Crit Care Med* 1998;**158**:700–5.

135. Elliot J, Vullermin P, Robinson P. Maternal cigarette smoking is associated with increased inner airway wall thickness in children who die of sudden infant death syndrome. *J Respir Crit Care Med* 1998; **158**:802–6.

136. Margraf LR, Tomashefski JFJ, Bruce MC, Dahms BB. Morphometric analysis of the lung in bronchopulmonary dysplasia. *Am Rev Respir Dis* 1991;**143**:391–400.

137. Coalson JJ, Winter VT, Siler-Khodr T, Yoder BA. Neonatal chronic lung disease in extremely immature baboons. *Am J Respir Crit Care Med* 1999;**160**:1333–46.

138. Openshaw PJ, Lemanske RF. Respiratory viruses and asthma: can the effects be prevented? *Eur Respir J* 1998;**11**(Suppl 27):35–39s.

139. Kumar A, Sorkness R, Kaplan MR, Castleman WL, Lemanske RF. Chronic episodic reversible airway obstruction after viral bronchiolitis in rats. *Am J Respir Crit Care Med* 1997;**155**:130–4.

140. Castleman WL, Sorkness RL, Lemanske RF, Grassee G, Suyemoto MM. Neonatal viral bronchiolitis and pneumonia induces bronchiolar hypoplasia and alveolar dysplasia in rats. *Lab Invest* 1988;**59**:387–96.

141. Coalson JJ, Gerstmann DR, Winter VT, Delemos RA. Bacterial colonization and infection studies in the premature baboon with bronchopulmonary dysplasia. *Am Rev Respir Dis* 1991;**144**:1140–6.

142. Abman SH, Groothius JR. Pathophysiology and treatment of bronchopulmonary dysplasia. Current issues. *Pediatr Clin North Am* 1994;**41**:277–315.

143. Gorenflo M, Vogel M, Herbst L, Bassir C, Kattner E, Obladen M. Influence of clinical and ventilatory parameters on morphology of bronchopulmonary dysplasia. *Pediatr Pulmonol* 1995;**19**:214–20.

144. Cherukupalli K, Larson JE, Rotschild A, Thurlbeck WM. Biochemical, clinical and morphologic studies on lungs of infants with bronchopulmonary dysplasia. *Paediatr Pulmonol* 1996;**22**:215–29.

145. Northway WH, Moss RB, Carlisle KB, Parker BR, Popp RL, Pitlock PT, Eichler I, Lamm RL, Brown BWJ. Late pulmonary sequelae of bronchopulmonary dysplasia. *N Eng J Med* 1990;**323**:1793–9.

146. Merkus PJFM. *Growth of Lungs and Airways in Asthma.* Leiden University, 1993, pp. 146–70.

147. Merkus PJFM, ten Have-Opbroek AAW, Quanjer PH. Human lung growth: a review. *Pediatr Pulmonol* 1996;**21**:383–97.

148. Coalson JL, Winter VT, Gerstman DR, Idell S, King RJ, Delemos RA. Pathophysiologic, morphometric and biochemical studies of the premature baboon with bronchopulmonary dysplasia. *Am Rev Respir Dis* 1992;**145**:872–81.

149. Thibault DW, Mabry S, Rezaiekhaligh M. Neonatal pulmonary oxygen toxicity in the rat and changes with aging. *Pediatr Pulmon* 1990;**9**:96–108.

150. Buch S, Han RNN, Liu J, Moore A, Edelson JD, Freeman BA, Post M, Tanswell AK. Basic fibroblast growth factor and growth factor receptor gene expression in 85% O_2-exposed rat lung. *Am J Physiol* 1995;**268**:455–64.

151. Moore AM, Buch S, Han RNN, Freeman BA, Post M, Tanswell AK. Altered expression of type I collagen TGFβ1 and related genes in rat lung exposed to 85% O_2. *Am J Physiol* 1995;**268**:178–84.

152. Davis JM, Dickerson B, Metlay L, Penney DP. Differential effects of oxygen and barotrauma on lung injury in the neonatal piglet. *Pediatr Pulmonol* 1991;**10**:157–63.

153. Han RNN, Buch S, Tseu I, Young J, Christie NA, Frndova H, Lye SJ, Post M, Tanswell AK. Changes in structure, mechanics and insulin-like growth factor-related gene expression in the lungs of newborn rats exposed to air or 60% oxygen. *Pediatr Res* 1996;**39**:921–9.

154. Hershenson MB, Garland A, Kelleher MD, Zimmermann A, Hernandez C, Solway J. Hyperoxia-induced airway remodelling in immature rats. Correlation with airway responsiveness. *Am Rev Respir Dis* 1992;**146**:1294–300.

155. Laitinen LA, Laitinen A. Modulation of bronchial inflammation: corticosteroids and other therapeutic agents. *Am J Respir Crit Care Med* 1994; **150**:S87–90.

156. Laitinen LA, Laitinen A. Remodeling of asthmatic airways by glucocorticosteroids. *J Allergy Clin Immunol* 1996;**97**:153–8.

157. Stewart AG, Fernandes D, Tomlinson PR. The effect of glucocorticoids on proliferation of human cultured airway smooth muscle. *Br J Pharm* 1995; **116**:3219–26.

158. Shiels IA, Blowler SD, Taylor SM. Homologous serum increases fibronectin expression and cell adhesion in airway smooth muscle cells. *Inflammation* 1996;**20**:373–87.

159. Cohen MD, Ciocca V, Panettieri RA Jr. TGF-beta 1 modulates human airway smooth-muscle cell proliferation induced by mitogens. *Am J Respir Cell Mol Biol* 1997;**16**:85–90.

160. Jaskoll T, Choy HA, Melnick M. The glucocorticoid–glucocorticoid receptor signal transduction pathway, transforming growth factor-b and embryonic mouse lung development in vivo. *Pediatr Res* 1996;**39**:749–59.

161. Melnick M, Choy HA, Jaskoll T. Glucocorticoids, tumor necrosis factor-alpha and epidermal growth factor regulation of pulmonary morphogenesis: a multivariate in vitro analysis of their related actions. *Dev Dyn* 1996;**205**:365–78.

162. Massaro GD, Massaro D. Formation of alveoli in rats: postnatal effect of prenatal dexamethasone. *Am J Physiol* 1992;**263**:37–41.

163. Pinkerton KE, Willet KE, Peake JL, Sly PD, Jobe AH, Ikegami M. Prenatal glucocorticoid and T4 effects on lung morphology in preterm lambs. *Am J Respir Crit Care Med* 1997;**156**:624–30.

164. Johnson JWC, Mitzner W, Beck JC, London WT, Sly DL, Lee PA, Kouzami VA, Cavalieri RL. Long-term effects of betamethasone on foetal development. *Am J Obstet Gynecol* 1981;**141**:1053–61.

165. Tschanz SA, Damke BM, Burri PH. Influence of postnatally administered glucocorticoids on rat lung growth. *Biol Neonate* 1995;**68**:229–45.

166. Burri PH. Structural aspects of prenatal and postnatal development and growth of the lung. In: JA McDonald, ed. *Lung Growth and Development*. Marcel Dekker, New York, 1997, pp. 1–35.

167. Burri PH, Hislop AA. Structural considerations. *Eur Respir J* 1998;**12**:59s–65s.

168. Laitinen LA, Laitinen A, Haahtela T. A comparative study of the effects of an inhaled corticosteroid, budesonide and a beta 2-agonist, terbutaline, on airway inflammation in newly diagnosed asthma: a randomized, double-blind, parallel-group controlled trial. *J Allergy Clin Immunol* 1992;**90**:32–42.

169. Tomlinson PR, Wilson JW, Stewart AG. Salbutamol inhibits the proliferation of human airway smooth muscle cells grown in culture: relationship to elevated cAMP levels. *Biochem-Pharmacol* 1995; **49**:1809–19.

170. Plotnick LH, Ducharme FM. Should inhaled anticholinergics be added to beta2 agonists for treating acute childhood and adolescent asthma? A systematic review. *BMJ* 1998;**317**:971–7.

171. Schittny JC, Miserocchi G, Sparrow MP. Spontaneous peristaltic airway contractions propel lung liquid through the bronchial tree of intact and foetal lung explants. *Am J Respir Cell Mol Biol* 2000;**23**:11–18.

172. Ulrik CS. Outcome of asthma:longitudinal changes in lung function. *Eur Respir J* 1999;**13**:904–18.

Developmental physiology

KAREN E WILLET AND PETER D SLY

INTRODUCTION

There is no doubt that environmental factors influence the expression of a genetic tendency to produce the wheezing illnesses that have been called asthma. In addition, the different expressions of asthma at different stages of life can be influenced both by aspects of normal anatomical and physiological development and by environmental factors.

Current thinking suggests that three patterns of wheezing lower respiratory illness (wLRI) occur during childhood: transient early wheezing, persistent wheezing and late-onset wheezing. Almost two-thirds of all children who wheeze during the first 3 years of life fit into the category of 'transient early wheezers' (Chapter 3). This group of infants is characterized by impaired pulmonary function prior to the onset of any wheezing illnesses, and lower lung function in later childhood, despite the absence of clinical wheeze or asthma. These children are thought to have inherently small airways, although this conjecture is based on studies that did not measure airway calibre directly. On the other hand, children who have persistent wheeze are more likely to have a family history of asthma and allergies and present with allergic symptoms early in life. Unlike transient early wheezers, children with persistent wheeze have, on average, normal lung function in early infancy but reduced lung function in later childhood. It is thought that chronic inflammation may lead to structural abnormalities in these children. The two most common causes of acute wLRI during early life are the respiratory syncytial virus (RSV) and parainfluenza. Infants hospitalized with RSV bronchiolitis have a very high rate of subsequent wheezing, but not necessarily of atopy. Debate exists as to whether this is due to asthma.

If these patterns of wheezing disorder are produced by differences in the normal pattern of physiological development of the respiratory system, some understanding of physiological development is necessary for those carrying out research in this area and for the rational treatment of childhood wheezing illnesses.

NORMAL INTRAUTERINE LUNG DEVELOPMENT

At the moment of birth, the lungs have to be capable of air breathing and gas exchange. In order to achieve this function, the lungs need to have developed a large surface area, consisting of thin walled alveoli containing a dense capillary network. There is now considerable evidence that the intrauterine environment has a profound influence on the growth and structural maturation of the lungs both before and after birth (Chapter 4a).

During development, fetal lungs are maintained in an expanded state by the active secretion of a lung liquid. Rate of secretion of lung liquid in fetal sheep increases from around 1.6 ml/kg/h in mid-gestation to 3–4 ml/kg/h during the last 30 days of gestation (term 150 days).[1] After entering the lung lumen, this fluid moves along the trachea into the pharynx of the fetus, where it is either swallowed or enters the amniotic sac, making a substantial contribution to amniotic fluid volume. The total fluid volume held in the lungs of fetal sheep increases from 3 ml/kg in mid-gestation to 50 ml/kg just prior to term, substantially more than the air-filled lung volume at end-expiration after birth (20–30 ml/kg).

Thus the lungs are hyper-expanded during late intrauterine life. The degree of lung expansion during development is a critical determinant of growth and structural maturation. Reduced lung expansion induced by gravitational drainage of lung liquid leads to lung hypoplasia and structural immaturity.[2] Conversely, sustained over-expansion, as a result of tracheal obstruction, results in lung hyperplasia and the formation of 'air-spaces' with thinner than normal walls.[2]

Fetal breathing movements (FBM) are coordinated, rhythmical contractions of the fetal respiratory muscles caused by brainstem neural activity. FBM occur in episodes of 20–60 min interspersed by periods of apnoea, and can be detected in mammalian fetuses throughout the final two-thirds of gestation. Individual FBM cause small reductions (3–4 mmHg) in intra-thoracic pressure, small changes (1–2%) in thoracic dimensions and small oscillations (<1 ml) of fluid flow in the trachea.[3–5] FBM are central to the control of fetal lung growth because they influence the movement of lung liquid. Episodes of FBM are associated with a net efflux of lung liquid, as a result of lowered upper airway resistance.[6] During the intervening apnoeic periods, the lungs become increasingly distended with newly secreted liquid, due to tonic contraction of laryngeal constrictor muscles and narrowing of the glottis. Abolition of FBM in the womb reduces the expansion of the fetal lungs by 25–30%.[7]

Our limited insight into the mechanical changes that occur in the developing lung during late gestation comes through studies in preterm infants. During the last weeks of gestation chest wall compliance decreases; chest wall stability in the presence of resistive loads improves and thoraco-abdominal asynchrony decreases; extrathoracic airway stability increases; dynamic lung compliance increases; and minute volume displacement of the diaphragm and diaphragmatic work decrease.[11–14] Studies in preterm sheep also indicate marked changes in the weeks preceding birth. Respiratory system elastance (Ers, inverse of compliance) decreases four-fold between 121 and 135 days gestation (term = 150 days)[15] and a further 2.5-fold between 135 days and term. The fall in Ers is due mainly to a fall in lung elastance (El), which corresponds to a 10-fold increase in lung volume. While chest wall elastance (Ew) falls slightly, its proportional contribution to Ers increases. Total respiratory system resistance (R_{rs}) decreases five-fold during this period, although it is likely this reflects mainly tissue resistance (R_{ti}), as our own estimates using the forced oscillation technique suggest there is little change in airway resistance (R_{aw}).

PERINATAL INFLUENCES ON POSTNATAL LUNG FUNCTION

Preterm birth

Primitive alveoli have been identified as early as 29–30 weeks and are uniformly present by around 36 weeks gestation.[16,17] At birth up to about half of the full adult complement are present.[16,17] The remaining alveoli are formed during the first two years after birth, with most being formed during the first 6 months of life. For infants born prematurely, alveolar development may be an entirely postnatal event. By contrast, airway branching is complete by the 16th week of gestation and cartilage and submucosal glands extend as far down the airways as they do in adults by 24 weeks gestation (Chapter 3a). Between 22 weeks gestation and 8 months of age, the normal infant has a linear increase in airway diameter with age and the growth of the airway tree is symmetrical, i.e. the relative growth of airways being similar at all generations.[18] The area of the airway wall occupied by muscle and submucosal glands also increases linearly with age, when related to the size of the airways.[18] Infants born prematurely have relatively small airways with relatively more bronchial smooth muscle and submucosal glands than infants born at term, when compared at the same postnatal age. These changes are exaggerated in infants born prematurely who required mechanical ventilation.[18] In addition, the development of the lung parenchyma is abnormal, with fewer alveoli and an increase in interstitial collagen and elastin. Throughout childhood the lungs of children who have been ventilated during the neonatal period have fewer alveoli and a lower surface area than expected for lung volume[19] or for airway size.[18]

There is unequivocal evidence that preterm birth and subsequent early postnatal events impact on lung function and respiratory health in childhood and beyond, although it is only recently that researchers have begun to identify the relative contribution of various perinatal factors to respiratory outcome. Prematurity (i.e. lung immaturity at birth) and low birth weight *per se* appear to have only a minor impact on long-term lung function.[20,21] However the development of respiratory distress syndrome (RDS) and progression to chronic neonatal lung disease (CLD) are associated with more prolonged impairment of lung function.[22–24] Prematurity is also associated with an increased incidence of recurrent wheeze and asthma.[25–27] It is difficult to distinguish between the effects of low birth weight (intrauterine growth retardation) and prematurity, as the two are often closely linked, but recent studies suggest that low birth weight is an independent risk factor for asthma and wheezing both in preterm and in term infants.[21,28,29] Schaubel et al. recently found that birth weight <1500 g, prematurity, the development of RDS and progression to CLD are all significant risk factors for physician diagnosed asthma.[30] In this and other studies it is clear that infants who develop CLD are at greatest risk for impaired lung function in later childhood[22,24] and for an increased incidence of asthma and wheeze.[30] The detrimental effects of CLD may relate to the injurious effect of hyperoxia, as duration of oxygen therapy appears to increase the risk of respiratory problems.[31]

It is important to identify and minimize any factors that threaten normal lung development during this critical period of rapid lung growth and development. Any perinatal event that increases the risk of preterm birth (e.g. intrauterine infection or maternal hypertension) or impairs normal lung growth and development, for example by impacting on fetal breathing movements (e.g. maternal smoking), can ultimately impact on lung function and respiratory health during childhood and beyond. Conversely, interventions that reduce the severity of neonatal respiratory disease (pre- and postnatal steroids, postnatal surfactant) can potentially minimize the risk of childhood respiratory problems.

Intrauterine smoking

One of the most harmful, yet totally avoidable agents to adversely affect the developing lung is maternal smoking during pregnancy. During the nine months of pregnancy, a woman who smokes 20 cigarettes a day will inhale toxic chemicals, capable of affecting growth and development of the fetus, more than 50 000 times.[32] The major components of cigarette smoke known to harm the developing mammalian fetus are nicotine and carbon monoxide. The major effects of nicotine on the fetus include: constriction of the utero-placental circulation, resulting in decreased uterine arterial blood flow with hypoxia and acidosis in the fetus; and release of catecholamines within the fetus. Carbon monoxide crosses the placenta and reaches a stable concentration in the fetus after 14–24 h at a level 10–15% higher than in the maternal circulation. The washout time required to reach half of the peak level is 2 h in the mother and 7 h in the fetus.[32]

The effects of intrauterine smoking on the fetus include: a reduction in birth weight by a mean of about 175–200 g; reduction in fetal head growth; increased risk of preterm birth, especially through an increased incidence of placenta praevia, placental abruption and premature rupture of membranes; and an increase in perinatal mortality.[32] Animal experiments have demonstrated that nicotine results in a decrease in FBM and fetal hypoxia.[33] A similar reduction in FBM following maternal smoking has been reported in humans.[34,35] *In utero* exposure to cigarette smoke leads to the formation of hypoplastic lungs with fewer, larger air spaces of reduced surface area in experimental animals.[36] Paradoxically, chronic intrauterine smoking is associated with a reduced incidence of respiratory distress syndrome and earlier maturation of lung surfactant,[37] possibly due to the increased fetal catecholamine levels. The net effect on postnatal lung function is therefore complex.

Numerous studies over the last decade have documented the detrimental effects of intrauterine smoke exposure on postnatal lung function (see also Chapter 7e). Impaired lung function is present in early infancy[38–41] and continues during childhood and into adolescence.[42] As well as impaired lung function, infants born to smoking mothers have reduced respiratory drive and blunted ventilatory response to hypoxia.[43] The impact of maternal smoking on lung function appears to be more pronounced in girls than in boys.[44] Importantly, prenatal smoke exposure has a more pronounced effect on postnatal lung function than does postnatal smoke exposure.[42] This observation highlights the extreme vulnerability of the lung to adverse influences during fetal development. In addition to impaired lung function, there is also a well-established link between *in utero* smoke exposure and the risk of developing asthma and other wheezing disorders during childhood.[45,46]

LUNG FUNCTION DURING CHILDHOOD

The first year of life

Advances in the knowledge of the postnatal development of the lungs have come about from studies measuring lung function in infants. The rapid thoracic compression (RTC) or 'squeeze' technique has been used extensively to measure forced expiration in infants.[47] The RTC technique produces forced expiratory flows by the sudden application of a pressure to the thorax and abdomen at the end of a tidal inspiration, using an inflatable thoraco-abdominal jacket connected to a positive pressure reservoir (Figure 6c.3, p. 147).

Prior to the RTC manoeuvre, a reproducible end-expiratory volume (FRC) is established from at least three tidal breaths. RTC, initiated at end-inspiration, then produces a partial expiratory flow–volume (PEFV) curve, with exhalation continuing to a volume below FRC. The maximal flow occurring at the previously established tidal FRC is known as V'_{max}, FRC (Chapter 6b). The RTC has several limitations: flows are measured only in the tidal range, flows at FRC are highly variable, and it is uncertain whether flow-limitation can be achieved in healthy infants. A later adaptation of the RTC, the raised volume RTC (RVRTC), measures expiratory flow over an extended volume range (by inflating the infant's lungs prior to jacket compression) and produces forced expiratory volume-time (FEV_t) measurements analogous to the FEV_1 in older subjects.[48] More recently Hall *et al.* measured lung mechanics in healthy infants using the forced oscillation technique (FOT).[49] The FOT involves the application of a composite sinusoidal signal either to the airway opening (input impedance) or to the thorax (transfer impedance). Responses derived from perturbations of the respiratory system provide detailed information about its mechanical behaviour. FOT data can be modelled to provide information on airway and tissue (parenchymal) damping and elastance.

Tissue damping, or frequency dependent resistance, describes the energy dissipated in moving the tissues of the lung parenchyma. As there is no bulk flow of gas at this level, this is not a true Newtonian resistance.

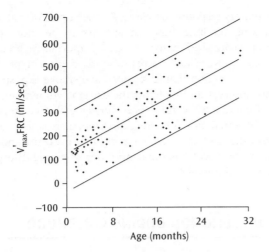

Figure 4b.1 *Forced expiratory flows at functional residual capacity (V'_{max}, FRC) vs age, for 112 infants, reported by Tepper et al. (ref. 51). The individual data points, together with the regression line and two standard deviation limits are shown.*

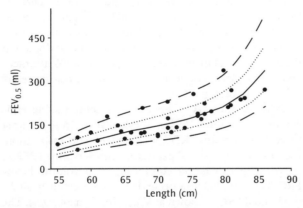

Figure 4b.2 *Forced expiratory volume in 0.5 s ($FEV_{0.5}$) vs length, for 28 infants, data adapted from Hall et al., (ref. 49). Solid line represents the fitted regression equation. Variation in data representing one (⋯⋯⋯) and two (— —) standard variants are shown. Points represent z-scores for each infant.*

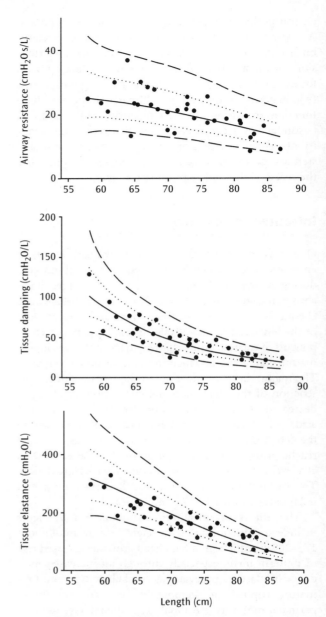

Figure 4b.3 *Airway resistance, parenchymal elastance and parenchymal damping versus length in 28 infants, data adapted from Hall et al., (ref. 49). Solid line represents the fitted regression equation. Variation in data representing one (⋯⋯⋯) and two (— —) standard variants are shown.*

Lung function, assessed by the RTC technique, shows an essentially linear increase with somatic growth and with lung volume throughout the first year of life[50,51,51a] (Figure 4b.1). In contrast to the wide variability of V'_{max}FRC measurements for a given length, FEV_t measurements are much less variable.[48] The relationship of $FEV_{0.5}$ to length is non-linear, this parameter increasing more rapidly than V'_{max}FRC during the same interval[49] (Figure 4b.2). Airway resistance decreases rapidly during the first year in an essentially linear fashion (Figure 4b.3). The decreases in parenchymal elastance and damping (resistance) with length are not linear (Figure 4b.3) and neither is the increase in lung volume (Figure 4b.4). Thus complex relationships exist between the flow-resistive and elastic properties of the lungs and airways to produce the apparently linear increase in V'_{max}FRC reported during the first year of life.

Childhood and adolescence

Lung size increases with increasing height in children and adolescents (Figure 4b.5); lung volume is generally reported to increase as a power function with height, with an exponent between about 2.75 and 3.[52,53] The increase

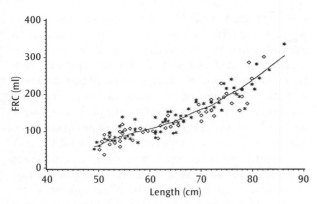

Figure 4b.4 *Functional residual capacity vs length for healthy infants from East Boston, reported by Hanrahan et al., (ref. 40). Data for both males (◇) and females (*) are shown.*

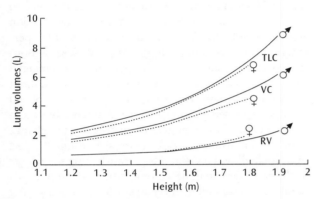

Figure 4b.5 *Changes in respiratory mechanics with age. Data adapted from Lanteri and Sly, (ref. 56).*

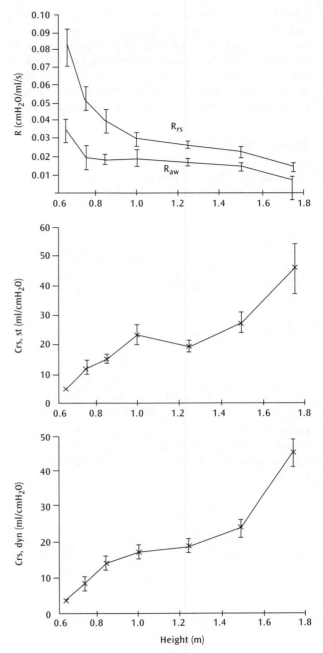

Figure 4b.6 *Plot of regression equations for the increase in lung volumes with height, reported by Hibbert et al., (ref. 53).*

in compliance with height has also been described by a power function, with exponents reported between 1.75 and 2.4.[54–56] The increase in compliance does not occur equally at all age ranges, the greatest increase occurs with increasing height in the youngest children[56] (Figure 4b.6). If the age range of the children studied is restricted to those under 2 years of age, the exponent of the power function increases to as high as 3.2.[57] The decrease in resistance, both of the airways and of the respiratory system, can also be described by a power function with increasing height, with exponents of −1.3 and −1.7, respectively[56] (Figure 4b.6).

Longitudinal estimates of lung growth demonstrate a high degree of 'tracking' within individuals, i.e. individuals tend to remain in their relative position within a population.[58–60] This means that those individuals who have low lung function at birth are likely to remain low, relative to their peers, and vice versa. Tracking remains high throughout adolescence, the period of most rapid growth.[59] When comparing growth in pulmonary function from one study to the next, one must realize that the

estimates of increase with height differ depending on whether the data have been collected longitudinally or cross-sectionally, with the estimated increase with height being greater from cross-sectional analyses.[61]

The symptoms and signs of asthma occur most commonly in the preschool and early school years. This timing has been attributed (partly) to an increase in the exposure to upper respiratory viruses due to increased social contact with other children. Symptoms typically become less severe and less frequent as children grow.

One explanation has been that children contract fewer viral infections as they become older. However, the rapid increase in lung size in children of this age group could also contribute to the decrease in wheezing. This is particularly prominent as children enter puberty, when lung growth is most rapid (Figure 4b.7). Changes in airway wall compliance may also contribute to the loss of symptoms.

Dysanaptic growth

Although the subject of some controversy, the lung parenchyma and airways are considered to grow at different

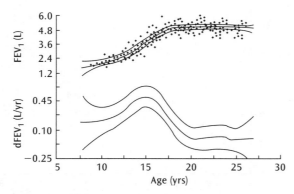

Figure 4b.7 *Changes in forced expiratory volume in one second (FEV₁) and in growth velocity with age for male subjects, reported by Sherrill* et al., Pediatr Pulmonol *1990;**8**:145–54.*

rates.[62] Hibbert *et al.*,[59] however, suggested that the rate of growth of different parts of the lung remain constant relative to one another, based on the demonstration of 'tracking' of measurements of forced expiratory flow, the good correlation of volume-corrected flow over time, and the consistency of the shape of forced expiratory flow–volume curves for an individual over time. Lanteri and Sly[56] concluded that the different rates of growth of airway resistance and compliance, measured at the same lung volume cross-sectionally in children between the ages of 3 weeks to 15 years, supported the concept of dysanaptic growth as the increase in compliance occurred at a greater rate than the decrease in resistance in this age range. A schematic representation of isotropic and dysanaptic growth is shown in Figure 4b.8.

The importance of dysanaptic growth is demonstrated by the differing patterns of wheezing illnesses seen at different ages. During the first year or two, viral LRI can cause widespread airway obstruction, hyperinflation and wheezing. In later childhood, the airway obstruction associated with viral LRI is usually less severe and hyperinflation is less common. Hogg and co-workers demonstrated that resistance of the central airways remained constant, when corrected for lung weight, throughout childhood.[63] However, the resistance of the peripheral airways (expressed the same way) fell dramatically around 5 years of age. They suggested this may be due to a change in the mechanism of increase in lung size around this age. In early childhood most of the increase in lung size occurs by the development of new alveoli, whereas later in childhood the predominant mechanism for increasing lung

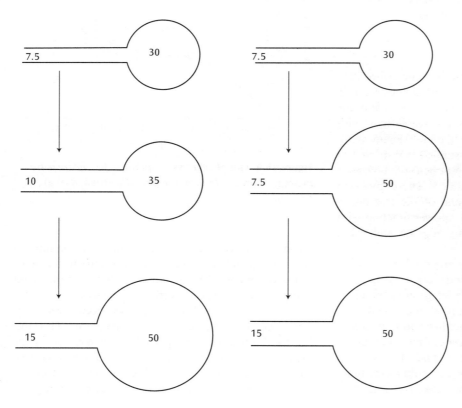

Figure 4b.8 *Schematic representation of isotropic and dysanaptic growth of airways and lung volumes. During isotropic growth, the airways and lung parenchyma grow in proportion with one another, such that at any given time the ratio of airway size to lung volume remains constant. By contrast, during dysanaptic growth the airways and lung parenchyma grow at different rates, and the relationship between airway size and lung volume may vary depending on when it is measured.*

size is an increase in the size of each alveolus. This could lead to an increased 'pull' on the small airways, via the mechanical interdependence of the airways and air spaces, resulting in an increase in small airway calibre. This suggestion would certainly fit with the clinical pattern of obstructive airway disease in children. If airways are relatively small for the air spaces they subtend, flow-limitation (Chapter 6b) is more likely to occur, particularly at times of increased ventilatory requirement, during forced expirations, or with acute lower respiratory infection, which results in mucosal oedema and further airway narrowing.

Gender differences in lung growth and development

Throughout childhood, male infants have a higher incidence of respiratory illnesses. In preterm boys, the incidence and severity of RDS and mortality due to respiratory complications are considerably higher than in girls.[64,65] There is some evidence in both humans and in experimental animals to suggest that *in utero* lung maturation is delayed in males compared with age matched females. Human amniotic fluid lecithin to sphingomyelin (L/S) ratio is higher in females than in males during the third trimester of pregnancy, the difference in degree of maturity being in the order of 1–2 weeks.[66,67] Similar developmental and functional differences have been reported in experimental animals.[68–70] Male sex hormones are thought to contribute, at least in part, to sex differences in fetal lung development.[71]

During infancy and childhood, boys are more likely than girls to develop wheeze[28] and asthma.[30,72,73] There is a widely held belief that boys are more susceptible to wheezing illnesses because they have smaller airways than their size-matched female counterparts, although this conjecture is based primarily on reports examining forced expiratory flows. Numerous studies measuring forced expiratory flow in infants[74,75] and in older children[76,77] have reported higher flows in girls than in size-matched boys, although in the majority of studies this is true only when flows are adjusted for lung volume. Both functional and anatomical studies have demonstrated that lung volume is smaller in girls than boys of the same length or height.[78,79] Interestingly, Taussig *et al.* found that $V'_{max}FRC$ derived from maximal expiratory flow–volume (MEFV) curves was higher in girls than boys, but when derived from partial expiratory flow–volume (PEFV) curves there was no difference, suggesting that girls, but not boys, are able to increase V'_{max} with deep inspiration.[80] In a later study, Landau *et al.* reported that boys had improved V'_{max} on partial flow–volume curves after atropine administration, suggesting that boys may have greater resting airway tone than girls.[81]

Forced expiratory flows, especially in the absence of expiratory flow-limitation, may not only reflect airway calibre, but other aspects of airway dynamics, as well as the elastic properties of the lungs. Therefore caution should be exercised when drawing inferences about airway size from forced expiratory flow measures, given the lack of confirmatory data from measurements more closely correlated with airway calibre, such as airway resistance. Most studies suggest that airway resistance is comparable in size-matched males and females during childhood[82–84] although there is some disagreement over this point. Hanrahan and co-workers reported that boys had higher respiratory resistances than girls at birth, but the rate of decline in resistance over the ensuing 18 months was more rapid in boys.[40] In contrast, Cuijpers *et al.* reported that below 140 cm, resistance was higher in girls than in boys, whereas above this height, the reverse was true.[85] There is no anatomical evidence to suggest that boys have smaller airways than girls. Hislop and Haworth examined airway size and structure in normal infants between 22 weeks gestation and 8 months postnatal age.[18] There were no gender differences in airway size, from main bronchus through to respiratory bronchioles. Tracheal volume and cross-sectional area also do not appear to differ between boys and girls.[86]

POSTNATAL INFLUENCES ON NORMAL GROWTH

The major adverse influences that have been reported on the growth and development of lung function in infants and children include active and passive smoking[87–89] (Chapter 7e) and family history of asthma.[44] Longitudinal studies, beginning in mid-childhood, have suggested that early childhood LRIs may alter growth potential.[58] However, prospective studies strongly suggest that low lung function precedes LRIs. Martinez *et al.* first documented this phenomenon, reporting that infants whose values for total respiratory conductance (inverse of resistance) were in the lowest third of the range for all infants had a 3.7-fold higher risk of having a wheezing illness.[90] Several investigators have also reported a link between the pattern of breathing (as a surrogate for airway mechanics) and subsequent wheeze.[45,91] More recently, Dezateux and colleagues demonstrated that specific airway conductance was significantly lower in infants who subsequently wheezed during the first year of life.[92] Of particular interest in this study, the authors found that the group of infants with low lung function were more likely to be born to mothers who smoked during pregnancy or to have a first degree relative with physician diagnosed asthma. The association between specific airway conductance and subsequent wheeze was greatly diminished after adjusting for these variables. Similar findings have been reported by Young *et al.*[93]

Asthma may be associated with a delay in the onset of puberty,[94–97] leading to apparent growth retardation

(Chapter 15). Most studies report catch-up growth, with children eventually reaching normal adult height.[95] Treatment with high doses of corticosteroids can lead to stunting, but treatment with moderate doses of inhaled steroids is unlikely to have any adverse effect on growth and is more likely to promote normal growth by controlling the underlying asthma. Longitudinal population studies have mainly shown that asthmatic children and adolescents exhibit growth of lung function parallel to but at a lower level than non-asthmatics.[98–100] Gold and colleagues studied the gender and race specific effects of asthma/wheeze on pulmonary function level and annual growth velocity in a cohort of 10 792 white and 944 black children aged 6–18 years.[100] In comparison with white boys who never reported wheeze, FEV_1 and FEF_{25-75} levels were 5.7% and 16.9% lower respectively for white boys with a diagnosis of asthma who had wheezed in the preceding 12 month period. Corresponding values for white girls were 3.4% and 13.6% lower. The prevalence of asthma was higher among blacks, but no race differences were found in the effect of asthma/wheeze on FEV_1 or FEF_{25-75}. In general, children with asthma did not have slower growth of lung function in *per cent* terms, but in *absolute* terms, growth of FEV_1 and FEF_{25-75} were slower for asthmatic boys with wheeze, and for girls with asthma and wheeze, growth of FEF_{25-75} was slower. The authors found no difference in associations between asthma/wheeze and growth deficits in the preadolescent and adolescent periods. It should be stressed that apparent growth of FEV_1 may differ from growth of lung volume (FVC) in asthmatic children, as demonstrated recently by Xuan *et al.*[77] Where FEV is not measured after administering a bronchodilator, as was the case in the study by Gold *et al.*,[73] it may reflect current reversible airflow obstruction.

The influence of treatment with corticosteroids on long-term outcome of asthma is difficult to assess, due to changes in treatment approaches over the years.[101–103] Agertoft and Pedersen[104] compared a group of children studied at 6-month intervals for 1–2 years without inhaled budesonide and then for 3–6 years on inhaled budesonide. A further group of children (controls) were treated with theophylline, β_2-agonists and sodium cromoglycate over the same period. Although both groups experienced a substantial improvement in the level of FEV_1, during the observation period, the improvement was greater in those children treated with budesonide. Furthermore, in those children not treated with budesonide, a small annual decrease in percentage predicted FEV_1 was seen. The authors also reported an inverse relationship between duration of asthma symptoms prior to budesonide treatment and the relative improvement in FEV. These findings suggest that earlier intervention with inhaled corticosteroids may prevent airway damage that could otherwise occur during the course of childhood asthma.[104–107] Studies in experimental animals clearly demonstrate that corticosteroid exposure during the early neonatal period can impair alveolar development.[108]

We do not yet know whether these observations might also apply to human infants.

CONCLUSIONS

Many factors can adversely affect lung function and respiratory health in childhood. Some can be modified, others cannot. Perinatal events and initiation of treatment early during the onset of asthma have the greatest potential to influence long-term lung health. Over the last decade we have become increasingly aware that the lung is especially vulnerable during perinatal development, therefore it is important, wherever possible, to minimize the risk of adverse influences during this critical time. Of no less importance, we have recently begun to appreciate the contribution of persistent airway inflammation to abnormal lung growth during childhood and adolescence, and to recognize that by reducing the degree of airway inflammation through early therapeutic intervention more favourable growth of lung function may be achievable.

Despite the considerable progress we have made in recent times, there remain many gaps in our knowledge of the normal pattern of the physiological development of the respiratory system. Perhaps the most glaring is our lack of understanding of the relative development of the different parts of the respiratory system and the effect this has on clinical disease. We know very little about the pattern of development of the mechanical properties of the chest wall and of the tissues of the pulmonary parenchyma. The influence of the pattern of development of the pulmonary and bronchial circulations on wheezing illnesses has been largely ignored. Better comprehension of these influences can only lead to a better understanding of the nature and mechanisms of wheezing illnesses and to more appropriate methods of treating them.

REFERENCES

1. Harding R, Hooper SB. Regulation of lung expansion and lung growth before and after birth. *J Appl Physiol* 1996;**81**:209–24.
2. Alcorn D, Adamson TM, Lambert TF, Maloney JE, Ritchie BC, Robinson PM. Morphological effects of chronic tracheal ligation and drainage in the foetal lamb lung. *J Anat* 1977;**123**:649–60.
3. Maloney JE, Adamson TM, Brodecky AV, Cranage S, Lambert TF, Ritchie BC. Diaphragmatic activity and lung liquid flow in the unanesthetized foetal sheep. *J Appl Physiol* 1975;**39**:423–8.
4. Clewlow F, Dawes GS, Johnston BM, Walker DW. Changes in breathing, electrocortical and muscle

activity in unanaesthetized foetal lambs with age. *J Physiol* 1983;**341**:463–76.

5. Harding R, Liggins GC. Changes in thoracic dimensions induced by breathing movements in foetal sheep. *Reprod Fert Devel* 1996;**8**:117–24.

6. Harding R, Sigger JN, Wickham PJD, Bocking AD. The regulation of flow of pulmonary fluid in foetal sheep. *Respir Physiol* 1984;**57**:47–59.

7. Miller AA, Hooper SB, Harding R. Role of foetal breathing movements in control of foetal lung distension. *J Appl Physiol* 1993;**75**:2711–17.

8. Sparrow MP, Weichselbaum M, McCray PB. Development of the innervation and airway smooth muscle in human foetal lung. *Am J Resp Cell Mol Biol* 1999;**20**:550–60.

9. McCray PB. Spontaneous contractility of human foetal airway smooth muscle. *Am J Respir Cell Mol Biol* 1993;**8**:573–80.

10. Sparrow MP, Warwick SP, Everett AW. Innervation and function of the distal airways in the developing bronchial tree of foetal pig lung. *Am J Resp Cell Mol Biol* 1995;**13**:518–25.

11. Gerhardt T, Bancalari E. Chestwall compliance in full-term and premature infants. *Acta Paediatr Scand* 1980;**69**:359–64.

12. Heldt GP. Development of stability of the respiratory system in preterm infants. *J Appl Physiol* 1988; **65**:441–4.

13. Deoras KS, Greenspan JS, Wolfson MR, Keklikian EN, Shaffer TH, Allen JL. Effects of inspiratory resistive loading on chest wall motion and ventilation: differences between preterm and full-term infants. *Pediatr Res* 1992;**32**:589–94.

14. Duara S, Silva Neto G, Claure N, Gerhardt T, Bancalari E. Effect of maturation on the extrathoracic airway stability of infants. *J Appl Physiol* 1992; **73**:2368–72.

15. Willet KE, Gurrin L, Burton P, *et al.* Differing patterns of mechanical response to direct foetal hormone treatment. *Respir Physiol* 1996;**103**:271–80.

16. Langston C, Kida K, Reed M, Thurlbeck WM. Human lung growth in late gestation and in the neonate. *Am Rev Respir Dis* 1984;**129**:607–13.

17. Hislop AA, Wigglesworth JS, Desai R. Alveolar development in the human foetus and infant. *Early Human Devel* 1986;**13**:1–11.

18. Hislop AA, Haworth SG. Airway size and structure in the normal foetal and infant lung and the effect of premature delivery and artificial ventilation. *Am Rev Respir Dis* 1989;**140**:1717–26.

19. Hislop AA, Wigglesworth JS, Desai R, Aber V. The effects of preterm delivery and mechanical ventilation on human lung growth. *Early Human Devel* 1987;**15**:147–64.

20. Jacob SV, Coates AL, Lands LC, *et al.* Long-term pulmonary sequelae of severe bronchopulmonary dysplasia. *J Pediatr* 1998;**133**:193–200.

21. Wjst M, Popescu M, Trepka MJ, Heinrich J, Wichmann HE. Pulmonary function in children with initial low birth weight. *Pediatr Allergy Immunol* 1998;**9**:80–90.

22. Parat S, Moriette G, Delaperche MF, Escourrou P, Denjean A, Gaultier C. Long-term pulmonary functional outcome of bronchopulmonary dysplasia and premature birth. *Pediatr Pulmonol* 1995;**20**:289–96.

23. Cano A, Payo F. Lung function and airway responsiveness in children and adolescents after hyaline membrane disease: a matched cohort study. *Eur Respir J* 1997;**10**:880–5.

24. Gross SJ, Iannuzzi DM, Kveselis DA, Anbar RD. Effect of preterm birth on pulmonary function at school age: a prospective controlled study. *J Pediatr* 1998; **133**:188–92.

25. Greenough A, Maconochie I, Yuksel B. Recurrent respiratory symptoms in the first year of life following preterm delivery. *J Perinat Med* 1990;**18**:489–94.

26. Kitchen WH, Olinsky A, Doyle LW, Ford GW, Murton LJ, Slonim L, Callanan C. Respiratory health and lung function in 8-year-old children of very low birth weight: a cohort study. *Pediatrics* 1992;**89**:1151–8.

27. Elder DE, Hagan R, Evans SF, Benninger HR, French NP. Recurrent wheezing in very preterm infants. *Arch Dis Child Fetal Neo Ed* 1996;**74**:F165–71.

28. Lewis S, Richards D, Bynner J, Butler N, Britton J. Prospective study of risk factors for early and persistent wheezing in childhood. *Eur Respir J* 1995;**8**:349–56.

29. Svanes C, Omenaas E, Heuch JM, Irgens LM, Gulsvik A. Birth characteristics and asthma symptoms in young adults: results from a population-based cohort study in Norway. *Eur Respir J* 1998;**12**:1366–70.

30. Schaubel D, Johansen H, Dutta M, Desmeules M, Becker A, Mao Y. Neonatal characteristics as risk factors for preschool asthma. *J Asthma* 1996;**33**:255–64.

31. Gregoire MC, Lefebvre F, Glorieux J. Health and developmental outcomes at 18 months in very preterm infants with bronchopulmonary dysplasia. *Pediatrics* 1998;**101**:856–60.

32. Newnham JP. Smoking in pregnancy. *Foetal Med Rev* 1991;**3**:115–32.

33. Manning F, Walker D, Feyerbend C. The effect of nicotine on foetal breathing movements in conscious pregnant ewes. *Obstetr Gynecol* 1978;**52**:563–8.

34. Gennser G, Marsal K, Brantmark B. Maternal smoking and foetal breathing movements. *Am J Obstet Gynecol* 1975;**123**:861–7.

35. Manning F, Pugh EW, Boddy K. Effect of cigarette smoking on foetal breathing movements in normal pregnancies. *BMJ* 1975;**1**:552–3.

36. Collins MH, Moessinger AC, Kleinerman J, Bassi J, Rosso P, Collins AM, James LS, Blanc WA. Foetal lung hypoplasia associated with maternal smoking: a morphometric analysis. *Pediatr Res* 1985;**19**:408–12.

37. Lieberman E, Torday J, Barbieri R, Cohen A, Van Vunakis H, Weiss ST. Association of intrauterine cigarette smoke exposure with indices of foetal lung maturation. *Obstet Gynecol* 1992;**79**:564–70.

38. Hanrahan JP, Tager IB, Segal MR, Tosteson TD, Castile RG, Van Vunakis H, Weiss ST, Speizer FE. The effect of maternal smoking during pregnancy on early infant lung function. *Am Rev Respir Dis* 1992;**145**:1129–35.

39. Brown RW, Hanrahan JP, Castile RG, Tager IB. Effect of maternal smoking during pregnancy on passive respiratory mechanics in early infancy. *Pediatr Pulmonol* 1995;**19**:23–8.

40. Hanrahan JP, Brown RW, Carey VJ, Castile RG, Speizer FE, Tager IB. Passive respiratory mechanics in healthy infants. Effects of growth, gender, and smoking. *Am J Respir Crit Care Med* 1996;**154**:670–80.

41. Milner AD, Marsh MJ, Ingram DM, Fox GF, Susiva C. Effects of smoking in pregnancy on neonatal lung function. *Arch Dis Child* 1999;**80**:F8–14.

42. Gilliland FD, Berhane K, McConnell R, Gauderman WJ, Vora H, Rappaport EB, Avol E, Peters JM. Maternal smoking during pregnancy, environmental tobacco smoke exposure and childhood lung function. *Thorax* 2000;**55**:271–6.

43. Ueda Y, Stick SM, Hall G, Sly PD. Control of breathing in infants born to smoking mothers. *J Pediatr* 1999; **135**:226–32.

44. Tager IB, Hanrahan JP, Tosteson TD, Castile RG, Brown RW, Weiss ST, Speizer FE. Lung function, pre- and post-natal smoke exposure, and wheezing in the first year of life. *Am Rev Respir Dis* 1993;**147**: 811–17.

45. Carlsen L, Carlsen KH, Nafstad P. Perinatal risk factors for recurrent wheeze in early life. *Pediatr Allergy Immunol* 1999;**10**:89–95.

46. Stein RT, Holberg CJ, Sherrill D, Wright AL, Morgan WJ, Taussig L, Martinez FD. Influence of parental smoking on respiratory symptoms during the first decade of life – The Tucson Children's Respiratory Study. *Am J Epidemiol* 1999;**149**:1030–7.

47. Adler SM, Wohl ME. Flow-volume relationship at low lung volumes in healthy term newborn infants. *Pediatrics* 1978;**61**:636–40.

48. Turner DJ, Stick SM, Lesouef KL, Sly PD, Lesouef PN. A new technique to generate and assess forced expiration from raised lung volume in infants. *Am J Respir Crit Care Med* 1995;**151**:1441–50.

49. Hall GL, Hantos Z, Petak F, Wildhaber JH, Tiller K, Burton PR, Sly PD. Airway and respiratory tissue mechanics in normal infants. *Am J Respir Crit Care Med* 2000;**162**:1397–402.

50. Taussig LM, Landau LI, Godfrey S, Arad I. Determinants of forced expiratory flows in newborn infants. *J Appl Physiol* 1982;**53**:1220–7.

51. Tepper RS, Reister T. Forced expiratory flows and lung volumes in normal infants. *Pediatr Pulmonol* 1993;**15**:57–61.

51a. Hoo AF, Dezateux C, Hanrahan JP, Cole TJ, Pepper RS, Stocks J. Sex-specific prediction equations for $V_{MAX}FRC$ in infancy. *Am J Resp Crit Care Med* 2002;**165**:1084–92.

52. Cook CD, Helliesen PJ, Agathon S. Relationship between mechanics of respiration, lung size, and body size from birth to young adulthood. *J Appl Physiol* 1958;**13**:349–52.

53. Hibbert ME, Lannigan A, Landau LI, Phelan PD. Lung function values from a longitudinal study of healthy children and adolescents. *Pediatr Pulmonol* 1989;**7**:101–9.

54. Nightingale DA, Richards CC. Volume-pressure relations of the respiratory system of curarized infants. *Anaesthesiol* 1965;**26**:710–14.

55. Sharp JT, Druz WS, Balagot RC, Badelin VR, Danon J. Total respiratory compliance in infants and children. *J Appl Physiol* 1970;**29**:775–9.

56. Lanteri CJ, Sly PD. Changes in respiratory mechanics with age. *J Appl Physiol* 1993;**74**:369–78.

57. Fletcher ME, Stack C, Ewart M, Davies CJ, Ridley S, Hatch DJ, Stocks J. Respiratory compliance during sedation, anesthesia, and paralysis in infants and young children. *J Appl Physiol* 1991;**70**:1977–82.

58. Lebowitz MD, Holberg CJ, Knudson RJ, Burrows B. Longitudinal study of pulmonary function development in childhood, adolescence, and early adulthood. Development of pulmonary function. *Am Rev Respir Dis* 1987;**136**:69–75.

59. Hibbert ME, Hudson IL, Lanigan A, Landau LI, Phelan PD. Tracking of lung function in healthy children and adolescents. *Pediatr Pulmonol* 1990;**8**:172–7.

60. Sherrill D, Holberg CJ, Lebowitz MD. Differential rates of lung growth as measured longitudinally by pulmonary function in children and adolescents. *Pediatr Pulmonol* 1990;**8**:145–54.

61. Pattishall EN, Helms RW, Strope GL. Noncomparability of cross-sectional and longitudinal estimates of lung growth in children. *Pediatr Pulmonol* 1989;**7**:22–8.

62. Mead J. Dysanapsis in normal lungs assessed by the relationship between maximal flow, static recoil, and vital capacity. *Am Rev Respir Dis* 1980;**121**:339–42.

63. Hogg JC, Williams J, Richardson JB, Macklem PT, Thurlbeck WM. Age as a factor in the distribution of lower-airway conductance and in the pathologic anatomy of obstructive lung disease. *N Engl J Med* 1970;**282**:1283–7.

64. Perelman RH, Palta M, Kirby R, Farrell PM. Discordance between male and female deaths due to the respiratory distress syndrome. *Am J Obstet Gynecol* 1986;**78**:238–44.

65. Luerti M, Parazzini F, Agarossi A, Bianchi C, Rocchetti M, Bevilacqua G. Risk factors for respiratory distress syndrome in the newborn. A multicenter Italian survey. *Acta Obstet Gynecol Scand* 1993;**72**: 359–64.

66. Torday JS, Nielsen HC, Fencl MdM, Avery ME. Sex differences in foetal lung maturation. *Am Rev Respir Dis* 1981;**123**:205–8.

67. Fleisher B, Kulovich MV, Hallman M, Gluck L. Lung profile: sex differences in normal pregnancy. *Obstet Gynecol* 1985;**66**:327–30.

68. Kotas RV, Avery ME. The influence of sex on foetal rabbit lung maturation and on the response to glucocorticoid. *Am Rev Respir Dis* 1980;**121**:377–80.

69. Adamson IY, King GM. Sex-related differences in cellular composition and surfactant synthesis of developing foetal rat lungs. *Am Rev Respir Dis* 1984;**129**:130–4.

70. Willet KE, Jobe AH, Ikegami M, Polk D, Newnham J, Kohan R, Gurrin L, Sly PD. Postnatal lung function after prenatal steroid treatment in sheep: effect of gender. *Pediatr Res* 1997;**42**:885–92.

71. Nielsen HC. Androgen receptors influence the production of pulmonary surfactant in the testicular feminization mouse foetus. *J Clin Invest* 1985;**76**:177–81.

72. Remes ST, Korppi M, Remes K, Pekkanen J. Prevalence of asthma at school age: a clinical population-based study in eastern Finland. *Acta Paediatr* 1996;**85**:59–63.

73. Gissler M, Jarvelin MR, Louhiala P, Hemminki E. Boys have more health problems in childhood than girls: follow-up of the 1987 Finnish birth cohort. *Acta Paediatr* 1999;**88**:310–14.

74. Taussig LM. Maximal expiratory flows at functional residual capacity: a test of lung function for young children. *Am Rev Respir Dis* 1977;**116**:1031–8.

75. Tepper RS, Morgan WJ, Cota K, Wright A, Taussig LM. Physiologic growth and development of the lung during the first year of life [published erratum appears in *Am Rev Respir Dis* 1987;**136**(3):800]. *Am Rev Respir Dis* 1986;**134**:513–19.

76. Hibbert ME, Couriel JM, Landau LI. Changes in lung, airway, and chest wall function in boys and girls between 8 and 12 years. *J Appl Physiol* 1984;**57**:304–8.

77. Schwartz J, Katz SA, Fegley RW, Tockman MS. Sex and race differences in the development of lung function. *Am Rev Respir Dis* 1988;**138**:1415–21.

78. Thurlbeck WM. Postnatal human lung growth. *Thorax* 1982;**37**:564–71.

79. Hibbert M, Lannigan A, Raven J, Landau L, Phelan P. Gender differences in lung growth. *Pediatr Pulmonol* 1995;**19**:129–34.

80. Taussig LM, Cota K, Kaltenborn W. Different mechanical properties of the lung in boys and girls. *Am Rev Respir Dis* 1981;**123**:640–3.

81. Landau LI, Morgan W, McCoy KS, Taussig LM. Gender related differences in airway tone in children. *Pediatr Pulmonol* 1993;**16**:31–5.

82. Stanescu D, Moavero NE, Veriter C, Brasseur L. Frequency dependence of respiratory resistance in healthy children. *J Appl Physiol* 1979;**47**:268–72.

83. Lodrup Carlsen KC, Magnus P, Carlsen KH. Lung function by tidal breathing in awake healthy newborn infants. *Eur Respir J* 1994;**7**:1660–8.

84. Klug B, Bisgaard H. Specific airway resistance, interrupter resistance, and respiratory impedance in healthy children aged 2–7 years. *Pediatr Pulmonol* 1998;**25**:322–31.

85. Cuijpers CE, Wesseling G, Swaen GM, Wouters EF. Frequency dependence of oscillatory resistance in healthy primary school children. *Respiration* 1993;**60**:149–54.

86. Griscom NT, Wohl ME, Fenton T. Dimensions of the trachea to age 6 years related to height. *Pediatr Pulmonol* 1989;**6**:186–90.

87. Sherrill DL, Martinez FD, Lebowitz MD, Holdaway MD, Flannery EM, Herbison GP, Stanton WR, Silva PA, Sears MR. Longitudinal effects of passive smoking on pulmonary function in New Zealand children. *Am Rev Respir Dis* 1992;**145**:1136–41.

88. Cook DG, Whincup PH, Papacosta O, Strachan DP, Jarvis MJ, Bryant A. Relation of passive smoking as assessed by salivary cotinine concentration and questionnaire to spirometric indices in children. *Thorax* 1993;**48**:14–20.

89. Rona RJ, Chinn S. Lung function, respiratory illness, and passive smoking in British primary school children. *Thorax* 1993;**48**:21–5.

90. Martinez FD, Morgan WJ, Wright AL, Holberg CJ, Taussig LM. Diminished lung function as a predisposing factor for wheezing respiratory illness in infants. *N Engl J Med* 1988;**319**:1112–17.

91. Yuksel B, Greenough A, Giffin F, Nicolaides KH. Tidal breathing parameters in the first week of life and subsequent cough and wheeze. *Thorax* 1996;**51**:815–18.

92. Dezateux C, Stocks J, Dundas I, Fletcher ME. Impaired airway function and wheezing in infancy: the influence of maternal smoking and a genetic predisposition to asthma. *Am J Resp Crit Care Med* 1999;**159**:403–10.

93. Young S, Arnott J, O'Keeffe PT, Le Souef PN, Landau LI. The association between early life lung function and wheezing during the first 2 years of life. *Eur Respir J* 2000;**15**:151–7.

94. Hauspie R, Susanne C, Alexander F. Maturational delay and temporal growth retardation in asthmatic boys. *J Allergy Clin Immunol* 1977;**59**:200–6.

95. Martin AJ, McLennan LA, Landau LI, Phelan PD. The natural history of childhood asthma to adult life. *BMJ* 1980;**280**:397–400.

96. Balfour-Lynn L. Growth and childhood asthma. *Arch Dis Child* 1986;**61**:1049–55.

97. Merkus PJ, van Essen-Zandvliet EE, Duiverman EJ, van Houwelingen HC, Kerrebijn KF, Quanjer PH. Long-term effect of inhaled corticosteroids on growth rate in adolescents with asthma. *Pediatrics* 1993;**91**:1121–6.

98. Kelly WJ, Hudson I, Raven J, Phelan PD, Pain MC, Olinsky A. Childhood asthma and adult lung function. *Am Rev Respir Dis* 1988;**138**:26–30.

99. Roorda RJ, Gerritsen J, van Aalderen WM, Schouten JP, Veltman JC, Weiss ST, Knol K. Follow-up of asthma from childhood to adulthood: influence of potential childhood risk factors on the outcome of pulmonary function and bronchial responsiveness in adulthood. *J Allergy Clin Immunol* 1994;**93**: 575–84.

100. Gold DR, Wypij D, Wang X, Speizer FE, Pugh M, Ware JH, Ferris BG Jr, Dockery DW. Gender- and race-specific effects of asthma and wheeze on level and growth of lung function in children in six US cities. *Am J Respir Crit Care Med* 1994;**149**: 1198–208.

101. Nakadate T, Kagawa J. Pulmonary function development in children with past history of asthma. *J Epidemiol Comm Health* 1992;**46**:437–42.

102. Borsboom GJ, Van Pelt W, Quanjer PH. Pubertal growth curves of ventilatory function: relationship with childhood respiratory symptoms. *Am Rev Respir Dis* 1993;**147**:372–8.

103. Mosfeldt Laursen EKKH, Backer V, Bach-Mortenson N, Prahl P, Koch C. Pulmonary function in adolescents with childhood asthma. *Allergy* 1993;**48**:267–72.

104. Agertoft L, Pedersen S. Effects of long-term treatment with an inhaled corticosteroid on growth and pulmonary function in asthmatic children. *Respir Med* 1994;**88**:373–81.

105. Haahtela T, Jarvinen M, Kava T, *et al.* Comparison of a beta 2-agonist, terbutaline, with an inhaled corticosteroid, budesonide, in newly detected asthma. *N Engl J Med* 1991;**325**:388–92.

106. Haahtela T, Jarvinen M, Kava T, *et al.* Effects of reducing or discontinuing inhaled budesonide in patients with mild asthma. *N Engl J Med* 1994;**331**:700–5.

107. Selroos O, Pietinalho A, Lofroos A, Riska H. Effect of early vs late intervention with inhaled corticosteroids in asthma. *Chest* 1995;**108**: 1228–34.

108. Massaro D, Teich N, Maxwell S, Massaro GD, Whitney P. Postnatal development of alveoli. Regulation and evidence for a critical period in rats. *J Clin Invest* 1985;**76**:1297–305.

Postnatal maturation of immune and inflammatory functions

PATRICK G HOLT

INTRODUCTION

Immuno-inflammatory mechanisms are acknowledged as major aetiological factors in wheezing disease. The clearest example is atopic asthma, a process which is driven by CD4$^+$ T helper 2 (Th2) cells responding to inhaled antigens from a variety of non-microbial sources. The cytokines secreted by CD4$^+$ T-cells recruit a variety of other cell populations, either directly through cytokine receptors on the secondary effector cells or indirectly via IgE antibody. This increasingly wide cascade of cells initially includes B-cells, neutrophils, mast cells, macrophages and also platelets and eventually eosinophils and the secreted products of these cells produce the airway tissue pathology characteristic of chronic asthma. However, it is clear that wheeze can also be produced by acute and chronic respiratory infection and in this situation the inflammation underlying the symptomology does not involve IgE and therefore must result from Th2-independent adaptive immunity and/or innate immuno-inflammatory mechanisms involving cells such as granulocytes, macrophages, etc. A wide range of cell-mediated inflammatory reactions represent potential avenues for airway tissue damage (Table 4c.1). A clear understanding of the functional capacity of these different classes of defence mechanisms in early postnatal life is accordingly a prerequisite to elucidation of the aetiology of wheezing disorders in infancy and early childhood. The review below focuses on aspects of innate and adaptive immune function in early life, in particular those mechanisms which are believed to be of direct relevance to the aetiology and pathogenesis of asthma.

Immune function in the fetal compartment: incompetence or tight regulation?

The transition from the protected intrauterine environment to the hostile outside world presents a major challenge to the developing immune system, and there is increasing evidence that the adaptation process set in motion in the newborn by early contact with antigenic stimuli can have far reaching consequences in relation to susceptibility to inflammatory diseases in later life.

It also appears possible that initial contacts between the developing immune system and antigens from the outside environment may occur *in utero,* and the general concept that responsiveness to exogenous antigens does not develop until after birth is now being challenged by an increasingly wide body of information. In particular, a variety of studies on cord blood have demonstrated the presence of putative memory T-cells which proliferate in response to dietary and inhalant allergens (see below), autoantigens,[1] bacterial and viral antigens,[2,3] and parasite antigens.[4,5] Moreover, the offspring of mothers infected by parasites express parasite-specific immunity at birth, evidenced by the presence of IgM antibodies in serum,[6] and tetanus-specific IgM also appears in the serum of newborns of vaccinated mothers.[7]

Table 4c.1 *Cell populations which potentially mediate direct tissue damage in the respiratory tract*

Cell population	Major receptors for 'triggering'	Effector mechanisms	Potential result(s) of local triggering in the respiratory tract
CD4$^+$ T-cells	Protein antigens	Cytokine secretion	Help for antibody synthesis (incl. IgE*); recruitment/activation of macrophages, PMN, eosinophils; direct triggering of mast cells (via cytokines); direct tissue damage (e.g. via TNF)
CD8$^+$ T-cells	Viral antigen	Lysis of infected cells; cytokines	Direct tissue damage
Gamma-delta T-cells	Heat shock (stress) proteins	Cytokines	Direct tissue damage; modulation of CD4/CD8 T-cell functions
Macrophages	FcR (IgG and IgE*) bacterial lipolysaccharide fungal ß-glucan viruses complement components cytokines; microbial DNA	Cytokines; chemotactic factors; leukotrienes; prostaglandins; PAF; cytotoxic enzymes; respiratory burst	Direct tissue damage; recruitment of granulocytic and mononuclear cells; platelet activation (via PAF); modulation of local T-cell activation
Polymorphonuclear leukocytes	FcR (IgG) cytokines (esp IL8)	Major basic protein; cytokines; respiratory burst	Direct tissue damage
Mast cells	High affinity IgE* receptor C5a; cytokines	Vasoactive amines; cytokines; leukotrienes; chemotactic factors; PAF; prostaglandins	Direct tissue damage
Eosinophils	IgG FcR; low affinity IgE* receptor; cytokines (esp. IL5*); PAF	Eosinophil cationic protein; major basic protein; respiratory burst	Direct tissue damage
Natural Killer Cells	Altered surface antigens on virus infected cells	Lysis of infected cells; cytokines	Direct tissue damage; modulation of T-cell activation

*Th-2-dependent allergy.

Given that IgM cannot cross the placenta, these latter findings imply that antigens experienced by the pregnant mother can cross the placenta and trigger primary immune responses in the fetus. However, it is also clear that there are significant limitations on the degree to which such fetal responses can mature e.g. there is no evidence of class switching in the tetanus-specific responses in the offspring of vaccinated mothers until the infants are themselves vaccinated.[7]

Accepting that the fetal immune system indeed develops at least partial competence before birth, the question arises as to how immune responses resulting from interactions between fetal and maternal bone marrow derived cells at the fetomaternal interface are regulated, particularly given that trafficking of fetal cells into the mother (which can potentially sensitize the maternal immune system against paternal HLA antigens expressed on fetal cells) is readily demonstrable.[8–12] This 'tolerance' process has intrigued experimental immunologists since Medwar's prediction 50 years ago that on the basis of the self–non-self model of the immune system, mothers should reject their fetuses.[13] However, recent studies[14] indicate that the maternal immune system maintains the capacity to eliminate fetal cells penetrating into the maternal circulation, while remaining 'tolerant' to the fetus. This suggests that tolerance in this context is a regionally controlled process, localized at the fetomaternal interface itself.

The mechanism(s) which maintain immunological homeostasis within this milieu are beginning to be understood. At one level, it is clear that generalized 'immunosuppression' is maintained firstly via constitutive production of high levels of IL-10 by placental trophoblasts[15] and by local production by both trophoblasts and macrophages of tryptophan metabolites generated via indoleamine 2,3-dioxygenase, which is highly suppressive to T-cell activation and proliferation.[16] A further level of suppression is provided via expression of FasL on fetal cells within the placenta as a means of elimination of activated T-cells which escape IL-10/tryptophan suppression.[17,18]

However, it is inevitable that occasional T-cell activation events will escape attrition via these pathways. Studies in the mouse model indicates that if such responses generate significant amounts of toxic Th1 cytokines locally, such as IFNγ, the likely result is placental detachment and/or fetal resorption.[19,20] To protect against this possibility, a further level of control operates at the fetomaternal interface, in the form of local production at high level within the placenta of a range of molecules which selectively antagonize Th1 responses or which are trophic for Th1-antagonistic Th2 responses. As well as IL-10 which essentially programs antigen presenting cells (APC) for selective Th2 priming,[21] these include IL-4[15] which is the specific growth factor for Th2 cells, prostaglandin E2 which selectively stimulates Th2 immunity via effects on APC,[21] and progesterone[22–24] which inhibits IFNγ gene expression. The constitutive production of this cocktail of mediators during fetal life effectively skews immune function towards the Th2 cytokine phenotype;[25] while this plays an important protective role in damping potentially toxic Th1 immunity in this microenvironment, it has certain downstream consequences in relation to postnatal development of immune competence, which may be significant in later disease expression (see discussion below).

GENERAL IMMUNE COMPETENCE DURING INFANCY

Resistance to bacterial and fungal infections[26] and in particular viral infections[27,28] is diminished relative to adults during infancy, suggesting deficiencies in both innate and adaptive immune mechanisms in early life. The capacity to generate virus-specific immunological memory following infection in infants is diminished[29] as is the expression of cellular immunity during the course of the infection.[30–32]

The cellular and molecular mechanism(s) underlying this apparent maturational deficiency in immune function are the subject of increasingly intensive research, driven by the expanding immunological literature indicating that in many countries the prevalence and severity of a range of immuno-inflammatory diseases is increasing, concomitant with progressively decreasing age of onset. Salient findings relating to the functional capacity of the principal immune effector cell populations during the perinatal period are summarized below.

Surface phenotype of lymphocyte populations in peripheral blood

Leukocyte populations (in particular lymphocytes) express a wide range of function-associated molecules which have been identified via generation of appropriate monoclonal antibodies. Flow cytometric analyses of the expression of these 'surface markers' on cord blood cells reveals the presence of a substantial proportion of lymphocytes in the neonate exhibiting phenotypic characteristics of fetal/immature cells. Within the T-cell compartment, the most noteworthy characteristics are frequent expression of CD1,[33] PNA antigen[34] and CD.[35,38] The latter, designated 'common thymocyte' antigen, is expressed on up to 95% of cord blood CD4[+] T-cells and is tenfold less frequent on CD4[+] T-cells in adults.[35] The presence of this surface antigen generally designates mature

thymocytes as opposed to adult naive peripheral T-cells,[33,34] and this suggestion is consistent with the finding that in vitro exposure to thymic hormones upregulates surface expression of CD38 on cord blood T-cells whereas adult T-cells are unresponsive.[36]

The rate at which these surface expression patterns change postnatally has not been investigated in detail for the full range of markers, however some have attracted particular interest. Of particular significance is the presence in neonates of a high proportion of T-cells which co-express both CD4 and CD8, which is characteristic of immature cells.[37,38] The proportion of circulatory T-cells which express IL-2R and HLA-DR, both indicative of previous activation, are low during infancy and do not move into the adult range until the early school years;[37] CD57 expression on T-cells, which marks non-MHC-restricted cytotoxic lymphocytes, is also low during infancy.[37]

T-cells emigrating from the thymus express the CD45RA isoform of the leukocyte common antigen CD45, and after antigen stimulation switch to expression of CD45RO. The majority of these activated CD45RA[−]RO[+] T-cells die within a few days, but a subset enters the long-lived recirculating T-cell compartment as 'memory' cells committed to recall responsiveness to their respective antigens.[39] CD45RA is expressed on approximately 90% of CD4[+] T-cells in cord blood, and these are progressively replaced with age by CD45RO[+] cells with accumulating antigen exposure.[39–44] The proportion of CD45RO[+] cells enters the adult range in the teen years[37,44] and the rates of increase are equivalent for TcR1 and TcR2 populations and are slightly higher for CD4[+] cells than CD8[+] cells.[44]

L-selectin is expressed on both T and B-cells and is a marker of naive cells. The percentage of CD4[+] L-selectin[+] T-cells is similar to that of CD4[+] CD45RA[+] cells.[35] CD19 and CD20 mark B-cells, and the percentage and absolute number of these in peripheral blood decline during infancy.[37] CD5 is expressed on the majority of B-cells during infancy while a lesser proportion express L-selectin and CD23; expression of the latter two markers increase in frequency with age whereas CD5 declines with maturation.[37]

NK cells are most frequent in the circulation when they comprise around 20% of circulating lymphocytes,[37] and the majority express the immature HNK[+]T3-M1-surface phenotype.[45] After an initial decline during early infancy the percentage of NK cells rapidly climbs to adult levels.[37]

T-LYMPHOCYTE FUNCTIONS DURING INFANCY AND EARLY CHILDHOOD

T-cell activation

Polyclonally induced T-cell proliferative responses in short term cultures are high at birth and decline to adult levels during later during infancy.[46,47] However, activation induced via TcR stimulation[48] or via stimulation through CD2,[49,50] is diminished. Studies from our laboratory suggest that this deficiency in CD2 signalling is secondary to a maturational defect in CD3 function,[51] and we have further established that while initial activation may proceed rapidly in T-cells from infants, proliferation is not sustained and their capacity to expand to generate stable clones is diminished relative to adults.[52] These deficiencies may be due in part to decreased capacity for IL-2 production following stimulation.[50,53]

It has also been observed that cord blood T-cells are more susceptible to tolerance/anergy induction in response to bacterial superantigen, employing stimulation protocols which do not tolerize adult-cells.[54]

These differences have also been linked to variations in IL-2 production,[54] but may also reflect defective activation of the Ras signalling pathway, which has been suggested to underlie the development of secondary unresponsiveness to alloantigen stimulation by neonatal T-cells.[55] Developmental aberrations in a range of signalling systems have been reported in neonatal T-cells including protein kinase C,[56] phospholipase C and associated Lck expression,[57] and CD28, the latter being associated with dysfunction in FasL-mediated cytotoxicity[58] and reduced production of NFκB.[59]

T-cell effector functions

Evidence from a variety of studies indicates that both cytotoxic effector[60,61] and B-cell helper functions[60–62] are deficient in infancy. These developmental deficiencies may be due to a combination of factors including reduced expression of cytokine receptors,[63,64] decreased production of a wide range of cytokines,[53,65–71] and decreased expression of costimulator molecules such as CD40L.[72,73]

Of particular relevance to discussions below is the finding that cord blood but not adult T-cells respond polyclonally to IL-4,[74] and their capacity to produce IFNγ appears to be reduced to a greater degree than capacity to secrete T-helper 2 (Th2) cytokines such as IL-4[52] i.e. their responses are 'skewed' to favour Th2 cytokine production.

It is also pertinent to note that development of Th-cell (in particular Th1) immunity to both vaccines[75] and natural viral infections such as measles[76] is diminished and/or Th2 skewed during infancy. Nevertheless, highly potent stimuli given during infancy[77] or even in utero[78] are capable of eliciting vigorous Th1 responses, indicating that the deficiency in Th1 function in neonates is not absolute. These findings are consistent with other observations which suggest that one of the principal differences between neonatal and adult naive T-cells may be a requirement for more powerful costimulator signals for effective activation in neonates.[71]

It has also been suggested that the disparity in T-cell function between adults and neonates may simply be a reflection of the differing proportion of CD45RA⁻ naive

Th⁻ cells in the two age groups, and that these differences disappear rapidly after activation and conversion to the CD45RO⁺ 'memory' phenotype. However, direct comparisons between purified CD45RA⁻ Th-cells from adults and cord blood indicate that following activation under identical conditions, the neonatal cells fail to achieve the same level of activation as the adult T-cells.[50] Moreover, even after expansion and cloning, a high proportion of Th-cells from infants still express the low cytokine-producing phenotype characteristic of the neonatal period.[52]

B-cell functions

Production of antibodies in neonates following vaccination or infection is reduced relative to adults,[29] and in vitro studies suggest that this is associated with reduced capacity for isotype switching from IgM to other immunoglobulin classes.[79] It has been widely debated as to the relative importance of deficiencies in the T-cell vs B-cell compartment in this context,[60,80–82] and recent studies suggest contributions from both cell types. In particular, it is evidence that while polyclonally induced Ig production by neonatal B-cells is low in the presence of neonatal T-helper cells, if mature T-cell help or soluble signals from them is provided, production levels markedly improve.[62,83,84] However, overall production remains below adult levels.[83,84]

One of the most critical signals in the induction of class switching involves the interaction between B-cell CD40 and its ligand expressed on activated T-cells.[85,86] As noted above, CD40L expression has generally been reported as low on neonatal T-cells,[72,73] and this may be a major factor in the reduced capacity for Ig production in this age group. However, in vitro hyperstimulation with anti-CD3 in the presence of IL-2 and IL-4 can induce sufficient CD40L expression on neonatal T-cells to promote isotype switching in neonatal B-cells,[87] but it is not clear how these findings relate to the in vivo situation.

In addition to their primary role in Ig production, B-cells are now recognized as important APC, particularly in secondary immune responses.[88,89] The APC functions of B-cells has not been studied in human neonates, but are reportedly deficient in infant mice and do not develop full competence until after weaning.[90]

Mononuclear phagocytic cells (MPC) and dendritic cells (DC)

It is evident from recent studies that MPC and DC represent two sides of the same cellular coin, and in some cases are virtually interchangeable, depending upon the balance of molecular differential signals present within the local tissue microenvironment. However the mature stage of these cell types are phenotypically and functionally distinct, the major role of MPC being the clearance of the bulk of incoming foreign antigens from challenge sites and the provision of antigen-specific activation signals to pre-primed 'memory T-cells', whereas the DC appear involved principally in the initial 'sensitization' of naive T-cells to individual antigens.

In relation to ontogenic studies in humans, the *MPC population* most studied are blood monocytes. They appear similar to their adult counterparts in the steady state with respect to numbers in blood and overall phagocytic capacity,[91,92] and also with respect to random migration characteristics, enzymatic profiles and bactericidal activity.[93] However, subtle differences in expression of function associated surface markers have been noted between adult and neonatal blood MPC, including decreased expression of CD16 (FcgR111) and CD62L on neonatal cells with a concomitant elevation in expression of CD36.[94]

It has also been noted, however, that neonates are susceptible to rapid depletion of mature phagocytes under conditions of stress such as overwhelming bacterial sepsis; this indicates developmentally immature myelopoiesis, and is associated with instability of mRNA specific for the key regulatory cytokines M-CSF and GM-CSF.[95]

Additionally, neonatal MPC express lower levels of HLA-DR than their adult counterparts,[96] and this is associated with diminished capacity to present viral and alloantigen[97] and to support polyclonal activation of T-cells leading to IFNγ production.[98,99] This deficiency in APC functions can be redressed to a degree by pretreatment of the neonatal MPC with IFNγ to upregulate HLA-DR,[96] however murine data suggests that this regulatory mechanism may be attenuated in neonates due to high level production by neonatal monocytes of IFNβ which inhibits the effects of IFNγ.[100]

MPC migration into inflammatory foci in peripheral tissues is delayed and attenuated,[101,102] due in part to reduced capacity for chemokine-induced expression of integrins (in particular Mac-1) required for adhesion to endothelium.[103] Neonatal MPC are also reportedly deficient in capacity to produce a range of cytokines including IL-10,[67,70] IL-6,[104] TNF,[105,106] and IL-12,[65] the latter being associated with a similar instability of mRNA as reported above for GM-CSF.

The decreased capacity of MPC in newborns to produce the acute phase cytokines TNF and IL-6 may underlie their diminished febrile responses to infection.[107] TNF secretion by neonatal MPC is also less susceptible to IFNγ-mediated stimulation,[105] and this may act in tandem with their decreased overall capacity for IFNγ production to limit the intensity and duration of acute inflammatory responses during infancy.

The function of specific MPC populations at peripheral tissue sites has been less intensely studied, with the exception of the pulmonary alveolar macrophage (AM) population. In experimental animals, these appear functionally deficient relative to adults by a variety of criteria, including chemotactic, phagocytic and bacteriostatic/fungistatic activities.[108–111] Studies in sheep

and in non-human primates suggest that functional maturation of this MPC population is relatively slow postnatally and takes at least 6 months for completion.[109,111] Studies in human neonates are very limited, but the available evidence does suggest a similar maturational deficiency in microbicidal activity during early infancy.[112]

Studies on the ontogeny of *DC populations* are even more limited, and restricted almost entirely to experimental animals. However, the tissue distribution and phenotypic properties of these important cells appear very similar between mammalian species, which may be expected in the light of recent information indicating the central role of these cells in host defence, as the essential link between the innate and adaptive arms of the immune response.[113–115] Additionally, comparative functional studies on mucosal tissue-derived DC populations from experimental animals and humans indicate very similar functions,[116] and hence cautious extrapolation from the animals studies appears justified.

On this basis, it appears that bone marrow derived DC precursors start to seed into peripheral tissues in late fetal life, and at birth the numbers of DC[117–120] and their expression of MHC II[120–122] are low relative to adults. This is particularly the case with respect to the airway mucosa.[120] Airway DC from infant rats express poor APC activity *in vitro*, and also exhibit markedly reduced capacity to upregulate this function in response to cytokine signals such as GM-CSF.[123] An important function of the airway mucosal DC population in adults is to respond rapidly to inhalation of inflammatory stimuli including soluble recall antigens, and the nature of the response involves rapid recruitment of fresh DC precursors to the challenge site (presumably to sample the incoming antigens) and their subsequent trafficking to draining lymph nodes.[114,124] This response is also markedly reduced in infant animals, and does not attain adult equivalent levels of activity until after weaning.[123]

We have recently demonstrated that in resting airways tissues, the resident DC selectively stimulate low level Th2 responses which is associated with production of IL-10 by the DC.[125] However, after receipt of GM-CSF maturation signals they switch functional phenotype (via up-regulation of production of Th1-trophic IL-12) and now prime for more Th1-skewed immunity[125] (Figure 4c.1). The finding that infant airway DC are relatively refractory to GM-CSF signals[123] implies that the capacity for these important APC to divert Th-cell responses to inhalant allergens away from the potentially pathogenic Th2 cytokine phenotype is relatively low, and this finding has implications in the aetiology of atopic asthma, as discussed below.

Polymorphonuclear leukocytes (PMN)

PMN represent the first line of cellular defence against incoming pathogens, in particular bacteria, and are

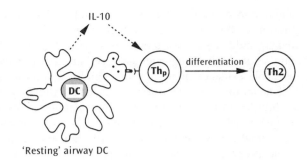

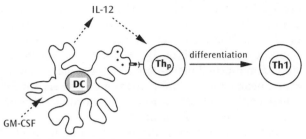

Figure 4c.1 *Antigen presentation by airway dendritic cells (DC) in regulation of Th1/Th2 responses. Antigen-bearing airway DC migrate to draining lymph nodes and present antigen (•) to precursor T-cells (Th$_p$) together with IL-10, inducing differentiation of primed T-cells down the Th2 pathway. If the DC receive a GM-CSF signal they switch to IL-12 production and instead stimulate Th1 differentiation.*

usually the first bone marrow derived cells to arrive at a challenge site. The impaired production and delivery of PMN to sites of infection[126] appears to be an important factor underlying the increased susceptibility of neonates to infection. This is partly due to a reduced PMN storage pool and a relative failure to increase the stem cell proliferative rate during sepsis.[127,128]

A recent report suggests that reduced production of GM-CSF (the principal cytokine stimulus for PMN production) by neonatal monocytes and T-cells in response to infectious challenge may contribute to this deficiency.[129] However, a much wider literature (reviewed in detail in ref. 130) indicates that functional deficiencies intrinsic to the PMN themselves are likely to play a much more important role. It is clear from work in many independent laboratories that neonatal PMN exhibit a variety of functional defects in adherence, aggregation, movement, phagocytosis, and intracellular killing, which are reflected in deficiencies in signal transduction, cell surface receptor up-regulation and mobility, cytoskeletal rigidity, microfilament contraction, oxygen metabolism, and antioxidant mechanisms.[130]

More recent reports also implicate deficiencies in regulation of expression of L-selectin and Mac-1 in the failure of neonatal PMN to efficiently 'home' to inflammatory foci,[103] and defective diapedesis associated with excessive plasma membrane fluidity[131] is also likely to play a

significant role in limiting the effective migration of these cells into tissues. PMN are now recognized to secrete the full gamut of cytokines previously thought to be restricted to mononuclear cells.[132,133] The reduced contribution of this potentially important source of cytokines at inflammatory sites in the neonate is likely to have significant, but as yet unknown, effects on local immunological homeostasis.

Mucosal lymphocyte populations in neonates

The mucosal tissues most studied in the neonate are those associated with the gastrointestinal tract. T-cells infiltrate human fetal small intestine from 14 weeks' gestation,[134,135] and by 19 weeks there are well defined Peyer's patches with primary B-cell follicles and T-dependent zones present.[135] There are also numerous T-cells in the epithelium and the underlying lamina propria.[135,136] The intraepithelial (IEL) T-cell population in the fetus ranges between 3–5 per 100 epithelial cells, compared with 6–27 per 100 in postnatal and adult tissue;[137] no data are available on the kinetics of the postnatal expansion of this population. Tgd cells comprise a significantly greater proportion of fetal IELs, being up to 20% of the overall CD3$^+$ population. In addition, a much higher percentage of fetal T-cells are CD4-8$^-$, the range being 35–70% in fetal intestine compared with 6% in postnatal tissue.[137]

It has been reported that activation of gastric mucosal T-cells during infancy in the rat, particularly associated with weaning onto solid food, is a normal phenomenon, and provides obligatory signals for growth and maturation of the small intestine[138,139]; indirect evidence suggests that a similar process is operative in human infants.[140]

Considerably less information is available concerning the respiratory tract. Lung parenchymal tissue in rodents demonstrates a steady accumulation of T-cells during the period birth-weaning, and a slower increase in corresponding populations in the lamina propria of the conducting airways.[120] No data are currently available on the distribution of T-cells in human neonatal lung tissue, and the limited information on airway tissue suggests a similar pattern of postnatal T-cell influx to that reported for rodents.[141]

The frequency of plasma cells, in particular those secreting IgA and IgM, increases rapidly in mucosal tissues of the gastrointestinal and respiratory tracts of human infants, in response to exogenous (especially microbial) antigen stimulation,[142–144] and this is reflected in the progressively increasing concentration of secretory IgA in saliva.[145,146]

The significance of organized lymphoid aggregates in mucosal tissues of the human respiratory tract is controversial, and their presence is now generally acknowledged to reflect a recent history of active local antigenic stimulation.[147] These structures, known as bronchus associated lymphoid tissue (BALT) are found frequently in heavy smokers but only rarely in healthy non-smokers.[148] However, they are also frequent in tissues from children with chronic or recurrent pneumonia.[149] BALT is rare in fetal tissue, but is present as small lymphoid aggregates in a large proportion of lung tissue samples from children under the age of 10 months;[149,150] given the fact that these structures are comparatively rare in the normal adult, their more frequent occurrence in infants suggests that they may have a transient role in local host defence in the respiratory tract during the early postnatal period.[148]

Postnatal maturation of mast cell (MC) populations

The expression of allergic reactions at mucosal surfaces requires the presence of functional mast cells, and adult GIT and respiratory tract tissues typically contain distinct mucosal mast cell populations (MMC) within the epithelium, plus connective tissue mast cells (CTMC) in the underlying lamina propria; these MCs exhibit unique enzymatic and mediator profiles and respond differently to anti-inflammatory drugs.

There is virtually no definitive information available on the postnatal maturation of these populations in human neonates, although some indirect evidence suggests that the GIT population seeds into local tissues as immature precursors during infancy, in response to local antigenic stimulation.[137] Information on the kinetics of postnatal development of these cells is limited to a single study from our laboratory on rats, which indicates that both MMC and CTMC populations in the respiratory tract are established entirely postnatally.[151] The populations develop slowly after an initial lag in early infancy, and do not resemble adults until after weaning.[151] Moreover, at around the time in late infancy that tissue seeding rates start to accelerate, significant levels of MC products (such as specific proteases) are transiently detected in serum, suggesting that the immature MC in the neonates are either spontaneously unstable or are undergoing local stimulation.[151] Similar observations have been reported for infant mice.[152]

Aetiology and pathogenesis of atopic asthma: the significance of postnatal development of immune function

The scheme depicted in Figure 4c.2 represents a working model for the aetiology and pathogenesis of atopic asthma, based upon recent findings from several laboratories (reviewed in refs 153, 154).

The salient findings upon which this model is based are as follows:

1 *Initial priming* of the human immune system against inhalant allergens can occur *in utero*,[155-158] stimulated by either transplacental transport of allergen to which the mother is exposed, or via cross-reacting antigens.

2 The resting *fetal Th-cell responses* are strongly Th2 polarized[159] due to the operation of Th1-inhibitory mechanisms at the fetomaternal interface[25] as detailed above.

3 During *early infancy*, the weak Th2 responses to inhalant allergens are subjected to Th-cell cross-regulation driven via direct allergen stimulation, resulting in either boosting/consolidation of Th2 reactivity (most commonly in children with positive atopic family history) or diversion towards Th1 polarized immunity in non-atopic subjects via 'low zone tolerance' or 'immune deviation' mechanisms.[153,160,161]

4 In contrast, the high levels of *dietary allergens* commonly encountered during infancy are sufficient to trigger a more potent set of regulatory mechanisms (T-cell deletion or induction of specific anergy) which in all but a small minority of subjects lead to the development of classical tolerance ('high zone tolerance' known in this context as 'oral tolerance') to the allergens.[153,162] During this process, Th2 responses are transiently induced, resulting in transient IgE production, often accompanied by positive skin-prick test reactivity and symptoms of food allergy.[162]

5 By the age of 5–6 years T-cell reactivity to dietary allergens is rare, whereas children display patterns of *inhalant* allergen-specific Th1 or Th2 polarized Th-cell memory identical to those seen in non-atopic or atopic adults, and these are associated with predictable patterns of skin-prick test reactivity to the inhalant allergens.[160,163]

6 *Persistent wheezing* symptoms, however, develop in only a subset of the atopic children,[154,164] in particular in those who manifest early sensitization to inhalants.[165,166]

7 Persistent wheeze is marked by characteristic *histopathological changes* in the airway wall indicative of excessive local Th2 cell activation and chronic, non-resolving inflammation;[167] the findings reported in (5) suggest that the occurrence of these events during active lung growth represents the worst case scenario with respect to long-term wheezing outcomes.

The fact that Th2 immunity to inhalant allergens results in persistent wheeze in only a subset of children and young adults, and yet >90% of those with wheeze are atopic,[164] suggests that atopy provides a 'matrix' for chronic disease development, but other cofactors are required.

We have argued earlier that the best candidates for the latter are agents which directly add to Th2-mediated airway inflammation such as virus infection,[154,168] or host factors which upregulate the intensity/duration of allergen-driven Th2-cell responses in the airway mucosa, in particular those associated with dysregulation of airway DC function.

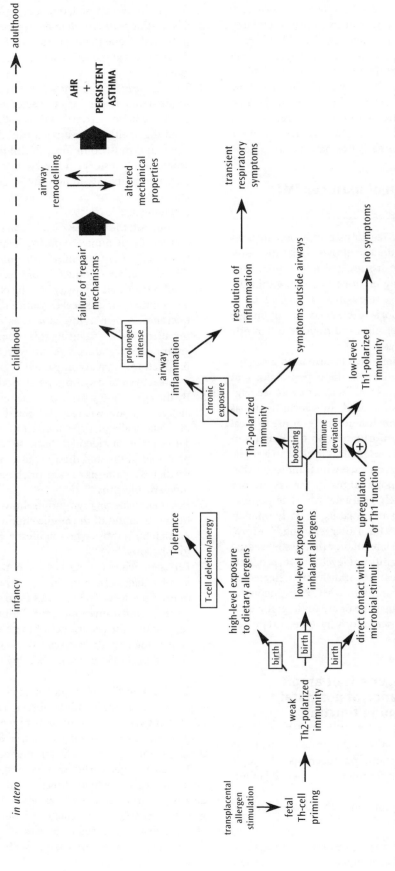

Figure 4c.2 *Two stage model for postnatal development of persistent atopic asthma. The two stage model envisages an initial phase in infancy/early childhood involving consolidation of Th2-polarized inhalant allergen-specific immunological memory, which in a subset of atopics in phase 2 results in chronic non-resolving airways inflammation, in turn producing phenotypic changes in airway tissue responsible for the manifestations of airways hyperresponsiveness (AHR).*

However, 'risk' for development of persistent atopic asthma may be determined largely by earlier developmental events in the scheme in Figure 4c.2, which precede the final compartmentalization of inhalant allergen-specific Th-cell immunity into Th1 vs Th2 memory.

We demonstrated several years ago[51] that genetic risk for atopy was associated with delayed postnatal maturation of CD4$^+$ Th-cell function, in particular capacity to generate the Th1 cytokine IFNγ, and several groups have subsequently confirmed these findings.[169–174] We hypothesize that diminished Th1 competence during the critical period in infancy early childhood during which fetally primed Th2 responses to allergen are normally 'immune deviated' towards non-pathogenic Th1-polarized immunity (see refs 160, 161) reduces the efficiency of this process, thus increasing the risk for boosting/consolidation of Th2 polarized memory.

The mechanism(s) underlying this genetically determined maturational defect have yet to be determined, but they may involve an exaggeration and/or prolongation of the normal fetal situation discussed above, in which Th2 polarization of immune function is the norm. That is, during infancy the balance between capacity to secrete Th1 vs Th2 cytokines progressively shifts in all children to eventually favour Th1, but the rate of transition from the fetal to adult-like phenotype proceeds slower in children at genetic risk of atopy.

As noted above, the immune deviation process which ultimately results in development of low level Th1 immunity to inhalant allergen in non-atopics is driven by direct exposure to allergen. The key APC which regulate this process are airway intraepithelial DC, and the available evidence indicates that these are also functionally immature at birth,[120,123] and variation in the rate at which they mature postnatally may be an additional determinant of risk for atopy/asthma.[175] It is well established that the impetus for postnatal maturation of Th1 function is provided via stimulation by microbial signals (such as bacterial LPS) which are unique to the extrauterine environment, from both pathogens and in particular commensal microflora.[153,162] In this regard it is pertinent to note the recent description of a polymorphism in the gene encoding the high affinity LPS receptor CD14, which is associated with intensity of atopy.[176,177] In this context irritant stimuli,[120] in particular microbial agents such as LPS,[178,179] provide potent activation/maturation signals for DC, which may account for recent findings suggesting that LPS present in house-dust protects against allergen sensitization in infants at high risk of asthma by enhancing Th1 immunity.[180]

It is interesting to speculate that the maturational defect in Th1 function in children at genetic risk of atopy may also influence asthma development via an alternative route. Thus, a further consequence of this deficiency appears to be attenuated capacity to respond efficiently during infancy to microbial vaccines such as BCG[181] or diphtheria–pertussis–tetanus.[182] However in addition, reduced capacity to generate the Th1 cytokines IL-12[183] and IFNγ,[184,185] is observed in subjects who develop severe bronchiolitis during infancy, suggesting that reduced Th1 immunity increases the intensity and/or duration of respiratory viral infection and hence increases risk for spread to the small airways. This finding is consistent with the recent suggestion that viral wheeze during infancy may be a 'flag' for an underlying maturation deficiency in Th1-mediated defence, rather than direct promoter of Th2 functions.[186] Thus it is conceivable that diminished capacity for expression of Th1-mediated immunity during the critical stage of rapid lung growth during early life may increase susceptibility to virus induced damage to airway tissue, which may synergize with that resulting from local allergen-induced Th2-mediated responses, setting in motion the second phase of the process described in the model in Figure 4c.2.

CONCLUSIONS

An increasing body of evidence implicates maturational deficiencies in adaptive immune function as an aetiologic factor in the development of atopy and atopic asthma. The cellular site(s) of the defect(s) are not established, and may include antigen presenting cells as well as the T-cell system. The molecular nature of the defect(s) also awaits elucidation, and it appears likely that several will be involved.

REFERENCES

1. Yu M, Fredrikson S, Link J, Link H. High numbers of autoantigen-reactive mononuclear cells expressing interferon-gamma, IL-4 and transforming growth factor-beta are present in cord blood. *Clin Exp Immunol* 1995;**101**:190–6.

2. Piccinni M-P, Mecacci F, Sampognaro S, Manetti R, Parronchi P, Maggi E, Romagnani S. Aeroallergen sensitization can occur during foetal life. *Int Arch Allergy Immunol* 1993;**102**:301–3.

3. Aase JM, Noren GR, Reddy DV, St Geme JW. Mumps-virus infection in pregnant women and the immunologic response of their offspring. *New Eng J Med* 1972;**286**:1379–82.

4. Novato-Silva E, Gazzinelli G, Colley DG. Immune responses during human schistosomiasis mansoni. XVIII. Immunologic status of pregnant women and their neonates. *Scand J Immunol* 1992;**35**:429–37.

5. Fievet N, Ringwald P, Bickii J. Malaria cellular immune responses in neonates from Cameroon. *Parasite Immunol* 1996;**18**:483–90.

6. Sanjeevi CB, Vivekanandan S, Narayanan PR. Fetal response to maternal ascariasis as evidenced by

anti-*Ascaris lumbricoides* IgM antibodies in the cord blood. *Acta Pediatr Scand* 1991;**80**:1134–8.

7. Gill TJ, Repetti CF, Metlay LA. Transplacental immunisation of the human foetus to tetanus by immunisation of the mother. *J Clin Invest* 1983; **72**:987–96.

8. Herzenberg LA, Bianchi DW, Schroder J, Cann HM, Iverson MG. Fetal cells in the blood of pregnant women: detection and enrichment by fluorescence-activated cell sorting. *Proc Natl Acad Sci USA* 1979;**76**:1453.

9. Lo Y-MD, Wainscoat JS, Gillmer MDG, Patel P, Sampietro M, Fleming KA. Prenatal sex determination by DNA amplification from maternal peripheral blood. *Lancet* 1989;**9**:1363.

10. Bianchi DW, Zickwolf GK, Yih MC, Flint A, Geifman OH, Erikson MS, Williams JM. Erythroid specific antibodies enhance detection of fetal nucleated erythrocytes in maternal blood. *Prenat Diagn* 1993;**13**:293.

11. Wachtel S, Elias S, Price J, Wachtel G, Phillips O, Shulman L, Meyers C, Simpson JL, Dockter M. Fetal cells in the maternal circulation: isolation by multiparameter flow cytometry and confirmation by polymerase chain reaction. *Hum Reprod* 1991;**6**:1466.

12. Shulman L, Phillips O, Meyers CM, Shook D, Simpson JL. Prenatal diagnosis with fetal cells isolated from maternal blood by multiparameter flow cytometry. *Am J Obstet Gynecol* 1994;**165**:1731.

13. Medawar PB. Some immunological and endocrinological problems raised by the evolution of viviparity in vertebrates. *Symp Soc Exp Biol* 1954;**7**:320.

14. Bonney EA, Matzinger P. The maternal immune system's interaction with circulating fetal cells. *J Immunol* 1997;**158**:40–7.

15. Roth I, Corry DB, Locksley RM, Abrams JS, Litton MJ, Fisher SJ. Human placental cytotrophoblasts produce the immunosuppressive cytokine interleukin 10. *J Exp Med* 1996;**184**:539–48.

16. Munn DH, Zhou M, Attwood JT, Bondarev I, Conway SJ, Marshall B, Brown C, Mellor AL. Prevention of allogeneic fetal rejection by tryptophan catabolism. *Science* 1998;**281**:1191–3.

17. Guller S, LaChapelle L. The role of placental Fas ligand in maintaining immune privilege at maternal–fetal interface. *Semin Reprod Endocrinol* 1999;**17**:39–44.

18. Hammer A, Blaschitz A, Daxbock C, Walcher W, Dohr G. Gas and Fas-ligand are expressed in the uteroplacental unit of first-trimester pregnancy. *Am J Reprod Immunol* 1999;**41**:41–51.

19. Krishnan L, Guilbert LJ, Wegmann TG, Belosevic M, Mosmann TR. T helper 1 response against *Leishmania major* in pregnant C57BL/6 mice increases implantation failure and foetal resorptions. *J Immunol* 1996;**156**:653–62.

20. Krishnan L, Guilbert LJ, Russell AS, Wegmann TG, Mosmann TR, Belosevic M. Pregnancy impairs resistance of C57BL/6 mice to *Leishmania major* infection and causes decreased antigen-specific IFN-responses and increased production of T helper 2 cytokines. *J Immunol* 1996;**156**:644–52.

21. Hilkens CM, Vermeulen H, Joost van Neerven RJ, Snijdewint FGM, Wierenga EA, Kapsenberg ML. Differential modulation of T helper type 1 (Th1) and T helper type 2 (Th2) cytokine secretion by prostaglandin E_2 critically depends on interleukin-2. *Eur J Immunol* 1995;**25**:59–63.

22. Piccinni M-P, Giudizi M-G, Biagiotti R, *et al*. Progesterone favours the development of human T helper cells producing Th2-type cytokines and promotes both IL-4 production and membrane CD30 expression in established Th1 cell clones. *J Immunol* 1995;**155**:128–33.

23. Szekeres-Bartho J, Faust Z, Varga P, Szereday L, Kelemen K. The immunological pregnancy protective effect of progesterone is manifested via controlling cytokine production. *Am J Reprod Immunol* 1996; **35**:348–51.

24. Szekeres-Bartho J, Wegmann TG. A progesterone-dependent immunomodulatory protein alters the Th1/Th2 balance. *J Reprod Immunol* 1996;**31**:81–95.

25. Wegmann TG, Lin H, Guilbert L, Mosmann TR. Bidirectional cytokine interactions in the maternal-foetal relationship: is successful pregnancy a Th2 phenomenon? *Immunol Today* 1993;**14**:353–6.

26. Miller ME. Phagocyte function in the neonate: selected aspects. *Pediatrics* 1979;**64**:709–12.

27. Wilson CB. Immunologic basis for increased susceptibility of the neonate to infection. *J Pediatr* 1986;**108**:1–12.

28. Burchett SK, Corey L, Mohan KM, Westall J, Ashley R, Wilson CB. Diminished interferon-γ and lymphocyte proliferation in neonatal and postpartum primary herpes simplex virus infection. *J Infect Dis* 1992; **165**:813–18.

29. Hayward AR, Groothuis J. Development of T-cells with memory phenotype in infancy. *Adv Exp Med Biol* 1991;**310**:71–6.

30. Friedmann PS. Cell-mediated immunological reactivity in neonates and infants with congenital syphilis. *Clin Exp Immunol* 1977;**30**:271–6.

31. Starr SE, Tolpin MD, Friedman HM, Paucker K, Plotkin SA. Impaired cellular immunity to cytomegalovirus in congenitally infected children and their mothers. *J Infect Dis* 1979;**140**:500–5.

32. Hayward AR, Herberger M, Saunders D. Herpes simplex virus-stimulated γ-interferon production by newborn mononuclear cells. *Pediatr Res* 1986;**20**:398–400.

33. Griffiths-Chu S, Patterson JAK, Berger CL, Edelson RL, Chu AC. Characterization of immature T cell subpopulations in neonatal blood. *Blood* 1984;**64**:296–300.

34. Maccario R, Nespoli L, Mingrat G, Vitiello A, Ugazio AG, Burgio GR. Lymphocyte subpopulations in the neonate: identification of an immature subset of OKT8-positive, OKT3-negative cells. *J Immunol* 1983;**130**:1129–31.

35. Clement LT, Vink PE, Bradley GE. Novel immunoregulatory functions of phenotypically distinct subpopulations of CD4+ cells in the human neonate. *J Immunol* 1990;**145**:102–8.

36. Gerli R, Bertotto A, Spinozzi F, Cernetti C, Battaglia A, Falchetti R, Grignani F, Rambotti P. Thymic hormone modulation of CD38 (T10) antigen on human cord blood lymphocytes. *Clin Immunol Immunopathol* 1987;**45**:323–32.

37. Hannet I, Erkeller-Yuksel F, Lydyard P, Deneys V, De Bruyere M. Developmental and maturational changes in human blood lymphocyte subpopulations. *Immunol Today* 1992;**13**:215–18.

38. Calado RT, Garcia AB, Falcao RP. Age-related changes of immunophenotypically immature lymphocytes in normal human peripheral blood. *Cytometry* 1999; **38**:133–7.

39. Hassan J, Reen DJ. Neonatal CD4+ CD45RA+ T-cells: precursors of adult CD4+ CD45RA+ T-cells? *Res Immunol* 1993;**144**:87–92.

40. Sanders ME, Makgoba MW, Shaw S. Human naive and memory T-cells; reinterpretation of helper-inducer and suppressor-inducer subsets. *Immunol Today* 1988;**9**:195–9.

41. Gerli R, Bertotto A, Spinozzi F, Cernetti C, Grignani F, Rambotti P. Phenotypic dissection of cord blood immunoregulatory T-cell subsets by using a two-color immunofluorescence study. *Clin Immunol Immunopathol* 1986;**40**:429–35.

42. Kingsley G, Pitzalis C, Waugh A, Panayi G. Correlation of immunoregulatory function with cell phenotype in cord blood lymphocytes. *Clin Exp Immunol* 1988;**73**:40–5.

43. Bradley L, Bradley J, Ching D, Shiigi SM. Predominance of T-cells that express CD45R in the CD4+ helper/inducer lymphocyte subset of neonates. *Clin Immunol Immunopathol* 1989;**51**:426–35.

44. Hayward A, Lee J, Beverley PCL. Ontogeny of expression of UCHL1 antigen on TcR-1+ (CD4/8) and TcR delta+ T-cells. *Europ J Immunol* 1989;**19**:771–3.

45. Abo T, Miller CA, Gartland GL, Balch CM. Differentiation stages of human natural killer cells in lymphoid tissues from fetal to adult life. *J Exp Med* 1983;**157**:273–84.

46. Pirenne H, Aujard Y, Eljaafari A, Bourillon A, Oury JF, Le GS, Blot P, Sterkers G. Comparison of T cell functional changes during childhood with the ontogeny of CDw29 and CD45RA expression on CD4+ T-cells. *Pediatr Res* 1992;**32**:81–6.

47. Stern DA, Hicks MJ, Martinez FD, Holberg CJ, Wright AL, Pinnas J, Halonen M, Taussig LM. Lymphocyte subpopulation number and function in infancy. *Dev Immunol* 1992;**2**:175–9.

48. Bertotto A, Gerli R, Lanfrancone L, Crupi S, Arcangeli C, Cernetti C, Spinozzi F, Rambotti P. Activation of cord T lymphocytes. II. Cellular and molecular analysis of the defective response induced by anti-CD3 monoclonal antibody. *Cell Immunol* 1990;**127**:247–59.

49. Gerli R, Agea E, Muscat C, Tognellini R, Fiorucci G, Spinozzi F, Cernetti C, Bertotto A. Activation of cord T lymphocytes. III. Role of LFA-1/ICAM-1 and CD2/LFA-3 adhesion molecules in CD3-induced proliferative response. *Cell Immunol* 1993;**148**:32–47.

50. Hassan J, Reen DJ. Cord Blood CD4+ CD45RA+ T-cells achieve a lower magnitude of activation when compared with their adult counterparts. *Immunology* 1997;**90**:397–401.

51. Holt PG, Sommerville C, Baron-Hay MJ, Holt BJ, Sly PD. Functional assessment of CD2, CD3 and CD28 on the surface of peripheral blood T-cells from infants at low versus high genetic risk for atopy. *Pediatr Allergy Immunol* 1995;**6**:80–4.

52. Holt PG, Clough JB, Holt BJ, Baron-Hay MJ, Rose AH, Robinson BWS, Thomas WR. Genetic 'risk' for atopy is associated with delayed postnatal maturation of T-cell competence. *Clin Exp Allergy* 1992;**22**:1093–9.

53. Hassan J, Reen DJ. Reduced primary antigen-specific T-cell precursor frequencies in neonates is associated with deficient interleukin-2 production. *Immunology* 1996;**87**:604–8.

54. Takahashi N, Imanishi K, Nishida H, Uchiyama T. Evidence for immunologic immaturity of cord blood T-cells. *J Immunol* 1995;**155**:5213–19.

55. Porcu P, Gaddy J, Broxmeyer HE. Alloantigen-induced unresponsiveness in cord blood T lymphocytes is associated with defective activation of Ras. *Proc Natl Acad Sci USA* 1998;**95**:4538–43.

56. Whisler RL, Newhouse YG, Grants IS, Hackshaw KV. Differential expression of the alpha and beta isoforms of protein kinase C in peripheral blood T and B cells from young and elderly adults. *Mech Ageing Develop* 1995;**77**:197–211.

57. Miscia S, Du Baldassarre A, Sabatino G, Bonvini E, Rana RA, Vitale M, Di Valerio V, Manzoli FA. Inefficient phospholipase C activation and reduced Lck expression characterize the signaling defect of umbilical cord T lymphocytes. *J Immunol* 1999;**163**:2416–24.

58. Sato K, Nagayama H, Takahasji TA. Aberrant CD3- and CD28-mediated signaling events in cord blood T-cells are associated with dysfunctional regulation of Fas ligand-mediated cytotoxicity. *J Immunol* 1999; **162**:4464–71.

59. Hassan J, O'Neill S, O'Neill LAJ, Pattison U, Reen DJ. Signalling via DC28 of human naive neonatal T lymphocytes. *Clin Exp Immunol* 1995;**102**:192–8.

60. Andersson U, Bird AG, Britten S, Palacios R. Human and cellular immunity in humans studied at the

cellular level from birth to two years. *Immunol Rev* 1981;**57**:5–19.

61. Hayward AR. Development of lymphocyte responses in humans, the foetus and newborn. *Immunol Rev* 1981;**57**:43–61.

62. Splawski JB, Lipsky PE. Cytokine regulation of immunoglobulin secretion by neonatal lymphocytes. *J Clin Invest* 1991;**88**:967–77.

63. Zola H, Fusco M, Macardle PJ, Flego L, Roberton D. Expression of cytokine receptors by human cord blood lymphocytes: comparison with adult blood lymphocytes. *Pediatr Res* 1995; **38**:397–403.

64. Zola H, Fusco M, Weedon H, MacArdle PJ, Ridings J, Roberton DM. Reduced expression of the interleukin-2-receptor chain on cord blood lymphocytes: relationship to functional immaturity of the neonatal immune response. *Immunology* 1996;**87**:86–91.

65. Lee SM, Suen Y, Chang L, Bruner V, Qian J, Indes J, Knoppel E, van de Ven C, Cairo MS. Decreased interleukin-12 (IL-12) from activated cord versus adult perioperal blood mononuclear cells and upregulation of interferon-γ, natural killer, and lymphokine-activated killer activity by IL-12 in cord blood mononuclear cells. *Blood* 1996;**88**:945–54.

66. Qian JX, Lee SM, Suen Y, Knoppel E, van de Ven C, Cairo MS. Decreased interleukin-15 from activated cord versus adult peripheral blood mononuclear cells and the effect of interleukin-15 in upregulating antitumor immune activity and cytokine production in cord blood. *Blood* 1997; **90**:3106–17.

67. Chheda S, Palkowetz KH, Garofalo R, Rassin DK, Goldman AS. Decreased interleukin-10 production by neonatal monocytes and T-cells: relationship to decreased production and expression of tumor necrosis factor-α and its receptors. *Pediatr Res* 1996;**40**:475–83.

68. Chalmers IMH, Janossy G, Contreras M, Navarrete C. Intracellular cytokine profile of cord and adult blood lymphocytes. *Blood* 1998;**92**:11–18.

69. Scott ME, Kubin M, Kohl S. High level interleukin-12 production, but diminished interferon-γ production, by cord blood monoculear cells. *Pediatr Res* 1997;**41**:547–53.

70. Kotiranta-Ainamo A, Rautonen J, Rautonen N. Interleukin-10 production by cord blood mononuclear cells. *Pediatr Res* 1997;**41**:110–13.

71. Adkins B. T-cell function in newborn mice and humans. *Immunol Today* 1999;**20**:330–5.

72. Durandy A, De Saint Basile G, Lisowska-Grospierre B, Gauchat J-F, Forveille M, Kroczek RA, Bonnefoy J-Y, Fischer A. Undetectable CD40 ligand expression on T-cells and low B cell responses to CD40 binding antagonists in human newborns. *J Immunol* 1995;**154**:1560–8.

73. Fuleihan R, Ahern D, Geha RS. Decreased expression of the ligand for CD40 in newborn lymphocytes. *Eur J Immunol* 1994;**24**:1925–8.

74. Early EM, Reen DJ. Antigen-independent responsiveness to interleukin-4 demonstrates differential regulation of newborn human T-cells. *Eur J Immunol* 1996;**26**:2885–9.

75. Rowe J, Macaubas C, Monger T, Holt BJ, Harvey J, Poolman JT, Sly PD, Holt PG. Antigen-specific responses to diphtheria–tetanus–acellular pertussis vaccine in human infants are initially Th2 polarized. *Infect Immunity* 2000;**68**:3873–7.

76. Gans HA, Maldonado Y, Yasukawa LL, Bweeler J, Audet S, Rinki MM, DeHovitz R, Arvin AM. IL-12, IFNγ, and T cell proliferation to measles in immunized infants. *J Immunol* 1999;**162**:5569–75.

77. Marchant A, Goetghebuer T, Ota M, *et al*. Newborns develop a Th1-type immune response to Mycobacterium bovis bacillus Calmette–Guerin vaccination. *J Immunol* 1999;**163**:2249–55.

78. Malhotra I, Ouma J, Wamachi A, *et al*. *In utero* exposure to helminth and mycobacterial antigens generates cytokine responses similar to that observed in adults. *J Clin Invest* 1997;**99**:1759–66.

79. Lewis DB, Wilson CB. In: JS Remington, JO Klein, eds. *Infectious Diseases of the Foetus and Newborn Infant*. WB Saunders, London, 1995, p. 20.

80. Conley ME, Cooper MD. Immature IgA B cells in IgA-deficient patients. *New Eng J Med* 1981;**317**:495–501.

81. Cooper MD. Current concepts. B lymphocytes, normal development and function. *N Eng J Med* 1987;**317**:1452–9.

82. Gathings WE, Kubagawa H, Cooper MD. A distinctive pattern of B cell immaturity in perinatal humans. *Immunol Rev* 1981;**57**:107–14.

83. Watson W, Oen K, Ramdahin R, Harman C. Immunoglobulin and cytokine production by neonatal lymphocytes. *Clin Exp Immunol* 1991;**83**:169–74.

84. Gauchat J-F, Gauchat D, De Weck AL, Stadler BM. Cytokine mRNA levels in antigen-stimulated peripheral blood mononuclear cells. *Eur J Immunol* 1989;**7**:804–10.

85. Stavnezer J. Antibody class switching. *Adv Immunol* 1996;**61**:79–146.

86. Grewal IS, Flavell RA. The role of CD40 ligand in costimulation and T-cell activation. *Immunol Respir* 1996;**153**:85–106.

87. Splawski JB, Lipsky PE. Prostaglandin E_2 inhibits T cell-dependent Ig secretion by neonatal but not adult lymphocytes. *J Immunol* 1994;**152**:5259–66.

88. Chesnut RW, Grey HM. Antigen presentation by B cells and its significance in T–B interactions. *Adv Immunol* 1986;**39**:51–82.

89. Pierce SK, Morris JF, Grusby MJ, Kaumaya P, van Buskirk A, Srinivasan M, Crump B, Smolenski LA.

Antigen-presenting function of B lymphocytes. *Immunol Rev* 1988;**106**:149–56.

90. Morris JF, Hoyer JT, Pierce SK. Antigen presentation for T cell interleukin-2 secretion is a late acquisition of neonatal B cells. *Eur J Immunol* 1992;**22**: 2923–8.

91. Van Tol MJD, Ziljstra J, Thomas CMG, Zegers BJM, Ballieux RE. Distinct role of neonatal and adult monocytes in the regulation of the *in vitro* antigen-induced plaque-forming cell response in man. *J Immunol* 1984;**134**:1902–8.

92. Weinberg AG, Rosenfeld CR, Manroe BL, Browne R. Neonatal blood cell count in health and disease. *J Pediatr* 1985;**106**:462–6.

93. Speer CP, Gahr M, Wieland M, Eber S. Phagocytosis-associated functions in neonatal monocyte-derived macrophage. *Pediatr Res* 1988;**24**:213–16.

94. Murphy FJ, Reen DJ. Differential expression of function-related antigens on newborn and adult monocyte subpopulations. *Immunology* 1996;**89**:587–91.

95. Buzby JS, Lee SM, Van Winkle P, DeMaria CT, Brewer G, Cairo MS. Increased granulocyte-macrophage colony-stimulating factor mRNA instability in cord versus adult mononuclear cells is translation-dependent and associated with increased levels of A + U-rich element binding factor. *Blood* 1996;**88**:2889–97.

96. Stiehm ER, Sztein MB, Oppenheim JJ. Deficient DR antigen expression on human cord blood monocytes: reversal with lymphokines. *Clin Immunol Immunopathol* 1984;**30**:430–6.

97. Clerici M, DePalma L, Roilides E, Baker R, Shearer GM. Analysis of T helper and antigen-presenting cell functions in cord blood and peripheral blood leukocytes from healthy children of different ages. *J Clin Invest* 1993;**91**:2829–36.

98. Taylor S, Bryson YJ. Impaired production of γ-interferon by newborn cells *in vitro* is due to a functionally immature macrophage. *J Immunol* 1985;**134**:1493–8.

99. Lewis DB, Yu CC, Meyer J, English BK, Kahn SJ, Wilson CB. Cellular and molecular mechanisms for reduced interleukin 4 and interferon-gamma production by neonatal T-cells. *J Clin Invest* 1991;**87**:194–202.

100. Inaba K, Kitaura M, Kato T, Watanabe Y, Kawade Y, Muramatsu S. Contrasting effect of alpha/beta- and gamma-interferons on expression of macrophage Ia antigens. *J Exp Med* 1986;**163**:1030–5.

101. Fowler R, Schubert WK, West CD. Acquired partial tolerance to homologous skin grafts in the human infant at birth. *Ann NY Acad Sci* 1960;**87**:403–28.

102. Uhr JW, Dancis J, Neumann CG. Delayed hypersensitivity in premature neonatal humans. *Nature* 1960;**187**:1130–1.

103. Török C, Lundahl J, Hed J, Lagercrantz H. Diversity in regulation of adhesion molecules (Mac-1 and L-selectin) in monocytes and neutrophils from neonates and adults. *Arch Dis Child* 1993;**68**:561–5.

104. Yachie A, Takano N, Ohta K, Uehara T, Fujita S, Miyawaki T, Taniguchi N. Defective production of interleukin-6 in very small premature infants in response to bacterial pathogens. *Infect Immun* 1992;**60**:749–53.

105. Burchett SK, Weaver WM, Westall JA, Larsen A, Kronheim S, Wilson CB. Regulation of tumor necrosis factor/cachectin and IL-1 secretion in human mononuclear phagocytes. *J Immunol* 1988;**140**:3473–81.

106. English BK, Burchett SK, English JD, Ammann AJ, Wara DW, Wilson CB. Production of lymphotoxin and tumor necrosis factor by human neonatal mononuclear cells. *Pediatr Res* 1988;**24**:717–22.

107. Klein JO, Remington JS, March SM. Current concepts of infection of the fetus and newborn infant. In: JS Remington, JO Klein, eds. *Infectious Diseases of the Fetus and Newborn Infant*. WB Saunders, Philadelphia, 1983, p. 14.

108. Bellanti JA, Nerurkar LS, Zeligs BJ. Host defenses in the fetus and neonate: studies of the alveolar macrophage during maturation. *Pediatrics* 1979;**23**(Suppl):726–39.

109. Weiss RA, Chanana AD, Joel DD. Postnatal maturation of pulmonary antimicrobial defense mechanisms in conventional and germ-free lambs. *Pediatr Res* 1986;**20**:496–504.

110. D'Ambola JB, Sherman MP, Taskin DP, Gong Jr. H. Human and rabbit newborn lung macrophages have reduced anti-candida activity. *Pediatr Res* 1988;**24**:285–90.

111. Kurland G, Cheung ATW, Miller ME, Ayin SA, Cho MM, Ford EW. The ontogeny of pulmonary defenses: alveolar macrophage function in neonatal and juvenile rhesus monkeys. *Pediatr Res* 1988;**23**:293–7.

112. Alenghat E, Esterly JR. Alveolar macrophages in perinatal infants. *Pediatrics* 1984;**74**:221–3.

113. Janeway CA. The immune response evolved to discriminate infectious nonself from noninfectious self. *Immunol Today* 1992;**13**:11–16.

114. McWilliam AS, Napoli S, Marsh AM, Pemper FL, Nelson DJ, Pimm CL, Stumbles PA, Wells TNC, Holt PG. Dendritic cells are recruited into the airway epithelium during the inflammatory response to a broad spectrum of stimuli. *J Exp Med* 1996;**184**:2429–32.

115. Matzinger P. Tolerance, danger, and the extended family. *Annu Rev Immunol* 1994;**12**:991–1045.

116. Holt PG, Stumbles PA. Regulation of immunological homeostasis in peripheral tissues by dendritic cells: the respiratory tract as a paradigm. *J Allergy Clin Immunol* 2000;**105**:421–9.

117. Brandtzaeg P, Halstensen TS, Huitfeldt HS, Krajci P, Kvale D, Scott H, Thrane PS. Epithelial expression of HLA, secretory component (poly-Ig receptor), and adhesion molecules in the human alimentary tract. *Ann NY Acad Sci* 1992;**664**:157–79.

118. Mayrhofer G, Pugh CW, Barclay AN. The distribution, ontogeny and origin in the rat of Ia-positive cells with dendritic morphology and of Ia antigen in epithelia, with special reference to the intestine. *Eur J Immunol* 1983;**13**:112–22.

119. McCarthy KM, Gong JL, Telford JR, Schneeberger EE. Ontogeny of Ia+ accessory cells in foetal and newborn rat lung. *Am J Respir Cell Mol Biol* 1992;**6**:349–56.

120. Nelson DJ, McMenamin C, McWilliam AS, Brenan M, Holt PG. Development of the airway intraepithelial dendritic cell network in the rat from class II MHC (Ia) negative precursors: differential regulation of Ia expression at different levels of the respiratory tract. *J Exp Med* 1994;**179**:203–12.

121. Mizoguchi S, Takahashi K, Takeya M, Naito M, Morioka T. Development, differentiation and proliferation of epidermal Langerhans cells in rat ontogeny studied by a novel monoclonal antibody against epidermal Langerhans cells, RED-1. *J Leukoc Biol* 1992;**52**:52–61.

122. Romani N, Schuler G, Fritsch P. Ontogeny of Ia-positive and Thy-1-positive leukocytes of murine epidermis. *J Invest Dermatol* 1986;**86**:129–33.

123. Nelson DJ, Holt PG. Defective regional immunity in the respiratory tract of neonates is attributable to hyporesponsiveness of local dendritic cells to activation signals. *J Immunol* 1995;**155**:3517–24.

124. McWilliam AS, Nelson D, Thomas JA, Holt PG. Rapid dendritic cell recruitment is a hallmark of the acute inflammatory response at mucosal surfaces. *J Exp Med* 1994;**179**:1331–6.

125. Stumbles PA, Thomas JA, Pimm CL, Lee PT, Venaille TJ, Proksch S, Holt PG. Resting respiratory tract dendritic cells preferentially stimulate Th2 responses and require obligatory cytokine signals for induction of Th1 immunity. *J Exp Med* 1998;**188**:2019–31.

126. Mease AD. Tissue neutropenia: the newborn neutrophil in perspective. *J Perinatal* 1990;**x**:55–9.

127. Christensen RD, MacFarlane JL, Taylor NL, Hill HR. Blood marrow neutrophils during experimental group B streptococcal infection: quantification of the stem cell, proliferative, storage and circulating pools. *Pediatr Res* 1982;**16**:49–53.

128. Erdmann SH, Christensen RD, Bradley PP, Rothstein G. Supply and release of storage neutrophils: a developmental study. *Biol Neonate* 1982;**41**:132–7.

129. English BK, Hammond WP, Lewis DB, Brown CB, Wilson CB. Decreased granulocyte-macrophage colony-stimulating factor production by human neonatal blood mononuclear cells and T-cells. *Pediatr Res* 1992;**31**:211–16.

130. Hill HR. Biochemical, structural, and functional abnormalities of polymorphonuclear leukocytes in the neonate. *Pediatr Res* 1987;**22**:375–82.

131. Wolach B, Dor MB, Chomsky O, Gavrieli R, Shinitzky M. Improved chemotactic ability of neonatal polymorphonuclear cells induced by mild membrane rigidification. *J Leukoc Biol* 1992;**51**:324–8.

132. Lloyd AR, Oppenheim JJ. Poly's lament: the neglected role of the polymorphonuclear neutrophil in the afferent limb of the immune response. *Immunol Today* 1992;**13**:169–73.

133. Spencer JM, Dillon SB, Isaacson PG, MacDonald TT. T cell subclasses in human fetal ileum. *Clin Exp Immunol* 1986;**65**:553–8.

134. Spencer JM, MacDonald TT, Isaacson PG. Development of the gut associated lymphoid tissue in human fetal gut. *Adv Exp Med Biol* 1987;**216B**:1421–30.

135. Spencer JM, MacDonald TT, Finn TT, Isaacson PG. Development of Peyer's patches in human fetal terminal ileum. *Clin Exp Immunol* 1986;**64**:536–43.

136. Monk TJ, Spencer J, Cerf-Bensussan N, MacDonald TT. Activation of mucosal T-cells *in situ* with anti-CD3 antibody phenotype of the activated T-cells and their distribution within the mucosal micro-environment. *Clin Exp Immunol* 1988;**74**:216–22.

137. Spencer J, Isaacson PG, Walker-Smith JA, MacDonald TT. Heterogeneity in intraepithelial lymphocyte subpopulations in fetal and postnatal human small intestine. *J Pediatr Gastroenterol Nutr* 1989;**9**:173–7.

138. Cummins AG, Thompson FM, Mayrhofer G. Mucosal immune activation and maturation of the small intestine at weaning in the hypothymic (nude) rat. *J Pediatr Gastroenterol Nutr* 1991;**12**:361–8.

139. Thompson FM, Mayrhofer G, Cummins AG. Dependence of epithelial growth of the small intestine on T cell activation during weaning in the rat. *Gastroenterology* 1996;**111**:37–44.

140. Cummins AG, Eglinton BA, Gonzalez A, Roberton DM. Immune activation during infancy in healthy humans. *J Clin Immunol* 1994;**14**:107–15.

141. Stoltenberg L, Thrane PS, Rognum TO. Development of immune response markers in the trachea in the foetal period and the first year of life. *Pediatr Allergy Immunol* 1993;**4**:13–19.

142. Bridges RA, Condie RM, Zak SJ, Good RA. The morphologic basis of antibody formation development during the neonatal period. *J Lab Clin Med* 1959;**53**:331–8.

143. Perkkio M, Savilahti E. Time of appearance of immunoglobulin-containing cells in the mucosa of the neonatal intestine. *Pediatr Res* 1980;**14**:953–5.

144. Thrane PS, Rognum TO, Brandtzaeg P. Ontogenesis of the secretory immune system and innate defence factors in human parotid glands. *Clin Exp Immunol* 1991;**86**:342–8.

145. Haworth JC, Dilling L. Concentration of gamma-A-globulin in serum, saliva, and nasopharyngeal secretions of infants and children. *J Lab Clin Med* 1966;**67**:922–9.

146. Selner JC, Merril DA, Claman HN. Salivary immunoglobulin and albumin. Development during the newborn period. *J Pediatr* 1968;**72**:685–95.

147. Holt PG. BALT development in human lung disease: a normal host defence mechanism awaiting therapeutic exploitation? *Thorax* 1993;**48**:1097–8.

148. Meuwissen HJ, Hussain M. Bronchus-associated lymphoid tissue in human lung: correlation of hyperplasia with chronic pulmonary disease. *Clin Immunol Immunopathol* 1982;**23**:548–61.

149. Emery JL, Dinsdale F. The postnatal development of lymphoreticular aggregates and lymph nodes in infants' lungs. *J Clin Pathol* 1973;**26**:539–45.

150. Gould SJ, Isaacson PG. Bronchus-associated lymphoid tissue (BALT) in human fetal and infant lung. *J Pathol* 1993;**169**:229–34.

151. Wilkes LK, McMenamin C, Holt PG. Postnatal maturation of mast cell subpopulations in the rat respiratory tract. *Immunology* 1992;**75**:535–41.

152. Cummins AG, Munro GH, Miller HRP, Ferguson A. Association of maturation of the small intestine at weaning with mucosal mast cell activation in the rat. *J Cell Biol* 1988;**66**:417–23.

153. Holt PG, Macaubas C. Development of long term tolerance versus sensitisation to environmental allergens during the perinatal period. *Curr Opin Immunol* 1997;**9**:782–7.

154. Holt PG, Macaubas C, Stumbles PA, Sly PD. The role of allergy in the development of asthma. *Nature* 1999;**402**:B12–17.

155. Kondo N, Kobayashi Y, Shinoda S, Kasahara K, Kameyama T, Iwasa S, Orii T. Cord blood lymphocyte responses to food antigens for the prediction of allergic disorders. *Arch Dis Child* 1992;**67**:1003–7.

156. Piastra M, Stabile A, Fioravanti G, Castagnola M, Pani G, Ria F. Cord blood mononuclear cell responsiveness to beta-lactoglobulin: T-cell activity in 'atopy-prone' and 'non-atopy-prone' newborns. *Int Arch Allergy Immunol* 1994;**104**:358–65.

157. Miles EA, Warner JA, Jones AC, Colwell BM, Bryant TN, Warner JO. Peripheral blood mononuclear cell proliferative responses in the first year of life in babies born to allergic parents. *Clin Exp Allergy* 1996;**26**:780–8.

158. Holt PG, O'Keeffe PO, Holt BJ *et al*. T-cell 'priming' against environmental allergens in human neonates: sequential deletion of food antigen specificities during infancy with concomitant expansion of responses to ubiquitous inhalant allergens. *Ped Allergy Immunol* 1995;**6**:85–90.

159. Prescott SL, Macaubas C, Holt BJ, Smallacombe T, Loh R, Sly PD, Holt PG. Transplacental priming of the human immune system to environmental allergens: universal skewing of initial T-cell responses towards the Th-2 cytokine profile. *J Immunol* 1998;**160**:4730–7.

160. Yabuhara A, Macaubas C, Prescott SL, Venaille T, Holt BJ, Habre W, Sly PD, Holt PG. Th-2-polarised immunological memory to inhalant allergens in atopics is established during infancy and early childhood. *Clin Exp Allergy* 1997;**27**:1261–9.

161. Prescott SL, Macaubas C, Smallacombe T, Holt BJ, Sly PD, Holt PG. Development of allergen-specific T-cell memory in atopic and normal children. *Lancet* 1999;**353**:196–200.

162. Holt PG. Environmental factors and primary T-cell sensitisation to inhalant allergens in infancy: reappraisal of the role of infections and air pollution. *Pediatr Allergy Immunol* 1995;**6**:1–10.

163. Macaubas C, Sly PD, Burton P, Tiller K, Yabuhara A, Holt BJ, Smallacombe TB, Kendall G, Jenmalm MC, Holt PG. Regulation of Th-cell responses to inhalant allergen during early childhood. *Clin Exp Allergy* 1999;**29**:1223–31.

164. Woolcock AJ, Peat JK, Trevillion LM. Is the increase in asthma prevalence linked to increase in allergen load? *Allergy* 1995;**50**:935–40.

165. Sherrill D, Stein R, Kurzius-Spencer M, Martinez F. Early sensitization to allergens and development of respiratory symptoms. *Clin Exp Allergy* 1999;**29**:905–11.

166. Peat JK, Salome CM, Woolcock AJ. Longitudinal changes in atopy during a 4-year period: relation to bronchial hyperresponsiveness and respiratory symptoms in a population sample of Australian schoolchildren. *J Allergy Clin Immunol* 1990;**85**:65–74.

167. Holgate S. The inflammation-repair cycle in asthma: the pivotal role of the airway epithelium. *Clin Exp Allergy* 1998;**28**(S5):97–103.

168. Johnston SL, Pattemore PK, Sanderson G *et al*. The relationship between upper respiratory infections and hospital admissions for asthma: a time-trend analysis. *Am J Respir Crit Care Med* 1996;**154**:654–60.

169. Rinas U, Horneff G, Wahn V. Interferon-γ production by cord-blood mononuclear cells is reduced in newborns with a family history of atopic disease and is independent from cord blood IgE-levels. *Pediatr Allergy Immunol* 1993;**4**:60–4.

170. Tang M, Kemp A, Varigos G. IL-4 and interferon-gamma production in children with atopic disease. *Clin Exp Immunol* 1993;**92**:120–4.

171. Martinez FD, Stern DA, Wright AL, Holberg CJ, Taussig LM, Halonen M. Association of interleukin-2 and interferon-γ production by blood mononuclear cells in infancy with parental allergy skin tests and with subsequent development of atopy. *J Allergy Clin Immunol* 1995;**96**:652–60.

172. Liao SY, Liao TN, Chiang BL, Huang MS, Chen CC, Chou CC, Hsieh KH. Decreased production of IFNγ

and increased production of IL-6 by cord blood mononuclear cells of newborns with a high risk of allergy. *Clin Exp Allergy* 1996;**26**:397–405.

173. Warner JA, Miles EA, Jones AC, Quint DJ, Colwell BM, Warner JO. Is deficiency of interferon gamma production by allergen triggered cord blood cells a predictor of atopic eczema? *Clin Exp Allergy* 1994;**24**:423–30.

174. Piccinni M-P, Beloni L, Giannarini L, Livi C, Scarselli G, Romagnani S, Maggi E. Abnormal production of T helper 2 cytokines interleukin-4 and interleukin-5 by T-cells from newborns with atopic parents. *Eur J Immunol* 1996;**26**:2293–8.

175. Holt PG. Dendritic cell ontogeny as an aetiological factor in respiratory tract diseases in early life. *Thorax* 2001;**56**:419–20.

176. Baldini M, Lohman IC, Halonen M, Erickson RP, Holt PG, Martinez FD. A polymorphism in the 5′-flanking region of the CD14 gene is associated with circulating soluble CD14 levels with total serum IgE. *Am J Respir Cell Mol Biol* 1999;**20**:976–83.

177. Gao P-S, Mao X-Q, Baldini M, Roberts MH, Adra CN, Shirakawa T, Holt PG, Martinez FD, Hopkin JM. Serum total IgE levels and CD14 on chromosome 5q31. *Clin Genet* 1999;**56**:164–5.

178. Holt PG, Sly PD, Björkstén B. Atopic versus infectious diseases in childhood: a question of balance? *Ped Allergy Immunol* 1997;**8**:53–8.

179. Martinez FD, Holt PG. The role of microbial burden in the aetiology of allergy and asthma. *Lancet* 1999;**354**:12–15.

180. Gereda JE, Leung DYM, Thatayatikom A, Streib JE, Price MR, Klinnert MD, Liu AH. Relation between house-dust endotoxin exposure, type 1 T-cell development, and allergen sensitisation in infants at high risk of asthma. *Lancet* 2000; **355**:1680–3.

181. Shirakawa T, Enomoto T, Shimazu S, Hopkin JM. Inverse association between tuberculin responses and atopic disorder. *Science* 1997;**275**:77–9.

182. Prescott SL, Sly PD, Holt PG. Raised serum IgE associated with reduced responsiveness to DPT vaccination during infancy. *Lancet* 1998; **351**:1489.

183. Blanco-Quirós A, González H, Arranz E, Lapeña S. Decreased interleukin-12 levels in umbilical cord blood in children who developed acute bronchiolitis. *Pediatr Pulmonol* 1999;**28**:175–80.

184. Renzi PM, Turgeon JP, Marcotte JE, Drblik SP, Bérubé D, Gagnon MF, Spier S. Reduced interferon-γ production in infants with bronchiolitis and asthma. *Am J Respir Crit Care Med* 1999;**159**: 1417–22.

185. Leech SC, Price JF, Holmes BJ, Kemeny BJ. Nonatopic wheezy children have reduced interferon-gamma. *Allergy* 2000;**55**:74–8.

186. Martinez FD, Stern DA, Wright AL, Taussig LM, Halonen M. Differential immune responses to acute lower respiratory illness in early life and subsequent development of persistent wheezing and asthma. *J Allergy Clin Immunol* 1998;**102**: 915–20.

4d

Genetics

PETER N LE SOUËF

INTRODUCTION

Asthma has been observed to run in families for many years, yet the mechanism of its inheritance remains unclear. Knowledge of how asthma is inherited should help clarify the relative contributions of genetics and environment in the aetiology of asthma, and also has the potential to allow different varieties of asthma to be identified as particular genetic entities. More practically, some genotypes are likely to be associated with specific responses to pharmacological therapy. Eventually, individuals may be targeted for therapy against particular environmental factors according to their genetic profile.

Whether any individual can develop asthma if environmental stimuli are strong enough remains unclear. The possibility remains that genes determine which individuals are susceptible, and environment determines whether or not asthma develops in susceptible individuals only.

EPIDEMIOLOGICAL EVIDENCE

Reviewing epidemiological evidence of the inheritance of asthma and asthma-related traits is useful, as this information can guide molecular genetic studies to gather relevant phenotypic data.

Family studies

Epidemiological data suggest that asthma has a genetic component, but inheritance does not usually follow simple Mendelian patterns.[1] This suggests that there may be many genes involved or that environmental differences between family members are strong enough to obscure the genetic component. The observation that asthma clearly runs in some families,[2] cannot be taken as proof of genetic transmission, since families share environment as well as genes. History taking does not reliably ascertain phenotypic status for families, as the family member interviewed is likely to have recall bias and be more likely to remember their own respiratory history than that of other family members. There are also problems in the change in perception of asthma over the last few decades, change in diagnostic labels used by doctors, and family size. Nonetheless, some studies demonstrate a consistent pattern of increased positive family history for allergic disease (of 40–80%) in those with allergic rhinitis or asthma compared with those without allergic disease (20% or less).[3] The risk of allergy developing in offspring is about 66% if both parents are allergic, 50% if one parent is allergic and about 20% in the general population.[2] Atopy (increased IgE-related responses such as total IgE, specific IgE and skin reactivity) also runs in families and history of atopy in the parents is a strong risk factor for atopy in children. In another study, if atopy was present in neither, one or both parents, the percentage of children with atopy increased from 0–20% to 30–50% and 60–100%, respectively.[4]

Twin studies

Studies comparing monozygotic (MZ) and dizygotic (DZ) twins have also shown that the environment exerts a stronger effect than genetics. MZ twins have an identical genetic make-up and DZ twins share only 50% of their genetic material. Studies of MZ and DZ twins assume that environment will be much the same for each pair of twins. For MZ versus DZ twins, concordance was higher for asthma,[5,6] serum IgE and skin reactivity,[7] but environment exerted a greater influence than genetics on total IgE level, skin reactivity and RAST responses.[8] Concordance for airway responsiveness was greater in MZ than DZ twins in some[7] but not all studies.[9] A genetic contribution to asthma as high as 68% has been recorded in one study of 4 year old twins.[9a] Thus, twin studies suggest that genes influence individual susceptibility for asthma and atopy, and perhaps for the level of airway responsiveness. High levels of discordance in some studies is strong evidence for important environmental influences.

Gender

In the first decade of life, boys appear more likely to develop asthma than girls.[2] In a longitudinal study in New Zealand, 1056 children were followed from soon after birth to 6 years of age and 14.3% of the boys and only 6.3% of the girls developed asthma during the study period.[10] The difference between the sexes disappears during the second decade when asthma prevalence is much the same in males and females.[11] Whether the gender differences are due to genetic or environmental factors has not been established, but data collected in early life in Tucson suggests that a genetic component is very likely. This group studied infants longitudinally and found an association between lower respiratory function measured soon after birth and wheeze in the first few years of life in males but not in females.[12–14] In those aged 3 to 6 years, this predictive effect of lower respiratory function was no longer evident.[14]

Why should male infants be predisposed to asthma? Several further lines of evidence suggest that boys are genetically predisposed to being born with smaller airways than girls, and that these small airways are the cause of their increased susceptibility to asthma in early life. Forced expiratory flows are lower in male infants than female infants,[15] whereas by late adolescence, flows are equal in the two sexes.[16] Both the incidence of respiratory illness[17] and the prevalence of atopy are greater in male than female infants.[18]

Race

Early studies examining the prevalence of asthma in racial groups in developing countries reported very low incidences of asthma. For example, in a study in Papua New Guinea, only 0.6% of children were observed to have asthma[19] and no asthma could be found in children in the Gambia in a report from 1975.[20] These low figures for prevalence may be related to a rural environment, as a more recent study of rural Australian Aboriginal people found a prevalence of only 0.5% in 8- to 12-year-old

children[21] and rural prevalence of asthma was half that for urban Aboriginal people in the Northern Territory.[22]

Data on the world-wide prevalence of asthma in different countries have recently become available. The International Study of Asthma and Allergies in Childhood[23] study has used questionnaire data to assess the prevalence of asthma in many different countries in the world.[23] These data have shown striking differences in prevalence between different countries,[23] but whether these differences are due to race or environment is not known. However, the very strong environmental effects, especially those related to a rural compared with an urban environment, are likely to account for much of the difference.

Nonetheless, studies of different racial groups living in the same country demonstrate differences in asthma-related parameters that could reflect genetic racial differences. An example is the study of 2053 Auckland school-children, in which correction was made for socio-economic status, smoking and other parameters. Bronchial hyperresponsiveness (BHR) was present in 20% of Europeans, 13% of Maoris and 9% of Pacific Islanders.[24] BHR rates for the groups contrasted with incidence of current wheeze, with the highest level of 22% in Maoris, compared with 16% in Europeans and Pacific Islanders.

In a UK study of young children, when all significant confounders were accounted for, the odds ratio for wheeze in South Asian compared with Caucasian children was 1.82.[25]

Airway responsiveness

The level of airway responsiveness in rats is strain dependent. Since rats within a strain are virtually identical genetically, inter-strain differences may be due to a genetic effect. Airway response to 5-hydroxytryptamine after exposure to aerosolized endotoxin varies between strains,[26] and strain dependent differences in airway response to intravenous substance P have been demonstrated.[27] In contrast, no difference was found between strains for response to inhaled methacholine, but wide variability in the level of response within strains was shown,[28] suggesting that airway responsiveness in these rats was mainly determined by environment.

Airway responsiveness in humans also appears to be determined by genetic factors. In children from families with asthma, a bimodal distribution of the levels of airway response to methacholine was reported, with a unimodal distribution being noted for those from normal families.[29] A segregation analysis was used to determine that the results could not be explained by genetic segregation at a single autosomal locus. It is unclear if the level of airway responsiveness in infants is set by genetic factors. Infants with a family history of atopy studied within a few weeks of birth were noted to have increased responsiveness compared with those without this history, but a subsequent larger analysis did not confirm these findings.[30]

Airway size

As noted above, boys may have smaller airways than girls in early life and the development of asthma-like respiratory symptoms in the first few years of life in boys may correlate with airway size. The reason that girls did not show the same relations between parameters reflecting airway size and respiratory symptoms[12] is not known.

MOLECULAR GENETICS

Molecular genetic research undertaken in the last decade into the genetics of asthma has established important new information.

Polygenic nature of asthma

Several extensive genome screens have been completed and these have shown that many regions of the human genome are linked to asthma or its associated phenotypic features.[31–39] While some regions have shown up consistently in different genome screens, many regions have been identified in only one of the studies.[1] Whether such unique regions are detected due to type I statistical errors or due to unique interactions between environment and genotype specific to that geographical location and population remains unclear.

Lack of dominant genes in determining genetic susceptibility

The lack of strong, consistent data linking genomic regions to asthma also shows that there are no powerful asthma susceptibility genes. Data obtained to date suggest that no single allele contributes more than 10% of the susceptibility to asthma in any given population.[40,41]

Extensive numbers of genes with polymorphisms associated with the asthma phenotype

Candidate gene studies have been completed on a large number of genes and in many of these, polymorphisms have been discovered that have been associated with asthma or its related attributes in population studies.[1,41] At this stage, many of the findings require confirmation in other populations, as some of them are likely to be the result of type II statistical errors.

Environmental interactions

Whether or not a genetically susceptible individual develops asthma is strongly dependent on environmental

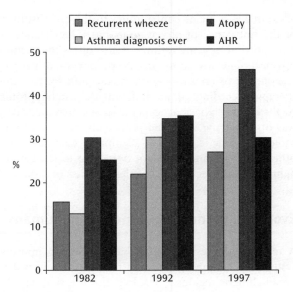

Figure 4d.1 *Wheeze in Wagga children aged 9 years 1982–1997. The same protocol was used to evaluate each group of children.[43] Recurrent wheeze, asthma diagnosis ever and atopy increased over the three study periods, but airway hyperresponsiveness (AHR) did not.*

factors. Changes in such factors over the last 20 or 30 years are likely to be responsible for the large increase in the prevalence of asthma that has been observed over this period. For example in an Australian study, the prevalence of wheeze in previous 12 months increased in Belmont, a coastal town, from 10.4% in 1982 to 27.6% in 1992 ($p < 0.001$)[42] and similar increases were noted in Wagga, an inland town in Australia[43] (Figure 4d.1). Despite extensive research, the most important epidemiological factors responsible for this observed increase in asthma prevalence are still not known. The strong environmental effects have the advantage of maximizing the phenotypic expression of a genetic susceptibility and this would assist the task of detecting genetic effects. On the other hand, the strength of the environmental effects is so great that identifying the smaller genetic effects for asthma susceptibility may have become especially difficult and the problem of determining interactions between environment and genetics even more complex.

Pharmacogenetics

A promising advance in the knowledge of asthma has come from studies in which response to a pharmacological agent has been compared with the presence or absence of an allele in a particular gene.[44] The most consistent data to date involve beta-2 sympathomimetic drugs and the beta-2 adrenoreceptor polymorphisms.[45,46] Asthma pharmacogenetics may provide key information on the basic mechanisms in acute asthma. If a strong response to treatment is seen for one allele and no response is seen for the other allele, this would suggest that the response allele makes a major contribution to the establishment of the imbalance of airway tone and inflammation in a proportion of acute asthma. It also offers the exciting prospect of greatly improving the proportion of patients responding to an anti-asthma medication by directing therapy according to an individual's genetic profile. In these ways, pharmacogenetic studies may provide a way of classifying acute and potentially chronic asthma. Molecular genetic studies in asthma to date have used other pathways and have not been able to shed much light on either mechanisms of classification of asthma.

Evolution of immune responses in humans

A recent hypothesis suggests that the human immune system has adapted genetically to improve survival in broad climatic regions.[47] The hypothesis is that populations originating in hostile tropical environments have immune responses with a more proinflammatory profile than populations that have moved and resided for many millennia in a temperate, cold or desert environment. The rationale for this hypothesis is as follows. When human ancestors emigrated from East Africa, their immune function would most likely have been relatively up-regulated or proinflammatory in order to cope with life in a tropical environment, where infective disease is common and parasitic infection, particularly helminthic infection, is endemic.[48] The proinflammatory responses one would expect to be most involved would be the T-helper 2 (Th2) lymphocyte and IgE-mediated responses, as these are important in anti-helminthic defences[49] (Table 4d.1). People moving to a temperate, cold or desert environment would not have needed such proinflammatory immune responses, as many infective organisms, including helminthic parasites, are less

aggressive, since they rely on both heat and humidity to thrive.[50] Proinflammatory responses would have caused a modest increase in mortality from allergy and autoimmune diseases and gradually been lost.

A great deal of data supports this hypothesis including: (i) the higher prevalence of proinflammatory alleles in inflammatory genes in population groups with an ancestral location over recent tens of thousands of years in a tropical versus a non-tropical location (Figure 4d.2),[50–59] and (ii) the increased prevalence of Th2-related diseases, including atopic disease and asthma, found in those relocating from a tropical to a temperate environment (Table 4d.2).[60–68] The populations in which there are most data are African–Americans, in whom asthma is approximately twice as common as in European–Americans.[47,61–65] In other words, at least half of the asthma seen in African–Americans may be explained by this population's tropical ancestry. Similar data have been published for other groups, including Asians living in Britain. For example, South Asian children in Blackburn had twice the admission rate for asthma compared with non-Asians (OR 2.03, 95%CI 1.32–3.12, $p < 0.01$)[67] and South Asian children in

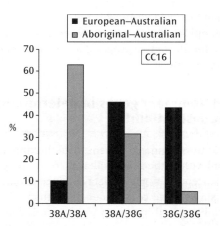

Figure 4d.2 *Proportion of individuals with the Clara cell 16 kDa protein (CC16) A38G polymorphism in two different populations in Australia. The proinflammatory 38A allele is much more common in the Aboriginal–Australian population than the European population ($p < 0.001$).[47]*

Table 4d.1 *Comparison of Ascaris infection and IgE in a two different tropical Venezuelan environments.[49]*

Ascaris infection	Location	
	Coche Island	**Caracas slums**
Prevalence (%)	51	57
Intensity (epg)[a]	1435 (6531)	7621 (20464)[b]
Anti-Ascaris IgE		
(%+ve)	61	37[b]
(Conc PRU/ml)	0.91 (2.48)	0.30 (0.90)[b]
Total IgE (IU/ml)[a]	941 (3126)	2172 (5649)[b]

The intensity of infection in Coche Island was lower with higher anti-Ascaris IgE levels but lower total IgE levels. These data suggest that the ability to mount a greater specific IgE response is associated with reduced parasitic infection and reduced polyclonal (non-specific) production of IgE (epg: egg count per gram of faeces; IU: international unit; PRU: Phadebas RAST units; SD: standard deviation).
[a]Geometric mean (SD).
[b]$p < 0.001$.

Table 4d.2 *Comparison of rates of asthma between African–American (AA) and European–American (EA) children. The former have more asthma than the latter*

	AA vs EA children
Asthma age 7–14 yr[58]	OR 1.57 (CI 1.17–2.10)
Asthma in children[59]	OR 2.9
Asthma in children[60]	12% vs 6%
Emergency admission rates[61]	4-fold higher

OR: odds ratio; CI: 95% confidence intervals.

Leicester had an odds ratio of 1.82 for wheezing.[25] Clearly, many of the world-wide differences in inflammatory disease susceptibility and prevalence may be due to relatively recent evolutionary effects on the immune system. Thus, the importance of the evolutionary data is that it has broad implications towards understanding the nature of the immune system and disease susceptibility.

FINDINGS FOR SPECIFIC GENES

Over the last ten years, asthma genetic studies have focused on examining either previously known or new genes, identifying polymorphisms that are associated with an increased risk of developing asthma. These studies have been highly successful in identifying associations between polymorphisms and the presence of asthma or asthma-related phenotypic features.[1] Several polymorphisms are known to be important as risk factors for asthma and there are many others for which a relationship is suspected.[1,69] The polymorphisms that are most strongly suspected of involvement in asthma are those that fulfil certain criteria.

Inflammatory function: the gene's product has a function related to inflammation.

Linkage data: exists for phenotypic attributes related to inflammation and the gene's location.

Site of polymorphism: the polymorphism is located in a part of the gene that is likely to significantly affect morphology, function or quantity of protein produced.

Functional data, tissue or fluid levels: the polymorphism has been shown to affect *in vitro* gene function, or tissue or serum levels of the gene's protein.

Association data: data from more than one cohort associates an allele with an attribute related to inflammation.

Allele frequency: alleles are in sufficient prevalence to allow differences between populations to be detected.

DATA FROM SELECTED CANDIDATE GENE STUDIES

Beta-2 adrenoreceptor gene, Arg→Gly16 (G46C) and Gln→Glu27 (G76C): These polymorphisms are common, functionally significant and associated with differences in asthma symptoms and severity in adults,[70] wheeze and AHR in children[71] and increased IgE in asthmatic families.[72] They have also been associated with specific IgE levels and parasite load in endemically parasitized Venezuelans, suggesting an important role in IgE regulation.[73] Allele frequencies in European–Australians were – arg16: 45.9%; gly16: 54.1%; gln27: 61.3%; glu27: 38.7%.[71]

Tumour necrosis factor alpha (TNFα) gene, G-308A: The TNFα gene is located on chromosome 6 within the class III region of the MHC. TNFα is a central mediator of inflammation and a −308 promoter polymorphism has been reported.[1] G-308A was associated with asthma in children[74] and, for the G and A alleles, frequencies were −308A 76.5% and −308G 23.5%.[74]

Interleukin-4 (IL-4), C-589T: IL-4 is important in IgE production and the −589T allele has been associated with raised serum IgE levels,[73] reduced $FEV_{1.0}$[54] and asthma severity.[55] Allele frequencies were −590C 73% and −590T 27%.[75]

IL-4 receptor (IL-4R) gene, Ile50: The Ile50 allele has been associated with atopic asthma and specific IgE.[56] Allele frequencies were Ile50 74% and Val50 26%.[57]

Clara cell 16 kDa protein (CC16), A38G: CC16 is secreted from the airway epithelium and has strong anti-inflammatory activity. An A38G polymorphism in the first exon was reported and an association noted between the 38A allele, asthma[76] and reduced serum levels of CC16, consistent with CC16's anti-inflammatory role.[77] Allele frequencies in European–Australians for 38A were 33.3% and 38G 66.7%.[76]

CD14, C-159T: This gene has a major role in directing whether a Th1 or Th2 response will occur and the promoter polymorphism has been associated with asthma severity.[78] Allele frequencies were −159C 51.4% and −159T 48.6%.[78]

Beta chain of the high affinity IgE receptor (Fcε R1-β), E237G: The 237G allele has been associated with skin allergy responses and airway hyperresponsiveness (AHR) in European–Australians.[79] Allele frequency for 237G was 20% in European–South Africans.[53]

RANTES promoter polymorphism: RANTES is a chemokine with increased activity in inflammatory lung disease and its gene is on chromosome 17q11.2, a region linked with asthma in African–American families.[58] A functional promoter polymorphism,[58,59] was associated with atopic dermatitis in German children.[59]

SUMMARY AND FUTURE DIRECTIONS

Asthma results from complex interactions between genetic and environmental influences. Data from epidemiological studies suggests that many genes could have the potential to contribute to the genetic susceptibility to asthma and these could include genes controlling airway size in infant boys, atopy, gender, and race. Over the last decade, molecular genetic studies have provided important information about the genetics of asthma:

- asthma is polygenic and there are no dominant genes in determining genetic susceptibility;
- many genes have polymorphisms that are associated with asthma;

- pharmacogenetic studies can improve the selection of responders to certain medications;
- immune responses in humans that currently cause asthma are likely to have arisen as defences against parasites;
- interracial differences in allergy and asthma susceptibility may be due to evolutionary pressures.

Molecular genetic studies have the potential to allow different varieties of asthma to be identified as particular genetic entities, but little progress has been made on this aspect to date, perhaps due to the predominant use of cross-sectional rather than longitudinal populations in association studies.[80] More practically, some genotypes are likely to be associated with specific responses to pharmacological therapy. Eventually, individuals may be targeted for therapy against particular environmental factors according to their genetic profile.

REFERENCES

1. Hall IP. Genetics and pulmonary medicine. *Thorax* 1999;**54**:65–9.
2. Ownby DR. Environmental factors versus genetic determinants of childhood inhalant allergies. *J Allergy Clin Immunol* 1990;**86**:279–87.
3. Blumenthal MN, Yunis E, Mendell N, Elston RC. Preventive allergy: genetics of IgE-mediated diseases. *J Allergy Clin Immunol* 1986;**78**:962–8.
4. Kaufman HS, Frick OL. The development of allergy in infants of allergic patients: a prospective study concerning the role of heredity. *Ann Allergy* 1976;**37**:410–15.
5. Lubs ML-E. Empiric risks for genetic counseling in families with allergy. *J Pediatr* 1972;**80**:26–31.
6. Duffy DL, Martin NG, Battistutta D, Hopper JL, Mathews JD. Genetics of asthma and hay fever in Australian twins. *Am Rev Respir Dis* 1990;**142**:1351–8.
7. Hopp RJ, Bewtra AK, Watt GD, Nair NM, Townley RG. Genetic analysis of allergic disease in twins. *J Allergy Clin Immunol* 1984;**73**:265–70.
8. Wuthrich B, Baumann E, Fries KH, Schnyder UW. Total and specific IgE (RAST) in atopic twins. *Clin Allergy* 1981;**11**:147–54.
9. Zamel N, Leroux M, Vanderdoelen JL. Airway response to inhaled methacholine in healthy nonsmoking twins. *J Appl Physiol* 1984;**56**:936–9.
9a. Koeppen-Schomerus G, Stevenson J, Plomin R. Genes and environment in asthma: a study of 4 year old twins. *Arch Dis Child* 2001;**85**:398–400.
10. Horwood LJ, Fergusson DM, Hons BA, Shannon FT. Social and familial factors in the development of early childhood asthma. *Pediatrics* 1985;**75**:859–68.
11. Martin AJ, McLennan LA, Landau LI, Phelan PD. The natural history of childhood asthma to adult life. *Br J Med* 1980;**1**:1397–1400.
12. Martinez FD, Morgan WJ, Wright AL, Holberg CJ, Taussig LM. Diminished lung function as a predisposing factor for wheezing respiratory illness in infants. *N Engl J Med* 1988;**319**:1112–17.
13. Martinez FD, Morgan WJ, Wright AL, Holberg CJ, Taussig LM. Initial airway function is a risk factor for recurrent wheezing respiratory illness during the first three years of life. *Am Rev Respir Dis* 991;**143**:312–16.
14. Martinez FD, Wright AL, Taussig LM, Holberg C, Halonen M, Morgan WJ. Asthma and wheezing in the first six years of life. *N Engl J Med* 1995;**332**:133–8.
15. Taussig LM, Landau LI, Godfrey S, Arad I. Determinants of forced expiratory flow in newborn infants. *J Appl Physiol* 1982;**53**:1270–7.
16. Polgar G, Weng TR. The functional development of the respiratory system. State of the Art. *Am Rev Respir Dis* 1979;**120**:625–95.
17. Gold DR, Tager IB, Weiss ST, Tosteson TD, Speizer FE. Acute lower respiratory illness in childhood as a predictor of lung function and chronic respiratory symptoms. *Am Rev Respir Dis* 1989;**140**:877–84.
18. Magnusson CGM. Cord serum IgE in relation to family history and as predictor of atopic disease in early infancy. *Allergy* 1988;**43**:241–51.
19. Woolcock AJ, Dowse GK, Temple K, Stanley H, Alpers MP, Turner KJ. The prevalence of asthma in the South-Fore people of Papua New Guinea. A method for field studies of bronchial reactivity. *Eur Respir Dis* 1983;**64**:571–81.
20. Godfrey RC. Asthma and IgE levels in rural and urban communities of The Gambia. *Clin Allergy* 1975;**5**:201–7.
21. Veale AJ, Peat JK, Tovey ER, Salome CM, Thompson JE, Woolcock AJ. Asthma and atopy in four rural Australian aboriginal communities. *Med J Aust* 1996;**165**:192–6.
22. Whybourne A, Lesnikowski C, Ruben A, Walker A. Low rates of hospitalization for asthma among Aboriginal children compared to non-Aboriginal children of the top end of the Northern Territory. *J Paediatr Child Health* 1999;**35**:438–41.
23. The International Study of Asthma and Allergies in Childhood (ISAAC) Steering Committee. Worldwide variation in prevalence of symptoms of asthma, allergic rhinoconjunctivitis, and atopic eczema: ISAAC. *Lancet* 1998;**351**:1225–32.
24. Pattemore PK, Asher MI, Harrison AC, Mitchell EA, Rea HH, Stewart AW. Ethnic differences in prevalence of asthma symptoms and bronchial hyperresponsiveness in New Zealand schoolchildren. *Thorax* 1989;**44**:168–76.
25. Kuehni C, Silverman M. Wheezing in two generations of South Asians and Caucasians living in the UK. *Am J Respir Crit Care Med* 2000;**161**:A499.
26. Pauwels R, Van Der Straeten M, Weyne J, Bazin H. Genetic factors in non-specific bronchial reactivity in rats. *Eur J Respir Dis* 1985;**66**:98–104.

27. Joos G, Kips J, Pauwels R, Van Der Straeten M. The effect of tachykinins on the conducting airways of the rat. *Arch Int Pharmacodyn* 1986;**280**(Suppl):176–90.

28. Wang CG, Dimaria G, Bates JHT, Guttmann RD, Martin JG. Methacholine-induced airway reactivity in inbred rate. *J Appl Physiol* 1986;**61**:2180–5.

29. Townley RG, Bewtra A, Wilson AF, Hopp RJ, Elston RC, Nair N, Watt GD. Segregation analysis of bronchial response to methacholine inhalation challenge in families with and without asthma. *J Allergy Clin Immunol* 1986;**77**:101–7.

30. Young S, Sherrill DL, Arnott J, Depeveen D, Le Souëf PN, Landau LI. Parental factors affecting respiratory function during the first year of life. *Pediatr Pulmonol* 2000;**29**:331–40.

31. Palmer LJ, Cookson WO. Genomic approaches to understanding asthma. *Genome Res* 2000;**10**:1280–7.

32. Ober C, Tsalenko A, Parry R, Cox NJ. A second-generation genomewide screen for asthma-susceptibility alleles in a founder population. *Am J Hum Genet* 2000;**67**:1154–62.

33. Bleecker ER, Postma DS, Meyers DA. Evidence for multiple genetic susceptibility loci for asthma. *Am J Respir Crit Care Med* 1997;**156**(4 Pt 2):S113–16.

34. CSGA. A genome-wide search for asthma susceptibility loci in ethnically diverse populations. The Collaborative Study on the Genetics of Asthma (CSGA). *Nat Genet* 1997;**15**:389–92.

35. Ober C, Cox NJ, Abney M, *et al*. Genome-wide search for asthma susceptibility loci in a founder population. The Collaborative Study on the Genetics of Asthma. *Hum Mol Genet* 1998;**7**:1393–8.

36. Dizier MH, Besse-Schmittler C, Guilloud-Bataille M, *et al*. Genome screen for asthma and related phenotypes in the French EGEA Study. *Am J Respir Crit Care Med* 2000;**162**:1812–18.

37. Daniels SE, Bhattacharrya S, James A, *et al*. A genome-wide search for quantitative trait loci underlying asthma. *Nature* 1996;**383**:247–50.

38. Wjst M, Fischer G, Immervoll T, *et al*. A genome-wide search for linkage to asthma. German Asthma Genetics Group. *Genomics* 1999;**58**:1–8.

39. Kurz T, Strauch K, Heinzmann A, *et al*. A European study on the genetics of mite sensitization. *J Allergy Clin Immunol* 2000;**106**:925–32.

40. Sandford A, Weir T, Pare P. The genetics of asthma. *Am J Respir Crit Care Med* 1996;**153**:1749–65.

41. Sandford AJ, Pare PD. The genetics of asthma. The important questions. *Am J Respir Crit Care Med* 2000;**161**:S202–6.

42. Peat JK, van den Berg RH, Green WF, Mellis CM, Leeder SR, Woolcock AJ. Changing prevalence of asthma in Australian children. *BMJ* 1994;**308**:1591–6.

43. Downs SH, Marks GB, Car NG, Belousova EG, Sporik R, Peat JK. Prevalence and severity of allergic disease in Wagga Wagga, Australia 1992–97. *Eur Respir J* 1999;**14**:216s [abstract].

44. Hall IP. Pharmacogenetics of asthma. *Eur Respir J* 2000;**15**:449–51.

45. Hall IP, Wheatley AP, Dewar JC. Genetic polymorphisms of adrenergic receptors. *Methods Mol Biol* 2000;**126**:117–26.

46. Tan S, Hall IP, Dewar J, Dow E, Lipworth B. Association between beta 2-adrenoceptor polymorphism and susceptibility to bronchodilator desensitisation in moderately severe stable asthmatics. *Lancet* 1997;**350**:995–9.

47. Le Souëf PN, Goldblatt J, Lynch NR. Evolutionary adaptation of inflammatory immune responses in humans. *Lancet* 2000;**356**:242–4.

48. Lynch NR, Goldblatt J, Le Souëf PN. The relation between parasite disease and asthma. *Thorax* 1999;**54**:659–60.

49. Lynch NR, Hagel IA, Palenque ME, *et al*. Relationship between helminthic infection and IgE response in atopic and non-atopic children in a tropical environment. *J Allergy Clin Immunol* 1998;**101**:217–21.

50. Stromberg BE. Environmental factors influencing transmission. *Vet Parasitol* 1997;**72**:247–56.

51. Eber E, Laing IA, Goldblatt J, Rye PJ, Musk AW, James AL, Ryan GF, Burton P, Le Souëf PN. CC16 genotype frequencies: differences between two Western Australian populations (abstract). *Eur Respir J* 1998;**12**:443s.

52. Hayden CM, Hurley D, Laing IA, Goldblatt J, Musk AW, James AL, Ryan GF, Le Souëf PN. β-2-adrenoreceptor genotype frequencies in two Western Australian populations (abstract). *Eur Respir J* 2000;**16**:24s.

53. Green SL, Gaillard MC, Song E, Dewar JB, Halkas A. Polymorphisms of the beta chain of the high-affinity immunoglobulin E receptor (FcERI-β) in South African black and white asthmatic and nonasthmatic individuals. *Am J Respir Crit Care Med* 1998;**158**:1487–92.

54. Burchard EG, Silverman EK, Rosenwasser LJ, *et al*. Association between a sequence variant in the IL-4 gene promoter and FEV(1) in asthma. *Am J Respir Crit Care Med* 1999;**160**:919–22.

55. Burchard EG, Silverman EK, Rosenwasser LJ, *et al*. Association between a sequence variant in the IL-4 gene promoter and asthma severity (abstract). *Am J Respir Crit Care Med* 1999;**159**:A645.

56. Diechmann K, Bardutzky J, Forster J, Heinzmann A, Kuehr J. Common polymorphisms in the coding part of IL-4 receptor gene. *Biochem Biophys Res Comm* 1997;**231**:696–7.

57. Pillari A, Lilly CM, Yandava CN, Drazen JM. Association of interleukin-4 receptor alpha gene mutations and asthma (abstract). *Am J Respir Crit Care Med* 1999;**159**:A645.

58. Nickel R, Beck LA, Stellato C, Schliemer RP. Chemokines and allergic disease. *J Allergy Clin Immunol* 1999;**104**:723–42.

59. Nickel R, Barnes KC, Sengler C, Casolaro V, Friedhoff LR, Weber P. Evidence for linkage of chemokine polymorphisms to asthma in populations of African descent (abstract). *J Allergy Clin Immunol* 1999;**103**(Suppl):S174.

60. Gold DR, Rotnitzky A, Domohosh AL, Ware JK, Speizer FE, Ferris BG, *et al.* Race and gender difference in respiratory illness prevalence and their relationship to environmental exposures in children 7 to 14 years of age. *Am Rev Respir Dis* 1993;**148**:10–18.

61. Litonjua AA, Carey VJ, Weiss ST, Gold DR. Race, socioeconomic factors, and area of residence are associated with asthma prevalence. *Pediatr Pulmonol* 1999;**28**:394–401.

62. Nelson DA, Johnson CC, Divine GW, Strachmann C, Joseph CLM, Ownby DR. Ethnic differences in the prevalence of asthma in middle class children. *Ann Allergy Asthma Immunol* 1997;**78**:21–6.

63. VonBehren J, Kreutzer R, Smith D. Asthma hospitalization trends in California, 1983–1996. *J Asthma* 1999;**36**:575–82.

64. Sarpong DR, Hamilton RG, Eggleston PA, Adkinson NF. Socioeconomic status and race as risk factors for cockroach allergen exposure and sensitization in children with asthma. *J Allergy Clin Immunol* 1996;**97**:1393–401.

65. Miller JE. The effects of race/ethnicity and income on early childhood asthma prevalence and health care use. *Am J Public Health* 2000;**90**:428–30.

66. Gillam SJ, Jarman B, White P, Law R. Ethnic differences in consultation rates in urban general practice. *BMJ* 1989;**299**:953–7.

67. Myers P, Ormerod LP. Increased asthma admission rates in Asian patients: Blackburn 1987. *Respir Med* 1992;**86**:297–300.

68. Gilthorpe MS, Lay-Yee R, Wilson RC, Walters S, Griffiths RK, Bedi R. Variations in hospitalization rates for asthma among black and minority ethnic communities. *Respir Med* 1998;**92**:642–8.

69. Drazen JM, Silverman EK. Genetics of asthma: conference summary. *Am J Respir Crit Care Med* 1997;**156**:S69–71.

70. Reishaus E, Innis M, MacIntyre N, Liggett SB. Mutations in the gene encoding for the beta-2 adrenergic receptor in normal and asthmatic subjects. *Am J Respir Cell Mol Biol* 1993;**8**:334–9.

71. Ramsay CE, Hayden CM, Tiller KJ, Burton PR, Goldblatt J, Le Souëf PN. Polymorphisms in the beta-2-adrenoreceptor gene are associated with decreased airway responsiveness. *Clin Exp Allergy* 1999;**29**:1195–203.

72. Dewar JC, Wilkinson J, Wheatley A, *et al.* The glutamine 27 beta2-adrenoreceptor polymorphism is associated with elevated IgE levels in asthmatic families. *J Allergy Clin Immunol* 1997;**100**:261–5.

73. Ramsay CE, Hayden CM, Tiller KJ, *et al.* Association of polymorphisms in the beta-2-adrenoreceptor gene with higher levels of parasitic infection. *Hum Genet* 1999;**104**:269–74.

74. Albuquerque RV, Palmer LJ, Hayden CM, Laing IA, Rye PJ, Gibson NA, Burton PR, Goldblatt J, Le Souëf PN. Association of polymorphisms within the tumour necrosis factor (TNF) genes and childhood asthma. *Clin Exp Allergy* 1998;**28**:578–84.

75. Rossenwasser LJ, Klemm DJ, Dresback JK, Inamura H, Klinnert K, Borish L. Promoter polymorphisms in the chromosome 5 gene cluster in asthma and atopy. *Clin Exp Allergy* 1995;**25**(Suppl 2):74–8.

76. Laing IA, Goldblatt J, Eber E, Rye PJ, Gibson NA, Palmer LJ, Burton PR, Le Souëf PN. A polymorphism of the CC16 gene is associated with increased risk of asthma. *J Med Genet* 1998;**35**:463–7.

77. Laing IA, Hermans C, Bernard A, Burton PR, Goldblatt J, Le Souëf PN. Association between plasma CC16 levels, the A38G polymorphism and asthma. *Am J Respir Crit Care Med* 2000;**161**:124–7.

78. Baldini M, Lohman IC, Halonen M, Erickson RP, Holt PG, Martinez FD. A polymorphism in the 5′ flanking region of the CD14 gene is associated with circulating soluble CD14 levels and with total serum immunoglobulin E. *Am J Respir Cell Mol Biol* 1999;**20**:976–83.

79. Hill MR, Cookson WO. A new variant of the beta subunit of the high-affinity receptor for immunoglobulin E (Fc epsilon R1-beta E237G): associations with measures of atopy and bronchial hyper-responsiveness. *Hum Mol Genet* 1996; **5**:959–62.

80. Le Souëf PN. Use of cohorts with extensive longitudinal data in investigating the molecular genetics of asthma. *Clin Exp Allergy* 1998;**28**(Suppl 1):46–50.

Remodelling and inflammation

WILLIAM R ROCHE AND PETER K JEFFERY

INTRODUCTION

Bronchial asthma has recently come to be defined as a chronic inflammatory disorder of the conducting airways,[1,2] with clinical expression in the form of recurrent breathlessness and wheeze. As such, asthma shares its differential diagnosis with a variety of obstructive disorders of the airway, in the adult chronic obstructive pulmonary disease (COPD) and in the child episodic viral lower respiratory illness, of which acute viral bronchiolitis is an extreme form. The clinical features of asthma are the end result of variable obstruction of the conducting airways by a variety of processes including: vascular congestion, airway wall oedema, smooth muscle contraction and accumulation of debris and mucus in the lumen. The relative contribution of each of these processes to thickening of the airway wall and the disease state is uncertain, even in adult disease.[3] The airway walls in asthma are thickened by the remodelling process by between 50 and 300% of normal and there is lumenal narrowing, which is further compromised by excessive mucus admixed with an inflammatory exudate. In cases of fatal asthma, the longer is the duration of asthma, the thicker becomes the airway wall.[4] However, it has been suggested that airway wall thickness *per se* is not a requirement for asphyxic fatality as a group of relatively young asthmatics (i.e. with a relatively short history of asthma) had an airway wall thickness not significantly different to that of non-asthma controls. Lumenal secretions and plugging are likely the greater contribution to asthmatic death in these young cases of fatal asthma.[4] All tissue structural components, as well as inflammatory cell infiltration and oedema, can contribute to the observed thickening, however in the last mentioned study it was thickening of the adventitial layers that was most pronounced in the older group with the longest duration of disease. The present chapter focuses on structural alterations that occur in the airway wall (now commonly referred to as 'remodelling') and on the associated chronic inflammation of asthma.

It should be born in mind that the inflammatory reaction, in its *acute* phase, is designed to protect the host and to restore tissue and its function to normal. One generally accepted proposal is that the accelerated decline in forced expiratory flow over time, which occurs in an important subset of asthmatics, is the direct result of a switch from acute, episodic, to *chronic* inflammation and to consequent airway and parenchymal remodelling.[5,6] The proposal is compelling but, as yet, there is no unequivocal evidence that the remodelling process is dependent upon the prior development of chronic inflammation. It is equally plausible that the processes responsible for the development of chronic inflammation are distinct to those responsible for remodelling.[7] The last consideration has important implications for the design of disease modifying therapy: those agents that are effective anti-inflammatory drugs may not necessarily prevent or attenuate the process of remodelling.

The concept of 'remodelling' implies that a process of 'modelling' must have preceded it. The lung, *in utero*, undergoes extensive modelling and remodelling yet these processes are entirely appropriate to the normal process of lung development. Many of the cytokines and growth factors thought to be proinflammatory in asthma and in COPD are also expressed normally without detriment to the *developing lung*: indeed they appear to be essential to it.[8] Accordingly the working definition of remodelling proposed herein recognizes that the process of remodelling *per se* is not of necessity abnormal. It is: 'An alteration in size, mass or number of tissue structural components that occurs during growth or repair, in response to injury and/or inflammation. It may be appropriate, as in normal lung development or that which occurs transiently during normal repair, or 'inappropriate' when it is chronic and associated with abnormally altered tissue structure and function as, for example, in asthma or COPD.[7]

In *wound healing* (in the skin) the components of an appropriate response include: formation of a clot, swelling/oedema, rapid restitution of the denuded areas by epithelial de-differentiation, proliferation and migration from the margins of the wound. These responses are normally associated with an inflammatory reaction: i.e. early infiltration of the injured tissue by neutrophils and later by lymphocytes and macrophages. Reticulin is deposited within days and this may mature to form collagen, a scar, within 2–3 weeks. In addition healing may involve contraction of the surrounding tissue (in the case of an open wound), by myofibroblasts that may proliferate transiently in relatively large numbers.[9] Thus, normal tissue architecture and function is restored consequent to an entirely appropriate inflammatory reaction with which there has been an associated remodelling process. Each of these stages in normal wound healing and many of the inflammatory cell types and cytokines involved appear also in asthma, but in contrast, both the inflammation and remodelling persist. The consequence of the persistence is exaggerated remodelling inappropriate to the maintenance of normal (airway) function. The reasons for the persistence of the inflammation in the airway wall are unknown but may be the result of repeated inhalation of allergen or exposure to high concentrations of allergen, persistent infection, a genetically influenced abnormal host inflammatory response or a defective repair process.

THE AIRWAY WALL

Two different approaches to the study of asthma in adults have focused attention on the importance of inflammatory processes in the airway wall in the pathogenesis of this condition. Firstly, pharmacological manipulation of the responses to allergens have shown that while the immediate asthmatic response is alleviated by β_2 agonists, the subsequent late phase response to allergen challenge is relatively refractory to these agents and instead responds to corticosteroids.[10] This would indicate that mechanisms other than simple mast-cell degranulation and smooth muscle contraction (which should be blocked by β_2 agonists) are involved in allergen-induced airway obstruction. Secondly, the cellular basis of asthma, the study of which was previously confined to autopsy material, has been revolutionized by the easier, safe access to the airway by application by experienced investigators of fibreoptic bronchoscopy, bronchoalveolar lavage and biopsy.[11]

Bronchial epithelium

The conducting airways are lined by a complex epithelium which, in the larger human airways, appears to be stratified with the most superficial ciliated and mucus-secreting goblet cells being, at least in part, dependent underlying basal cells for their attachment and structural support.[12,13]

The presence of *goblet cells* is confined to larger airways except in asthma and chronic infective disorders where they extend to the bronchioles and contribute to the secretion of mucus which aggravates airway obstruction.[14] The majority of the mucus is secreted into the bronchial lumina from glands deep in the walls of the bronchi which develop from buds of the epithelium (Plate 1). These glands have ducts lined by ciliated epithelium which connect to collecting ducts that drain the secretory acini. The necks of these glands may become enlarged in asthma and have been described as bronchial diverticula or bronchial duct ectasia. Rupture of the ducts has been associated with the development of interstitial emphysema in adult patients with asthma.[15]

The bronchial epithelium has a number of important roles to play in airway homeostasis: to act as a barrier to infective and noxious agents; to actively contribute to host defence mechanisms; to warm and humidify inspired air; and to play a role in inflammatory and neural networks. This major interface between the host and the environment is exposed to a wide variety of insults, including inhaled allergens, viruses and pollutants. The shedding of the bronchial epithelium in asthmatics has been recognized by the presence in the sputum of epithelial clusters such as Creola bodies[16] and the observation that only residual basal cells remain attached to the basement membrane in postmortem histology with the accumulation of sloughed epithelial cells in the bronchial lumen.

The assessment of *epithelial damage* in mild asthma awaited the development of endoscopic biopsies and lavage (Figure 5.1). Although biopsies can be difficult to assess because of forceps-induced damage, the use of rigid bronchoscopy allowed for the demonstration of intraepithelial oedema in the relatively large biopsies taken by this technique.[17] Similar findings were subsequently reported in fibreoptic bronchoscopy biopsies and correlated with the number of eosinophil leukocytes which infiltrated the epithelium.[18] Other workers produced evidence from biopsy, bronchoalveolar lavage and bronchial washings of correlations between epithelial shedding and bronchial hyperreactivity.[11,19,20] There is recent evidence that epithelial disruption may be less severe in non-atopic (intrinsic) asthma.[21]

Loss of superficial epithelium is accompanied by mitotic activity in the remaining epithelial cells in normal healthy individuals.[22] There is repeated epithelial regeneration in the form of simple and then stratified cells prior to restoration of the normal ciliated and goblet-cell phenotypes: experimental studies indicate the

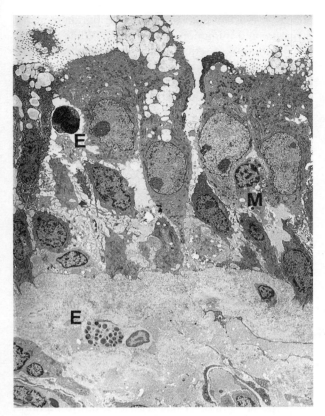

Figure 5.1 *Bronchial biopsy from an asthmatic subject showing intraepithelial oedema, cell separation and inflammatory cells. E: eosinophils; M: mast cell (electron microscopy, ×2200).*

The mechanism of epithelial cell damage can only really be understood in the light of a model of the bronchial epithelium as a truly stratified structure. Bronchoalveolar lavage fluid from asthmatic subjects contains superficial epithelial cells and is usually devoid of basal cells (Plate 2): this is in keeping with autopsy findings of the shedding of superficial columnar epithelial cells with the presence of residual cells on the basement membrane.[27] Furthermore, cells shed into bronchial lavage are viable, as demonstrated by persistent ciliary activity, suggesting that epithelial loss may be related to a specific failure of intercellular adhesion mechanisms rather than generalized cell death.[28] The desmosome is the principal intercellular adhesion structure present at the site of basal-suprabasal cell adhesion and in asthma, epithelial loss may be due to specific loss of desmosomal function.

The pattern of epithelial loss in asthma is consistent with experimental studies involving the exposure of guinea pig epithelium to purified eosinophil leukocyte-derived major basic protein. This induces intraepithelial separation at the basal-suprabasal cell junction at concentrations less than those which cause epithelial cell death.[29] Furthermore, the separation between basal and suprabasal cells is also seen in virus[30] and pollutant-induced epithelial cell damage.[31] In asthma, the eosinophil leukocyte is the most likely effector cell to be involved in this damage and the secretion of granule-derived cationic proteins into the epithelium has been detected by the immunohistochemical demonstration of their persistence in postmortem samples from patients dying of acute severe asthma.[32]

Basement membrane, collagen and elastic tissue

One of the most characteristic histological features of bronchial asthma is an apparent thickening of the bronchial epithelial 'basement membrane'. This is an early event in asthma and occurs in patients with a short clinical history, mild disease and also in children (Figure 5.2 and Plate 3).[33,34,35]

The epithelial reticular basement membrane, to which the epithelium is attached and which has been referred to as the 'true' basement membrane, is about 80 nm thick (i.e. below the resolution of the light microscope) and is composed of non-fibrillar collagen IV, non-collagenous proteins such as laminin and fibronectin, and proteoglycans.[33] The true basement membrane is anchored to underlying connective tissue by fibres that immunostain for collagen VII similar to the arrangement found in skin.[36] Additionally, in humans and primates (but absent from the airways of many laboratory animals used to model asthma) the true basement membrane is supported by an adjacent thicker fibrillary layer, the lamina reticularis or 'reticular basement membrane', normally about 8 μm in thickness (albeit estimates vary dependent

entire process normally takes approximately two weeks.[23] However there are reports that such mitotic activity is deficient in asthma and this has led to the suggestion that there may be defective repair of epithelium in asthma.[24,22] Aggregations of platelets together with fibrillary material, thought to be fibrin have been observed in association with the damaged surface.[25] Such fibrin deposits are also seen during the late phase response following allergen challenge (personal observation). The greater the loss of surface epithelium in biopsy specimens the greater appears to be the degree of airways hyperresponsiveness.[11,25] It is recognized that there is inevitably artefactual loss of surface epithelium during the taking and preparation of such small biopsy pieces, even normally, which makes interpretation of the epithelial loss seen in bronchial biopsies both difficult and controversial.[26]

Such damage to the epithelium may have a number of physiological consequences including the loss of modulation of smooth muscle function, induction of endothelin synthesis, increased permeability to antigens and proinflammatory cytokine production by the epithelium. All of these factors can potentially contribute to the abnormal bronchial microenvironment and find clinical expression as airway obstruction.

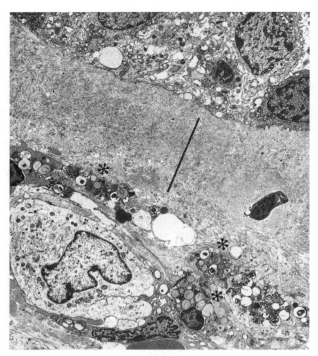

Figure 5.2 *Bronchial biopsy showing subepithelial fibrosis (bar) and eosinophil leukocytes (*) in the mucosa of an asthmatic subject (electron microscopy, ×6000).*

on the technique used to measure it and the processing schedule used to prepare the tissue for analysis) composed largely of reticulin. The thickening remains even when asthma is mild and well controlled by anti-asthma treatment[37] and is present in patients with a long history of asthma but who have not died of their asthma.[38] The thickening is not progressive (as in fibrosis): it is maximal early on in childhood when asthma frequently develops and does not appear to increase significantly with age, duration or with severity of disease.[39]

As with interstitial collagens the reticular basement membrane immunostains for epitopes associated with collagens III and V, and, to a lesser extent, collagen I and this has led to the term 'subepithelial fibrosis' being applied to the layer.[40] Whether or not this represents an ongoing fibrotic process in asthma is much debated. Additionally the reticular basement membrane immunostains for tenascin and fibronectin.[41] The increase and addition of these and other proteins may be responsible for the glassy (hyaline) appearance that also characterizes this layer in asthma. This profile of extracellular matrix deposition indicates a mesenchymal origin for this matrix.

Increased numbers of specialized fibroblasts, referred to as 'bronchial myofibroblasts' have been associated external to the reticular basement membrane.[42] These cells have both secretory and contractile cytoplasmic organelles and increase in number in association with the thickening of the reticular basement membrane.[42] As these fibroblasts can secrete both connective tissue and cytokines relevant to the inflammatory response they

may be important both for their contribution to airway structure and immunopathologically.[43] While the clinical significance of reticular basement membrane thickening in the larger airways (bronchi) has yet to be appreciated, the extension of its thickening to small distal airways (i.e. bronchioles) may be of greater functional significance.

There is no consensus as to whether there is increased interstitial collagen in asthma nor whether it increases with disease severity or duration. A recent study of bronchial biopsies obtained from asthmatics of varying severity reports increased collagen[44] whereas another reports no difference in collagen content.[45] Electron microscopic quantitative assessment of interstitial collagen in biopsies of mild asthmatics found no difference in the area of the mucosa occupied by collagen fibres.[46] There is similar controversy over loss of elastic tissue in asthma, one study demonstrating there is not[46] and others indicating that there is either elastolysis or altered ultrastructure of elastic tissue.[5,47]

Smooth muscle

Bronchial smooth muscle bundles surround the airways as two opposing spirals, forming a perforated network rather than the continuous muscle sheet as seen in the bowel wall. Whether the increase in muscle mass in asthma (Plate 1) is due to muscle fibre proliferation (i.e. hyperplasia)[48] or hypertrophy is at present unclear. Two patterns of distribution of increased muscle mass have been described in asthma: one in which the increase occurs throughout the airways and another in which the increase is restricted to the largest airways:[49,50] it is suggested that in the former there is muscle fibre hypertrophy throughout the bronchial tree, in the latter hyperplasia alone.

A newly proposed mechanism involves de-differentiation of existing smooth muscle bundles. Cells that have ultrastructural features of both a contractile and secretory phenotype have been found in substantial numbers in the late phase response to allergen challenge. It has been suggested that, with repeated exposure to allergen, these may contribute to the increased mass of bronchial smooth muscle by a process of differentiation of existing smooth muscle and its migration to a subepithelial site where new muscle is formed.[51] The mechanisms involved in this response are likely to be similar to those occurring in atherosclerosis where there is vascular smooth muscle de-differentiation and migration to form a neo-intima composed of increased vascular smooth muscle.[52,7]

The extent of airway smooth muscle plasticity and the secretory potential and role of muscle in airway inflammation and remodelling has recently become apparent. Not only can the contractile form release proinflammatory mediators[53] but reversion of muscle to a 'secretory' phenotype may promote increases of extracellular matrix.[54,55]

The increase in muscle mass is associated with increased airway responsiveness to histamine or methacholine in asthma (see Chapter 6c). Careful computer modelling of the response to bronchial challenge in asthma has shown that the loss of the plateau exhibited by normal subjects and the continued narrowing of the airways with increasing doses of provocant can be predicted by a model which takes two factors into account – airway thickening and a loss of pulmonary recoil.[56] These factors may operate by uncoupling airway and parenchymal structures leading to unopposed shortening of airway smooth muscle which acting upon a thickened airway wall results in excessive airway narrowing (Figure 6c.11). Thus, bronchial wall thickening may be of considerable importance in determining not only the degree of bronchial hyperreactivity but also its potentially fatal nature. Mast-cell infiltration of ASM may be a unique feature of asthma.[57]

Inflammation may spill over to affect adjacent arteries and alveoli.[58] Peribronchial inflammation likely disrupts the normal interdependence of the airways and their adjacent lung parenchyma, lead to 'uncoupling' of the airways, so that the elastic force opposing airway smooth muscle shortening is reduced leading to excessive maximal airway narrowing. Experimentally, this sort of uncoupling has been demonstrated in guinea pigs exposed *in utero* to passive smoking.[59]

Airway wall vessels

The increase in thickness of the bronchial wall in severe asthma is not accounted for by the increase in bronchial smooth muscle and mucous gland mass alone. Dilatation of bronchial mucosal blood vessels, congestion and wall oedema are also consistently reported features of fatal asthma and these can account for considerable swelling of the airway wall that encroaches on the lumen.[60,61,62] Vasodilatation, congestion and mucosal oedema in response to a variety of mediators of inflammation[63] can be rapid and, equally, probably can also be relatively rapidly reversed. There are indications that there may also be new growth of bronchial vessels that contributes to an increase in vascularity of the airway wall, particularly in severe asthma.[64,65] It is from these vessels that inflammatory cells are recruited to the wall, many of which migrate through the mucosa and its epithelium to enter the airway lumen.

INFLAMMATION

The bronchi have a constitutive population of mast cells, T-lymphocytes, B-lymphocytes and occasional granulocytes which clearly contribute to normal host defence. The cellular infiltrate in asthma is composed of an augmented T-cell population, markedly increased numbers of eosinophils[66] and in some circumstances, an influx of neutrophils.[67] Although the accumulation of inflammatory cells in the bronchial mucosa has long been associated with fatal asthma,[27] there is consistent evidence from recent studies that a similar inflammatory population is present even in mild disease. For good clinical and ethical reasons, relatively little is known of the nature and development of the inflammatory process in the asthmatic airway in childhood, although there are some data to indicate that processes similar to adult disease are active in established asthma in childhood.[34]

T-lymphocytes

The constitutive T-lymphocyte population in the adult bronchus shows at most a small increase in asthma.[66,67] These cells are CD3$^+$ (Plate 4), CD45RO$^+$ and are mainly CD4$^+$, indicating that they are helper T-cells that have had previous exposure to antigen. There is evidence that in asthma the T-cell population is activated to a greater extent than in non-asthmatic subjects, as evidenced by the expression of the interleukin-2 receptor marker CD25.[66] The T-lymphocytes are not confined to the lamina propria but also infiltrate the epithelium, which may enhance their exposure to antigen and also be important in the generation of chemotactic gradients for other cells in the inflammatory infiltrate.

Many of the functions of T-lymphocytes are mediated by cytokines which are produced by gene transcription and translation in response to antigenic stimulation. There is increasing evidence for the division of the cytokine secretion profile of human helper T-cells into two categories – the Th1 cell pattern with the secretion of IL-2, TNF-α, IFN-γ, GMCSF, and the Th2 pattern with the secretion of IL-4, IL-5, IL-6, TNFα and GMCSF[68] (see Chapter 4c).

The Th2 phenotype would appear to be relevant to allergic bronchial asthma, as the range of cytokines secreted favours the production of IgE by the effect of interleukin-4 on B cells,[69] eosinophil leukocyte production, recruitment, survival and activation by the combined effects of GMCSF and interleukin-5.[70,71] *In situ* hybridization for m-RNA in bronchoalveolar lavage cells has shown an excess of cells positive for interleukin-2, -3, -4, -5 and GMCSF in asthmatic subjects and no difference in cells with interferon-γ message.[72] Thus, the observed range of T-cell cytokines associated with asthma does not entirely fit the proposed Th2 phenotype but the data are clearly in accordance with the view that the T-lymphocyte plays an important role in the pathogenesis of the mucosal inflammation of the bronchi.

Biopsy data indicate that there is a correlation between T-cell number and eosinophil leukocyte infiltration of the airways,[66] suggesting either that eosinophil recruitment is T-lymphocyte dependent or that these cells share common recruitment mechanisms in order to enter the airways.[73] Studies of atopic non-asthmatic individuals have shown T-lymphocyte number and activation and eosinophil recruitment at levels between those found in normal and asthmatic subjects, suggesting that there may be a critical threshold above which these allergen-mediated events find clinical expression.[66,67] The time and site of selection of the T-lymphocytes for the observed range of cytokine messages is uncertain and this knowledge is central to any proposed intervention to reduce sensitization to aeroallergens or to attempt to treat disease early in life in order to prevent the subsequent development of asthma.

Mast cells

The application of the tools of modern biology has greatly expanded the knowledge of the human mast cell (MC). Human mast cells may be divided into two types, based on the content of neutral proteases in their granules.[74] Mast cells which contain tryptase, a tetrameric trypsin-like protease, in their granules are termed MC_T while those which also possess chymase, carboxypeptidase-A and cathepsin-G are called MC_{TC}. The biological role of these proteases is uncertain but tryptase is present in large amounts in the mast cell (10 pg/cell in lung) and can enhance the effect of histamine on smooth muscle,[75] activate the collagenase system and enhance fibroblast proliferation.[76] Chymase can generate angiotensin II from angiotensin I, inactivate bradykinin, enhance mucus production and degrade basement membranes.[77,78,79]

Both types of mast cell are present in the bronchus and they secrete potent inflammatory mediators such as histamine, prostaglandin D_2 and leukotriene C_4 in response to antigen stimulation and also release proteoglycan heparin which stabilizes the tryptase tetramer and promotes the action of fibroblast growth factors. Mast cells can also contribute to the cytokine network in the mucosa by the synthesis of tumour necrosis factor-α and interleukin-3, -4, -5, and -6 (Plate 5).[80] Thus, the mast cell must now be regarded as both a rapid response cell and a contributor to the chronic inflammation and airway remodelling which are characteristic of asthma.

The evidence for mast-cell activation in asthma is based on the detection of histamine in lavage fluid[81] and ultrastructural and immunohistochemical studies. Mast cells do not increase in number in the bronchial wall in asthma but in the disease state they infiltrate the bronchial epithelium.[82] This relocation of cells is accompanied by a characteristic ultrastructural appearance of the mast-cell granules which show dissolution of their electron-dense cores and partial degranulation. Little is known of the mechanisms of reconstitution of human mast-cell granules and the biological interpretation of the ultrastructural appearances in asthma is uncertain, as are the relative proportion of mediators and the absolute composition of granules with this appearance. The

location of mast cells within sensitized smooth muscle bundles has also been described in asthma and may contribute to the bronchial hyperresponsiveness of the atopic asthmatic.[57,83]

The control of mast-cell phenotype appears to be largely governed by the cytokine stem cell factor, which regulates the production of mast-cell precursors from stem cells and their subsequent differentiation into MC_{TC}.[84] This is largely a fibroblast-derived cytokine and there may be an interplay between mast cells and their surrounding mesenchymal cells with the production of trophic factors essential for mutual survival and function.[85,86] In contrast, the MC_T-cell is largely dependent on T-lymphocyte function[87] and again, the capacity for cytokine secretion by the mast cell may mean that this interaction is also based on a two-way exchange of signals.

Eosinophils

The infiltration of the bronchial mucosa by eosinophilic polymorphonuclear leukocytes is characteristic of asthma in all ages. However, there is a large range in the number of eosinophils detected by immunohistology in tissues from cases of fatal asthma suggesting there is heterogeneity of the asthma phenotype or that the eosinophils have degranulated extensively.[88,89] These cells are practically absent from the mucosa of normal subjects but can form an almost uniform sheet of cells in the mucosa of patients with severe asthma (Figure 5.2). This finding has clinical relevance in that there appears to be a relationship between the number of eosinophils and the severity of disease as measured by symptom scores and drug usage.[90] In contrast, there appear to be fewer neutrophils in the mucosa of stable asthmatics than are seen in normal individuals.[11,25]

The pathogenetic mechanisms of the eosinophil are due to the secretion of *mediators* which can be divided into three classes: the lipid-derived mediators which induce acute inflammatory responses; the cytotoxic granule components; and the proinflammatory cytokines. Eosinophils secrete platelet-activating factor (PAF), which is in itself an eosinophil chemoattractant and activator. PAF also increases vascular permeability and induces smooth muscle spasm and may thus contribute to airway obstruction. Eosinophils are also major producers of leukotriene C_4 and also produce prostaglandin E_2 and 15-lipoxygenase products, including 15-HETE, which contribute to further inflammation and secretion of mucus.[91]

The characteristic granules of eosinophils contain high concentrations of toxic proteins, including eosinophil cationic protein, major basic protein, eosinophil-derived neurotoxin and eosinophil peroxidase. Major basic protein, which forms the characteristic cores of eosinophil granules, is toxic to a variety of cells, including bronchial epithelial cells, at concentrations that are achieved *in vivo* and has been detected in association with epithelial damage in asthmatics.[32] Eosinophil cationic protein (Plate 6) is also toxic to epithelial cells and this protein shares with major basic protein and eosinophil peroxidase the capacity to induce histamine release from mast cells.[92] Eosinophil peroxidase induces oxidative damage to cells in the presence of hydrogen peroxide and a halide and may also contribute to the cell damage seen in asthma. Eosinophils express message for a range of cytokines, including tumour necrosis factor-α, transforming growth factors α and β, interleukin-1 and GMCSF.[93,94,95] The secretion of these cytokines can directly and indirectly by interactions with other cells in the mucosal cytokine network, enhance eosinophil recruitment, survival and activation, leading to the perpetuation of the allergic inflammatory process.

Neutrophils

Neutrophil infiltration, which has hitherto been neglected in asthma, is now seen also as a major feature of acute exacerbations of asthma[96] and is a predominant cell type in severe steroid resistant asthma[97,98] and acute sudden onset fatal asthma.[89] It is uncertain whether this pattern of cellular infiltrate is the result of corticosteroid treatment *per se* or the result of virus or allergen exposure which may have induced a neutrophilic response.

Cellular recruitment

The presence of an excessive number of cells within a biopsy specimen is not necessarily evidence of increased cellular recruitment. The histological appearances of an inflammatory cell infiltrate may be the result of increased numbers of circulating cells, up-regulation or newly expressed chemoattractants or their cell surface receptors, increased survival within the tissue compartment or decreased traffic into another compartment, i.e. the bronchial lumen. Equally, increased recruitment but with increased traffic through the tissue will not be detectable in a biopsy specimen.

Nevertheless, there is considerable evidence for increased inflammatory cell recruitment into the bronchial mucosa in asthma. Ultrastructural studies have identified increased contact between intravascular leukocytes and the endothelium in asthma.[11] This probably reflects the rolling of leukocytes along the endothelium which is mediated by the vascular selectins.[99] P selectin is stored in Weibel–Palade granules in endothelial cells and is expressed on the surface within minutes of stimulation, while the expression of E selectin is slower due to the need to induce synthesis prior to expression.[100] The selectin-mediated contact allows for further steps, including the interaction of leukocyte integrins with the immunoglobulin supergene family of adhesion molecules (ICAM-1, ICAM-2 and VCAM-1) on the endothelium and the action of chemoattractants which promote migration through the endothelium and within the extravascular compartment.[101]

The selective accumulation of eosinophils in allergic asthma is the result of a variety of processes. The expression of VCAM-1 on the endothelium allows for the selective binding of cells which express the β_2 integrin VLA-4 and thus enhances the recruitment of eosinophils; T-cells and basophils.[73] Although VCAM-1 can be selectively induced on the endothelium by interleukin-4, it is also expressed in response to the pleiotropic cytokines such as tumour necrosis factor-a which also induce the non-specific ligands E selectin and ICAM-1 which have been demonstrated in the bronchial mucosa *in vivo*.[102] Further selective mechanisms include the capacity of platelet-activating factor to selectively induce the migration of eosinophils and not neutrophils through the vascular endothelium by a mechanism which does not require selective adhesion mechanisms.[103] Similarly, the highly potent chemokine family includes chemoattractants which are selective for CD4$^+$ cells, including eosinophils, but not neutrophils. The presence of neutrophils (and also of monocytes) in response to an acute severe exacerbation is likely due to the upregulation of cell surface (CXCR2) receptors associated with increased expression of neutrophil chemoattractants such as IL8.

Once present in the tissues, the eosinophils (or other cell types) accumulate beneath the bronchial basement membrane in large numbers and from this site infiltrate the epithelium. This accumulation of eosinophils may be in part due to the potential for both fibroblast and epithelial-derived cytokines to enhance cell survival at this site. The subsequent migration into the epithelium may be the result of chemoattractants secreted by either epithelial cells or the intraepithelial T-lymphocytes and mast cells.[101,104,105]

CHILDHOOD, INFANCY AND LUNG DEVELOPMENT

There are three salient questions concerning the pathogenesis of asthma in early life. Firstly, are the cellular mechanisms underlying atopic asthma in these children identical to those encountered in adults? Secondly, if so, when do the structural airway changes which contribute to the pathogenesis occur and when do they become irreversible? Thirdly, how do these mechanisms differ from those which contribute to non-atopic wheeze (such as viral episodic wheeze in infancy)?

Lung development

The reticular basement membrane appears to be absent in the fetus (at least up to 18 weeks of gestation)[106] but develops even in normal, healthy non-smoking individuals, presumably during early childhood. Its thickening in asthma begins early,[39] even before asthma is diagnosed.[107] The increased thickening in adult asthma involves increases in tenascin and certain laminins and tenascin are involved in normal lung development but are down-regulated in the adult lung. It is possible that abnormal persistence of these basement membrane-associated molecules could underlie some of the pathogenic processes in early asthma.[108]

The number of alveoli increases rapidly in the first two years of extrauterine life to reach near-adult values followed by a further lower rate of increase until 8 years of age, accompanied by a similar increase in the number of small airways.[109] Studies of airway conductance, based on morphometric analysis of lungs obtained at post mortem, suggest that in the first four years of life the diameter of the small airways and hence their conductance is relatively low but this increases after five years.[110,111]

Taken together, these studies would appear to indicate that the distal (peripheral), but not central, airway conductance in infants and preschool children is not due to smaller numbers of airways but to the relatively low cross-sectional area of the bronchioles. This anatomical pattern of development is probably the structural basis of the observation that in the first five years of life inflammation in the airways is likely to predispose to bronchiolar obstruction and may explain some of the difficulties in the distinction between classic asthma and episodes of viral lower respiratory tract wheeze in this group. In addition, events at birth may also influence the remodelling process: e.g. prematurity and mechanical ventilation are associated with increases of bronchial smooth muscle and of mucus-secreting elements.[112]

Preschool child and infancy

Little is known of the cellular and molecular pathophysiology of wheezing illnesses in the preschool child and infant. Bronchial lavages from persistently wheezy young children (mean age 15 months) show mark hypercellularity, but no excess of eosinophils or mast cells. Episodic viral wheezers also differ from atopic preschool wheezers in having no excess of eosinophils.[113] It would seem that eosinophilic infiltration may be less prominent in the airways of children than adults with asthma.[113,114,115]

The importance of the conducting airways as a site of disease in early life is emphasized by the virtual restriction of the occurrence of episodic viral lower respiratory illness to childhood. The overlapping features of acute viral bronchiolitis and asthma are not confined to the clinical presentation but have a biological basis in both the pulmonary anatomy and the inflammatory reactions which occur in the bronchi. There is evidence from both human and experimental virus infections that the inflammatory response to lower respiratory tract infection may involve both mast cells and eosinophils. Sendai virus infection of neonatal rats has been reported to induce persistent increases in airway mast cells and hyperresponsiveness to methacholine.[116] Respiratory syncytial virus (RSV) infections with associated wheezing have been reported to be associated with levels of eosinophil cationic protein in nasopharyngeal secretions that are four- to five-fold in excess of the levels found in upper or lower respiratory RSV infections without wheeze.[117] This may be explained by the bias in selection of patients with severe RSV infections, towards the atopic phenotype and could relate simply to atopy.

Such responses may be the result of inappropriate selection of the T-cell cytokine repertoire in response to viral infection with the secretion of a Th2 pattern of cytokines and the initiation of a pattern of inflammation in the airways that is normally associated with allergic disease rather than the T-lymphocyte-mediated response to a pathogen. If so, the inappropriate response may be a reflection of delayed maturation of the immune system. But whether viral infections can thus imprint an abnormal response on the airway mucosa and contribute to the development of asthma has yet to be established. Nevertheless, the combination of such inflammation with the documented anatomical vulnerability of the bronchiole to obstruction in young children may explain the difficulty in differentiating between infectious and allergic wheezing in infancy.

Childhood

The morphological features of atopic asthma in children of school-going age are probably similar to those encountered in adults, with mucus plugging, inflammatory cell infiltration, mast-cell degranulation and thickening of the reticular basement membrane in both open lung biopsy and autopsy specimens.[34] Epithelial damage is also reported in asthmatic children.[34,114,118] Schoolchildren with asthma symptoms tend to have greater numbers of eosinophils and mast cells in induced sputum samples than normal children or children with asymptomatic bronchial hyperresponsiveness,[119] suggesting that these cells also play a role in the pathogenesis of mild asthma in childhood. Bronchoalveolar lavage of asthmatic children in this age group has shown statistical associations between bronchial responsiveness to inhaled histamine and eosinophil numbers and mast-cell tryptase concentrations in lavage fluid.[120]

SUMMARY AND CONCLUSIONS

Bronchial asthma is a chronic inflammatory disorder of the conducting airways in which T-helper lymphocytes predominate. The clinical features of asthma are the end result of variable obstruction of the conducting airways by varying combinations of inflammation, vascular congestion, airway wall oedema, increased mass of bronchial smooth muscle and its contraction and accumulation of debris and mucus in the lumen. Many of the cytokines and growth factors thought to be proinflammatory in asthma are also expressed normally but transiently without detriment to the developing lung: indeed they appear to be essential to it. It is the persistence of inflammation that characterizes asthma. The process of 'remodelling' *per se*, which may or not be a consequence of chronic inflammation, is not necessarily abnormal. It may be appropriate when transient and in response to injury during lung development or 'inappropriate' when it is chronic and associated with abnormally altered tissue structure and function, as in asthma. There is fragility and shedding of the bronchial epithelium in asthma, thickening of the epithelial reticular basement membrane and an increase in the mass of airway smooth muscle. Whether the increase in muscle mass in asthma is due to muscle fibre proliferation (i.e. hyperplasia) or hypertrophy is at present unclear. There may also be a process of differentiation of existing smooth muscle and its migration to a subepithelial site where new muscle is formed. Dilatation of bronchial mucosal blood vessels, congestion and wall oedema are also consistently reported features of fatal asthma and these can account for considerable swelling of the airway wall that reduces lumenal patency. The cellular infiltrate in asthma is composed of an augmented T-cell population, markedly increased numbers of eosinophils and, in severe disease and exacerbations, an influx of neutrophils.

The limited data that are available indicate that the morphological features of atopic asthma in children of school-going age are similar to those encountered in adults, with mucus plugging, inflammatory cell infiltration, mast-cell degranulation and thickening of the reticular basement membrane. Thickening of the reticular basement membrane in asthmatics begins early even before asthma is diagnosed. Little is known of the cellular and molecular pathophysiology of wheezing illnesses in the preschool child and infant. New data from biopsies, BAL and sputum in this early age group are beginning to be published and will prove to be invaluable in unravelling the origins of asthma and, no doubt, its relationship to atopy and infection.

REFERENCES

1. Barnes PJ. A new approach to the treatment of asthma. *New Engl J Med* 1989;**321**:1517–27.
2. Global Initiative for Asthma. *Global strategy for asthma management and prevention.* NHLBI/WHO workshop report (based on a March 1993 meeting). National Heart, Lung and Blood Institute, 1995, p. 1.
3. Djukanovic R, Roche WR, Wilson JW, *et al.* Mucosal inflammation in asthma. *Am Rev Respir Dis* 1990;**142**:434–57.
4. Bai TR. Abnormalities in airway smooth muscle in fatal asthma. *Am Rev Respir Dis* 1990;**141**:552–7.
5. Bousquet J, Jeffery PK, Busse WW, Johnson M, Vignola AM. Asthma. From bronchoconstriction to airways inflammation and remodelling. *Am J Respir Crit Care Med* 2000;**161**:1720–45.
6. Pare PD, Roberts CR, Bai TR, Wiggs BJ. The functional consequences of airway remodelling in asthma. *Monaldi Arch Chest Dis* 1997;**52**:589–96.
7. Jeffery PK. Remodelling in asthma and COPD. *Am J Respir Crit Care Med* 2001;**164**:2220–8.
8. Warburton D, Schwarz M, Tefft D, Flores-Delgado G, Anderson KD, Cardoso WV. The molecular basis of lung morphogenesis. *Mech Dev* 2000;**92**:55–81.
9. Serini G, Gabbiani G. Mechanisms of myofibroblast activity and phenotypic modulation. *Exp Cell Res* 1999;**250**:273–83.
10. Cockcroft DW, Murdock KY. Comparative effects of inhaled salbutamol, sodium cromoglycate, and beclomethasone dipropionate on allergen-induced early asthmatic responses, late asthmatic responses, and increased bronchial responsiveness to histamine. *J All Clin Immunol* 1987;**79**:734–40.
11. Beasley R, Roche WR, Roberts JA, Holgate ST. Cellular events in the bronchi in mild asthma and after bronchial provocation. *Am Rev Respir Dis* 1989;**139**:806–13.
12. Evans MJ, Cox RA, Shami SG, Wilson B, Plopper CG. The role of basal cells in attachment of columnar cells to the basal lamina of the trachea. *Am J Respir Cell Mol Biol* 1989;**1**:463–9.
13. Evans MJ, Plopper CG. The role of basal cells in adhesion of columnar epithelium of airway basement membrane. *Am Rev Respir Dis* 1989;**138**:481–3.
14. Thurlbeck WM, Malaka D, Murphy K. Goblet cells in the peripheral airways in chronic bronchitis. *Am Rev Respir Dis* 1975;**112**:65–9.
15. Cluroe A, Holloway L, Thomson K, Purdie G, Beasley R. Bronchial gland duct ectasia in fatal bronchial asthma: association with interstitial emphysema. *J Clin Pathol* 1989;**42**:1026–31.
16. Naylor B. The shedding of the mucosal of the bronchial tree in asthma. *Thorax* 1962;**7**:69–72.
17. Laitinen LA, Heino M, Laitinen A, Kava T, Haahtela T. Damage to the airway epithelium and bronchial reactivity in patients with asthma. *Am Rev Respir Dis* 1985;**131**:599–606.
18. Ohashi Y, Motojima S, Fukuda T, Makino S. Airway hyperresponsiveness, increased intracellular spaces of bronchial epithelium, and increased infiltration of eosinophils and lymphocytes in bronchial mucosa in asthma. *Am Rev Respir Dis* 1992;**145**:1469–76.
19. Wardlaw AJ, Dunnette S, Gleich GJ, Collins JV, Kay AB. Eosinophils and mast cells in bronchoalveolar lavage in subjects with mild asthma. *Am Rev Respir Dis* 1988;**137**:62–9.

20. Jeffery PK, Wardlaw AJ, Nelson FC, Collins JV, Kay AB. Bronchial biopsies in asthma. An ultrastructural, quantitative study and correlation with hyperreactivity. *Am Rev Respir Dis* 1989;**140**:1745–53.

21. Amin K, Ludviksdottir D, Janson C *et al*. Inflammation and structural changes in the airways of patients with atopic and nonatopic asthma. *Am J Respir Crit Care Med* 2000;**162**:2295–301.

22. Holgate ST. Epithelial damage and response. *Clin Exp Allergy* 2000;**30**(Suppl 1):37–41.

23. Wilhelm DL. Regeneration of tracheal epithelium. *J Pathol* 1953;**65**:543–50.

24. Holgate ST, Lackie PM, Davies DE, Roche WR, Walls AF. The bronchial epithelium as a key regulator of airway inflammation and remodelling in asthma. *Clin Exp Allergy* 1999;**29**(Suppl 2):90–5.

25. Jeffery PK, Wardlaw A, Nelson FC, Collins JV, Kay AB. Bronchial biopsies in asthma: an ultrastructural quantification study and correlation with hyperreactivity. *Am Rev Respir Dis* 1989;**140**:1745–53.

26. Ordonez C, Ferrando R, Hyde DM, Wong HH, Fahy JV. Epithelial desquamation in asthma. Artifact or pathology? *Am J Respir Crit Care Med* 2000;**162**:2324–9.

27. Dunnill MS. The pathology of asthma, with special reference to changes in the bronchial mucosa. *J Clin Pathol* 1960;**13**:27–33.

28. Montefort S, Roberts JA, Beasley R, Holgate ST, Roche WR. The site of disruption of the bronchial epithelium in asthmatic and non-asthmatic subjects. *Thorax* 1992;**47**:499–503.

29. Frigas SE, Loegering DA, Gleich GJ. Cytotoxic effects of the guinea pig major basic protein on tracheal epithelium. *Lab Invest* 1980;**42**:35–43.

30. Hers JFP. Disturbances of the ciliated epithelium due to the influenza virus. *Am Rev Respir Dis* 1966;**93**:162–71.

31. Abdi S, Evans MJ, Cox RA, *et al*. Inhalation injury to tracheal epithelium in an ovine model of cotton smoke exposure. Early phase (30 minutes). *Am Rev Respir Dis* 1990;**142**:1436–9.

32. Filley WV, Holley KE, Kephart GM, Gleich GJ. Identification by immuno-fluorescence of eosinophil major basic protein in lung tissues of patients with bronchial asthma. *Lancet* 1982;**i**:11–16.

33. Roche WR, Beasley R, Williams JH, Holgate ST. Subepithelial fibrosis in the bronchi of asthmatics. *Lancet* 1989;**i**:520–4.

34. Cutz E, Levison H, Cooper DM. Ultrastructure of airways in children with asthma. *Histopathology* 1978;**2**:407–21.

35. Saetta MJ, Di Stefano A, Maestrelli P, *et al*. Airway mucosal inflammation in occupational asthma induced by toluene diisocyanate. *Am Rev Respir Dis* 1992;**145**:160–8.

36. Wetzels RHW, Robben HCM, Leigh AM, *et al*. Distribution patterns of type VII collagen in normal and malignant tissues. *Am J Pathol* 1991;**139**:451–9.

37. O'Shaughnessy TC, Ansari TW, Barnes NC, Jeffery PK. Reticular basement membrane thickness in moderately severe asthma and smokers' chronic bronchitis with and without airflow obstruction. *Am J Respir Crit Care Med* 1996;**153**:A879 (abstract).

38. Sobonya RE. Quantitative structural alterations in long-standing allergic asthma. *Am Rev Respir Dis* 1984;**130**:289–92.

39. Payne D, Rogers A, Adelroth E, Guntapaldi K, Bush A, Jeffery PK. Reticular basement membrane thickness in children with difficult asthma. *Am J Respir Crit Care Med* 2001;**163**:A19 (abstract).

40. Roche WR, Beasley R, Williams JH, Holgate ST. Subepithelial fibrosis in the bronchi of asthmatics. *Lancet* 1989;**1**:520–3.

41. Laitinen A, Altraja A, Kampe M, Linden M, Virtanen I, Laitinen L. Tenascin is increased in airway basement membrane of asthmatics and decreased by an inhaled steroid. *Am J Respir Crit Care Med* 1997;**56**(3 Pt 1):951–8.

42. Brewster CEP, Howarth PH, Djukanovic R, *et al*. Myofibroblasts and subepithelial fibrosis in bronchial asthma. *Am J Respir Cell Mol Biol* 1990;**3**:507–11.

43. Roche WR. Fibroblasts and asthma. *Clin Exp Allergy* 1991;**21**:545–8.

44. Minshall EM, Leung DYM, Martin RJ, *et al*. Eosinophil-associated TGF-beta1 mRNA expression and airways fibrosis in bronchial asthma. *Am J Respir Cell Mol Biol* 1997;**17**:326–33.

45. Chu HW, Halliday JL, Martin RJ, Leung DYM, Szefler SJ, Wenzel SE. Collagen deposition in large airways may not differentiate severe asthma from milder forms of the disease. *Am J Respir Crit Care Med* 1998;**158**:1936–44.

46. Jeffery P, Godfrey RWA, Adelroth E, Nelson F, Rogers A, Johansson S-A. Effects of treatment on airway inflammation and thickening of reticular collagen in asthma: a quantitative light and electron microscopic study. *Am Rev Respir Dis* 1992;**145**:890–9.

47. Mauad T, Xavier AC, Saldiva PH, Dolhnikoff M. Elastosis and fragmentation of fibers of the elastic system in fatal asthma. *Am J Respir Crit Care Med* 1999;**160**:968–75.

48. Heard BE, Hossain S. Hyperplasia of bronchial muscle in asthma. *J Pathol* 1983;**110**:319–31.

49. Ebina M, Yaegashi H, Chiba R, Takahashi T, Motomiya M, Tanemura M. Hyperreactive site in the airway tree of asthmatic patients revealed by thickening of bronchial muscles. *Am Rev Respir Dis* 1990;**141**:1327–32.

50. Ebina M, Takahashi T, Chiba T, Motomiya M. cellular hypertrophy and hyperplasia of airway smooth muscles underlying bronchial asthma – a 3-D morphometric study. *Am Rev Respir Dis* 1993;**148**:720–6.

51. Gizycki MJ, Adelroth E, Rogers AV, O'Byrne PM, Jeffery PK. Myofibroblast involvement in the allergen-induced late response in mild atopic asthma. *Am J Respir Cell Mol Biol* 1997;**16**:664–73.

52. Jeffery PK. Structural changes in asthma. In: C Page, J Black, eds. *Airways and Vascular Remodelling in Asthma and Cardiovascular Disease*. Academic Press, London, 1994, pp. 3–19.

53. John M, Hirst JS, Jose PJ, *et al*. Human airway smooth muscle cells express and release RANTES in response to T helper 1 cytokines. *J Immunol* 1997;**158**:1841–7.

54. Halayko AJ, Camoretti-Mercado B, Forsythe SM, *et al*. Divergent differentiation paths in airway smooth muscle culture: induction of functionally contractile myocytes. *Am J Physiol* 1999;**276**:L197–L206.

55. Hirst SJ. Airway smooth muscle cell culture: application to studies of airway wall remodelling and phenotype plasticity in asthma. *Eur Respir J* 1996;**9**:808–20.

56. Wiggs BR, Bosken C, Pare PD, James A, Hogg JC. A model of airway narrowing in asthma and in chronic obstructive pulmonary disease. *Am Rev Respir Dis* 1992;**145**:1251–8.

57. Brightling CE, Bradding P, Symon FA, Holgate ST, Wardlaw AJ, Parord ID. Mast cell infiltration of airway smooth muscle in asthma. *NEJM* 2002; **346**:1699–705.

58. Saetta M, Di Stefano A, Rosina C, Thiene G, Fabbri LM. Quantitative structural analysis of peripheral airways and arteries in sudden fatal asthma. *Am Rev Respir Dis* 1991;**143**:138–43.

59. Elliot J, Caroll N, Bosco M, McCrohan M, Robinson P. Increased airway responsiveness and decreased alveolar attachment points following in utero smoke exposure in the guinea pig. *Am J Respir Crit Care Med* 2001;**163**:140–4.

60. Carroll NG, Cooke C, James AL. Bronchial blood vessel dimensions in asthma. *Am J Respir Crit Care Med* 1997;**155**:689–95.

61. Kuwano K, Bosken CH, Pare PD, Bai TR, Wiggs BR, Hogg JC. Small airways dimensions in asthma and in chronic obstructive pulmonary disease. *Am J Respir Crit Care Med* 1993;**148**:1220–3.

62. Lambert RK, Wiggs BR, Kuwano K, Hogg JC, Pare PD. Functional significance of increased airway smooth muscle in asthma and COPD. *J Appl Physiol* 1991;**74**:2771–81.

63. Widdicombe J. New perspectives on basic mechanisms in lung disease: 4. Why are the airways so vascular? *Thorax* 1998;**48**:290–5.

64. Vrugt B, Wilson S, Bron A, Holgate ST, Djukanovic R, Aalbers R. Bronchial angiogenesis is severe glucocorticosteroid-dependant asthma. *Eur Respir J* 2000;**15**:1014–21 (abstract).

65. Charan NB, Baile EM, Pare PD. Bronchial vascular congestion and angiogenesis. *Eur Respir J* 1997;**10**:1173–80.

66. Bradley BL, Azzawi M, Jacobson M, *et al*. Eosinophils, T-lymphocytes, mast cells, neutrophils and macrophages in bronchial biopsy specimens from atopic subjects with asthma: comparison with biopsy specimens from atopic subjects without asthma and normal control subjects and relationship to bronchial hyperresponsiveness. *J All Clin Immunol* 1991;**88**:661–74.

67. Djukanovic R, Lai CWK, Wilson JW, *et al*. Bronchial mucosal manifestations of atopy: a comparison of markers of inflammation between atopic asthmatics, atopic non-asthmatics and healthy controls. *Eur Respir J* 1992;**5**:538–44.

68. Romagnani S. Human Th1 and Th2 sub-sets: doubt no more. *Immunol Today* 1991;**12**:256–7.

69. Del Prete G, Maggi E, Parronchi P, *et al*. IL-4 is an essential factor for the IgE synthesis induced *in vitro* by human T-cell clones and their supernatants. *J Immunol* 1988;**140**:4193–8.

70. Silberstein DS, Owen WF, Gasson JC, *et al*. Enhancement of human eosinophil cytotoxicity and leukotriene synthesis by biosynthetic (recombinant) granulocyte-macrophage colony-stimulating factor. *J Immunol* 1986;**137**:3290–4.

71. Lopez AF, Sanderson CJ, Gamble JR, *et al*. Recombinant human interleukin 5 is a selective activator of human eosinophil function. *J Exp Med* 1988;**167**:219–24.

72. Robinson DS, Hamid Q, Sun Y, *et al*. Predominant Th2-like bronchoalveolar T-lymphocyte population in atopic asthma. *New Engl J Med* 1992;**326**:298–304.

73. Dobrina A, Menegazzi R, Carlos TM, *et al*. Mechanisms of eosinophil adherence to cultured vascular endothelial cells. Eosinophils bind to the cytokine-induced endothelial ligand vascular cell adhesion molecule-1 via the very late activation antigen-4 integrin receptor. *J Clin Invest* 1991;**88**:20–6.

74. Irani AA, Schwartz LB. Neutral proteases as indicators of human mast cell heterogeneity. *Monogr All* 1990;**27**:146–62.

75. Sekizawa K, Caughey GH, Lazarus SC, Gold WM, Nadel JA. Mast cell tryptase causes airway smooth muscle hyperresponsiveness in dogs. *J Clin Invest* 1989;**83**:175–9.

76. Ruoss SJ, Hartmann T, Caughey GH. Mast cell tryptase is a mitogen for cultured fibroblasts. *J Clin Invest* 1991;**88**:493–9.

77. Reilly CF, Tewksbury DA, Schechter NM, Travis J. Rapid conversion of angiotensin I to angiotensin II by neutrophil and mast cell proteinases. *J Biol Chem* 1982;**257**:8619–22.

78. Briggaman RA, Schechter NM, Fraki J, Lazarus GS. Degradation of the epidermal–dermal junction by a proteolytic enzyme from human skin and human polymorphonuclear leukocytes. *J Exp Med* 1984;**160**:1027–42.

79. Sommerhoff CP, Caughey GH, Finkbeiner WE, *et al.* Mast cell chymase. A potent secretagogue for airway gland serous cells. *J Immunol* 1989;**142**:2450–6.

80. Bradding P, Roberts JA, Britten KM, *et al.* Interleukin-4, -5, and -6 and tumour necrosis factor-α in normal and asthmatic airways: evidence for the human mast cell as a source of these cytokines. *Am J Respir Cell Mol Biol* 1994;**10**:471–80.

81. Agius RM, Godfrey RC, Holgate ST. Mast cell and histamine content of human bronchoalveolar lavage fluid. *Thorax* 1985;**40**:760–7.

82. Djukanovic R, Wilson JW, Britten KM, *et al.* Quantitation of mast cells and eosinophils in the bronchial mucosa of symptomatic atopic asthmatics and healthy control subjects using immunohistochemistry. *Am Rev Respir Dis* 1990;**142**:863–71.

83. Ammit AJ, Bekir SS, Johnston PR, Armour CL, Black JL. Mast cell numbers are increased in the smooth muscle of human sensitized isolated bronchi. *Am J Respir Crit Care Med* 1997;**155**:1123–9.

84. Nocka K, Buck J, Levi E, Besmer P. Candidate ligand for the c-kit trans-membrane kinase receptor: KL, a fibroblast derived growth factor stimulates mast cells and erythroid progenitors. *EMBO J* 1990;**9**:3287–94.

85. Jordana M. Mast cells and fibrosis – who's on first? *Am J Respir Cell Mol Biol* 1993;**8**:7–8.

86. Roche WR. Mast cells and tumors. The specific enhancement of tumour proliferation *in vitro*. *Am J Pathol* 1985;**119**:57–64.

87. Irani AM, Craig SS, de Blois G, *et al.* Deficiency of the tryptase-positive, chymase-negative mast cell type in gastrointestinal mucosa of patients with defective T-lymphocyte function. *J Immunol* 1987;**138**:4381–6.

88. Azzawi M, Johnston PW, Majumdar S, Kay A, Jeffery PK. T-lymphocytes and activated eosinophils in asthma and cystic fibrosis. *Am Rev Respir Dis* 1992;**145**:1477–82.

89. Sur S, Crotty TB, Kephart GM, *et al.* Sudden onset fatal asthma: a distinct entity with few eosinophils and relatively more neutrophils in the airway submucosa? *Am Rev Respir Dis* 1993;**148**:713–19.

90. Bousquet J, Chanez P, Lacoste JY, *et al.* Eosinophilic inflammation in asthma. *New Engl J Med* 1990;**323**:1033–9.

91. Gleich GJ. The eosinophil and bronchial asthma: current understanding. *J All Clin Immunol* 1990;**85**:422–36.

92. Henderson WR, Chi EY, Klebanoff SJ. Eosinophil peroxidase-induced mast cell secretion. *J Exp Med* 1980;**152**:265–79.

93. Kita H, Onhishi T, Okubo Y, *et al.* Granulocyte/macrophages colony-stimulating factor and interleukin-3 release from human peripheral blood eosinophils and neutrophils. *J Exp Med* 1991;**174**:745–8.

94. Costa JJ, Matossian K, Resnik MB, *et al.* Human eosinophils can express the cytokine tumour necrosis factor-α and macrophage inflammatory protein-1α. *J Clin Invest* 1993;**91**:2673–84.

95. Wong DTW, Elovic A, Matossian K, *et al.* Eosinophils from patients with blood eosinophilia express transforming growth factor β1. *Blood* 1991;**78**:2702–7.

96. Fahy JV, Kim KW, Liu J, Boushey HA. Prominent neutrophilic inflammation in sputum from subjects with asthma exacerbation. *J Allergy Clin Immunol* 1995;**95**:843–52.

97. Jatakanon A, Uasuf C, Maziak W, Lim S, Chung KF, Barnes PJ. Neutrophilic inflammation in severe persistent asthma. *Am J Respir Crit Care Med* 1999;**160**:1532–9.

98. Sur S, Crotty TB, Kephart GM, *et al.* Sudden-onset fatal asthma: a distinct entity with few eosinophils and relatively more neutrophils in the airway mucosa. *Am Rev Respir Dis* 1993;**148**:713–19.

99. Lawrence MB, Springer TA. Leukocytes roll on a selectin at physiologic flow rates: distinction from and prerequisite for adhesion through integrins. *Cell* 1991;**65**:859–73.

100. Geng J, Bevilacqua MP, Moore KL, *et al.* Rapid neutrophil adhesion to activated endothelium mediated by GMP-140. *Nature* 1990;**343**:757–60.

101. Resnick MB, Welter PF. Mechanisms of eosinophil recruitment. *Am J Respir Cell Mol Biol* 1993;**8**:349–55.

102. Montefort S, Roche WR, Howarth PH, *et al.* Intercellular adhesion molecule-1 (ICAM-1) and endothelial leukocyte adhesion molecule-1 (ELAM-1) expression in the bronchial mucosa of normal and asthmatic subjects. *Eur Respir J* 1992;**5**:815–23.

103. Morland CM, Wilson SJ, Holgate ST, Roche WR. Selective eosinophil recruitment by transendothelial migration and not by leukocyte–endothelial cell adhesion. *Am Rev Respir Dis* 1992;**6**:557–66.

104. Humbles AA, Conroy DM, Marleau S, *et al.* Kinetics of eotaxin generation and its relationship to eosinophil accumulation and the late reaction in allergic airway disease: analysis in a guinea pig model *in vivo*. *J Exp Med* 1997;**186**:601–12.

105. Li D, Wang D, Griffiths-Johnson DA, Wells TNC, Williams TJ, Jose PJ, Jeffery PK. Eotaxin protein gene expression in guinea-pigs: constitutive expression and upregulation after allergen challenge. *Eur Respir J* 1997;**10**:1946–54.

106. Jeffery PK. The development of large and small airways. *Am J Respir Crit Care Med* 1998;**157**:S174–80.

107. Pohunek P, Roche WR, Turzikova J, Kurdman J, Warner JO. Eosinophilic inflammation in the bronchial mucosa of children with bronchial asthma. *Eur Respir J* 1997;**11**:160s (abstract).

108. Laitinen A, Karjalainen E-M, Altraja A, Laitinen LA. Histopathologic features of early and progressive asthma. *J Allergy Clin Immunol* 2000;**105**:S509–S513.

109. Thurlbeck WM. Postnatal human lung growth. *Thorax* 1982;**37**:564–71.

110. Hogg JC, Williams J, Richardson JB, Macklem PT, Thurlbeck WM. Age as a factor in the distribution of lower airway conductance and in the pathologic anatomy of obstructive lung disease. *New Eng J Med* 1970;**282**:1283–7.

111. Jeffery PK. Early childhood asthma: anatomic development. *Am J Respir Crit Care Med* 1995;**151**:S7–S9.

112. Jeffery PK, Gaillard D, Moret T. Human airway secretory cells during development and in mature epithelium. *Eur Respir J* 1991;**5**:93–104.

113. Stevenson EC, Turner G, Heaney LG, Schock BC, Taylor R, Gallagher T, Ennis M, Shields MD. Bronchoalveolar lavage findings suggest two different forms of childhood asthma (see comments). *Clin Exp Allergy* 1997;**27**:1027–35.

114. Cokugras H, Akcakaya N, Camcioglu Y, Sarimurat N, Aksoy F. Ultrastructural examination of bronchial biopsy specimens from children with moderate asthma. *Thorax* 2001;**56**:25–9.

115. Krawiec ME, Westcott JY, Chu HW, Balzar S, Trudeau JB, Schwartz LB, Wenzel SE. Persistent wheezing in very young children is associated with lower respiratory inflammation. *Am J Respir Crit Care Med* 2001;**163**:1338–43.

116. Castleman WL, Sorkness RL, Lemanske RF, McAllister PK. Viral bronchiolitis during early life induces increased numbers of bronchiolar mast cells and airway hyperresponsiveness. *Am J Pathol* 1990;**137**:821–31.

117. Garofalo R, Kimpen JLL, Welliver RC, Ogra P. Eosinophil degranulation in the respiratory tract during naturally acquired respiratory syncytial virus infection. *J Pediatr* 1992;**120**:28–32.

118. Konradova V, Copova C, Sukova B, Houstek J. Ultrastructure of the bronchial epithelium in three children with asthma. *Pediatr Pulmonol* 1985;**1**:182–7.

119. Pin I, Radford S, Kolendowicz R, *et al*. Airway inflammation in symptomatic and asymptomatic children with methacholine hyperresponsiveness. *Eur Respir J* 1993;**6**:1249–56.

120. Ferguson AC, Whitelaw M, Brown H. Correlation of bronchial eosinophil and mast cell activation with bronchial hyperresponsiveness in children with asthma. *J All Clin Immunol* 1992;**90**:609–13.

The clinical features and their assessment

SHEILA McKENZIE

SYMPTOMS AND SIGNS

The classical clinical features of asthma are wheeze, cough and breathlessness. These terms are used in a number of questionnaires used to describe the prevalence of asthma[1] but there is a great deal of variation in the wording and definitions used in questionnaires. There are further problems: doctors' and families' perceptions of 'wheeze' may change over time;[2] the use of 'asthma' as a label for wheezy any illness;[3] and a lower threshold for reporting symptoms[4] that may also be inaccurate.[5] Assuming that 'wheeze' could be considered a homogenous symptom, there are no exact equivalents of 'wheeze' in some languages.[6,7]

In recent years there has been a better awareness of cough as a presenting complaint of asthma[8] but the most recent British asthma guidelines state '... criteria for defining asthma in the presence of chronic or recurrent cough have not been adequately defined'.[9] Recurrent cough is a common complaint in childhood and it is important to consider how it relates to wheeze and to asthma (Table 6a.1). Previously practitioners were very

Table 6a.1 *Recurrent cough*

Sensitive but not specific for asthma
Poorly predicts wheeze/asthma
Isolated chronic coughers no more atopic than
  healthy children
Nocturnal cough: parents know whether there is
  coughing but not how much
Cannot identify which children will be helped by
  asthma therapy

ready to ascribe cough to bronchitis,[10] but now there is some anxiety that too many children who cough are being diagnosed asthmatic and treated inappropriately.[11–13] Whereas all that wheezes probably coughs, all that coughs certainly does not wheeze. In asthma, cough may be the only complaint because the child and his parents are unaware of wheeze.[14] There has been no real evaluation of the third symptom of the triad: how many children with the complaint of breathlessness have asthma?

'Doctor-diagnosed' asthma is a term sometimes used by epidemiologists.[15] If the epidemiology of asthma based on reported symptoms is to have any meaning it is crucial that subjects with non-specific respiratory symptoms are not classified as asthmatic and that doctors and patients understand the terms each uses.[16,17]

Relationship between cough and wheeze

Hypotheses about the relationship between cough and wheeze[18] are based mainly on animal and adult human studies. Cough receptors in the airways are sited both in the mucosa and in smooth muscle (Figure 6a.1). It has been proposed that viruses and other agents associated with wheezing illnesses strip away mucosal epithelium to expose sub-epithelial cough receptors[19] thereby increasing the sensitivity of the cough reflex. Patients with acute viral infections have increased cough receptor sensitivity (CRS) to agents such as citric acid which returns to normal when recovery has taken place.[20] Only children who have cough as a prominent feature with acute asthma have increased CRS with an acute attack.[21] Increased amounts of locally active mediators also increase CRS.[22] This could be the reason that asthmatics cough. A primary and

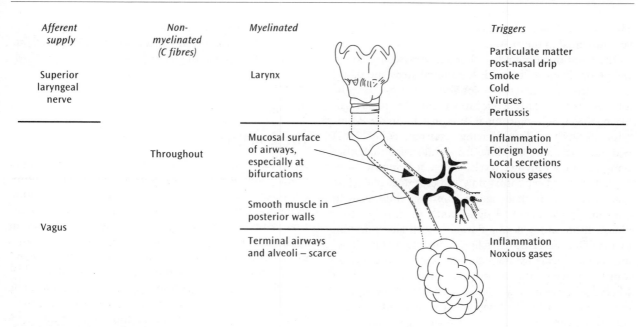

Afferent supply	Non-myelinated (C fibres)	Myelinated		Triggers
Superior laryngeal nerve		Larynx		Particulate matter Post-nasal drip Smoke Cold Viruses Pertussis
	Throughout	Mucosal surface of airways, especially at bifurcations		Inflammation Foreign body Local secretions Noxious gases
		Smooth muscle in posterior walls		
Vagus		Terminal airways and alveoli – scarce		Inflammation Noxious gases

Figure 6a.1 *Cough receptors.*

fundamental increase in CRS is another hypothesis for the cough of asthma but in both adults and children whose asthma is controlled there is no such increase in sensitivity.[21,23,24] Change in airway size does not appear to alter CRS in either normal or asthmatic subjects.[20,23,25] Cough receptors are sparse in peripheral airways. McFadden[26] has proposed that airflow obstruction in the small airways – deduced from pulmonary function studies – results in breathlessness rather than cough and wheeze, since the receptors for cough are located mainly in the large airways and airflow obstruction is too mild to cause wheeze. At the moment it seems that the cough of asthma is more likely to be related to airway inflammation, mucous in the airways and direct sensitivity to triggers than to an increase in CRS or airway calibre.

Coughing is a well-described trigger for wheezing in asthmatics[27] possibly by similar mechanisms to exercise. Histamine and methacholine both produce cough and bronchoconstriction and while these are closely related the evidence suggests that they can be triggered independently.[28] Disodium cromoglycate blocks the bronchoconstriction induced by nebulized water,[29] but not the cough, whilst lignocaine (lidocaine) blocks the cough but not bronchoconstriction. Cough appears to be related to respiratory water loss after exercise[30] while bronchoconstriction is related to both water[31] and respiratory heat losses.[32] These observations suggest that the mechanisms of cough and wheeze in asthma are related but can be independently triggered.

Is recurrent cough a marker for asthma?

Epidemiological evidence supports the observation that recurrent coughing is a poor marker for wheeze. Only half of a large group of children who coughed were also reported to wheeze.[33] Recurrent cough affected about 20% of 7-year-olds and 9% of 11-year-olds, a difference probably reflecting the incidence of respiratory infection in the two age groups. There was no difference in the prevalence of wheeze, 12% in both groups. In another large study of 7 and 8-year-olds[34] cough was reported in 22% and wheeze in 15%. Thirteen percent coughed without wheezing. Of those who coughed about a third were atopic and one third demonstrated bronchial hyperresponsiveness (BHR). Of those with cough, no wheeze and who were not atopic, only eight demonstrated BHR. Thus cough is a poor predictor of wheeze and atopic status.

Whilst it is true that most patients with moderate and severe atopic asthma have very reactive airways, in a study in New Zealand,[35] only 50% of children with mild asthma were shown to have reactive airways, 26% of children with cough and no wheeze and 8% of children with no symptoms at all were reactive. Non-specific testing of BHR has been shown not to distinguish children with recurrent cough who eventually become asthmatic.[36] Children with cough but without wheeze have increased BHR but are no more likely to be atopic than children with no respiratory symptoms.[37] Increased BHR during coughing episodes is significantly less during cough-free periods.[38] Thus, as far as BHR is concerned coughers seem to be intermediate between controls and wheezers. This has also been shown for bronchodilator responsiveness.[39,40]

Does airway pathology differ between coughers and wheezers? In a study of cellular content in bronchoalveolar lavage in children with atopic and non-atopic wheeze, cough and controls, the cell profile of children with chronic cough was similar to that of control children.[41]

This suggests that the pathology associated with cough is very proximal in the airway.

In a questionnaire study,[42] children with isolated cough were more likely to live in dust polluted areas and damp houses, whereas the triad of cough, wheeze, and breathlessness was related to allergic history and preterm birth. In the prospective, longitudinal Tucson Children's Respiratory Study,[43] children having recurrent cough (RC) without wheeze did not differ from children with neither symptom in serum IgE levels, skin test response, size-corrected forced expiratory flow, or percentage of decline following cold air challenge. In contrast, children with both RC and wheeze had significantly more respiratory illness, more atopy, lower flow at end-tidal expiration (V'maxFRC), and greater declines in lung function following cold air challenge than children with neither symptom. Current parental smoking was a risk for RC without wheeze, whereas male gender, maternal allergy, wheezing lower respiratory tract illness in early life, and high IgE were significant risks for RC with wheeze, compared with children having neither symptom.

Why do parents worry about nocturnal cough? Sleeplessness and fear of choking are two main concerns. However the relationship of cough to time spent asleep and restlessness is very poor.[44] Parents are proxy reporters of symptoms and it has been demonstrated that both parents'[37] and children's[45] records of nocturnal cough compare very poorly with recordings on voice-activated tapes. One third of parents of primary school-children complain that their children have night cough but only 9.6% have cough and wheezing.[46] It has been shown that some coughers respond in the laboratory to bronchodilator,[39] but in two studies where coughing was recorded, neither night-time cough in a small group of children who definitely had asthma nor recurrent isolated coughers benefited from the use of asthma medication.[47,48] In an unselected group of children with recurrent isolated cough inhaled corticosteroids benefited some of the children.[49] Some may be suffering from the recently described adult 'eosinophilic bronchitis'.[50] Whether a child with chronic cough and no wheeze will respond to medication cannot be predicted by current testing.

Thus, children presenting with chronic cough and no wheeze have many epidemiological and clinical differences from those with asthma.[43] Very few turn out to have asthma, probably no more than a control group. More work needs to be done in understanding why coughers have other features of asthma such as BHR and bronchodilator responsiveness (BDR) while they are coughing. Epithelial damage, mediator release, and increased sensitivity of parasympathetic receptor reflexes, which include the cough reflex, are known to occur in rhinoviral infection.[51] These mechanisms could all explain the increase in airways responsiveness, both BHR and BDR, and the increased CRS during rhinoviral infection in sensitive individuals. Rhinovirus replication persists for up to 3 weeks, long enough to cause persistent symptoms, at least in some subjects. What is now needed, short of a vaccine to prevent rhinovirus replication, is medication which will suppress cough receptor sensitivity.

Wheeze

THE SYMPTOM

Diagnosing childhood asthma is largely dependent upon parental symptom reporting. There are a number of difficulties: some parents confuse croup, stridor, dyspnoea, and nocturnal snoring with wheeze,[52] nighttime symptoms are difficult to quantify,[44] recollection of symptoms may change,[53] parents' and children's reports of symptom frequency may be discordant,[54] clinicians' and parents' words for symptoms[55] and definitions[1,16,17] may differ and, lastly, 'wheeze' does not translate into some languages.[56] Non-English speaking parents report symptoms less accurately.[16] It has been shown that at least 20% of parents misclassify both wheeze and other respiratory sounds, such as stridor, and that parents of asthmatics are no better than parents of children with no respiratory problems. In addition parents are better at locating respiratory sounds than labelling them.[16] It may be that wheeze is for much of the time a sound heard on auscultation or that if there are two sounds, for instance wheeze and upper airway noise due to nasal secretions, parents become confused. Another factor which may affect symptom reporting is the relative weighting assigned to different symptoms. Among adult patients, cough and breathlessness were rated as of greater importance than wheeze (or chest tightness or sleep disturbance).[57] There are no similar data for parents or children.

THE SIGNS

Forgacs' classical text on lung sounds[58] explains wheezing and crackling and their relationship. *Breath sounds* are believed to be generated by turbulent flow in the large airways and their intensity varies directly with the flow rate. The smaller the child the less distance between the large airways and the chest wall and the longer sound will be heard through expiration. This is particularly true over the upper lobes where sound is filtered least. Breath sounds are heard very faintly when there is hyperinflation. This is believed to be due to reflection of sound at the pleural surface.

Crackling is believed to result from explosive equalization of gas pressure between two compartments of the lung when a closed section of the airway separating them suddenly opens. In primary airway disease, such as asthma and bronchiolitis, where airways are swollen and narrowed, generalized medium or coarse crackling can be heard throughout both phases of respiration. The crackling originates anywhere along the airways which open and close at different times. Whether or not these crackles are easy to hear depends on whether they are obscured by wheezing, are damped by hyperinflation or by the thicker chest wall in older patients. Chronic suppurative disease of large airways, such as bronchiectasis or in cystic fibrosis, leads to very coarse sounds which merge into wheezes. They may be focal and exaggerated by coughing. The fine inspiratory crackling associated with lobar pneumonia or pulmonary oedema originates in small airways and is high pitched in both.

Wheeze is a musical sound produced by oscillation of the bronchial wall at points of flow limitation (choke points). (See Chapter 6b.) The total cross-sectional area of the small airways of the lung is much greater than the total cross-sectional area of the large airways. The linear velocity of gas flowing in small airways is usually too slow to cause turbulent oscillations of narrowed airways. Wheeze may originate in large airways which have been narrowed by compression or by intrabronchial or intraluminal obstructions, which cause an increase in flow velocity of gas through them with resultant oscillation. This in turn determines the pitch of the wheeze. In localized disease, such as that caused by a bronchogenic cyst, bronchomalacia or an inhaled foreign body, airway narrowing results in a wheeze whose pitch although different in inspiration and expiration is fixed and constant and usually located to one side of the chest. The nearer the larynx the more resonance there will be in the supralaryngeal area and the inspiratory wheeze may take on the quality of stridor. Because noise is conducted well in a small chest it may be difficult to be certain about the site of a lesion on the basis of added sounds. Differences in the quality of the breath sounds are probably better indicators of the site of a lesion.

When small airways are narrowed by mucosal oedema, secretions or bronchospasm, the intrathoracic pressure rises in expiration in order to expel gas through them. The pressure outside the large airways exceeds that inside and the large airways collapse downstream of the 'equal pressure point' as a result. This is known as dynamic compression of the large airways (Chapter 6b) and is contributory to the wheezing in generalized small airways disease, such as in bronchiolitis, and in asthma. Intraluminal narrowing caused by mucosal swelling and mucous plugging are the other contributory factors to the wheeze. Airways close at different points along their length causing wheezing of different pitch and at different times in expiration (Chapter 6b).

Thus, on auscultation, wheeze of 'fixed' pitch occurring in inspiration and expiration suggests a localized abnormality. Wheezes of 'varying' pitch occurring predominantly throughout expiration reflect the narrowing of airways of different calibre, the result of dynamic compression associated with widespread airways disease. In practice children with localized disease, e.g. caused by an impacted foreign body, will have retained secretions, peripherally, and hence a 'mixed' pattern of wheezing may be heard or if the object has produced complete occlusion, no wheezing at all.

Wheeze is best heard at the throat not over the chest where there is damping of sound transmission.[59]

Nocturnal wheezing

One of the first acknowledgements that nocturnal wheezing could be a problem for children as well as adults was embodied in the original asthma diary card.[60] In epidemiological studies of asthma in children before the introduction of drugs for regular use in asthma, there is no readily identifiable documentation of night-time cough or wheeze. It is difficult now to know how common classical nocturnal airway narrowing is in children. Laboratory based studies have shown that selected asthmatic school-children waken during the night with symptoms.[61,62] Nocturnal wheezing is a real problem in adolescents with troublesome asthma but the younger the child the more difficult it is to know how much wheeze, as distinct from cough, there is at night.

It is not known whether the mechanisms which operate in adults and older children with nocturnal asthma[63] operate in the wheezy infant or preschool child and it is not known how soon the circadian variation in airway calibre develops. Delayed hypersensitivity to allergens causing airway narrowing 4–6 hours after exposure and a similar response to exercise can certainly be demonstrated in school-children.[64,65] These may amplify the circadian rhythm of airway calibre to cause nocturnal symptoms.

Recurrent attacks of asthma have been cited as a potential cause of sleep disturbance and are related to poor performance during the day.[66] A community study has suggested that children with asthma have no more sleep difficulties than other children, 38%.[67] However, the results of this study should not obscure the very real and potentially dangerous symptom of nocturnal wheeze. Compared with matched controls, children with asthma have significantly more disturbed sleep, tend to have more psychological problems, and perform less well on some tests of memory and concentration. In general, improvement of nocturnal asthma symptoms by changes in treatment is followed by improvement in sleep and psychological function in subsequent weeks.[68]

Shortness of breath

In the older studies of the symptoms of asthma,[69] in adult asthmatics,[57] and more recently in epidemiological studies, shortness of breath is cited.[1] It is difficult to know what is meant by parental reporting of shortness of breath in a child, as this is a subjective symptom. In a study of clinical-physiological correlations in acute asthma, dyspnoea has been defined as 'the investigator's impression of the degree of the child's breathlessness'.[70] Children who reported dyspnoea demonstrated severe airway obstruction. On the other hand severe airway obstruction was present in some who did not report dyspnoea. Clifford[37] defined breathlessness for parents as 'out of breath or puffed'. The increased work of breathing associated with bronchoconstriction and breathing at increased lung volumes is probably what is expressed in the term 'breathless'. Difficulty in breathing is probably a better term and is how many parents know their child is wheezy.[1] As this is a difficult symptom to define, it is probably not appropriate to include it in a questionnaire which is to be used as a research tool. 'Breathlessness on exercise' is not a symptom of respiratory disease, as everybody will be breathless in response to enough exercise. 'Undue breathlessness on exercise' is something that can only be validated using appropriate laboratory testing. Breathlessness due to asthma should be distinguished from poor physical fitness, due to obesity or lack of exercise, or a disinclination to take part in sport. Coughing and/or wheezing on exercise is more likely to discriminate between asthmatic and non-asthmatic children.

Rapid and difficult breathing

In a recent study of infants with bronchiolitis respiratory rate did not correlate with severity as assessed by poor oxygen saturation values measured by oximetry.[71] The counting of respirations and its meaning is still debated.[72,73] Tachypnoea is no indicator of the severity of an attack in older children with acute asthma.[70,74] A raised respiratory rate is more in keeping with pneumonia.

Work of breathing is directly proportional to airway resistance and breathing rate and inversely related to lung compliance. In some very ill infants, presumably where there is a markedly increased airways resistance, there is a slowing of breathing and hypercapnoea.[75] The younger the infant the more compliant the chest wall and so the more inefficient is the work of breathing in maintaining alveolar ventilation. Intercostal and sternal recession reflect both this and the large negative intrathoracic pressures which are needed to sustain minute ventilation.[76] When the respiratory muscles tire, respiration fails.[77]

Chest tightness

This is a subjective sensation very infrequently mentioned in studies of children's complaints. Parents when proxy reporting do not use the term, preferring difficulty in breathing or breathing hard. In a group of adults with asthma symptoms who underwent bronchial challenge, chest tightness correlated significantly with the fall in FVC but not with the fall in FEV_1.[78] These subjects could have an enhanced perception of small changes in lung function. In another adult study, whose aim was to identify the best words to use in a questionnaire for asthma, chest tightness identified asthma better than breathlessness,[79] although adult asthmatics may not rate it of more importance.[57]

General clinical examination

GROWTH

Growth in children with asthma can be affected by both poor control or by drug treatment (Chapter 15). Even when control is good puberty is commonly delayed.[80]

Infants with wheezing associated with disorders such as CF and BPD grow poorly for reasons which are not just related to the chest disorder but to problems such as malabsorption and feeding difficulties. When a wheezy infant presents with poor growth other conditions need to be considered.

CHEST DEFORMITY

Children with chest deformity – a prominent sternum with depression over the lower ribs (Harrison's sulci) – are at the very end of the spectrum of severe, troublesome asthma.[81] Chest deformity correlates well with radiographic features of hyperinflation.[82] Nowadays it is a rare clinical sign and suggests that asthma is very poorly controlled. In addition, it is a reflection of hyperinflation in severe chest disease in children with cystic fibrosis (CF) and chronic lung disease of prematurity. Right ventricular hypertrophy and congenital abnormalities of the muskuloskeletal system are also associated with chest deformity. Finally, pigeon chestedness in the absence of symptoms is not uncommon. A proper history should avoid the need for extensive investigations and associated anxiety.

OTHER ATOPIC FEATURES

The incidence of eczema, hay fever and urticaria in asthmatic children under the age of 14 years is much higher than in controls,[83] in proportion to the severity of asthma. The first appearance of and subsequent variation in some of the allergic manifestations often does not correspond to the clinical course of the asthma. Eczema is particularly troublesome during the first two years, and usually predates wheeze. There is a significant correlation between the severity of the asthma and the severity of the eczema. On the other hand symptoms of hay fever usually have their onset after wheezing, often many years after, and their severity does not correlate with the severity of the asthma. In all children who have eczema 80% will wheeze at some time.[84]

QUESTIONNAIRES AND DIARIES

Questionnaires are for diagnosing asthma and so determining its prevalence or for monitoring its severity, or both.[85] Burr[11] has highlighted the advantages and difficulties with this. Definitions of symptoms and items included are inconsistent.[1] Wheeze can mean different things in different languages and different cultures[56] and could make international comparisons of prevalence problematic. In the UK, 10% of the adult population have a reading age of <11 years. Few questionnaires (if any) are marked with a reading age.

To remove bias as far as possible, a health questionnaire, which asks about many aspects of health and so removes the focus on asthma symptoms, may be preferable to an asthma or respiratory questionnaire.[86] Questionnaires ask parents about wheeze. The World Health Organisation (2000)[86a] suggests that wheeze may be heard at the mouth or using a stethoscope. If wheeze can only be heard by a stethoscope, parents who respond positively to a question about their child's wheeze either understand something different to a sound or could be reporting something different together. There is ample room for confusion.

Questionnaires have been developed for monitoring asthma[87,88] and these seem more promising. The Paediatric Asthma Diary seems to be the most rigorously tested in children in whom there has been a full asthma workup, including all recommended testing for the diagnosis.[88] (The methodology of questionnaire evaluation is very well explained in this reference.)

Symptom reporting and objective testing

There are large differences between reported symptoms in children and results of bronchial challenge. In two Australian studies undertaken at about the same time, the relationships were quite different. In one, 6.7% of children had BHR but no symptoms and 5.6% had a diagnosis of asthma but no BHR.[89] In the second, 53% of those with BHR had no asthma diagnosis and 48% of those with diagnosed asthma did not have BHR.[90] The definition of BHR was similar. This calls into question the validity of the reported symptoms. The validity of questionnaires used on their own to measure prevalence must be rigorously defended.[91] For epidemiology studies, calls have now been made for objective testing.[92]

Diaries are used for both clinical and research purposes. For a score-based diary to be a useful tool for either purpose there should be validation of the symptoms which it records. It has been shown that cough at night recorded on a voice activated tape did not correlate with what parents recorded on diaries.[93] Thus the documentation of cough at night does not necessarily indicate that asthma is poorly controlled or that a child has asthma at all (see above). Night-time cough is not used in a questionnaire for adults[94] and perhaps it is time it was removed from children's diaries. Documentation of the early morning PEF which reflects night-time broncho-constriction is potentially more useful.

A criticism of diaries is that they are poorly kept.[44,95] Entries are often made in batches. Simultaneous recording in written diaries and electronic diaries suggested that

about one fifth of diaries kept by adults have errors.[96] Electronic diaries recording drug usage[97] or spirometry seem more promising[98] but, with time, there is increasingly poor recording adherence.[99]

Diaries used for recording symptoms, PEF and drug usage have been used in countless clinical trials. It is important to ensure that these are scored properly. Usually night-time symptoms, daytime symptoms and symptoms on exercise are documented on a scale of 0–3. Total scores can be used simply to give some idea of whether the subject(s) did or did not have asthma during the period. This may be entirely appropriate as it was in Johnston's study.[100] There the variability of PEF throughout the day in a group of symptomatic children was all that was to be measured. However, counting total symptom scores recorded by a parent before and after treatment may be a coarse way of discovering how well asthma is controlled or if a treatment is of value. The rules of using ordinal scales for this purpose state that categories must be mutually exclusive.[101,102] In asthma trials they rarely are. If cough, wheeze and difficulty in breathing scores 3, is this worse, than, say, where only difficulty in breathing is scored? Sometimes mean scores are at the lower end of the possible total, indicating little room for improvement, at least using these symptoms. More information could be gained by assessing the score for each symptom separately or for each time of day. It may be better to define a clinically relevant improvement over the whole period of investigation. Should it be a reduction in the number of episodes of wheezing, an improvement in night-time symptoms or less exercise-induced wheeze? Or simply, asthma 'yes' or asthma 'no', night and day.

Changes in *PEF variation* over time show poor concordance with changes in other parameters of asthma severity. When only PEF is monitored, clinically relevant deteriorations in symptoms, FEV_1, or bronchial responsiveness may be missed.[103] Home spirometry or PEF monitoring seems to add little to symptom-based management protocols.[104,105] This suggests that home recording of PEF alone may not be sufficient to monitor asthma severity reliably in children.

Extra treatment for symptoms is also recorded in diaries. What relationship this bears to what is actually taken requires examination. In any event this further confounds the meaning of symptom scores. If the treatment is taken to prevent symptoms then the total number of doses will be discordant with the symptom scores. If taken after symptoms have developed then the two will be concordant.

One of the many difficulties of evaluating drugs in the long-term treatment of wheezy infants (<2 years) is that symptom scores and extra drug usage are all that can be used to measure day to day control at the moment. Change in lung function would be a more objective measure of efficacy. Some of the new lung function studies appropriate for young children where only passive co-operation is required are now of help[106,107] (Chapter 6b).

For both clinical purposes and intervention studies, it should be clear whether improvement in lung function, airway inflammation, BHR, or control of symptoms is the principal goal. This cannot be answered until it is known if, in the long term, good lung function with control of airway inflammation is as important as symptom control.

ACUTE WHEEZING – SIGNS AND SCORING SYSTEMS

Do the physical signs in acute wheezing disorders reflect the severity of an attack and thus help to decide about hospital admission, treatment and progress? (Table 6a.2).

Table 6a.2 *Signs of severity in acute wheezing*

Too breathless to feed, talk or play
Cyanosis; unreliable; oximetry more useful
Tachycardia
Nasal flaring
Use of accessory muscles
Head retraction and 'nodding'
Pulsus paradoxicus >15 mmHg
  • difficult to measure and insensitive
(Wheezing, dyspnoea and tachypnoea not useful for judging severity)

Infants

Several studies have considered signs such as *chest indrawing, cyanosis, crackles* and *pulse rate* and have derived clinical scores from them.[71,75,108] Cyanosis and the presence of crackles predict severity but these signs are neither very sensitive nor specific. There is poor agreement between physicians about the degree of retraction and wheezing. Nasal flaring and tachycardia together predict low oxygen saturation and all three predict length of stay in hospital.[108] One physical sign which has not been formally considered is '*pausing*'. If a distressed infant who is working hard to breathe develops irregular respirations with pauses, then it seems very likely that exhaustion is impending.

Most studies agree that *scoring systems* for the wheezy infant have little to commend them and that objective measures of gas exchange such as blood gas analysis and pulse oximetry are better reflections of severity. What is important is that it is possible for an infant to score low even when he is already needing oxygen and hospital admission. The likely course of a mildly wheezy infant at the beginning of an illness cannot be predicted with current techniques, either scoring systems or oximetry measurements. This is unlike the position for children with asthma where it is possible early in the

attack to know whether hospital admission is necessary (Chapter 12).

Head retraction is seen in severely distressed infants and is not unique for wheezy infants.[109] It reflects the fixing of the neck in extention in order to fix the origin of the sternomastoid and scalene muscles so that they can work as efficiently as possible. Contraction of the accessory muscles will then only move the chest and not the head as well, although head-nodding is seen commonly in acutely wheezy infants. It has been proposed that extension of the neck splints the infants' compliant, cartilage-deficient airways and thus minimizes collapse on inspiration.

Children

In the case of older children with asthma, the position is little different. Kerem[70] confirmed what others have shown previously.[110] *Pulsus paradoxicus* and the *use of the accessory muscles of respiration* when present are related to severe asthma as determined by both lung function and oxygen saturation but severe hypoxaemia can be present in the absence of these signs. Reduced FEV_1 on spirometry could indicate severe airways obstruction in the absence of hypoxaemia and almost certainly precedes it.[70]

The use of accessory muscles contributes to the increased work of breathing at high lung volumes. Pulsus paradoxicus, the amount the blood pressure decreases during inspiration, reflects the high negative intrathoracic pressures created during inspiration which increase left ventricular afterload which in turn reduces systolic pressure. This is not easy to measure in practice in small children as it may not be easy to relate the systolic pressure to the phases of respiration. When deflating the blood pressure cuff there is an interval between the point when the Korotkoff sounds are first heard at a rate slower than the heart rate and when they are heard at the same rate as the heart rate and at equal amplitude. This interval is the measurement of pulsus paradoxicus. When paradox exceeds 15 mmHg asthma is severe.[111]

Scoring systems have been based on these signs as well as respiratory rate, heart rate, wheeze, and dyspnoea. High scores certainly suggest severe airway obstruction but low scores do not rule it out.

DIFFERENTIAL DIAGNOSES

Recurrent wheezing is such a common problem that it seems unreasonable to investigate every child for underlying disease unless there are additional clinical features. In addition to the wheezing which follows bronchiolitis and accompanies non-viral infections, the main disorders to be considered are cystic fibrosis, congenital lung disorders and foreign body aspiration (Table 6a.3). Unusual causes of wheezing are considered in Chapter 13a and

Table 6a.3 *Conditions other than asthma and bronchiolitis which can cause wheezing*

Infection

Wheeze rare in infants with non-viral infections
M. pneumoniae infection causes acute wheezing in 30%
Tuberculosis: focal wheezing; CXR changes

Genetic Disorder

Cystic fibrosis: rarely uncomplicated wheezing
Immune deficiencies: cause bacterial infections, but rarely wheeze
Primary ciliary dyskinesia:
- symptoms from early infancy
- wheeze not prominent

Congenital Abnormalities

Tracheo-oesophageal fistula: CXR changes
Other airway abnormalities:
- early onset; unusual noises such as biphasic stridor
- radiology helpful

Miscellaneous

Gastro-oesophageal reflux: wheeze with or without aspiration
Foreign body aspiration
- suggestive history in 80%; focal signs; radiology

gastro-oesophageal reflux is considered in Chapter 7c. Wheezing whose onset is in early infancy should be investigated thoroughly (Chapter 9). Dry cough often accompanies wheeze in children with asthma. A persistent wet cough should ring alarm bells, and always calls for further investigation.

Infections

NON-VIRAL

The symptoms of *Chlamydia trachomatis* infection in the young infant are cough and tachypnoea. The chest radiograph shows patchy areas consistent with collapse and consolidation. The clinical picture is one of pneumonia rather than a wheezing illness. Chlamydial infection in older children appears to imitate asthma[92] which does not respond to bronchodilators. *Chlamydia pneumoniae* was identified in 1986. Its relationship with wheezing illnesses in childhood has still to be clarified. In one study,[93] children with asthma symptoms who reported multiple episodes of asthma-like symptoms were those with persistently high *C. pneumoniae* antibody titres. It is not known whether treatment with a macrolide is beneficial. It has been suggested that *C. pneumoniae* infection causes asthma in adults,[94] but *C. pneumoniae* infection when diagnosed by microimmunofluorescence serology is not a major risk factor for the development of asthma in children.[96]

A *Mycoplasma pneumoniae* chest infection is an acute illness in which cough and fever are the major features.

Wheezing may be heard on auscultation in about one third.[112] The chest radiograph may show patchy consolidation, unilateral in about 85% and most commonly in a lower lobe. Pleural effusions and/or hilar adenopathy feature in 20–30%.

Tuberculosis is on the increase in the West and will need to be considered more often in children. Obstruction of a bronchus because of compression by a large, swollen hilar node or, more commonly, by erosion of such a node into the bronchus can cause wheezing. The changes on the chest radiograph reflect bronchial compression and result in lobar or segmental hyperinflation or consolidation. These features can imitate the classical radiographic appearances of an inhaled foreign body.[113] The diagnosis is made at bronchoscopy when material can be collected for culture.

Post-bronchiolitic wheezing

Wheezing and cough often continue for days or weeks after the acute illness of bronchiolitis in a very young infant and represent slow resolution of airway inflammation,[114] persistence of virus[115] and interindividual differences in host response.[116] This diagnosis is made on clinical grounds and by exclusion of underlying disorders. Most infants who suffer bronchiolitis develop episodic wheeze with further viral infections. The long-term consequences of viral wheezing illnesses in infants and young children are reviewed in Chapters 3, 7b, and 9.

Obliterative bronchiolitis and other post-viral disorders

These are rare complications of viral wheezing illnesses of infancy. They usually follow infections with specific adenovirus subtypes, especially in conjunction with measles.[117] Changes consistent with reduced peripheral perfusion of the lungs and persistent overinflation on the chest radiograph together with a disabling respiratory illness characterized by prolonged hyperinflation and persistent wheeze with fine crackles distinguish this illness from the very frequent post-bronchiolitic wheezing.[118] Response to treatment is unrewarding.

Small numbers of children with structural damage to the lungs assumed to have resulted from damage by viral infections have been described in case reports. The aetiology is probably multifactorial. Most are associated with intractable wheeze and respiratory failure. Bronchiectasis and the Swyer–James–McLeod syndrome are two conditions included in this group.[119] The latter is the name given to a small hyperlucent lung seen on the chest radiograph. The peripheral bronchi are narrow and show chronic inflammatory changes. The hyperlucency is caused by alveolar overdistension and reduced pulmonary vascularity. Measles, adenovirus and mycoplasma have been incriminated.

Cystic fibrosis

Infants with cystic fibrosis may present with severe clinical illnesses indistinguishable from viral bronchiolitis. Such infants have a particularly severe illness with a high morbidity and slow recovery.[120] Most infants with cystic fibrosis presenting with respiratory symptoms have had them for months and have in addition features of undernutrition. Thus, a severe wheezing illness requiring prolonged hospitalisation is a strong indication for further investigation. A history of respiratory symptoms, together with a persistently abnormal chest radiograph and poor growth are also suggestive of cystic fibrosis.

Disorders of host defence

PRIMARY CILIARY DYSKINESIA

Buchdahl and colleagues[121] reviewed the clinical features of 18 children with this disorder. All those with ultrastructural abnormalities or absence of cilia had been symptomatic in the first week of life. Three of seven with normal ultrastructure but low ciliary beat frequency also had symptoms in the first week of life. This was an important distinguishing feature between the group and other children with chronic respiratory symptoms. Although chronic cough was described as a symptom in these children wheeze was not. In a recent review[122] atypical asthma is cited as a differential diagnosis. A properly taken history of associated features such as persistent nasal discharge or recurrent otitis media should point to the diagnosis.

IMMUNOGLOBULIN SUBCLASS DEFICIENCY

This group of disorders is particularly associated with chronic bacterial chest infection and failure to thrive. IgG3 deficiency is associated with atopic disease[123] but is not a deficiency that needs to be remedied. When immunoglobulin subclasses in children with asthma were compared with controls[124] all major subclasses in young asthmatics were reduced. However, no child was deficient in any subclass according to the reference ranges of Schur.[125] The authors postulate that delayed maturation of subclass production is associated with asthma. More recently, this has been confirmed in Asian children who have neither major immunoglobulin deficiency nor subclass deficiency.[126] Estimation of subclass concentrations therefore does not need to be undertaken routinely in children with uncomplicated wheezing disorders.

CELL MEDIATED OR COMBINED IMMUNE DEFICIENCY

Recurrent wheezing is not a prominent feature of these disorders which are associated with bacterial infection and failure to thrive.

Gastro-oesophageal reflux (GOR)

This topic is dealt with in Chapter 7c. Reflux can contribute to asthma either by a vagally mediated reflex mechanism or, rarely, by aspiration.[127] In infants who wheeze recurrently the question of aspiration arises more frequently. Simpson[128] has reviewed this difficult topic. In a study of 38 children under 18 months with recurrent respiratory symptoms[129] 33 were wheezy. There was no association between indices which described the amount of GOR and measures which described the degree of abnormality in lung function. What matters may be the individual responsiveness to GOR, not how much GOR there is. Whilst treatment of reflux is associated with improvement in certain groups of patients, particularly those with pneumonia, the evidence is less convincing with asthma and with wheezing disorders in infants. Where there is radiographic evidence supporting a diagnosis of aspiration, then appropriate investigations for GOR are justified. There is however no good radiological technique which reliably demonstrates aspiration. There is at present nothing to support the routine investigation for GOR in infants and children with recurrent wheezing, unless they have troublesome symptoms unresponsive to anti-asthma treatment.

Congenital abnormalities

LESIONS CAUSING COMPRESSION OR OBSTRUCTION OF AIRWAYS

Rare intrabronchial or mediastinal lesions can cause wheezing in infants by direct large-airway narrowing. Abnormal vessels and intrathoracic masses such as bronchogenic cyst, teratoma, neuroblastoma, sequestration and even cardiomegaly can cause extrabronchial compression and tachypnoea in early infancy. Isolated wheezing is very unusual. Intrabronchial lesions include bronchomalacia and bronchial stenosis. Some are associated with congenital lobar emphysema. Chest radiography in an infant who has unexplained respiratory symptoms will show focal signs, often hyperinflation, and further radiographic studies will help to clarify the abnormality (Figures 6a.2 and 6a.3).

TRACHEO-OESOPHAGEAL FISTULA (TOF)

Children with the H-type fistula can present with recurrent chestiness. Chest radiographs will demonstrate abnormalities consistent with atelectasis and pneumonia, identical to those in children with recurrent aspiration due to GOR. Abdominal distention with an elevated diaphragm is common.

Foreign body aspiration

This is the most important consideration in children beyond infancy. In a review of 25 children who had

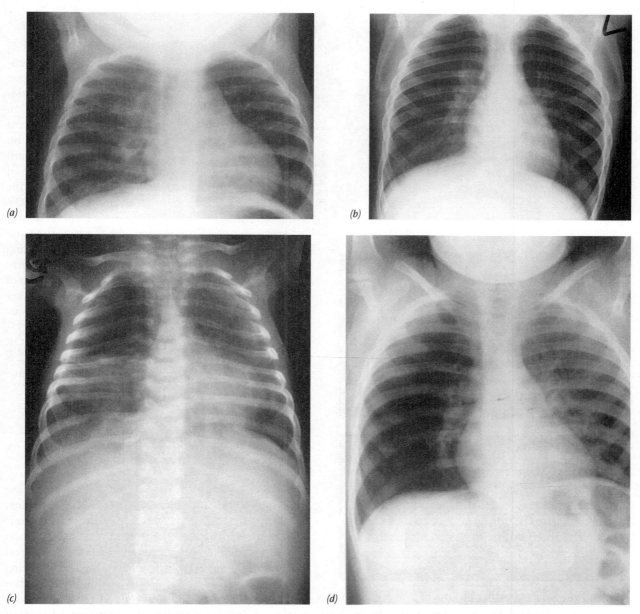

Figure 6a.2 *The plain chest radiograph in some wheezy conditions. (a) Bronchiolitis. The patchy radio-opaque areas in the upper right zone suggest segmental collapse. (b) Obliterative bronchiolitis. This radiograph was obtained several months after an adenoviral infection. It shows gross hyperinflation and pruning of vessels in the peripheral lung fields. (c) Cystic fibrosis. The bilateral lower zone shadows are consistent with consolidation. There is consolidation of both upper zones. This child presented with wheezing. (d) Inhaled foreign body. This child had been mistakenly treated for asthma. Note the hyperlucent right lung. A nut was removed from the right main bronchus at bronchoscopy.*

aspirated, in 21 there was a positive history.[130] Wheezing unresponsive to bronchodilators and focal signs on auscultation such as reduced breath sounds on one side should point to the possibility. Chest radiography will usually confirm a focal abnormality, usually hyperinflation of one lung or lobe, depending on the site of impaction. Complete occlusion is nearly always secondary to prolonged impaction with local inflammation, and leads to radiographic signs of collapse distally. Impaction on the left is not infrequent (about 40%) but there is often delay

in recognizing radiographic signs associated with a foreign body in the left lower lobe bronchus.[131]

On the rare occasion where the chest radiograph does not give a clear indication of abnormality in spite of the clinical picture, an isotope lung scan will help to locate a segment or lobe which is particularly poorly ventilated. Paediatric bronchoscopy is a straightforward procedure in experienced hands, used for diagnostic as well as therapeutic purposes. Foreign bodies are usually removed using a rigid bronchoscope.

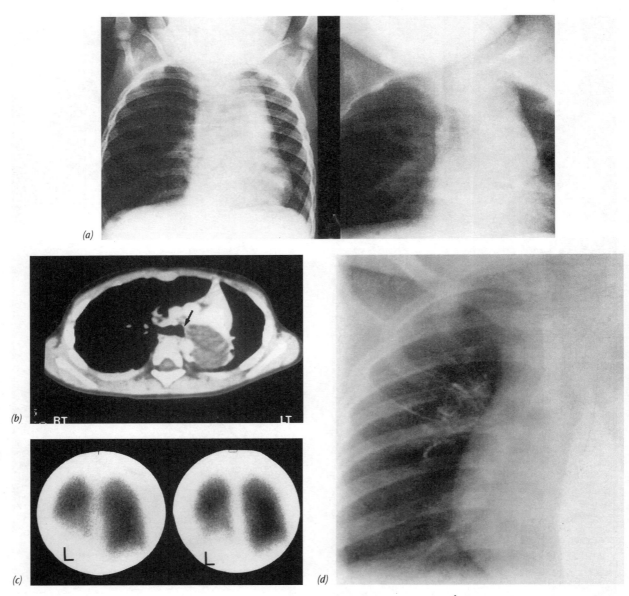

Figure 6a.3 *Specialized radiology techniques. (a) Penetrated chest radiograph in an 18-month-old child who presented with wheeze and stridor. The plain radiograph (left) shows the mediastinum deviated to the left. The penetrated film (right) shows a normal trachea and carina but the left main bronchus is not seen. There is a suggestion of a mass in relationship to it. (b) Computed tomogram at the level of the carina in the same child. This shows the mass in the left hemithorax closely apposed to the left main bronchus (arrow). A bronchogenic cyst was removed at surgery. (c) Ventilation and perfusion lung scanning (posterior views). Both perfusion (right) and ventilation (left) scans show a matched segmental defect in the left lower and mid-zones in a child with bronchiectasis. (d) Barium swallow. This shows gross gastroesophageal reflux. Contrast is seen in the lung. This child presented with wheezing on two occasions with consolidation on the plain radiograph. The investigation demonstrated a large hiatus hernia with gastroesophageal reflux and pulmonary aspiration.*

Bronchiectasis

Bronchiectasis should be considered when there is persistent wheezing associated with a persistent wet cough or purulent sputum. Ventilation/perfusion scans will help to define whether disease is limited to one lobe or more (Figure 6a.3) and computed tomography of the chest should be routine.[118,132] Children with lesions isolated to one lobe often benefit from surgery. A history of recurrent infections suggests underlying undiagnosed conditions such as immunoglobulin deficiencies and the very rare possibility of a late presentation of cystic fibrosis with bronchiectasis should not be forgotten. Neither of these conditions presents with exclusive wheeze. Chronic and rare disorders in children who have lived in countries where they are less likely to be diagnosed in infancy may come to notice only following migration.

INVESTIGATIONS

There is poor agreement between physicians and parents about what is wheeze in their child, when the 'gold standard' is wheeze heard on auscultation of the chest.[17] There is also poor agreement among adult physicians about signs elicited on physical examination of the chest.[133] The case for objective testing for the diagnosis of asthma and wheezing disorders is compelling.[92,134,135]

Chest radiology

ACUTE WHEEZING

Routine chest radiology in series of children with acute asthma does not provide useful information for children's care plans.[136,137] Patchy collapse and sometimes lobar collapse together with hyperinflation are the usual findings. Lobar collapse generally improves with the asthma. Air leaks are usually identified clinically and, as is usual, in the spontaneously breathing asthmatic do not require treatment. In the very few asthmatics who require assisted ventilation, chest radiology is essential not only to ascertain the correct positioning of the endotracheal tube but also to know of the presence of air leaks (Chapter 12).

Chest radiology has been evaluated in a group of infants with acute bronchiolitis.[138] It is the clinical status which determines management not the appearance of the chest radiograph. As in asthma, hyperinflation with patchy areas of collapse (in 25%) is usual. Imaging is only useful when intensive care is considered, when there is sudden deterioration or in infants with an underlying cardiac or chronic pulmonary disorder.

RECURRENT AND CHRONIC COUGH AND WHEEZE

There is no information about how often useful information is obtained from the chest radiograph in thriving infants with a diagnosis of post-bronchiolitic wheeze. Unless the findings on chest radiology will influence the course of management it can be argued that there is little point in undertaking them. A child with previous lobar collapse during an acute illness should have a follow-up chest radiograph. There are no guidelines about when this should be done but if the lobe has not re-expanded after the acute phase of the illness then bronchoscopy should be considered. Recurrent segmental or lobar collapse in an infant would be a strong indication for further investigation for GOR or TOF. Once such abnormalities have been excluded then further radiographs need to be justified.

Congenital abnormalities in infants with prolonged respiratory symptoms need to be considered, but these are rarely present with solely uncomplicated cough and wheeze. Children who are not thriving and in whom underlying chronic disorders are being considered will need chest radiology as part of the overall evaluation (Figure 6a.2). In otherwise healthy older children who have a clear history consistent with asthma, routine chest radiography is not indicated.

SPECIAL RADIOLOGICAL PROCEDURES (FIGURE 6A.3)

A *filter view* of the mediastinum with magnification – or 'penetrated' chest radiograph – is useful to define mediastinal structures especially the trachea, carina and major bronchi. This procedure has largely been replaced by computed tomography (CT) scanning of the chest.

Fluoroscopy of the chest to look for mediastinal movement is sometimes used to aid in the diagnosis of a foreign body. When the foreign body causes air trapping then, on expiration, the mediastinum moves away from the abnormal side. With a good history and careful examination screening should not be needed very often. In cases where there is no trapping (for example when there are small fragments of foreign material on both sides) screening could be unhelpful. Indications for barium swallow include the identification of lesions causing extrinsic pressure on the oesophagus, aberrant vessels for example which may also cause pressure on the airways, gastro-oesophageal reflux and aspiration. Barium swallow has also been largely replaced by CT scanning for compression and pH monitoring for GOR.

CT scanning gives an excellent anatomical description of the intrathoracic structures, masses and the lung parenchyma, is especially useful in defining the extent of bronchiectasis and may be useful to asses airway wall thickness in difficult asthma.[139] There is however a high radiation burden from a CT scan.

Ventilation/perfusion scanning gives a functional description of the lungs. In a wheezy child who has a hyperlucent or small lung identified on the chest radiograph it is important to know whether it is normally ventilated and normally perfused. Normally functioning but small lungs are not especially rare. In MacLeod's syndrome the small lung is poorly ventilated and poorly perfused and in children who have a hypoplastic pulmonary artery the lung is poorly perfused but well ventilated. In all cases it is important to describe the function of the 'normal' lung if surgery is being considered. In bronchiectasis if only one lobe or segment is affected then the clinical result of surgery should be very good.

Skin-prick testing and other allergy tests

The role of routine skin testing in the management of asthma is controversial. It can be argued that demonstrating positive skin tests are useful in persuading patients to take measures to reduce house dust exposure or to part with pets. Evidence to support these measures is still being gathered. A more persuasive argument would be that such measures should be taken before children are sensitized! Skin testing is not difficult to perform properly and to interpret provided the tester has been trained. The interpretation of total and specific serum IgE assays can be problematic. If specific allergen testing is to drive management, then methods of testing need to be easier and, in the case of specific IgE measurements, cheaper. Their roles in epidemiology and research and their clinical usefulness are discussed in Chapter 7a. Severe asthma in a non-atopic schoolchild is unusual and calls for careful assessment. Recent evidence suggests that inhaled corticosteroids benefit only preschool wheezers who are sensitized to aeroallergens.[107]

Bronchodilator responsiveness, exercise and bronchial provocation testing

The USA asthma guidelines[140] suggest that all patients with respiratory symptoms suggestive of asthma have *BDR testing* and if the diagnosis is in doubt to proceed to tests of bronchial responsiveness to non-specific agents. Current British guidelines do not suggest this for children.[9] Until the sensitivity and specificity of BDR testing studies in children are known they cannot be promoted as diagnostic tests. BDR testing in preschool children, using the measurement of airway resistance by the interrupter technique before and 15 minutes after bronchodilator, has an 80% sensitivity and 80% specificity for wheeze in the previous 6 weeks.[39] A sensitivity and specificity profile is not available for change in FEV_1 in response to bronchodilator in children, although this can be derived from the data available[141] and seems to be excellent for the identification of children with moderate or severe asthma. The change quoted in the US guidelines, 12% of expected, is based on the BDR expected in adult controls. The only equivalent figure available for children is 9%[141] which is the change demonstrated in healthy children plus two standard deviations of the change. A fall in Rint of upto 46% could be normal in young children.[153] Anything in excess of this could be considered BDR.

The interpretation of tests of *bronchial responsiveness*, whether to exercise or to the inhalation of agents such as methacholine, is similarly problematic. How-ever, if an exercise test causes a child's PEF or FEV_1 to drop by over 15% expected and especially if wheezing is heard then there is little doubt that he/she has asthma. However, only a proportion of asthmatics have exercise-induced wheezing (Chapter 6c). Metacholine responsiveness alone is not specific or sensitive for asthma in children.

Lung function testing in the assessment of wheezing

Lung function testing in wheezy infants is at the moment a research and not a diagnostic tool (Chapter 6b).

For older children where a diagnosis of asthma is certain, *routine spirometry* on a 'one-off' clinic visit has limited value and is difficult to justify as a routine, unless the child has difficult asthma where response to interventions are being monitored.[142] Information from spirometry can be used in several ways: to learn more about the child's perception of asthma by matching symptoms to function; to evaluate bronchodilator response (Chapter 6b); and to better describe the nature of the obstructive pattern which may be evident on spirometry. Many asthmatic children who are free of symptoms and have normal measurements of PEF and FEV_1 continue to demonstrate abnormal flow–volume curves and abnormal mid-expiratory rates, suggestive of small airways narrowing. These findings are of increasing clinical relevance.[143,144] Detailed pulmonary function can be very useful in the assessment of the child who is being kept away from school because of 'asthma' and who may have either only non-specific cough or other social and emotional problems. Repeated normal pulmonary function tests (especially in the absence of increased bronchial responsiveness) make it very unlikely that asthma is problematic.

The *measurement of PEF at home* using portable peak flow meters is widely accepted and recommended as a useful way of assessing control. However, the use of PEF recording for routine management is of unproven efficacy in children and there are many pitfalls.[145] In a group of asthmatic children, most of whom were symptomatic, variability of PEF throughout the day has been shown not to be a good indicator of poor control in children.[100,95,104,105] Only a few children demonstrated the variability of 20% expected in symptomatic adults. Each child should know their own best PEF. The fall in PEF which would predict or reflect a deterioration in control should be calculated and recorded on the self-management plan.

It is unfortunate that, until recently, normal population charts (from 1970) have been supplied with the mini-peak flow meters. The interpretation of normal values for height, and their range, is often misunderstood. Whilst relating individual readings to population means for height might be appropriate for epidemiological studies and for following individuals' progress, it is quite inappropriate and even dangerous for day to day use. For example, if a child's best PEF lies on the 95th centile for height s/he may be significantly wheezy when it drops to the 10th centile, a value which although still inside the normal population range is not normal for the child. Failure to understand this can result in symptoms being dismissed and appropriate treatment not given.

Handheld *electronic spirometers* should allow more detailed information about lung function to be collected at home. In practice, children seem to lose interest in making recordings and so the value of monitoring with a portable spirometer is also limited.[95,99]

SEVERITY AND PATTERNS OF ILLNESS

Two of the earliest studies of childhood asthma, one in Aberdeen and one in Melbourne[146,147] classified asthma according to severity. Both studies graded severity according to frequency of attacks and status between attacks. Both considered 15% of asthmatics had severe asthma. There is no modern comparable study to judge what proportion of childhood asthmatics belong to each group. Severity relates to treatment and may change with season and with time. The adequacy of the treatment reflects both the experience of the physician caring for the child and the parental supervision. Practice varies enormously and this is reflected in the patterns of hospital admissions with acute asthma.[148] Nowadays, then, the 'step' of the asthma treatment guidelines at which control is gained, is regarded as the measure of severity. The difficulty with this is that prescribing of treatment does not always follow guidelines. Children with recurrent cough are often considered for treatment with corticosteroids[13] and there is anecdotal evidence that up to 13% of all children, from preschool age to adolescence, have been prescribed inhaled corticosteroids at some time in the UK.

For practical purposes the following classification is a guideline.

Mild

Symptoms or drops in PEF which occur once or twice a week and are easily controlled with a bronchodilator are classed as mild. In the preschool child symptoms may occur only during respiratory tract infections and there may be long intervals when the child has no symptoms.

Moderate

Children with symptoms which would occur almost every day without treatment but whose asthma is easy to control with daily prophylactic medication up to the level of low-dose steroids have moderately severe asthma. They will need extra medication to prevent symptoms during an upper respiratory tract infection, but rarely miss school or need hospital treatment for an acute attack.

Severe

Those who need daily treatment with high-dose (>400 µg/day) inhaled steroids, who often need additional treatment with extra steroids and bronchodilators have severe asthma. Careful management and education in preventative treatment should allow children in this category to continue in relatively uninterrupted education. Very few children whose treatment is closely supervised are unable to participate in exercise or need frequent inpatient treatment. Many will still have abnormal lung function when tested by spirometry, even when symptom free.

Difficult

The European Respiratory Society has defined 'difficult asthma' in children as 'patients with symptoms requiring rescue bronchodilator on >3 days/week, despite treatment with ≥1500 µg/day of inhaled budesonide (or equivalent), as well as regular long-acting β_2-agonist (or a previous unsuccessful trial of long-acting β_2-agonist), and/or regular oral prednisolone'.[142] These patients are truly difficult in spite of treatment or are not being given treatment. At least this definition highlights a problem in a group where there is real risk of sudden death. Broadly, using this definition there are three subgroups: true difficult asthma which satisfies the definition, apparent difficult asthma where there is non-adherence to treatment, and symptoms related to an alternative diagnosis.[149]

This classification has some shortcomings. It takes no account of the cardinal features of symptom pattern and atopic status, and it is simply determined by the level of therapy to control reported symptoms. It includes no definition of lung function. Not all children will fall easily into one of these groups. A very few who do not need continuous treatment may be at risk of sudden severe attacks. This pattern is especially evident in the preschool age group. At school age the pattern may be indicative of a high degree of sensitivity to a particular allergen. Although asthmatics who die in an attack are generally poorly controlled and poorly supervised,[150] there are certainly a few who have a pattern of illness which would be classified as mild.[151]

Development of a validated method for asthma severity categorization is essential for using a stepped care approach to asthma pharmacotherapy.[152]

REFERENCES

1. Cane RS, Ranganathan SC, McKenzie SA. What do parents understand by 'wheeze'? *Arch Dis Child* 2000;**82**:327–32.
2. Anderson HR. Is the prevalence of asthma changing? *Arch Dis Child* 1989;**64**:172–5.
3. Strachan DP, Anderson HR, Limb ES, O'Neill A, Wells N. A national survey of asthma prevalence, severity, and treatment in Great Britain. *Arch Dis Child* 1994;**70**:174–8.
4. Whincup PH, Cook DG, Strachan DP, *et al*. Time trends in respiratory symptoms in childhood over a 24 year period. *Arch Dis Child* 1993;**68**:729–34.
5. Britton J. Symptoms and objective measures to define the asthma phenotype. *Clin Exp Allergy* 1998;**28**(Suppl 1):2–7.

6. Burney P, Chinn S. Developing a new questionnaire for measuring the prevalence and distribution of asthma. *Chest* 1987;**91**:79s–83s.
7. Woolcock A. Epidemiologic methods for measuring prevalence of asthma. *Chest* 1987;**91**:89s–92s.
8. Spelman R. Two year followup of the management of children with chronic or recurrent cough in children according to an asthma protocol. *Br J Gen Prac* 1991;**41**:406–9.
9. British Thoracic Society, National Asthma Campaign Royal College of Physicians of London *et al*. British Guidelines on Asthma Management. Review and Position Statement. *Thorax* 1995;**52**(Suppl 1).
10. Jones A. Coughing, wheezing and the diagnosis of asthma. *Practitioner* 1990;**234**:274–6.
11. Burr ML. Diagnosing asthma by questionnaire in epidemiological surveys. *Clin Exp Allergy* 1992;**22**:509–10.
12. Silverman M WN. Asthma – time for a change in name? *Arch Dis Child* 1997;**77**:62–4.
13. Picciotto A, Hubbard M, Sturdy P, Naish J, McKenzie SA. Prescribing for persistent cough in children. *Respir Med* 1998;**92**:638–41.
14. Boner AL, de Sefano G, Piacentini GL, *et al*. Perception of bronchoconstriction in chronic asthma. *J Asthma* 1992;**295**:323–30.
15. Luyt DK, Burton PR, Simpson H. Epidemiological study of wheeze, doctor diagnosed asthma, and cough in preschool children in Leicestershire. *BMJ* 1993;**306**:1386–90.
16. Cane RS, McKenzie SA. Parents' interpretations of children's respiratory symptoms on video. 2001;**84**:31–4.
17. Elphick HE, Sherlock P, Foxall G, Simpson EJ, Shiell NA, Primhak RA, Everard ML. Survey of respiratory sounds in infants. *Arch Dis Child* 2001;**84**:35–9.
18. Editorial. Cough and wheeze in asthma: are they interdependent? *Lancet* 1988;**i**:447–8.
19. Higgenbottom T. Cough induced by changes of ionic composition of airway surface liquid. *Bull Eur Physiopathol Respir* 1984;**20**:553–62.
20. Pounsford JC, Birch MJ, Saunders KB. Effect of bronchodilators on the cough response to inhaled citric acid in normal and asthmatic subjects. *Thorax* 1985;**40**:662–7.
21. Chang AB, Phelan PD, Robertson CF. Cough receptor sensitivity in children with acute and non-acute asthma. *Thorax* 1997;**52**:770–4.
22. Choudry NB, Fuller RW, Pride NB. Sensitivity of the human cough reflex. *Am Rev Respir Dis* 1989;**140**:137–41.
23. Fujimura M, Sakamoto S, Matsuda T, Kamio Y. Cough receptor sensitivity and bronchial responsiveness in normal and asthmatic subjects. *Eur Respir J* 1992;**5**:291–5.
24. Chang AB, Phelan PD, Sawyer SM, Del Brocco S, Robertson CF. Cough sensitivity in children with asthma, recurrent cough, and cystic fibrosis. *Arch Dis Child* 1997;**77**:331–4.
25. Fujimura M, Sakamoto S, Kamio Y, Matsuda T. Effects of methacholine induced bronchoconstriction and procaterol induced bronchodilation on cough receptor sensitivity to inhaled capsaicin and tartaric acid. *Thorax* 1992;**47**:441–5.
26. McFadden ERJ. Exertional dyspnea and cough as preludes to acute attacks of bronchial asthma. *N Engl J Med* 1975;**292**:555–9.
27. Young S, Bitsakou H, Caric D, McHardy GJ. Coughing can relieve or exacerbate symptoms in asthmatic patients. *Respir Med* 1991;**85**(Suppl A):7–12.
28. Chausow AM, Banner AS. Comparison of the tussive effects of histamine and methacholine in humans. *J Appl Physiol* 1983;**55**:541–6.
29. Sheppard D, Rizk NW, Boushey HA, Bethel RA. Mechanism of cough and bronchoconstriction induced by distilled water aerosol. *Am Rev Respir Dis* 1983;**127**:691–4.
30. Banner AS, Green J, O'Connor M. Relation of respiratory water loss to coughing after exercise. *N Engl J Med* 1984;**311**:883–6.
31. Argyros GJ, Phillips YY, Rayburn DB, Rosenthal RR, Jaeger JJ. Water loss without heat flux in exercise-induced bronchospasm [published erratum appears in *Am Rev Respir Dis* 1993 Jul;**148**(1):following 264]. *Am Rev Respir Dis* 1993;**147**:1419–24.
32. Deal ECJ, McFadden ERJ, Ingram RHJ, Strauss RH, Jaeger JJ. Role of respiratory heat exchange in production of exercise-induced asthma. *J Appl Physiol* 1979;**46**:467–75.
33. Clifford RD, Radford M, Howell JB, Holgate ST. Prevalence of respiratory symptoms among 7 and 11 year old schoolchildren and association with asthma. *Arch Dis Child* 1989;**64**:1118–25.
34. Clough JB, Williams JD, Holgate ST. Profile of bronchial responsiveness in children with respiratory symptoms. *Arch Dis Child* 1992;**67**:574–9.
35. Sears MR, Jones DT, Holdaway MD, *et al*. Prevalence of bronchial reactivity to inhaled methacholine in New Zealand children. *Thorax* 1986;**41**:283–9.
36. Galvez RA, McLaughlin FJ, Levison H. The role of the methacholine challenge in children with chronic cough. *J Allergy Clin Immunol* 1987;**79**:331–5.
37. Clifford RD, Howell JB, Radford M, Holgate ST. Associations between respiratory symptoms, bronchial response to methacholine, and atopy in two age groups of schoolchildren. *Arch Dis Child* 1989;**64**:1133–9.
38. Chang AB, Phelan PD, Sawyer SM, Robertson CF. Airway hyperresponsiveness and cough-receptor sensitivity in children with recurrent cough. *Am J Respir Crit Care Med* 1997;**155**:1935–9.
39. McKenzie SA, Bridge PD, Healy MJR. Airways resistance in preschool children with wheeze and cough. *Eur Respir J* 1999;**15**:533–8.

40. McKenzie SA, Mylonopolou M, Bridge PD. Bronchodilator responsiveness and atopy in 5–10 year old coughers. *Eur Respir J* 2001;**18**:977–81.

41. Marguet C, Jouen-Boedes F, Dean TP, Warner JO. Bronchoalveolar cell profiles in children with asthma, infantile wheeze, chronic cough, or cystic fibrosis. *Am J Respir Crit Care Med* 1999;**159**:1533–40.

42. Kelly YJ, Brabin BJ, Milligan PJ, Reid JA, Heaf D, Pearson MG. Clinical significance of cough and wheeze in the diagnosis of asthma. *Arch Dis Child* 1996; **75**:489–93.

43. Wright AL, Holberg CJ, Morgan WJ, Taussig LM, Halonen M, Martinez FD. Recurrent cough in childhood and its relation to asthma. *Am J Respir Crit Care Med* 1996;**153**:1259–65.

44. Fuller P, Picciotto A, Davies M, McKenzie SA. Cough and sleep in inner-city children. *Eur Respir J* 1998; **12**:426–31.

45. Falconer A OCHP. Poor agreement between reported and recorded nocturnal cough in asthma. *Ped Pulmonol* 1993;**15**:209–11.

46. Hill RA, Standen PT, Tattersfield AE. Asthma, wheezing and absence in primary schools. *Arch Dis Child* 1989;**64**:246–51.

47. Hoskyns EW, Beardsmore CS, Simpson H. Chronic night cough and asthma severity in children with stable asthma. *Eur J Pediatr* 1995;**154**:320–5.

48. Chang AB, Phelan PD, Carlin JB, Sawyer SM, Robertson CF. A randomised, placebo controlled trial of inhaled salbutamol and beclomethasone for recurrent cough. *Arch Dis Child* 1998;**79**:6–11.

49. Davies MJ, Fuller P, Picciotto A, McKenzie SA. Persistent nocturnal cough: randomised controlled trial of high dose inhaled corticosteroid. *Arch Dis Child* 1999;**81**:38–44.

50. Brightling CE, Ward R, Goh KL, Wardlaw AJ, Parord ID. Eosinophilic bronchitis is an important cause of chronic cough. *Am J Resp Crit Care Med* 1999;**160**:406–10.

51. Gwaltney JMJ. Rhinovirus infection of the normal human airway. *Am J Respir Crit Care Med* 1995; **152**:S36–9.

52. Lee DA, Winslow NR, Speight AN, Hey EN. Prevalence and spectrum of asthma in childhood. *BMJ (Clin Res Ed)* 1983;**286**:1256–8.

53. Peat JK, Salome CM, Toelle BG, Baumna A, Wollcock AJ. Reliability of a respiratory history questionnaire and effect of mode of administration on classification of asthma in children. *Chest* 1992;153–7.

54. Wong TW, YTS, Liu JLY, Wong SL. Agreement on responses to respiratory illnesses questionnaire. *Arch Dis Child* 1998;**78**:379–80.

55. Ostergaard MS. Childhood asthma: parents' perspectives – a qualitative interview study. *Fam Pract* 1998;**15**:153–7.

56. Pararajasingam CD, Sittampalam L, Damani P, Pattemore PK, Holgate ST. Comparison of the prevalence of asthma among Asian and European children of Southampton. *Thorax* 1992;**47**:529–32.

57. Osman LM, McKenzie L, Cairns J, Friend JA, Godden DJ, Legge JS, Douglas JG. Patient weighting of importance of asthma symptoms. *Thorax* 2001;**56**:138–42.

58. Forgacs P. *Lung Sounds*. Baillière Tindall, London, 1975.

59. Meslier N, Charbonneau G, Racineux JL. Wheezes. *Eur Respir J* 1995;**8**:1942–8.

60. Connelly N, Godfrey S. Assessment of the child with asthma. *J Asthma Res* 1970;**8**:31.

61. Kales A, Kales JD, Sly RM, Scharf MB, Tan TL, Preston TA. Sleep patterns of asthmatic children: all-night electroencephalographic studies. *J Allergy* 1970;**46**:300–8.

62. Smith TF, Hudgel DW. Arterial oxygen desaturation during sleep in children with asthma and its relation to airway obstruction and ventilatory drive. *Pediatrics* 1980;**66**:746–51.

63. van Aalderen WM, Postma DS, Koeter GH, Knol K. Nocturnal airflow obstruction, histamine, and the autonomic central nervous system in children with allergic asthma. *Thorax* 1991;**46**:366–71.

64. Price JF, Hey EN, Soothill JF. Antigen provocation to the skin, nose and lung, in children with asthma; immediate and dual hypersensitivity reactions. *Clin Exp Immunol* 1982;**47**:587–94.

65. Boner AL, Vallone G, Chiesa M, Spezia E, Fambri L, Sette L. Reproducibility of late phase pulmonary response to exercise and its relationship to bronchial hyperreactivity in children with chronic asthma. *Pediatr Pulmonol* 1992;**14**:156–9.

66. Fitzpatrick MF, Engleman H, Whyte KF, Deary IJ, Shapiro CM, Douglas NJ. Morbidity in nocturnal asthma: sleep quality and daytime cognitive performance. *Thorax* 1991;**46**:569–73.

67. Tirosh E, Scher A, Sadeh A, Jaffe M, Lavie P. Sleep characteristics of asthmatics in the first four years of life: a comparative study. *Arch Dis Child* 1993;**68**: 481–3.

68. Stores G, Ellis AJ, Wiggs L, Crawford C, Thomson A. Sleep and psychological disturbance in nocturnal asthma. *Arch Dis Child* 1998;**78**:413–19.

69. Commey JOO, Levison H. Physical signs in asthmatic children. *Pediatrics* 1976;**58**:537–41.

70. Kerem E, Canny G, Tibshirani R, *et al. Pediatrics* 1991;**87**:481–6.

71. Wang EE, Milner RA, Navas L, Maj H. Observer agreement for respiratory signs and oximetry in infants hospitalized with lower respiratory infections. *Am Rev Respir Dis* 1992;**145**:106–9.

72. Morley C. Respiratory rate and severity of illness in babies under six months. *Arch Dis Child* 1990; **65**:234–7.

73. Berman S, Simoes EAF, Laneta C. Respiratory rate and pneumonia in infancy. *Arch Dis Child* 1991;**66**:81.

74. Kesten S, Maleki-Yazdi MR, Sanders BR. Respiratory rate during acute asthma. *Chest* 1990;**97**:535–6.

75. Mulholland EK, Olinsky A, Shann F. Clinical findings and severity in acute bronchiolitis. *Lancet* 2000; **335**:1259–61.

76. Milner A. Changing concepts in asthma. *Arch Dis Child* 1978;**53**:535–6.

77. Lebel MH, Gauthier M, Lacroix J, Rousseau E, Buiteau M. Respiratory failure in severe bronchiolitis. *Arch Dis Child* 1989;**64**:1431–7.

78. Salome CM, Xuan W, Gray EJ, Belooussova E, Peat JK. Perception of airway narrowing in a general population sample. *Eur Respir J* 1997;**10**:1052–8.

79. Bai J, Peat JK, Berry G, Marks GB, Woolcock AJ. Questionnaire items that predict asthma and other respiratory conditions in adults. *Chest* 1998; **114**:1343–8.

80. Balfour-Lynn L. Growth and childhood asthma. *Arch Dis Child* 1986;**61**:1049–55.

81. McNicol KN, Williams HE, Gillam GL. Chest deformity, residual airways obstruction and hyperinflation, and growth in children with asthma. *Arch Dis Child* 1970;**45**:783–9.

82. Gillam GL, McNicol KN, Williams HE. Chest deformity, residual airways obstruction and hyperinflation, and growth in children with asthma. 2. Significance of chronic chest deformity. *Arch Dis Child* 1970;**45**:789–99.

83. McNicol KN, Williams HE. Spectrum of asthma in children. 2. Allergic components. *BMJ* 1973; **4**:12–16.

84. Rajka G. *Essential Aspects of Atopic Dermatitis*. Springer-Verlag, Berlin, 1989.

85. Asher MI, Keil U, Anderson HR, *et al*. International Study of Asthma and Allergies in Childhood (ISAAC): rationale and methods. *Eur Respir J* 1995;**8**:483–91.

86. Asmussen L, Olson LM, Grant EN, Landgraf JM, Fagan J, Weiss KB. Use of the child health questionnaire in a sample of moderate and low-income inner-city children with asthma [in process citation]. *Am J Respir Crit Care Med* 2000;**162**:1215–21.

86a. World Health Organisation (2000) Management of the Child with a Serious Infection or Severe Malnutrition Chapter 3. Cough or Difficult Breathing Section 3.3.

87. Usherwood TP, Scrimgeour A, Barber JH. Questionnaire to measure perceived symptoms and disability in asthma. *Arch Dis Child* 1990; **65**:779–81.

88. Santanello NC, Davies G, Galant SP, *et al*. Validation of an asthma symptom diary for interventional studies. *Arch Dis Child* 1999;**80**:414–20.

89. Salome CM, Peat JK, Britton WJ, Woolcock AJ. Bronchial hyperresponsiveness in two populations of Australian schoolchildren. I. Relation to respiratory symptoms and diagnosed asthma. *Clin Allergy* 1987;**17**:271–81.

90. Pattemore PK, Asher MI, Harrison AC, Mitchell EA, Rea HH, Stewart AW. The interrelationship among bronchial hyperresponsiveness, the diagnosis of asthma, and asthma symptoms [see comments]. *Am Rev Respir Dis* 1990;**142**:549–54.

91. Kuehni CE, Davis A, Brooke AM, Silverman M. Are all wheezing disorders in very young (preschool) children increasing in prevalence? *Lancet* 2001;**357**:1821–5.

92. Peat JK, Toelle BG, Marks GB, Mellis CM. Continuing the debate about measuring asthma in population studies. *Thorax* 2001;**56**:406–11.

93. Archer LN, Simpson H. Night cough counts and diary card scores in asthma. *Arch Dis Child* 1985; **60**:473–4.

94. Venables KM, Farrer N, Sharp L, Graneek BJ, Newman Taylor AJ. Respiratory symptoms questionnaire for asthma epidemiology: validity and reproducibility. *Thorax* 1993;**48**:214–24.

95. Kamps AW, Roorda RJ, Brand PL. Peak flow diaries in childhood asthma are unreliable. *Thorax* 2001; **56**:180–2.

96. Hyland ME KCARHP. Diary keeping in asthma: comparison of written and electronic methods. *BMJ* 1993;**306**:487–9.

97. Gibson NA, Ferguson AE, Aitchison TC, Paton JY. Compliance with inhaled asthma medication in preschool children. *Thorax* 1995;**50**:1274–9.

98. Pelkonen AS, Nikander K, Turpeinen M. Reproducibility of home spirometry in children with newly diagnosed asthma [in process citation]. *Pediatr Pulmonol* 2000;**29**:34–8.

99. Wensley DC, Silverman M. The quality of home spirometry in school children with asthma. *Thorax* 2001;**56**:183–5.

100. Johnston IDA, Anderson HA, Patel S. Variability in peak flow in wheezy children. *Thorax* 1984;**39**:583–7.

101. MacKenzie CR, Charlson ME. Standards for the use of ordinal scales in clinical trials. *BMJ* 1986; **292**:40–3.

102. Forrest M, Anderson B. Ordinal scales and statistics in medical research. *BMJ* 1986;**292**:537–8.

103. Brand PL, Duiverman EJ, Waalkens HJ, van Essen-Zandvliet EE, Kerrebijn KF. Peak flow variation in childhood asthma: correlation with symptoms, airways obstruction, and hyperresponsiveness during long-term treatment with inhaled corticosteroids. Dutch CNSLD Study Group. *Thorax* 1999;**54**:103–7.

104. Mortimer KM, Redline S, Kattan M, Wright EC, Kercsmar CM. Are peak flow and symptom measures good predictors of asthma hospitalisations and unscheduled visits? *Ped Pulmol* 2001;**31**:190–7.

105. Wensley D, Silverman M. Peak flow-based self management for children with asthma. *Thorax* 2002 (in press).

106. Nielsen KG, Bisgaard H. The effect of inhaled budesonide on symptoms, lung function, and cold air and methacholine responsiveness in 2- to 5-year-old asthmatic children [in process citation]. *Am J Respir Crit Care Med* 2000;**162**:1500–6.

107. Pao CS, McKenzie SA. Inhaled corticosteroids for persistent wheeze in preschool children. *Am J Respir Crit Care Med* 2001;**163**:1278.

108. Simpson H, Matthew DJ, Inglis JM, George EC. Virological findings and blood gas tensions in acute lower respiratory tract infections in children. *BMJ* 1974;**2**:629–32.

109. Chidiac P, Alexander IS. Head retraction and respiratory disorders in infancy. *Arch Dis Child* 1990;**65**:567–8.

110. McKenzie SA, Edmunds AT, Godfrey S. Status asthmaticus: a one year study. *Arch Dis Child* 1979;**54**:486.

111. Rebuck AS, Tamarken JL. Pulsus paradoxicus in asthmatic children. *Can Med Assoc J* 1975; **112**:710–11.

112. Broughton RA. Infections due to Mycoplasma pneumoniae in childhood. *Pediatr Infect Dis* 1986; **5**:71–85.

113. Irving RM, Richards A, Fisher EW. Pulmonary tuberculosis presenting as suspected foreign body aspiration. *J Laryngol Otol* 2000;**106**:453–6.

114. Smyth RL, Fletcher JN, Thomas HM, Hart CA. Immunological responses to respiratory syncytial virus infection in infancy. *Arch Dis Child* 1997;**76**:210–14.

115. Riedel F, Oberdieck B, Streckert HJ, Philippou S, Krusat T, Marek W. Persistence of airway hyperresponsiveness and viral antigen following respiratory syncytial virus bronchiolitis in young guinea-pigs. *Eur Respir J* 1997;**10**:639–45.

116. Openshaw PJ. Potential mechanisms causing delayed effects of respiratory syncytial virus infection. *Am J Respir Crit Care Med* 2001;**163**:S10–13.

117. Sly PD, SotoQuiros S, Landau LI, Hudson I, Newton John H. Factors predisposing to abnormal pulmonary function after adenovirus type 7 pneumonia. *Arch Dis Child* 1984;**59**:935–9.

118. Chang AB, Masel JP, Masters B. Post-infectious bronchiolitis obliterans: clinical, radiological and pulmonary function sequelae. *Pediatr Radiol* 1998;**28**:23–9.

119. Reid L, Simon G, Zorab RA, Seidelin R. The development of unilateral hypertransradiancy of the lung. *Br J Dis Chest* 1967;**61**:190–2.

120. Accurso FJ. Early respiratory course in infants with cystic fibrosis. *Ped Pulmonol* 1991;**7**(Suppl):42–5.

121. Buchdahl RM, Reiser J, Ingram N, Rutman A, Cole PJ, Warner JO. Ciliary abnormalities in respiratory disease. *Arch Dis Child* 1988;**63**:238–43.

122. Bush A, Cole P, Hariri M, *et al.* Primary ciliary dyskinesia: diagnosis and standards of care. *Eur Respir J* 1998;**12**:982–8.

123. Morgan G, Seymour ND, Turner MW, Strobel S, Levinsky RJ. Heterogenicity of clinical syndromes associated with selective subclass IgG deficiency. *Prog Immunodef Res Ther* 1986;**11**:229–33.

124. Loftus BG, Price JF, Lobo-Yeo A, Vergani D. IgG subclass deficiency in asthma. *Arch Dis Child* 1988;**63**:143–7.

125. Schur PH. IgG subclasses: a review. *Ann Allergy* 1987;**58**:899–999.

126. Chan G, Seah CC, Yap HK, Goh DY, Lee BW. Immunoglobulin (Ig) and IgG subclasses in Asian children with bronchial asthma. *Ann Trop Paediatr* 1995;**15**:280–4.

127. Orenstein SR, Orenstein DM. Gastroesophageal reflux and respiratory disease in children. *J Pediatr* 1988;**112**:847–58.

128. Simpson H. Gastro-oesophageal reflux and the lung. *Arch Dis Child* 1991;**66**:277–8.

129. Hampton FJ, McFadyen UM, Beardsmore CS, Simpson H. Gastro-oesophageal reflux and respiratory function in infants with respiratory disease. *Arch Dis Child* 1991;**66**:848–53.

130. Puterman S, Gorodischer R, Leiberman A. Tracheobronchial foreign bodies: the impact of a postgraduate educational program on diagnosis, morbidity and treatment. *Pediatr* 1982; **70**:96–8.

131. Davies H, Gordon I, Matthew D, *et al.* Longterm followup after inhalation of foreign bodies. *Arch Dis Child* 1990;**65**:619–21.

132. Kuhn JP. High-resolution computed tomography of pediatric pulmonary parenchymal disorders. *Radiol Clin North Am* 1993;**31**:533–51.

133. Spiteri MA, Cook DG, Clarke SW. Reliability of eliciting physical signs in examination of the chest. *Lancet* 1988;**1**:875.

134. Britton J, Lewis S. Objective measures and the diagnosis of asthma. We need a simple diagnostic test – but don't yet have one [editorial]. *BMJ* 1998;**317**:227–8.

135. von Mutius E. Air pollution and asthma – fact or artifact? A plea for inclusion of objective measures in environmental epidemiology [editorial; comment]. *Pediatr Pulmonol* 1998;**25**:297–8.

136. Canny GJ, Reisman J, Healy R, *et al.* Acute asthma: observations regarding management of a pediatric emergency room. *Pediatrics* 1989;**83**:507–12.

137. Rushton AR. The role of the chest radiograph in the management of childhood asthma. *Clin Pediatr* 1982;**21**:325–8.

138. Dawson KP, Long A, Kennedy J, Mogridge N. The chest radiograph in acute bronchiolitis. *J Paediatr Child Health* 1990;**26**:209–11.

139. Awad LN, Muller NL, Park SC, Abboud RT, Fitzgerald JM. Airway wall thickness in patients with near fatal asthma and control groups: assessment with HRCT scanning. *Thorax* 1998;**53**:248–53.

140. US Department of Health and Human Services. National asthma education program: executive summary: guidelines for the diagnosis and management of asthma. Publication no 91-3042A, 1991. NIH, Bethesda, MA.

141. Dales RE, Spitzer WO, Tousignant P, Schechter M, Suissa S. Clinical interpretation of airway response to a bronchodilator. Epidemiologic considerations. *Am Rev Respir Dis* 1988;**138**:317–20.

142. Chung KF, Godard P, Adelroth E, *et al.* Difficult/therapy-resistant asthma: the need for an integrated approach to define clinical phenotypes, evaluate risk factors, understand pathophysiology and find novel therapies. ERS Task Force on Difficult/Therapy-Resistant Asthma. European Respiratory Society [in process citation]. *Eur Respir J* 1999;**13**:1198–1208.

143. Supplement. The role of small airways in asthma: a review and key questions. *Am J Respir Crit Care Med* 1998;**157**:S173–203.

144. Kraft M. The distal airways: are they important in asthma? *Eur Respir J* 1999;**14**:1403–17.

145. Sly PD, Flack F. Is home monitoring of lung function worthwhile for children with asthma? *Thorax* 2001;**56**:164–5.

146. Dawson B, Horobin G, Illsley R, Mitchell R. A survey of childhood asthma in Aberdeen. *Lancet* 1969;**1**:827–30.

147. Williams H, McNicol KN. Prevalence, natural history and relationship of wheezy bronchitis and asthma in children: an epidemiological study. *BMJ* 1969;**4**:321–5.

148. Hewer SL, Hambleton G, McKenzie S, *et al.* Paediatric asthma audit: a multicentre pilot study. *Arch Dis Child* 1993;**64**:167–9.

149. Ranganathan RS, Jaffe A, Payne DNR, McKenzie SA. Difficult asthma: defining the problems. *Ped Pulmonol* 2001;**31**:114–20.

150. McKenzie SA. Sudden death in asthma. *Arch Dis Child* 1989;**64**:1450–1.

151. Robertson C, Rubinfield A, Bowes G. Pediatric asthma deaths in Victoria: the mild are at risk. *Ped Pulmonol* 1992;**13**:95.

152. Colice GL, Burgt JV, Song J, Stampone P, Thompson PJ. Categorizing asthma severity. *Am J Respir Crit Care Med* 1999;**160**:1962–7.

153. Beydon N, Amsallem F, *et al.* Pre-post brochodilator interrupter resistance values in healthy young children. *Am J Resp Crit Care Med* 2002;**165**:1388–94.

Lung function

PETER D SLY AND FELICITY S FLACK

INTRODUCTION

The most important function of the lungs is to supply oxygen to the body and to remove carbon dioxide. The mechanical properties of the airways, lung tissues and chest wall and the dynamics of breathing influence the efficiency of gas exchange during breathing. Pulmonary function measurement is a routine part of the management of respiratory disease in adults and children over the age of 6 to 8 years. Infant lung function testing up to 18 months or so is becoming increasingly sophisticated and more widespread and we now have tools to investigate the pre-school child. Many advances in our understanding of the pathogenesis of respiratory diseases have come through an understanding of physiological disturbances demonstrated by pulmonary function tests. Knowledge of the physiological principles behind the tests and of the techniques used for making the measurements is necessary to understand the changes that occur in lung function during disease, the appropriate use of lung function testing, and the interpretation of the data produced.

The *conditions* under which measurements of lung function are made can have major influences on the results produced. To achieve reliable results in children, the technician requires patience, special training and experience to obtain the child's maximum cooperation. This requirement means that laboratories not routinely dealing with children may not be able to produce reliable data. Preliminary coaching, which is often time-consuming, is frequently required to achieve consistent results. It is equally important to provide a pleasant environment, separate from areas where invasive or painful procedures are performed, as a child's fear may cause poor results. Studies in children under 6–8 years old rarely produce reliable or repeatable results except in laboratories with special expertise. While it may be appropriate for simple spirometry to be performed in doctor's surgeries (after appropriate staff training), more complicated tests should be carried out in specialist, paediatric lung function laboratories. The conditions in which we have least control, the child's home, render domiciliary measurements of PEF or spirometry the least reliable.

Measurement conditions are even more likely to influence the outcome of tests in *infants*. Most methods require the infant to be sleeping in the supine position. This is necessary for reproducible results. In general, infants cannot be relied upon to sleep naturally on demand, or to remain asleep long enough to allow pulmonary function to be measured. The majority of infant lung function tests occur with the infant sedated, most commonly with chloral hydrate or a similar sedative. Sedating infants for pulmonary function testing is considered safe, with no reported serious adverse effects despite many thousands of tests having been performed throughout the world. However, a fall in arterial oxygen saturation has been reported in wheezy infants sedated for pulmonary function testing[1] and continuous monitoring of oxygen saturation is considered mandatory. Other factors, which may influence the results of the infant lung function tests, include environmental temperature and humidity, posture, the time since the last feed and sleep state. The importance of these factors has been reviewed.[2]

For all lung function tests a *record* must be kept with at least name, date of birth, height, gender, and date of test. Other information that may be important, depending on the clinical situation, includes perinatal history, environmental tobacco smoke exposure, family and personal history of atopy, racial origin and past medical history, including drug and radiation exposure. For all lung function tests inspection of the raw data is an essential step in quality control. Inspection of raw curves may indicate poor cooperation with the testing procedures.

Results from computerized lung function testing equipment should not be accepted without the ability to monitor, and preferably adjust the raw data. It is better to have no data than erroneous and misleading data that lead to inaccurate diagnosis or management.

CLINICAL PHYSIOLOGY

Lung volumes

The measurement of lung volume, the amount of gas within the lungs at any given point in the breathing cycle, provides important information in its own right about the state of the respiratory system. Also, because the value of many parameters of lung function, such as resistance, compliance, and forced expiratory flows, is dependent on the lung volume at which they are measured, a knowledge of lung volume assists in the interpretation of other measures of lung function.

The commonly used terms to subdivide lung volume are illustrated in Figure 6b.1. By convention, each subdivision is called a 'volume', while any combination of two or more volumes is called a 'capacity'. Tidal volume (Vt) is the volume of gas breathed in and out with each breath. Vital capacity (VC) is the maximal volume that can be exhaled following a maximal inspiration. Functional residual capacity (FRC) is the amount of gas remaining in the lungs at the end of expiration (ERV + RV). Total lung capacity (TLC) is the total amount of gas contained within the lungs following a maximal inspiration. Residual volume (RV) is the amount of gas left in the lungs following a maximal expiration.

MAINTENANCE OF LUNG VOLUME

During normal tidal breathing in *adults and older children*, the end-expiratory lung volume, FRC, coincides with the elastic equilibrium volume (EEV) of the respiratory system. This EEV occurs where the inward elastic recoil of the lungs balances the outward elastic recoil of the chest wall (Figure 6b.2). The EEV is the volume the respiratory system would assume if all the breathing muscles were relaxed during passive expiration. This normally occurs at approximately 40% of VC. Tidal breathing then begins from this relaxation volume. This volume is thought to be an 'efficient' volume from which to breathe as the inspiratory muscles are close to the optimal position on their length-tension curves. However, FRC does not always coincide with EEV. At times of increased ventilatory requirements, such as during exercise or with lung disease, active expiration can push FRC below EEV (Figure 6b.1). Breathing from volumes below EEV is less efficient and uses more energy and may contribute to the development of respiratory failure.

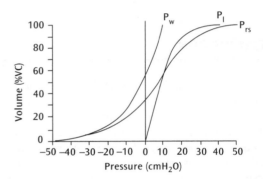

Figure 6b.2 *The static volume-pressure relationships of the chest wall (P_w), lungs (P_l) and respiratory system (P_{rs}). The elastic equilibrium volume (EEV) of the respiratory system is the volume where the inward recoil of the lungs (represented by a positive recoil pressure) is balanced by the outward recoil (represented by a negative recoil pressure) of the chest wall. This occurs at approximately 40% of vital capacity (VC) in normal adults and older children.*

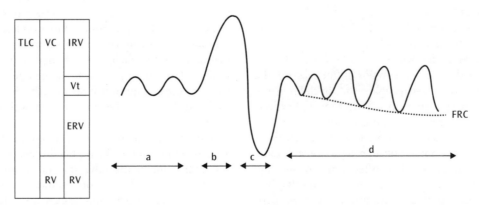

Figure 6b.1 *Schematic representation of the commonly used subdivisions of lung volumes. TLC: total lung capacity; VC: vital capacity; RV: residual volume; IRV: inspiratory reserve capacity; Vt: tidal volume; ERV: expiratory reserve volume. FRC (functional residual capacity) is the volume left in the lungs at the end of expiration, whether that occurs at the end of a normal tidal breath or at times of increased ventilatory requirements. a: tidal breathing; b: maximal inspiration; c: maximal expiration; d: period of tidal breathing during which FRC is changing.*

The chest wall of *newborn infants* is less stiff than that of older children and has a reduced recoil pressure. Also, the neonatal lung is relatively stiff. This combination results in EEV occurring at a relatively low lung volume, where there is risk of closure of small airways. This situation is even worse in infants born prematurely and in those who develop respiratory distress syndrome (RDS). Breathing from low lung volumes is inefficient because extra force is required to open airways that close during expiration. Under these circumstances FRC is usually actively elevated above EEV by increasing respiratory rate, thus beginning the next inspiration before EEV has been reached and by slowing down the rate of expiration by contracting the inspiratory muscles or the adductor muscles of the glottis. In extreme cases, such as with neonatal RDS, this 'expiratory braking' can be heard as 'grunting' during expiration.

Maintenance of lung volume is unlikely to present a problem in *asthmatics*. A reduction in static recoil pressure has been reported in some adults with long-standing asthma,[3] resulting in a shift of the static volume–pressure curve to the left. Similar data are lacking for children, however, most children with asthma are likely to have normal static elastic recoil pressures.

MEASUREMENT OF LUNG VOLUMES

Thoracic gas volume at functional residual capacity (Vtg, FRC) is measured directly in a *plethysmograph*, using techniques based on Boyle's law. Details of these techniques and discussion of the assumptions on which they are based are published elsewhere.[4] TLC and RV are calculated from Vtg combined with measurements of inspiratory capacity (IC = Vt + IRV, Figure 6b.1) and VC. RV may be falsely elevated if the child does not exhale fully. RV is one of the most variable of all lung function values in children[5] and values must be interpreted with caution.

Caution must also be exercised in the measurement and interpretation of lung volumes by plethysmography in the presence of severe airway obstruction. Under these circumstances, changes in mouth pressure are likely to under-represent changes in alveolar pressure during occluded breathing efforts, leading to an overestimation of lung volume.

Whole body plethysmography has been adapted for use in infants. Most commonly, constant mass 'pressure' plethysmographs are used. Much technical expertise is required to produce reliable results in infants. Again, the assumption that equilibration of mouth and alveolar pressures during the occluded breathing efforts, is unlikely to be justified in infants with airway obstruction.[6]

Alternatively, lung volumes can be measured by *gas dilution*. In theory these techniques are simple, involving the measurement of the dilution of a known concentration of gas by an unknown volume (the Vtg). By measuring the final gas concentration, it is possible to calculate Vtg.

Although the helium-dilution method is simple to perform and is relatively inexpensive,[7] it is time-consuming, potentially limiting cooperation, and is likely to under-estimate the Vtg significantly in the presence of airway obstruction. Gas dilution techniques measure that proportion of lung volume that is in free communication with the airway opening and are likely to miss poorly ventilated or non-communicating lung units. In addition, these techniques are extremely sensitive to leaks. Leaks result in a falsely low final indicator gas concentration and a falsely elevated estimate of lung volume. The nitrogen washout technique can also be used, where 100% O_2 is used to wash the nitrogen from the alveoli.

New techniques for measuring lung volume are being developed using, for example, an ultrasonic time-of-flight flow sensor that can calculate the molecular mass of the gas passing through it. This has been used to measure lung volume during the wash in of a heavy gas such as SF_6. Such measurements may permit the simultaneous assessment of lung volumes and gas mixing indices during other infant lung function tests but should be considered as research tools at present.

CHANGES IN LUNG VOLUMES SEEN DURING ASTHMA

Mild to moderate episodes of asthma are rarely associated with alterations in lung volume. As asthma becomes more severe, the volume of gas in the lungs increases, i.e. hyperinflation develops. In the short term, TLC does not usually change, but FRC and RV increase, resulting in a reduction in VC.[8] The mechanisms behind this hyperinflation are complex, but seem to include both active components, entailing persistent tonic activity of the inspiratory muscles, as well as passive components due to increases in airway resistance which prolong the expiratory time constant leading to incomplete expiration.[9] Expiratory flow-limitation (EFL) has been suggested as a trigger for hyperinflation during bronchoconstriction. However, Tantucci *et al.*[10] showed that 7 out of 10 subjects had an increase in end-expiratory lung volume following methacholine challenge before EFL was achieved. This suggests that other factors, as yet unexplained, are responsible for this phenomenon.

The elastic properties of the respiratory system

The elastic properties of the respiratory system are determined by its structure. When a force is applied to an elastic structure, it resists deformation by producing an opposing force to return it to the relaxed state. This opposing force is known as the elastic recoil pressure (P_{el}). The force that is required to stretch a purely elastic structure depends on how far it is stretched, not on how rapidly it is being stretched. Similarly, the pressure required to overcome the elastic recoil of the lung and chest wall depends on the lung volume above (or below) EEV (Figure 6b.2). The elastic recoil pressure divided by the lung volume gives a measure of the elastic properties of the respiratory system and is called elastance (E):

$$E = \Delta P_{el}/\Delta V$$

The reciprocal of elastance is known as the compliance (C), and describes how much the respiratory system will be inflated for a given change in applied pressure:

$$C = \Delta V/\Delta P_{el}$$

When lung volume is plotted on the ordinate and P_{el} is plotted on the abscissa, the slope of the volume-pressure curve at any point, is equivalent to the compliance (Figure 6b.2).

In most children with asthma, the elastic properties of the respiratory system are unlikely to change. However, if gross hyperinflation develops, the respiratory system may be moved to a volume where the volume–pressure curve begins to plateau and the system becomes very stiff. Under these circumstances further inflation of the lungs is difficult.

Dynamics of respiration

Breathing involves motion of the respiratory system, which is produced by forces required to overcome the elastic, flow-resistive, and inertial properties of the lungs and chest wall. Under normal circumstances the respiratory muscles produce these forces.

The force required to move a block of wood over a surface is determined by the friction between the block of wood and the surface, and by its velocity. It is not, however, determined by its position. Similarly, the pressure required to produce a flow of gas between the atmosphere and the alveoli must overcome the frictional resistance of the airways. This pressure is proportional to the flow (V'), the rate at which volume is changing. Thus:

$$Pm - Pa = Pfr \propto V'$$

where Pm is pressure at the mouth (usually atmospheric pressure) and Pfr the pressure required to overcome frictional resistance. The pressure required to produce a unit of flow is known as the flow resistance (R):

$$R = Pfr/V'$$

Most commonly used tests of pulmonary function model the respiratory system as a single compartment, with a single resistance and a single elastance. The equation describing the balance of forces acting on the system during ventilation is often referred to as the equation of motion of the respiratory system. It can be written as follows:

$$P = EV + RV' + IV''$$

where P is the applied pressure and I, the co-efficient of acceleration, represents the inertance of the respiratory system. Under most circumstances, especially in obstructive airway disorders, the inertance is negligible and therefore ignored. During spontaneous breathing, the applied pressure is produced by the respiratory muscles and can be measured as the transpulmonary pressure (Ptp). During normal tidal respiration, about 90% of the applied pressure is required to overcome the elastic forces and about 10% is required to overcome the frictional or flow-resistive forces. In asthma, this distribution of forces may alter. More pressure is likely to be required to overcome flow-resistive forces as airway narrowing occurs. However, relatively minor increases in FRC could result in marked increases in the pressure required to overcome elastic forces. Changes in the inertive properties are unlikely. Thus the resultant balance of forces is difficult to predict and could change rapidly during acute asthma.

The lungs do not behave like a simple balloon on a pipe. In reality there is not a single value for Raw but rather a continuous distribution of Raw throughout the bronchial tree. Any ventilation inhomogeneity will affect this distribution. In addition, energy is dissipated moving the tissues of the lungs and chest wall.

Traditionally it is thought that most of the force required to overcome the flow resistive forces of the respiratory system moves gas through the airways, with little energy dissipated by the tissues of the respiratory system. The contribution of tissue visco-elasticity to the behaviour of the respiratory system has become increasingly apparent. The energy expended moving the tissues has been called tissue viscance, or tissue resistance. When measured during inspiration, tissue resistance increases with increasing lung volume[11,12] while airway resistance (Raw) falls. Tissue resistance contributes about 65% of respiratory system resistance at FRC in mechanically ventilated animals, and increases to as much as 95% at higher lung volumes.[12,13] Studies in human infants have confirmed these results.[14]

Elegant studies[15,16] have demonstrated that changes in the lung periphery are important determinants of responsiveness to methacholine. These studies have measured both small airways (<3 mm diameter) and tissue properties. The well-recognized phenomenon of bronchodilation induced by taking a big breath, seen in normal adults, has also been attributed to a relaxation of ASM tone. This effect is not always seen in asthmatics and is thought to be due to an excess of parenchymal hysteresis over airway hysteresis. These effects can be quantified by comparing the forced flow at a fixed lung volume produced on forced expirations from end-tidal inspiration (partial manoeuvre) with that from TLC (maximal manoeuvre); this is known as the M:P ratio and a value >1 indicates bronchodilation following a deep inspiration resulting from a decrease in ASM tone. These measurements are difficult in younger children and have not been attempted in infants. Indirect studies have compared the expiratory flows from partial flow–volume loops to those from maximal flow–volume loops as an indication of the relative importance of tissue and airway hysteresis. These studies suggest that the chronic inflammation seen in asthma, increases the relative contribution of tissue hysteresis to lung function.[17,18] This area is attracting considerable research attention, which should clarify the importance of the tissue properties to diseases such as asthma.

Measurement of resistance and compliance

Airway resistance (Raw) is usually measured in children by plethysmography. When a subject breathes within a sealed plethysmograph (box), pressure changes within the plethysmograph are recorded as a result of variations in alveolar pressure (P_A) which lead to small changes (ΔV) in alveolar gas volume. Provided pressure changes due to other influences, such as change in gas conditions from BTPS within the lungs to ATPS within the box, and gas exchange with the blood can be eliminated, the relationship between change in P_A and flow at the mouth can be used to determine the Raw.

This technique has been standardized for use in adults and older children and includes the following steps:

1 The relationship between change in P_A and change in P_{box} is determined during respiratory effort against an occluded airway.
2 The subject breathes from the plethysmograph or from a gas conditioning circuit through a flow meter while supporting the cheeks with the hands. Panting efforts are usually made at a frequency of 1–3 Hz with a Vt of 50–150 ml, giving a mouth flow of 0.3–3.0 l/s peak-to-peak.

Precise details of the technique are published elsewhere.[4] Repeatability is generally poor in younger children.

Raw is difficult to measure by whole body plethysmography in awake young children. However, a method of measuring specific airway resistance, sRaw, in a single step with an accompanying adult has been developed.[19,20]

Measurement of *compliance* in spontaneously breathing subjects either requires the subject to relax their respiratory muscles against an occluded airway at various points during tidal breathing, or depends on the insertion of an oesophageal balloon to measure changes in intrathoracic pressure. These techniques measure compliance of the respiratory system (Crs) or lung (Cl) respectively and are not commonly used in children. Examination of the volume–pressure curve of the respiratory system (Figure 6b.2) reveals a substantial volume range over which compliance is essentially constant. However, both at high lung volumes and at low lung volumes the respiratory system becomes stiffer, i.e. compliance decreases.

A number of techniques are available for measuring resistance and compliance in spontaneously breathing infants. Techniques invoking the Hering–Breuer reflex

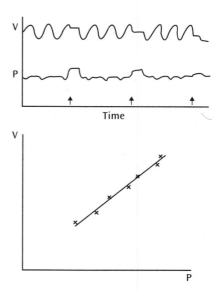

Figure 6b.3 *Schematic representation of data collected during the multiple occlusion test and the resultant 'static' volume–pressure (V–P) relationship that can be constructed in order to determine the compliance ($\Delta V/\Delta P$). The arrows indicate where occlusions are made.*

rely on the assumption that inflation produces complete relaxation of both inspiratory and expiratory respiratory muscles and that it can be elicited during airway occlusion. Airway opening pressure is assumed to equilibrate with alveolar pressure during the occlusion. There are two main variants of these occlusion techniques. In the *multiple occlusion technique* pressure is measured at the mouth during brief expiratory airway occlusions, performed on multiple breaths, or even during a single expiration. Occlusions are performed at different volumes above FRC and the individual measurements are plotted as volume versus pressure. The slope of the line of best fit is the compliance of the respiratory system (Figure 6b.3). In the *single breath technique*, the airway is occluded at end-inspiration, with the subsequent expiration occurring passively. A passive expiratory flow–volume curve is then constructed and a line fitted to the linear portion (Figure 6b.4). Compliance is calculated by dividing the total exhaled volume by the mouth pressure recorded during the occlusion. The slope of the linear part of the passive flow–volume curve is equal to the reciprocal of the expiratory time constant (τrs). Resistance (Rrs) can be calculated as follows: Rrs = τrs/Crs, by analogy with simple electrical circuit theory.

The main problems with these techniques are ensuring relaxation of the respiratory muscles following airway occlusion and equilibration of mouth and alveolar pressures. Generally, the presence of a plateau in mouth pressure is evidence that both of these assumptions have been satisfied. There are no firm recommendations as to how long a plateau should be maintained. It has been suggested that the duration of the airway occlusion can influence the values of Crs calculated from the subsequent expiration.[21]

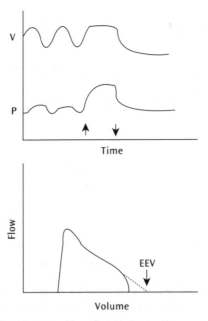

Figure 6b.4 *Schematic representation of data collected during the single breath technique and the 'passive' expiratory limb of the flow–volume relationship constructed following release of occlusion. The slope of the line fitted to the 'linear' portion of the flow–volume curve is equal to the reciprocal of the expiratory time-constant. The arrows indicate where the occlusion is applied and released. EEV is the theoretical elastic equilibrium volume.*

Despite their widespread use, there are no currently agreed standards for performing these tests.

Measurement of Raw by whole body plethysmography has been modified for *infants* by the inclusion of a re-breathing bag, containing heated, humidified, oxygen-enriched gas at BTPS, to avoid the need for 'panting'. This is a sophisticated technique that requires a large amount of expertise and training, but has the advantage of producing simultaneous measurements of lung volume and Raw. However, this technique is less reliable in the presence of airway obstruction, particularly in the youngest infants, due their very compliant upper airways.[22] In addition, because infants normally breathe through the nose, the value of Raw includes a major component of upper airway resistance which is affected by nasal obstruction.

In recent years a series of oscillatory techniques have been developed for measuring resistance and compliance in *infants and preschool children*. The advantage of these techniques is that they are non-invasive and can be performed during normal tidal breathing. The forced oscillation technique (FOT) determines pulmonary resistance by imposing known variations of flow at the mouth and measuring the pressure changes that result. A continuous sinusoidal signal (>4–6 Hz) generated by a loudspeaker is used. The frequency of the oscillations is higher than that of the patient's spontaneous breathing so the effects of the normal breathing cycle can be subtracted. Paediatric

reference values have been published for respiratory resistance measured by FOT at 8, 12 and 16 Hz.[23]

Tissue resistance comprises a significant proportion of the total respiratory resistance at normal breathing frequencies and bronchoconstriction is associated with increases in parenchymal resistance and elastance. Therefore it is important to be able to measure both airway and tissue resistance. Measurement of pulmonary resistance at low oscillation frequencies (0.5–20 Hz) is a non-invasive way of estimating the airway and tissue parameters separately. These measurements can only be taken during suspension of breathing. Infants must be sedated and measurements are taken during the end-inspiratory occlusion apnoea initiated by the Hering–Breuer reflex.[24]

Impulse oscillometry (IOS) is a similar method to FOT except brief pulses of pressure generated by a loudspeaker instead of a continuous sinusoidal signal are used. The data from several 'impulses' are analysed to give Rrs and Xrs in the frequency range 5–35 Hz.[25] Because of technical limitations, the frequency resolution is limited and data are only available in 5 Hz intervals (5 Hz, 10 Hz, etc).

Another non-invasive method of measuring respiratory resistance is called the *interrupter technique (Rint)*. Following a brief interruption to airflow, alveolar pressure equilibrates with mouth pressure. Respiratory resistance can be estimated by calculating the ratio of pressure change at the mouth to flow at the time of occlusion. The Rint device is small in size and simple to use making it an appropriate method for use in preschool children.[26]

The *high-speed interrupter technique* was described by Frey *et al.*[27] as a method of estimating changes in airway wall mechanics in infants. In this technique airflow at the mouth is interrupted several times within 0.15 s by a fast rotating shutter whilst normal breathing continues. This allows high frequency (32–1300 Hz) impedance measurements to be performed. Frey showed that the first anti-resonance is a function of airway wall compliance and is independent of airway diameter. While further validation is required, this technique holds the promise of being able to study the mechanical properties of airway walls *in situ*.

CHANGES IN RESISTANCE AND COMPLIANCE SEEN IN ASTHMA

Changes in resistance and compliance may occur in asthma. The airway narrowing encountered during an episode of asthma results in an increase in Raw, despite the partly compensatory increase in lung volume seen (which should limit the increase in Raw). Compliance is unlikely to change acutely in most asthmatics, although a decrease in Crs has been reported in symptomatic children.[28] A loss of elastic recoil has been reported in some adults with a long history of persistent asthma.[3] This results in an increase in responsiveness to natural and chemical stimuli, as the elastic recoil of the lung tissues is thought to limit the degree to which airway smooth muscle can shorten *in vivo*.[29,30] In infants, studies of the response to methacholine challenge show increases in Raw as well as tissue damping. These responses are increased if the infant has a history of respiratory disease.[31]

Forced expiration

Forced vital capacity manoeuvres from which PEF, FEV_1 and maximum expiratory flow–volume curves can be derived are the basis of the most common and most useful tests of lung function in children. Forced expiratory manoeuvres, as used to stress the respiratory system in lung function testing, are not 'natural' phenomena. Cough is a natural forced expiration and, as such, provides valuable information about the respiratory system, in particular about the state of the airways.

PHYSIOLOGY OF WHEEZING

Gas flows into and out of the lungs along pressure gradients. During inspiration alveolar pressure is lowered below atmospheric pressure, due to the actions of the inspiratory muscles expanding the thorax. This results in a pressure gradient between the mouth and the alveoli. Gas flows into the lungs along this gradient. As the pressure surrounding the intra-thoracic airways is essentially alveolar pressure, a pressure gradient also exists across the airway wall, which tends to expand the airways during inspiration. At the end of inspiration when the inspiratory muscles relax, the lungs are inflated to a volume above the elastic equilibrium volume of the respiratory system. At this volume, the inward recoil of the lungs and chest wall produce a positive alveolar pressure, relative to atmospheric pressure, and provide the driving force necessary to produce expiration. Contraction of expiratory muscles can contribute to this driving pressure. The airway transmural pressure gradient is reversed and the intra-thoracic airways tend to narrow during expiration. The higher the expiratory driving pressure, the greater the tendency to narrow the intra-thoracic airways.

During forced expiration, expiratory flow is independent of the driving pressure over most of the expired vital capacity, once a threshold value of driving pressure is exceeded. This phenomenon is known as *expiratory flow-limitation*. The mechanism for expiratory flow-limitation is complex.[32] In fluid dynamic terms, a system cannot carry a greater flow than the flow for which fluid velocity equals wave speed at some point in the system. The wave speed is the speed at which a small disturbance travels in a compliant tube filled with fluid. The speed of a pressure wave is determined by the elasticity of the wall of the tube and the density of the fluid within. In the arteries this is the speed at which the pulse propagates. In the airway the speed is higher than this, mainly because the fluid density (i.e. gas density) is lower. The wave speed (c) in a compliant tube with an area A that depends on a lateral

pressure P, filled with a fluid of density ρ, is given by:

$$c = (AdP/\rho dA)^2$$

where dP/dA is the slope of the pressure-area curve for the airway, an expression of airway wall elasticity. Maximal flow is the product of the fluid velocity at wave speed and airway area,

$$V'_{max} = cA$$

Flow-limitation occurs in the airways when actual flow equals V'_{max}, at any site within the airway tree. At high lung volumes the flow-limiting site in the human airways is typically in the second and third generations. As lung volume decreases, airway calibre decreases, the flow-limiting site moves peripherally and V'_{max} decreases. This is the explanation for the observation that the tail of the maximum expiratory flow–volume curve provides information about small airway function. At low lung volumes the density dependence of maximal flow is small and the viscosity dependence is large and becomes the predominant mechanism limiting expiratory flow.

Flow-limitation in a compliant tube is accompanied by flutter of the walls at the site of flow-limitation.[33,34] This can be modelled simply in a child's party balloon, by filling the balloon and then releasing it to let it empty spontaneously. The flutter balances the energy in the system, as the driving pressure in excess of that required to produce V'_{max} is dissipated in causing wall flutter. In the presence of airway obstruction, this flutter may become large enough to generate sound, heard as *wheezing*. Thus expiratory wheezing is a sign of expiratory flow-limitation.[35] Note, wheezing always implies flow-limitation, but flow-limitation can occur without producing a wheeze.[35] In children with mild asthma, wheeze may be heard during forced expiration (including during a cough) but be absent during tidal breathing. This implies that flow-limitation is occurring during forced expiration but not during tidal breathing. As the severity of the asthma increases and airway narrowing worsens, flow-limitation may occur during tidal expiration and wheezes may be heard during tidal breathing. Focal wheeze, for instance unilateral wheeze in the presence of an inhaled foreign body implies focal obstruction with focal flow-limitation.

Measurements of forced expiration have long been used to detect the presence of obstructive lung disease. They are useful because expiratory flow is independent of the force driving flow over most of the expired vital capacity, so long as reasonable effort is made.[32] This observation led directly to the description of the maximal expiratory flow–volume (MEFV) curve, which emphasized that, at most lung volumes, there was a limit to maximal expiratory flow (V'_{max}). The peak expiratory flow is discussed below. Flows near RV may be effort dependent, as expiratory muscle contraction may not be able to provide sufficient force to maintain flow-limitation at this low lung volume.

FORCED EXPIRATORY MANOEUVRES

Most children can accomplish forced expiratory manoeuvres by the age of 7 years and sometimes as young as 3 years. To produce reliable measurements, children need to be able to give a maximal effort, without hesitation, preferably for three seconds. However, healthy children empty their forced vital capacity in less than 3 seconds, some in less than 1 second. In young children, a learning effect may be operative and more than the standard two practice and three definitive tests may be required to obtain consistent, representative data. The expiratory limb of a normal child's maximal flow–volume curve is slightly convex to the volume axis. The curve from a child with airway obstruction becomes concave to the volume axis (Figure 6b.5). The shape of the expiratory limb gives a good indication of the presence and degree of airway obstruction, but this visual impression has proven very difficult to reproduce with a 'number' or 'index'.

In 1994 the American Thoracic Society (ATS) published standard procedures for spirometry.[36] The criteria for end of test require that there be a minimum change in volume of 0.03 l over a 1 second period given a forced expiratory time of at least 6 seconds. While children usually meet the ATS criteria for reproducibility after some coaching, they often do not meet all the test criteria. Therefore it is recommended that test criteria for children is based on proportional and not absolute criteria.[37,38]

The variables usually calculated from the *forced expiratory manoeuvre* are the forced vital capacity (FVC), the forced expiratory volume in 1 second (FEV_1), and the forced expiratory flow between 25% and 75% of the FVC (FEF_{25-75}). The FEF_{25-75} is a measure of the average flow over the middle 50% of FVC. The FVC and FEV_1 are the most robust measurements of airway obstruction. The FEV_1 gives a good balance between reproducibility and the ability to detect airway obstruction. An FEV_1/FVC ratio of <75% is indicative of airway obstruction. Forced expiratory flows at lower lung volumes are more sensitive to minor degrees of airway obstruction. There is a widely held belief that flows at low lung volumes reflect obstruction of the small airways. However, the MEFV curve represents the 'integrated output' of the entire respiratory system and is not easily partitioned into components reflecting different anatomical areas. While the site of flow-limitation generally does move toward the smaller airways in a smooth fashion as lung volume decreases, this peripheral progression cannot be determined from the flow–volume curve. Furthermore, flows at low lung volume are particularly sensitive to changes in absolute lung volume, which increases the variability of these measurements particularly when interpreting responses to challenge tests or bronchodilator therapy. The effect of change in volume is an underestimation of change in lung function.

Forced expiration can also be measured in infants using the *rapid thoracic compression technique* (RTC). The RTC technique produces forced expiratory flows by suddenly applying a pressure to the thorax and abdomen at the end of a tidal inspiration (Figure 6c.3, p. 147). This is achieved using an inflatable thoraco-abdominal jacket connected to a positive pressure reservoir. Flow is measured at the mouth with an appropriately sized pneumotachograph attached to a mask sealed around the infant's nose and mouth, and a flow–volume curve constructed. Prior to the RTC manoeuvre, a reproducible FRC is established from at least three tidal breaths. RTC, initiated at end-inspiration, then produces a partial expiratory flow–volume (PEFV) curve, with exhalation continuing to a volume below the previous FRC. RTC manoeuvres are performed with increasing jacket pressures until the pressure that produces the highest expiratory flows is determined. The maximal flow occurring at the previously established tidal FRC known as $V'_{max}FRC$ reported (Figure 6b.6). A joint task force of the American Thoracic and European Respiratory Societies has recently published methods for standardizing the RTC between centres.[39]

Use of the RTC has led to major advances in the understanding of the normal growth and development

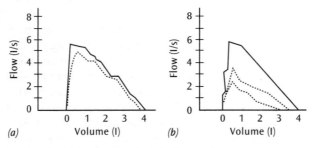

(a)   *(b)*

Figure 6b.5 *Maximal expiratory flow–volume curves showing (a) a normal pattern and (b) the presence of airway obstruction (lower dashed curve), together with the response to inhaled bronchodilator (upper dashed curve). Solid line: reference curve.*

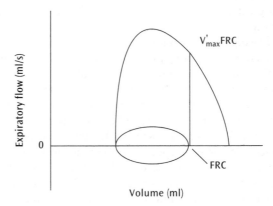

Figure 6b.6 *Schematic representation of the forced expiratory flow–volume curve produced by the rapid thoracic compression test. The 'forced' curve is laid over the previous tidal curve and the maximal flow at the previous FRC position ($V'_{max}FRC$) calculated.*

of the respiratory system and of respiratory diseases. For example, Seidenberg et al. [40] demonstrated that lung function abnormalities persist for up to three months, in the absence of clinical symptoms, following an episode of acute viral bronchiolitis. See also Chapters 3 and 9.

However, the RTC technique has not proved to be the key to understanding intrathoracic airway function that it initially promised to be. Useful measurements of forced expiration rely on expiratory flow-limitation being achieved. While this may be the case with the RTC technique in infants with airway obstruction, flow-limitation is unlikely to be achieved in healthy infants. Furthermore, FRC is notoriously variable in infants, even over short time periods. This leads to substantial variability in the values of $V'_{max}FRC$. Many studies have consistently failed to demonstrate a bronchodilator response following single doses of inhaled sympathomimetics, yet clinical studies have shown that some infants appear clinically to benefit from inhaled bronchodilators. They breathe more easily and have less wheezing. One possible reason for this discrepancy is that bronchodilators alter FRC, possibly reducing hyperinflation. Because of the dependence of $V'_{max}FRC$ on lung volume, this decrease in FRC would have the effect of reducing any change in the $V'_{max}FRC$ measured by RTC thus masking the expected improvement following bronchodilator treatment (Chapter 9).

In an attempt to overcome many of the problems with the RTC technique, the *raised volume rapid thoraco-abdominal compression* (RVRTC) technique has been developed. In this technique the infant's lungs are inflated to a pre-set pressure using an external gas source prior to the RTC.[41, 42] The advantage of RVRTC is that the lung volume from which the forced expiration occurs can be standardized to a given pressure. This technique appears to be more sensitive in wheezy infants and in infants with cystic fibrosis than the conventional RTC technique (Figure 6b.7).

In older children and adults, flow-limitation is achieved during forced expiratory manoeuvres. This allows reproducible measurements of lung function to be taken. One of the concerns about the RTC technique is whether flow-limitation is achieved in infants, particularly healthy ones. Feher and colleagues found that several rapid lung

inflations immediately before a rapid compression manoeuvre in infants inhibited inspiration and enabled flow-limitation to be achieved.[42] They also demonstrated the presence of expiratory flow-limitation during forced expiration by applying brief 'pulses' of negative pressure at the airway opening during the forced expiration and showing that expiratory flow does not increase with the increase in airway pressure.[43] This provides a relatively easy method for assessing whether expiratory flow-limitation has indeed been achieved in an individual infant.

PEAK EXPIRATORY FLOW

Measurement of peak expiratory flow (PEF) is of value in identifying and assessing the degree of airflow-limitation in epidemiological studies and in clinical practice, where it can be helpful in monitoring the progress of disease and the effects of treatment. PEF is the maximum flow achieved during a forced expiration starting from the level of maximal lung inflation.[44]

Traditionally, PEF has not been thought to be flow-limited because a plateau is not seen on isovolume pressure flow (IVPF) curves, presumably because of inability of the respiratory muscles to generate sufficient force. However, Kano et al.[45] demonstrated that performing the forced expiration following a breath hold at TLC decreased PEF. They proposed that the breath hold allowed viscoelastic energy in the airway wall to be dissipated, resulting in a reduction of airway wall stiffness. This would result in more compressible airways and a reduction in the maximal flow sustainable. These observations are consistent with flow-limitation being achieved at PEF.

This does not, however, mean that PEF is independent of effort. The magnitude of PEF depends on how this maximal flow is reached. If expired volume from TLC at which PEF is reached is small, PEF will be higher because, at higher lung volume the higher elastic recoil pressure and lower upstream resistance result in greater wave speed and a higher PEF (Figure 6b.8). In any interpretation of changes in PEF, the magnitude of effort and the volume at which PEF is reached are critical.

In the past significant errors have been identified in the PEF measured with mini-flow meters[46] (Figure 6b.9).

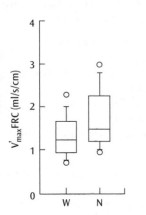

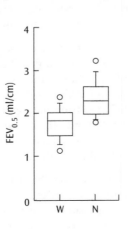

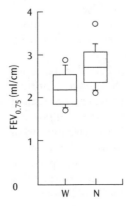

Figure 6b.7 *Box and whisker plots showing the median interquartile range of $V'_{max}FRC$, $FEV_{0.5}$, and $FEV_{0.75}$ in a group of recurrently wheezy infants (W) and matched normal controls (N). The data are taken from Turner DJ. Assessment of forced expiration from raised lung volumes in infants. Doctor of Philosophy thesis, University of Western Australia, 1994.*

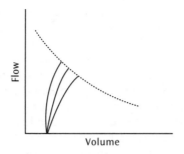

Figure 6b.8 *Schematic representation of how peak expiratory flow (PEF) can be 'effort-dependent' and still reach the maximal achievable speed, i.e. wave speed (represented by the dotted line).*

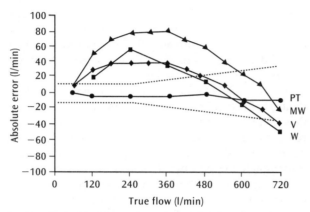

Figure 6b.9 *Absolute error plots for three full range peak flow meters and a pneumotachograph. The dotted lines indicate the American Thoracic Society guidelines for accuracy. PT: pneumotachograph, MW: mini-Wright, V: Vitalograph, W: Wright. (Reproduced with permission from* Thorax 1992;**47**:904–9.)

These errors arose previously because of non-linearities in the meters themselves due to the physics involved in recording PEF. However mini-flow meters currently on the market have had these errors corrected by adjusting the measurement scale. The values of PEF produced by an individual asthmatic child are likely to differ from one type of mini-flow meter to another. The same is probably true for different meters of the same type. Thus it is important that every asthmatic who is going to use a mini-flow meter, should have a personal one. Furthermore, they should be encouraged to take their own meter with them when they visit their physician.

Although PEF increases with height during childhood, at any given height there is a wide range of normal values. This limits the usefulness of expressing a measured PEF as a per cent of predicted normal, based on population studies. Thus, each child needs to determine what their 'personal best' PEF is by monitoring PEF for one to two weeks at a time when they are well. This 'personal best' can then be used as a base for comparison during exacerbations of asthma, assuming the 'best' is not a spurious value produced, for example, during a cough.

In summary, measurements of forced expiration have been the basis of the physiological assessment of asthma and contributed to the clinical management for many years. There are, however, limitations with some of the measurements. As long as these limitations are understood and taken into account when interpreting the results of tests based on forced expiration, valuable clinical information can be obtained.

Measurement of lung function in preschool children

Measurements of lung function are important tools in the management of asthma and other respiratory diseases. However, it is difficult to obtain reliable measurements in preschool children using standard methods such as PEF or FEV_1 although interactive computer-based animation helps.[47]

The oscillatory techniques have been shown in several studies to be suitable techniques for measuring lung function in this group. A study of lung function tests in an emergency department showed that FOT could be used to measure lung function in untrained, acutely ill asthmatics. Successful tests were completed in 19% of 3-year-olds, 40% of 4-year-olds and 83% of 5-year-olds.[48] Another study showed that airway obstruction and bronchodilator responses could be measured in children as young as 3 years by FOT.[49]

Several studies have evaluated the use of the interrupter technique to measure lung function in preschool children. These studies show that this technique can also be used to measure airway resistance in normal children and those with lung disease as young as two.[25,26,50] This technique is useful for detecting responses to bronchodilators however it may not be able to detect responses to bronchoprovocation.[50]

The sRaw (plethysmographic) technique can be used in children as young as 3 years old.[19,20]

Gas exchange

The main function of the respiratory system is to supply oxygen to the body and to remove excess carbon dioxide. There are five basic steps involved in this process:

1 ventilation, the exchange of gas between the atmosphere and the alveoli;
2 diffusion across the alveolar-capillary membranes;
3 transport of gases in the blood;
4 diffusion from the capillaries of the systemic circulation to the cells of the body;
5 the use of O_2 and production of CO_2 within the cells – internal respiration.

Ventilation has been covered in the section dealing with lung mechanics.

Gas diffusion is a passive process: gases diffuse from a site of high partial pressure to a site of low partial pressure.

The flux is proportional to the area available for diffusion and to the difference in partial pressure per unit length of the diffusion pathway. Conditions that thicken the alveolar wall, which is the main blood–gas barrier, have the potential to interfere with diffusion. Fortunately, these conditions are rare in children with wheezing disorders and will not be considered.

GAS TRANSPORT

Gas is transported in the blood by two main means: dissolved in plasma or combined with haemoglobin. Approximately 98% of O_2 transported in the blood is bound to haemoglobin. In the lung, where the O_2 partial pressure is high, O_2 combines loosely with the haem portion of haemoglobin forming oxyhaemoglobin. When the oxyhaemoglobin reaches the tissues, where oxygen partial pressure is low, the O_2 is released and diffuses to the cells. The binding of O_2 to haemoglobin is a non-linear process, as demonstrated by the sigmoid-shaped oxygen-haemoglobin dissociation curve (Figure 6b.10). When haemoglobin is 100% saturated with O_2, large changes in the partial pressure of O_2 (PaO_2) are required before the arterial oxygen saturation (SaO_2) falls much. However, below an SaO_2 of about 90%, the relationship between fall in PaO_2 and in SaO_2 becomes steeper. Increases in both body temperature and in arterial pH shift the haemoglobin–oxygen dissociation curve to the right, facilitating the peripheral unloading of O_2. Normal lungs have sufficient reserve capacity to overcome the increased difficulty in loading of O_2 under these circumstances. However, in the presence of marked ventilation/perfusion imbalance (see below) right shifts in the haemoglobin–O_2 dissociation curve may become more significant.

Carbon dioxide is transported more readily in the blood than O_2, because CO_2, being a non-polar molecule, is highly lipid soluble. Carbon dioxide is transported in the blood in three ways, all of which begin with CO_2 being dissolved in the plasma after it has diffused into the systemic capillaries from the tissues:

1 as bicarbonate ions (60–70%);
2 combined with haemoglobin to form carbamino-haemoglobin (15–30%);
3 dissolved in plasma and red blood cells (7–10%).

Carbon dioxide does not bind to haemoglobin at the same site as O_2. It binds directly with some of the amino groups that form the haemoglobin molecule. The carbon dioxide-haemoglobin dissociation curve is less curvilinear (Figure 6b.10b).

VENTILATION/PERFUSION IMBALANCE IN THE LUNGS

Heterogeneity of the ventilation/perfusion (V/Q) balance in the lungs most commonly occurs with conditions that produce ventilation heterogeneity, such as obstructive

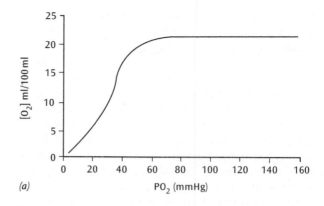

(a)

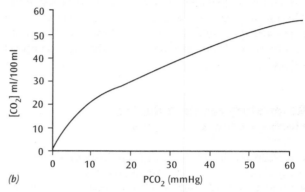

(b)

Figure 6b.10 *The relationship between (a) the arterial partial pressure of oxygen (PaO_2) and the whole blood oxygen content ([O_2]), assuming a haemoglobin concentration of 15 g/100 ml, and (b) The relationship between the arterial partial pressure of carbon dioxide ($PaCO_2$) and the whole blood carbon dioxide content ([CO_2]).*

airway diseases like asthma. V/Q mismatch causes a decrease in the transfer of O_2 to arterial blood and a decrease in CO_2 elimination. However, the end result is a lowering of arterial PO_2, with a lesser increase in arterial PCO_2. Several factors contribute to this phenomenon. The gas tensions in an individual alveolar-capillary unit depend on the ratio of ventilation to perfusion in that unit. Well-ventilated units tend to raise the O_2 tension towards that of the inspired gas (about 150 mmHg when breathing air) whereas well perfused units tend to lower oxygen tension towards that of the mixed venous blood (normally about 40 mmHg). For the same reasons, the PCO_2 is higher in over-perfused units and lower in over-ventilated units. The extreme case of over-ventilation and under-perfusion results in an increase in deadspace, whereas the converse (V/Q = O) results in intrapulmonary shunt. Mixing of the blood from units with different V/Q balance does not compensate for the different O_2 and CO_2 tensions, because, by definition, relatively more blood comes from the under-ventilated, over-perfused units. This results in a difference between the gas tensions in the mixed pulmonary venous blood (which becomes the arterial gas tension) and the mixed alveolar gas (in reality the average tension), and is expressed as an alveolar − arterial (A − a) difference. The A − a difference is greater for O_2 than for CO_2.

A lowering of the arterial PO_2, or an increase of arterial PCO_2, results in an increase in respiratory rate via chemoreceptor stimulation. This increase in respiratory rate is able to lower the $PaCO_2$ but cannot raise the PaO_2 to the same extent. This is because of the different shapes of the blood gas content–tension curves (Figure 6b.10). Because the oxyhaemoglobin dissociation curve is almost flat at high blood O_2 contents, increasing ventilation to well ventilated units cannot increase blood O_2 content. Whereas increasing ventilation will remove extra CO_2 from the blood passing through the well-ventilated units. This means that increasing ventilation, in the face of V/Q heterogeneity results in a lowering of the $PaCO_2$ towards or below normal, but does not increase the PaO_2 to normal values.

Respiratory function during sleep – circadian rhythms

Circadian rhythms have long been recognized to be an integral part of nature. In humans, the circadian rhythms are under the basic control of 'pacemakers' located in the suprachiasmic nuclei of the hypothalamus. The 24-hour period of the circadian rhythms comes from an interaction between environmental factors, such as the diurnal variation in illumination, and the intrinsic output of the pacemakers.

Diurnal variations have been described in lung mechanics, gas exchange and transport, and in bronchial responsiveness. Airway calibre, as judged from measurements of FEV_1, and Raw has been demonstrated to be smaller at night than during the day. A circadian rhythm with a peak at about 16.00 h and a trough at about 03.00–04.00 h has been described in normal adults. Hetzel and Clark,[51] measuring PEF demonstrated that the 'peak to trough' amplitude was about 8% for normal adults and about 50% for asthmatics. They suggested that an amplitude of >20% was highly suggestive of asthma. However, their asthmatic subjects all had moderately severe asthma and were in the recovery phase following an acute exacerbation of their asthma. The reported diurnal variation appears to be much higher in children,[52,53] with the upper confidence intervals of a normal population being approximately 30%. Thus measurement of diurnal variation in airway calibre does not appear to be a useful aid to the diagnosis of asthma in children. A diurnal variation in bronchial responsiveness has also been reported,[54–56] however, the precise timing of the rhythm depends on the agonist used.[56] The mechanisms underlying these diurnal variations have not been identified with certainty. They are not a function of sleep *per se*, or of the recumbent posture, as they continue if sleep is prevented.[57] Variations in vagal tone,[58] in cortisol secretion,[59] or in catachol levels[60] do explain the diurnal variations in airway calibre or in bronchial responsiveness.

Recent studies in which bronchial and transbronchial biopsies have been performed at 16.00 and 14.00 h have demonstrated a diurnal variation in parenchymal inflammation in nocturnal asthmatics. Diurnal variations in lung function in nocturnal asthmatics were found to correlate with the diurnal variation in parenchymal inflammation. In contrast, epithelium did not vary significantly from 16.00 to 04.00 h and as such did not correlate with the nocturnal falls in lung function.[61]

An understanding of these diurnal variations in airway calibre, bronchial responsiveness and parenchymal inflammation will allow a better understanding of the nature of asthma and lead to improved management. In general, airways are narrower and more sensitive at night. Thus they may be less able to cope with exposures to adverse environmental exposures, e.g. cigarette smoke, house-dust mite, or cold air, during the night than during the day. Interpretation of changes in lung function needs to include an allowance of the changes to be expected if the tests are performed at different times of the day. This is particularly important in clinical trials.

PHYSIOLOGICAL MEASUREMENT IN CLINICAL SITUATIONS

Pulmonary function testing in the management of childhood asthma

TESTS USED IN THE CLINIC OR SURGERY

Correct assessment of the severity of asthma is central to determining medication requirements and to individualizing a treatment plan. Physical examination and lung function testing, in children old enough to perform the tests, are integral parts of this assessment. The absence of physical signs does not exclude significant asthma and there may be a poor correlation between physical signs and spirometry in some children with asthma.

Children with troublesome asthma should have their pulmonary function measured at each visit, provided they are old enough to perform the tests reliably. Measurement of forced expiration, using a machine that produces a flow–volume loop, provides the most valuable information for assessing asthma control. In many settings such equipment is not available and the doctor relies on measurement of PEF using a mini-flow meter. 'One-off' measures of PEF are unlikely to produce useful results, particularly in children who are not experienced in using a mini-flow meter. If PEF is to be measured, the child should use its own mini-flow meter. The PEF value should be compared with the child's 'personal best' and not assessed as a per cent of predicted.[44]

The most useful time to measure pulmonary function is when the child's asthma is thought to be under control.

Persistent abnormalities of lung function after an adequate dose of a short acting β-agonist at this time need to be taken seriously and asthma treatment intensified.

HOME MONITORING OF PEAK EXPIRATORY FLOW

Monitoring of PEF has become an integral part of current asthma management. Asthma management plans that have been developed in many parts of the world include regular monitoring of PEF as an indication of when to increase medication. This position has arisen because of the demonstration that many asthmatics, especially children, are not able to adequately perceive their degree of airway obstruction.[62] An objective measure of asthma severity should allow, in theory, for more effective asthma management, with a reduction in both mortality and morbidity. Only one study to investigate the usefulness of incorporating home monitoring of PEF into 'asthma management plans' has been reported in children, with entirely negative results.[63]

When using PEF monitoring to assess lung function in a community setting changes in PEF do not necessarily correspond to changes in 'true' lung function, measured with a spirometer in children with asthma.[64] Clinically significant falls in PEF can occur in the absence of changes in spirometric lung function and vice versa[64] (Figure 6b.11). Furthermore, when daily symptom diaries are recorded in parallel with PEF, symptoms of asthma generally preceded falls in PEF and were acted upon in preference to PEF.[65] Although children are capable of maintaining the technical quality of their expiratory manoeuvres, over time their compliance with regular home monitoring declines rapidly.[66] Home monitoring of lung function has not been shown to improve asthma management. Therefore, it should not be used as a surrogate for a well-developed asthma management plan, based on a combination of respiratory symptoms, the results of PEF monitoring and regular medical review.[67]

Clinical anecdotes do suggest that regular monitoring of PEF can be helpful in managing children with troublesome asthma, especially those with life-threatening attacks. The position adopted by the Respiratory Paediatricians in Australia and New Zealand[70] is as follows: regular monitoring of PEF is not warranted in children with mild or infrequent asthma but children who require continuous

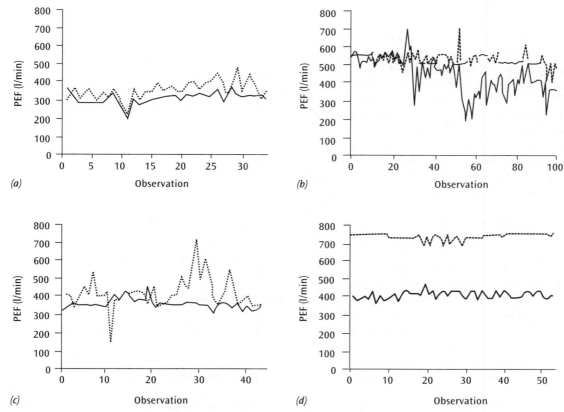

Figure 6b.11 *Selected data to demonstrate particular clinically important patterns. In all panels the spirometer data are depicted by the solid line and that from the mini-flow meter by the dotted line. (a) Despite a difference in mean PEF, the mini-flow meter (Ferraris) accurately reflected the only important fall in lung function. (b) The mini-flow meter (mini-Wright) failed to reflect marked falls in lung function. (c) A 'false-positive' fall in PEF measured with the mini-flow meter (Vitalograph). (d) No relationship between the PEF measured with the spirometer and mini-flow meter (Vitalograph). The mini-flow meter recordings are almost certainly produced by the 'spitting' manoeuvre.*[64]

maintenance treatment with inhaled steroids may benefit from monitoring PEF, provided they are able to produce reliable measurements.

Ultimately, the decision as to whether an individual child is likely to benefit from home PEF monitoring must be made by the paediatrician, taking into account all clinical factors, including: age; ability to perform the manoeuvre; pattern of asthma; severity of symptoms; perception of symptoms and likely compliance.

Acute severe asthma and respiratory failure

The first step in the management of an acute asthma attack is an adequate assessment of the severity of the airway obstruction. In the majority of children clinical assessment will determine the initial management. Clinical signs of severe asthma are described in Chapters 6a and 12.

The most useful measurement of pulmonary function in the assessment of acute asthma is *arterial oxygen saturation (SaO$_2$)* by pulse oximetry. Geelhoed et al.[68] have demonstrated that children presenting to the emergency room with an SaO$_2$ <92% are likely to require admission (odds ratio 10.0), whereas those presenting with an SaO$_2$ >95% are very unlikely to require admission (odds ratio 0.29) (Figure 6b.12). Measurement of arterial blood gases is not routinely necessary in the management of acute asthma. However, measurement of time trends in PaCO$_2$ and PaO$_2$ is usually indicated in severe asthma, when initial aggressive therapy has failed or when the child is critically ill at the time of presentation. Blood gases will usually be normal in children with mild asthma. With moderate asthma, PaO$_2$ will usually be normal or slightly low, and PaCO$_2$ will be low, due to hyperventilation (as discussed above). As the severity of the asthma increases and the V/Q heterogeneity worsens, PaO$_2$ falls and PaCO$_2$ increases towards normal, then becomes elevated. The finding of a normal or elevated PaCO$_2$ in a child with moderate-to-severe asthma should be regarded as an indication of developing respiratory failure, and appropriate management steps instituted without delay.

Measurement of the *degree of airway obstruction* (PEF or FEV$_1$) does not predict which children require admission[69] but values below 25–30% of predicted value after adequate bronchodilation suggest severe or life-threatening airway obstruction. Children need to be experienced in performing forced expiratory manoeuvres to produce reliable results and during an acute attack of asthma is not an appropriate time to teach a child how to measure lung function. Peak expiratory flow readings may be helpful in children who are experienced in using a peak flow meter, particularly during the recovery phase, provided one can be sure that the child's technique is adequate. Admission to hospital is likely to be necessary if the postbronchodilator PEF is less than 50% of the child's previous best after bronchodilator therapy.[70]

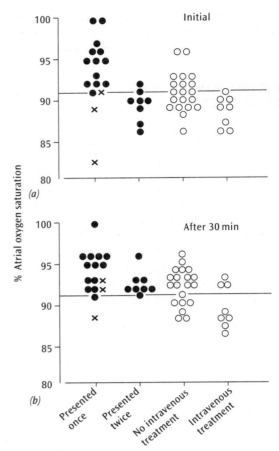

Figure 6b.12 *Arterial oxygen saturation of 52 children (a) before and (b) 30 minutes after nebulization. Symbols: ● : children send home; ✕ : parents unhappy with decision to send home; ○ : children admitted. (From: ref. 68, with permission.)*

Where comparisons have been made, airway obstruction appears to improve more rapidly than does V/Q heterogeneity in both adults[71] and in children.[72] Improvement in clinical symptoms appears to be more closely related to improvement in airway obstruction than to improvement in V/Q matching.

Clinical trials

Trials of new medications for the treatment of paediatric asthma usually include at least one objective outcome variable, commonly multiple daily PEF recordings or spirometry at times of laboratory visits. Within-day peak expiratory flow variability (PEFV) is correlated with measures of bronchial responsiveness[53,73] and to severity of asthma, as judged by medication requirements and mean lung function.[53]

However, the relationship between asthma symptoms and measurements of PEF, either mean PEF or PEFV, have not been well established in children. In a population survey, Quackenboss et al.[52] demonstrated that the risk of symptoms consistent with asthma was 2.3 times greater for those with excessive PEFV. In an attempt to investigate the relationship between asthma symptoms and measurements of PEF 80 children, aged 6–16 years, were studied[74] during a 2-week baseline period prior to commencing a drug trial. There was a weak but statistically significant relationship between mean symptom score and PEFV (r = 0.35, $p < 0.01$). There was no relationship between mean symptom score and FEV_1 or $PD_{20}FEV_1$ to inhaled histamine measured at the laboratory visit at the end of the baseline period. The implication of these data is that clinical trials of asthma medication should not rely on measurements of PEF or of PEFV as primary outcome variables. In fact, one could question the value of making these measurements at all.

Bronchodilator response

The measurement of the acute effects of a bronchodilating drug serves two main purposes: to support the clinical diagnosis of reversible airway obstruction and to demonstrate the potential benefit of bronchodilator therapy.

In the literature there appears to be a discrepancy between clinical and physiological studies examining bronchodilator responsiveness in infants and preschool children. Some clinical studies demonstrate statistically significant improvements in the signs of airway obstruction with inhaled bronchodilator treatment,[75–77] although in most of these studies the improvement is small. Mallol et al.[75] demonstrated that children admitted to hospital with acute wheezing illnesses in the first year of life had a more rapid reduction of symptoms and a shorter hospital stay if they received nebulized bronchodilators when compared with a group receiving nebulized normal saline.

In contrast, physiological studies have not produced convincing evidence of improved lung function following inhaled bronchodilators. In 1978, Lenny and Milner[78] reported that children less than 12 months of age did not show a fall in respiratory system resistance, using a forced oscillation technique. Prendiville et al.[79] studied recurrently wheezy infants using the RTC technique and body plethysmography and found no changes in specific resistance or in Vtg following bronchodilator, but a fall in group mean $V'_{max}FRC$. A more recent randomized crossover clinical trial of salbutamol in infants found no effect on either symptoms or pulmonary function.[80] Similarly arterial oxygen saturation has been reported to increase,[77,81] decrease,[82] or to show no change[83] following bronchodilator treatment in wheezy infants.

All of the above studies have used grouped data to assess response and have not compared the results to a control group. To overcome some of these problems 22 wheezy infants, less than 6 months old, were studied during the acute phase of bronchiolitis, using a double-blind, placebo-controlled protocol.[84] Despite using both individual and grouped data to assess the response, no differences were found between the active and placebo groups. Some infants in both groups had an increase in $V'_{max}FRC$, some had a decrease, and most showed no change.

A bronchodilator response would be expected to include some or all of: a decrease in FRC; a decrease in airway resistance; a decrease in respiratory rate. Each of these factors may influence the values of lung function measured, for technical reasons, and may obscure a true, beneficial change in lung function.

Recent studies using low frequency forced oscillation have shown that both healthy infants and those with recurrent wheeze can respond to bronchodilators.[85] These data give the promise of a future rational approach to the use of bronchodilators in infants. There is also promising data that shows FOT or the interrupter technique can be used to evaluate bronchial obstruction and it's reversibility in preschool children.[26,49,86]

Measurement of bronchodilator response in schoolchildren is essentially the same as the measurement in adults. The most commonly used measurements are FEV_1 or PEF. Usually, the change in FEV_1 or PEF following a bronchodilator is expressed as a percentage of the prebronchodilator baseline. However, the changes in FEV_1 after bronchodilator drugs have consistently been shown to be independent of the magnitude of the FEV_1.[86] Thus, it is statistically inappropriate to express change in FEV_1 as a percentage of baseline, or indeed as a proportion of the predicted value; change in FEV_1 should be expressed in absolute terms.[87] Similar conclusions were reached from a study in healthy children, reported by Hutchinson et al.[5] A more recent study[88] suggested that statistically the most appropriate method of expressing bronchodilator response in children was to express the change in FEV_1 as a proportion of the predicted value. These authors found that this index was independent of age, stature and initial FEV_1. Unfortunately, the number of subjects in this study was too small to distinguish between the additive model (absolute change) and the multiplicitave model (ΔFEV_1 %predicted). Therefore a sensible approach to reporting bronchodilator response would be to assess the response as both an absolute change in FEV_1 (>190 ml is significant in an adult) or in PEF (>60 l/min is significant in an adult)[87] and as change in FEV_1 %predicted (>9% appears to be an appropriate cut-off for bronchodilator response in children),[88] and examine whether either of these is independent of age, stature, and baseline airway calibre in the population under study.

There are no data addressing the usefulness of measuring bronchodilator response as part of the diagnosis of asthma. While the presence of a significant bronchodilator response (see above) in a child with low lung function is compatible with a diagnosis of asthma it is not diagnostic. More importantly, the lack of a bronchodilator response in the presence of low lung function does not exclude a diagnosis of asthma.

The precise details of how to test for bronchodilator responsiveness depend on the reason for performing the test. If the aim is to determine the child's maximal lung function, then a maximal dose of bronchodilator should be given. Most laboratories would use 5 mg of salbutamol (or equivalent) delivered by a jet nebulizer driven with compressed air at 8 l/min, with the child breathing through a mouthpiece. This technique ensures the maximum delivery of bronchodilator to the lungs. An alternative to using a nebulizer is to use a large volume holding chamber ('spacer') and a metered dose inhaler. Delivering five puffs, one at a time, over a 5-minute period is likely to achieve equivalent bronchodilation. If, however, the aim of the test is to determine how much bronchodilator response occurs with the child's usual bronchodilator therapy, then the child should be asked to take their bronchodilator in their usual manner. Individual clinical circumstances will determine which determine which test is most appropriate.

Following β-agonist therapy 80–90% of the maximal improvement in lung function occurs within ten minutes. Therefore, the measurement of lung function should be repeated ten minutes after completing the bronchodilator treatment. About 20 minutes should be allowed after the anticholinergic agent ipratropium bromide. Lack of a bronchodilator response in a child with marked airway obstruction does not necessarily indicate fixed airway obstruction. A large proportion of the airway obstruction may be due to mucosal swelling and oedema and to mucous obstruction of the airway lumen. These factors will limit the ability of the bronchodilator to reach the airway smooth muscle and are also less likely to respond acutely to bronchodilator therapy. In these circumstances a course of oral or high-dose inhaled steroids may be necessary before one can demonstrate acute bronchodilator responsiveness.

In which children should bronchodilator responsiveness be measured? Any asthmatic child with baseline airway obstruction, defined as a FEV_1/FVC ratio of <75% or a concave expiratory flow–volume curve, should have bronchodilator response measured. A child presenting for assessment for the first time, with no obvious baseline airway obstruction should also have bronchodilator responsiveness measured as apparently normal pulmonary function, defined on per cent of predicted normal, may not be the child's maximal lung function. On subsequent assessments, measurement of bronchodilator response is not necessary in children without airway obstruction and with lung function at their personal best.

REFERENCES

1. Mallol J, Sly PD. Effect of chloral hydrate on arterial oxygen saturation in wheezy infants. *Pediatr Pulmonol* 1988;**5**:96–9.
2. Stocks J, Sly PD, Tepper RS, Morgan WJ (eds). Infant respiratory function testing. Chichester: Wiley-Liss, 1996.
3. Gold WM, Kaufman HS, Nadel JA. Elastic recoil of the lungs in chronic asthmatic patients before and after therapy. *Appl Physiol* 1967;**23**:433–8.
4. Peslin R. Body plethysmography. In: AB Otis, ed. *Techniques in Respiratory Physiology Part II. Techniques in the Life Sciences.* Elsevier, County Clare, Ireland, 1984.
5. Hutchinson AA, Erben A, McLennan LA, Landau LI, Phelan PD. Intrasubject variability of pulmonary function testing in healthy children. *Thorax* 1981;**36**:370–7.
6. Castile RG, Brown R. More problems with Boyle's law – or, 'Vtg or not Vtg, that is the question' [editorial]. *Am Rev Respir Dis* 1986;**133**:184–5.
7. Clausen JL. *Pulmonary Function Testing in Children: Guidelines and Controversies.* Grane and Stratton, NY, 1984.
8. McFadden ER, Kiser R, deGroot WJ. Acute bronchial asthma: relations between clinical and physiological manifestations. *N Engl J Med* 1973;**288**:221–5.
9. Macklem PT. Hyperinflation [editorial]. *Am Rev Respir Dis* 1984;**129**:1–2.
10. Tantucci C, Ellaffi M, Duguet A, et al. Dynamic hyperinflation and flow limitation during methacholine-induced bronchoconstriction in asthma. *Eur Respir J* 1999;**14**:295–301.
11. Sly PD, Brown KA, Bates JHT, Macklem PT, Milic-Emili J, Martin JG. The effect of lung volume on interrupter resistance in cats challenged with methacholine. *J Appl Physiol* 1988;**64**:360–6.
12. Ludwig MS, Dreshaj I, Solway J, Munoz A, Ingram RH. Partitioning of pulmonary resistance during constriction in the dog: effects of volume history. *J Appl Physiol* 1987;**62**:807–15.
13. Sly PD, Lanteri CJ. Differential responses of the airways and pulmonary tissues to inhaled histamine in young dogs. *J Appl Physiol* 1990;**68**:1562–7.
14. Petak F, Hayden MJ, Hantos Z, Sly PD. Volume dependence of respiratory impedance in infants. *Am Respir Crit Care Med* 1997;**156**:1172–7.
15. Sekizawa K, Yanai Y, Shimizu H, Sasaki H, Takishima T. Serial distribution of bronchoconstriction in normal subjects. *Am Rev Respir Dis* 1988;**134**:1182–9.
16. Ohuri T, Sekizawa K, Yanai M, et al. Partitioning of pulmonary responses to inhaled methacholine in subjects with asymptomatic asthma. *Am Rev Respir Dis* 1992;**146**:1501–5.
17. Burns CB, Taylor WR, Ingram RH. Effects of deep inhalation in asthma: relative airway and parenchymal hysteresis. *J Appl Physiol* 1985;**59**:1590–6.
18. Julia-Serda G, Molfino NA, Chapman KR, et al. Heterogenous airway tone in asthmatic subjects. *J Appl Physiol* 1992;**73**:2328–32.

19. Klug B, Bisgaard H. Measurement of the specific airway resistance by plethysmography in young children accompanied by an adult. *Eur Respir J* 1997;**10**:1599–605.

20. Lowe L, *et al*. Specific airway resistance in 3-year old children: a prospective cohort study. *Lancet* 2002;**359**:1904–8.

21. Mallol J, Willet K, Burton P, Sly PD. Influence of duration of occlusion time on respiratory mechanics measured with the single-breath technique in infants. *Pediatr Pulmonol* 1994;**17**:250–7.

22. ATS/ERS. Respiratory mechanics in infants: physiologic evaluation in health and disease. *Am Rev Respir Dis* 1993;**147**:474–96.

23. Ducharme FM, Davis M, Ducharme GR. Paediatric reference values for respiratory resistance measured by forced oscillation. *Chest* 1998;**113**:1322–8.

24. Sly PD, Hayden MJ, Petak F, Hantos Z. Measurement of low-frequency respiratory impedance in infants. *Am Respir Crit Care Med* 1996;**154**:161–6.

25. Bisgaard H, Klug B. Lung function measurement in awake young children. *Eur Respir* 1995;**8**:2067–75.

26. Bridge PD, Ranganathan S, McKenzie SA. Measurement of airway resistance using the interrupter technique in preschool children in the ambulatory setting. *Eur Respir* 1999;**13**:792–6.

27. Frey U, Silverman M, Kraemer R, Jackson AC. High-frequency respiratory input impedance measurements in infants assessed by the high speed interrupter technique. *Eur Respir* 1998;**12**:148–58.

28. Greenough A, Loftus BG, Pool J, Price JF. Abnormalities of lung mechanics in young children. *Thorax* 1987;**42**:500–5.

29. Macklem PT. Bronchial hyperresponsiveness. *Chest* 1985;**85**(Suppl 1):58S–159S.

30. Ding DJ, Martin JG, Macklem PT. The effects of lung volume on maximal methacholine-induced bronchoconstriction in normal humans. *J Appl Physiol* 1987;**62**:1324–30.

31. Hall GL, Hantos Z, Wildhaber JH, Petak F, Sly PD. Methacholine responsiveness in infants assessed with low-frequency forced oscillation and forced expiration techniques. *Thorax* 2001;**56**:42–7.

32. Macklem PT, Mead J. The Respiratory System, Section 3. In: *Handbook of Physiology. Part 1. Mechanics of Breathing,* AP Fishman, Section Ed. American Physiological Society, Bethesda, 1986.

33. Meslier N, Charbonneau G, Racineux JL. Wheezes. *Eur Resp J* 1995;**8**:1942–8.

34. Webster PM, Sawatzky RP, Hoffstein V, Leblanc R, Hinchey MJ, Sullivan PA. Wall motion in expiratory flow imitation: choke and flutter. *J Appl Physiol* 1985;**59**:1304–12.

35. Gavriely N, Kelly KB, Grotberg JB, Loring SH. Forced expiratory wheezes are a manifestation of airway flow limitation. *J Appl Physiol* 1987;**62**:2398–403.

36. Anonymous. Standardization of Spirometry, 1994 Update. American Thoracic Society. *Am J Respir Crit Care Med* 1995;**152**:1107–36.

37. Desmond KJ, Allen PD, Demizio DL, Kovesi T, Coates AL. Redefining end of test (EOT) criteria for pulmonary function testing in children. *Am J Respir Crit Care Med* 1997;**156**:542–5.

38. Arets HGM, Brackel HJL, Van der Ert CK. Forced expiratory manoeuvres in children: do they meet ATS and ERS criteria for spiremetry. *Eur Resp J* 2001;**18**:655–60.

39. Sly PD, Tepper R, Henschen M, Gappa M, Stocks J. Standards for infant respiratory function testing: tidal forced expirations. *Eur Respir J* 2000;**16**:741–8.

40. Seidenberg J, Masters IB, Hudson I, Olinsky A, Phelan PD. Disturbance in respiratory mechanics in infants with bronchiolitis. *Thorax* 1989; **44**:660–7.

41. Turner DJ, Stick SM, Lesouef KL, Sly PD, Lesouef PN. A new technique to generate and assess forced expiration from raised lung volume in infants. *Am J Respir Crit Care Med* 1995;**151**(5):1441–50.

42. Feher A, Castile R, Kisling J, *et al*. Flow limitation in normal infants: a new method for forced expiratory manoeuvres from raised lung volumes. *Appl Physiol* 1996;**80**:2019–25.

43. Jones MH, Davis SD, Kisling JA, Howard JM, Castile R, Tepper RS. Flow limitation in infants assessed by negative expiratory pressure. *Am J Respir Crit Care Med* 2000;**161**(3 Pt 1):713–17.

44. Quanjer PH, Lebowitz MD, Gregg I, Miller MR, Pedersen OF. Peak expiratory flow: conclusions and recommendations of a Working Party of the European Respiratory Society. *Eur Respir J Suppl* 1997;**24**:2S–8S.

45. Kano S, Burton DL, Lanteri CJ, Sly PD. Determination of peak expiratory flow. *Eur Respir J* 1993;**6**: 1347–52.

46. Miles JF, Tunnicliffe W, Cayton RM, Ayres JG, Miller MR. Potential effects of correction of inaccuracies of the mini-Wright peak expiratory flow meter on the use of an asthma self-management plan. *Thorax* 1996;**51**(4):403–6.

47. Vilozni D, Barker M, *et al*. An interactive, computer-animated system (Spiro Game) facilitates spirometry in preschool children. *Am J Resp Crit Care Med* 2001;**164**:2200–5.

48. Ducharme FM, Davis GM. Measurement of respiratory resistance in the emergency department: feasibility in young children with acute asthma. *Chest* 1997;**111**:1519–25.

49. Delacourt C, Lorino H, Herve-Guillot M, Reinert P, Harf A, Housset B. Use of the forced oscillation technique to assess airway obstruction and reversibility in children. *Am Respir Crit Care Med* 2000;**161**:730–6.

50. Phagoo SB, Wilson NM, Silverman M. Evaluation of a new interrupter device for measuring bronchial responsiveness and the response to bronchodilator in 3 year old children [see comments]. *Eur Respir* 1996;**9**:1374–80.

51. Hetzel MR, Clark TJH. Comparison of normal and asthmatic circadian rhythms in peak expiratory flow rate. *Thorax* 1980;**35**:732–8.

52. Quackenboss JJ, Lebowitz MD, Krzyzanowski M. The normal range of diurnal changes in peak expiratory flow rates: relationship to symptoms and respiratory disease. *Am Rev Respir Dis* 1991;**143**:323–30.

53. Sly PD, Hibbert ME, Landau LI. Diurnal variation of peak expiratory flow rate in asthmatic children. *Pediatr Pulmonol* 1986;**2**:141–6.

54. DeVries K, Goei JT, Booy-Noord H, Orie NGM. Changes during 24 hours in the lung function and histamine hyperreactivity of the bronchial tree in asthmatic and bronchitic patients. *Int Arch Allergy* 1962;**20**:93–101.

55. Gervais P, Reinberg A, Gervais C, Smolensky M, DeFrance O. Twenty-four-hour rhythm in the bronchial hyperreactivity to house dust in asthmatics. *J Allergy Clin Immunol* 1977;**59**:207–13.

56. Sly PD, Landau LI, Olinsky A. Failure of ipratropium bromide to modify the diurnal variation of asthma in asthmatic children. *Thorax* 1987;**42**:357–60.

57. Heztel MR, Clark TJH. Does sleep cause nocturnal asthma? *Thorax* 1979;**34**:749–54.

58. Sly PD, Landau LI. Diurnal variation in bronchial responsiveness in asthmatic children. *Paediatric Pulmonol* 1986;**2**:344–52.

59. Soutar CA, Costello J, Ijaduola O, Turner-Warick M. Nocturnal and morning asthma. Relationship to plasma corticosteroids and response to cortisol infusion. *Thorax* 1975;**30**:436–40.

60. Postma DS, Koeter GH, Keyzer JJ, Muers H. Influence of slow-release terbutaline on the circadian variation of cathecholamines, histamine and lung function in non-allergic patients with partially reversable airflow obstruction. *J Allergy Clin Immunol* 1986;**77**:471–7.

61. Kraft M, Martin RJ, Wilson S, Djukanovic R, Holgate ST. Lymphocyte and eosinophil influx into alveolar tissue in nocturnal asthma. *Am Respir Crit Care Med* 1999;**159**:228–34.

62. Sly PD, Landau LI, Weymouth R. Home recording of peak expiratory flow rates and perception of asthma. *Am J Dis Child* 1985;**139**:479–82.

63. Uwyyed K, Springer C, Avital A, Bar-Yishay E, Godfrey S. Home recording of PEF in young asthmatics: does it contribute to management? *Eur Respir J* 1996;**9**(5):872–9.

64. Sly PD, Cahill P, Willet K, Burton P. Accuracy of mini peak flow meters following changes in lung function in children with asthma. *Br Med J* 1994; **308**:572–4.

65. Clough JB, Sly PD. Can peak expiratory flow be used as a predictor or lower respiratory symptoms? *Am Rev Respir Dis* 1993;**147**:A267.

66. Wensley D, Silverman M. The quality of home spirometry in school children with asthma. *Thorax* 2001;**56**:183–5.

67. Sly PD, Flack F. Is home monitoring of lung function worthwhile for children with asthma? *Thorax* 2001;**56**:164–5.

68. Geelhoed GC, Landau LI, LeSouef PN. Predictive value of oxygen saturation in emergency evaluation of asthmatic children. *Br Med J* 1988;**297**:395–6.

69. Kerem E, Tibshirani R, Canny G, *et al.* Predicting the need for hospitalization in children with acute asthma. *Chest* 1990;**98**:1355–61.

70. Henry RL, Robertson CF, Asher I, *et al.* Management, of acute asthma. Respiratory paediatricians of Australia and New Zealand. *Paediatr Child Health* 1993;**29**:101–3.

71. Roca J, Ramis LI, Rodrituez-Roisin R, Ballester E, Montserrat JM, Wagner PD. Serial relationships between ventilation-perfusion inequality and spirometry in acute severe asthma requiring hospitalization. *Am Rev Respir Dis* 1988; **137**:1055–61.

72. Mihatsch W, Geelhoed GC, Landau LI, LeSeouf PN. Time course of change in oxygen saturation and peak expiratory flow in children admitted to hospital with acute asthma. *Thorax* 1990;**45**:438–41.

73. Ryan G, Latimer KM, Dolovich J, Hargreave FE. Bronchial responsiveness to histamine: relationship to diurnal variation of peak flow rate, improvement after bronchodilator, and airway calibre. *Thorax* 1982;**37**:423–9.

74. Sly PD. Peak flow monitoring in children. *Monaldi Arch Chest Dis* 1993;**48**:662–7.

75. Mallol J, Barrueto L, Girardi G, *et al.* Use of nebulized bronchodilators in infants under 1 year of age: analysis of four forms of therapy. *Pediatr Pulmonol* 1987;**3**:298–303.

76. Lowell DI, Lister G, Von Koss H, McCarthy P. Wheezing in infants: the response to epinephrine. *Pediatrics* 1987;**79**:939–45.

77. Schweich PJ, Hurt TL, Walkley EI, Mullen N, Archibald LF. The use of nebulized albuterol in wheezing infants. *Pediatr Emergency Care* 1992; **8**:184–8.

78. Lenny W, Milner AD. At what age do bronchodilator drugs work? *Arch Dis Child* 1978;**53**:532–5.

79. Prendiville A, Green S, Silverman M. Paradoxical response to nebulized salbutamol in wheezy infants assessed by partial expiratory flow–volume curves. *Thorax* 1987;**42**:86–91.

80. Chavasse RJ, Bastian-Lee Y, Richter H, Hilliard T, Seddon P. Inhaled salbutamol for wheezy infants: a randomised controlled trial. *Arch Dis Childhood* 2000;**82**(5):370–5.

81. Schuh S, Canny G, Reisman JJ, *et al.* Nebulized albuterol in acute bronchiolitis. *Pediatrics* 1990;**117**:633–7.

82. Ho L, Collis G, Landau LI, Le Souef PN. Effect of salbutamol on oxygen saturation in bronchiolitis. *Arch Dis Childhood* 1991;**66**:1061–4.

83. Klassen TP, Rowe PC, Sutcliffe T, Ropp LJ, McDowell IW, Li MM. Randomized trial of salbutamol in acute bronchiolitis [published erratum appears in *J Pediatr* 1991 Dec;119(6):1010]. *Pediatr* 1991;**118**:807–11.

84. Sly PD, Lanteri CJ, Raven JM. Do wheezy infants recovering from bronchiolitis respond to inhaled salbutamol? *Pediatr Pulmonol* 1991;**10**:36–9.

85. Hayden MJ, Petak F, Hantos Z, Hall G, Sly PD. Using low-frequency oscillation to detect bronchodilator responsiveness in infants. *Am Respir Crit Care Med* 1998;**157**:574–9.

86. Beydon N, Amsallen F, *et al.* Pre- post bronchodilator interrupter resistance values in healthy young children. *Am J resp Crit Med* 2002;**165**:1388–94.

87. Anon. Reversibility of airflow obstruction FEV1 vs peak flow. *Lancet* 1992;**340**:85–6.

88. Waalkens HJ, Merkus PJFM, van Essen-Zandvliet EEM, *et al.* Assessment of bronchodilator response in children with asthma. *Eur Respir J* 1993;**6**:645–51.

6c

Bronchial responsiveness

NICOLA WILSON AND MICHAEL SILVERMAN

INTRODUCTION

The stimulus-response concept

The concept of bronchial responsiveness (BR) has had a central role in the theory and management of asthma for 25 years. In spite of this, there is agreement on neither the relationship between increased bronchial responsiveness and asthma nor on the place of bronchial responsiveness testing in its diagnosis or management. At its most general, the term implies a particular degree of airflow obstruction (sometimes called bronchoconstriction) which is induced by a standardized stimulus; to many people, the concept is envisaged as an *in vivo* 'organ bath' (Figure 6c.1). While this is an attractive shorthand way of conceptualizing BR, the analogy has many shortcomings. BR has different implications for pulmonologists from different scientific disciplines (Figure 6c.1).

This chapter will discuss briefly the practical aspects of the measurement of bronchial responsiveness, with particular reference to young children and infants. Possible mechanisms for an increased level will be considered along with a review of environmental influences and an assessment of its relationship to symptoms and other clinical features. Unless otherwise stated, the term bronchial responsiveness will be used to denote the degree of sensitivity to the stimulus and not the maximum level of constriction induced. BR should be distinguished from the term bronchial hyperresponsiveness (BHR) which has been used to indicate bronchoconstriction occurring below a particular threshold level of stimulus. This threshold has been used to define a state of increased responsiveness in particular studies. Threshold levels are somewhat arbitrary and may vary from study to study.

In real life, the *stimulus* may not be easily quantifiable at target level because of immeasurable factors affecting administration, deposition in the lungs or rate of removal. These unknowns will be compounded by the type of stimulus (aerosol compared with exercise, for instance), the age of the subject, the route of breathing (nasal or oral) and the underlying lung pathology. Measuring the *response* is equally problematic in life. It may depend on the type of lung function test, the technique used and even the particular model of equipment. The measurement technique may itself influence the airflow obstruction, which is the object of measurement. The 'big breath' controversy is an example of this: under resting conditions, a maximum inspiration may enhance airway obstruction in an asthmatic subject, whereas after induced airway narrowing, it may cause transient relief. Finally, the *analysis* of what is inevitably a complex relationship between stimulus and response (even in an organ bath) presents many more potential variables. Many of these shortcomings will be considered in this chapter.

Increased bronchial responsiveness (sometimes referred to as bronchial hyperreactivity or hyperresponsiveness, BHR) implies an exaggerated bronchoconstrictor response to a stimulus. The term can describe either the response to a low level of stimulus or too great a response to a standard stimulus (or both). It can be quantified either by inhalation of a pharmacological aerosol or by applying non-pharmacological stimuli such as antigen, exercise,

1. Basic physiologist – organ bath

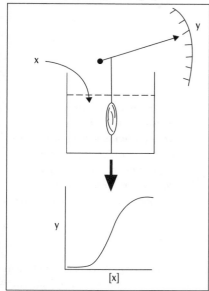

2. Clinical physiologist – organ *in situ*

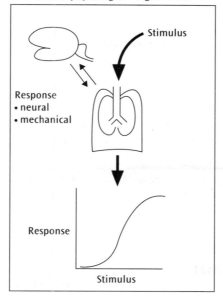

3. Clinician – patients

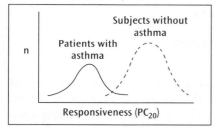

4. Epidemiologist – population

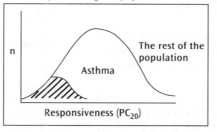

Figure 6c.1 *The concept of BR depends on view point.*

cold air or an osmotic load. The term non-specific responsiveness is sometimes applied when it has been assessed by a constrictor agent, which, unlike allergens or certain industrial chemicals, does not imply specific sensitization. It is this aspect of bronchial responsiveness that will be discussed in this chapter, with only passing reference to the response to sensitizing agents.

Asthma and bronchial responsiveness

Early studies in selected populations of adults comparing those without symptoms to atopic asthmatics showed a distinction between the two groups.[1] A good correlation between the degree of response to methacholine and histamine and asthma medication was shown in most but not all studies.[1–5] So the term increased bronchial responsiveness was included into the definition of asthma used by the American Academy of Respiratory Diseases[6] and has been incorporated into the definition of asthma for epidemiological purposes.[7] However, the relationship between the two is now known to be more complex than was first considered. Studies have shown that increased bronchial responsiveness is not synonymous with asthma and it has been found in other disorders as well as in asymptomatic individuals[8–13] and has a continuous

unimodal population distribution (Figure 6c.2). Nonetheless, the consideration of the measurement of BR in asthma has led to some important insights. For example, the association of increased responsiveness and airway inflammation following exposure to allergens, toxic gases and viral infections, all major precipitants of asthmatic symptoms, has focused attention on the role of the inflammatory process in asthma and the use of bronchial responsiveness as a possible marker.

Broadly speaking, challenge tests can be divided into two categories.

1 Direct tests are those in which pharmacological stimuli, methacholine or histamine for example, act by direct action on receptors on smooth muscle.
2 Indirect tests may be more specific for asthma, as indicators of underlying inflammation; stimuli, such as exercise, isocapnic hyperventilation or inhalation of hypo- or hyper-osmolar aerosols, probably act by interaction with inflammatory cells or via a neural pathway, rather than acting directly on smooth muscle.[14–18a]

Because of the number of factors potentially involved in determining the response to a constrictor agent, this classification is likely to prove an oversimplification.

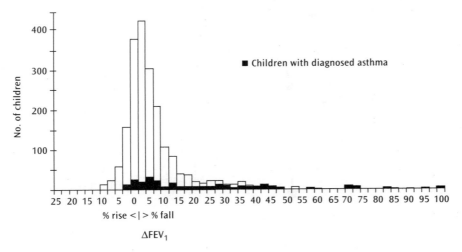

Figure 6c.2 *Frequency distribution of change in FEV$_1$ after an inhaled cumulative dose of 3.9 μmol histamine in a population of New Zealand children (total n = 2045, asthma = 294) (from ref. 8 with permission).*

MEASUREMENT OF BRONCHIAL RESPONSIVENESS

Bronchial challenge procedures

A number of different methods have been used to measure non-specific bronchial responsiveness in children (Table 6c.1). Guidelines for the conduct of challenge procedures have been published.[19,19a]

The measurement of BR in school-children is straightforward but infants and preschool children are especially challenging. Below the age of 2, studies can only be performed during sleep after sedation (Figure 6c.3). Aerosol challenge is the only feasible method, although cold-air hyperventilation induced by CO_2 has been used.[20] In nasal breathing infants, much of the aerosol cannot reach the lungs.[21,22] In this age group measurement of the airway response to challenge is constricted by the types of test available and their limitations in nose-breathing infants, in whom the greater part of the challenge has been deposited in the nose. Between 2 and 5 years of age, limited forms of challenge procedure are possible in the majority of children and great technical advances have been made in this area in recent years.[23–26]

Direct challenge with constrictor aerosols

The most commonly used stimuli to determine bronchial responsiveness are aerolized constrictor agents such as methacholine or histamine, which act directly on smooth muscle. The agent is given in increasing (usually doubling) concentrations until a predetermined change in lung function, measured after each step, occurs. Three methods are in common use and their relative merits are shown in Table 6c.2. The age of the child, availability of equipment and the size of the study determine the choice of method.

Inhaled sulphur dioxide, metabisulphite, prostaglandins, leukotrienes and other mediators can be given using this method but are not frequently used in clinical or epidemiological practice in children, although they may have a role in research protocols.

Analysis of results

THRESHOLD RESPONSE

Using a dosimeter, the delivered dose of the agonist can be calculated as concentration × output; for the tidal breathing method, the delivered concentration is used. Conventionally, the dose or concentration causing a predetermined change in lung function is calculated from the log dose–response curve and called the provocative concentration (PC) or dose (PD); it describes the sensitivity to the stimulus. This index of PC or PD is the most frequently used and straightforward to calculate (Figure 6c.4). The problem with its use in population studies is that many subjects do not achieve the required change in lung function, which results in censored data. To some extent this can be overcome by using regression methods for extrapolation. Another solution recommended by some workers is the calculation of the slope of the dose–response curve (reactivity) which applies even to subjects whose change in lung function is only marginal.[30] A review of the two approaches based on statistical considerations concludes that there is little to gain from this more cumbersome approach.[31] With the use of a random effects model, in which all the available challenge data for the individual are compared to the total population data, covariates known to influence the response can be included.[13]

MAXIMAL AIRWAY RESPONSE

It has been claimed that, irrespective of the sensitivity of the stimulus, the maximal amount of airway narrowing is the critical feature which distinguishes severe or moderate asthma from mild or episodic asthma and normals.[32,33] The distinguishing feature is the development of a plateau in maximal constriction (Figure 6c.5) which occurs in

Table 6c.1 *Types of challenge used to measure bronchial responsiveness in children*

Stimulus	Mode of action	Comment
Direct challenge[19]		
Histamine	H_1 receptors on smooth muscle (small component local reflex)	Systemic side effects such as flushing and local effects such as cough at high concentrations
Methacholine (carbachol, acetylcholine)	Muscarinic receptors (M_3) on smooth muscle; may also affect other receptor types	Minimal side effects, so can be used in high concentrations in normal subjects
Indirect challenge[15,19a]		
Airway epithelial challenge by osmotic change in ELF and/or cooling of epithelium	Indirect challenge probably mediated by interaction with inflammatory cells (e.g. mast cells) and neural reflexes	Refractoriness to repeated challenges in majority of subjects is a feature
Exercise	Increased ventilation results in cooling and evaporative water loss which increase in ELF osmotic pressure	Physiological but single-dose challenge; stimulus can be increased by inspiration of (cold) dry air during exercise; affected by ambient air conditions
Isocapnic hyperventilation (Cold/dry air)	Mimics hyperventilation of exercise. Stimulus increased by cooling and drying of inspired air	Equipment cumbersome, little advantage over exercise in airconditioned surroundings; dry air adequate; cooling probably unnecessary
'Osmotic' challenge: distilled water, hypertonic saline (usually 3–4.5%)	Hypo or hypertonic stimuli have similar constrictor effect	Easiest 'indirect' challenge to obtain dose-response relationship; refractoriness to repeat challenge; Cl^- free solutions induce cough
Dry powder mannitol test[16,43]	Hyperosmotic stimulus	Convenient preparation for epidemiological studies; simpler than aerosols
Adenosine 5-monophosphate[17,18]	Acts via mast cell to release histamine and other autocoid mediators	Convenient 'indirect' challenge; few clinical studies reported

ELF: epithelial lining fluid.

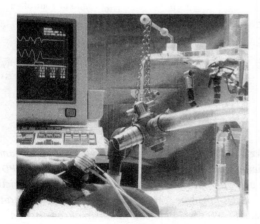

Figure 6c.3 *Infant undergoing bronchial challenge. The response is measured by the rapid thoracic compression ('squeeze') technique.*

healthy adults and children, when big-breath tests of lung function (such as FEV_1) are used (see below). Since the degree of maximal constriction of the airway determines the potential severity of asthma and hence the risk,

restoration or limitation in maximal constriction has been advocated as a therapeutic goal.[33,34]

Indirect challenge

EXERCISE TEST

Exercise can be performed by free running or on a treadmill or exercise bicycle; standardized protocols for each method are available.[35,36] The degree of induced bronchoconstriction is related to the relative humidity and the temperature of inspired air, which therefore should ideally be controlled.[37] To obtain a maximal constrictor response the exercise should be continued for 6–10 minutes at a level which increases the heart rate to 90% maximum for age (>180 beats/min is a rough guide). The ideal environmental conditions are (a) about 21°C and (b) 45% relative humidity (giving a water content of 10 mg/l air). By giving dry air (via a Douglas bag) during exercise, a more potent stimulus is achieved with about a 10% greater fall in FEV_1. As the maximum bronchoconstriction occurs about five minutes after the end of the exercise

Table 6c.2 *Methods of delivering constrictor aerosols*

Method	Delivery of aerosol	Lung function measurement and index of BR	Comment
Standard tidal breathing method[1]	2 min tidal breathing via jet nebulizer; agonist doubled every 5 min after saline inhalation	90 and 180 s lowest value used and compared to post saline value; PC	Cheap, simple; time consuming; high output nebulizer can be used but will give different results
Modified tidal breathing method[26]	1 min tidal breathing; quadrupling increases in concentration; no saline inhalation	180 s value compared to baseline; PC	Shortened protocol for preschool children; risk of adverse response to increased step change
Dosimeter method[27]	Aerosol inhaled during 5 maximal inspirations; saline followed by doubling doses	90 s compared to post saline values; cumulative PD	Expensive equipment; quick to perform; suitable for children ≥7 years
Handheld dosimeter[28]	Saline followed by varying number of maximal inhalations and concentrations doubling doses	90 s; cumulative PD	Cheap and mobile; quick to use; suitable for epidemiological studies
Reservoir method[23]	Aerosol contained in large volume reservoir	PC or PD can be calculated	Advantage in small children as inspired dose is independent air entrainment
Ultrasonic nebulizer: hypertonic saline (usually 4.5%), distilled water[29]	Aerosol inhaled for doubling durations (e.g. 0.5, 1, …, 8 min); high output nebulizer (i.e. 1.0–2.3 ml/min)	60 + 180 s; PD (ml of water) or time-based analysis of response	Tendency to cough with distilled water, usually wears off; occasional severe response; long duration

PD: cumulative provocation dose; PC: provocative concentration; BR: bronchial responsiveness.

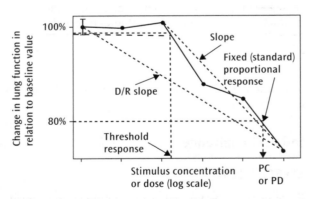

Figure 6c.4 *Theoretical dose–response curve to constrictor agent demonstrating ways of assessing response. PC or PD derived by interpolation of the last two points, using a regression line or a threshold response and the dose–response (D/R) slope.*

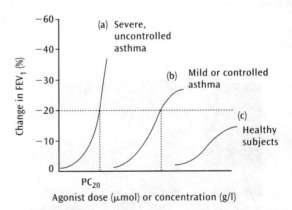

Figure 6c.5 *Three typical dose–response curves to histamine or methacholine representing (a) severely reduced PC/PD with a steep slope and no limitation to bronchoconstriction (plateau) as might be seen in severe asthma; (b) moderately reduced PC/PD with a plateau in maximal constriction suggestive of mild or episodic asthma; (c) response at high concentration of agonist with low plateau response in a normal subject (after ref. 32).*

period, lung function should be measured serially for at least 10 minutes (Figure 6c.6), or until spontaneous recovery occurs if the 'area under the curve' is sought as a measure of the response. A refractory period which lasts up to 2 hours, when the response to repeated exercise is attenuated, has been described in over 50% of responders[38] possibly due to a leukotriene and prostaglandin-dependent mechanism.[39] There is no late response.[40]

HYPERVENTILATION AND COLD AIR CHALLENGE

Methods which involve hyperventilation with dry air or with subfreezing air probably give equivalent results.

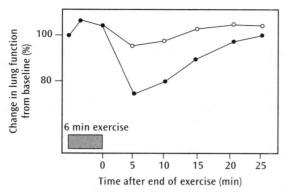

Figure 6c.6 *The result of an exercise test in an asthmatic child (•) showing protection by pretreatment with a bronchodilator (○). A small increase in PEF during exercise is followed by a sharp fall after its cessation, and slow, spontaneous recovery.*

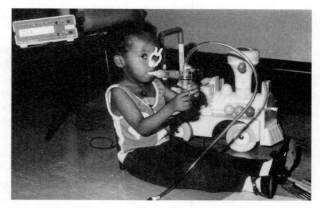

Figure 6c.7 *A 5-year-old child performing a hypertonic saline challenge.*

They are not appropriate for children under 7 years of age whereas free running exercise challenge has been used in children as young as 3 years old.[41]

The results of exercise or other challenge tests in which a single 'dose' stimulus is used depend simply on the measurement of the maximum change in lung function from baseline value (Figure 6c.6). For this reason, results from a multiple dose protocol such as histamine and methacholine challenge are not strictly comparable with the results of tests using a single level of stimulus such as exercise. However, it is possible to match them for statistical purposes by choosing the methacholine dose that produces a response closest to the response on exercise.[42]

OSMOTIC CHALLENGE

Both hypotonic and hypertonic aerosols act as bronchoconstrictor agents. Thus, inhalation of distilled water or hypertonic saline (4.5%) can be used.[29] In order to deliver a sufficient volume the use of a high output ultrasonic nebulizer with a large two-way valve is recommended. Instead of increasing the dose of the stimulus at each step, it is usual to double the inhalation time from 0.5–8 minutes. Coughing during inhalation can initially be troublesome with distilled water but it is less marked with hypertonic saline and tends to resolve as the test proceeds. Children as young as 5 years can perform hypertonic saline challenges (Figure 6c.7).

The dose of the osmotic aerosol from each step is calculated by weighing the container and tubing before and at the end of each step of the challenge procedure to determine the mean output/min and multiplying by the duration of the inhalation. Alternatively, a dose related to the total aerosol inhalation time can be used. The PD is then calculated from the log dose–response curve, as in Figure 6c.4.

An ingenious method to alter airway osmolality using dry mannitol powder is effective and repeatable in adults.[43] Inhaled in doubling doses from pre-prepared capsules,

the response correlates well with methacholine challenge in children, in both degree and rate of recovery.[44] The test promises to supersede other forms of indirect challenge for clinical and epidemiological studies.

MEASUREMENT OF THE RESPONSE TO CHALLENGE

With the development of infant lung function testing and indirect methods to measure the response to challenge in preschool children, bronchial responsiveness can be assessed in children of all ages (Table 6c.3).

Direct observation of airway narrowing (by high resolution CT) is not ethical in children, but has been carried out experimentally in adult subjects.[64]

FACTORS AFFECTING THE MEASUREMENT OF BRONCHIAL RESPONSIVENESS

Correlation between different protocols

METHODS OF AEROSOL DELIVERY

Several methods have been well standardized (Table 6c.2). Despite more peripheral aerosol deposition occurring with the tidal breathing method, there was no difference between it and the dosimeter method in adults. In young children, the tidal breathing method has been found to be more repeatable and easier to use. When nebulizers with very different outputs and aerosol characteristics are used, absolute values of PC or PD are not comparable; however, this should not alter the relative distribution of results in population studies.

LUNG FUNCTION TESTS TO ASSESS THE RESPONSE

The choice of lung function test has a greater effect on the measured response than the choice of aerosol delivery system.[46] When using FEV_1 to assess the response there is a much clearer separation between normal subjects and

Table 6c.3 *Lung function tests*

10 years and over	
Specific conductance (SG_{aw})	The most sensitive, therefore a lower level of stimulus can be used; not very repeatable so 35–40% change considered significant
FEV_1	Easy to perform; sensitivity reduced because the maximal inspiration reduces airway tone so abolishes mild bronchoconstriction;[45] effect magnified by repeated manoeuvers;[46] reproducible so 20% change significant
7–10 years	
FEV_1 Peak expiratory flow	Frequently used; both are affected by maximal manoeuvres
5–7 years	
Forced oscillation technique[47,48]	Needs expensive equipment; problems in detecting induced bronchoconstriction in younger children due to distortion of the signal and associated changes in lung volume, time-consuming and needs more cooperation from the young child than earlier studies suggest
15 months – 6 years	
Direct	
Interrupter technique (R_{int})[49,50]	Easy to use; underestimates degree of bronchoconstriction, particularly in small children;[49] useful for bronchodilator challenge.[50]
Plethysmography[24,51]	Needs expensive equipment; sRaw can be measured in young children on parent's knee
Indirect measure of lung function	
Transcutaneous oxygen[26,50,52–3] (Figure 6c.6)	Reproducible reflection of changes during induced bronchoconstriction;[26] time-consuming; possibly affected by coughing and respiratory pattern; concerns raised[55].
Auscultation of the chest or trachea[54–7]	Easy to perform and controversially more reliable than transcutaneous oxygen;[55] detection of bronchoconstriction may depend on method of aerosol delivery
Up to 18 months	
Rapid thoracic compression technique[58–9] (Figure 6c.3)	May be as sensitive as FEV_1 in older children; raised volume method allows FEV_t to be measured (see Chapter 6b) increasing sensitivity; heavy sedation needed
Plethysmography	Technically demanding; sedation needed; upper (nasal) airway included in measure of resistance
Respiratory impedance[60–62]	Analogous to forced oscillation; permits tissue and airway wall properties to be studied, as well as airway calibre
Transcutaneous oxygen[63]	Seems to work only for wheezy infants, not normal infants

patients with asthma than when airway resistance is used.[45] This difference may be explained by a differential effect of maximal inspiration between normals and asthmatics if deep inspiration is more likely to abolish mild degrees of bronchoconstriction in normal subjects.[45] If normal adults are prevented from taking deep breaths during challenge, their response to methacholine resembles that of asthmatic subjects (Figure 6c.8).[64–66]

TACHYPHYLAXIS (REFRACTORWESS)

Exercise tests should not be repeated within 2–3 hours, as there is a partial refractory period.[38] Tachyphylaxis, lasting as long as 7 days, occurs after methacholine challenge in normal adults, but not those with asthma.[67] The difference between the two groups is probably due to the much greater lung dose inhaled by normal subjects.

COMPARISON OF DIRECT AND INDIRECT TESTS

Both histamine and methacholine have been widely used in population studies and have been found to give equivalent results when dose is expressed in molar units.[67] The correlation in individuals is not exact. When the results of direct challenge (histamine or methacholine) have been compared to indirect challenge (exercise, hyperventilation, cold air, non-isotonic stimulus) only a weak or no correlation has been found.[14,68] The difference may be especially marked where BR is used as a clinical trial outcome measure.[42] Inhaled corticosteroids had a prompt effect on exercise-induced asthma (anti-inflammatory), but the effect on methacholine response was incomplete after 6 months treatment (remodelling). It has been argued that the response to an indirect stimulus may be more relevant in asthma as induced bronchoconstriction is the

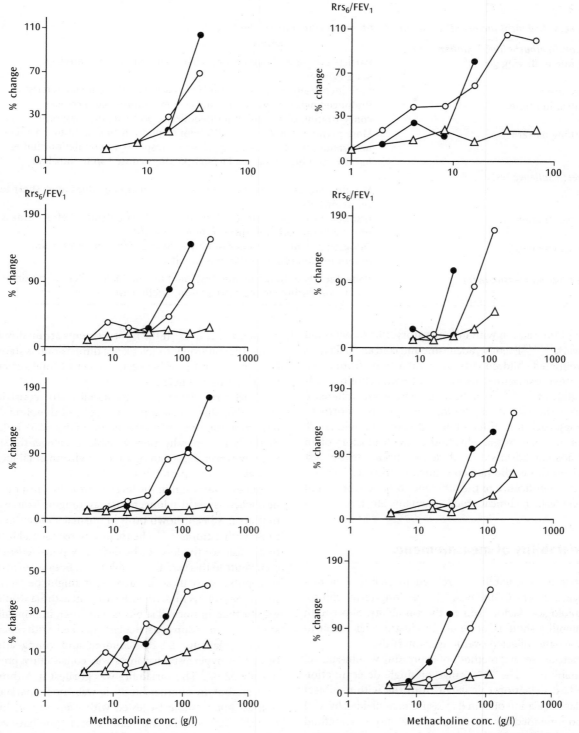

Figure 6c.8 *Comparison of methacholine dose–response curves in eight healthy adult subjects performed on three days in random order. On one day (●), the methacholine challenge was performed without any big breath manoeuvres, the response being measured by the forced oscillation technique, as respiratory resistance at 6 Hz (Rrs_6). On another day (○), the response was measured by Rrs_6, but FEV_1 was also measured at baseline, so that a big breath manoeuvre was performed once, at the start of the challenge procedure. On the third day (△), the response was measured by FEV_1. The within-subject differences between these curves illustrate the immediate and longer (>5 min) effect of big breaths on induced bronchoconstriction in normal subjects. In all eight subjects, there is a marked reduction in methacholine-induced bronchoconstriction when the response is assessed by FEV_1, compared to when it is measured by Rrs_6 in the absence of any big breath manoeuvres (note left shift of solid compared with open circle curves). A plateau response is clearly seen in 4/8 subjects using FEV_1 but in none using Rrs_6. The dose–response curves assessed by Rrs_6, when an FEV_1 was performed just once, at the start of the procedure, are intermediate. (From ref. 66.)*

Table 6c.4 *Technical factors affecting the short-term repeatability of challenge tests*

Aerosols (methacholine, histamine, etc.)	
Flow rate of driving gas	Particle size, site of deposition; $>5 \mu g$ rain out in upper airways; $<1 \mu$ exhaled
Device used	Even identically made jet-nebulizers may have different characteristics
Nebulization time	Prolonged nebulization time reduces temperature and increases concentration of aerosol in jet-nebulizers; both enhance response
Breathing pattern	More peripheral deposition with tidal respiration compared to maximal inspiration; this has negligible effect on response in population studies; nasal vs oral breathing (via face-mask) affects dose two to four-fold
Indirect challenge tests	
Exercise	Minute ventilation, duration of exercise, ambient air conditions; short-term refractoriness
Hyperventilation	Inspired air temperature and humidity all affect outcome; refractoriness limits determination of short-term repeatability
Osmotic challenge	Duration and tonicity of aerosol (hypo or hyper); refractoriness limits determination of short-term repeatability
Lung function measurement	Repeatability of lung function test and bronchodilator effect of maximal inhalation during induced bronchoconstriction are critical

result of interaction with inflammatory cells or neuronal pathways.[14,69,70] Exercise, adenosine and cold air challenges differentiated children with clear-cut asthma from those with other respiratory disorders but methacholine challenge did not.[17,18,71,72] On the other there was no difference between the two in separating asthma from normals, although each test differentiated different individuals.[70] Furthermore, in 5-year-old children, with a history of an early hospital admission with acute wheeze, neither test identified those who had continued to wheeze.[73] Therefore, the significance of the difference between direct and indirect tests in clinical practice remains blurred.

Repeatability of measurements

Short-term repeatability is related to technical factors in measurement (Table 6c.4). In the long-term, clinical and biological factors add to the variability. Short-term repeatability should not be used to justify trial size or to analyse data collected over longer intervals.

There are several methods of expressing within-subject repeatability.[74] The 95% range of single determination (standard deviation calculated from the within-subject standard deviation of paired measurement divided by $\sqrt{2}$) is recommended for assessing repeatability of a method and the 95% confidence interval for change (calculated directly from the within-subject standard deviation) for determining change in BR within subjects. In tests of bronchial responsiveness comprising a dose–response relationship, it is usual to use a log conversion for the concentration of agonist. Repeatability is often expressed in terms of doubling dilutions, which can be derived by dividing the 95% range of within-subject SD by $\log_{10}2$. When the repeatability of different methods is being compared, Bland and Altman have recommended plotting the difference between the two methods against their mean and calculating the limits of agreement (mean

difference ± 2 SD).[75] If the measurements are on different scales, the solution is to calculate a dimensionless statistic, by using the ratio of between-subject to total variance, the intraclass coefficient.

Short-term technical repeatability to constrictor aerosols in children is in the range of 1–2 doubling dilutions for histamine and methacholine (Table 6c.5). Indirect methods are generally more variable. Even over the short term, however, some biological or environmental factors may also affect repeatability (see below).

Marked variation in the level of bronchial responsiveness when assessed at longer intervals ranging from weeks to years has been shown both in normal subjects and in those with asthma.[82–84] The many environmental factors that influence the level of bronchial responsiveness will contribute to this variation (Table 6c.6). Because of greater susceptibility to these influences, it might be thought that variation in children with clear-cut asthma would be greater than in normal subjects. However, in population studies the variation is particularly marked: with repeated cold-air challenge in 287 children and young adults, bronchial hyperresponsiveness was consistently present in only 12%.[83] The variability was greatest in asthmatic subjects but in another study it was more marked in non-asthmatic subjects, tested with exercise and histamine.[84] Changes in airway calibre over time have some effect on BR within subjects.[83,85] Dirksen *et al.* found that 20% of the variation in PC_{20} with time was due to change in FEV_1 and only 11% of the difference in PC_{20} *between* subjects was due to differences in FEV_1.[85]

Environmental influences on bronchial responsiveness (Table 6c.6)

ALLERGEN EXPOSURE

Allergen exposure in sensitized subjects affects the level of bronchial responsiveness as shown by an increase in

Table 6c.5 *Repeatability of bronchial challenge tests*

Test	Lung function test	Study population Age	Nature	No. of subjects	Interval between tests	Repeatability CoV (%)	95% CI (doubling dilutions)
Histamine							
Tidal breathing[76]	PEF	Child	Asthma	22	4 h	8	–
				22	24 h	36	–
Handheld dosimeter[77]	FEV$_1$	Child	Asthma	44	2–3 h	–	<1
		Child	Normal	28	2–3 h	–	<1
Methacholine							
Tidal breathing[78]	FEV$_1$	Child	Random	14	2 m	–	1.43
Tidal breathing[26] (shortened protocol)	FEV$_1$ PtcO$_2$	Child	Asthma	9	24 h	–	0.8 0.96
Tidal breathing[79]	sRaw	Child	Asthma	22	24 h	–	2.3
	sRaw	3.6	Mixed	20	7 days		1.9
	sRaw Rint				<3 weeks		
Aerosol reservoir[23]	Rrs$_5$ Pt$_c$o$_2$	Young child	Asthma	16			1.92 3.19 3.34
					8 weeks	–	1.23
Cold air[25]	sRaw	Young child	Asthma	13			9.5 SDs 'poor'
						–	
Exercise							
Treadmill[36]	PEF	Child	Asthma	8	2 h	31	–
Hyperventilation[80]	PEF	Child	Asthma	11	2 h	8	–
Osmotic challenge[81]	FEV$_1$	Child	Asthma	17	Within 10 days	–	1.7

CoV: coefficient of variation.

Table 6c.6 *Biological and environmental risk factors for increased bronchial responsiveness*

Long-term determinants	Short-term determinants
Perinatal	Allergen exposure
Low birth weight	Diet
Maternal smoking	Viral infection
Place of birth	Airway calibre
Month of birth	Medication
Ethnic group	Gastroesophageal
Infancy	reflux
Allergen exposure	Time of day
house-dust mite	(diurnal variation)
pets	
Passive smoking	
Early viral infection?	
Childhood	
Passive smoking	
Allergen exposure/sensitization	
Air pollution	

BR in grass-sensitive subjects during the pollen season.[86] Approximately 50% of atopic asthmatic subjects demonstrate both an immediate bronchoconstrictor response to experimental allergen challenge and a delayed response which occurs 3–8 hours later (Figure 6c.9). Attention has focused on this late response as it is associated with a sustained increase in bronchial responsiveness which may persist for several days and is associated with inflammatory changes in the airways[88–90] and increase in circulating eosinophils and basophils.[91] It has often been thought to be an appropriate model for the study of atopic asthma. Recently, repeated low levels of inhaled allergen have been shown to increase bronchial responsiveness markedly for up to 6 weeks even in the absence of an early response.[92–93] This obviously has great clinical significance as well as helping to explain variability in BR when measured from time to time. Not only does allergen exposure influence the level of BR, but the level of BR will affect the response to other stimuli. For example, sensitization to house-dust mite has been shown to be a significant factor in the constrictor response to exercise.[94]

VIRUS INFECTIONS

Virus infections are frequently cited as being inducers of increased bronchial responsiveness and thus implicated in the pathogenesis of asthma.[95–96] Virus infections are very commonly associated with acute exacerbations of wheezing, both in atopic childhood asthma and independently of atopy in infants and preschool children.[97–99]

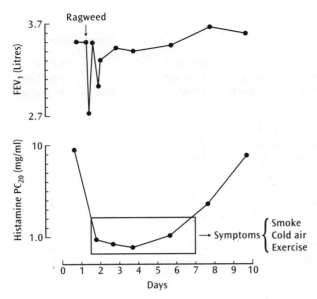

Figure 6c.9 *Prolonged increase in bronchial responsiveness (reduction in histamine PC_{20}) following a dual reaction to ragweed pollen extract in a sensitive adult asthmatic (from ref. 87 with permission). This study was performed outside the pollen season. Thus, allergen avoidance for several months did not prevent a prolonged response to a single exposure (albeit to a high dose).*

However, there is very little evidence to support the contention that virus infections are implicated in inducing any long-term inflammatory process or in sustained increases in the level of responsiveness, which are responsible for subsequent recurrent symptoms.

There have been two lines of reasoning linking viral infections to a state of increased bronchial responsiveness. The first is the finding that in normal subjects, a period of increased responsiveness can be induced by experimental viral infections.[100] This has not been confirmed in all studies,[101–102] nor shown in asthmatics. But it has recently been demonstrated in adults with a history of virus-induced wheeze, independently of atopy and unrelated to baseline lung function.[103] The second considers the observation that following RSV bronchiolitis in early infancy, children have increased levels of responsiveness when assessed later in childhood.[104–105] Such children frequently exhibit a tendency to episodic wheezing, particularly in association with further viral infections. This tendency is often imputed to a state of hyperresponsiveness induced by the initial infection. It is more likely that BHR precedes, and is a risk factor for, the development of viral wheezing illnesses in the first two years of life[106–107] although this does not necessarily preclude an additional contribution from viral illnesses themselves. However, there is no relationship between BHR and the continued tendency to wheeze in the preschool period.[107–110] Furthermore, in many epidemiological studies, no association

with recent viral infections and increased responsiveness has been found,[77,111] although it is seen in experimental viral infection in those with a history of viral wheeze.[103] In clinical practice, it is clear that there is a large subgroup of children who wheeze, some very severely, solely in association with viral infections but who are completely free of respiratory symptoms between these episodes. This is not a pattern suggestive of a chronic inflammatory process nor has inflammation been detected in such children, in contrast to those considered to have asthma.[112] Also, treatment with inhaled corticosteroids had no effect on histamine responsiveness in preschool children with wheeze related to clinical virus infections.[112a]

SMOKING

The effect of smoking can occur both *in utero* and also in childhood from passive inhalation. It is usually impossible to separate the two effects. Studies in newborn infants initially claimed that the airways of those whose mothers smoked were more responsive to histamine that those whose mothers did not.[113] With a more complete picture of the situation, it seems that this no longer holds true.[107] In older children with smoking mothers, responsiveness was increased in both asthmatic and normal children independently of the presence of atopy, particularly in boys.[114] In another study, acute cigarette smoke challenge induced prolonged increases in bronchial responsiveness without necessarily causing bronchoconstriction in a population of both asthmatic and normal children.[115] Thus smoking has a dual effect by independently increasing both the risk of atopic sensitization and the level of bronchial responsiveness.

LOCATION AND ETHNIC GROUP

The reported prevalence of asthma varies widely throughout the world. Because of differences in study techniques and populations studied, it is difficult to make accurate comparisons of the level of bronchial responsiveness in different geographical areas. The place of birth should be taken into consideration as well as the area of residence.[116] In addition to location, ethnicity may affect the relationship between bronchial responsiveness and symptoms. In New Zealand, after allowing for other confounding factors, it was found that Maori children had more asthma-like symptoms than Europeans or Pacific Islanders, but Maoris and Pacific Islanders with asthma had less bronchial responsiveness than Europeans.[117] Geographical differences in responsiveness are therefore likely to result from a large number of interacting environmental and genetic factors.

POLLUTION

Experimentally, many toxic gases such as oxides of nitrogen and ozone lead to airway inflammation and increased responsiveness.[89,118] The detrimental effect of pollutant gases in the atmosphere on the level of bronchial responsiveness and lung function is less easy to demonstrate, and some of the results have been conflicting. In children without respiratory symptoms, bronchial responsiveness was found to be increased in those living in a highly polluted area compared with those who did not.[119,120] Other studies have shown no such difference.[121–122] However, in Hong Kong, reduction in the sulphur content of fuels was associated with a significant fall in the BHR rate in non-asthmatic children.[123]

Increased responsiveness associated with airway inflammation following sensitization to a variety of industrial chemicals has been widely reported. It is of little direct relevance to children but it illustrates the principle that a large number of substances can induce a chronic inflammatory process in previously healthy people, who become sensitized. This raises the question of whether allergen avoidance in infancy in high-risk groups will prevent or simply postpone sensitization.

Effect of medication on bronchial responsiveness

Medication can have a short-term effect by blocking the pathway of bronchoconstriction induced by a stimulus, a medium-term effect by modulating airway inflammation, or a long-term effect by modifying the underlying structural pathology (remodelling).

SHORT-TERM EFFECTS

Interest in the short-term effect of drugs is mainly directed to the study of specific pathways and to consideration of the effect of recent medication on the results of responsiveness tests.

Methylxanthines and β_2-agonists are functional antagonists of direct stimuli by direct action on smooth muscle and may antagonize indirect stimuli both by effects on inflammatory cells and action on smooth muscle. There is heterogeneity of protection.[124] Anticholinergic agents act by inhibition of vagal neural pathways at muscarinic receptors; their effects are not always predictable because of the complexity of the muscarinic subtypes.[125] Nedocromil sodium and cromoglycate (cromolyn sodium) protect against indirect challenges such as exercise, sulphur dioxide and osmolar challenge stimuli, which probably act through activated inflammatory cells or by excitation of sensory nerves. They have little effect against histamine or methacholine inhalation, although a sensoneural effect for cromoglycate has been proposed.[126] Corticosteroids have no immediate (<1 h) effect on induced bronchoconstriction, including the response to exercise and the early response to inhaled allergen. Leukotriene antagonists (LTRAs) are specific to those forms of response which involve cysteinyl leukotrienes, such as exercise- and aspirin-induced asthma.[127–128a]

MEDIUM AND LONG-TERM EFFECTS

Medium-term effects have been studied in two ways: as a change in responsiveness, allowing for the duration of any acute drug effect, and by the attenuation of increased responsiveness associated with the late allergen reaction.

Long-term use of β_2-agonists leads to a small but significant increase in responsiveness, especially to antigen challenge, in most studies.[129–131] This tolerance was associated with a loss of protection to allergen, methacholine[129] and histamine[130] challenge, without a reduction of bronchodilator effect. Long-acting β_2-agonists have a similar effect, the loss of protection being demonstrable after as few as 2 days.[124] There is marked loss of degree and duration of protection against exercise-induced asthma within one month if regular salmeterol is used in teenagers.[132] Down-regulation of mast cell β_2-receptors is the most likely mechanism[133] although increased allergen access to the lower airways, following bronchodilation has been suggested to contribute to increased allergic responsiveness.[134] The clinical significance of this modest increase in responsiveness is the subject of continuing debate but it has been incriminated as a factor in increasing asthma severity and prevalence. Of greater clinical importance is loss of protection against natural challenge, and with it, a loss of protection by β-agonists as well.[135]

Methylxanthines, antimuscarinic agents and antihistamines do not have any significant medium-term effect on bronchial responsiveness. In theory, *LTRAs* should do so, by virtue of their effects on eosinophil recruitment and activation, but this has not yet been demonstrated, although montelukast causes significant inhibition of exercise-induced airway obstruction in children.[127,128]

Cromoglycate (cromolyn sodium), in contrast to its efficient protection against the increased responsiveness associated with a late reaction to allergen exposure, has minimal additional effect on BR in clinical asthma after continuous use.[136–138] Conflicting results have been reported with *nedocromil*.[136] The discrepancy between these two situations is of interest when considering the role of the drugs as anti-inflammatory agents in asthma and the possible relationship between late allergen-induced increased responsiveness and clinical asthma.

Corticosteroids by inhalation reduce allergen-provoked increases in responsiveness as well as baseline BR.[124,130,131,136,139–142] This effect is probably both dose and duration-related. A small reduction in methacholine responsiveness has been demonstrated two hours after a single dose of budesonide 800 μg but reduction continued progressively over several months of treatment.[130] With doses above 1 mg/day, a maximal reduction has been shown within a month in adult asthmatics.[136] In one long-term study of children, a plateau of benefit of a mean

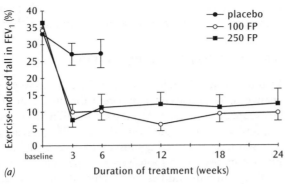 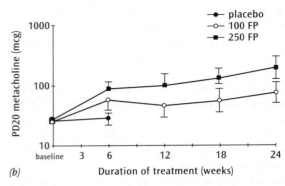

Figure 6c.10 *Effect of treatment with placebo, fluticasone 100 μg bd or fluticasone 250 μg bd on (a) the severity of exercise-induced bronchoconstriction expressed as maximal % fall in FEV$_1$ (geometric mean ± SEM) and (b) methacholine PC$_{20}$ (geometric mean ± doubling doses) (from ref. 42 with permission).*

of 2.1 doubling histamine dilutions was seen after 20–26 months.[131] This improvement was considered to be suboptimal. This beneficial effect on responsiveness is not an artificial effect of increase in airway calibre, as improvement in lung function and PC$_{20}$ are not related[139,140] and differences in PC$_{20}$ remain after allowing for changes in lung function.[141] The reduction in responsiveness is not permanent and levels return to pretreatment values within 2–3 weeks of withdrawal of steroid therapy.[140,142] Of particular interest is the finding that even after prolonged therapy, in the majority of subjects responsiveness to methacholine was not reduced to the normal range. The maximal reduction is small, up to about three doubling dilutions;[136] this is in contrast to the greater than 15 doubling dilution difference seen between severe asthma and some healthy subjects. Wide intra-subject variation in improvement has been noted.

The slow and incomplete effect of inhaled corticosteroids on BR in childhood asthma contrasts with the rapidity (3 weeks) with which they achieve a maximal effect on exercise-induced asthma[42] (Figure 6c.10). Given what is known of the dependency of exercise-induced asthma on an inflammatory milieu, this rapid effect is probably anti-inflammatory. The prolonged effect on 'direct' BR may be brought by the slower process of structural remodelling of the airway, leaving an intractable irreversible element of bronchial responsiveness. Such a line of reasoning has raised interest in more vigorous anti-inflammatory treatment in early childhood in order to prevent such a scenario in later life, but this remains purely speculative. The reduction of bronchial responsiveness following treatment with inhaled steroids is not seen in other situations.[143–145] Airway inflammation or a particular type of inflammation and consequent remodelling may therefore be specific for the increased bronchial responsiveness seen in asthma.

Oral steroids, in contrast to the inhaled route, have generally produced a small effect on responsiveness, suggesting that the site of action is in the airway epithelium rather than the endothelium or interstitium.[136,146]

MECHANISMS OF INCREASED BRONCHIAL RESPONSIVENESS

The precise mechanism of increased bronchial responsiveness is unknown. It involves a complex interaction of different factors which may vary between individuals and even in the same individual at different times (Figure 6c.11).[147]

Increased airways smooth muscle responsiveness

A number of clinical observations suggest that airway smooth muscle is important in bronchial responsiveness; the transient nature of bronchoconstriction after challenge and the prompt response to β$_2$-agonists clearly implicates a muscular mechanism. Furthermore, mathematical modelling of airway narrowing suggests that the increase in smooth muscle mass or changes in the smooth muscle contractile properties, characteristic of asthma, may be the most important factor in excessive airway narrowing.[148] Theoretically, there may be an increased capacity to shorten rapidly, and to a greater degree. Decreased pulmonary elastance with uncoupling of the airway smooth muscle from the surrounding parenchyma would reduce the load against which muscle contraction takes place, so increasing the amount of unimpeded shortening and hence airway narrowing which is possible.[149] This may be a major factor in the increased bronchial responsiveness seen in emphysema, but peripheral lung involvement in asthma is increasingly being recognized.[150]

The dynamic properties of airway smooth muscle[149,151–152] may be dependent on cyclical stretching during tidal breathing and sighing, which, by allowing a fluid relationship between actin and myosin filaments, maintains the muscle in an ideal force-length relationship. Uncoupling of the airway from the forces, which maintain this dynamic state, leads to shorter, stiffer smooth muscle

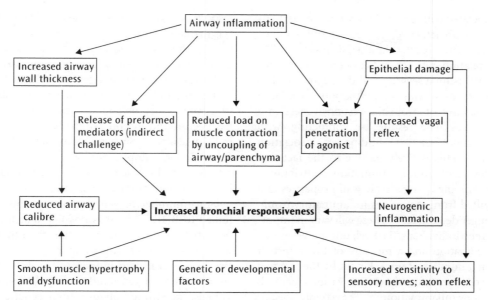

Figure 6c.11 *Interaction of different pathological factors resulting in increased bronchial responsiveness.*

with the capacity to generate excessive force. Conversely, big breath effects may be able to ameliorate these effects, during bronchial challenge in healthy subjects and during natural airway narrowing in asthmatics. This does not preclude important additional genetic factors, the effect of inflammation on smooth muscle cell phenotype and (fetal) developmental factors.[106,107,113]

Geometric considerations: airway calibre; remodelling

Resistance to laminar airflow is inversely proportional to the fourth power of the radius, so reduction of airway calibre has an exponential effect on airway resistance. The response to stimuli is usually expressed as a percentage change of resting value. With reduced airway calibre a smaller absolute change in diameter is required to produce an equivalent percentage change. On the other hand, in the presence of bronchoconstriction the potential for increasing muscle tone will be reduced. In some population studies reduced starting lung function has been found to be a small but significant independent determinant of the level of bronchial responsiveness.[83,85] Of course, both reduced lung function and airway responsiveness could be independently associated with asthma.

However, it has been postulated that airway wall thickness resulting from an increase in the tissue element, due to oedema and cellular inflammation on the luminal side of smooth muscle, as well as structural remodelling of the sub-epithelial region, will significantly increase airway resistance for a given amount of smooth muscle contraction. This will have a minimal effect on resting lung function[148,153–154] (Figure 6c.12). This effect will be exaggerated if there is an infolding of the airway wall. The lumen diameter can be reduced still further by liquid

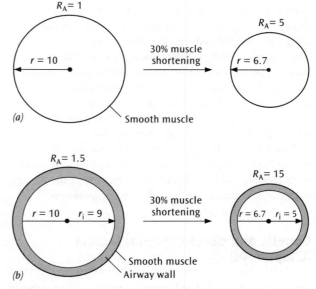

Figure 6c.12 *Effect of increasing wall thickness upon airway resistance (R_A). The addition of a tissue element inside smooth muscle (b) magnifies the increase in R_A for the same 30% smooth muscle contraction because the internal radius (r_i) is affected disproportionately (from ref. 154 with permission).*

in-filling of the interstices of the folds of the presence of mucus.[154–155]

Airway inflammation

Results of bronchial biopsy, bronchoalveolar lavage and examination of cells in induced sputum provide ample evidence that even mild asthma in adults and older children is associated with airway inflammation, particularly infiltration with activated eosinophils and lymphocytes, together with patchy epithelial loss.[88,89,156-60] However, the relation between indices of airway inflammation and both asthma severity and the degree of BR is complex. Indices of airway inflammation have been related to a measure of bronchial responsiveness in a number of studies. The results are conflicting, with some,[161-162] but not all[163-164] finding an association between the two. This is likely be due to the fact that many processes, apart from inflammation, contribute to BR (Figure 6c.12), including airway wall properties that may have resulted from a previous inflammatory insult, which is no longer detectable.[147] These will vary in importance in different individuals. The relation between evidence of inflammation and a measure of BR is further complicated in a number of ways. Firstly, by the fact that little or no correlation is found between various methods of assessing airway inflammation.[165-166] Secondly, specific inflammatory methods do not relate in the same way to different tests of BR. For example in one study, eosinophils in induced sputum related to BR assessed by inhaled hypertonic saline but not methacholine.[161] Response to therapeutic agents may further confound the issue, by producing differing effects on inflammation and remodelling.[42] So conflicting results between studies that consider the correlation between BR with airway inflammation are not surprising. There is also disagreement between findings in those with hay fever but not asthma. One study found that evidence of inflammation in the lower airways was related to BHR[167] but another did not.[168]

Inhalation of irritant gases, industrial chemicals and particularly allergens in susceptible individuals causes both demonstrable inflammatory changes in the airway with parallel increase in bronchial responsiveness.[89]

Genetic and developmental factors (Chapter 4d)

There are several inbred mouse strains which exhibit BHR and which can be used to study non-inflammatory mechanisms for BHR.[169]

From twin studies, the inheritability of asthma has been calculated as upto 68%.[170] There is clear evidence that multiple genes are involved.[171] A number of studies have demonstrated a genetic link between atopy and BHR, but not all people with atopy have BHR.[171] Several other lines of reasoning suggest that there may be separate genetic influences on the inheritance of atopy and BHR.[172-174] A family history of asthma increases the likelihood of bronchial responsiveness in atopic but not non-atopic children.[175] Bronchial responsiveness had been reported as greater in the new born offspring of asthmatic mothers,[113] but this observation has recently been retracted.[107] Two cohort studies have shown that for girls, in whom wheezing is less common than in boys, pre-morbid bronchial

responsiveness measured in the first few weeks after birth was markedly greater in those who subsequently wheezed than in those who did not.[106,107] Such an observation is compatible with a genetic basis for responsiveness.

Further evidence for a genetic influence in BR is suggested by family studies in which, in contrast to population studies (see below), a bimodal distribution of BR has been found in non-asthmatic relatives of asthmatic individuals.[176-177] Since a similar bimodal distribution is found in non-atopic, non-asthmatic individuals from asthmatic and atopic families[178] a genetic effect which is independent of atopy is suggested.

Since number of genetic polymorphisms have been linked to BHR,[179-181] it is possible that there are many potential genetic influences, other than those associated with atopy, each of which may exert a minor influence. Because many genetic influences are likely, with different combinations of genes influencing BR in different individuals, the strong polymorphous genetic influence on BR which is apparent in family studies, may weaken when single genes considered in a group of unrelated individuals.

EPIDEMIOLOGY

Distribution in population

Different methods used to describe bronchial responsiveness (including the actual or extrapolated fall in FEV_1, the slope of the dose–response curve to histamine or methacholine, and the response to cold air), have all indicated a skewed unimodal distribution, with no distinct separation between symptomatic and asymptomatic people[8-12,182-3] (Figure 6c.2). A particular cut-off point to define increased bronchial hyperresponsiveness (BHR) is therefore somewhat arbitrary. It is often taken as a change of FEV_1 of at least 20% to a concentration of methacholine/histamine of <8 g/l or a dose of <7.8 µmol. For exercise and cold-air challenge the definitive fall in FEV_1 varies between 12% and 15%.[35,36,184] There is no apparent difference in population distribution between adults and school-age children for the different types of test used.

Since the methods that have been used in different surveys have varied, different studies are not strictly comparable. A lack of separation between normal and abnormal is not altogether surprising as in reality airways are bombarded by a large number of different types of stimuli to which there is likely to be a range of intra-individual susceptibility, whereas a particular challenge test provokes only one pathway. The large number of factors which can influence both the measurement and the actual level explains the lack of a tight correlation with asthma. Moreover, it is clear that asthma is not a single disorder but rather encompasses a range of patterns of symptoms which in children includes chronic cough and episodic wheeze and a precise definition remains elusive.[185]

Association with asthma

INFANCY AND PRESCHOOL AGE

Challenge tests are time-consuming in those under 7 years of age, so there are insufficient population data in this young age group. In small random samples of infants, as well as infants of atopic parents, no association has been found between lower respiratory symptoms and responsiveness beyond the neonatal period.[107–109] Similarly, in a selected group of 3-year-olds with a past history of wheeze, there was no correlation with current symptoms.[110]

However, one study of slightly older preschool children, using an indirect challenge technique, reported BHR to isocapnic hyperventilation in 26/38 'asthmatic' children compared to 2/29 controls.[25]

SCHOOL-AGE CHILDREN AND ADULTS

One study compared the correlation between asthma (undefined) and BHR, measured by different types of challenge test and using different methods of analysis from a number of population studies.[186] A single challenge test to assess BHR gave a median positive predictive value (the likelihood of a person with a positive test having the condition) of only 26% (range 9–75%) for asthma and between 11–76% for other respiratory symptoms. In contrast the negative predictive value for asthma was 86–100%. Similarly, a recent attempt was made to find the optimal level of bronchial responsiveness (methacholine and exercise) that could be used alone to diagnose asthma in those with clear-cut disease versus those with no history of respiratory disease[184] (Figure 6c.13). This approach has the disadvantage in epidemiological studies that, although the sensitivity and specificity are acceptable, the positive predictive value is low. This is because asthma is

a relatively uncommon condition compared to the absolute number of normal subjects with a positive result.

Variation in environmental factors (Table 6c.6) could explain the discrepancy between the result of a single challenge and a history of respiratory symptoms. Although one study of selected atopic adult asthmatics found an overall relationship between change in PD_{20} and symptoms,[187] other workers following children aged 7–8 years and subjects 8–66 years with 3–4 weekly methacholine challenge tests and continuous home-based symptom and peak flow measurements showed dissociation between exacerbation of symptoms and the level of bronchial responsiveness.[4,68] These observations confirm data collected by the authors from a cohort of children with asthma some 30 years ago suggesting that BR (the response to exercise) was independent of lung function and current symptoms.

As there is good short-term repeatability for challenge protocols, this suggests that varying environmental factors affect symptoms, lung function and bronchial responsiveness differently. One important factor may be the imprecision of the diagnostic term 'asthma'. Different patterns of wheezing may have different pathogeneses and thus different relationships to increased bronchial responsiveness. In school-age children, wheeze as opposed to a diagnosis of asthma does not predict BHR,[188] which suggests that the pathogenesis of wheezing in childhood is multifactorial with differing associations with BHR and atopy (see below). Nonetheless, taken as a group, asthmatic adults and school-age children show a greater degree of bronchial responsiveness than the rest of the population.

Relation to atopy

Several observations link increased bronchial responsiveness to atopy. The first concerns experimental allergen inhalation[87] (Figure 6c.9). Second is the finding that

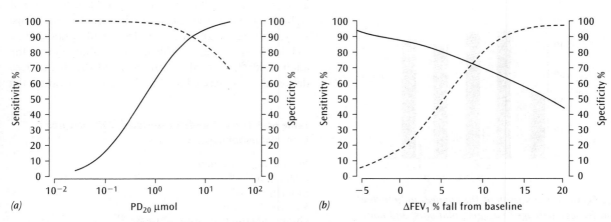

Figure 6c.13 *Cut-off points for distinguishing normal children from asthmatics (a) for histamine/methacholine PD_{20} and (b) for change in FEV_1 following an exercise test (ΔFEV_1). The balanced optimal value occurs where sensitivity and specificity are equal. (----): specificity; (—): sensitivity (from ref. 184 with permission).*

responsiveness is increased during seasonal exposure to allergen and can be reduced following avoidance in susceptible individuals.[86,189] Thirdly, in a number of population studies, atopy has been found to be strongly related to increased bronchial responsiveness even in asymptomatic subjects.[190–191] One longitudinal study has shown that children in whom atopy was demonstrable by 8–10 years were three times more likely to show BHR at 12–14 years than those who became atopic later.[116] In another, atopic sensitization in infancy has been shown to predict increased levels of bronchial responsiveness at 7 years.[192] The development of BHR may therefore depend on the duration of atopic sensitization. In a population study of 13-year-old children, the correlation of atopy with lung function has been shown to occur primarily as a result of the relationship between atopy and bronchial responsiveness.[193]

The cross-sectional study of a population of children in New Zealand by Crane and colleagues (Figure 6c.14) suggests that the association develops beyond the age of 7 years, as the level of responsiveness of non-atopic children declines while that of atopic children is retained.[175]

In population studies, the association between atopy and BHR has been shown to be greatest in older children and young adults, declining in older age.[191] From the limited evidence available, this relationship does not seem to hold in very young children: no correlation has been found with either maternal, or cord IgE and BR measured soon after birth[113] or between IgE and BR at 5 years[194] or in a selected group of children assessed at three years of age.[110] In contrast to findings in older children and adults, the level of responsiveness in these 3-year-olds was significantly greater in non-atopic than atopic children and was not related to the frequency of symptoms. In a number of studies of children with a history of RSV bronchiolitis in infancy, the level of bronchial responsiveness when assessed between seven and ten years was unrelated to atopy or subsequent wheezing.[104–105] In another population of school-children 7–11

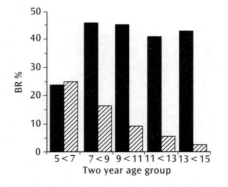

Figure 6c.14 *A comparison of the changes in bronchial responsiveness with age in atopic (solid bars) and non-atopic (hatched bars) children. Beyond the 7–9 age group, the gap between atopic and non-atopic children widens with increasing age (from ref. 175 with permission).*

years of age, wheeze was unrelated to bronchial responsiveness in the absence of atopy.[195]

Together these observations indicate that in large population studies of subjects over 7 years of age, bronchial responsiveness is strongly influenced by atopy even in the absence of symptoms. There also exists a subpopulation of childhood wheezers and ex-wheezers in whom, in contrast to those with asthma, BHR is independent of both atopy and symptoms.

Other disorders

Increased bronchial responsiveness has been described in a number of respiratory disorders apart from asthma (Table 6c.7). Studies suggest that abnormal baseline lung function plays a greater role than in asthma[77,196–198] and that these conditions are better distinguished from asthma with an exercise test rather than methacholine challenge.[71]

Bronchial responsiveness and age

It has been clear for many years that, given the many variables involved, crude values of BR cannot be compared between age groups,[202] but in spite of this, there is a fairly widely held view that bronchial responsiveness (BR) decreases with age. This view comes from a number of reports, demonstrating that most apparently normal infants respond to inhaled provocation tests[20,106,107,203–204] and that the dose of inhaled agonist required to produce a given fall in lung function increases with age.[205–207]

Recent studies have cast serious doubt on the validity of the fall in BR with age. Collis *et al.*[208] demonstrated that children over the age of 6–12 months have inspiratory flows that exceed the flows commonly used to drive jet-nebulizers and are thus likely to receive similar doses from the nebulizer regardless of their size. These predictions were confirmed by *in vivo* studies measuring pulmonary deposition of radiolabelled aerosols.[209] Le Souëf has estimated that the size-corrected dose of agonist delivered by a jet nebulizer to a child 1 year of age is likely to be about eight times that delivered to an adult; a child 5 years of age is likely to receive about four times the adult dose; while a child 10 years of age is likely to receive about double the adult dose.[202] He further demonstrated that if the dose delivered was corrected for the size of the individual, the

Table 6c.7 *Other disorders associated with increased bronchial responsiveness*

Inflammatory disorders
Cystic fibrosis[196–7]
Bronchiectasis[198–9]
Recurrent croup[200]
Chronic obstructive airways disease[201]

Developmental disorders
Prematurity[77,145]

age effect on BR reported in two studies either disappeared or was reversed.[208–209] Similarly, Stick and colleagues demonstrated than an apparent age effect, suggesting that infants responded to a lower concentration of inhaled histamine than did older children, disappeared if the inhaled dose was corrected for air entrainment.[210] An ingenious experiment by Tepper *et al.*[211] continues the controversy. They compared the bronchial response to methacholine in 13-year-old girls and 42-year-old women of identical body size. The children had significantly greater responsiveness. The increased rate of shortening in the young may explain greater BR.[149]

Relative responsiveness can be measured by a system of ranking individual results or alternatively a relative change of different subgroups of the population can be compared at different ages (for example, atopic, non-atopic; symptomatic, asymptomatic) if similar growth rates are assumed.

An additional factor complicating the reported decrease in BR with age is the fact that aerosols are delivered to infants and young children via a face-mask, whereas aerosols tend to be delivered to older children and adults via a mouthpiece. The dose of aerosol depositing in children's lungs has been shown to be 2–5 times higher for inhalation via the oral route when compared to nasal inhalation.[22] Thus, the use of a mouthpiece is likely to produce a lower provocation concentration than a face-mask with nasal inhalation. Many studies do not adequately control or report the route of aerosol inhalation, making comparison between individuals, or between studies, impossible.

In the final analysis, therefore, we may never know whether bronchial responsiveness really does change with age.

Natural history

Several prospective population studies of bronchial responsiveness are ongoing and their results, which could be expressed by a ranking procedure to overcome the effect of growth on the absolute response, will be of great value. Meanwhile, the natural history of bronchial responsiveness throughout childhood is speculative, based on limited information. Lower respiratory symptoms in infancy (largely related to respiratory viral infections) are known to be independent of the level of bronchial responsiveness.[107–109] However, children admitted to hospital with RSV bronchiolitis were found to have increased levels in most studies, when assessed at 7–11 years of age, independently of current symptoms and atopy.[104–105] This could mean that increased responsiveness predisposed to hospital admission, that severe early lower respiratory viral infection induced increased levels, or both. On the other hand, atopic sensitization, a strong determinant of bronchial responsiveness, increases through childhood.

It is therefore possible that two distinct factors determine the level of bronchial responsiveness throughout childhood. One unrelated to atopy, which operates in younger children, perhaps due to diminished lung function either as a consequence of intranterine developmental influences or due to some other unspecified genetic influence. The other is linked to atopic sensitization. Evidence for this is obtained from a New Zealand cross-sectional study in which the prevalence of BHR was the same in atopic and non-atopic children of 5–7 years, but thereafter increased with age in atopics and decreased in non-atopics[175] (Figure 6c.14). The progress of BHR into adult life from longitudinal population studies of children assessed over an 18–27 year period is somewhat conflicting. One suggested that the prevalence of BHR decreased in both symptomatic and asymptomatic subjects.[213] Unlike atopy, BHR in childhood was not a predictor of adult symptoms but was associated with reduced lung function. In a recent study, reduced FEV_1 but not FVC in early adult life was associated with BHR.[214] Another study found that levels of BR remained high and were unaffected by age in symptomatic subjects but decreased in those who because asymptomatic.[215]

CLINICAL APPLICATIONS (TABLE 6C.8)

A screening for asthma

The observation that asthma in children is characteristically associated with atopy and increased bronchial responsiveness is based on hospital-based populations. Wheezing, responsive to bronchodilator therapy, in hospital-based preschool children and in the community of older children is often independent of atopy and BHR as discussed above. Is this therefore not asthma? The argument is circular as it depends on the definition of asthma, which cannot be agreed upon. Since neither an abnormal level of responsiveness nor a precise definition of asthma is available, it is not surprising that a test of bronchial responsiveness, by any method, has proved to be unsatisfactory as a screening test for asthma in the population. In the community as a whole there are numerically more asymptomatic than asthmatic children who have BHR (assessed by histamine or methacholine); a positive test therefore has a low (around 55%) positive predictive value (the likelihood of a person with a positive test having the condition).[184]

Also, in the community (as opposed to hospital populations) a significant number of children with a physician diagnosis of asthma (undefined) have a negative result, so the test has a low negative predictive value (the likelihood of a person with a negative result not having the condition).[186] Some success in the use of a free-range exercise test detecting widespread asthma has been demonstrated,[216] but this has been shown to be no better

Table 6c.8 *Applications of tests of bronchial responsiveness*

Purpose	Comment
Population for screening for asthma	Very poor positive predictive value because of modest specificity and relatively low prevalence rate for asthma
Diagnosis of asthma	Unhelpful in the borderline cases where diagnosis is in doubt; absence of BHR casts doubt on diagnosis
Assessing asthma severity	The correlation between responsiveness and severity (judged by the level of treatment) holds only for large groups; there is too much overlap for clinical use; extreme responsiveness may be a risk factor for sudden death in asthma[225]
Clinical management	Confirmatory tests for exercise- or diet-related symptoms are occasionally valuable; it is sometimes useful to confirm the relative efficacy of drugs or their duration of protective effect
Research	Epidemiology (clues to risk factors); mechanisms of airway obstruction; studies of the efficacy of drugs or devices; natural history and genetic basis of asthma and airway disorders in children; outcome of environmental interventions

than a symptom-based questionnaire.[217] Strictly speaking, a screening program should seek the public health outcome; a study in Nottingham failed to show any beneficial effect from referral to their general practitioners, of newly diagnosed cases of childhood asthma identified by screening.[218]

Diagnosis of asthma

Similarly a test of bronchial responsiveness is unlikely to be helpful in making the diagnosis of asthma in an individual where there is any doubt. In children, when clear-cut cases of asthma were compared to other chronic respiratory disorders, exercise tests gave better discrimination between the two groups than methacholine.[71,72] However, claims made in the press for the discriminant powers of bronchial challenge tests are generally based on a comparison of barn-door cases of asthma with supernormal, non-atopic controls.[25,184] Real life is not so clear cut. Adding BHR to symptomatic diagnosis reduces the sensitivity from 0.78 to about 0.3.[218a]

Prognostic marker

Despite its limitations in screening for asthma, BHR may be a useful prognostic marker, permitting the identification of symptom-free children at risk of subsequent overt disease. Two groups have studied neonatal cohorts, showing that neonatal histamine responsiveness is a risk factor for wheezing in infancy and the preschool period.[106,107] In the Perth cohort, neonatal responsiveness predicted asthma at age 6,[219] but not atopy, IgE or eosinophilia. This observation reinforces the hypothesis that an innate, possibly constitutional form of airway responsiveness contributes independently of atopy, to the development of asthma.

Most studies have shown that symptom-free schoolchildren hyper-responsive to pharmacological or exercise challenge are at a greater risk of subsequent symptomatic asthma.[220–222] An exercise challenge test gave conflicting results, one study showing good prediction 6 years after a positive test,[223] while the other showed poor prediction after 10 years.[224] The prognostic sensitivity is low and there is interaction with atopy, so that bronchial challenge alone is unlikely to identify subjects suitable for intervention with anti-inflammatory drugs. A prognostic index combining BHR with other risk factors (such as allergy) may be more sensitive.

Assessment of the severity of asthma

In populations of atopic asthmatic school-children and adults, the level of responsiveness has been shown to correlate with severity and drug requirements.[1–3,5] In contrast, in 3-year-old children, those requiring prophylactic therapy were actually less responsive to methacholine than those who did not.[110] One possible explanation for this discrepancy is that in young children, the level of bronchial responsiveness is more easily reversed by therapy. A finding of severely increased levels of responsiveness indicates a need for more vigorous preventer therapy, although it is probable that the same information would be apparent from an appropriate history. It has been suggested, but not proved, that extreme responsiveness is a risk factor for sudden death from asthma.[225] This risk may be more related to the maximal attainable degree of airway narrowing than the sensitivity to the constriction stimulus, because it reflects the potential severity of airway obstruction and may also be an indication of chronic airway inflammation.[226] Although a lack of a plateau in maximal constriction can be demonstrated in asthmatic children[33] and this excessive airway narrowing can be modified by treatment with inhaled steroids in adults,[34] the relationship between maximal airway narrowing and severity of asthma has not yet been well explored in childhood asthma.

Management of asthma

When serial measurements of responsiveness and symptoms were monitored over a prolonged period, a clear dissociation between the two was apparent,[4,137] even after steroid treatment.[140] Nonetheless, in adult asthma, when current guideline recommendations were compared to a strategy to additionally reduce methacholine responsiveness, clinical control, lung function and bronchial biopsy evidence of airway remodelling and inflammation, were all significantly better when BR was the target for therapy than when it was not,[227] albeit at the cost of higher doses of inhaled corticosteroids. This approach has not yet been reported in children, but the study of Hofstra and colleagues[42] would suggest that methacholine responsiveness is not appropriate, and that its use in this way could lead to massive over-treatment. An exercise-test-based management plan might be more appropriate, especially since higher doses of inhaled corticosteroids are needed to treat exercise-induced asthma than other asthma symptoms.[228]

EXERCISE-RELATED SYMPTOMS

There are circumstances when it might be helpful to know whether exercise-induced asthma is being either exaggerated or under-reported. Care has to be taken in interpretation because the result is highly dependent on inspired air conditions and the response is known to vary greatly from time to time.

DIET-RELATED SYMPTOMS

Ingested substances are often incriminated as inducing symptoms.[229] It has been shown that it is frequently difficult to confirm the history by double-blind challenge when lung function alone is used in the assessment. In a number of studies, a significant increase in responsiveness was demonstrated in the absence of changes in resting lung function following ingestion of the incriminated substance (Chapter 7d). Substances that have been shown temporarily to increase responsiveness in selected individuals include cola drinks, tartrazine, sodium metabisulphite, egg, peanuts, food cooked in oil, dilute hydrochloric acid and ice.

Research

While imperfect as a model of asthma, airway obstruction induced by bronchial challenge procedures has taught us much about the physiology of airway obstruction and about individual differences in airway function, which probably have clinical significance. Examples include work of Permutt and colleagues on the effect of deep inspiration in the amelioration of airway obstruction;[64,65] that of Fredberg and colleagues on the dynamics of smooth muscle contraction in asthma,[152] and that of Milic-Emili and

co-workers on the relationship of flow-limitation, hyperinflation and the perception of dyspnoea.[230–231] The link between genetics and molecular biology, and cell biology, organ physiology and disease is nowhere better illustrated than in relation to the study of airway smooth muscle.

Despite exhortations in the recent past[232–233] which fly in the face of clinical experience, bronchial responsiveness testing has of little proven value for the diagnosis and management of childhood asthma. Perhaps the major application of bronchial responsiveness tests has been in clinical research. Epidemiological applications have provided important information on risk factors for disease[191] and secular trends.[234] We understand the mechanics of airway obstruction in children better as a result of pharmacological challenge in infants,[235] while evidence for different types of wheezing disorder in early childhood is emerging as a result of the contrast between data in young children and older subjects.[107–110,175] However, BHR is a marker for asthma and may be less sensitive in survey work than a valid questionnaire.[14,218a,236]

The observation that airway inflammation induced by inhalation of toxic gases increased bronchial responsiveness[89] contributed a great deal to our current understanding of asthma as a chronic inflammatory disease. Therapeutic interventions which block the process involved in the generation of allergen-induced increased responsiveness at a molecular level are eagerly awaited.

Therapeutic trials incorporating challenge techniques provide information about the efficacy and duration of the protective action of bronchodilators[237] and the effectiveness of the devices used to administer drugs.[238] The number of subjects required to demonstrate an effect on exercise-induced asthma under well controlled conditions is quite small: nine for a crossover and 15 for a parallel study, detecting a 50% reduction.[239] The efficacy of environmental interventions have also been successively assessed by incorporating a test of BR.[123,240] Finally, it is hoped that some of the cohorts, incorporating bronchial challenge from birth, will provide the data needed for studies of the molecular genetic basis for increased responsiveness.

CONCLUSIONS

An enormous range of airway responsiveness to constrictor stimuli is found in the population, both in terms of sensitivity and the size of the response. Undoubtedly, the severest end of this continuous distribution contains the majority of cases of moderate to severe asthma, a fact which reflects the ease with which bronchoconstriction can be induced. All the same, it is quite apparent that responsiveness, however measured, is not synonymous with asthma and cannot as such be used as a screening tool. The many factors which are involved in its determination, the imprecision of a diagnosis of asthma and the presence in the population of clearly asthmatic subjects, particularly children, who are not responsive makes this often held assumption absurdly simplistic.

Many interesting questions and issues which have clear practical importance have been raised by the large number of studies undertaken. The relevance of asymptomatic BHR is one. Does this reflect an abnormality of airway function, which is a risk factor for disease, and is it a consequence of early airway damage or genetically determined? Another issue is the finding that there are elements of responsiveness that are amenable to treatment with inhaled steroids and others that are not. Does this resistant component represent scarring which could have been prevented by either rigorous early treatment or a different therapeutic approach altogether? This question clearly has great implications when considering the management of wheezing in young children, in whom prognosis is often good and prediction of long-term future morbidity imprecise. The assumed causal association between bronchial responsiveness and airway inflammation has been questioned[241] on the grounds that the two are not invariably associated nor do they necessarily respond similarly to treatment with inhaled steroids, as discussed above.

A picture emerges of a condition of airway responsiveness that has many facets. A large component relates to atopy or a reaction to allergen, in both those with and without asthma. This allergic element in responsiveness seems to increase in importance during middle childhood. In older children and adults, it correlates strongly to symptoms of asthma. Other factors clearly determine the level of responsiveness found in other disorders, which may reflect airway damage. Much remains unknown but clearer understanding of the natural history and pathogenesis of BR in different situations and at different ages will lead to a more rational basis for the management of asthma and hopefully to prevention of morbidity in a wide range of conditions.

REFERENCES

1. Cockroft DW, Killan DN, Mellon JJA, Hargreave FE. Broncheal reactivity to inhaled histamine: a method and clinical survey. Clin Allergy 1977;7:235–43.
2. Juniper EF, Frith PA, Hargreave FE. Airway responsiveness to histamine and methacholine: relationship to minimum treatment to control symptoms of asthma. Thorax 1981;36:575–9.
3. Avital A, Noviski N, Bar-Yishay E, Springer C, Godfrey S. Non-specific bronchial reactivity in asthmatic children depends on severity but not on age. Am Rev Respir Dis 1991;144:36–8.
4. Joseph LK, Gregg L, Mulle MA, Holgate ST. Non-specific bronchial reactivity and its relationship to clinical expression of asthma: a longitudinal study. Am Rev Respir Dis 1989;140:350–7.
5. Avital A, Godfrey S, Springer C. Exercise, methacholine, and adenosine 5′-monophosphate challenges in children with asthma: relation to severity of the disease. Pediatr Pulmonol 2000;30:207–14.
6. American Thoracic Society Standards for the diagnosis and care of patients with chronic obstructive pulmonary disease (COPD) and asthma. Am Rev Respir Dis 1987;136:225–43.
7. Toelle BG, Peat JK, van den Berg RH, Dermand J, Woolcock AJ. Comparison of three definitions of asthma: a longitudinal perspective. J Asthma 1997;34:161–7.
8. Pattemore PK, Asher MI, Harrison AC, et al. The interrelationship among bronchial hyperresponsiveness, the diagnosis of asthma and asthma symptoms. Am Rev Res Dis 1990;142:549–54.
9. Rijcken B, Schouten JP, Weiss ST, et al. The distribution of bronchial responsiveness to histamine in symptomatic and asymptomatic subjects. Am Rev Respir Dis 1989;140:615–23.
10. Cockcroft DW, Gerscheid A, Murdock KY. Unimodal distribution of bronchial responsiveness to inhaled histamine in a random human population. Chest 1983;83:751–4.
11. Salome CM, Peat JK, Britton WJ, Woolcock AJ. Bronchial responsiveness in two populations of school children. Relationship to respiratory symptoms and diagnosed asthma. Clin Allergy 1987;17:271–81.
12. Weiss ST, Tager IG, Weiss JW, et al. Airways responsiveness in a population sample of adults and children. Am Rev Respir Dis 1984;129:898–902.
13. Sherrill DC, Martinez FD, Sears MR, Lebowitz MD. An alternative method for comparing and describing methacholine response curves. Am Rev Respir Dis 1993;148:116–22.
14. Pauwels R, Joos G, van der Straeten M. Bronchial responsiveness is not asthma. Clin Allergy 1988;8:317–21.
15. Van Schoor J, Joos GF, Pauwels RA. Indirect bronchial hyperresponsiveness in asthma: mechanisms, pharmacology and implications for clinical research. Thorax 2000;16:514–33.
16. Anderson SD, Brannan JD, Spring JF. A new method for bronchial provocation testing in asthmatic subjects using a dry powder of mannitol. Am J Respir Crit Care Med 1997;156:758–65.
17. Avital A, Picard E, Uwyyed K, Springer C. Comparison of adenosine 5′-monophosphate and methacholine for the differentiation of asthma from chronic airway diseases with the use of the auscultative method in very young children. J Pediatr 1995;127:438–40.
18. Van Den Berge M, Kerstjens HA, Meijer RJ, De Reus DM, Koeter GH, Kauffman HF, Postma DS. Corticosteroid-induced improvement in the PC$_{20}$ of adenosine monophosphate is more closely

associated with reduction in airway inflammation than improvement in the PC_{20} of methacholine. *Am J Respir Crit Care Med* 2001;**164**:1127–32.

18a. Holgate ST, Adenosine provocation: a new test for allergic type airway inflammation. *Am J Resp Crit Care Med* 2002;**165**:317–9.

19. Sterk PJ, Fabbri LM, Quanjer PH, *et al*. Airway responsiveness. Standardized challenge testing with pharmacological physical and sensitising stimuli in adults. Report Working Party Standardization of Lung Function Tests, European Community for Steel and Coal. Official Statement of the European Respiratory Society. *Eur Respir J* (Suppl) 1993:53–83.

19a. Joos GF, O'Connor BJ. ERS Task force on indirect airway challenges. *Eur Resp J* 2002; in press.

20. Geller DE, Morgan WJ, Cota K, Wright AL, Taussig LM. Airway responsiveness to cold, dry air in normal infants. *Pediat Pulmonol* 1998;**4**:90–7.

21. Becquemin MH, Swift DH, Bouchickhi N, Roy M, Teillac A. Particle deposition and resistance in the noses of adults and children. *Eur Respir J* 1991;**4**:694–702.

22. Everard M, Hardy JG, Milner AD. Comparison of nebulized aerosol deposition in the lungs of healthy adults following oral and nasal inhalation. *Thorax* 1993;**48**:1045.

23. Klug B, Bisgaard H. Measurement of lung function in awake 2–4 year old asthmatic children during methacholine challenge and acute asthma: a comparison of the impulse oscillation technique, the interrupter technique, and transcutaneous measurement of oxygen versus whole-body plethysmography. *Pediatr Pulmonol* 1996;**21**:290–300.

24. Klug B, Bisgaard H. Measurement of the specific airway resistance by plethysmography in young children accompanied by an adult. *Eur Respir J* 1997;**10**:1599–605.

25. Nielsen KG, Bisgaard H. Lung function response to cold air challenge in asthmatic and healthy children of 2–5 years of age. *Am J Respir Crit Care Med* 2000;**161**:1805–9.

26. Phagoo SB, Wilson NM, Silverman M. Repeatability of methacholine challenge in asthmatic children measured by change in transcutaneous oxygen tension. *Thorax* 1992;**47**:804–8.

27. Chai H, Far RS, Froehlick LA, *et al*. Standardisation of bronchial inhalation challenge procedures. *J Allergy Clin Immunol* 1975;**56**:323–7.

28. Yan K, Salome C, Woolcock AJ. Rapid method for measuring bronchial responsiveness. *Thorax* 1983;**38**:760–5.

29. Smith CH, Anderson SD. Inhalation provocations using non-isotonic aerosols. *J Allergy Clin Immunol* (1989);**84**:781–90.

30. Peat JK, Salome CM, Berry G, Woolcock AJ. Relation of dose-response slope to respiratory symptoms and lung function in a population study of adults living in Busselton, Western Australia. *Am Rev Respir Dis* 1992;**146**:860–5.

31. Chinn S, Burney PG, Britton JR, Tattersfield AE, Higgins BG. Comparison of PD20 with two alternative measures of response to histamine challenge in epidemiological studies. *Eur Respir J* 1993;**6**:670–9.

32. Woolcock AJ, Salome CM, Yan K. The shape of the dose response curve to histamine in asthmatic and normal subjects. *Am Rev Respir Dis* 1984;**13**:71–3.

33. De Pee S, Timmers MC, Hermans J, Duiverman EJ, Sterk PJ. Comparison of maximal airway narrowing to methacholine between children and adults. *Eur Respir J* 1991;**4**:421–8.

34. Bel EH, Timmers MC, Zwinderman AH, Dijkman JH, Sterk PJ. The effect of inhaled corticosteroids on maximal degree of airway narrowing to methacholine in asthmatic subjects. *Am Rev Respir Dis* 1991; **143**:109–13.

35. Tsanakas JN, Milner RDG, Banister OM, Boon AW. Free running asthma screening test. *Arch Dis Child* 1988; **63**:261–5.

36. Silverman M, Anderson S. Standardisation of exercise test in asthmatic children. *Arch Dis Child* 1972;**47**:882–9.

37. McFadden ER. Respiratory heat and water exchange: physiological and clinical implications. *J Appl Physiol* 1983;**54**:331–6.

38. Edmunds AT, Tooley M, Godfrey S. The refractory period following exercise-induced asthma, its duration and relation to severity of exercise. *Am Rev Respir Dis* 1978;**117**:247–54.

39. Manning PJ, Watson RM, O'Byrne P. Exercise-induced refractoriness in asthmatic subjects involves leukotrienes and prostaglandin interdependent mechanisms. *Am Rev Respir Dis* 1993;**148**:950–4.

40. Hofstra WB, Sterk PJ, Neijens HJ, Kouwenberg JM, Mulder PG, Duiverman EJ. Occurrence after late response to exercise in asthmatic children. *Eur Resp J* 1996;**9**:1348–55.

41. Lenney W, Milner AD. Recurrent wheezing and the preschool child. *Arch Dis Child* 1978;**53**:468–73.

42. Hofstra WB, Kouwenberg JMP, Kuethe MC, Sterk PJ. Dose response over time to inhaled fluticasone proprionate treatment of exercise and methacholine induced bronchoconstriction in children with asthma. *Pediatr Pulmonol* 2000;**29**:415–23.

43. Anderson SD, Spring J, Moore B, *et al*. The effect of inhaling a dry powder of sodium chloride on the airways of asthmatic subjects. *Eur Respir J* 1997;**10**:2465–73.

44. Subbarao P, Brannan JD, Ho B, Anderson SD, Chan HK, Coates AL. Inhaled mannitol identifies methacholine-responsive children with active asthma. *Pediatr Pulmonol* 2000;**29**:291–8.

45. Orehek J, Gaynard P, Grimend C, Charpin J. Effect of maximal respiratory manoeuvres on bronchial

sensitivity of asthmatic patients as compared to normal people. *Br Med J* 1975;**1**:123–5.

46. Knox AJ, Coleman HE, Britton JR, Tattersfield AE. A comparison of three measures of the response to inhaled methacholine. *Eur Respir J* 1989;**2**:736–40.

47. Duiverman EJ, Neijens HI, van Strik R, *et al*. Comparison of forced oscillometry and forced expirations for measuring dose-related responses to inhaled methacholine in asthmatic children. *Bull Eur Physiopathol Respir* 1986;**27**:133–6.

48. Wilson NM, Bridge P, Phagoo SB, Silverman M. The measurement of methacholine responsiveness in 5 year old children: three methods compared. *Eur Respir J* 1995;**8**:364–70.

49. Phagoo SB, Wilson NM, Silverman M. Evaluation of the interrupter technique for measuring change in airway resistance in 5-year-old asthmatic children. *Pediatr Pulmonol* 1995;**20**:387–95.

50. Beydon N, Trang-Pham H, Bernard A, Gaultier C. Measurements of resistance by the interrupter technique and of transcutaneous partial pressure of oxygen in young children during methacholine challenge. *Pediatr Pulmonol* 2001;**31**:238–46.

51. DeBaets F, Van Daele S, Franckx H, Vinaimont F. Inhaled steroids compared with disodium cromoglycate in preschool children with episodic viral wheeze. *Pediatr Pulmonol* 1998;**25**:361–6.

52. Mochizuki H, Mitsuhashi M, Tokuyama K, *et al*. A new method of measuring bronchial hyperresponsiveness in younger children. *Ann Allergy* 1985;**55**:162–6.

53. Wilson NM, Phagoo SB, Silverman M. The use of transcutaneous oxygen tension and pulse oximetry in the assessment of the response to inhaled methacholine. *Thorax* 1991;**46**:433–7.

54. Avital A, Bar-Yishay E, Springer C, Godfrey S. Bronchial provocation tests in young children using tracheal auscultation. *J Pediatr* 1988;**112**:591–4.

55. Yong SC, Smith CM, Wach R, Kurian M, Primhak RA. Methacholine challenge in preschool children: methacholine-induced wheeze versus transcutaneous oximetry. *Eur Respir J* 1999;**14**:1175–8.

56. Sprikkelman AB, Schouten JP, Lourens MS, Heymans HS, van Aalderen WM. Agreement between spirometry and tracheal auscultation in assessing bronchial responsiveness in asthmatic children. *Respir Med* 1999;**93**:102–7.

57. Spence DPS, Bentley S, Evans DH, Morgan MDL. Effects of methacholine-induced bronchoconstriction on the spectral characteristics of breath sounds in asthma. *Thorax* 1992;**47**:680–3.

58. Prendiville A, Green S, Silverman M. Bronchial responsiveness to histamine in wheezy infants. *Thorax* 1987;**42**:92–9.

59. Hayden M, Sly PD, Devadason SG, Gurrin LC, Wildhaber JH, le Souef PN. Influence of driving pressure on raised-volume forced expiration in infants. *Am J Respir Crit Care Med* 1997;**156**:1876–83.

60. Frey U, Silverman M, Kraemer R, Jackson AC. High frequency respiratory input impedance measurements in infants assessed by the high speed interrupter technique. *Eur Respir J* 1998;**12**:148–58.

61. Frey U, Jackson AC, Silverman M. Differences in airway wall compliance as a possible mechanism for wheezing disorders in infants. *Eur Respir J* 1998;**12**:136–42.

62. Hall GL, Hantos Z, Wildhaber JH, Petak F, Sly PD. Methacholine responsiveness in infants assessed with low frequency forced oscillation and forced expiration techniques. *Thorax* 2001;**56**:42–7.

63. Clarke JR, Reese A, Silverman M. Comparison of the squeeze technique and transcutaneous oxygen tension for measuring the response to bronchial challenge in normal and wheezy infants. *Pediatr Pulmonol* 1993;**15**:244–50.

64. Brown RH, Croisille P, Mudge B, Diemer FB, Permutt S, Togias A. Airway narrowing in healthy humans inhaling methacholine without deep inspirations demonstrated by HRCT. *Am J Respir Crit Care Med* 2000;**161**:1256–63.

65. Skloot G, Permutt S, Togias A. Airway hyperresponsiveness in asthma: a problem of limited smooth muscle relaxation with inspiration. *J Clin Invest* 1995;**96**:2393–403.

66. Wilson NM, Phagoo SB, Silverman M. FEV_1 measures persistently attenuate the response to methacholine challenge in normal subjects. *Am Rev Respir Dis* 1991;**143**(Suppl):A410.

67. Fujimura M, Myou S, Kamio Y, Hashimoto T, Matsuda T. Duration of tachyphylaxis in response to methacholine in healthy non-asthmatic subjects. *Respirology* 1999;**4**:47–51.

68. Clough JB, Hutchinson SA, Williams JD, Holgate ST. Airway response to exercise and methacholine in children with respiratory symptoms. *Arch Dis Child* 1991;**66**:579–83.

69. Joos GF, Kips JC, Pauwels RW. Direct and indirect bronchial responsiveness for epidemiological studies of asthma in children: comparison with histamine responsiveness. *Respir Med* 1993;**87**(Suppl B):31–6.

70. Haby MM, Anderson SD, Peat JK, *et al*. An exercise challenge protocol for epidemiological studies of asthma in children comparison with histamine challenge. *Eur Respir J* 1994;**7**:43–5.

71. Godfrey S, Springer C, Noviski N, Maayan C, Avital A. Exercise but not methacholine differentiates asthma from chronic lung disease in children. *Thorax* 1991;**46**:488–92.

72. Carlsen KH, Engh G, Mork M, Schroder E. Cold air inhalation and exercise-induced bronchoconstriction in relationship to methacholine bronchial responsiveness: different patterns in asthmatic

children and children with other chronic lung diseases. *Respir Med* 1998;**92**:308–15.

73. Wilson NM, Bridge P, Silverman M. Bronchial responsiveness and symptoms in 5–6 year old children: a comparison of a direct and indirect challenge. *Thorax* 1995;**50**:339–45.

74. Chinn S. Statistics in respiratory medicine 2. Repeatability and method comparison. *Thorax* 1991;**46**:454–6.

75. Bland JM, Altman DG. Statistical methods for assessing agreement between two methods of clinical measurement. *Lancet* 1986;**I**:307–10.

76. Hariparsad D, Wilson N, Dixon C, Silverman M. Reproducibility of histamine challenge tests in asthmatic children. *Thorax* 1983;**38**:258–60.

77. Chan KN, Elliman A, Bryan EM, Silverman M. Clinical significance of airway responsiveness in children of low birth weight. *Pediatr Pulmonol* 1989;**7**:251–8.

78. Sears MR, Jones DT, Holdaway MD. Prevalence of bronchial reactivity to inhaled methacholine in New Zealand children. *Thorax* 1986;**41**:283–9.

79. Badier M, Guillot C, Dubus JC. Bronchial challenge with carbachol in 3–6 year old children: body plethysmography assessments. *Pediat Pulmonol* 1999;**27**:117–23.

80. Wilson N, Dixon C, Silverman M. Bronchial responsiveness to hyperventilation in children with asthma: inhibition by ipratropium bromide. *Thorax* 1984;**39**:588–93.

81. Reidler J, Reade T, Robertson CF. Repeatability of response to hypertonic saline aerosol in children with mild to severe asthma. *Pediatr Pulmonol* 1994;**18**:330–6.

82. Clough JB, Williams JD, Holgate ST. Profile of bronchial responsiveness in children with respiratory symptoms. *Arch Dis Child* 1992;**67**:574–9.

83. Redline S, Tager IB, Speizer FE, Rosher R, Wiess ST. Longitudinal variability in airway responsiveness in a population-based sample of children and young adults. *Am Rev Respir Dis* 1989;**140**:172–8.

84. Backer V, Groth S, Dirksen A. Spontaneous changes in bronchial responsiveness in children and adolescents: an 18 month follow-up study. *Pediatr Pulmonol* 1991;**11**:22–8.

85. Dirksen A, Madsen F, Engel T, *et al.* Airway calibre as a confounder in interpreting bronchial responsiveness in asthma. *Thorax* 1992;**47**:702–6.

86. Boulet LP, Cartier A, Thomson NL, *et al.* Asthma and increases in bronchial responsiveness from seasonal pollen exposure. *J Allergy Clin Immunol* 1983;**71**:399–406.

87. Cockroft DW. Mechanisms of perennial asthma. *Lancet* 1993;**ii**:253–6.

88. Beasley R, Roche WR, Roberts A, Holgate ST. Cellular events in the bronchi of asthmatics. *Am Rev Respir Dis* 1989;**139**:806–17.

89. Chung KF. Role of inflammation in the hyperactivity of the airways in asthma. *Thorax* 1986;**411**:657–62.

90. Pin I, Freigag AP, O'Byrne PM, *et al.* Changes in the cellular profile of induced sputum after allergen-induced asthmatic responses. *Am Rev Respir Dis* 1991;**145**(6):1265–9.

91. Gibson PG, Manning PJ, O'Byrne, P, *et al.* Allergen induced asthmatic responses: relationship between increases in airway responsiveness and increases in circulating eosinophils, basophils and their progenitors. *Am Rev Respir Dis* 1992;**143**:331–5.

92. Thre E, Zetterstrom B. Increase in non-specific bronchial responsiveness after repeated inhalations of low doses of allergen. *Clin Exp Allergy* 1993;**23**:298–306.

93. Sulakzvelide I, Inman MD, Rerecich T, O'Byme PM. Increases in airway eosinophils and interleukins with minimal bronchoconstriction during repeated low-dose allergen challenge in atopic subjects. *Eur Resp J* 1998;**11**:821–7.

94. Frischer TH, Kuehr J, Meinert R, Karmaus W, Urbanek R. Relationship between exposure to dust mite allergen and bronchial response to exercise in schoolchildren sensitised to dust mites. *Pediatr Pulmonol* 1993;**16**:13–18.

95. Sterk PJ. Virus-induced airway hyperresponsiveness in man. *Eur Respir J* 1993;**6**:894–902.

96. Pattemore PK, Johnston SL, Bardin PG. Viruses as precipitants of asthma symptoms I. *Epidemiol Clin Exp Allergy* 1992;**22**:325–6.

97. Wright A, Taussig L, Ray C, *et al.* The Tucson Children's Respiratory Study II. Lower respiratory tract illness in the first year of life. *Am J Epidemiol* 1989;**126**(6):1232–46.

98. Johnston SL, Pattemore PK, Sanderson G, *et al.* A community study of the role of virus infections in exacerbations of asthma in 9–11 year old children. *Br Med J* 1995;**311**:629–30.

99. Horn ME, Brain EA, Gregg L, *et al.* Respiratory viral infection and wheezy bronchitis in childhood. *Thorax* 1979;**34**:23–8.

100. Empey DW, Laitinen LA, Jacobs L, Gold WM, Nadel JA. Mechanisms of bronchial hyperreactivity in normal subjects after upper respiratory tract infections. *Am Rev Respir Dis* 1976;**113**:131–9.

101. Jenkins CR, Breslin ABX. Respiratory tract infections and airway reactivity in normal and asthmatic subjects. *Am Rev Respir Dis* 1984;**130**:879–83.

102. Summers QA, Higgins PG, Burrow IG, Tyrrell DAJ, Holgate ST. Bronchial reactivity to histamine and bradykinin is unchanged after rhinovirus infection in normal subjects. *Eur Respir J* 1992;**5**:313–17.

103. McKean M, *et al.* Adult experimental model of viral wheeze. *Eur Respir J* 2001;**18**:23–32.

104. Pullan CR, Hey EN. Wheezing asthma and pulmonary dysfunction 10 years after infection with respiratory syncytial virus. *Br Med J* 1992;**284**:1665–9.

105. Sly PD, Hibbert ME. Childhood asthma following hospitalisation with acute viral bronchiolitis in infancy. *Pediatr Pulmonol* 1989;**7**:153–8.

106. Clarke J, Salmon B, Silverman M. Bronchial responsiveness in the neonatal period as a risk factor for recurrent respiratory illness in infancy. *Am J Respir Crit Care Med* 1995;**151**:1434–40.

107. Young S, Arnott J, O'Keefe PT, Le Souef PN, Landau LI. The association between early life lung function and wheezing during the first 2 years of life. *Eur Respir J* 2000;**15**:151–7.

108. Stick SM, Arnoll J, Turner DJ, et al. Bronchial responsiveness and lung function in recurrently wheezy infants. *Am Rev Respir Dis* 1991;**144**:1012–15.

109. Clarke JR, Reese A, Silverman M. Bronchial responsiveness and lung function in infants with lower respiratory tract illness over the first 6 months of life. *Arch Dis Child* 1992;**67**:1454–8.

110. Wilson NM, Phagoo SB, Silverman M. Atopy, bronchial responsiveness and symptoms in wheezy 3 year olds. *Arch Dis Child* 1992;**67**:492–5.

111. Woolcock AJ, Peat JK, Salome CM, et al. Prevalence of bronchial hyperresponsiveness in a rural adult population. *Thorax* 1986;**42**:361–8.

112. Stevenson EC, Turner G, Heaney LG, et al. Bronchoalveolar lavage findings suggest two different forms of childhood asthma. *Clin Exp Allergy* 1997;**27**:1027–35.

112a. De Baets F, van Daeles, Frankx H, Vinaimont F. Inhaled steroids compared with disodium cromoglycate in children with episode viral wheeze. *Pediatr Pulmol* 1998;**25**:361–6.

113. Young S, Le Souëf PN, Geelhoed GC, et al. The influence of a family history of asthma and parental smoking on airway responsiveness in early infancy. *New Eng J Med* 1991;**324**:1168–73.

114. Martinez FD, Awognoni G, Marci F, et al. Parental smoking enhances bronchial responsiveness in 9 year old children. *Am Rev Respir Dis* 1988;**138**:518–23.

115. Menon P, Rando RJ, Stankins RP, Salveggio JE, Lehrer SB. Passive cigarette smoke challenge studies: increase in bronchial hyperreactivity. *J Allergy Clin Immunol* 1992;**89**:560–6.

116. Peat JK, Salome CM, Woolcock AJ. Longitudinal changes in atopy during a 4 year period; relation to bronchial hyperresponsiveness and respiratory symptoms in a population of Australian school children. *J Allergy Clin Immunol* 1990;**85**:60–74.

117. Pattemore PK, Asher M, Harrison AC, et al. Ethnic differences in prevalence of asthma symptoms and bronchial hyperresponsiveness in New Zealand school children. *Thorax* 1989;**44**:168–76.

118. Molfino NA, Wright SC, Katz I, et al. Effect of low concentrations of ozone on inhaled allergen responses in asthmatic subject. *Lancet* 1990;**338**:199–203.

119. Molfino NA, Slutsky AS, Zamel N. The effects of air pollution on allergic bronchial responsiveness. *Clin Exp Allergy* 1992;**22**:667–72.

120. Wang JY, Isine TR, Chen HI. Bronchial responsiveness in an area of air pollution resulting from wire reclamation. *Arch Dis Child* 1992;**67**:488–90.

121. Ware JH, Feins BG, Dockery DW, et al. Effects of ambient sulphur oxides and suspended particles on respiratory health of pre-adolescent children. *Am Rev Res Dis* 1986;**133**:834–42.

122. Von Mutius E, Martinez FD, Fritzsch C, et al. Prevalence of asthma and atopy in two areas of West and East Germany. *Am J Respir Crit Care Med* 1994;**149**:358–64.

123. Wong CM, Lam TH, Peters J, et al. Comparison between two districts of the effects of an air pollution intervention on bronchial responsiveness in primary school children in Hong Kong. *J Epidemiol Commun Health* 1998;**52**:571–8.

124. Bisgaard H. Long-acting beta-2 agonists in the management of childhood asthma. *Pediatr Pulmonol* 2000;**29**:221–4.

125. Barnes PJ. Muscarinic receptor subtypes: implication for lung disease. *Thorax* 1989;**44**:161–7.

126. Page CP. Sodium cromoglycate, a tachykinin antagonist? *Lancet* 1994;**343**:70.

127. Pearlman DS, Ostrom NK, Bronsky EA, Bonuccelli CM, Hanby LA. The leukotriene D4-receptor antagonist Zafirlukast attenuates exercise-induced bronchoconstriction in children. *J Pediatr* 1999;**134**:273–9.

128. Kemp JP, Dockham PJ, Shapiro GG, et al. Montelukast once daily inhibits exercise-induced bronchochonstriction in 6–14 year old children with asthma. *J Pediatr* 1998;**133**:424–8.

128a. Yoshida S, Saktamoto H, Ishazaki Y, et al. Efficacy of leukotriene receptor antagonist in bronchial hyperresponsiveness and hypersensitivity to analgesics in aspirin intolerant asthma. *Clin Exp Allergy* 2000;**30**:64–79.

129. Cockcroft DW, McParland CP, Britto SA, Swystun VA, Rutherford BC. Regular inhaled salbutamol and airway responsiveness to allergen. *Lancet* 1993;**342**:833–7.

130. Vathenan AS, Knox AJ, Wisniewski A, Tattersfield AE. The course of change in bronchial reactivity with an inhaled corticosteroid in asthma. *Am Rev Respir Dis* 1991;**143**:1317–21.

131. Kerrebijn KF, van Essen-Zandvliet EEM, Niejens HJ. Effect of long-term treatment with inhaled corticosteroids and beta-agonists on the bronchial responsiveness in children with asthma. *J Allergy Clin Immunol* 1987;**79**:653–9.

132. Simons FE, Gerstner TV, Cheang MS. Tolerance to the bronchoprotective effect of salmeterol in

adolescents with exercise-induced asthma using concurrent inhaled glucocorticoid treatment. *Pediatrics* 1997;**99**:655–9.

133. O'Connor BJ, Aikman SL, Barnes PJ. Tolerance to the bronchodilator effects of beta agonists in asthma. *New Engl J Med* 1992;**327**:1204–8.

134. Lai CKW, Twentyman OP, Holgate ST. The effect of an increased inhaled allergen dose after inhaled rimeterol hydro-bromide and the occurrence and magnitude of the late asthmatic response and the associated changes in nonspecific bronchial responsiveness. *Am Rev Respir Dis* 1987;**140**:917–23.

135. Lipworth BJ, Aziz I. A dose of albuterol does not overcome bronchoprotective subsensitivity in asthmatic subjects receiving regular salmeterol or formoterol. *J Allergy Clin Immunol* 1999;**103**:88–92.

136. Fuller RW. Do prophylactic asthma drugs alter airway hyperresponsiveness? In: CP Page, PJ Gardiner, eds. *Bronchial Responsiveness.* Blackwell Scientific, Oxford, 1993, pp. 297–315.

137. Silverman M, Connolly NM, Balfour-Lynn L, Godfrey S. Long-term trial of disodium cromoglycate and isoprenaline in children. *Br Med J* 1972;**3**:378–81.

138. Reques FG, Sanz CC, Sanchez CS, *et al.* Long-term modification of histamine-induced bronchoconstriction by disodium cromoglycate and ketotifen versus placebo. *Allergy* 1985;**40**:242–9.

139. Dutoit JL, Salome CM, Woolcock AJ. Inhaled corticosteroids reduce the severity of bronchial responsiveness in asthma but oral theophylline does not. *Am Rev Respir Dis* 1987;**136**:1174–8.

140. Van Essen-Zadvliet EE, Hughes MD, Waalkens HJ, Duiverman EJ, Kerrebijn, K. Remission of childhood asthma after long-term treatment with an inhaled corticosteroid (budesonide): can it be achieved? *Eur Respir J* 1994;**7**:63–8.

141. Ryan G, Latimer KM, Juniper EF, Roberts RS, Hargreave FE. Effect of beclomethasone dipropionate on bronchial responsiveness to histamine in controlled nonsteroid dependent asthma. *J Allergy Clin Immunol* 1985;**75**:25–30.

142. De Baets FM, Gokeyn M, Kerrebijn KF. The effect of two months of treatment with inhaled budesonide on bronchial responsiveness to histamine and house dust mite antigen in asthmatic children. *Am Rev Respir Dis* 1990;**142**:581–6.

143. Bel EH, van der Veen H, Dijkman JH, Sterk PH. The effect of inhaled budesonide on the maximal degree of airway narrowing in leukotriene D_4 and methacholine in normal subjects *in vivo. Am Rev Respir Dis* 1989;**139**:427–31.

144. Watson A, Li TK, Joyce H, Pride NB. Trial of the effect of inhaled corticosteroids on bronchoconstrictor and bronchodilator responsiveness in middle aged smokers. *Thorax* 1988;**43**:231P.

145. Chan KN, Silverman M. Increased airway responsiveness in children of low birthweight at school age: effect of topical corticosteroids. *Arch Dis Child* 1993;**69**:120–4.

146. Jenkins CR, Woolcock AJ. Effect of prednisone and beclomethasone dipropionate on airway responsiveness in asthma: a comparative study. *Thorax* 1988;**43**:378–84.

147. Haley KJ, Drazen JM. Inflammation and airway function in asthma: what you see is not necessarily what you get. *Am J Respir Crit Care Med* 1998;**157**:1–3.

148. Martin JG, Dureot A, Eidelman DH. The contribution of smooth muscle to airway narrowing and airway hyperresponsiveness. *Eur Respir J* 2000;**16**:349–54.

149. Que CL, *et al.* Homeokinesis and short term variability of human airway calibre. *J Appl Physiol* 2001;**91**:1131–41.

150. Kraft M. The distal airways: are they important in asthma? *Eur Respir J* 1999;**14**:1403–17.

151. Gunst SJ, Tang DD. The contractile apparatus and mechanical properties of airway smooth muscle. *Eur Respir J* 2000;**15**:600–16.

152. Fredberg JJ. Airway obstruction in asthma: does the response to a deep inspiration matter? *Respir Res* 2001:**2**:273–5.

153. Schellenberg RR. Mechanisms of airway hyperresponsiveness. In: CP Page, PJ Gardiner, eds. *Airway Hyperresponsiveness: Is It Really Important For Asthma?* Blackwell Scientific, Oxford, 1993, pp. 33–54.

154. James AL, Pare PD, Hogg JC. The mechanics of airway narrowing in asthma. *Am Rev Respir Dis* 1989;**139**:242–6.

155. Seow CY, Wang L, Pare PD. Airway narrowing and internal structural constraints. *J Appl Physiol* 2000;**88**:527–33.

156. Pin I, Radford S, Kolendowicz R, *et al.* Airway inflammation in symptomatic and asymptomatic children with methacholine hyperresponsiveness. *Eur Respir J* 1993;**6**:1249–56.

157. Lundgren R, Sodenberg M, Horstedt P, Stenling R. Morphological studies of mucosal biopsies from asthmatics before and after ten years treatment with inhaled steroids. *Eur Respir J* 1988;**1**:883–9.

158. Ferguson AC, Whitelaw M, Brown H. Correlation of bronchial eosinophil and mast cell activation with bronchial hyperresponsiveness in children with asthma. *J Allergy Clin Immunol* 1992;**90**:609–13.

159. Jeffrey PK, Wardlaw J, Nelson FC, Collins JV, Kay AB. Bronchial biopsies in bronchial asthma: an ultrastructural quantitative study and correlation with hyperreactivity. *Am Rev Respir Dis* 1989;**140**:1745–53.

160. Cai Y, Carty K, Henry RL, Gibson PG. Persistence of sputum eosinophilia in children with controlled asthma when compared with healthy children. *Eur Respir J* 1998;**11**:848–53.

161. Gibson PG, Saltos N, Borgas T. Airway mast cells and eosinophils correlate with clinical severity and airway hyperresponsiveness in corticosteroid-treated asthma. *J Allergy Clin Immunol* 2000;**105**:752–9.

162. Jatakanon A, Lim S, Kharitonov SA, Chung KF, Barnes PJ. Correlation between exhaled nitric oxide, sputum eosinophils and methacholine responsiveness in patients with mild asthma. *Thorax* 1988;**53**:91–5.

163. Crimi E, Spanevello A, Neri M, Ind PW, Rossi GA, Brusasco V. Dissociation between airway inflammation and airway hyperresponsiveness in allergic asthma. *Am J Respir Crit Care Med* 1998;**157**:4–9.

164. Iredale MJ, Wanklyn SA, Phillips IP, Krausz T, Ind PW. Non-invasive assessment of bronchial inflammation in asthma: no correlation between eosinophilia of induced sputum and bronchial responsiveness to inhaled hypertonic saline. *Clin Exp Allergy* 1994;**24**:940–5.

165. Wilson NM, James A, Uasuf C, *et al.* Asthma severity and inflammation markers in children. *Pediatr Allergy Immunol* 2001;**12**:125–32.

166. Lim S, Jakakanon A, Meah S, Oates T, Chung KF, Barnes PJ. Relationship between exhaled nitric oxide and mucosal eosinophilic inflammation in mild to moderately severe asthma. *Thorax* 2000;**55**:184–8.

167. Foresi A, Leone C, Pelucchi A, *et al.* Eosinophils, mast cells, and basophils in induced sputum from patients with seasonal allergic rhinitis and perennial asthma: relationship to methacholine responsiveness. *J Allergy Clin Immunol* 1997;**100**:58–64.

168. Djukanovic R, Lai CKW, Wilson JW, *et al.* Bronchial mucosal manifestations of atopy: a comparison of markers of inflammation between atopic asthmatics, atopic nonasthmatics and healthy controls. *Eur Respir J* 1992;**5**:538–44.

169. Duguet A, Biyah K, Minshall E, Gomes R, Wang CG, Taoudi-Benchekroun M, Bates JH, Eidelman DH. Bronchial responsiveness among inbred mouse strains. Role of airway smooth muscle shortening velocity. *Am J Respir Crit Care Med* 2000;**161**:839–48.

170. Koeppen-Schomerus G, Stevenson J, Plomin R. Genes and environment: a short study of 4 year old twins. *Arch Dis Child* 2001;**85**:398–400.

171. Los H, Koppelmann GH, Postma DS. The importance of genetic influence in asthma. *Eur Respir J* 2000;**14**:1210–27.

172. Welty C, Weiss ST, Tager IB, *et al.* The relationship of airway responsiveness to cold air, cigarette smoking and atopy, to respiratory symptoms and pulmonary function in adults. *Am Rev Respir Dis* 1984;**130**:198–203.

173. Von Mutius E, Nicolai T. Familial aggregation of asthma in a South Bavarian population. *Am J Respir Care Med* 1996;**153**:1266–72.

174. Gray L, Peat JK, Belousova E, Xuan W, Woolcock AJ. Family patterns of asthma, atopy and airway hyperresponsiveness: an epidemiological study. *Clin Exp Allergy* 2000;**30**:393–9.

175. Crane J, O'Donnell TV, Prior IA, Waste DA. The relationships between atopy, bronchial hyperresponsiveness and a family history of asthma: a cross-sectional study of migrant Tokelauan children in New Zealand. *J Allergy Clin Immunol* 1989;**84**:768–72.

176. Longo G, Strinati R, Poli F, Fumi F. Genetic factors in nonspecific bronchial hyperreactivity. *Am J Dis Child* 1987;**141**:331–4.

177. Hopp RJ, Bewtra AK, Bivan R, Nair NM, Townley RG. Bronchial reactivity pattern in nonasthmatic parents of asthmatics. *Ann Allergy* 1988;**61**:184–6.

178. Townley RG, Bewtra AK, Nair NM, *et al.* Methacholine inhalation challenge studies. *J Allergy Clin Immunol* 1979;**64**:569–74.

179. Trabetti E, Cusin V, Malerba G, *et al.* Association of the Fc epsilon RI-beta gene with bronchial hyper-responsiveness in an Italian population. *J Med Genet* 1998;**35**:680–1.

180. Li-Kam-Wa TC, Mansur AH, *et al.* Association between 308 tumour necrosis factor promoter polymorphism and bronchial hyperreactivity in asthma. *Clin Exp Allergy* 1999;**29**:1204–8.

181. Hill MR, James AL, Faux JA, *et al.* Fc epsilon RI-beta polymorphism and risk of atopy in a general population sample. *BMJ* 1995;**311**:776–9.

182. O'Connor G, Sparrow D, Taylor D, Segal M, Weiss S. Analysis of dose response curves to methacholine. *Am Rev Respir Dis* 1987;**136**:1412–17.

183. Peat JK, Salome CM, Benny C, Woolcock AJ. Relation of dose–response slope to respiratory symptoms in a population sample of adults and children. *Am Rev Respir Dis* 1991;**144**:663–7.

184. Godfrey S, Springer C, Bar YE, Avital A. Cut-off points defining normal and asthmatic bronchial reactivity to exercise and inhalation challenges in children and young adults. *Eur Respir J* 1999;**14**:659–68.

185. Silverman M, Wilson N. Asthma – time for a change of name? *Arch Dis Child* 1997;**77**:62–4.

186. Pattemore PK, Holgate ST. Bronchial hyperresponsiveness and its relationship to asthma in childhood. *Clin Exp Allergy* 1993;**23**:886–900.

187. Britton JR, Burney PGJ, Chinn S, Papacosta AO, Tattersfield A. The relation between changes in airway reactivity and change in respiratory symptoms and medication in a community study. *Am Rev Respir Dis* 1988;**138**:530–4.

188. Burrows B, Sears MR, Flannery EM, Habison P, Holdaway MD. Relationship of bronchial responsiveness assessed by methacholine to serum IgE, lung function, symptoms and diagnoses in 11 year old New Zealand children. *J Allergy Clin Immunol* 1992;**90**:376–85.

189. Platts-Mills TAE, Mitchell EB, Mozzoro H, Nock P, Wilkins SR. Reduction of bronchial hyperreactivity during prolonged allergen avoidance. *Lancet* 1982;**2**:675–8.

190. Sears MR, Burrows EM, Flannery EM, *et al*. Relation between airway responsiveness and serum IgE in children with asthma and apparently normal children. *New Engl J Med* 1991;**325**:1067–71.

191. Peat JK, Salome CM, Woolcock AJ. Factors associated with bronchial hyperresponsiveness in Australian adults and children. *Eur J Respir Dis* 1992;**5**:921–9.

192. Van Asperen PP, Kemp AS, Mukhi A. Atopy in infancy predicts the severity of bronchial hyperresponsiveness in late childhood. *J Allergy Clin Immunol* 1990;**85**:790–5.

193. Sears MR, Burrows B, Herbison GP, *et al*. Atopy in childhood III. Relationship with pulmonary function and airway responsiveness. *Clin Exp Allergy* 1993;**3**:957–63.

194. Wilson NM, Dore CJ, Silverman M. Factors relating to the severity of symptoms at 5 years in children with severe wheeze in the first 2 years of life. *Eur Respir J* 1997;**10**:346–53.

195. Clifford RD, Radford M, Howell JB, Holgate ST. Prevalence of atopy and range of bronchial response to methacholine in 7 and 11 year old school children. *Arch Dis Child* 1989;**64**:1120–32.

196. Mellis CM, Levison H. Bronchial reactivity in cystic fibrosis. *Pediatrics* 1978;**61**:446–50.

197. Silverman M, Hobbs FOR, Gordon IRS, Carswell F. Cystic fibrosis, atopy and airways liability. *Arch Dis Child* 1978;**53**:873–7.

198. Varpela E, Laitenan LA, Keskinen H, Korhola O. Asthma, allergy and bronchial hyperreactivity to histamine in patients with bronchiectasis. *Clin Allergy* 1978;**8**:273–80.

199. Pang J, Chan HS, Sang JV. Prevalence of asthma, atopy and bronchial hyperreactivity in bronchiectasis: a controlled study. *Thorax* 1989;**44**:948–51.

200. Zach M, Erben A, Olinsky A. Croup, recurrent croup and airway hyperreactivity. *Arch Dis Child* 1981;**56**:336–41.

201. Ramsdale EH, Morris MM, Roberts AS, Hargreave FE. Bronchial responsiveness to methacholine in chronic bronchitis: relationship to airflow obstruction and cold air responsiveness. *Thorax* 1984;**39**:912–18.

202. Le Souëf PN. Can measurements of airway responsiveness be standardised in children? *Eur Respir J* 1993;**6**:1085–7.

203. Tepper RS. Airway reactivity in infants: a positive response to methacholine and metaproterenol. *J Appl Physiol* 1987;**62**:1155–9.

204. Le Souëf PN, Geelhoed GC, Turner DJ, Morgan SEG, Landau LI. Response of normal infants to inhaled histamine. *Am Rev Respir Dis* 1989;**139**:62–6.

205. Gerritsen J, Koeter GH, Postma DS, Schouten JP, Knol K. Prognosis of asthma from childhood to adulthood. *Am Rev Respir Dis* 1989;**140**:1325–30.

206. Montgomery GL, Tepper RS. Changes in airway reactivity with age in normal infants and young children. *Am Rev Respir Dis* 1990;**142**:1372–6.

207. Hopp RJ, Bewtra A, Nair NM, Townley RG. The effect of age on methacholine response. *J Allergy Clin Immunol* 1985;**76**:609–13.

208. Collis GG, Cole CH, Le Souëf PN. Dilution of nebulised aerosols by air entrainment in children. *Lancet* 1990;**336**:341–3.

209. Chua HL, Collis GG, Newbury AM, *et al*. The influence of age on aerosol deposition in children. *Eur Respir J* 1994;**7**:2185–91.

210. Stick SM, Turnbull S, Chua HL, Landau LI, Le Souëf PN. Bronchial responsiveness to histamine in infants and older children. *Am Rev Respir Dis* 1990;**142**:1143–6.

211. Tepper RS, Stevens J, Eigen H. Heightened airway responsiveness in normal female children compared with adults. *Am J Respir Crit Care Med* 1994;**149**:678–81.

212. Duguet A, Wang CG, Gomes R, Ghezzo H, Eidelman DH, Tepper RS. Greater velocity and magnitude of airway narrowing in immature than in mature rabbit lung explants. *Am J Resp Crit Care Med* 2001;**164**:1728-33.

213. De Gooijer A, Brand PLP, Gerritsen J, *et al*. Changes in respiratory symptoms and airway hyperresponsiveness after 27 years in a population-based sample of school children. *Eur Respir J* 1993;**6**:848–54.

214. Xuan W, Peat JK, Toelle BG, Marks GB, Berry G, Woolcock AJ. Lung function growth and its relation to airway hyperresponsiveness and recent wheeze. Results from a longitudinal population study. *Am J Respir Crit Care Med* 2000;**161**:1820–4.

215. Rijcken B, Shouten JP, Weiss ST, *et al*. Long term variability of bronchial responsiveness to histamine in a random population sample of adults. *Am Rev Respir Dis* 1993;**148**:944–9.

216. Williams D, Briton J, Wilson I. Screening a state middle school for asthma using the free running asthma screen. *Arch Dis Child* 1993;**69**:667–9.

217. Ninan TK, Russell G. Is exercise testing useful in a community-based asthma survey? *Thorax* 1993;**48**:1218–21.

218. Hill R, Williams S, Britton J, Tattersfield A. Can morbidity associated with untreated asthma in primary school children be reduced? A controlled intervention study. *Br Med J* 1991;**303**:1169–74.

218a. Remes ST, Pekkanen J, Remes K, Salonen RO, Korppi M. In search of childhood asthma: questionnaire, tests of bronchial hyperresponsiveness and clinical evaluation. *Thorax* 2002;**57**:120–6.

219. Palmer L, Rye PJ. Airway responsiveness in early infancy predicts asthma, lung function and respiratory symptoms by school age. *Am J Respir Crit Care Med* 2001;**163**:37–42.

220. Burrows B, Sears MR, Flannery ED. Relation of the course of bronchial responsiveness from age 9 to 15 to allergy. *Am J Respir Crit Care Med* 1995;**152**:1302–6.

221. Carey VJ, Weiss ST, Tager IB, Leeder SR, Speizer FE. Airways responsiveness, wheeze onset, and recurrent asthma episodes in young adolescents: the East Boston Childhood Respiratory Disease Cohort. *Am J Respir Crit Care Med* 1996;**153**: 356–61.

222. Lombardi E, Morgan WT, Wright AL. Cold air challenge at age 6 and subsequent incidence of asthma: a longitudinal study. *Am J Respir Crit Care Med* 1997;**156**:1863–9.

223. Jones A, Bowen P. Screening for childhood asthma using an exercise test. *Br J Gen Pract* 1994; **44**:127–31.

224. Rasmussen F, Lambrechtsen J, Siersted HC, Hansen HS, Hansen NC. Asymptomatic bronchial hyperresponsiveness to exercise in childhood and the development of asthma-related symptoms in young adulthood: the Odense Schoolchild Study. *Thorax* 1999;**54**:587–9.

225. Zach MS, Karner V. Sudden death in asthma. *Arch Dis Child* 1989;**64**:1446–51.

226. Macklem PT. A hypothesis linking bronchial hyperreactivity and airway inflammation implications for therapy. *Ann Allergy* 1990;**64**:113–16.

227. Sont JK, Willems LN, Bel EH, van Krieken JH, Vandenbroucke JP, Sterk PJ. Clinical control and histopathologic outcome of asthma when using airway hyperresponsiveness as an additional guide to long-term treatment. The AMPUL Study Group. *Am J Respir Crit Care Med* 1999;**159**:1043–51.

228. Pedersen S, Hansen OR. Budesonide treatment of moderate and severe asthma in children: a dose–response study. *J Allergy Clin Immunol* 1995;**90**:29–33.

229. Wilson NM. Food related asthma: a difference between two ethnic groups. *Arch Dis Child* 1985;**60**:861–5.

230. Sulc J, Volta CA, Ploysongsang Y, Eltayara L, Olivenstein R, Milic EJ. Flow limitation and dyspnoea in healthy supine subjects during methacholine challenge. *Eur Respir J* 1999;**14**:1326–31.

231. Tantucci C, Ellaffi M, Duguet A, *et al.* Dynamic hyperinflation and flow limitation during methacholine-induced bronchoconstriction in asthma. *Eur Respir J* 1999;**14**:295–301.

232. Woolcock AJ. Assessment of bronchial responsiveness as a guide to prognosis and therapy in asthma. *Med Clin North Am* 1990;**74**:753–65.

233. Cockcroft DWJ, Hargreave FE. Airway hyperresponsiveness: relevance of random population data to clinical usefulness. *Am Rev Respir Dis* 1990;**142**:497–500.

234. Burr ML, Portland MK, King S, Vaughan-Williams E. Changes in asthma prevalence: two surveys 13 years apart. *Arch Dis Child* 1989;**64**:1452–6.

235. Prendiville A, Green S, Silverman M. Airway responsiveness in wheezy infants: evidence for functional β adrenergic receptors. *Thorax* 1987;**42**:100–4.

236. Pearce N, Perkinsen J, Beasley R. Role of bronchial responsiveness testing in asthma prevalence surveys. *Thorax* 2000;**55**:352–4.

237. Ahrens HC, Bonham AC, Maxwell GA, Weinberger MM. Method for comparing the peak intensity and duration of action of aerosolized bronchodilators using bronchoprovocation with methacholine. *Am Rev Respir Dis* 1984;**129**:903–6.

238. Clarke JR, Aston H, Silverman M. Delivery of salbutamol by metered dose inhaler and valved spacer to wheezy infants: effect on bronchial responsiveness. *Arch Dis Child* 1993;**69**:125–9.

239. Dahlen B, O'Byrne PM, Watson RM, Roquet A, Larsen F, Inman MD. The reproducibility and sample size requirements of exercise-induced bronchoconstriction measurements. *Eur Respir J* 2001;**17**:581–8.

240. Gruber W, Eber E, Mileder P, Modl M, Weinhandl E, Zach MS. Effect of specific immunotherapy with house dust mite extract on the bronchial responsiveness of paediatric asthma patients. *Clin Exp Allergy* 1999;**29**:176–81.

241. Chapman ID, Foster A, Morley J. The relationship between inflammation and hyperreactivity of the airways in asthma. *Clin Exp Allergy* 1993; **23**:168–71.

6d

Inflammation

JONATHAN GRIGG

INTRODUCTION

Inflammation is a non-specific protective reaction of vascularized tissue. Usually, it resolves completely leaving tissue both structurally and functionally normal.[1] Stimuli that trigger inflammation may either be immunological or non-immunological, but both result in an accumulation of effector cells such as neutrophils, lymphocytes and eosinophils. In the lung, as in other tissues, pro-inflammatory stimuli trigger the release of proteins (mediators) which act on blood vessels to recruit and activate systemic effector cells (Figure 6d.1). Disruption of this process, by stimuli persistence or genetically pre-programmed alternations in mediator expression, may lead to abnormal resolution (sometimes referred to as remodelling: see Chapter 5) and persistence of disease. There is a large degree of redundancy in the actions of pro-inflammatory mediators and effector cells. Thus a single mediator can be a major determinant of symptoms under some circumstances, but in other contexts, symptoms may persist in its absence.

Measuring inflammation in the lung[2,3] serves two functions. First, insights are gained into the key mediators and cells underlying clinical disease, which guide the development of specific therapies. Second, clinically relevant information may be obtained using inflammatory markers that is not apparent by symptom history, and clinical examination.

SAMPLING METHODS AND THEIR APPLICATIONS

Bronchial tissue

Bronchial inflammation is directly sampled by mucosal biopsy via a fibreoptic bronchoscope. Bronchoscopy is performed after local anaesthesia of the upper airways and larynx. The bronchoscope is passed through the nose into the trachea, and several subsegmental biopsy samples (usually from the right middle and lower bronchi) taken using alligator forceps. For immunocytochemistry and *in situ* hybridization, biopsies need to be fixed immediately in 4% paraformaldehyde and embedded in optimum cutter temperature (OCT) compound, before storage at $-80°C$. Sections ($6\,\mu m$) are cut from the frozen biopsies for processing.

Bronchial biopsy has shown that the core abnormality underlying the inflammatory substrate of adult atopic asthma is abnormal activation of pulmonary Th2 lymphocytes (Figure 6d.1). Thus over 60% of bronchial CD3+ T-cells are positive for interleukin (IL)-5 mRNA (a prototypic Th2 cytokine) compared with 10% positivity for both atopic and non-atopic controls.[4] IL-5 promotes the terminal differentiation of committed eosinophil precursors, activates mature eosinophils, enhances eosinophil adhesion to vascular endothelium.[5] Since the number of pulmonary tissue T-cells is relatively small, their activation

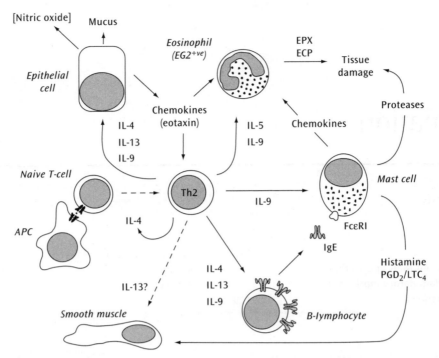

Figure 6d.1 *Pleiotropic activities of T-helper type 2 (Th2)-type cytokines in allergic asthma. Upon recognition of the antigen and activation by antigen presenting cells (APC), naive T-cells differentiate into Th2 cells, a process that is promoted by interleukin 4 (IL-4). Activated Th2 cells stimulate B-cells to produce IgE antibodies in response to IL-4, and to a lesser extent to IL-13 or IL-9. IgE binds the high affinity IgE receptor at the surface of mast cells, the proliferation and differentiation of which is promoted by IL-9, in synergy with other factors such as fibroblast derived mast-cell growth factor. At contact with antigen, mast cells release the contents of their granules, including histamine, which will induce a bronchospasm, together with newly synthesized prostaglandins and leukotrienes (PGD₂, and LTC₄). Mast cells also release chemotactic factors that contribute to the recruitment of inflammatory cells, particularly eosinophils, whose proliferation and differentiation from bone marrow progenitors is promoted by IL-5 and IL-9. Finally, epithelial cells up-regulate their production of mucus and chemokines in responses to Th2 cytokines such as IL-4, IL-13 and IL-9. The presence of the IL-13 receptor at the surface of smooth muscle cells suggests that this factor can also directly affect smooth muscle contractility, but this remains to be demonstrated. (From ref. 56.)*

state is difficult to assess directly. Emphasis has therefore been on the amplified downstream effects of Th2 cell activation such as pulmonary eosinophilia, which have the potential to effect other tissue compartments. Eosinophilia in bronchial mucosal biopsies can be identified by monoclonal antibodies (mAb). The mAb EG2 identifies activated eosinophils expressing eosinophil cationic protein (ECP).[1] ECP is localized in the matrix of the specific granule of eosinophils and induces a wide range of proinflammatory effects.[6] Stimuli that initiate ECP secretion include IgE and IL-5 (Figure 6d.1). Compared with healthy atopic and non-atopic controls, steroid-naive adults with active asthmatic symptoms have increased numbers of EG2-positive eosinophils in the bronchial mucosa.[7] The link between pulmonary Th2 lymphocyte activation and tissue eosinophilia is the increased expression of a group of proteins, the C–C chemokines (e.g. eotaxin), which specifically recruit and activate eosinophils.[8] Increased C–C chemokine expression occurs in both atopic and non-atopic asthma (measured after steroid withdrawal), and

can be detected in a wide range of pulmonary tissue cells including epithelial cells, fibroblasts and macrophages[7] (Figure 6d.2).

In asthmatic adults, levels of bronchial tissue eosinophilia are associated with increased symptom severity. For example, adults with persistent wheeze have higher numbers of bronchial EG2 positive cells compared with those with intermittent symptoms only[9] (Figure 6d.3). Indeed, a third of asthmatic adults with intermittent symptoms have tissue eosinophils within the range for normal controls.[9] Bronchial biopsy has been shown to be safe in children with difficult asthma.[10] Bronchial biopsies from children with moderate atopic asthma show submucosal infiltration with lymphocytes and degranulating mast cells, but not eosinophils.[11] A similar paucity of intraepithelial eosinophils and increased numbers of mast cells, has been found in symptomatic adults receiving high-dose corticosteroids.[12] One explanation for the low eosinophil numbers and symptoms is that eosinophil-associated symptoms are removed by steroids, but a proportion of

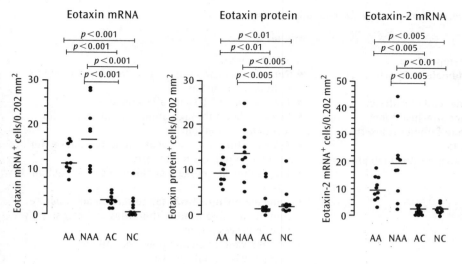

Figure 6d.2 *EG2 positive eosinophils and eotaxin mRNA positive cells in bronchial biopsies from adults with atopic asthma (AA), non-atopic asthma (NAA), atopic controls (AC), and non-atopic controls (NC). Tissue eosinophilia and C–C chemokine activation is present in both asthmatic groups. (From ref. 7 with permission.)*

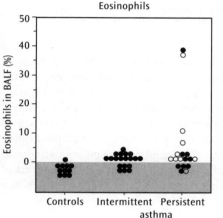

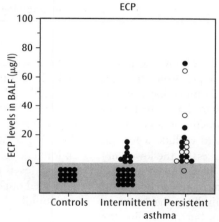

Figure 6d.3 *Changes in bronchoalveolar lavage fluid eosinophil (%) and ECP in intermittent and persistent adult atopic asthma, compared with non-atopic controls. ○: atopic; ●: non-atopic patients with persistent asthma. (From ref. 9 with permission.)*

disease is driven by products of other cells remain, such as mast cell-derived leukotrienes (see below). However in general, bronchial biopsy can identify a pattern of inflammation that is strongly associated with asthma i.e. tissue eosinophilia and increased C–C chemokine expression. These data suggest that the role of tissue eosinophils in asthma symptoms is 'context dependent', i.e. inflammatory markers must be interpreted in the light of symptoms on the day of sampling, ongoing corticosteroid therapy, and duration of disease.[13] The essential role of eosinophils in asthma implies that indirect monitoring of tissue eosinophil levels could help clinical management, particularly as anti-inflammatory agents are the mainstay of therapy. The key questions are whether indirect makers reflect ongoing tissue inflammation, and whether monitoring inflammation changes practice within the pragmatic clinical setting.

Airway

There is a complex relationship between asthmatic inflammation in the tissue and in the airway. Repeat bronchial biopsies in asthmatic adults after allergen challenge[14] show that by two hours tissue and airway eosinophils remain at baseline levels, but bronchial C–C chemokine transcription has increased. At 4 hours, a 'late' fall in FEV_1 develops, associated with persistent increased expression of C–C chemokines, and a four-fold increase in the number of tissue EG2-positive eosinophils. The fall in FEV_1 correlates strongly with the total number of tissue eosinophils and tissue eotaxin reactivity. Subsequently, tissue EG2-positive eosinophils spill over into the airway. Thus at 24 hours, whilst tissue eotaxin levels and EG2-positivity decline, the number of EG2-positive cells in the airway increase further. These data show that (i) inflammatory cells in pulmonary tissue move into the airway in asthma; and (ii) airway cellularity does mirror tissue inflammation, but not necessarily at the same time point.

BRONCHOALVEOLAR LAVAGE

Airway eosinophils and mediators can be directly sampled by bronchoalveolar lavage (BAL). BAL is a less invasive technique than bronchial biopsy, and is an important tool

Table 6d.1 *Non-bronchoscopic bronchoalveolar lavage for intubated children*

Materials	Methods
• Normal sterile saline at room temperature • Suction catheter with single end hole (6 French <1 yr, 8 FG 1–5 yr, 10 FG >5 yr) • 3-way tap inserted onto proximal end of catheter • Bronchoscopic connector for endotracheal tube (to allow partial ventilation while catheter is inserted) • Suction trap attached to 3-way tap • Low pressure suction pressure adaptor (too high pressure reduces fluid return)	After intubation • Turn child's head to the left (so that catheter enters right main bronchus) • Pre-oxygenate (100% for a few breaths) • Insert catheter through bronchoscopic connector (continue ventilation) • Ask anaesthetist to stop ventilation (ventilation during instillation reduces fluid return) • Instil saline at 1 ml/kg. For children over 20 kg limit to 20 ml • Immediately turn 3-way tap to suction and aspirate into suction trap while withdrawing catheter slightly (this improves return) • Resume ventilation and re-wedge catheter • Repeat twice (total 3 ml/kg) • Transport lavage fluid on ice (not necessary for microbiological samples)

for validating more practical and ethically acceptable sampling techniques. In adults, BAL is performed through a fibreoptic bronchoscope inserted under local anaesthesia. Recruiting asthmatic children for fibreoptic BAL in order to measure inflammation is unethical, unless there are other clinical indications (e.g. to exclude a foreign body). In contrast, serendipitous access to the lower airway can be obtained in children of all ages prior to elective surgery. In this circumstance, most researchers instil and aspirate normal saline via a blindly wedged suction catheter (Table 6d.1). For children, but not adults, the instilled volume is indexed to body weight.[15,16] Although site of BAL is unknown when using a suction catheter, the procedure is quick, and the plastic components are cheap and disposable. In general, small instilled volumes sample cells from the large airways (bronchial wash), whereas larger instilled vol-umes sample cells and solutes from both the bronchi and alveoli (BAL).

BAL and bronchial biopsy in adult asthmatics not receiving steroids, give very similar results. The percentage of eosinophils and the concentration of ECP in BAL fluid (BALF) mirrors the stepwise increase in the eosinophils and activated T-cells in the bronchial submucosa as asthma severity increases[9] (Figure 6d.3). Ennis and colleagues have applied non-bronchoscopic BAL to a large number of asthmatic and non-asthmatic children and found a similar BALF pattern to that of adult asthmatics, namely increased numbers of BALF eosinophils[17] and concentration of ECP[18] compared with atopic controls. These researchers also found that 75% of children with only intermittent viral-wheeze had BALF–ECP levels within the normal range for atopic healthy children,[17] a finding that mirrors the biopsy studies in asthmatic adults with intermittent symptoms.[9] BAL has also been useful in excluding asthmatic inflammation in the context of active symptoms. For example, children with chronic non-productive cough

without wheeze, have a significantly lower percentage of BALF eosinophils when compared with atopic asthmatics,[19] and an increased percentage of BALF neutrophils when compared with non-asthmatic controls.[19] In summary, eosinophils and eosinophil products in the BALF that are above the range for atopic healthy children do reflect eosinophilic tissue inflammation, and normal levels of eosinophils/products in the context of untreated ongoing symptoms can exclude chronic tissue eosinophilia.

INDUCED SPUTUM

Induced sputum offers the best compromise between practicality and invasiveness for direct sampling of the lower airway. Sputum can be induced in children from 7 years of age using nebulized saline, with a success rate of approximately 70%.[20] The technique has been shown to be safe in adults whose lung function is severely impaired (FEV_1 40–60% of predicted).[21] Hypertonic saline may be used either as a 4.5% solution, or as increasing concentrations of saline. A problem with induced sputum is how to remove or identify salivary contamination. Two techniques are in current use: the 'whole sputum' method, where sputum and saliva is collected together and results corrected for contamination, and the 'selected' method, where the mucocellular parts of the sputum are removed before processing. In atopic asthmatics, there is a good correlation between the percentage of induced sputum eosinophils and the percentage of eosinophils in bronchial washings within the same individual.[22] The relationship within individuals between the percentage of eosinophils in induced sputum and the number of tissue EG2-positive cells (per mm^2 of lamina propria) is statistically significant, but not as strong.[22] This loss of precision is not surprising since (i) eosinophils move out of

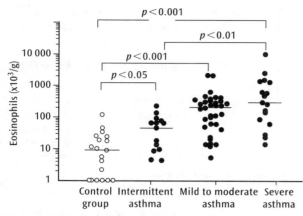

Figure 6d.4 *Eosinophil counts in induced sputum in adult atopic asthmatics and non-atopic controls showing that airway eosinophilia increases with increased asthma severity. (From ref. 23 with permission.)*

lung tissue into the airway; and (ii) steroid therapy may selectively attenuate tissue, but not airway eosinophilia.[12] Overall, eosinophilia in one lung compartment is a reflection of eosinophilia in an adjacent compartment (induced sputum vs bronchial wash, bronchial wash vs tissue eosinophilia), but the strength of association decreases when non-adjacent compartments are compared. In the clinical setting, these technical considerations may be less important, since sputum eosinophils in adult asthmatics still increase with increasing asthma severity, and this pattern appears to be relatively unaffected by ongoing use of inhaled corticosteroids[23] (Figure 6d.4).

Analysis of induced sputum of asthmatic children will be clinically useful, if it identifies a disassociation between reported symptoms and eosinophilic inflammation. In adults who are clinically well controlled on corticosteroids, those with high sputum eosinophils are at increased risk of relapse on steroid withdrawal compared to those with normal levels.[24] However in children, Wilson *et al.*[20] found no correlation between induced sputum eosinophils and asthma severity in both mild and moderate asthmatics. Furthermore she found a wide overlap in the percentage of eosinophils between normals and asthmatics, and suggests either 1) a single induced sputum sample has a limited role for the diagnosis of paediatric asthma, or 2) induced sputum eosinophils are highly context dependent (e.g. low numbers if no symptoms on the day of sampling). The latter may explain why there is a good association between the severity of airflow obstruction and the percentage of eosinophils (EG2-positive) in induced sputum[25] in acute paediatric asthma exacerbations. In adults, when current guidelines were compared with a strategy to reduce sputum eosinophils, better clinical control was achieved overall with no additional steroid use.[25a] In summary, pulmonary eosinophil inflammation can be detected indirectly using induced sputum, and this

technique is repeatable, relatively non-invasive, and provides additional information that is not readily discernible by normal clinical practice.

Markers of inflammation in the breath

Nitric oxide (NO) is a gas that is present in exhaled breath, and can be measured by chemiluminescence. NO diffuses from the airway wall enriching NO-free alveolar air travelling to the mouth during expiration.[26] Exhaled NO (eNO) concentrations are therefore flow dependent.[27] NO is also generated in the nose, paranasal sinuses and oropharynx, and a fixed positive mouth pressure is often used to close the soft palate. There are two methods of sampling eNO. In the 'on-line' method exhaled gas is sampled at a fixed flow from a side port in the exhalation circuit. In 'off-line' sampling, exhaled air is collected in a NO-inert storage bag and analysed later. Since NO remains stable for several hours, off-line sampling can be performed outside the clinical setting. Both methods appear to give similar results.[26]

eNO has the potential to be the perfect marker of tissue inflammation in asthmatic children. It is easily measured, it can be regarded as a direct lower airway sample, is increased in atopic asthmatics when compared with non-atopic controls, and repeated measurements are possible. The events regulating the synthesis of NO by the asthmatic epithelium have been defined.[28] Normal human airway epithelium expresses NO synthase II (NOSII, the enzyme that converts L-arginine to NO and L-citrulline), due to continuous transcription activation of the gene *in vivo*. The increase levels of NO in the breath of atopic asthmatics is due to an inflammatory cytokine-driven increase in activity of the Stat1 activation pathway, which directly up-regulates NOSII expression. The airway of atopic asthmatics also has increased amounts of L-arginine, which also provides additional fuel for NO production.[28] Corticosteroids directly inhibits NOII expression at the level gene transcription.[29,30] Thus a decrease in eNO during corticosteroid treatment reflects either a decrease in tissue cytokines, inhibition of NO *per se*, or a combination of both.

Frank *et al.*[31] compared eNO in children with atopic asthma, non-atopic asthma, atopic normals and non-atopic normals. Although children with physician-diagnosed asthma had an increased eNO (8.3 p.p.b.) compared with non-asthmatic controls (3.4 p.p.b.), atopy was a major confounder. Thus eNO levels of non-atopic asthmatics (who also have eosinophilic pulmonary inflam- mation and C–C chemokine activation) were no different from non-atopic healthy controls (Figure 6d.5). Similarly in adult asthmatics, eNO correlates with the number of positive skin-prick tests, but not with functional markers of airway pathology.[32] In atopic children, one study reported raised eNO in recent wheezers and those with BHR.[32a] If high levels of eNO cannot always distinguish asthmatics

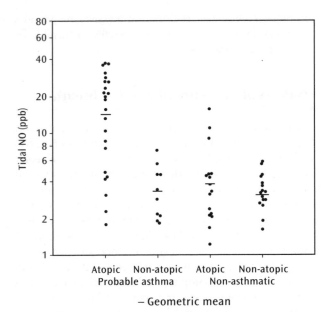

Figure 6d.5 *Scatter plot of tidal nitric oxide in children with physician-diagnosed asthma and normal controls. There is a wide overlap in eNO values between atopic asthmatics and atopic controls. Non-atopic asthmatics have eNO levels in the normal range. (From ref. 31 with permission.)*

Table 6d.2 *Correlation between markers of eosinophil activation in the serum and urine in 28 children with atopic asthma (modified from ref. 40)*

	Serum EPX	**Urine EPX**
Serum		
ECP	$r = 0.798$	$r = 0.510$
	$p < 0.001$	$p < 0.04$
EPX	–	$r = 0.596$
		$p < 0.01$

r = Spearman's rank correlation.

Inflammatory markers in the blood and urine

EOSINOPHIL MARKERS

ECP and EPX can be measured in blood samples. The half-life of ECP in the circulation is 45 minutes and the levels in blood collected into EDTA (which inactivates eosinophils) are very low. In contrast, the serum from a blood sample that has been allowed to clot in a tube without additives contains detectable levels of ECP and EPX. The serum level therefore reflects the propensity of eosinophils to release granule proteins, rather than the blood level *in vivo*. EPX (but not ECP) is excreted unchanged in the urine,[39] and there is a moderately good correlation between serum EPX and urinary EPX corrected for creatinine[40] (Table 6d.2). In asthma, increased release of cationic proteins by serum eosinophils is thought to be due to priming by pro-inflammatory mediators released from the abnormal lung. Priming of systemic eosinophils to release granule proteins not only occurs with asthma, but with many other conditions such as asymptomatic atopy, hay fever, and eczema.[41] The resulting wide overlap in serum ECP values between asthmatic and non-asthmatic children due to the confounding effect of atopy and atopic disease excludes its use as a diagnostic test for asthma. However when limited to asthmatics, there is a good relationship between airway eosinophil percentage and serum ECP,[42,43] and bronchial tissue EG2 positivity and serum ECP.[44] This relationship in asthmatics should mean that serum ECP, like sputum eosinophils,[24] should provide predictive data on risk of relapse/exacerbation. Indeed, in adults with stable well controlled asthma, an increased risk of mild exacerbation over 12 months is associated with a 'baseline' blood ECP of >20 mg/mL (relative risk 2.5).[45] However, not all children with elevated percentage of airway eosinophils have elevated levels of serum ECP,[46] and the ability of serum ECP to predict relapse/exacerbation in paediatric asthma remains unclear. In the future it may be possible to improve predictive accuracy for tissue eosinophilia by combining ECP and an independent marker such as eNO.

Serum ECP/EPX may help to identify those children with preschool wheeze who will eventually become

defined by symptoms, can it identify those patients reporting minimal symptoms but with significant eosinophilic tissue inflammation? Lim *et al.*[33] did bronchial biopsy and measured eNO in a range of adult atopic asthmatics (some of whom were receiving inhaled steroids), but found no correlation between the number of tissue eosinophils and eNO. In contrast, Piacentini and colleagues[34] found a reasonable correlation between sputum eosinophilia and eNO in steroid-naive asthmatic children, but not in a steroid treated subgroup. eNO is therefore not a specific test for asthma and is not an accurate way of assessing tissue inflammation during steroid therapy. However, high eNO levels may be useful as a *positive* test for tissue eosinophil inflammation, since in the study of Piacentini *et al.*[34] five out of six steroid-naive asthmatic children with eNO >20 parts per billion (p.p.b.) had sputum eosinophils outside the normal range ($>20\%$). At the other end of the spectrum, very low levels of eNO are a hallmark of primary ciliary dyskinesia, and can be used as a screening test for this condition.[35]

Markers of inflammation can also be detected in breath condensate, obtained by passing exhaled air though a glass tube cooled to 0°C.[3] These include hydrogen peroxide,[36] leukotrienes,[37] and markers of oxidative damage.[38] There is no current data on the clinical applicability of breath condensate analysis, but it offers an opportunity to describe patterns of many types of markers originating directly from the lower airway; an approach that could overcome the problems of specificity and sensitivity associated with single marker analysis.

asthmatic. The prevailing paradigm is that 'transient' preschool wheeze (defined post hoc) is not a result of atopic pulmonary inflammation, but is the response of a structurally vulnerable lung to viral colds (see Chapters 3 and 9). By contrast, preschool children with wheeze who will become asthmatics ('persistent' wheezers), may have airway cells that are already primed to release broncho-constricting mediators to a variety of environmental agents, including viral colds. Currently paediatricians are unable to identify these phenotypes using normal history and examination. However, Koller and co-workers[47] found that young infants presenting with wheeze (7–9 months of age), and a serum ECP level of greater than 20 mg/L, were more likely to develop more than three wheezing attacks in the following 12 months (odds ratio 12.4). Whether this predictive ability of ECP reflects ongoing pulmonary eosinophilic inflammation, or a genetic predisposition of systemic eosinophils to release ECP remains unclear.

LEUKOTRIENES

Leukotriene (LT) C_4 is a potent bronchoconstrictor. It is the major metabolite of arachidonic acid released in the pulmonary milieu. LTC_4 is rapidly converted into LTD_4, which in turn is converted to LTE_4, which is excreted unchanged in the urine. In the past laborious, pre-processing of the urine sample by high performance liquid chromatography was required to measure LTE_4, but pre-processing has recently been found to be no longer necessary.[48] The evidence of a relationship between urinary and pulmonary LT levels in asthma has not been directly determined. Urinary LTE_4 is increased in asthma,[49] and increases after allergen-challenge,[50] indirectly suggesting that LTs generated within the lung, do spill over into the urine.

Selective cysteinyl LT blocking therapy is now available, but can urinary LT levels provide predictive information on clinical response? In adult asthmatics, clinical response to LT blocker therapy was not associated with greater pre-treatment urinary LTE_4,[51] but responders had a lower ratio of LTE_4 to prostaglandin F_{1a} (0.32 ± 0.04 vs 0.78 ± 0.1). Currently, there are no similar data in children with asthma or with preschool wheeze. In one study, no difference was found in urinary LTE_4 between children with mild (steroid-naive) asthma and severe asthma,[49] but is unclear whether the severe group had evidence of eosinophil activation. In summary, LTs are the only mediator of asthmatic symptoms for which a specific blocking therapy is available. Urinary LT measurements could indicate in which children corticosteroids and LT blockade would be synergistic, but no clear data is available to date.

RELATIONSHIP OF INFLAMMATORY MARKERS TO PHYSIOLOGICAL MARKERS

There is no correlation between serum ECP and other functional measures of asthma such as bronchial responsiveness to histamine and cold air.[52] Similarly the relationship between sputum ECP with PC_{20} is very weak in adults with mild to severe asthma.[44] These finding are hardly surprising since physiological measurements in asthma have problems of their own for diagnosis and outcome prediction. The assessment of inflammation has however, provided new insights into what drives the physiological markers. For example, symptom free adults with airway hyperresponsiveness (AHR) to methacholine have increased levels of bronchial EG1 and EG2 positivity compared with healthy subjects with no AHR.[53] At the clinical level, inflammatory markers may provide different and synergistic information on the state of the asthmatic lung than physiological variables, but the clinical niches best suited to the combined use of mediator and physiological remain to be explored.

FUTURE DEVELOPMENTS

Information on thousands of potential mediators can now be derived from small volumes of biological fluids and tissues using proteomic and gene microarray technology. *Proteomics* allows the efficient analysis of thousands of proteins at a time, subsequent sequencing of femtomole quantities of proteins, and can be applied to the analysis of human sera,[54] urine and BALF. Making use of two-dimensional gel electrophoresis, high-throughput robotics and sophisticated image analysis the whole set of proteins of a body fluid can be separated, stained, single proteins identified on the image and punched out from the gel. The gels can identify not only up- and down-regulations of proteins, but changes in posttranslational modifications as well (Figure 6d.6). Peptides characteristic for the proteins can be eluted from the gel and sequenced by modern electrospray mass spectrometry, which allows detailed structural analysis of the amino acid backbone and posttranslational modifications (e.g. phosphorylation and glycosylation). The expectation is that form of inflammatory protein profiling will overcome the limitations of single mediator analysis.

There have been few attempts to extract clinically useful information from clinical and mediator variables using the *multivariate statistical techniques* that will be necessary for analysis of data from proteomic and genomic technology. An example of this statistical approach is provided by Clough et al.,[55] who studied 3 to 36-month-old children ($n = 107$) within 12 weeks of first wheeze. A range of variables were determined including parental IgE, serum soluble IL-2 receptor (sIL-2R), and proliferation and release of interferon gamma by the child's peripheral blood mononuclear cells. After testing several models, the one offering the best prediction of persistent wheeze with least risk of including asymptomatic subjects was: age at presentation + sIL-2R (56% sensitivity, 84% specificity, 76% positive predictive value, and 68% negative predictive value).

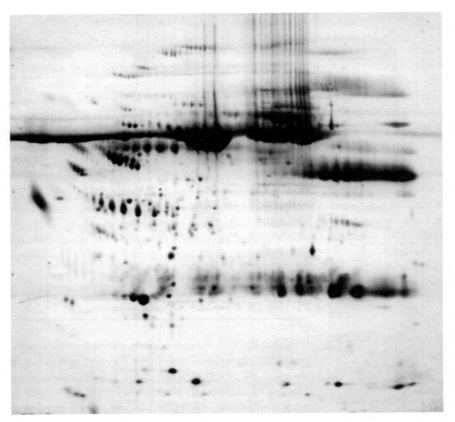

Figure 6d.6 *Serum proteome of a healthy 4-year-old child (with permission Dr H Hebestreit, Oxford Glycobiology Institute). 150 μl of serum were applied to an IPG strip in sample buffer. Isoelectric focusing was carried out using 70 000 Vh. The IPG strip was then transferred onto a 9–16% PAGE gradient gel, and SDS–PAGE performed under standard conditions. The gel was stained with a fluorescent dye and scanned into software for protein identification. Individual proteins appear as single dots with high molecular weight proteins appearing at the bottom of the gel.*

CONCLUSIONS

New methods for assessing lung inflammation in asthmatics have been developed over the last two decades. Nearly all have a predictable course: (i) a 'novelty' period where data derived from a small number of patients promises to increase understanding of the pathology of wheezing and identify children with asthma; (ii) a 'consolidation' period when data is generated by many researchers; and (iii) disillusionment, when the marker is found to add little to clinical management. The factors contributing to this cycle are that the relationship between an inflammatory mediator/cell in the lung and its marker is poorly defined at the outset, the independent effect of atopy is ignored, and a definitive diagnosis of asthma is expected from a single measurement of an inflammatory marker in dynamic process where inflammation waxes and wanes. Clinicians need to first ask whether inflammatory markers truly reflect inflammation in lung tissue that is specific to clinical picture of asthma (validation), and then consider if the valid marker provides information that changes clinical practice. Recent advances in induced sputum analysis offer the best combination of sensitivity, ease of use, and clinical applicability, at least for the older child. For the young child, indirect assessment of pulmonary inflammation, with its associated loss of accuracy, is the only practical and ethical option. For direct and indirect markers of inflammation, crossover to the clinical sphere will only occur when measurements add to the information gathered in normal clinical practice. As yet, this has not proved to be the case.

REFERENCES

1. Tai PC, Spry CJ, Peterson C, Venge P, Olsson I. Monoclonal antibodies distinguish between storage and secreted forms of eosinophil cationic protein. *Nature* 1984;**309**:182–4.
2. Silverman M, Pedersen S, Grigg J. Measurement of airway inflammation in young children. *Am J Respir Crit Care Med* 2000;**162**:1–57.
3. Gibson PG, Henry RL, Thomas P. Noninvasive assessment of airway inflammation in children: induced sputum, exhaled nitric oxide, and breath condensate. *Eur Respir J* 2000;**16**:1008–15.
4. Ying S, Durham SR, Corrigan CJ, Hamid Q, Kay AB. Phenotype of cells expressing mRNA for TH2-type (interleukin 4 and interleukin 5) and TH1-type (interleukin 2 and interferon gamma) cytokines in bronchoalveolar lavage and bronchial biopsies from atopic asthmatic and normal control subjects. *Am J Respir Cell Mol Biol* 1995;**12**:477–87.
5. Walsh GM, Hartnell A, Wardlaw AJ, Kurihara K, Sanderson CJ, Kay AB. IL-5 enhances the *in vitro* adhesion of human eosinophils, but not neutrophils,

in a leucocyte integrin (CD11/18)-dependent manner. *Immunology* 1990;**71**:258–65.

6. Venge P, Bystrom J, Carlson M, *et al.* Eosinophil cationic protein (ECP): molecular and biological properties and the use of ECP as a marker of eosinophil activation in disease. *Clin Exp Allergy* 1999;**29**:1172–86.

7. Ying S, Meng Q, Zeibecoglou K, *et al.* Eosinophil chemotactic chemokines (eotaxin, eotaxin-2, RANTES, monocyte chemoattractant protein-3 (MCP-3, and MCP-4), and C–C chemokine receptor 3 expression in bronchial biopsies from atopic and non-atopic (Intrinsic) asthmatics. *J Immunol* 1999;**163**:6321–9.

8. Sallusto F, Lanzavecchia A, Mackay CR. Chemokines and chemokine receptors in T-cell priming and Th1/Th2-mediated responses. *Immunol Today* 1998;**19**:568–74.

9. Vignola AM, Chanez P, Campbell AM, *et al.* Airway inflammation in mild intermittent and in persistent asthma. *Am J Respir Crit Care Med* 1998;**157**:403–9.

10. Payne D, McKenzie SA, Stacey S, Misra D, Haxby E, Bush A. Safety and ethics of bronchoscopy and endobronchial biopsy in difficult asthma. *Arch Dis Child* 2001;**84**:423–6.

11. Cokugras H, Akcakaya N, Seckin D, Camcioglu Y, Sarimurat N, Aksoy F. Ultrastructural examination of bronchial biopsy specimens from children with moderate asthma. *Thorax* 2001;**56**:25–9.

12. Gibson PG, Saltos N, Borgas T. Airway mast cells and eosinophils correlate with clinical severity and airway hyperresponsiveness in corticosteroid-treated asthma. *J Allergy Clin Immunol* 2000;**105**:752–9.

13. Martinez FD. Context dependency of markers of disease. *Am J Respir Crit Care Med* 2000;**162**: S56–7.

14. Brown JR, Kleimberg J, Marini M, Sun G, Bellini A, Mattoli S. Kinetics of eotaxin expression and its relationship to eosinophil accumulation and activation in bronchial biopsies and bronchoalveolar lavage (BAL) of asthmatic patients after allergen inhalation. *Clin Exp Immunol* 1998;**114**:137–46.

15. Grigg J, Riedler J, Robertson CF, Boyle W, Uren S. Alveolar macrophage immaturity in infants and young children. *Eur Respir J* 1999;**14**:1198–205.

16. Riedler J, Grigg J, Stone C, Tauro G, Robertson CF. Bronchoalveolar lavage cellularity in healthy children. *Am J Respir Crit Care Med* 1995;**152**:163–8.

17. Stevenson EC, Turner G, Heaney LG, *et al.* Bronchoalveolar lavage findings suggest two different forms of childhood asthma. *Clin Exp Allergy* 1997;**27**:1027–35.

18. Ennis M, Turner G, Schock BC, *et al.* Inflammatory mediators in bronchoalveolar lavage samples from children with and without asthma. *Clin Exp Allergy* 1999;**29**:362–6.

19. McGarvey LP, Forsythe P, Heaney LG, MacMahon J, Ennis M. Bronchoalveolar lavage findings in patients with chronic nonproductive cough. *Eur Respir J* 1999;**13**:59–65.

20. Wilson NM, Bridge P, Spanevello A, Silverman M. Induced sputum in children: feasibility, repeatability, and relation of findings to asthma severity. *Thorax* 2000;**55**:768–74.

21. Fahy JV, Boushey HA, Lazarus SC, *et al.* Safety and reproducibility of sputum induction in asthmatic subjects in a multicenter study. *Am J Respir Crit Care Med* 2001;**163**:1470–5.

22. Grootendorst DC, Sont JK, Willems LN, *et al.* Comparison of inflammatory cell counts in asthma: induced sputum vs bronchoalveolar lavage and bronchial biopsies. *Clin Exp Allergy* 1997;**27**:769–79.

23. Louis R, Lau LC, Bron AO, Roldaan AC, Radermecker M, Djukanovic R. The relationship between airways inflammation and asthma severity. *Am J Respir Crit Care Med* 2000;**161**:9–16.

24. Jatakanon A, Lim S, Barnes PJ. Changes in sputum eosinophils predict loss of asthma control. *Am J Respir Crit Care Med* 2000;**161**:64–72.

25. Norzila MZ, Fakes K, Henry RL, Simpson J, Gibson PG. Interleukin-8 secretion and neutrophil recruitment accompanies induced sputum eosinophil activation in children with acute asthma. *Am J Respir Crit Care Med* 2000;**161**:769–74.

25a. Green RH, Brightling CE, *et al.* Reduced asthma exacerbations with management strategy directed at normalising the sputum eosinophil count. *Am J Resp Crit Care Med* 2002;**165**(8):A320.

26. de Jongste JC, Alving K. Gas analysis. *Am J Respir Crit Care Med* 2000;**162**:S23–7.

27. Jobsis Q, Raatgeep HC, Hop WC, de Jongste JC. Controlled low flow off line sampling of exhaled nitric oxide in children. *Thorax* 2001;**56**:285–9.

28. Guo FH, Comhair SA, Zheng S, *et al.* Molecular mechanisms of increased nitric oxide (NO) in asthma: evidence for transcriptional and post-translational regulation of NO synthesis. *J Immunol* 2000;**164**:5970–80.

29. Radomski MW, Palmer RM, Moncada S. Glucocorticoids inhibit the expression of an inducible, but not the constitutive, nitric oxide synthase in vascular endothelial cells. *Proc Natl Acad Sci USA* 1990;**87**:10043–7.

30. Di Rosa M, Radomski M, Carnuccio R, Moncada S. Glucocorticoids inhibit the induction of nitric oxide synthase in macrophages. *Biochem Biophys Res Commun* 1990;**172**:1246–52.

31. Frank TL, Adisesh A, Pickering AC, *et al.* Relationship between exhaled nitric oxide and childhood asthma. *Am J Respir Crit Care Med* 1998;**158**:1032–6.

32. Ho LP, Wood FT, Robson A, Innes JA, Greening AP. Atopy influences exhaled nitric oxide levels in adult asthmatics. *Chest* 2000;**118**:1327–31.

32a. Leuppi JD, Downs SH, Dounie SR, Marks GB, Salome CM. Exhaled nitric oxide levels in atopic children: relation to specific sensitisation, AHR and symptoms. *Thorax* 2002;**57**:518–23.

33. Lim S, Jatakanon A, Meah S, Oates T, Chung KF, Barnes PJ. Relationship between exhaled nitric oxide and mucosal eosinophilic inflammation in mild to moderately severe asthma. *Thorax* 2000;**55**:184–8.

34. Piacentini GL, Bodini A, Costella S, *et al*. Exhaled nitric oxide, serum ECP and airway responsiveness in mild asthmatic children. *Eur Respir J* 2000;**15**:839–43.

35. Karadag B, James AJ, Gultekin E, Wilson NM, Bush A. Nasal and lower airway level of nitric oxide in children with primary ciliary dyskinesia. *Eur Respir J* 1999;**13**:1402–5.

36. Jobsis Q, Raatgeep HC, Schellekens SL, Kroesbergen A, Hop WC, de Jongste JC. Hydrogen peroxide and nitric oxide in exhaled air of children with cystic fibrosis during antibiotic treatment. *Eur Respir J* 2000;**16**:95–100.

37. Reinhold P, Becher G, Rothe M. Evaluation of the measurement of leukotriene B4 concentrations in exhaled condensate as a noninvasive method for assessing mediators of inflammation in the lungs of calves. *Am J Vet Res* 2000;**61**:742–9.

38. Nowak D, Kalucka S, Bialasiewicz P, Krol M. Exhalation of H_2O_2 and thiobarbituric acid reactive substances (TBARs) by healthy subjects. *Free Radic Biol Med* 2001;**30**:178–86.

39. Cottin V, Deviller P, Tardy F, Cordier JF. Urinary eosinophil-derived neurotoxin/protein X: a simple method for assessing eosinophil degranulation *in vivo*. *J Allergy Clin Immunol* 1998;**101**:116–23.

40. Koller DY, Halmerbauer G, Frischer T, Roithner B. Assessment of eosinophil granule proteins in various body fluids: is there a relation to clinical variables in childhood asthma? *Clin Exp Allergy* 1999;**29**:786–93.

41. Remes S, Korppi M, Remes K, Savolainen K, Mononen I, Pekkanen J. Serum eosinophil cationic protein (ECP) and eosinophil protein X (EPX) in childhood asthma: the influence of atopy. *Pediatr Pulmonol* 1998;**25**:167–74.

42. Ronchi MC, Piragino C, Rosi E, *et al*. Do sputum eosinophils and ECP relate to the severity of asthma? *Eur Respir J* 1997;**10**:1809–13.

43. Reimert CM, Ouma JH, Mwanje MT, *et al*. Indirect assessment of eosinophiluria in urinary schistosomiasis using eosinophil cationic protein (ECP) and eosinophil protein X (EPX). *Acta Trop* 1993;**54**:1–12.

44. Hoshino M, Nakamura Y. Relationship between activated eosinophils of the bronchial mucosa and serum eosinophil cationic protein in atopic asthma. *Int Arch Allergy Immunol* 1997;**112**:59–64.

45. Belda J, Giner J, Casan P, Md JS. Mild exacerbations and eosinophilic inflammation in patients with stable, well-controlled asthma after 1 year of follow-up. *Chest* 2001;**119**:1011–17.

46. Shields MD, Brown V, Stevenson EC, *et al*. Serum eosinophilic cationic protein and blood eosinophil counts for the prediction of the presence of airways inflammation in children with wheezing. *Clin Exp Allergy* 1999;**29**:1382–9.

47. Koller DY, Wojnarowski C, Herkner KR, *et al*. High levels of eosinophil cationic protein in wheezing infants predict the development of asthma. *J Allergy Clin Immunol* 1997;**99**:752–6.

48. Kumlin M. Analytical methods for the measurement of leukotrienes and other eicosanoids in biological samples from asthmatic subjects. *J Chromatogr A* 1996;**725**:29–40.

49. Severien C, Artlich A, Jonas S, Becher G. Urinary excretion of leukotriene E4 and eosinophil protein X in children with atopic asthma. *Eur Respir J* 2000;**16**:588–92.

50. Reiss TF, Hill JB, Harman E, *et al*. Increased urinary excretion of LTE_4 after exercise and attenuation of exercise-induced bronchospasm by montelukast, a cysteinyl leukotriene receptor antagonist. *Thorax* 1997;**52**:1030–5.

51. Tanaka H, Igarashi T, Saitoh T, *et al*. Can urinary eicosanoids be a potential predictive marker of clinical response to thromboxane A2 receptor antagonist in asthmatic patients? *Respir Med* 1999;**93**:891–7.

52. Gruber W, Eber E, Pfleger A, *et al*. Serum eosinophil cationic protein and bronchial responsiveness in pediatric and adolescent asthma patients. *Chest* 1999;**116**:301–5.

53. Laprise C, Laviolette M, Boutet M, Boulet LP. Asymptomatic airway hyperresponsiveness: relationships with airway inflammation and remodelling. *Eur Respir J* 1999;**14**:63–73.

54. Grigg J, McKean MC, Silverman M, *et al*. Downregulation of serum proteins during experimental coronavirus colds identified by proteome analysis. *Eur Respir J* 1999;**14**(Suppl 30):398S(abstract).

55. Clough JB, Keeping KA, Edwards LC, Freeman WM, Warner JA, Warner JO. Can we predict which wheezy infants will continue to wheeze? *Am J Respir Crit Care Med* 1999;**160**:1473–80.

56. Renauld J-C. New insights into the role of cytokines in asthma. *J Clin Pathol* 2001;**54**:577–89.

Impact of asthma on child and family

LIESL M OSMAN

INTRODUCTION

Asthma is the most common chronic illness of children.[1,2] In the 1995 ISAAC study, of 79 000 UK school-children aged 12–14 years, 33% reported some wheeze in the past 12 months, 20% reported having been ever diagnosed with asthma, 20% reported using asthma medication the past 12 months and 10% reported four or more asthma attacks.[3]

There is a high incidence of morbidity and poor control among children with diagnosed asthma. This means a significant number of children and their families must manage an illness whose course is difficult to predict, which can be life threatening, and is treated by medication which arouses fears of side effects, and of 'becoming addicted'.

Impact of asthma

Asthma impacts on children and families as a result of asthma symptoms, the need to manage medication to control symptoms, and child and family self-identification as having asthma. There are immediate health status and quality of life consequences of these factors; there may be long-term effects on psychological functioning of the child and family. In order to assess benefits of treatment for patients we need to be able to assess these psychological and quality of life outcomes as well as changes in purely clinical parameters such as lung function.

Patterns of asthma

A characteristic of asthma and wheezing illness is that for many children it is an intermittent condition with periods of high morbidity interspersed with periods of normal or near normal function.[4] In the long-term there can be partial or complete remisson[5–7] (Figure 6e.1).

Only 5% of children had continuing, persistent asthma to age 33 years. About 35% who had asthma at some stage had complete remission. Thus, asthma is unlike other chronic childhood illness such as diabetes or cystic fibrosis. Management by regular medication may cease to be necessary as children grow older and symptoms

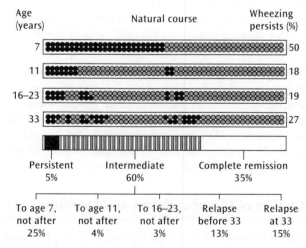

Figure 6e.1 *Prognosis for children who developed asthma or wheezy bronchitis by age 7. Each symbol represents 1% of such children, and the natural course of each 1% subsample can be traced vertically. Filled circles represent subjects reporting asthma or wheezy bronchitis in the previous year at ages 7 and 11, those reporting asthma or wheezy bronchitis since their 16th birthday at age 23, and those reporting wheezing in the previous year at age 33. (From ref. 5.)*

may remit, either partially or completely. It may be because of this that long-term studies have found weak or little effect of asthma on ultimate scholastic achievement, employment and social class.[8,9] This contrasts with the finding that obesity in late adolescence is significantly negatively related to social class 12 years later, controlling for parental social class, IQ and education.[11]

In the short term, however, asthma is likely to have significant impact on child and family quality of life. In measurement of symptom impact we are usually looking at short time spans of the last 4 weeks to the last 12 months. Broader measures of psychological factors such as child self-esteem or family functioning may not have a definite time span, but will be focused on a medium-term life stage of the child or family. We want to measure these short and medium-term outcomes in order to assess whether clinical improvement translates into quality of life improvement.

ASSESSING ASTHMA IMPACT ON THE CHILD AND FAMILY

There are three broad areas of impact of asthma:

1 *Quality of life impact*: assessing the effect of morbidity on everyday activities and social relationships and the degree of distress associated with symptoms and their management.
2 *Psychological impact*: assessing psychological status, for instance, child and/or parent anxiety and depression, presence of behaviour problems, child self-esteem.
3 *Family process impact*: assessing styles of normal family functioning and management of problems (for instance rigidity vs openness), specific illness management styles.

Quality of life assessment is increasingly used to assess immediate benefits of therapeutic intervention. Psychological assessment, and family process measurement, is most commonly explored in order to increase our understanding of factors which underlie good or poor self-management, and to help us in designing effective behavioural and information interventions.

Quality of life of children and families

It is well known that clinical measures of lung function have only weak relationships to symptom severity or to psychological and social impact of asthma.[12,13] As well, because asthma is episodic, as discussed above, clinical measurements, when a child is between episodes, may be normal or near normal. For very young children, physiological measurements can be difficult and often not pragmatic for routine care. For all these reasons, in order to effectively assess benefit of interventions, quality of life and health status measures are increasingly used.[14] It has

been shown that family and caregiver quality of fluctuate as symptoms vary in preschool children.[15]

Quality of life questionnaires (also described as health status questionnaires and health related quality of life questionnaires) can be generic or asthma specific. Generic scales look at impact of health status on physical, social and emotional functioning, without limiting health impact to respiratory symptoms. Asthma specific scales evaluate impact of respiratory symptoms.

Generic quality of life scales for children and families include the Child Health Questionnaire,[16] Adolescent Child Health and Illness Profile CHIP-AE[17] and the Functional Status Scale: FSIIR.[18] Asthma specific quality of life scales include the Paediatric Asthma Quality of Life Questionnaire,[19] the Paediatric Asthma Caregivers Quality of Life Questionnaire,[20] the HAY questionnaire[21] and the Quality of Life of Parents of Asthmatic Children (QOL–PAC).[22]

Psychological impact

Quality of life differences are only one aspect of impact of asthma. Children with asthma might show particular psychological characteristics, such as lower self-esteem, behavioural problems, or have difficulties in social relationships (Chapter 13c). Studies which suggest that this is so include Mullins,[23] where higher asthma uncertainty in adolescents was related to poorer psychological adjustment and Graetz[24] who found no differences overall between children with asthma and controls, but children with frequent hospitalization felt more lonely and were less preferred as playmates. Forero[25] found, among 4000 Australian adolescents, that the 18% with asthma more often reported feeling lonely. (These results are similar to those for teenagers with diabetes, who report more social isolation than a group of healthy controls.[26])

Silverglade[27] compared three groups of asthmatic adolescents ($N = 129$) classified on the basis of severity of illness with a fourth group of 74 healthy, non-asthmatic adolescents. Adolescents with mild asthma closely resembled the physically healthy comparison group; adolescents with moderate and severe asthma had irrational beliefs in the importance of approval and higher self-reported anxiety, depression, or hostility.

Bussing et al.[28] found that compared with a non-asthmatic control group, the children with asthma had significantly more anxiety disorders. Another study by Bussing[29] compared the frequency of current behaviour problems in 184 children with mild to moderate asthma, 41 children with severe asthma and 6927 children with no chronic conditions. Behaviour problems were assessed with the Behaviour Problem Index (BPI), an index developed by Zill[30] from Achenbach's Child Behaviour Check List (CBCL).[31–33] Bussing found that both the moderate and severe asthma group missed significantly more school days than the children with no chronic conditions, but only the 18% of children classified as having severe asthma had higher frequency of current behavioural problems.

Perrin et al.[34] conducted a controlled trial of a combined education and stress management program among children ages 6–14 years with asthma. Psychological status was assessed by the Child Behavior Checklist (CBCL) before and after the intervention. Children in the intervention group had a significant improvement in the total Behavior Problems Score ($p < 0.04$) and Internalizing Scale ($p < 0.01$) on the CBCL.

Not all studies have found psychological differences between children with and without asthma. Wjst et al.[35] surveyed parents of 2634 German children with a mean age of 10 years. Asthmatic children slept significantly less well than non-asthmatic children, but there were no significant differences in parent ratings of sociability (68% children with asthma vs 68% of children without asthma), playing with others (46% vs 42%), being 'always active' (54% vs 56%) and being 'mostly happy' (70% vs 74%).

Nassau et al.[36] found that 19 children (aged 8–10) with asthma, did not differ from matched children with diabetes ($N = 25$) or no chronic condition ($N = 24$) in social adjustment, social performance or social skills, on child, parent and teacher rating scales. Vazquez et al.[37] compared 48 children (8–13 years) with asthma (mild to moderate) with 41 children without asthma, using Harter's Self Perception Profile,[38,39] intended to measure self-esteem. He found no difference between children with asthma and control children in scholastic competence, social acceptance, athletic competence, physical appearance or global self-worth.

Austin et al.[40] found that 111 adolescents with asthma scored significantly better on Achenbach's Child Behaviour Check List than 117 adolescents with epilepsy, active and inactive. Asthma severity was not related to worse behavioural problems scores.

As part of the process of developing the Juniper Child Quality of Life and Caregiver Quality of Life, Townsend et al.[41] investigated perception among 100 patients and children of what were the major areas of burden from asthma for children and parents. Townsend concluded that children with moderate asthma perceived themselves as having some limitation in the level of activity they could perform, but not the type of activity. On the whole, bother from symptoms was greater than emotional distress caused by symptoms. Townsend concluded that although the children in the study found their respiratory symptoms troublesome, asthma did not cause major disruption in their lives.

Twenty years ago Staudenmayer[42] studied 175 children with asthma, taken from hospitalized inpatients, outpatients, and private practice. He identified five psychosocial factors among these groups. Three of these were: 'despair over social debilitation', 'quality of life' and 'dread of illness'. Two further factors identified were 'orientation towards compliance' and 'family communication' (in reality, mother child communication, which measured the child's level of communication about asthma with his or her mother). The incidence of high anxiety scores and low compliance scores was greatest among the inpatient (most severe) group and least in the private practice (mildest) group. However, Staudenmayer followed up his groups for 6 months and found that anxiety declined in the admitted group after hospital treatment and discharge. He concluded that the anxiety measured during admission was in part the consequence of a history of poor control resulting from poor medical manageability. As control improved anxiety decreased, and hence anxiety did not cause, but was a consequence of poorly controlled asthma.

These studies suggest that adverse behavioural and quality of life impact of asthma may be related to failure to control attacks, and high use of medication, and that psychological and social impairment is only found among a minority of children with severe and poorly controlled asthma. The best validated measures of psychological problems are behavioural, such as Achenbach's CBCL[31] or Zill's PBI,[30] a shortened form of the CBCL.

Family process impact

Until recently, most of the measures of the impact of asthma on the child, described above, have been based on parent report. Measures of child quality of life by parent report may as much reflect parental response to the child's asthma as actual child effect. Studies show that respiratory symptoms, such as persistent cough, are particularly worrying for parents.[41,43–45] Hopton[46] identified that parents' fear about child symptoms was often linked to past situations when their child had been diagnosed by doctors to be more seriously ill than they had thought. This 'fright' reduced parents' confidence in their own ability to judge the state of their child's health.

A number of studies have directly assessed parents' attitudes and the effect of asthma on family functioning. Donnelly et al.[47] found that among 100 parents of children with asthma who had been admitted to hospital, 64% of asthma parents believed that 'parents can't cope as well (with asthma) as they wish'. Among Donnelly's parents, 96% said they gave their child all their medications as prescribed, and 89% that the advantages of medication outweighed the disadvantages, but 86% also said that children shouldn't be given medication for long periods of time, 31% said children's bodies are too small to cope with medication, 71% said they changed the time for medication if the schedule was inconvenient, 60% said they sometimes forgot to give medication to their child, and 16% said they sometimes dispensed more medication than was prescribed.

Using a newly designed questionnaire to assess the 'bother' caused by asthma on children and families, Townsend et al.[41] studied 100 children with asthma and their families. Items with highest bother scores for parents were concern about long-term effects of drugs, side effects, feeling helpless when child had attack. Parents expressed highest bother on emotional impact of the child's asthma, and lower bother on items to do with impact on family day-to-day activity. That is, parents were more worried about the possibility of disruption than disturbed by actual disruption. 'Emotional items scored higher than did interference with daily activity', 'the inability of a parent to relieve the annoying symptoms of their child's asthma appears to be part of this burden'. The children however appeared to generally feel less emotional burden than their parents – most bother was caused by specific asthma symptoms, with the exception of 'feeling frightened by asthma attack'. Children were asked what they most wished they could do, which their asthma interfered with. Townsend noted that wishes were focused on doing better in activities they already did, such as swimming or running faster.

We see that parental concerns frequently revolve around the difficulties of making decisions about seriousness of symptoms and managing unexpected illness events. Parents are also concerned about giving regular medication to children. In the previous section we saw that some studies suggest that some children with asthma may have a higher than average incidence of behavioural problems. All of these factors will form a web of interactive influences on overall attitudes and asthma management in the family.

Gustafsson et al.[48,49] followed 100 families with children with a history of allergy, from birth to 18 months. At 3 months Gustafsson classified families (from videotaped interviews) on their own ability to adapt to demands of a situation (adaptability) and balance between emotional closeness and distance (cohesion). About one third of families had poor functioning at 3 months. Children were classified at 18 months as healthy, or having recurrent wheezing, chest infections or eczema. Family dysfunction at 3 months did not predict the later occurrence of wheezing illness in the child, but if the child acquired anxiety provoking symptoms, families were more likely to continue or begin dysfunctional interaction patterns.

Gustaffson concluded that the occurrence of wheezing symptoms increases the chance of family dysfunction. Comparing Gustaffson's findings with those of Staudenmayer, we can conclude that the presence of wheezing symptoms and attacks in children is a stress on families and the stress is exacerbated if symptoms are not brought under control. Studies in other illnesses, such as child cancer, have found similar family consequences.[50]

Perhaps surprisingly, we can conclude there is little evidence that for most children with asthma, the disease has much impact on family processes. Symptoms may limit a child's activities, but children often appear to accommodate to their symptoms, and do not feel much emotional bother from symptoms. Most families have some concerns about asthma medication, and about the need for regular medication, but they do not see their children as much different from children without asthma. However, the situation alters when symptoms frighten the child or its parents, and if at the same time parents do not have confidence that they know how to fully control the symptoms. In this case, a vicious circle may be entered, where sub-optimal family functioning results from the stress of being unable to control illness events, but this in turn increases the likelihood of poor family management of the illness.

FAMILY MANAGEMENT STYLES

Meijer[51,52] compared 20 families with a child with 'controlled' asthma to 20 families with a child with 'uncontrolled' asthma. He found that families with 'controlled' asthma were more cohesive and more structured than families with a child with 'uncontrolled' asthma. Families with a structured style of management had more rules of behaviour, and were more likely to emphasize the importance of compliance. Meijer concluded that a distinction between controlled and uncontrolled asthma is more strongly related to psychosomatic variables than a distinction on the basis of the severity of the asthma.

Studies have attempted to classify family asthma management styles. Wilson et al.[53] interviewed 117 physicians and 112 parents and identified 130 ineffective and effective asthma management behaviours falling into five areas of responsibility: symptom intervention, symptom prevention, use of medical and educational resources, communication among caregivers, and family relationships. However, Wilson did not demonstrate prospectively that behaviours rated as ineffective were related to worse observed clinical outcomes.

Taylor et al.[54] developed a set of 'management scenarios' from which children and caregivers could be scored on their self-management competency. They report that 'patients selected by physicians to be good or bad managers produced high or low scores respectively on the scenarios', but do not give further details of the relationship between scores and clinical outcomes.

More recently Zimmerman et al.[55] carried out a study among 102 predominantly Latino families. Children had a median age of 7 years, with one third below 5 years. Families were classified by their 'asthma self-regulation phase' and rankings were related to measures of asthma severity. Asthma self-regulation stage was assessed by answers to 11 structured questions (Table 6e.1). Higher (better) self-regulation phases were significantly associated with lower morbidity in days wheezing and sleep disturbance and home restrictions in the past month and emergency department visits in the past year. English speaking families were likely to be higher in self-regulation phase, and families higher in self-regulation phase rated higher their physician's care and involvement. Zimmerman[55] also found that families at higher stage levels had higher self-efficacy beliefs more highly.

Table 6e.1 *Modified version of Zimmerman's phase description and morbidity relationship (From ref. 55)*

Phase	No (%) of families	Wheezing days past month	Description
1	38	6.6	Asthma Symptom Avoidance: Family perceives child wheezes or coughs periodically but don't attribute symptoms to inherent physiological vulnerability.
2	47	4.3	Asthma Acceptance: Family accepts asthma as health threatening disease, but respond reactively, primarily with bronchodilator. Not aware or convinced of importance of preventive treatment.
3	15	3.1	Asthma Compliance: Family seeks to control symptoms by following physician's treatment recommendations which they are convinced will reduce asthma exacerbations. However, they are unaware of how to shift medications in response to dynamic symptom conditions, and are not confident about managing asthma on their own.
4	2	2.5	Asthma Self-Regulation: Family consults with physician to develop an adaptable treatment plan to manage symptoms. Using peak flow or symptom recognition family can recognize early warning signs and adjust medical regimes. They are confident of their ability to implement the plan and are able to contact their doctor when modifications are needed.

Hanson[43] carried out a study among 303 children with moderate to severe asthma, with an intervention programme aimed at increasing parental efficacy in managing their child's asthma. At the end of two years, efficacy had increased in both control and intervention groups, but efficacy was not related to scores on a management skills scale. Parents remained more likely to treat asthma episodically than preventively.

Some structured interventions to improve family management of asthma have been successful. Madge et al.[56] showed that a nurse-led intervention, providing a management plan, education and telephone support after discharge, to parents of children admitted to hospital with acute asthma, successfully reduced hospital re-admissions. Wesseldine et al.[57] found that a nurse-led intervention for children admitted to hospital with acute asthma, providing parents with a management plan, successfully reduced re-admission. However, Gebert et al.[58] did not achieve significant clinical improvement for families of children taking part in a 6-month education programme, although family management attitudes changed.

We can conclude that families do differ in their styles of asthma management, and the strongest evidence seems to be that families which are better organized and more structured in their handling of the tasks associated with managing the child's asthma, do better in controlling symptoms. It appears that aiding families by developing a structured management plan with them can be effective for children with more severe or poorly controlled asthma, who have had a hospital admission, but programmes with children with moderate asthma, in primary care, have not been successful in producing clinical benefits.

MEASURING THE IMPACT OF ASTHMA

The studies described above show that the impact of asthma can be measured by a very large number of methods and tools. Many of these studies have used measures that were not validated outside the study itself. This section describes and discusses tools that have been validated. All of these tools are structured questionnaires, which give easily summarized indicators and a small number of values. Some are generic instruments and some are asthma specific. Structured closed response questionnaires are sometimes criticized for not capturing the complexity of asthma impact on children and families. This is true, but a properly designed and validated questionnaire will have been shown to give scores which impact on quality of life, will be able to discriminate between 'healthy' and 'asthmatic' individuals, will show differences in scores between high and low asthma severity groups, and will be responsive to change in morbidity. Most quality of life and family functioning impact measurement tools give scores on several subscales (for instance, symptom bother, emotional distress, and activity limitation) and the variation between subscale scores can itself enrich our understanding of asthma impact.

Issues in measurement

VALIDITY AND RELIABILITY

Any validated quality of life, health status, psychological functioning or impact measurement questionnaires will have been constructed in consultation with potential respondents (parents and children) and health professionals. Usually preliminary studies identify a pool of items which all groups agree are relevant to those that are being measured. Studies then test the reliability and validity of the initial items. As a result of this process items will be discarded if they are found to be unreliable (a high level of non-consistent answers are given when the questionnaire is repeated), or insensitive (failing to discriminate between subgroups).

When a measure (generic or asthma specific) is reliable we expect good internal consistency; so that clusters of items which evaluate similar areas show consistent patterns of response. For instance we would expect answers on different activity limitations due to breathlessness to somewhat correlate with each other. Items will be discarded if responses within clusters are inconsistent with overall cluster scores, and are likely to also be discarded if they show no relation to total score. Internal reliability is often measured by the 'alpha co-efficient'. A value of 0.6 or higher is expected in a reliable scale. We also seek test–retest consistency in stable groups, although defining 'stability' can be difficult. Stability in physiological indicators such as lung function may not be appropriate indicators of stability in quality of life. For instance, a change in treatment regimen may not lead to a change in lung function, but might have impact on patient quality of life. Hence, in testing for reliability over time in stable groups, physician and patient self-report of 'no experienced change' are often used to define stability.[19] That is, we expect quality of life scores not to change in individuals who globally self assess that their quality of life has not changed, which can seem circular.

We need to be aware that reliability is not a completely inherent characteristic of a scale. A scale that is reliable with one population may be less consistent with another population, and a scale that discriminates in one population may be less sensitive to change in another population.

Validity is the extent to which a measurement tool is appropriate for a particular use. A valid instrument should be able to discriminate between populations in a consistent way. If a measurement instrument has not yet been shown to consistently discriminate between populations prospectively expected to be different, then we cannot be fully confident in its validity. For instance, French and Christie's Child Asthma Questionnaire[59] is interesting because it is the only attempt to create a self-report tool for children under 7 years, but although the scale has internal consistency and reliability it did not discriminate children with asthma from non-asthmatic children in the first, UK, study. A later Australian study has found differences in scores between asthmatic and non-asthmatic children.[60] Juniper's PAQLQ[19] and LeCoq's HAY scale[21,61] have been able to discriminate children with asthma from non-asthmatic children and children with higher levels of symptoms from those with lower levels, as has Bukstein's Integrated Therapeutics Group Child Asthma Questionnaire.[62]

Since validity and reliability are dependent on appropriate use of a scale, we may query the appropriateness of the wide age range suggested for many child quality of life questionnaires. Tables 6e.2 and 6e.3 show that several child questionnaires are supposedly usable from primary school entry to late adolescence. The age ranges quoted may be misleading. Closer examination of the validation studies for these questionnaires shows that there is usually a large median age group, with a few older or younger outliers. Although the PAQLQ is in theory usable from age 7 years, most children in the original validation study were aged at least 10 years, and Guyatt has suggested that age 10–11 is the age at which it is appropriate to take only child self-report rather than parent and child report.

PROXY REPORT

It is still the case that most quality of life scales and child psychological ratings are answered by parents. The exceptions are Juniper et al.'s PAQLQ[19] which is child self-report, to be used from age 7 years and French and Christie's Child Asthma Questionnaire with scales for children from 4 years.[59,60] Christie[60] found a moderate relationship between children's rating of asthma severity and parents' rating (0.5) but a lesser relationship between parental severity rating and child distress rating. Edelbrock[64] found that reliability of children's reports of clinical symptoms increased with child age, comparing children in age groups 6–9 years, 10–13 years and 14–18 years. Parent report was more reliable for the 6–9 year group but less reliable for the 10 years and older groups.

Comparing 81 children with asthma with 22 healthy controls, Klinnert et al.[65] found that maternal report indicated significantly more behavioural problems among the asthmatic children, but no differences were found when children were assessed by clinician interview and observation.

In children younger than 11, Guyatt et al.[66] found that children's global rating of change in symptoms correlated strongly with changes in quality of life (0.54–67) but not with measures of airway calibre or asthma control, while parents' global ratings did not correlate with children's quality of life but showed moderate correlations with airway calibre (0.29–48) and asthma control (0.50). In children over the age of 11, correlations with all clinical variables were higher for their own than their parents' global ratings. Guyatt[66] concluded that in children under 11, clinicians could gain complementary information from questioning children and parents. For children over 11, parents can provide little if any information beyond that obtained through questioning the child.

Thus studies suggest that children aged 10 and over are likely to be more reliable reporters of symptoms than their parents, and that parents become less aware of quality of life impact of asthma on their child as children reach puberty. Using parent report is valid for exploring

Table 6e.2 *Generic impact scales*

Measure	Age (years)	Timescale	Respondent	Items	Domains
Child Health Questionnaire PF-50[16]	5–15	4 weeks for most items	Parent	50	Global health, physical activities, social relationships, mental health emotions
Child Health Questionnaire PF-87[16]	10–17	4 weeks for most items*	Child	87	Emotional impact on family, interference with family activities
Adolescent Child Health and Illness Profile – CHIPAE[17]	11–17	4 weeks/1 year/ 2 years (depending on domain)	Child	153	Activity limitation, satisfaction with health, achievement, resilience, social functioning
Functional Status: FSIIR Stein, 1990[18]	4–16	4 weeks	Parent	43 (or 14)	Communication, mobility, mood, energy, sleeping, eating
Child Behaviour Check List (CBCL)[32]	5–14	3 months	Parent	133	
Behaviour Problems Index (PBI) derived from CBCL[30]	5–11 12–17	3 months	Parent	28	Subscales: **depression, antisocial, headstrong, hyperactive, immature/dependent, and peer conflict
Harter Self Esteem Scale[38]	8–16	Indeterminate	Child	36	Scholastic competence, athletic competence, social acceptance, physical appearance, and behavioural conduct, global self-worth

*Except family cohesion, general health perception and change in health.
**Each subscale includes between four to six questions.

Table 6e.3 *Asthma specific impact scales*

Measure	Age (years)	Timescale	Respondent	Items	Domains
Integrated Therapeutics Group Child Asthma Short Form[62]	4–14	4 weeks	Parent	8	Daytime symptoms, night-time symptoms activity limitation
Children's Health Survey for Asthma[75]	5–12	2, 4 or 8 weeks	Parent	48	Child activity, family activity, child emotional health, family emotional health
HAY scale[61]	8–12	'last few weeks'	Child	72	General: physical activity, cognitive activity, social activity, physical complaints. Asthma specific: symptoms, emotions, self concept, self management
Paediatric Asthma Quality of Life Questionnaire[19]	7–17	4 weeks	Child	23	Symptoms, limitations of activity, emotional 'bother'
Paediatric Caregivers Quality of Life Questionnaire[20]	0–17	4 weeks	Parent	13	Family activity limitations, parental distress, family disruption
Childhood Asthma Questionnaire[59]	A:4–7	Not specified e.g. 'recently'	Child	14	Interference with activity, bother
	B:8–11		Child	22/19*	Interference with activity, distress, severity
	C:12–16		Child	31/24*	Activities, distress, severity, general QoL
QOL–PAC[22]	0–16	Not specified e.g. 'recently'	Parent	48	Burden, subjective norms, social, financial, physician, effect of medication

*Australian version.

whole family impact of the child's asthma, but is not reliable for assessing actual frequency or impact of symptoms for the child itself. There seems no good reason for using parent report for children over the age of 12 years.

ADOLESCENTS

Children aged 12 and over are commonly included in studies evaluating therapeutic intervention which use adult quality of life/health status scales[67] but it is argued that important aspects of adolescent life are less well-covered in adult measures such as social contact. Qualitative studies find that adolescents feel that their views are often not listened to by adults, particularly in assessing their needs in healthcare.[68]

Using a Swiss version of the ISAAC questionnaire, Braun-Fahrlander[69] found that adolescents' self-reported prevalence rates of current asthma symptoms and 'asthma ever' were significantly higher than those obtained from questionnaires completed independently by parents. When parents and adolescents completed the questionnaire jointly prevalence rates were more similar to adolescent self-reported rates.

Generic adolescent quality of life scales, which have been developed, include the Child Health Questionnaire PF-87 for children aged 10–17 years, and the Adolescent Child Health and Illness Profile (CHIP-AE). The only asthma specific scale is the Juniper PAQLQ.[19]

So far, these adolescent scales have not been much used. Studies are needed to demonstrate whether they offer advantages over adult scales, which evidence suggests can validly be used for children from 12 years onwards.

IMPORTANT MEASURES OF ASTHMA IMPACT

The following section and Tables 6e.2 and 6e.3 review the measures that have either been well validated, or have been shown to discriminate as an outcome measure in therapeutic interventions in asthma.

Generic measures

The Child Health Questionnaire PF-50 (Parent form) and the Child Health Questionnaire PF-87 (Child form)[16] have recently been developed by the Medical Outcomes Study group, who developed the SF-36 Quality of Life questionnaire, the most widely used adult generic QoL scale. They are in the process of being internationally validated.[16]

The Functional Status IIR[18] is a non-asthma specific scale which measures health status of children with any chronic disorder. The 14-item short form (parent completed) assesses child eating and sleeping patterns, mood, attention to energy and behaviour in the previous 4 weeks. Mahajan *et al.*[70] found that scores on the FS II

discriminated between placebo and intervention groups in a therapeutic trial of effects of fluticasone propionate on children aged 4–11 years.

The Behavior Problem Index (BPI)[30] is a modification of the Achenbach Child Behavior Checklist and other instruments compiled by Peterson and Zill for the National Study of Children. Five subscales can be derived (Table 6e.2). It has been used, as described earlier, in evaluating asthma impact on children.[29,71]

The Harter Self-Esteem Scale[38,39] was devised by Harter to ascertain a child's competence. There is one version for children 4–7 years of age (parent report), and another for 8 to 16-year-olds (self-report). The younger version assesses four independent dimensions: cognitive competence, physical competence, peer acceptance, and maternal acceptance. The older version assesses five specific domains (Table 6e.2). It has been used in comparative studies[37] and a study evaluating intervention for asthmatic children.[72] There is a British version.[73]

Asthma specific measures

Integrated Therapy Group Child Asthma Short Form[62] is an 8-item parent completed scale which was derived from the earlier Usherwood scale.[74] It has been validated among families with children aged 4–14 years, with mean age 9 years. It has three domains: daytime symptoms (two items), night-time symptoms (two items), activity limitations (four items). Scores discriminated between physician classified mild and severe cases, but were not significantly related to FEV_1.

Children's Health Survey for Asthma[75] has been validated for the UK in 5 to12-year-olds in two cross-sectional studies and one longitudinal study, with 275 parents in total, showing good ability to discriminate between children with different recent levels of symptom activity, moderate discriminatory power for medication use and low relationship to lung function. No use of this scale has been reported for evaluation studies.

The HAY questionnaire[21,61] has recently been developed in the Netherlands. It is child self-complete, with a generic section that can be answered by non-asthmatic children. It discriminated between 80 children with asthma and 296 children without diagnosed asthma, and between children with different levels of recent asthma symptoms.

The Paediatric Asthma Quality of Life Questionnaire[19] was designed for self-report, for children from 7 to 17 years. However, in younger children (7–11 years) interviewer support is likely to be necessary for completion. As discussed above, the wide range of ages raises questions about discriminatory validity. The PAQLQ has been shown to discriminate over time between children rated as 'improved asthma control' and 'worsened control'. The PAQLQ assess degree distress and activity limitations.

The Paediatric Asthma Caregivers Quality of Life Questionnaire[20] was developed to assess the impact of asthma on family emotion and functioning, and resembles these components in the parent report Children's Health Survey for Asthma. The initial validation study showed change in scores was related to change in physician assessed change in asthma control. One other study has shown change in symptom scores over three months in preschool children was significantly related to change in PACQLQ scores.[15]

The QOL–PAC questionnaire[22] has detected improvement in family functioning after therapeutic intervention using the QOL–PAC.[70]

Childhood Asthma Questionnaire[63] has three forms for children aged from 4 years to 16 years, all to be self-reported. Younger children are asked to rate their feelings about asthma using 'smiley face' diagrams. The domains covered are not fully compatible between different age group forms. In early trials, the questionnaires did not discriminate between asthmatic and non-asthmatic children, but a recent Australian study by French[60] has reported discrimination by the scale.

UTILITY MEASURES AND 'QUALYS'

Utility values for health states are intended to measure the absolute value that people give to a particular health state, on a scale from 0–1, where 0 equals death, or the worst imaginable health state, and 1 equals perfect health.[76] Utility values are determined either by asking general population samples to rate a range of health states and then averaging their ratings, or by asking specific patient populations to compare their current health state to other health states. Once utility values have been determined they can be used to calculate QALYs: Quality Adjusted Life Years which represent the relative value of time spent in that state compared with a 'perfect health' year.

The advantage of utility measures is that they offer health economists a potential way to quantify benefits of treatment and to compare qualitative cost-effectiveness between treatments. The disadvantage of utility based methodologies and measures is that even in adults they are complex to use as a measure of quality of life change, and utility measures appear to be less sensitive to change than standard quality of life measures.[77]

Utility measures can be derived by using a utility based questionnaire, such as the Euroquol or Health Utilities Index (HUI), where responses are scored according to utility values derived from an original population study, as described above. However, the HUI[78] has not been found to be sensitive to respiratory symptom change in children.

Alternatively, utility can be derived directly from patient preferences by using methods such as Standard Gamble or Time Trade Off. These methods ask patients how much they would risk some adverse event, or trade some life benefit, in order to improve their present state. These techniques again were not found to be sensitive to

symptom change in children and needed quite high levels of reading and comprehension skills.[78]

At present there do not seem to be utility based measures suitable for use with children. Guyatt *et al.*'s Feeling Thermometer, asking children to rate their present state against theoretical perfect health was able to show change related to global assessment of change by clinicians, but is not a true utility measure, since it is not based on probabilistic trade offs by participants.[78]

CLINICAL IMPLICATIONS AND APPLICATIONS

Can these scales be used in every day clinical practice? The generic scales are too long, and too non-asthma specific to be of much use in an individual assessment. The asthma specific symptom oriented scales are more likely to be relevant to clinical practice. The advantage of using a validated scale is that it allows a picture to be built up over time of symptoms and quality of life for a child, using a consistent set of questions, which can be compared with norms for other children, and to the child's own scores.

To be useful, a scale should be quick to give, and should refer to a short time span, ideally about one month. The scale which best fits these criteria is the Child Asthma Short Form Scale.[62] This has only eight items, and refers to the last 4 weeks. However, since it is a parent report scale it is not suitable for children over 12 years.

The Paediatric Asthma Quality of Life Scale[19] is designed to be answered by the child. However, it has 23 items, and scoring is complex. A short form is currently under development. The corresponding scale designed to assess asthma impact on parents (the Paediatric Asthma Caregivers' Quality of Life Scale,[20] 13 items) is more straightforward to give and to score, but probably only rarely would a clinician want a formal assessment of impact of asthma on the parent, as provided by this scale.

However, these longer scales, and scales which are most oriented to psychological and quality of life assessment can be very relevant to clinics in planning new services, such as educational interventions. A pilot study of child and parent quality of life, and impact of asthma allows us to build up a picture of the patient group, and can give a clearer understanding of their needs. Administering these scales is likely to be an educational experience for clinicians and nurses, and can encourage open discussion with children and parents about their views of their asthma management.

It is sometimes said that quality of life/psychological assessment scales cannot be used on an individual basis, and that only group comparisons are valid. This view appears to be based on a misunderstanding of the measurement criteria in quality of life scales. All these scales have wide error margins, are essentially very 'fuzzy' measurements, and become less reliable as the group size in which they are used diminishes. The larger the group to which a scale score refers, the smaller the likely standard error in measurement and the more reliable the result. This means that a scale score for an individual must be used with caution, keeping in mind all these issues. Nonetheless, inherently all patient report of symptoms is subjective, and this is what the normal clinical interview accepts. Using a structured scale will not increase the unreliability inherent in patient self-report, and will allow consistent comparison between one point in time and the next.

As commented at the beginning of this section, the generic scales are the least likely to be of use in a normal clinical setting. Their value is in large-scale assessment in controlled trials of interventions. The studies described in this chapter show that both generic and asthma specific scales can be used in large trials although there have been insufficient studies yet for us to feel confident that all these scales are equally sensitive to quality of life change after therapeutic intervention. For children, the generic Child Health Questionnaire will be of interest. It is designed by the Medical Outcomes Study, the leaders in validated generic quality of life measures, is being widely validated, and will provide useful norms for children with and without chronic conditions, but with 87 items it is too long to be of use in every day assessment or in pilot studies for service planning.

In trials which aim to assess psychological outcomes (after specialized interventions), studies suggest that standard psychological tools are most suitable (such as the CBCL or PBI) and can be used effectively to discriminate psychological effects among children with poorly controlled or severe asthma. Broader psychological tools may also be useful in exploring psychological issues that may need addressing for some children, but are unlikely to be relevant to most children with asthma.

REFERENCES

1. Ait-Khaled N, Anabwani G, Anderson HR, et al. Worldwide variations in the prevalence of asthma symptoms: The International Study of Asthma and Allergies in Childhood (ISAAC). Eur Respir J 1998;**12**:315–35.
2. Robertson CF, Dalton MF, Peat JK, et al. Asthma and other atopic diseases in Australian children. Australian arm of the International Study of Asthma and Allergy in Childhood. Med J Aust 1998;**168**:434–8.
3. Kaur B, Anderson HR, Austin A, et al. Prevalence of asthma symptoms, diagnosis, and treatment in 12–14 year old children across Great Britain (International study of asthma and allergies in childhood, ISAAC UK). Br Med J 1998;**316**:118–24.
4. Wilson NM, Dore CJ, Silverman M. Factors relating to the severity of symptoms at 5 years in children with severe wheeze in the first 2 years of life. Eur Respir J 1997;**10**:346–53.
5. Strachan DP, Butland BK, Anderson HR. Incidence and prognosis of asthma and wheezing illness from early childhood to age 33 in a national British cohort. Br Med J 1996;**312**:1195–9.
6. Ross S, Godden D, Friend J, Legge J, Douglas G. Incidence and prognosis of asthma to age 33. Asthma or wheezy bronchitis in childhood is independent risk factor for wheezing symptoms in adulthood. Br Med J 1996;**313**:815.
7. Jenkins MA, Hopper JL, Bowes G, Carlin JB, Flander LB, Giles GG. Factors in childhood as predictors of asthma in adult life. Br Med J 1994;**309**:90–3.
8. Ross S, Godden D, McMurray D, et al. Social effects of wheeze in childhood: a 25 year follow up. Br Med J 1992;**305**:545–8.
9. Sibbald B, Anderson HR, McGuigan S. Asthma and employment in young adults. Thorax 1992;**47**:19–24.
10. Gibson PG, Henry RL, Vimpani GV, Halliday J. Asthma knowledge, attitudes, and quality of life in adolescents. Arch Dis Child 1995;**73**:321–6.
11. Sonne-Holm S, Sorensen TI. Prospective study of attainment of social class of severely obese subjects in relation to parental social class, intelligence, and education. Br Med J (Clin Res Ed) 1986;**292**:586–9.
12. Jones PW. Quality of life, symptoms and pulmonary function in asthma: long-term treatment with nedocromil sodium examined in a controlled multicentre trial. Nedocromil Sodium Quality of Life Study Group. Eur Respir J 1994;**7**:55–62.
13. Jones PW, Quirk FH, Baveystock CM. Why quality of life measures should be used in the treatment of patients with respiratory illness. Monaldi Arch Chest Dis 1994;**49**:79–82.
14. Juniper EF. Quality of life in adults and children with asthma and rhinitis. Allergy 1997;**52**:971–7.
15. Osman LM, Baxter-Jones ADJ, Helms PJ. Parents' quality of life and respiratory symptoms in young children with mild wheeze. Eur Respir J 2001;**17**:254–8.
16. Landgraf JM, Maunsell E, Speechley KN, et al. Canadian–French, German and UK versions of the Child Health Questionnaire: methodology and preliminary item scaling results. Qual Life Res 1998;**7**:433–45.
17. Forrest CB, Starfield B, Riley AW, Kang M. The impact of asthma on the health status of adolescents. Pediatrics 1997;**99**:E1.
18. Stein RE, Jessop DJ. Functional status II(R). A measure of child health status. Med Care 1990;**28**:1041–55.
19. Juniper EF, Guyatt GH, Feeny DH, Ferrie PJ, Griffith LE, Townsend M. Measuring quality of life in children with asthma. Qual Life Res 1996;**5**:35–46.
20. Juniper EF, Guyatt GH, Feeny DH, Ferrie PJ, Griffith LE, Townsend M. Measuring quality of life in the parents of children with asthma. Qual Life Res 1996;**5**:27–34.

21. le Coq EM, Colland VT, Boeke AJ, Boeke P, Bezemer DP, van Eijk JT. Reproducibility, construct validity, and responsiveness of the 'How Are You?' (HAY), a self-report quality of life questionnaire for children with asthma. *J Asthma* 2000;**37**:43–58.

22. Schulz RM, Dye J, Jolicoeur L, Cafferty T, Watson J. Quality-of-life factors for parents of children with asthma. *J Asthma* 1994;**31**:209–19.

23. Mullins LL, Chaney JM, Pace TM, Hartman VL. Illness uncertainty, attributional style, and psychological adjustment in older adolescents and young adults with asthma. *J Pediatr Psychol* 1997;**22**:871–80.

24. Graetz B, Shute R. Assessment of peer relationships in children with asthma. *J Pediatr Psychol* 1995;**20**:205–16.

25. Forero R, Bauman A, Young L, Booth M, Nutbeam D. Asthma, health behaviors, social adjustment, and psychosomatic symptoms in adolescence. *J Asthma* 1996;**33**:157–64.

26. Lloyd CE, Robinson N, Andrews B, Elston MA, Fuller JH. Are the social relationships of young insulin-dependent diabetic patients affected by their condition? *Diabet Med* 1993;**10**:481–5.

27. Silverglade L, Tosi DJ, Wise PS, D'Costa A. Irrational beliefs and emotionality in adolescents with and without bronchial asthma. *J Gen Psychol* 1994;**121**:199–207.

28. Bussing R, Burket RC, Kelleher ET. Prevalence of anxiety disorders in a clinic-based sample of pediatric asthma patients. *Psychosomatics* 1996; **37**:108–15.

29. Bussing R, Halfon N, Benjamin B, Wells KB. Prevalence of behavior problems in US children with asthma. *Arch Pediatr Adolesc Med* 1995; **149**:565–72.

30. Peterson JL, Zill N. Marital disruption, parent-child relationships and behavior problems in children. *Marriage Fam* 1986;**48**:295–307.

31. Achenbach TM, Edelbrock CS. Behavioral problems and competencies reported by parents of normal and disturbed children aged four through sixteen. *Monogr Soc Res Child Dev* 1981;**46**:1–82.

32. Achenbach TM, Verhulst FC, Baron GD, Althaus M. A comparison of syndromes derived from the Child Behavior Checklist for American and Dutch boys aged 6–11 and 12–16. *J Child Psychol Psychiat* 1987;**28**:437–53.

33. Achenbach TM, Hensley VR, Phares V, Grayson D. Problems and competencies reported by parents of Australian and American children. *J Child Psychol Psychiat* 1990;**31**:265–86.

34. Perrin JM, MacLean WEJ, Gortmaker SL, Asher KN. Improving the psychological status of children with asthma: a randomized controlled trial. *J Develop Behav Pediatr* 1992;**13**:241–7.

35. Wjst M, Roell G, Dold S, *et al*. Psychosocial characteristics of asthma. *J Clin Epidemiol* 1996;**49**:461–6.

36. Nassau JH, Drotar D. Social competence in children with IDDM and asthma: child, teacher, and parent reports of children's social adjustment, social performance, and social skills. *J Pediat Psychol* 1995;**20**:187–204.

37. Vazquez MI, Fontan-Bueso J, Buceta JM. Self-perception of asthmatic children and modification through self-management programmes. *Psychol Rep* 1992;**71**:903–13.

38. Harter S. *Manual for the Self-Perception Profile for Children*. University of Denver, Denver, CO, 2000.

39. Harter S. The perceived competence scale for children. *Child Develop* 1982;**53**:87–97.

40. Austin JK, Huster GA, Dunn DW, Risinger MW. Adolescents with active or inactive epilepsy or asthma: a comparison of quality of life. *Epilepsia* 1996;**37**:1228–38.

41. Townsend M, Feeny DH, Guyatt GH, Furlong WJ, Seip AE, Dolovich J. Evaluation of the burden of illness for pediatric asthmatic patients and their parents. *Ann Allergy* 1991;**67**:403–8.

42. Staudenmayer H. Medical manageability and psychosocial factors in childhood asthma. *J Chronic Dis* 1982;**35**:183–98.

43. Hansen BW. Acute illnesses in children. A description and analysis of parents' perception of illness threat. *Scand J Prim Health Care* 1994;**12**:15–19.

44. Cornford CS, Morgan M, Ridsdale L. Why do mothers consult when their children cough? *Fam Pract* 1993;**10**:193–6.

45. Kai J. What worries parents when their preschool children are acutely ill, and why; a qualitative study. *Br Med J* 1996;**313**:983–6.

46. Hopton J, Hogg R, McKee I. Patients' accounts of calling the doctor out of hours: qualitative study in one general practice. *Br Med J* 1996;**313**:991–4.

47. Donnelly JE, Donnelly WJ, Thong YH. Parental perceptions and attitudes toward asthma and its treatment: a controlled study. *Social Sci Med* 1987;**24**:431–7.

48. Gustafsson PA, Bjorksten B, Kjellman NI. Family dysfunction in asthma: a prospective study of illness development. *J Pediatr* 1994;**125**:493–8.

49. Gustafsson PA. Family dysfunction in asthma: results from a prospective study of the development of childhood atopic illness. *Pediatr Pulmonol* (Suppl) 1997;**16**:262–4.

50. Mastroyannopoulou K, Stallard P, Lewis M, Lenton S. The impact of childhood non-malignant life-threatening illness on parents: gender differences and predictors of parental adjustment. *J Child Psychol Psychiat* 1997;**38**:823–9.

51. Meijer AM, Oppenheimer L. The excitation-adaptation model of paediatric chronic illness. *Fam Process* 1995;**34**:441–54.

52. Meijer AM, Griffioen RW, van Nierop JC, Oppenheimer L. Intractable or uncontrolled asthma: psychosocial factors. *J Asthma* 1995;**32**:265–74.

53. Wilson SR, Mitchell JH, Rolnick S, Fish L. Effective and ineffective management behaviors of parents of infants and young children with asthma. *J Pediatr Psychol* 1993;**18**:63–81.

54. Taylor GH, Rea HH, McNaughton S, *et al.* A tool for measuring the asthma self-management competency of families. *J Psychosom Res* 1991; **35**:483–91.

55. Zimmerman BJ, Bonner S, Evans D, Mellins RB. Self-regulating childhood asthma: a developmental model of family change. *Health Educ Behav* 1999;**26**:55–71.

56. Madge P, McColl J, Paton J. Impact of a nurse-led home management training programme in children admitted to hospital with acute asthma: a randomised controlled study [see comments]. *Thorax* 1997;**52**:223–8.

57. Wesseldine LJ, McCarthy P, Silverman M. Structured discharge procedure for children admitted to hospital with acute asthma: a randomised controlled trial of nursing practice. *Arch Dis Child* 1999;**80**:110–14.

58. Gebert N, Hummelink R, Konning J, *et al.* Efficacy of a self-management program for childhood asthma – a prospective controlled study. *Patient Educat Counsel* 1998;**35**:213–20.

59. French DJ, Christie MJ, Sowden AJ. The reproducibility of the Childhood Asthma Questionnaires: measures of quality of life for children with asthma aged 4–16 years. *Qual Life Res* 1994;**3**:215–24.

60. French DJ, Carroll A, Christie MJ. Health-related quality of life in Australian children with asthma: lessons for the cross-cultural use of quality of life instruments. *Qual Life Res* 1998;**7**:409–19.

61. le Coq EM, Boeke AJ, Bezemer PD, Bruil J, van Eijk JT. Clinimetric properties of a parent report on their offspring's quality of life. *J Clin Epidemiol* 2000;**53**:139–46.

62. Bukstein DA, McGrath MM, Buchner DA, Landgraf J, Goss TF. Evaluation of a short form for measuring health-related quality of life among paediatric asthma patients. *J Allergy Clin Immunol* 2000; **105**:245–51.

63. French DJ, Christie MJ, West A. Quality of Life in Childhood Asthma: development of the Childhood Asthma Questionnaire. In: MJ Christie, DJ French, eds. *Assessment of Quality of Life in Childhood Asthma*. Harwood, Chur, Switzerland, 1995.

64. Edelbrock C, Costello AJ, Dulcan MK, Kalas R, Conover NC. Age differences in the reliability of the psychiatric interview of the child. *Child Dev* 1985;**56**:265–75.

65. Klinnert MD, McQuaid EL, McCormick D, Adinoff AD, Bryant NE. A multimethod assessment of behavioral and emotional adjustment in children with asthma. *J Pediatr Psychol* 2000;**25**:35–46.

66. Guyatt GH, Juniper EF, Griffith LE, Feeny DH, Ferrie PJ. Children and adult perceptions of childhood asthma. *Paediatrics* 1997;**99**:165–8.

67. Nelson HS, Busse WW, deBoisblanc BP, *et al.* Fluticasone propionate powder: oral corticosteroid-sparing effect and improved lung function and quality of life in patients with severe chronic asthma. *J Allergy Clin Immunol* 1999; **103**:267–75.

68. Slack MK, Brooks AJ. Medication management issues for adolescents with asthma. *Am J Health-Syst Pharm* 1995;**52**:1417–21.

69. Braun-Fahrlander C, Gassner M, Grize L, *et al.* Comparison of responses to an asthma symptom questionnaire (ISAAC core questions) completed by adolescents and their parents. SCARPOL-Team. Swiss Study on Childhood Allergy and Respiratory Symptoms with respect to Air Pollution. *Pediatr Pulmonol* 1998;**25**:159–66.

70. Mahajan P, Pearlman D, Okamoto L. The effect of fluticasone propionate on functional status and sleep in children with asthma and on the quality of life of their parents. *J Allergy Clin Immunol* 1998;**102**:19–23.

71. McCormick MC, Workman-Daniels K, Brooks-Gunn J. The behavioral and emotional well-being of school-age children with different birth weights. *Paediatrics* 1996;**97**:18–25.

72. Pless IB, Feeley N, Gottlieb L, Rowat K, Dougherty G, Willard B. A randomized trial of a nursing intervention to promote the adjustment of children with chronic physical disorders. *Paediatrics* 1994;**94**:70–5.

73. Hoare P, Mann H. Self-esteem and behavioural adjustment in children with epilepsy and children with diabetes. *J Psychosom Res* 1994;**38**:859–69.

74. Asmussen L, Olson LM, Grant EN, Fagan J, Weiss KB. Reliability and validity of the Children's Health Survey for Asthma. *Paediatrics* 1999;**104**:e71.

75. Usherwood TP, Scrimgeour A, Barber JH. Questionnaire to measure perceived symptoms and disability in asthma. *Arch Dis Child* 1990; **65**:779–81.

76. Rutten-van Molken MP. Health State Preference Estimation in Asthma. In: KB Weiss, AS Buist, SD Sullivan, eds. *Asthma's Impact on Society: The Social and Economic Burden*. Basel Dekker, New York, 2000, pp. 331–50.

77. Rutten-van Molken MP, Custers F, *et al.* Comparison of performance of four instruments in evaluating the effects of salmeterol on asthma quality of life. *Eur Respir J* 1995;**8**:888–98.

78. Juniper EF, Guyatt GH, Feeny DH, Griffith LE, Ferrie PJ. Minimum skills required by children to complete health-related quality of life instruments for asthma: comparison of measurement properties. *Eur Respir J* 1997;**10**:2285–94.

7a

Allergy

JILL A WARNER AND JOHN O WARNER

INTRODUCTION

Allergy in this chapter will refer to immediate IgE mediated hypersensitivity to ostensibly harmless environmental antigens often known as allergens. The term 'atopy' refers to the inherent susceptibility to developing allergy but is often confusingly used as a term synonymous with allergy.

The presence of allergy to common environmental allergens is very frequently associated with the presence of asthma. Epidemiological evidence would suggest that about 50% of asthma may be attributable to allergy.[1] However, there is a very strong association between the presence of allergy, as demonstrated either by raised IgE antibodies or positive skin-prick tests, and asthma. Thus up to 90% of children with asthma have allergies as compared with only 25–30% of the whole population.[2] Furthermore, the majority of children who become sensitized to aeroallergens during the first few years of life will develop asthma, whereas those children who become sensitized beyond the age of 8–10 have no greater risk of developing asthma than children who do not develop any allergy whatsoever.[3]

All diseases associated with allergy have increased in the population over the last 30–50 years with parallel rises in asthma, eczema, hay fever and even specific allergies such as that to peanuts[4,5,6] (Figure 7a.1). However, there is no evidence that this increase is a consequence of increased exposure of the population to allergens. Despite the association between allergy and asthma in childhood, the nature of the relationship is still a matter of some dispute. There is no direct evidence to establish whether allergy acts as an inducer of disease in the first place or is merely genetically linked and aggravates the condition once it has already developed.

Does allergy cause asthma?

There is no doubt that exposure to allergens is a risk factor for the development of allergic sensitization to those allergens.[7] Furthermore, exposure to allergens in sensitized individuals is a risk factor for exacerbations of asthma and indeed the persistence of asthma symptoms.[8] There is also very strong evidence that allergen exposure in sensitized subjects acts as a trigger for acute attacks.[9]

Many studies have implied that allergic sensitization and subsequent allergen exposure are causally associated with the development of bronchial hyperreactivity and the development of asthma. However, these are based on cross-sectional studies and there has yet to be a truly prospective longitudinal study which substantiates the relationship.[10] One group has suggested that by taking

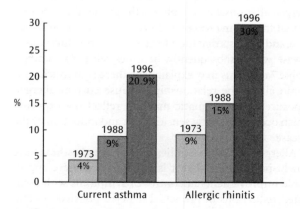

Figure 7a.1 *Prevalence rates for asthma and allergic rhinitis in 12 to 13-year-olds in the UK in 1973/1988/1996 from two studies (refs 4 and 5) using very similar ascertainment methods.*

Table 7a.1 *Lessons from occupational asthma: influences on asthma outcome after cessation of allergens exposure*

	Continuing asthma	Asymptomatic
Duration of exposure before onset of symptoms	Long	Short
Duration of symptoms before avoidance commenced	Long	Short
Associated tobacco smoke exposure	Present	Absent
Lung function at diagnosis	Abnormal	Normal or near normal
Sensitivity to allergen on bronchial challenge	High	Low
Eosinophilia in bronchial lavage/sputum	Present	Absent

into account the biases inherent in cross-sectional studies which relate allergy and allergen exposure to the induction of asthma, the contribution of allergy and allergen exposure to the development of asthma is less than 10%.[11] These observations must be balanced against studies which have shown a strong relationship between early sensitization to house mite, such that high levels of exposure in early life are associated with an over-four-fold greater risk of having continuing asthma at the age of 11,[12] and that sensitization to cockroach allergens is an important risk factor for asthma particularly in North American inner city dwellers.[13] The risk of allergically sensitized children developing airway hyperresponsiveness doubles with every doubling exposure to house-dust mite.[14]

This issue is discussed further in the chapter on preventing asthma, but the great difficulty in finally establishing a causal link between allergy and asthma is that no environment is truly allergen-free. Thus even in the absence of house-dust mite, such as at high altitude or in arid desert regions, there is still a significant prevalence of asthma and also of allergic sensitization to other environmental factors such as alternaria mould, animals and pollens.[15,16]

The only area where there is perhaps more compelling evidence of allergen exposure, allergy and asthma being causally related is in the occupational environment where there is a cause and effect relationship between exposure to the sensitizing agent and the development of asthma. Furthermore, the longer the duration of exposure to the allergen after onset of symptoms, the greater the probability that the asthma will persist even after long-term avoidance, and suggests that the allergen acts as an inducer of the disease which subsequently, becomes self-perpetuating[17] (Table 7a.1). This may explain why there is so much confusion about the relationship, because current allergen exposure in an asthmatic may not reflect the exposure which occurred during sensitization and induction of the disease.

Allergen avoidance studies in established asthma have conclusively shown that it is possible to achieve appreciable improvements in control of symptoms with associated reductions in bronchial hyperresponsiveness and need for concomitant anti-asthma therapy. This perhaps provides the most compelling reason for making a thorough assessment of the allergic status of asthmatic individuals.[18]

CLINICAL EVALUATION OF ALLERGY AND ASTHMA

Clinical history

The most obvious precipitant of acute episodes of asthma is *viral infection*. As a consequence, many families are unable to identify allergy as an obvious cause of their child's problem. However, occasional patients will quite clearly have acute episodes of coughing and wheezing on exposure to animal allergens, particularly if the animal is not present in their own home. Chronic exposure within the patient's own home may indeed contribute to chronicity of disease but there will not be obvious associations between exposure and exacerbation. Seasonal variations in symptoms may be associated with changes in pollen and/or mould counts but this is much more obvious in relation to allergic rhinoconjunctivitis than asthma.

There is no typical pattern of asthma in relation to *house-dust mite sensitivity*. Nocturnal symptoms are common in all asthmatics and no more likely in those with house mite sensitivity. However, profuse sneezing on arising in the mornings is a common association with house mite sensitivity. Furthermore, aggravation of asthma during domestic cleaning activities such as vacuuming may provide a clue to the specific allergy diagnosis.[19]

In taking a history, it is important to have details of the domestic environment. This should include the age and structure of the property, proximity to waterways, type of heating, carpeting, furniture and bedding, all of which can have an influence on house mite levels. The presence of double glazing and other energy saving strategies has appreciably reduced the number of air exchanges which occur in homes and thereby affects the accumulation of allergens as well as non-specific irritants. Such strategies also tend to be associated with higher indoor humidity which in turn will increase house-dust mite and mould exposure.

Hitherto, it has been felt that the use of *feather bedding* would have an adverse effect, both in relation to house mite sensitivity and also, of course, feather allergy. However latterly, studies have suggested that possession of feather pillows is associated with fewer problems, perhaps because such bedding is enclosed in more impermeable covers than when foam is employed.[20]

The presence of *pets in the home* should be carefully recorded and a similar note made of any pet contacts in the homes of relatives or friends. However, exposure to cat and dog allergen is ubiquitous and may be equally important even in schools. Indeed, it has been estimated that if a significant percentage of the children in any classroom come from cat or dog containing homes, they will transport sufficient allergen on their clothing into the classroom to have an adverse effect on cat- or dog-sensitized asthmatics.[21] It is also important to establish the parents' occupations. Occupational allergens may be transported back into the home and this has clearly been demonstrated in relation to the asthmatic children of laboratory workers who have a higher prevalence of sensitization to laboratory animals.[22]

It is generally considered that *food allergy* is a rare phenomenon in children with isolated asthma (see also Chapter 7d). Indeed a study investigating 140 children, aged 2–9 years, with histories of food induced wheezing, suggested on double-blind placebo controlled food challenge that only eight (6%) had reproducible reactions. Only one of the latter children had wheezing as the sole manifestation of food allergy.[23] However in other populations of children, where diseases more commonly associated with food intolerance co-exist with asthma, significantly higher percentages of children do show positive challenge responses to the foods with wheezing as one of a number of symptoms. Thus in a study of 410 children with asthma, 279 (68%) had a history of food associated wheezing.[24] All underwent double-blind food challenges and 60% had positive responses. The symptoms were diverse and manifest in the gastrointestinal tract, skin and respiratory tract. Of the positive food responders on challenge, 40% experienced wheezing as one of the symptoms but only 3% had wheezing as the sole symptom.

At the level of clinical history taking, it is highly improbable that food associated wheezing will occur in isolation. However, food allergy may be a contributory factor in asthmatic children who also have atopic dermatitis and/or gastrointestinal symptoms. It is also true to say that the younger the child, the higher the probability that food will be involved.[25] However, in considering food-associated wheezing overall, it is important to be aware that recurrent aspiration syndrome may be a far more probable explanation rather than food allergy.

One important presentation of food allergy, for which it is imperative that the clinician makes an accurate diagnosis, is food associated *anaphylaxis*. Laryngospasm and/or bronchospasm can sometimes be the only manifestation of food-associated anaphylaxis. Furthermore, any child with a clear-cut history of an acute reaction to foods such as peanut, tree nut, crustaceans, fish and seeds who also has asthma should be considered at risk of life-threatening allergic reactions and appropriately provided with epinephrine (adrenaline).[26]

Family history

It is clear that a tendency to mount allergic reactions (i.e. atopy) is often familial. Thus concordance for atopy amongst monozygotic twins is high. However, the concordance for developing asthma is quite low.[27] Nevertheless, the presence of a family history of atopic disease in an infant presenting with persistent cough and/or wheezing for the first time significantly increases the probability that that child will indeed have asthma. However, the use of family history as a means of predicting which children will develop asthma is neither sensitive nor specific.

Investigations

There is considerable confusion about the relative value of allergy investigations in asthma. As the majority of children will respond to pharmacotherapy irrespective of their allergic status, many individuals have considered allergy investigations to be superfluous. However, many families would rightfully believe that it is incumbent on the physician to search for provokers of disease. Furthermore, families increasingly question the use of pharmacotherapy without review of alternative approaches. Thus at the very least, it is likely that compliance with therapeutic recommendations will improve by more thorough initial investigation. However, there are other very compelling reasons why allergy investigation should be conducted. There are circumstances in which identification of allergens will facilitate recommendation of avoidance measures which can at the very least reduce requirement for concomitant pharmacotherapy. At best, identification of a key allergen may actually produce very appreciable clinical improvements. Furthermore, there are rare occasions where allergen immunotherapy may be recommended as part of the therapeutic strategy. Finally, the identification of allergy in an infant who has begun to show some clinical symptoms suggestive of asthma contributes significantly to the positive diagnosis of the disease and will certainly provide additional support for the early introduction of preventive asthma pharmacotherapies.

There are two components to investigation. The first is to confirm that a patient has a specific allergy which may be achieved by allergen skin testing, the measurement of IgE antibodies in the circulation or by direct allergen challenge, by inhalation for inhalant allergens and by ingestion for food allergens. The second component of the investigation is to substantiate that the child also has significant exposure to the allergen in question in their normal environment. Neglect of the second component of the investigation has often led to quite inappropriate recommendations.

ALLERGY SKIN TESTS (PLATES 7–9)

Allergy skin tests remain the principle aid to allergy diagnosis. There are several techniques, however it is only

Table 7a.2 *Aeroallergens around the world*

Region	Allergen
Temperate climates	House mite: *Dermatophagoides pteronyssinus* and *farinae*
	Cat/dog
	Grass pollen: rye/timothy/cocksfoot
	Tree pollen: silver birch (Scandinavia)
	Moulds: *Cladosporium, Aspergillus*
	Weeds, etc.: pareitaria, nettle, ragweed (USA)
	Cockroach (USA)
Sub-Arctic/Alpine	Tree pollen: birch (Scandinavia)
	Grass pollen (alpine areas)
Desert areas	Tree pollen: olive (Middle East)
	Mould: Alternaria (USA, Australia)
Tropical areas	House mite: *Blomia tropicalis*
	Cockroach (Fiji)
	Grass pollen: Bermuda/Bahia grass
	Weed pollen: *Parietaria*
	Insects: Nimity midge (Sudan), citrus red mite (Korea)

skin-prick testing that has stood the test of time. It is the least traumatic method and also the least likely to give systemic or non-specific reactions. Nevertheless, great care is required in performing the tests. Antihistamines will inhibit responses and may lead to false-negative results. The duration of effect of different antihistamines must be taken into account in recommending their withdrawal before performing the tests. Allergen preparations must be of known potency and there should always be a positive control with histamine solution and a negative control with the diluent. The diameter of the skin weal (not the flare) should be measured 15 minutes after testing. The mean of 2 diameters at right angles should be recorded in millimetres and can be compared with the positive histamine control provided there is no response to the diluent. The latter can occur occasionally, for example in children with dermographism. Under such circumstances, it becomes impossible to interpret the skin test result.

In general the larger the weal reaction, the greater the probability that the allergen is of relevance to the disease. Furthermore, a late skin reaction with a red or livid, itchy indurated area appearing 4–6 hours after testing at the site of the immediate response, is indicative of clinically relevant sensitivity.[28] However, the relative sensitivity and specificity of skin-prick test reactions in relation to asthma depends on the quality of the extract, its concentration, the skill of the investigator and the allergens employed. It is important also to recognize that a positive skin test does not confirm a diagnosis of allergy but merely identifies that there is IgE antibody present to that allergen. In other words, it demonstrates sensitization but not its relevance to disease. Indeed, 22% of randomly tested children under 5 have positive skin reactivity to one or more allergens. Although some remain asymptomatic, others will subsequently develop any combination of several diseases including asthma, rhinitis and eczema. Amongst asthmatic children, 90% have positive tests.[2]

In order to make a diagnosis of atopy alone, where this is being used to aid the diagnosis of asthma in an infant with respiratory symptoms, it may only be necessary to use a very small panel of allergens. In the UK, this can be restricted to house-dust mite, cat, grass pollen and the standard 2 controls. However, extension of the testing will depend on the environment from which the patient originates, the known allergen exposures, and clues picked up from careful history taking (Table 7a.2).

Coupled with a carefully taken clinical history, skin tests can be used to support recommendations of simple allergen avoidance. However, more extreme measures such as elimination of the much loved family pet or immunotherapy require more accurate diagnostic techniques as even with large skin test reactions, up to 15% may prove to be falsely positive when compared with direct organ challenge. It would, however, be true to say that a correctly performed negative skin-prick test in the presence of an appropriate positive response to histamine virtually always rules out allergy with false-negative results being rare, at least in children over 3 years of age. This is certainly true for the major inhalant and ingestant allergens, including house-dust mite, cat, grass and tree pollens, milk, egg, wheat, peanut and tree nuts. Unfortunately, however, for most fruits and vegetables, skin testing with commercial materials almost invariably produces false-negatives. Under such circumstances, only the use of fresh foods using the so-called prick to prick method will accurately identify a potentially relevant fruit or vegetable allergen[29,30,31] (Plates 8 and 9).

Hitherto, skin-prick testing has relied on the use of whole allergen extracts which were mainly characterized on the basis of the quantity of protein present in a weight for volume ratio. However, progressively more sophisticated techniques have identified the major allergenic proteins in allergen mixtures which have allowed characterization of extracts by the concentration of specific major allergens. Latterly, molecular cloning techniques have facilitated the development of recombinant allergens which can be used both to standardize extracts or can even be employed directly for skin-prick testing. Clearly the recombinant allergens can also be used in immunoassays.[32] Indeed, skin testing of allergic individuals with recombinant allergens from a range of sources is now beginning to show promising results and this may well improve both the sensitivity and specificity of testing.[33]

A good rule of thumb in interpreting allergy skin-prick test results is that any skin weal to an allergen, which is equal to or larger than the histamine control, which would be expected to induce a weal of around 5 mm in diameter, has an 80–85% probability of indicating that the allergen is relevant to asthma and will produce a positive response on bronchial challenge. If this reaction is followed by an additional late response, the probability increases further. If there is also a clear-cut history of reaction directly related to exposure, then a large positive skin test supporting the history provides as close to a 100% certainty of relevance as is ever possible in clinical medicine. Once the weal diameter is smaller than the histamine control, there is a progressively diminishing probability of the allergen being relevant, being only 25% with a weal of 3 mm or less. With appropriate controls, if the skin test response is negative, there is only a 5% or less chance that the allergen is relevant to the disease.

IgE ANTIBODY ASSAYS

For many decades, it has been possible to employ *in vitro* testing to identify specific allergies by the radioallergosorbent test (RAST). Such tests may be assumed to be about as sensitive as skin testing but are also more expensive and there is a delay before results are available. There are now new highly automated, enzyme-based assay systems which can give rapid results on tiny quantities of serum. They all work on the common principle. The allergen, usually on a solid phase, is incubated with the patient's serum and captures any specific antibodies. Subsequently, the complex is incubated with an antibody against human IgE which is linked either to a radio-label or an enzyme which can then be used to quantitate the amount of (specific) IgE fixed to the allergen on the solid phase (Figure 7a.2). It must be clear from this description that much like skin-prick testing, the assay relies entirely on the quality of the allergen and how well it is incorporated onto the solid phase. As for skin testing, the use of molecular techniques to develop recombinant allergens has improved quality of the assays very considerably.[34] The results of IgE antibody measurements are expressed either as units per ml or as a grade, often on a scale of 0–4. A grade 3 positive can be considered as being equivalent to a skin test response which is equal to the histamine control, while a grade 4 is greater than the histamine control. Such reactions may again be considered to indicate a high probability that the allergen is relevant, where

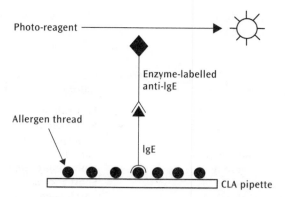

Figure 7a.2 *Diagrammatic representation of a form of IgE antibody testing, the MAST-CLA. Allergen is incorporated on a 'string' which combines with specific antibody from the patient. This is then complexed with anti-human IgE thus detecting only specific IgE. The marker is an enzyme label which when incubated with a photo-reagent produces light which can be detected on a photographic plate.*

grades 2 and 1 are probably indicative only of sensitization but not necessarily of disease. False-negative results are rather more frequent with *in vitro* assays than with accurately performed skin-prick tests.

Most recently, the value of *in vitro* testing has also been studied in relation to food allergy. It has been found that for four foods, milk, egg, peanut and fish, the negative and positive predictive values are high.[35] These latter studies, however, have been in children with atopic dermatitis rather than asthma. It remains to be established whether the same predictive value will be achieved in children with isolated asthma.

Specific *in vitro* allergy diagnosis is most useful where skin testing is inappropriate because patients have either extensive eczema or other skin problems such as dermatographism, which makes interpretation of the skin test results difficult. In patients needing to take continuous antihistamines, skin testing is also impossible. As with skin-prick testing, it is inappropriate to use a large panel of allergens but attention should be focused on those that appear relevant in relation to the child's environment and clinical history.

Inhalation challenge

The final arbiter of an accurate allergy diagnosis is direct organ provocation or challenge with the relevant allergen. In asthma, this clearly is primarily by direct bronchial provocation tests. However in routine clinical practice, these tests are only marginally more accurate than a well taken clinical history supplemented by relevant skin-prick tests and/or *in vitro* IgE antibody measurement.[36] Furthermore, there is the potential for inhalation challenges to produce prolonged and severe reactions. At least three-quarters of asthmatic children will have not only

Table 7a.3 *Comparison of characteristics of natural allergen exposure and bronchial allergen challenge responses*

	Natural	Induced Immediate reaction	Late reaction
Allergen	Particulate	Soluble	
Exposure time	Prolonged or repeated	Short	
Other factors involved	Varied i.e. infection/exercise	Partially controlled	
Response	Short and/or prolonged	Short-lived self-limiting	Prolonged
Effect of β-agonists	Variable	100% effective	Poor
Effect of steroids	Good	No short-term effect	Good
Effect on bronchial hyperresponsiveness	Enhanced	None	Enhanced

an immediate response to the allergen, which is predominantly bronchospasm lasting for 30–45 minutes and easily reversible with inhaled β-agonist, but also a late reaction. This occurs 3–4 hours after recovery from the immediate response and may last for many hours or even days. Not only can this late reaction be severe and prolonged but it is less easily reversed with inhaled β-agonists and it is almost always associated with an increase in bronchial hyperresponsiveness which can last for several weeks after the challenge[37] (Table 7a.3).

The principles of allergen bronchial challenge are the same as for the measurement of bronchial responsiveness, namely initially using the diluent and then subsequently after a 30-minute observation period, commencing with a very low concentration of allergen and increasing by doubling concentrations until a just significant drop in lung function, either by spirometry or peak flow, is measured. Usually the nadir of the lung function occurs 20 minutes after the challenge which is a little longer than the responses to pharmacological agents. However given the frequency of late reactions and the duration of the responses, such challenges are not relevant for routine clinical purposes and are usually only used for research.

FOOD CHALLENGES

The double-blind, placebo-controlled food challenge (DBPCFC) has been established as the gold standard for the investigation of adverse reactions to foods. However, in situations where the association is relatively vague and uncertain, it may be possible at least to establish whether or not a food is a cause of problems by an open challenge. For most other standard clinical purposes, a single-blind food challenge is probably sufficient. However whatever technique is employed, it must be performed in a safe environment. Given that food allergy associated with asthma has the potential to lead to severe and even

life-threatening anaphylaxis, such challenges should only be performed in hospital where full resuscitation facilities are available.

Many protocols have been suggested for challenges, of which probably the best is to have a single day of active challenge and a separate day of placebo exposure. However, time constraints sometimes dictate that it is necessary to conduct both components on a single day. The gap between increasing doses will be dictated by the history of the gap between exposure and response. The initial dose should be well below that which might normally be expected to produce a response, with doubling doses thereafter. While encapsulation of food might allow more objective double-blind procedures, this negates the potential effect of the food on the upper respiratory tract. The closer the exposure is to a normal domestic situation, the better. Imaginative preparation by dietitians (nutritionists) is required to provide appropriate materials for blinded challenges. Monitoring includes regular measurement of lung function as for bronchial challenges, and careful recording of any other symptoms, particularly focused on the gastrointestinal tract and skin.[38]

Other *in vitro* techniques

EOSINOPHIL PROTEINS

There has recently been a major commercial enterprise to develop *in vitro* techniques for diagnosing and monitoring allergic disease. The primary focus has been on the eosinophil as a key effector cell in allergic reactions. In many respects, asthma may be defined histopathologically as eosinophilic bronchitis. A number of proteins are released from activated eosinophils including eosinophil cationic protein (ECP), eosinophil peroxidase (EPO), eosinophil protein X (EPX) which used to be known as eosinophil derived neurotoxin, and major basic protein (MBP). All have been measured in plasma during the course of provoked asthma and, to a greater or lesser extent, are increased in active asthmatics.[39]

Most studies have shown some correlation between levels of eosinophil proteins and disease severity based on lung function and bronchial hyperresponsiveness but the relationship is relatively weak.[40] Longitudinal studies have shown that changes in levels of the eosinophil activation proteins mirror changes in lung function and clinical manifestations.[41] However, the eosinophil markers are also increased in relation to atopic eczema which may confound the observations in relation to asthma.[42] The degree to which measurement of such proteins will predict the outcome of asthma in infants with wheezing illnesses remains to be established by longitudinal study. However, results hitherto have been conflicting with both negative[43] and positive[44] associations with continuing symptoms in infant wheezers. One intriguing study has shown a correlation between levels of ECP and bronchodilator responsiveness in infant wheezers which would strongly point to such children as having asthma and might well promote the use of more aggressive anti-asthma therapy.[45]

EPX is the only eosinophil granule protein which can be accurately measured in urine with levels correlating both with blood and bronchoalveolar lavage eosinophil counts.[46] Urine sampling is clearly a much less invasive procedure and, therefore, much to be preferred. Furthermore, the serum sampling for measurement of the other eosinophil proteins requires precise conditions with separation of the serum from the blood clot within 1–2 hours of sampling and then deep freezing, preferably to −80°C, until assayed. However, current evidence would suggest that as is the case for serum eosinophil proteins, there is a considerable overlap in urinary EPX levels between children with asthma, with or without associated atopy and controls.[47]

The value of measuring either total eosinophil counts or eosinophil proteins in either serum or urine are very strictly limited because of a marked overlap between different patient groups, but there may be some value in utilizing the measurement as a component of monitoring individual asthmatic children longitudinally. Whether or not therapeutic strategies should be modified as a consequence of observing variations in levels remains to be established by study. It also remains to be established whether raised eosinophil protein levels in infants with early respiratory symptoms is a reliable predictor of future asthma which might, therefore, guide early intervention strategies.

LYMPHOCYTE MARKERS

When lymphocytes are activated, they express the interleukin-2 receptor as a prelude to proliferating. A portion of the receptor is detectable in the serum as a soluble component whose levels directly relate to the degree of lymphocyte activation. Measurement of soluble IL-2 receptor (sIL-2R) has been used as a marker of inflammation in a number of diseases including asthma.[48] Amongst infants who have presented with wheezing for the first time, a raised level of sIL-2R is to a certain extent predictive of subsequent persistent wheezing requiring anti-asthma therapy.[49] Furthermore, a very high sIL-2R level may be a feature of the fatality-prone asthmatic child.[50] Much as for all other serum markers of immunological activation and allergy, a great deal more work is required to establish whether the measurement of sIL-2R will have any clinical utility for individual patients or merely be a component of research.

Predictors of asthma in infancy

Much effort has been expended in identifying tests which might predict subsequent asthma in infants at various stages in the evolution of atopic disease. Thus skin-prick test positivity to egg,[51] house-dust mite,[52] and cat or grass pollen positivity by RAST[53] by 1–2 years of age are significant risk factors for later asthma, particularly when found in association with atopic eczema. Furthermore, even a raised cord-blood total IgE has some predictive value, since it is highly specific for the early development of atopic disease (including asthma) but very insensitive in that the majority of future asthmatics have normal total IgE levels early in life.[54]

In an attempt to provide more sensitive indicators of allergic sensitization which might predict later asthma, many studies have examined peripheral blood mononuclear cell responsiveness to allergen. Studies have shown that even in cord blood, there are differences in the degree of responsiveness to allergen and in the cytokine profiles from stimulated cells amongst those who subsequently go on to develop atopic disease. The balance of cytokine profiles in the future atopics is much more biased to the Th2 variety with low IFN-γ and higher production if IL-4, -10 and -13.[55,56] However as with other *in vitro* and *in vivo* allergy tests, there is much overlap between those who subsequently develop asthma and those who do not. Indeed, a recent study that has compared various markers of early sensitization in relation to later atopic disease has suggested that a combination of atopic dermatitis and evidence of food allergy by skin-prick test or specific IgE at 12 months of age provides the strongest combination risk for asthma by 24 months of age.[57] Measurement of total IgE, peripheral blood mononuclear cell responsiveness to allergen, blood eosinophil count or the measurement of the expression of an adhesion molecule marker of inflammation, soluble E-selectin did not improve the prediction.

MEASUREMENT OF EXPOSURE

It is self-evident that the detection of allergy in patients is only likely to be relevant if there is continuing exposure to the relevant allergen (Table 7a.2). This, however, is an area that is frequently neglected in clinical practice. There

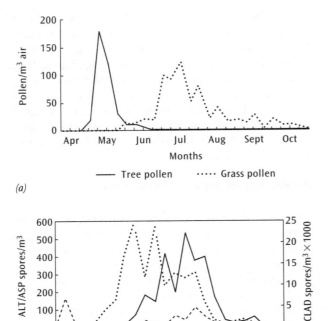

Figure 7a.3 *(a) A typical N. Europe season with pollen counts. (b) A typical N. Europe season with fungal spore counts.*

major allergens. Molecular recombinant technology has facilitated the development of highly sensitive enzyme-linked immunoassays for the accurate measurement of major-allergen concentrations in source materials such as household dust. Many trials have investigated the value of allergen avoidance techniques by measurement of such allergens but rarely, if ever, have the techniques been employed as part of clinical practice. It would, however, seem entirely appropriate to utilize such measurements prior to making any recommendations on allergen avoidance. Indeed, it would be perfectly appropriate to suggest that measurements should be made before and after employment of any avoidance techniques. This could lead to far more beneficial outcomes. Certainly as a result of measuring cat and dog allergen levels in dust from various sources, it has been possible to establish that the allergens from these animals are far more ubiquitous than has hitherto been appreciated. Thus, significant quantities can be detected in homes and also, indeed, schools where the animals are not themselves housed.[58]

Clearly there is a need to provide an evidence base for the use of allergen concentration monitoring in clinical practice but the concept that this could be of significant value is certainly highly credible.

are now relatively straightforward techniques available for measuring allergen concentration in dust or in the air.

Allergen source counting

It has long been established policy to measure and publicize the grass and tree pollen and mould spore counts through the spring, summer and autumn in many countries around the world. This has been of considerable value to seasonal allergy sufferers who have been able to modify their therapy according to variation in the counts. Clearly having access to the data can aid the clinician's assessment of individual patients by associating symptom scores day by day with the counts (Figure 7a.3). However for perennial allergens, rather less attention has been paid to exposure.

Direct measurement of allergenic proteins

Hitherto, most skin test and IgE antibody assays have used relatively crude extracts from whole allergen source such as house-dust mite or pollen. However, it is now possible to characterize individual proteins from the source material which have high allergenic potential and are associated with high specific IgE antibodies in >50% of those allergic to the crude extract. These are known as

REFERENCES

1. Pearce N, Pekkanen JRB. How much asthma is really attributable to atopy? *Thorax* 1999;**54**:268–72.
2. Van Asperen PP, Mukhi A. Role of atopy in the natural history of wheeze and bronchial hyperresponsiveness in children. *Pediatr Allergy Immunol* 1994;**5**:178–83.
3. Martinez FD. Viruses and atopic sensitization in the first years of life. *Am J Respir Crit Care Med* 2000;**162**:S95–9.
4. Burr ML, Butland BH, King S, Vaughan-Williams E. Changes in asthma prevalence: 2 studies 15 years apart. *Arch Dis Child* 1989;**64**:1452–6.
5. Kaur B, Anderson HR, Austin J, Burr M, Harkins L, Strachan DP, Warner JO. Prevalence of asthma symptoms, diagnosis and treatment in 12–14 year old children across Great Britain (International Study of Asthma and Allergies in Childhood, UK). *Br Med J* 1998;**316**:118–24.
6. Hourihane JO'B, Dean TP, Warner JO. Peanut allergy in relation to heredity, maternal diet and other atopic diseases: results of a questionnaire survey, skin-prick testing and food challenges. *Br Med J* 1996;**313**:6–9.
7. Wahn U, Lau S, Bergmann R, *et al.* Indoor allergen exposure is a risk factor for sensitization during the first 3 years of life. *J Allergy Clin Immunol* 1997;**99**:763–9.

8. Peat JK, Salome CM, Sedgwick CS. A prospective study of bronchial hyperresponsiveness and respiratory symptoms in a population of Australian school children. *Clin Exp Allergy* 1989;**19**:299–306.

9. Gelber LE, Seltzer LH, Bouzokis JK, *et al.* Sensitization and exposure to indoor allergens as risk factors for asthma among patients presenting to hospital. *Am Rev Respir Dis* 1993;**147**:573–8.

10. Sporik R, Squillace SP, Ingram JM, *et al.* Mite, cat, and cockroach exposure, allergen sensitization, and asthma in children: a case control study of 3 schools. *Thorax* 1999;**54**:675–80.

11. Pearce N, Douwes JRB. Is allergen exposure the major primary cause of asthma? *Thorax* 2000;**55**:424–31.

12. Sporik R, Holgate ST, Platts-Mills TAE, *et al.* Exposure to house-dust mite allergen (Der p 1) and the development of asthma in childhood. *New Engl J Med* 1990;**323**:502–7.

13. Platts-Mills TAE, Vervloet D, Thomas WR, *et al.* Indoor allergens and asthma: report of the 3rd International Workshop. *J Allergy Clin Immunol* 1997;**100**:S3–24.

14. Sherrill D, Stein R, Curzius-Spencer M, Martinez F. On early sensitization to allergens and development of respiratory symptoms. *Clin Exp Allergy* 1999; **29**:905–11.

15. Charpin D, Birnbaum J, Haddi E, *et al.* Altitude and allergy to house-dust mites. A paradigm of the influence of environmental exposure on allergic sensitization. *Am Rev Respir Dis* 1991;**143**:983–6.

16. Halonen M, Stern DA, Wright A, *et al.* Alternaria as the major allergen for asthma in children raised in a desert environment. *Am J Respir Crit Care Med* 1997;**155**:1356–61.

17. Montanaro A. Prognosis of occupational asthma. *Am Allergy Asthma Immunol* 1999;**83**:593–6.

18. Boner AL, Bodini A, Piacentini GL. Environmental allergens and childhood asthma. *Clin Exp Allergy* 1998;**5**:76–81.

19. Warner JO, Price JF. House mite sensitivity in childhood asthma. *Arch Dis Child* 1978;**53**:710–13.

20. Strachan DP, Carey IM. Home environment and severe asthma in adolescence: a population based case control study. *Br Med J* 1995;**311**:1053–6.

21. Lonnkvist K, Hallden G, Dahlen SE, *et al.* Markers of inflammation and bronchial reactivity in children with asthma exposed to animal dander in school dust. *Pediatr Allergy Immunol* 1999;**10**:45–52.

22. Krakowiak A, Szulc B, Gorski P. Allergy to laboratory animals in children of parents occupationally exposed to mice, rats and hamsters. *Eur Respir J* 1999;**14**:352–6.

23. Novembre E, de Martino J, Vierucci A. Foods and respiratory allergy. *J Allergy Clin Immunol* 1988;**81**:1059–65.

24. Bock SA. Respiratory reactions induced by food challenges in children with pulmonary disease. *Pediatr Allergy Immunol* 1992;**3**:188–94.

25. Hill DJ, Shelton MJ, Hosking CS. Manifestations of milk allergy in infancy. Clinical and immunological findings. *J Pediatr* 1986;**109**:270–6.

26. Sampson HA, Mendelson L, Rosen JP. Fatal and near-fatal food-induced anaphylaxis in children. *New Engl J Med* 1992;**327**:380–4.

27. Edfors-Lubs M. Allergy in 7000 twin pairs. *Acta Allergol* 1974;**26**:249–85.

28. Warner JO. The significance of late reactions following bronchial challenge with house-dust mite. *Arch Dis Child* 1976;**51**:905–11.

29. Dreborg S. *The Skin-prick Test. Methodological Studies and Clinical Applications*. Linkoping University Medical Dissertation No. 239, 1987.

30. Eigenmann PA, Sampson HA. Interpreting skin-prick tests in the evaluation of food allergy in children. *Pediatr Allergy Immunol* 1998;**9**:186–91.

31. Rance F, Juchet A, Bremont F, Dutau G. Correlations between skin-prick tests using commercial extracts and fresh foods, specific IgE and food challenges. *Allergy* 1997;**52**:1031–5.

32. Chapman MD, Smith AM, Vailes LD, Arruda LK. Recombinant allergens. New technologies for the management of patients with asthma. *Allergy* 1997;**52**:374–9.

33. Laffer S, Spitzauer S, Susani M, *et al.* Comparison of recombinant timothy grass pollen allergens with natural extract for diagnosis of grass pollen allergy in different populations. *J Allergy Clin Immunol* 1996; **98**:652–8.

34. Van Ree R, van Leeuwen WA, Aalberse RC. How far can we simplify *in vitro* diagnosis for grass pollen allergy? A study with 17 whole pollen extracts and purified natural and recombinant major allergens. *J Allergy Clin Immunol* 1998;**102**:184–90.

35. Sampson HA, Ho DG. Relationship between food specific IgE concentrations and the risk of positive food challenges in children and adolescents. *J Allergy Clin Immunol* 1997;**100**:444–51.

36. Warner JO. Bronchial provocation tests. *Arch Dis Child* 1977;**52**:750–1.

37. Cartier A, Thomson NC, Frith PA, *et al.* Allergen-induced increase in bronchial responsiveness to histamine: relationship to the late asthmatic response and change in airway calibre. *J Allergy Clin Immunol* 1982;**70**:170–7.

38. Sicherer SH. Food allergy: when and how to perform oral food challenges. *Pediatr Allergy Immunol* 1999;**10**:226–34.

39. Dahl R, Venge P, Olsson I. Variations in blood eosinophils and eosinophil cationic protein in serum of patients with bronchial asthma. *Allergy* 1978; **33**:211–15.

40. Rao KR, Frederick JM, Enander I, *et al.* Airway function correlates with circulating eosinophil but not mast cell markers of inflammation in childhood asthma. *Clin Exp Allergy* 1996;**26**:789–93.

41. Coller DY, Herouy Y, Gotz M, *et al*. Clinical value of monitoring eosinophil activity in asthma. *Arch Dis Child* 1995;**73**:413–17.

42. Carlsen K-H, Halvorsen R, Pettersen M, Lodrup-Carlsen KC. Inflammation markers and symptom activity in children with bronchial asthma. Influence of atopy and eczema. *Pediatr Allergy Immunol* 1997;**8**:112–20.

43. Oymar K, Bjerknes R. Is serum eosinophil cationic protein in bronchiolitis a predictor of asthma? *Pediatr Allergy Immunol* 1998;**9**:204–7.

44. Villa JR, Garcia G, Rueda S, Nogalas A. Serum eosinophil cationic protein may predict clinical cause of wheezing in young children. *Arch Dis Child* 1998; **78**:448–52.

45. Lodrup-Carlsen KC, Ragnhild H, Ahlstedt S, Carlsen K-H. Eosinophil cationic protein and tidal flow volume loops in children 0–2 years of age. *Eur Respir J* 1995;**8**:1148–54.

46. Cottin V, Deviller P, Tardy F, Cordier JF. Urinary eosinophil derived neurotoxin/protein X. A simple method for assessing eosinophil degranulation *in vivo*. *J Allergy Clin Immunol* 1998;**101**:116–23.

47. Oymar K. High levels of urinary eosinophil protein X in young asthmatic children predict persistent atopic asthma. *Pediatr Allergy Immunol* 2001;**12**:312–17.

48. Jones AC, Besley CR, Warner JA, Warner JO. Variations in serum soluble IL-2 receptor concentration. *Pediatr Allergy Immunol* 1994;**5**:230–4.

49. Clough JB, Keeping KA, Edwards LC, *et al*. Can we predict which wheezy infants will continue to wheeze? *Am Respir Crit Care Med* 1999;**160**:1473–80.

50. Warner JO, Nikolaizik WH, Besley CR, Warner JA. A childhood asthma death in a clinical trial; potential indicators of risk. *Eur Respir J* 1998;**11**:229–33.

51. Tariq SM, Matthews SM, Hakim E, Arshad SH. Egg allergy in infants predicts respiratory allergic disease by 4 years of age. *Pediatr Allergy Immunol* 2000;**11**:162–7.

52. Delacourt C, Labbe D, Vassault A, *et al*. Sensitization to inhalant allergens in wheezing infants is predictive of the development of infantile asthma. *Allergy* 1994;**49**:843–7.

53. ETAC Study Group. Allergic factors associated with the development of asthma and the influence of cetirizine in a double blind randomised placebo controlled trial: first results of ETAC. *Pediatr Allergy Immunol* 1998;**9**:116–24.

54. Croner S, Kjellman N-IM. Development of atopic disease in relation to family history and cord blood IgE levels – 11 year follow-up of 1654 children. *Pediatr Allergy Immunol* 1990;**1**:14–21.

55. Warner JA, Miles EA, Jones AC, *et al*. Is deficiency of IFN-γ production by allergen triggered cord blood cells a predictor of atopic eczema? *Clin Exp Allergy* 1994;**24**:423–30.

56. Kondo N, Kobayashi Y, Shiroda S, *et al*. Reduced interferon-gamma production by antigen-stimulated cord blood mononuclear cells is a risk factor of allergic disorders – a 6 year follow-up. *Clin Exp Allergy* 1998;**28**:1340–4.

57. Laan MP, Baert MRM, Bijl AMH, *et al*. Markers for early sensitization and inflammation in relation to clinical manifestations of atopic disease up to 2 years of age in 133 high risk children. *Clin Exp Allergy* 2000;**30**:944–53.

58. Warner JA. Controlling indoor allergens. *Pediatr Allergy Immunol* 2000;**11**:208–19.

Viral infection

IAN BALFOUR-LYNN AND PETER OPENSHAW

INTRODUCTION

Most parents of wheezy infants and young children report that the wheezing episodes start with a simple cold – a runny nose and mildly raised temperature, perhaps a sore throat and cough. Within a day or so, this is usually followed by a pronounced cough and wheeze. These symptoms may then last for several days, even weeks. By then the child has often caught another cold, and so the cycle repeats throughout the winter so that some children are virtually never free of symptoms. In older asthmatic children this pattern still occurs, although other factors (such as allergen exposure and exercise) now play an increasingly important part. Such asthmatic children, like their adult counterparts, also suffer from postviral exacerbations. When acute wheezing illnesses are associated with respiratory tract infection, viruses rather than bacteria cause the vast majority, particularly in infants. Unfortunately, many patients are said to have 'chest infections' and are then given antibiotics rather than bronchodilators. This could have implications for the future as recurrent antibiotic use in infancy has been associated with an increased risk of later asthma.[1]

This chapter highlights the importance of the multi-factorial association between viral respiratory infection and childhood wheezing (Figure 7b.1). The two major (overlapping) forms of viral wheeze will be highlighted, as discussed in Chapter 3: viral episodic wheeze in infants and young children and viral episodes in atopic asthma of older children. The relationship between viral respiratory tract infection and wheeze and asthma has been the subject of several recent reviews.[2–6]

EPIDEMIOLOGY

Epidemiological studies have provided evidence of the close relationship between viral upper respiratory tract infections (URTIs) and acute episodes of wheezing in all ages.[2] Viruses are commonly associated with wheezing illnesses in populations, in individuals, and in time, but are rarely found during asymptomatic periods. The recent use of molecular biology techniques, and in particular polymerase chain reaction (PCR) assays, has provided further evidence, particularly by implicating rhinoviruses, which had previously proved difficult to detect. Using these techniques, a community study of 9- to 11-year-old children showed that viral URTIs were associated with 80–85% of asthma exacerbations in school-age children.[7] There is a strong relationship between seasonal patterns of viral URTI and hospital admission for asthma,[8] especially for paediatric admissions which peak soon after children return to school after the vacation.

It is uncertain whether wheezy infants and children are more susceptible to viral infection or to URT symptoms, or whether colds are simply more noticeable in them, because of the additional symptoms of cough and wheeze. Work in the 1970s found that asthmatic children had a greater incidence of viral infection compared with their non-asthmatic siblings, due mainly to rhinovirus.[9] However, among children with rhinovirus infection, asthmatic children were also found to have a higher incidence of symptoms than other children.[10] It would seem, therefore, that both factors apply.

Several respiratory viruses are implicated and the greatest influence over the pattern of isolation is age (Table 7b.1).

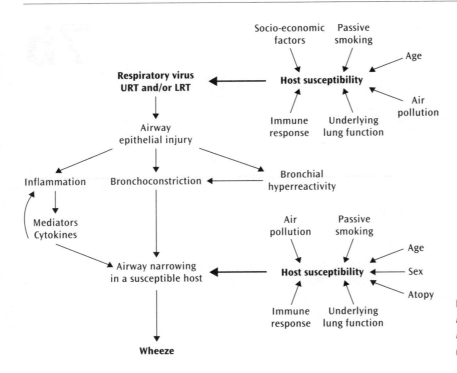

Figure 7b.1 *The interaction between respiratory viruses and a susceptible host that results in wheezing. (Adapted from ref. 3.)*

Table 7b.1 *Commonest respiratory viruses associated with URTI and wheezing in different age groups*

Infants	Preschool and school-children	Adolescents and young adults
RSV	Rhinovirus	Rhinovirus
Rhinovirus	Coronavirus	Coronavirus
Parainfluenza I–III	Influenza A & B	Influenza A & B
Adenovirus	Parainfluenza I–III	Parainfluenza I–III
	RSV	

Respiratory syncytial virus (RSV) most commonly occurs in infancy whilst rhinovirus predominates in older children. To put into context the size of the problem, figures from upstate New York reveal that 80% or more of all infants are infected with RSV in the first year of life.[11] About 40% have a clinically evident lower respiratory illness, but only 1% are hospitalized and 0.1% require intensive care (Figure 7b.2).

Risk factors

Several factors in the host predispose to a susceptibility to wheeze during viral respiratory infections, and together they determine the viral responsiveness of an individual.[3] It should be stressed here that risk factors are statistical concepts, and although an association may be implied, it is not necessarily causal. Age is important, viral wheezing being commonest in young infants but unusual under 8 weeks of age; rates tend to decline after 2 years. Males are more susceptible, probably because of differences in lung function and relative airway size. There are several socio-economic factors: low family

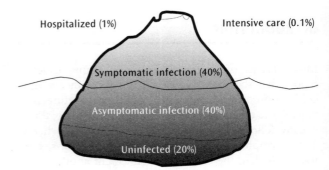

Figure 7b.2 *Putting RSV infection in the first year of life into context. Most research is carried out on the 1% of infants who are hospitalized with acute bronchiolitis, whilst so-called normal controls include the 40% of infants who have had subclinical RSV infection. (From ref. 11.)*

income, overcrowded homes and large families increase the risk of viral URTI. Attendance at day care centres is also a risk although apparently protective if the mother is a heavy smoker. The increased risk of wheezing at 2 years seen with larger families or day-care attendance in the first 6 months of life reverses, so that increased early exposure to other children is protective against development of asthma at 6–13 years of age,[12] evidence on which the 'Hygiene Hypothesis' for the protective effect of early infection was based (see later). Passive smoking is important in that it leads to an increase in viral respiratory infections and an increased risk of these infections becoming symptomatic. The risk is particularly associated with maternal smoking for two reasons: the greater contact time with mothers and the effect of smoking during pregnancy on lung growth and early infant lung function.

Indoor air pollution by oxides of nitrogen similarly increases the likelihood of wheezing in asthmatic children during a URTI. Bottle-feeding is a risk factor, as breast-feeding seems to reduce the severity of viral respiratory illnesses although it has no apparent effect on primary prevention of atopic asthma in high-risk children.

The role of *atopy* is less clear, mainly due to difficulties in defining and diagnosing atopy in the very young. It seems likely that atopy affects viral wheezing in children over 2 years rather than during infancy. The issue of whether early viral infections have a protective role against the development of atopy later in life is discussed later in this chapter.

Underlying *pulmonary function* is also important; infants with diminished airway conductance (measured before they had contracted their first respiratory illness) have an increased risk of wheezing for at least the first three years of life[13] (Chapters 3 and 9). *Preterm* infants, particularly if they required mechanical ventilation or if they developed bronchopulmonary dysplasia, are at high risk of recurrent viral wheezing (Chapter 13b). An alteration in the host *immune response* to viral infections is also a major risk factor and this is discussed later in the chapter. It should be pointed out however that about 20% of 3-year-old wheezy children have none of the known risk factors so there must be other important factors that are not yet understood.[3]

The influence of age

The contribution of viral respiratory tract infection (RTI) to wheezing remains important throughout life.[2,7,14] However its relative importance lessens over time due to the emergence of other factors that become more important in later childhood, in particular atopy (Figure 7b.3). The reduced impact of viral RTI is partly because they are less common in the older child. Another factor is the change in prevalence with age that occurs with some respiratory viruses (Table 7b.1). For example, rhinovirus is important in older asthmatics.[15] In these older atopic children the interaction between rhinovirus and airway inflammation may facilitate infection with rhinovirus, and exacerbate the underlying airway inflammation (see later). This aspect is less relevant in infants where atopy has little or no role in wheezing. Individual viruses may have age-dependent effects. RSV is a good example of this. Several factors, many of which are not understood, lead to acute infantile bronchiolitis in an 8-week-old, whilst an 8-month infant develops a straightforward viral wheeze, and an 8-year-old child has an asthma exacerbation. Of course, most children have a simple cold or remain asymptomatic. In the case of very young infants, where RSV predominates, the virus invades the epithelium of the lower respiratory tract and thus probably causes disease by obstructing small airways. Some of these infants may already have congenitally small or hyperreactive airways. Overall,

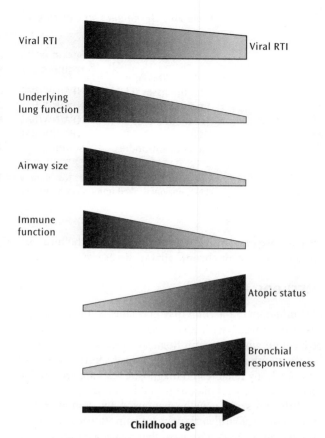

Figure 7b.3 *The influence of age on the relative importance of some of the factors associated with childhood wheezing. Viral respiratory tract infection (RTI) remains important throughout childhood. (Adapted from ref.128.)*

however, from what is known, many of the mechanisms by which viruses trigger wheezing in infants are probably very similar to those described in older asthmatics. Viral responsiveness is certainly age-dependent.

Viral diagnosis

Viral diagnosis is valuable for epidemiological studies, clinical management and prognosis. It will guide therapy as antivirals become available. Particularly during RSV seasonal outbreaks, cohorting of infants with proven RSV should be practised; infants who are RSV-negative or still awaiting confirmation of diagnosis should be kept in isolation. Cohort nursing needs to be combined with scrupulous hand-washing by nursing and medical attendants to reduce nosocomial infection; wearing gowns and gloves is also recommended.[16] Viral diagnosis may also be useful as an indication of prognosis for individual patients. For example, it is known that up to 75% of infants admitted to hospital with RSV-bronchiolitis will have recurrent episodes of cough and wheeze over the succeeding 2 years. Rarely, adenovirus infection can lead to the later development of obliterative bronchiolitis.

Table 7b.2 *Techniques for isolating RSV*

	Specimen required	Result < 24 hours	Available in clinical laboratories	Clinically useful
Immunoassay (ELISA)	NPA/NW/BAL	✓	✓	✓
Immunofluorescence	NPA/NW/BAL	✓	✓	✓
Tissue culture	NPA/NW/BAL	✗	✓	✗
PCR	NPA/NW/BAL	?	✗	?
Specific antibodies	Serum	✗	✓	✗

NPA: nasopharyngeal aspirate; NW: nasal washings; BAL: bronchoalveolar lavage; ELISA: enzyme-linked immunosorbent assay; PCR: polymerase chain reaction.

Persistence of adenoviral DNA in airway epithelium may be a risk factor for chronic airway disease.[16a]

METHODS

Examination of the child may give clues to the cause. For example, infants with RSV-bronchiolitis have a distinctive cough whereas parainfluenza-infected patients often present with a croupy illness. However, clinical diagnosis is not wholly reliable and diagnostic tests are required to give a specific viral diagnosis (Table 7b.2).

Infections are usually diagnosed by demonstrating the *presence of viral antigen* by immunofluorescent staining or immunoassay on nasopharyngeal aspirate (NPA). Rapid detection of viral antigen by immunoassay is by far the simplest, cheapest and most effective single method to diagnose viral respiratory infection. *Enzyme-linked immunosorbent assays* (ELISA) are available as commercial kits and monoclonal antibodies for use with these kits are available for most respiratory viruses, with the important exception of rhinovirus. ELISA measures free antigen so does not require the presence of intact respiratory epithelial cells. The test is simple and quick, and minimal training is required to perform it. Specimens can be kept in the refrigerator overnight or even sent to the laboratory by mail. Direct or indirect *immunofluorescent assays* are also available and their sensitivity and specificity is comparable to those of ELISA. However it takes trained personnel around 2 hours to process the samples, and it also requires the presence of intact exfoliated epithelial cells in the specimen.

Detecting the virus by *tissue culture* is also possible but results are rarely available in time to be of clinical value. The diagnosis can also be made by demonstrating a significant increase in *specific antibodies* in serum (usually two doubling dilutions or more) after the acute phase of the illness. Again, this has little practical value and taking a second blood sample when the child is recovered and has gone home is rarely acceptable in paediatric practice.

The use of *PCR* to detect viral RNA or DNA is now possible for all the common respiratory viruses but this service is not routinely offered in hospital microbiology departments. PCR has been of great value as a research tool, especially for detection of rhinovirus and coronavirus, which are poorly identified by standard methods.[17] However as the reliability, specificity and simplicity of PCR based methods improve, so it is likely that it will become more widely offered as a routine diagnostic tool. In one study, 108 children were surveyed for a one year period and nasal aspirates were taken during periods of respiratory symptoms.[17] Samples were also taken from asymptomatic children and adults. Rhinovirus was detected in 46 of 292 symptomatic episodes by culture (16% detection rate), but 146 of 292 episodes by PCR (50% detection rate). In asymptomatic individuals, 12% of children and 4% of adults were positive by PCR, but only one specimen from a child was positive by culture. It is clear from studies of this type that PCR is much more sensitive than viral culture. The significance of viral detection in asymptomatic individuals is uncertain. It may be wrong to dismiss this form of viral detection as 'false-positive'; it may indeed be that some asymptomatic individuals are undergoing acute infections, or that long-term viral shedding occurs from some individuals. There have been reports of persistence of viral genome (adenovirus in particular) in children and adults with chronic lung disease, particularly with chronic severe asthma and chronic bronchitis. Again, the significance of detection of genomic virus by PCR is unknown. It may be that persistent infection with some common viruses leads to chronic inflammation and disease. Alternatively, it may be that the inflammatory processes responsible for chronic disease allow viral persistence to occur. These intriguing questions will undoubtedly be answered in the near future.

COLLECTION OF SPECIMENS

Proper collection and handling of respiratory secretions are critical to viral diagnosis. Samples are usually collected by *NPA* in which the suction catheter is introduced into the nostril until it reaches the posterior wall of the nasopharynx. However NPA is not always successful, with inadequate samples sometimes collected if the nasopharynx is relatively dry. Furthermore, NPA may be associated with local trauma as well as coughing spasms, vagal bradycardia and transient hypoxaemia, especially in sick infants with bronchiolitis. This, not unnaturally, leads to a reluctance to carry out this procedure which further delays the diagnosis.

Nasal lavage is an under-utilized technique that has been shown to be useful and give comparable results to NPA in infants.[18] With the infant held in a supine position, 2 ml of room temperature saline are gently instilled into a nostril, whilst being simultaneously suctioned back from the anterior nares. The procedure can be repeated in the other nostril if necessary. It is free of adverse effects such as bradycardia, probably because the suction catheter need only be placed just inside the nose rather than in the nasopharynx, thus avoiding vagal stimulation. There is also less discomfort to the infant. Simultaneous suction avoids the infant aspirating the lavage fluid and insufficient 'dry' specimens are never obtained as lavage provides a better cell yield than NPA.

Other methods of collecting infected respiratory epithelial cells have been reported but are not routinely used in the UK in clinical practice. These include nasopharyngeal and throat swabs (which are poor methods), nasal washing with a rubber aspiration bulb, nasal brushing with a cytology brush, and nasal curettage. Naturally produced or induced sputum can be used. Finally, viral diagnosis can also be made on bronchoalveolar lavage specimens, although this invasive technique would not be employed solely for this purpose as upper airway specimens are usually sufficient.

VIRUS INFECTION IN INFANCY AND THE NATURAL HISTORY OF ASTHMA

Several longitudinal studies have shown a clear association between respiratory viral infections in infancy and respiratory abnormalities later in life. Whether these common infections have a role in the pathogenesis of childhood asthma and adult chronic obstructive pulmonary disease is however unclear. Two major hypotheses explain the association.[11,19] In the first, it is postulated that early viral infections directly damage the developing lung or alter the host immunity, and this causes subsequent symptoms and airway dysfunction. In the second, it is postulated that the initial symptomatic respiratory infection simply unmasks an inherent susceptibility to long-term respiratory abnormalities. The hypotheses are not mutually exclusive, and is likely that both account for subsequent problems, although to a differing degree in each individual (Figure 7b.4).

Evidence that early respiratory infections predispose to atopy and asthma

Sigurs *et al.* followed up 47 infants who had been hospitalized for RSV-bronchiolitis, over 3 years.[20] They found

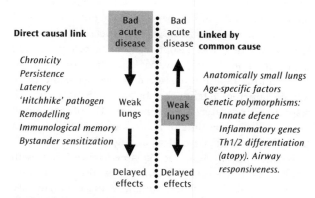

Figure 7b.4 *Hypotheses for the association between acute respiratory viral infections and late wheezing. Bad initial infection alters the host (lungs or immunity) leading to future wheeze; or bad initial infection unmasks an underlying tendency to wheeze. There is evidence to support both theories.*

that, compared with 93 matched controls, the patients had a higher rate of asthma diagnosis (23% vs 1%, a very low rate) and greater evidence of specific sensitisation against common allergens (32% vs 9%). RSV bronchiolitis was the most important risk factor for the development of asthma, and acted independently of a family history of (and by implication the inherited tendency for) asthma, although a family history of atopy did increase the risk. The same trends held true when the children were assessed again aged 7½ years.[21] In another long-term study, 61 children were followed for 9–10 years after hospital admission for bronchiolitis (66% were RSV-positive).[22] Compared with 47 matched controls, there was an excess of cough (odds ratio 4.0), wheeze (odds ratio 3.6), and bronchodilator usage (33% vs 3%). The index cases had significant reductions in measure of airflow but there were no differences in lung size, and there was no difference in skin-prick test response or in family history of atopy. A recent study has compared 29 infants, 4–12 months after they were hospitalized for acute RSV bronchiolitis, with 29 matched controls who had not had asthma, wheezing, or any LRI.[23] With minor exceptions, pulmonary function was similar in the two groups, suggesting a better prognosis for infant lung function after acute RSV bronchiolitis than previously reported. These studies (and others[24]) might at first sight imply a causal link, but they do not rule out a developmental or genetic predisposition to both severe bronchiolitis and to subsequent asthma. Most of the longitudinal studies are observational, and one of the problems is that RSV infection is almost universal in the first year of life, so that it is almost impossible to find an uninfected control group (Figure 7b.2). In reality therefore, controls consist of children selected on the basis of suffering mild RSV infection or of being over 6–8 months old in the RSV season.

Both genetic and acquired immunological factors also play a part in determining future wheezing after bronchiolitis. In 43 children with an RSV-positive LRI in the first 6 months of life, persistent wheeze at the age of 7–8 years was directly related to the level of RSV-specific IgE measured in the nasopharyngeal secretions during their initial illness.[25] However, this did not result in reduced lung function measured at 7–8 years, and there was no apparent relationship between RSV-specific IgE responses and later lung function. Peripheral blood eosinophilia at the time of acute bronchiolitis has been shown to be predict-ive of wheezing at 7 years of age.[26] This latter finding was not explained by differences in gender, family history of asthma or exposure to passive smoking. In addition, wheezy infants who went on to have persistent episodes of wheeze later in life were found to have higher serum levels of eosinophilic cationic protein (ECP) during their first acute LRI (not necessarily caused by RSV), compared with those who had less than three subsequent wheezing episodes in the next year.[27] Another study of infants, with at least one atopic parent, showed that (later) age at pre-sentation together with the serum level of soluble interleukin (IL)-2R offered the best model of prediction of persistent wheezing requiring treatment for at least one year after initial presentation.[28] Finally, in a study of infants hospitalized with bronchiolitis, monocyte IL-10 production measured 3–4 weeks after the acute illness, was signifi- cantly raised in those with recurrent wheezing over the next year compared with those without recurrent wheeze.[29] There was no association with either interferon-gamma (IFN-γ) or IL-4 levels however.

Evidence from animal studies supports the possibility of causal links between viral bronchiolitis and asthma. In guinea pigs, RSV infection causes increased sensitivity to inhaled histamine for at least 6 weeks, associated with persistence of RSV in the lungs.[30] Also, Brown Norway rats develop chronic, episodic and reversible airway obstruction after bronchiolitis.[31] In this latter model, a strong CD4+ T-cell response was present with reduced IFN-γ production, and a combination of persistent inflammation, fibrosis and deposition of extracellular matrix material led to airway remodelling. Further mechanisms by which viral infections could affect later development of lung disease include virus chronicity, persistence or latency[32] and provision of a local foothold for other infections.[33]

There is also strong evidence from animal models that viral infections interact with inhaled allergens to promote the development of airway inflammation and atopy. Uninfected mice develop no IgE antibody against inhaled antigen (ovalbumin), but during acute influenza infection, sensitization takes place.[34] When antigen exposure coincides with influenza infection, airway responsiveness to inhaled methacholine increases and serum IgE rises, while neither influenza A virus nor ovalbumin alone cause these changes.[35] Furthermore, nebulized ovalbumin induces systemic sensitization if the protein is inhaled in the presence (but not in the absence) of acute viral infections. This sensitization is sufficient to cause acute anaphylactic collapse during subsequent cutaneous challenge with ovalbumin.[36] These data suggest that viral inflammation allows inhaled antigen to penetrate the barrier of the respiratory mucosa, promoting systemic sensitization.

Evidence that prior risk leads to both viral LRTI and later atopic asthma

Underlying immunological, physiological or structural differences in the airways, present before they have been affected by their first lower respiratory illness (LRI) may predispose some infants to wheeze. Using the chest compression technique to obtain partial flow–volume loops in sedated babies, several studies have looked at lung function in pre-symptomatic infants.[37–40] Indirect measurements of airway function were lower in infants who later developed wheezing with presumed viral RTI or needed hospitalization for bronchiolitis, compared with those who did not. This pre-existing situation might be responsible for subsequent anomalies in lung function rather than direct viral damage.[41] This implies an underlying susceptibility to both symptomatic viral respiratory infection and later respiratory morbidity. The nature of this underlying airway condition is still unknown. The possibility that bronchial hyperresponsiveness (BHR) could be the relevant factor is suggested by some studies, showing that pre-symptomatic BHR is associated with subsequent wheeze.[40,42] However this is confounded by follow-up studies of lung function and BHR in the first year of life, showing no difference in BHR between wheezy infants and controls.[43–45]

Martinez has postulated that at least two different infant asthma-like syndromes may co-exist during the first years of life.[46] 'Transient infant wheeze', is not associated with family or personal atopy, but the infants may have diminished lung function before their first LRI which persists,[41] 'persistent wheeze' continues to be symptomatic beyond the early years, and there is a high prevalence of family history of asthma and personal atopy. Children in this group show deteriorating (pre-bronchodilator) lung function. Longer term follow-up of the Tuscon cohort, which was drawn from the community, showed that RSV LRI in early childhood was an independent risk factor for subsequent wheezing, but that the risk decreased with age and was lost by 13 years.[47] In addition, the association was not caused by an increased risk of allergic sensitization. In these studies, it would seem that the evidence is against direct viral damage being the cause of future respiratory morbidity.

HYGIENE HYPOTHESIS: IS EARLY VIRAL INFECTION PROTECTIVE?

There has been considerable recent interest in the role of infection in promoting immune maturation. In a completely clean environment, perhaps our immune system does not develop in an appropriate way and produces aberrant (allergic) responses. The possibility that common childhood infections could play a protective role in the development of allergic disease was suggested by British cohort studies showing a consistent relationship between birth order and the risk of atopy, the presence of older children appearing to protect their younger siblings.[48,49] More recently, a study from Guinea-Bissau showed that children with a clinical history of measles (at an average age of over 3 years) were less likely to develop atopy than measles-vaccinated children.[50] A similar effect is also reported in the UK.[51] The increase in atopic disease in industrialized countries has been ascribed to the decreased cross-infection rates due to decreased family size, now often referred to as the 'hygiene effect'.

Martinez and colleagues examined the relationships between LRIs in the first three years of life and atopy/serum IgE levels. Non-wheezing LRIs were associated with lower IgE levels and less skin test reactivity than wheezing LRIs and absent LRIs. At the age of 9 months, children with non-wheezing LRIs had higher IFN-γ production from mononuclear cells than the other groups. Martinez argues that the immune response to respiratory viral infections that do not induce wheeze promotes the Th1 development cells while suppressing the Th2 system.[52] Von Mutius et al. conducted surveys soon after reunification of East and West Germany, and showed a higher frequency of respiratory symptoms in the East German children (42% vs 27%) but a lower prevalence of asthma (3.8% vs 5.4%).[53] These findings have been used to support the argument that communal living, pollution and respiratory infections protect against asthma and atopy. The apparent protective effects of tuberculin sensitization[54] (subsequently unverified) and hepatitis virus infection[55] could also be explained in this way. The role of bacterial products may be greater than that of virus (Chapters 2 and 3).

There are plausible immunological mechanisms for the protective effect of infections in the development of atopic disease. Atopy is related to the expression of allergen-specific responses with production of Th2 cytokines such as IL-4 and IL-5, which promote IgE production and eosinophilia[56] (see Chapter 4c). In non-atopic individuals, following an uncommitted period in early infancy, the T-cell system is biased towards the Th1 phenotype with production of IFN-γ and inhibition of Th2 development. Fetally-derived allergen-reactive T-cells exhibiting a Th2 phenotype exist, which indicates intrauterine T-cell priming.[57] The continuation of these fetal allergen-specific Th2 responses during infancy, with a decreased capacity to produce IFN-γ has been demonstrated in subsequently atopic neonates.[58] Environmental factors such as microbial agents (viruses, other intracellular organisms, including mycobacteria, and bacterial products) may then exert their effects during early life by promoting the maturation of adaptive immune responses, including Th1 cell development. Activated macrophages and dendritic cells produce IL-12, which induces natural killer cells and Th1 cells to produce IFN-γ. IFN-γ provides the environment for the differentiation of antigen-specific CD4+ T-cells into Th1 cells and CD8+ T-cells into Tc1 cells with even higher IFN-γ production. In the absence of such stimuli, it seems that Th2-biased neonatal immune responses could persist and that allergen-specific Th2 responses become entrenched. Normal maturation may be slow and inefficient in children predisposed to atopy,[58] but it may be promoted by repeated exposure to ingested and inhaled bacteria as well as childhood viral infections. The epidemiological evidence favouring the protective role of 'dirt' is covered in detail in Chapter 2. It seems that normal maturation of the immune system is promoted by a rich gut flora. The situation for viral infections, as discussed above, is still controversial, and may differ between viruses.

MECHANISMS OF VIRAL WHEEZING

Acute effects on lung function and airway reactivity

Viral URTIs have been shown to cause small airway obstruction with no alteration to large airway function in normal adults; the changes may not always be clinically evident, but may persist for up to 8 weeks.[59] Although more difficult to study in young children, alterations in lung function have been found in infants hospitalized with acute bronchiolitis, as well as infants and children with simple URTI (reviewed in ref. 3). Some of these changes include alterations in flow, airway resistance and lung volumes. In those with bronchiolitis, some of the changes persisted for over a year, although as described above, pre-existing lung function abnormalities rather than consequences of bronchiolitis may have been responsible. In infants with a simple URTI, lung function returns to normal within 1 month.[60] It seems that although respiratory viruses transiently affect lung function in adults and children of all ages, the effects usually remain subclinical. However if lung function is already compromised, for instance in those prone to wheezing, then the effects may be greater even in the absence of chronic inflammation.[61]

Whether all respiratory viral infections can lead to bronchial hyperresponsiveness (BHR) in normal individuals is controversial. Both natural and experimental viral infections may lead to increased airway responsiveness to a number of agents, although not in all studies.[62] This is a particularly difficult area to study in small children. The increase in BHR is further enhanced if there is pre-existing BHR, as is the case in asthmatic children and adults. In an adult experimental model of viral wheeze, BHR lasting for up to 17 days was found only in those with a history of viral wheeze (independently of atopic status and without baseline BHR) and not at all in healthy subjects (whether or not atopic).[63] BHR usually begins early during the acute infection and may last for several weeks after an URTI,[63] even in normal individuals.[64] It is therefore unrelated to atopy, underlying inflammation or pre-existing BHR.

There are several potential mechanisms for viral enhancement of bronchial responsiveness:

BHR may result from direct viral injury to airway epithelium by a number of mechanisms, including increased permeability to antigen, changes in osmolarity of the epithelial lining fluid and loss of proposed epithelial-derived relaxant factors.[3]

Epithelial damage by the virus may also result in exposure and sensitization of cholinergic sensory nerve fibres normally protected by the epithelium. The M_2 muscarinic receptors on vagal nerve endings are markedly dysfunctional during viral infections, although the M_3 receptors on the airway smooth muscle function normally.[65] This leads to substantial increases in acetylcholine release and potential reflex bronchoconstriction. Repair of this damaged epithelium would account for the return to normal airway reactivity after 6 weeks.

The *function of β-adrenoreceptors* on airway smooth muscle is also impaired by viral infections thus reducing adrenergic relaxation, and in addition, non-adrenergic relaxation of the airways may be reduced by viral infection.[65]

Immune mechanisms are also a factor and are dealt with later in this chapter. Distant effects of (mainly) URT inflammation may affect the lower airways, by mechanisms which are not clear but are presumed to involve nerves, or circulating or inhaled agents.[15]

Overall, although virus-induced alteration in airway reactivity accounts for exacerbations in older children with established atopic asthma, this has not been shown in viral wheeze in young children.

INFLAMMATION

Epithelial cells which are the principal target for respiratory viruses, can trigger the initial immune response by secreting a range of proinflammatory cytokines, chemokines and mediators. Although it helps our understanding to split virus-induced inflammation into its various components, the different cell types, mediators and cytokines involved do not act in isolation – they all interact together to form the inflammatory cascade. The resultant inflammation is manifest by smooth muscle contraction, vascular engorgement, cellular infiltration within airway walls, oedema of the mucosal and submucosal layers and mucous secretion. This leads to airway narrowing and symptoms of cough and wheeze. The immunohistology has been studied in experimental and natural infections by bronchial mucosal biopsy[66,67] and in fatal cases of asthma.

CELLS

Alveolar macrophages are likely to be involved in the early immune response to respiratory viruses throughout the respiratory tract. Once activated, they release several pro-inflammatory cytokines, and infection of these macrophages by RSV leads to increased secretion of tumour necrosis factor-alpha (TNF-α), IL-6 and IL-8. However, they are also activated by stimuli that do not provoke airway obstruction so their relative role in precipitating wheezing is uncertain.[68]

Neutrophils are well-recognized as important inflammatory cells in viral URTIs, even those uncomplicated by bacterial infection. There may also be peripheral blood neutrophilia, an increase in nasal lavage neutrophil counts and neutrophil infiltration in nasal mucosa.[69] Neutrophils have also been found to be the predominant inflammatory cell in bronchial secretions of children with severe LRI due to RSV infection,[70] as well as in a human experimental model of viral wheeze in young adults.[71] Neutrophils display enhanced adhesion to airway epithelial cells infected with RSV or parainfluenza virus. They release a number of toxic reactive metabolites, which are damaging to airway tissues and could lead to airway inflammation, obstruction and BHR.

The main neutrophil chemoattractant is the chemokine, IL-8. It has been shown to be present and active in nasal aspirates of children who had naturally occurring colds causing asthma exacerbations.[69] Furthermore, the IL-8 levels correlated with increased levels of the neutrophil enzyme myeloperoxidase (MPO), which in turn correlated with the severity of upper respiratory symptoms in these children.

Eosinophils release a large number of mediators such as cysteinyl-leukotrienes and platelet-activating factor, but also release basic proteins such as major basic protein (MBP) and eosinophilic cationic protein (ECP), which are toxic to airway epithelium. MBP acts as an M_2 muscarinic receptor antagonist, which causes M_2 receptor dysfunction and subsequent BHR.[65] The association of eosinophilic infiltration and asthma is well documented, and this includes adult asthmatics infected with rhinovirus.

Eosinophils may also play a part in viral wheezing in children. *In vitro* work has shown that RSV activates human eosinophils and a study measuring the concentration of ECP in nasopharyngeal secretions of infants found significantly higher levels in those with RSV-induced wheezing compared with infants with URTI alone.[72] Increased levels of MBP, and the eosinophil chemoattractants RANTES and macrophage-inhibitory protein 1α (MIP-1α) have been found in the nasal aspirates of children with naturally-occurring virus-induced asthma exacerbations, compared with when they were asymptomatic.[73] MIP-1α and RANTES have also been found in lower airway secretions of infants ventilated with RSV-bronchiolitis together with ECP and eosinophil-derived neurotoxin (EDN) to a greater degree than in ventilated controls.[74] MIP-1α levels correlated with ECP concentrations suggesting a role for eosinophil degranulation products in the pathogenesis of RSV bronchiolitis. Non-bronchoscopic bronchoalveolar lavage studies have

Colour plates

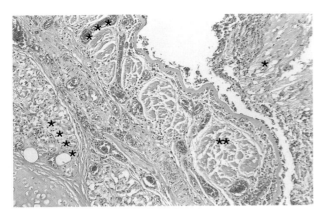

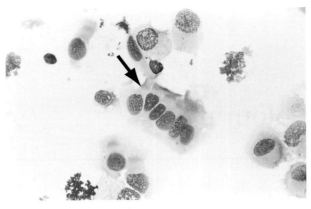

Plate 1 *Bronchial wall in fatal acute severe asthma, showing debris in the lumen (*), bundles of hyperplastic smooth muscle (**), vascular congestion (***), and mucus glands (****) (haematoxylin and eosin, ×32).*

Plate 2 *Bronchial washings from an asthmatic subject showing epithelial cell shedding, including a cluster of ciliated cells (May–Grunwald–Giemsa, ×200).*

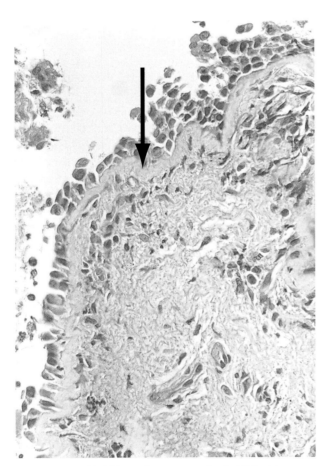

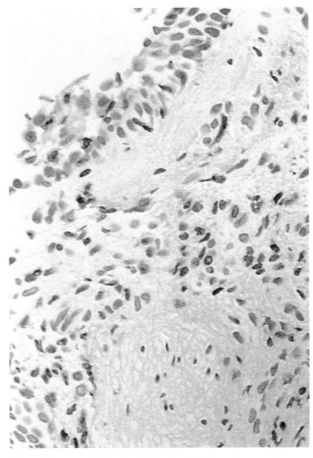

Plate 3 *Bronchial biopsy from a preschool child with asthma showing subepithelial fibrosis (arrow) and inflammatory cell accumulation in the underlying mucosa (haematoxylin and eosin, ×32).*

Plate 4 *Immunohistochemistry for CD3 showing T-lymphocytes infiltrating the bronchial mucosa and epithelium in asthma (immunoperoxidase, paraffin-embedded, ×128).*

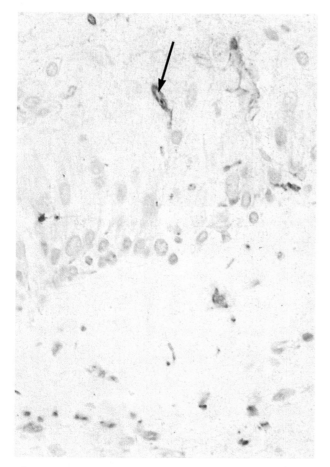

Plate 5 *Mast cells in the bronchial mucosa and epithelium in asthma showing immunoreactivity for interleukin 4 (immunoperoxidase, glycol methacrylate-embedded, ×128).*

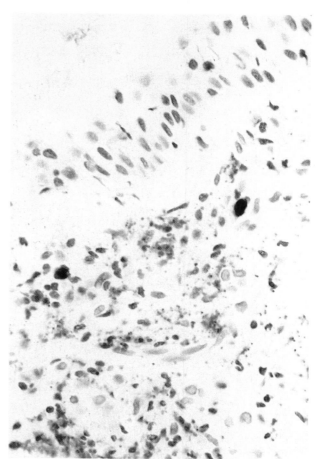

Plate 6 *Immunohistochemistry for eosinophil cationic protein showing eosinophils and extracellular material derived from eosinophil degranulation in the bronchial mucosa in asthma (immunoperoxidase, paraffin-embedded, ×128).*

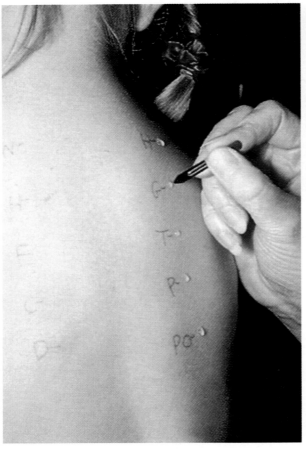

Plate 7 Prick skin tests being performed with a standard lancet on an infant's back – on the left the two lower tests, C: cat, D: dog, are already developing a positive response with a weal and flare.

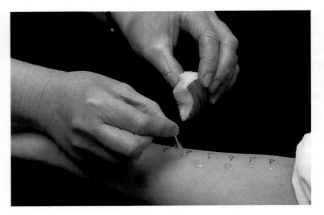

Plate 8 Prick to prick skin test with apple on the volar surface of a child's forearm.

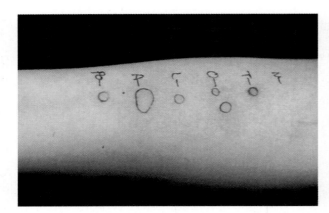

Plate 9 Weal responses outlined of a prick to prick for N: negative control; T: tree pollen; O: orange; L: lemon; A: apple; PO: histamine positive control in a child with oral allergy syndrome.

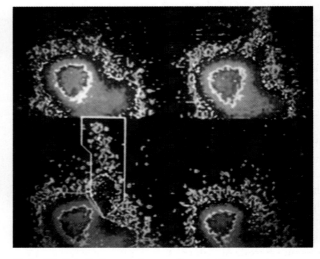

Plate 10 Detail of a one-hour reflux scintigraphy study.

shown that eosinophil (and mast cell) counts and ECP were not elevated in children prone to viral wheezing whilst they were asymptomatic, compared with non-atopic normal controls. Nor are eosinophils involved in exacerbations of (symptomatic) viral wheeze in an adult experimental model.[71] In contrast, atopic asthmatics had elevated cell counts and ECP even when well.[61,75] In conclusion, it seems that eosinophilic inflammation is a feature of viral wheezing during acute episodes but not at other times, in contrast to asthma where eosinophilic inflammation may be chronic.

T-lymphocytes have an important role in the pathogenesis of both adult and childhood asthma, particularly in terms of immunoregulation and cytokine production. Two types of T-helper (Th) cells have been identified, defined by their cytokine secretion patterns: Th1 cells secrete IL-2, IFN-γ and lymphotoxin, whereas Th2 cells secrete IL-4, IL-5, IL-6 and IL-10; several other cytokines are secreted by both types. Some features of the allergic asthmatic response are mediated by Th2 cytokines, particularly IgE production, eosinophil and mast cell activity. The balance of Th1 and Th2 responses is likely to be important in coordinating both cytotoxic and antibody responses to viral infection, which together provide antiviral activity and immunity against reinfection.[62,76]

T-helper cells are a common lymphocyte subtype found in the airways of individuals with RSV and rhinovirus-induced wheezing.[68] Although it is the Th1 response classically associated with antiviral immunity, in an animal model, the RSV G-protein primarily promoted a Th2 response,[77] which could account for some of the RSV lower airway symptomatology. The mouse model of RSV bronchiolitis also shows that enhanced T-cell responses are associated with increased severity of disease.[78] In particular, prior sensitization with a formalin inactivated RSV vaccine, or the attachment G protein (expressed by recombinant vaccinia virus) leads to Th2 cell driven augmented disease, contrasting to the usual Th1 response seen in primary viral infections. An exaggerated lymphocyte response may play a role in the pathogenesis of viral wheezing although it will also contribute to the eradication of these viral infections.[68] Once present in the airways, T-lymphocytes amplify and upregulate other inflammatory cells by the release of proinflammatory cytokines. Examples include IFN-γ, RANTES and MIP-1α, each one of which attracts and activates mast cells, basophils and eosinophils.[68]

There is intriguing evidence that pulmonary inflammation may be surprisingly prolonged in children with bronchiolitis. Smyth *et al.* used soluble interleukin-2 receptor (sIl2R) in serum to monitor T-cell activation in children with RSV bronchiolitis. Compared with control children, concentrations in both acute and convalescent samples were high. Although their levels do fall with time, high concentrations were found up to five months after the acute episode of bronchiolitis.[79] In contrast, levels are also increased in acute measles infection, but they decline

rapidly and are often normal one month after infection. Direct evidence for persisting pulmonary inflammation is hard to obtain from children who are clinically recovered from RSV infection.

Studies in the mouse model suggest that severe RSV bronchiolitis is sometimes associated with enhanced IL-4 responses to RSV. To test this hypothesis in man, Openshaw and colleagues studied the cohort of 7- to 8-year-old Swedish children described earlier.[21] They measured single cell production of IFN-γ and IL-4, and proliferative responses to RSV antigens and non-viral allergens in peripheral blood cells. Antigen-specific enhancement of IL-4 production was found in children with a history of bronchiolitis, both to whole RSV and purified cat antigen (Fel d); there was however no generalized bias towards IL-4 production to all antigens.[80] These results are compatible with the hypothesis that viral bronchiolitis in infancy enhances the risk of asthma/recurrent wheezing in later childhood by increasing the chance of Th2 sensitization to subsequent respiratory infections and to inhaled antigen. Alternatively, it is possible that children who suffer from bronchiolitis have an inherent predisposition to enhanced IL-4 responses. This is unlikely for two reasons: first, family history of asthma or atopy was not a risk factor for bronchiolitis in this study population;[21] secondly, there was no general trend towards enhanced IL-4 production to all antigens in these children, suggesting that the propensity to enhanced IL-4 production is specific and acquired.

In rhinovirus infection, peripheral blood lymphopaenia occurs during the acute phase of the illness (implying migration to the respiratory tract) and the degree of lymphopaenia correlates with the increase in airway reactivity.[81] This may represent selective accumulation of relevant cells in the lung during acute disease. Peripheral depletion of relevant cells would clearly make them less accessible to study during acute disease.

Mast cells may be central to the process as they release both histamine and leukotriene C_4. Both these mediators have been shown to be elevated in respiratory secretions of infants with viral wheeze.[82,83] Furthermore, animal studies have shown that viral infection can lead to mast cell hyperplasia and increased activity with associated bronchial hyperresponsiveness. As discussed above, mast cell counts were not elevated in bronchoalveolar fluid of children prone to viral wheezing when asymptomatic.[61]

MEDIATORS

Lipoxygenase products of arachidonic acid refer to the *cysteinyl-leukotrienes*, which are a group of lipid inflammatory mediators, that are released by all the principal inflammatory cells involved in lung inflammation as well as pulmonary endothelial and epithelial cells. Leukotriene C_4 and D_4 (LTC_4 and LTD_4) are the most active compounds and are potent bronchoconstrictors, affecting both small and large airways. Leukotrienes have also been shown to increase vascular permeability and increase mucus production. Certain respiratory viruses (RSV, parainfluenza 3 and influenza A) have been shown to induce release of LTC_4 into nasopharyngeal secretions.[84] LTC_4 release was particularly enhanced during RSV infection and was detected more often and in higher concentrations in those infants who developed bronchiolitis with wheezing rather than upper respiratory symptoms alone.[83,85] However, a study measuring systemic leukotriene production, found no alteration in urinary LTE_4 levels during acute episodes of viral wheezing in infants.[86] The role of cysteinyl leukotrienes in viral wheeze could be evaluated experimentally using leukotriene receptor antagonists, and it is tempting to speculate that they might have a beneficial effect in infant viral wheezing.

Cyclooxygenase products of arachidonic acid include the *prostaglandins and thromboxane*. Both prostaglandins D_2 and F_{2a} are potent bronchoconstrictors. Plasma levels of the primary metabolite of PGF_{2a} are elevated in infants with RSV bronchiolitis, and those with recurrent wheezing after the infection had the highest initial levels.[87] It has also been shown that RSV antibody complexes enhance neutrophil release of thromboxane, another bronchoconstrictor.[88] Prostaglandin E_2, on the other hand, seems to have an inhibitory effect and may protect the airways from bronchoconstriction. Viral damage of the epithelium may result in loss of some of these protective prostaglandins.

Histamine has been found in increased amounts in the nasopharyngeal secretions and plasma of infants with RSV infection.[82,87] Elevated histamine concentrations have also been found in bronchoalveolar fluid of children with viral wheezing when asymptomatic compared to normal controls, in levels comparable with those found in atopic asthmatics, which is surprising.[75] Persistent lack of therapeutic success with anti-histamines however throws some doubt on the relevance of these findings.

CYTOKINES

Cytokines are extracellular signalling proteins secreted by many different cell types with the ability to modify the behaviour of other closely adjacent cells, via specific receptors on the target cells. There are many different cytokines and new ones are being recognized and classified all the time. They interact through a complex network, influencing the inflammatory and immune responses, so the effects of combinations of cytokines cannot always be predicted based on knowledge of the action of individual ones. Many cytokines have an integral role in promoting and maintaining the chronic airway inflammation found in asthma, mainly due to their influences on eosinophil activity and IgE synthesis. This has been extensively reviewed recently.[89]

Cytokines also participate in the acute inflammatory changes seen during asthma exacerbations, and may be involved in viral wheezing, although there is less direct evidence. We will review some recent studies.

Nasal lavage interleukins (IL-1β, IL-8, IL-6 and TNF-α) are markedly elevated in children with naturally-occurring acute viral URTIs, and with the exception of TNF-α, the levels decreased significantly within 2–4 weeks.[90] The children studied were aged 3–54 months and subjects with a history of mild recurrent wheezing were not excluded. It is not clear how many of the children were also wheezing at the time of lavage, but it certainly implies that these cytokine elevations do not cause wheezing in all children, and therefore other host factors need to be present. Another study has shown that nasal TNF-α levels were significantly increased and present in three-quarters of infants during acute wheezy episodes associated with respiratory tract infections, and this was particularly associated with RSV.[86] However TNF-α was still present in the infants 1 week after they were symptom-free and also detected in more than half of their non-wheezy siblings during a simple URTI. TNF-α contributes to airway obstruction, again other host factors are necessary. IL-11 has been shown to produce airway inflammation and BHR. Its production is stimulated by RSV, parainfluenza and rhinovirus, and it has been detected in nasal aspirates of children with URTI, its levels correlating with clinically detectable wheeze.[91] As mentioned earlier, other nasal lavage work has shown that the eosinophil chemoattractants RANTES and MIP-1α may be important mediators of virus-induced asthma exacerbations.[73] However the same study failed to show a role for IL-5 which would have been expected from its known role in eosinophil regulation and asthma. Using induced sputum, another study has shown that asthmatic patients with confirmed viral infections had increased levels of IL-8 (as well as neutrophil count, ECP and fibrinogen levels) compared with non-asthmatic patients.[92] An experimental model referred to earlier, also showed increased IL-8 in induced sputum, but no increase in ECP, in atopic and non-atopic young adults with viral wheeze.[71]

Interferons (IFNs) may well have a role in viral wheezing.[3] Some may enhance IgE-mediated histamine release after exposure to several respiratory viruses, while others prevent Th2 responses. Whilst RSV has been shown to be acutely sensitive to both IFN-α and IFN-γ *in vitro*, clinical studies show that IFN production seems to be suppressed by RSV, particularly when compared with infection with influenza or parainfluenza viruses. A recent study found increased quantities of IFN-γ in the respiratory tract of infants with RSV bronchiolitis compared with healthy infants and those with RSV-induced URTI alone.[85] In addition, levels of IFN-γ were positively correlated with levels of cysteinyl-leukotrienes. This would imply that those who wheeze with RSV are mounting a Th1 response whilst those with URTI alone a Th2 response. This may appear to be at odds with some of the animal data presented earlier in the section on T-lymphocytes in mice, but in reality it is not. In different inbred strains of mice, there are clear genetic determinants of Th1 or Th2 responses in similarly sensitized RSV infected animals.[93] These studies emphasize the likely variability in the pathogenesis of bronchiolitis in genetically diverse species. For instance, in some infants, a syndrome of 'shock lung' with polymorphonuclear cell efflux may parallel the effects of overexuberant Th1 or cytotoxic T-lymphocyte responses shown in mice,[94] while in others it may represent overactive Th2 cells.[77]

In infants hospitalized with bronchiolitis, decreased production of IFN-γ by blood mononuclear cells correlates with reduced pulmonary function and increased histamine responsiveness 5 months after the acute illness, implying low IFN-γ production may be associated with the later development of asthma.[95] Whether the RSV induces lower levels or whether poor IFN-γ production is a predisposing factor is unknown. Indeed, it seems likely that low IFN-γ production is in truth a reflection of increased production of IL-4 and other type 2 cytokines. Low IFN-γ may therefore be a marker for increased Th2 activity, which itself is hard to determine directly.

ADHESION MOLECULES

Adhesion molecules are receptors located on vascular endothelium and airway epithelium with the corresponding ligands located on circulating leukocytes. ICAM-1 has been shown to act as a neutrophil and eosinophil receptor on airway epithelial cells and induces antigen-induced BHR. It has been shown by several investigators that the majority of rhinoviruses attach to the surface of cells via a receptor identified as ICAM-1.[96] If infection with rhinovirus leads to upregulation of ICAM-1 expression in the lower airways, this could account for rhinovirus-induced neutrophil influx, hyperresponsiveness and wheeze. In addition, upper and lower airway cells infected with RSV or parainfluenza virus, express increased levels of ICAM-1, which will in turn lead to enhanced levels of eosinophil and neutrophil adhesion. Certainly increased levels of soluble ICAM-1 (sICAM-1) have been detected in bronchoalveolar lavage fluid of children with trivial colds, and the elevated levels were still present 1 week after complete resolution of symptoms.[97] Serum levels of sICAM-1 were increased in children with RSV bronchiolitis compared with normal controls, and remained elevated 10 or more days later when the children were well; there was however marked overlap with the normal levels.[98] Another study, however, showed that levels of soluble vascular cell adhesion molecule-1 (VCAM-1) and soluble L-selectin but not ICAM-1, were elevated in infants with acute bronchiolitis, and the RSV status had no influence.[99] The exact nature of any association of levels of adhesion molecules with viral wheezing is not yet clear. However ICAM-1 expression is increased by several cytokines, for example IL-1β and TNF-α, and it is likely that adhesion molecules have a role in the pathogenesis of airway inflammation and viral wheezing.

Host immune responses

The role of host immune responses in protection and disease pathogenesis has been well studied for RSV and influenza virus infections, but less so for other respiratory viruses. Of these, RSV is clearly of major importance for paediatricians.

CELL-MEDIATED IMMUNITY

Cellular immune responses are capable of eliminating viruses before their release from infected cells, but are necessary for an effective protective antibody response to be mounted. To achieve viral elimination, a fine balance between over exuberant reactions and appropriate and rapid elimination of infected cells needs to be achieved. In influenza A infections, cellular immune responses are capable of limiting infection and preventing spread, although antibody responses are also clearly important.

In RSV infection, CMI is also important in antiviral defence, but there is good evidence that it also contributes to the pathological process. Children with impaired CMI show a prolonged shedding of RSV, 40–112 days compared with the usual mean of 7 days.[100] These children also develop RSV pneumonia at an age when this is otherwise uncommon (over 3 years old). Although a 10-year prospective study did not find any evidence that CMI contributed significantly to the outcome of RSV infection,[101] virus-specific cellular cytotoxic activity has been demonstrated in infants with acute RSV infection, usually within 1 week.[102] Chiba et al. found the activity was age-dependent with the response found in 65% of those aged 6–24 months, but in only 35–38% of those aged 5 months or less; this may, in part, account for the severity of the disease in the younger age group.[103]

The reason for the relatively poor CMI response in the young may be immunological immaturity, but it is more likely that the greater response seen in older children is a reflection of previous RSV infection. The enhanced response in older children may simply represent booster effects secondary to stimulation of memory cells.

HUMORAL IMMUNITY

The humoral immune response has an important role in protection against respiratory viruses, which is confirmed by the beneficial effect on incidence and severity of RSV bronchiolitis in children given prophylactic RSV immune globulin or humanized monoclonal antibody,[104] and by the evident serotype-specific protection conferred by influenza vaccination. Passive antibody therapy that delays respiratory viral infection to later childhood may even reduce the frequency and severity of pulmonary disease in later childhood.[105,106]

In a similar way to the CMI response, age has an important effect on humoral immunity. Infants under 6–8 months mount a poor antibody response to respiratory viral infections compared with older infants, and there is often a failure to develop a protective secretory IgA or neutralizing IgG response.[107] This poor antibody response is thought to be due to immaturity of the immune system. While this may account for the general age distribution of the disease, it does not account for the differences in disease severity seen amongst individuals of the same age. Concurrent or preceding infection and host genetics may play an important part.[108]

It has been argued that the presence of passively acquired maternal antibody may have an immunosuppressive effect on the development of the infant's own immune response. It seems that it is the response to the G glycoprotein of RSV that is particularly affected by maternal antibodies.[109] There is contrasting evidence as to whether these maternal antibodies are harmful or helpful. It has been hypothesized that due to lack of specific secretory IgA during the initial challenge with RSV, maternal IgG could diffuse to the lumen of the infant airways and form immune complexes.[110] Phagocytosis of these RSV:IgG immune complexes has been shown to stimulate release of inflammatory mediators by neutrophils, which could contribute to the pathological process.[111] Conversely, there is good evidence that maternal antibodies have a protective role in the first month of life and passive antibody therapy is effective in preventing disease in high-risk children.[112] RSV infection is commonest under the age of 6 months when these antibody titres are at their highest. As well as this, infants with the highest titres of transplacentally acquired RSV-specific IgG tend to develop less severe RSV pneumonia than those with lower titres and have significantly fewer infections.[113] Although high levels of passive antibody are protective, maternal antibody is detectable in infants up to 5 months and yet fails to protect children with the highest incidence of disease.

MUCOSAL IMMUNITY

The common respiratory viral infections enter the host via the airways, and some will then progress distally to the parenchyma of the lung. It is for this reason, that mucosal immunity has such an important role in the fight against these viruses, as it provides the host's first line of defence.

IgA is the predominant immunoglobulin in respiratory secretions, where it is found in its dimeric form known as secretory IgA (sIgA). Levels of nasal sIgA may determine susceptibility to respiratory infection. It has been shown that infants who mount a greater nasal non-specific IgA response have fewer respiratory infections, although the frequency of infection was not associated with the baseline nasal IgA level.[114] However a more recent study has shown that wheezy infants mount a normal nasal IgA response to viral infection when compared to their non-wheezing siblings with simple URTIs.[115]

Local IgE production may have a role in the pathogenesis of viral-wheezing (reviewed in ref. 116). Significantly higher titres of RSV-specific IgE in naso-pharyngeal secretions were found in those who wheezed compared with those with non-wheezing RSV infection; similar results were found in parainfluenza infection. The original specific-IgE response was found to be predictive of future wheezing at both 4 and 7–8 year follow-up.[25] This work suggests an association between the production of RSV-IgE and wheezing, although it is possible that virus-specific IgE antibody becomes mast cell bound and interacts with viral antigen, leading to the release of vasoactive and inflammatory mediators, which cause airway narrowing. The bronchoconstrictor mediator leukotriene C_4, detected in the nasopharyngeal secretions of infants with RSV bronchiolitis was positively correlated with RSV-IgE titres.[83] Other groups have found these studies hard to replicate, being unable to detect RSV-specific IgE.

The reason why certain children seem prone to a hyperactive IgE response may be related to abnormal T-cell regulatory mechanisms. Welliver has shown a reduced number of CD8 positive cells (suppressor/cytotoxic T-lymphocytes) during convalescence in those who wheezed with RSV compared with those with upper respiratory illness alone.[117] There was also an inverse correlation between RSV-IgE in nasopharyngeal secretions and CD8 positive cells in peripheral blood and it is suggested that these cells may include some that are responsible for suppression of IgE production. It is unknown whether this abnormal IgE regulation is virus-induced or constitutionally determined. Host factors, which regulate the response of T-lymphocytes to RSV, may be critical in determining the clinical outcome of RSV infection. CD8 T-cells and NK cells are an abundant source of IFN-γ, which inhibits the development of CD4 T-cells making IL-4 and IL-5, and it is these latter cytokines which are responsible for IgE production and eosinophilia.[118]

PROSPECTS FOR PREVENTION AND TREATMENT

New insights into the pathogenesis of respiratory viral infections suggest that a duel approach to treatment may be necessary. Prevention of infection by vaccination or antiviral therapy may clearly be beneficial. But in addition, it may also be beneficial to reduce the severity of the immune response, since much of the disease that results from respiratory viral infection is due to an exuberant inflammatory response.

With regard to *vaccination*, progress is being made with protein subunit vaccines, live attenuated vaccination, DNA vaccination and possibly synthetic vaccines based on know-ledge of antigenic peptides.[119,120] Clinical trials have been performed with purified fusion protein from RSV in children with bronchopulmonary dysplasia,[121] and cystic fibrosis,[122] both with promising results. There is also considerable interest in the potential to protect neonates by vaccination of pre-pregnant women, and pregnant or breast-feeding mothers. This may indeed by a good approach for some respiratory viral infections.[123] Since age appears to be a critical factor in the long-lasting effect of viral infections in childhood, a vaccine which delays infection until a later stage may have substantial later beneficial effects. It may indeed be possible to reduce the burden of viral wheeze in preschool children if effective vaccines are introduced. Such vaccines have the potential to affect the later development of asthma.

In terms of *passive immunotherapy*, the introduction of humanized monoclonal antibody to prevent RSV disease in high-risk children constitutes a major milestone.[124,125] It is possible that administering the antigen-binding fragment of antibody (Fab) by inhalation may be even more effective,[126] although this awaits testing in man. At present, the cost of passive immunotherapy has to be balanced against the likely benefits, and the treatment advantage is not always clear.[127]

New *antiviral therapies* are also promising, and many are under development. The use of anti-influenza drugs has not been universally adopted, despite their quite remarkable efficacy. These drugs have to be administered either prophylactically or within the first 48 hours of infection to have a significant effect on the duration of disease. It is probable that effective antivirals against specific respiratory viruses will become generally available during the next 5 years. Improved diagnostics are essential if they are to be targeted on those most likely to benefit.

An additional approach may be to treat the viral infection at the same time as using *immunomodulators* that reduce the severity of the immune reaction. Immune modulation based on elimination of T-cell subsets, anti-cytokines, anti-chemokines and the inhibition of antigen presentation all may have promise for the future. The advantage of these approaches to therapy is that they may be beneficial regardless of the type of virus that has initiated the inflammatory response. The drawback that immunotherapy causes immunosuppression may be overcome by the introduction of more selective agents.

REFERENCES

1. Wickens K, Pearce N, Crane J, Beasley R. Antibiotic use in early childhood and the development of asthma. *Clin Exp Allergy* 1999;**29**:766–71.
2. Pattemore PK, Johnston SL, Bardin PG. Viruses as precipitants of asthma symptoms. I. Epidemiology. *Clin Exp Allergy* 1992;**22**:325–36.
3. Balfour-Lynn IM. Why do viruses make infants wheeze? *Arch Dis Child* 1996;**74**:251–9.
4. Corne JM, Holgate ST. Mechanisms of virus induced exacerbations of asthma. *Thorax* 1997;**52**:380–9.
5. Johnston SL. Viruses and asthma. *Allergy* 1998; **53**:922–32.
6. Openshaw PJM, Hewitt C. Protective and harmful effects of viral infections in childhood on wheezing disorders and asthma. *Am J Respir Crit Care Med* 2000;**162**:S40–3.
7. Johnston SL, Pattemore PK, Sanderson G, *et al.* Community study of role of viral infections in exacerbations of asthma in 9–11 year old children. *Br Med J* 1995;**310**:1225–9.
8. Johnston SL, Pattemore PK, Sanderson G, *et al.* The relationship between upper respiratory infections and hospital admissions for asthma: a time-trend analysis. *Am J Respir Crit Care Med* 1996;**154**:654–60.
9. Minor TE, Baker JW, Dick EC, DeMeo AN, Ouellette JJ, Cohen M, Reed CE. Greater frequency of viral respiratory infections in asthmatic children as compared with their nonasthmatic siblings. *J Pediatr* 1974;**85**:472–7.
10. Horn MEC, Gregg I. Role of viral infection and host factors in acute episodes of asthma and chronic bronchitis. *Chest* 1973;**63**(Suppl):S44–8.
11. Long CE, McBride JT, Hall CB. Sequelae of respiratory syncytial virus infections. A role for intervention studies. *Am J Respir Crit Care Med* 1995;**151**:1678–81.
12. Ball TM, Castro-Rodriguez JA, Griffith KA, Holberg CJ, Martinez FD, Wright AL. Siblings, day-care attendance and the risk of asthma and wheezing during childhood. *New Engl J Med* 2000;**343**:538–43.
13. Martinez FD, Morgan WJ, Wright AL, Holberg C, Taussig LM, Group Health Medical Associates. Initial airway function is a risk factor for recurrent respiratory illnesses during the first three years of life. *Am Rev Respir Dis* 1991;**143**:312–16.
14. Nicholson KG, Kent J, Ireland DC. Respiratory viruses and exacerbations of asthma in adults. *Br Med J* 1993;**307**:982–6.
15. Gern JE, Busse WW. Association of rhinovirus infections with asthma. *Clin Micro Rev* 1999;**12**:9–18.
16. Madge P, Paton JY, McColl JH, Mackie PL. Prospective controlled study of four infection-control procedures to prevent nosocomial infection with respiratory syncytial virus. *Lancet* 1992;**340**:1079–83.
16a. Hogg JC. Role of latent viral infections in chronic obstructive pulmonary disease and asthma. *Am J Resp Crit Care Med* 2001;**164**(10 pt 2):571–5.
17. Johnston SL, Sanderson G, Pattemore PK, Smith S, Bardin PG, Bruce CB, Lambden PR, Tyrrell DAJ, Holgate ST. Use of polymerase chain reaction for diagnosis of picornavirus infection in subjects with and without respiratory symptoms. *J Clin Micro* 1993;**31**:111–17.
18. Balfour-Lynn IM, Girdhar DR, Aitken C. Diagnosing respiratory syncytial virus by nasal lavage. *Arch Dis Child* 1995;**72**:58–9.
19. Openshaw PJM, Hewitt CR. Protective and harmful effects of viral infections in childhood on wheezing disorders and asthma. *Am J Respir Crit Care Med* 2000;**162**:S40–3.

20. Sigurs N, Bjarnason R, Sigurbergsson F, Kjellman B, Bjorksten B. Asthma and immunoglobulin E antibodies after respiratory syncytial virus bronchiolitis: a prospective cohort study with matched controls. *Pediatrics* 1995;**95**:500–5.

21. Sigurs N, Bjarnason R, Sigurbergsson F, Kjellman B. Respiratory syncytial virus bronchiolitis in infancy is an important risk factor for asthma and allergy at age 7. *Am J Respir Crit Care Med* 2000;**161**:1501–7.

22. Noble V, Murray M, Webb MSC, Alexander J, Swarbrick AS, Milner AD. Respiratory status and allergy nine to 10 years after acute bronchiolitis. *Arch Dis Child* 1997;**76**:315–19.

23. Dezateux C, Fletcher ME, Dundas I, Stocks J. Infant respiratory function after RSV-proven bronchiolitis. *Am J Respir Crit Care Med* 1997;**155**:1349–55.

24. Openshaw PJM, Walzl G. Infections prevent the development of asthma – true, false or both? *J Roy Soc Med* 1999;**92**:495–9.

25. Welliver RC, Duffy L. The relationship of RSV-specific immunoglobulin E antibody responses in infancy, recurrent wheezing, and pulmonary function at age 7–8 years. *Pediatr Pulmonol* 1993;**15**:19–27.

26. Ehlenfield DR, Cameron K, Welliver RC. Eosinophilia at the time of respiratory syncytial virus bronchiolitis predicts childhood reactive airway disease. *Pediatrics* 2000;**105**:79–83.

27. Koller DY, Wojnarowski C, Herkner KR, Weinlander G, Raderer M, Eichler I, Frischer T. High levels of eosinophil cationic protein in wheezing infants predict the development of asthma. *J Allergy Clin Immunol* 1997;**99**:752–6.

28. Clough JB, Keeping KA, Edwards LC, Freeman WM, Warner JA, Warner JO. Can we predict which wheezy infants will continue to wheeze? *Am J Respir Crit Care Med* 1999;**160**:1473–80.

29. Bont L, Heijnen CJ, Kavelaars A, van Aalderen WMC, Brus F, Draaisma JThM, Geelen SM, Kimpen JLL. Monocyte IL-10 production during respiratory syncytial virus bronchiolitis is associated with recurrent wheezing in a one-year follow-up study. *Am J Respir Crit Care Med* 2000;**161**:1518–23.

30. Robinson PJ, Hegele RG, Schellenberg RR. Allergic sensitization increases airway reactivity in guinea pigs with respiratory syncytial virus bronchiolitis. *J Allergy Clin Immunol* 1997;**100**:492–8.

31. Kumar A, Sorkness RL, Kaplan MR, Lemanske RF, Jr. Chronic, episodic, reversible airway obstruction after viral bronchiolitis in rats. *Am J Respir Crit Care Med* 1997;**155**:130–4.

32. Dakhama A, Vitalis TZ, Hegele RG. Persistence of respiratory syncytial virus (RSV) infection and development of RSV-specific IgG1 response in a guinea-pig model of acute bronchiolitis. *Eur Respir J* 1997;**10**:20–6.

33. Openshaw PJM. When we sneeze, does the immune system catch a cold? *Br Med J* 1991;**303**:935–6.

34. Sakamoto M, Ida S, Takishima T. Effect of influenza virus infection on allergic sensitization to aerosolized ovalbumin in mice. *J Immunol* 1984;**132**:2614–17.

35. Suzuki S, Suzuki Y, Yamamoto N, Matsumoto Y, Shirai A, Okubo T. Influenza A virus infection increases IgE production and airway responsiveness in aerosolized antigen-exposed mice. *J Allergy Clin Immunol* 1998;**102**:732–40.

36. O'Donnell DR, Openshaw PJM. Anaphylactic sensitization to aeroantigen during respiratory virus infection. *Clin Exp Allergy* 1998;**28**:1501–8.

37. Martinez FD, Morgan WJ, Wright AL, Holberg CJ, Taussig LM, 'Group Health Medical Associates' personnel. Diminished lung function as a predisposing factor for wheezing respiratory illness in infants. *New Engl J Med* 1988;**319**:1112–17.

38. Tager IB, Hanrahan JP, Tosteson TD, Castile RG, Brown RW, Weiss ST, Speizer FE. Lung function, pre- and post-natal smoke exposure, and wheezing in the first year of life. *Am Rev Respir Dis* 1993;**147**:811–17.

39. Young S, O'Keefe PT, Arnott J, Landau LI. Lung function, airways responsiveness, and respiratory symptoms before and after bronchiolitis. *Arch Dis Child* 1995;**72**:16–24.

40. Clarke JR, Salmon B, Silverman M. Bronchial responsiveness in the neonatal period as a risk factor for wheezing in infancy. *Am J Respir Crit Care Med* 1995;**151**:1434–40.

41. Martinez FD, Wright AL, Taussig LM, Holberg CJ, Halonen M, Morgan WJ. Asthma and wheezing in the first six years of life. The Group Health Medical Associates. *New Engl J Med* 1995;**332**:133–8.

42. Young S, Arnott J, O'Keefe PT, Le Souef PN, Landau LI. The association between early lung function and wheezing during the first 2 years of life. *Eur Respir J* 2000;**15**:151–7.

43. Stick SM, Arnott J, Turner DJ, Young S, Landau LI, LeSouef PN. Bronchial responsiveness and lung function in recurrently wheezy infants. *Am Rev Respir Dis* 1991;**144**:1012–15.

44. Clarke JR, Reese A, Silverman M. Bronchial responsiveness and lung function in infants with lower respiratory tract illness over the first six months of life. *Arch Dis Child* 1992;**67**:1454–8.

45. Young S, O'Keefe PT, Arnott J, Landau LI. Lung function, airway responsiveness, and respiratory symptoms before and after bronchiolitis. *Arch Dis Child* 1995; **72**:16–24.

46. Martinez FD. Role of respiratory infection in onset of asthma and chronic obstructive pulmonary disease. *Clin Exp Allergy* 1999;**29**(Suppl 2):53–8.

47. Stein RT, Sherrill D, Morgan WJ, Holberg CJ, Halonen M, Taussig LM, Wright AL, Martinez FD. Respiratory syncytial virus in early life and risk of wheeze and allergy by age 13 years. *Lancet* 1999;**354**:541–5.

48. Butland BK, Strachan DP, Lewis S, Bynner J, Butler N, Britton J. Investigation into the increase in hay fever

and eczema at age 16 observed between the 1958 and 1970 British birth cohorts. *Br Med J* 1997;**315**:717–21.

49. Strachan DP, Taylor EM, Carpenter RG. Family structure, neonatal infection, and hay fever in adolescence. *Arch Dis Child* 1996;**74**:422–6.

50. Shaheen SO, Aaby P, Hall AJ, Barker DJ, Heyes CB, Shiell AW, Goudiaby A. Measles and atopy in Guinea-Bissau. *Lancet* 1996;**347**:1792–6.

51. Bodmer C, Anderson WJ, Reid TS, Godden DJ on behalf of the WHEASE Study Group. Childhood exposure to infection and the risk of adult onset wheeze and atopy. *Thorax* 2000;**55**:383–7.

52. Martinez FD, Stern DA, Wright AL, Taussig LM, Halonen M. Association of non-wheezing lower respiratory tract illnesses in early life with persistently diminished serum IgE levels. Group Health Medical Associates. *Thorax* 1995;**50**:1067–72.

53. Von Mutius E, Martinez FD, Fritzsch C, Nicolai T, Roell G, Thiemann HH. Prevalence of asthma and atopy in two areas of West and East Germany. *Am J Respir Crit Care Med* 1994;**149**:358–64.

54. Shirakawa T, Enomoto T, Shimazu S, Hopkin JM. The inverse association between tuberculin responses and atopic disorder. *Science* 1997;**275**:77–9.

55. Matricardi PM, Rosmini F, Ferrigno L, Nisini R, Rapicetta M, Chionne P, Stroffolini T, Pasquini P, D'Amelio R. Cross sectional retrospective study of prevalence of atopy among Italian military students with antibodies against hepatitis A virus. *Br Med J* 1997;**314**:999–1003.

56. Romagnani S. Induction of TH1 and TH2 responses: a key role for the 'natural' immune response? *Immunol Today* 1992;**13**:379–81.

57. Prescott SL, Macaubas C, Holt BJ, Smallacombe TB, Loh R, Sly PD, Holt PG. Transplacental priming of the human immune system to environmental allergens: universal skewing of initial T cell responses toward the Th2 cytokine profile. *J Immunol* 1998;**160**:4730–7.

58. Prescott SL, Macaubas C, Smallacombe T, Holt BJ, Sly PD, Holt PG. Development of allergen-specific T-cell memory in atopic and normal children. *Lancet* 1999;**353**:196–200.

59. Busse WW. Respiratory infections: their role in airway responsiveness and the pathogenesis of asthma. *J Allergy Clin Immunol* 1990;**85**:671–83.

60. Martinez FD, Taussig LM, Morgan WJ. Infants with upper respiratory illnesses have significant reductions in maximal expiratory flow. *Pediatr Pulmonol* 1990; **9**:91–5.

61. Stevenson EC, Turner G, Heaney LG, Schock BC, Taylor B, Gallagher T, Ennis M, Shields MD. Bronchoalveolar lavage findings suggest two different forms of childhood asthma. *Clin Exp Allergy* 1997; **27**:1027–35.

62. Folkerts G, Busse WW, Nijkamp FP, Sorkness R, Gern JE. Virus-induced airway hyperresponsiveness and asthma. *Am J Respir Crit Care Med* 1998;**157**:1708–20.

63. McKean MC, Leech M, Lambert PC, Hewitt C, Myint S, Silverman M. A model of viral wheeze in non-asthmatic adults: symptoms and physiology. *Eur Respir J* 2001;**18**:23–32.

64. Empey DW, Laitinen LA, Jacobs L, Gold WM, Nadel JA. Mechanisms of bronchial hyperreactivity in normal subjects after upper respiratory tract infection. *Am Rev Respir Dis* 1976;**113**:131–9.

65. Jacoby DB, Fryer AD. Interaction of viral infections with muscarinic receptors. *Clin Exp Allergy* 1999;**29**(Suppl 2):59–64.

66. Fraenkel DJ, Bardin PG, Sanderson G, Lampe F, Johnston SL, Holgate ST. Lower airways inflammation during rhinovirus colds in normal and in asthmatic subjects. *Am J Respir Crit Care Med* 1995; **151**:879–86.

67. Trigg CJ, Nicholson KG, Wang JH, Ireland DC, Jordan S, Duddle JM, Hamilton S, Davies RJ. Bronchial inflammation and the common cold: a comparison of atopic and non-atopic individuals. *Clin Exp Allergy* 1996;**26**:665–76.

68. Welliver RC. Immunologic mechanisms of virus-induced wheezing and asthma. *J Pediatr* 1999;**135**:S14–20.

69. Teran LM, Johnston SL, Schröder J-M, Church MK, Holgate ST. Role of nasal interleukin-8 in neutrophil recruitment and activation in children with virus-induced asthma. *Am J Respir Crit Care Med* 1997;**155**:1362–6.

70. Everard ML, Swarbrick A, Wrightham M, McIntyre J, Dunkley C, James PD, Sewell HF, Milner AD. Analysis of cells obtained by bronchial lavage of infants with respiratory syncytial virus infection. *Arch Dis Child* 1994;**71**:428–32.

71. McKean MC, Hewitt C, Lambert PC, Myint S, Silverman M. An adult model of viral wheeze: inflammation in the upper and lower respiratory tracts. *Clin Exp Allergy* 2002; in press.

72. Garofalo R, Kimpen JL, Welliver RC, Ogra PL. Eosinophil degranulation in the respiratory tract during naturally acquired syncytial virus infection. *J Pediatr* 1992; **120**:28–32.

73. Teran LM, Seminario MC, Shute JK, Papi A, Compton SJ, Low JL, Gleich GJ, Johnston SL. RANTES, macrophage-inhibitory protein 1α, and the eosinophil product major basic protein are released into upper respiratory secretions during virus-induced asthma exacerbations in children. *J Infect Dis* 1999;**179**:677–81.

74. Harrison AM, Bonville CA, Rosenberg HF, Domachowske JB. Respiratory syncytial virus-induced chemokine expression in the lower airways: eosinophil recruitment and degranulation. *Am J Respir Crit Care Med* 1999;**159**:1918–24.

75. Ennis M, Turner G, Schock BC, Stevenson EC, Brown V, Fitch PS, Heaney LG, Taylor B, Shields MD. Inflammatory mediators in bronchoalveolar lavage samples from children with and without asthma. *Clin Exp Allergy* 1999;**29**:362–6.

76. Openshaw PJM, Pala P, Sparer T, Matthews S, Pennycook A, Hussell T. T-cell subsets and lung inflammation: lessons from respiratory syncytial virus. *Eur Respir Rev* 2000;**10**:108–11.

77. Alwan WH, Kozlowska WJ, Openshaw PJM. Distinct types of lung disease caused by functional subsets of antiviral T cells. *J Exp Med* 1994;**179**:81–9.

78. Openshaw PJM. Immunopathological mechanisms in respiratory syncytial virus disease. *Sem Immunopathol* 1995;**17**:187–201.

79. Smyth RL, Fletcher JN, Thomas HM, Hart CA, Openshaw PJM. Sustained immune activation following bronchiolitis in infancy. *Lancet* 1999;**354**:1997–8.

80. Pala P, Bjarnason R, Sigurbergsson F, Metcalfe C, Sigurs N, Openshaw PJM. Enhanced IL-4 responses in children with a history of respiratory syncytial virus bronchiolitis in infancy. *Eur Resp J* 2002; in press.

81. Levandowski RA, Ou DW, Jackson GG. Acute-phase decrease of T lymphocyte subsets in rhinovirus infection. *J Infect Dis* 1986;**153**:743–8.

82. Welliver RC, Wong DT, Sun M, Middleton Jr E, Vaughan RS, Ogra PL. The development of respiratory syncytial virus-specific IgE and the release of histamine in nasopharyngeal secretions after infection. *New Engl J Med* 1981;**305**:841–6.

83. Volovitz B, Welliver RC, De Castro G, Krystofik DA, Ogra PL. The release of leukotrienes in the respiratory tract during infection with respiratory syncytial virus: role in obstructive airway disease. *Pediatr Res* 1988; **24**:504–7.

84. Volovitz B, Faden H, Ogra PL. Release of leukotriene C4 in respiratory tract during acute viral infection. *J Pediatr* 1988;**112**:218–22.

85. Van Schaik SM, Tristram DA, Nagpal IS, Hintz K, Welliver RC II, Welliver RC. Increased production of interferon gamma and cysteinyl leukotrienes in virus-induced wheezing. *J Allergy Clin Immunol* 1999; **103**:630–6.

86. Balfour-Lynn IM, Valman HB, Wellings R, Webster ADB, Taylor GW, Silverman M. Tumour necrosis factor-α and leukotriene E$_4$ production in wheezy infants. *Clin Exp Allergy* 1994;**24**:121–6.

87. Skoner DP, Fireman P, Caliguiri L, Davis H. Plasma elevations of histamine and a prostaglandin metabolite in acute bronchiolitis. *Am Rev Respir Dis* 1990;**142**:359–64.

88. Faden H, Kaul TN, Ogra PL. Activation of oxidative and arachidonic acid metabolism in neutrophils by respiratory syncytial virus antibody complexes: possible role in disease. *J Infect Dis* 1983; **148**:110–16.

89. Chung KF, Barnes PJ. Cytokines in asthma. *Thorax* 1999;**54**:825–57.

90. Noah TL, Henderson FW, Wortman IA, Devlin RB, Handy J, Koren HS, Becker S. Nasal cytokine production in viral acute upper respiratory infections of childhood. *J Infect Dis* 1995;**17**:584–92.

91. Einarsson O, Geba GP, Zhu Z, Landry M, Elias JA. Interleukin-11: stimulation *in vivo* and *in vitro* by respiratory viruses and induction of airways hyperresponsiveness. *J Clin Invest* 1996;**97**:915–24.

92. Pizzichini MM, Pizzichini E, Efthimiadis A, Chauhan AJ, Johnston SL, Hussack P, Mahony J, Dolovich J, Hargreave F. Asthma and natural colds. Inflammatory indices in induced sputum: a feasibility study. *Am J Respir Crit Care Med* 1998;**158**: 1178–84.

93. Hussell T, Georgiou A, Sparer TE, Matthews S, Pala P, Openshaw PJM. Host genetic determinants of vaccine-induced eosinophilia during respiratory syncytial virus infection. *J Immunol* 1998;**161**: 6215–22.

94. Cannon MJ, Openshaw PJM, Askonas BA. Cytotoxic T cells clear virus but augment lung pathology in mice infected with respiratory syncytial virus. *J Exp Med* 1988;**168**:1163–8.

95. Renzi PM, Turgeon JP, Marcotte JE, Drblik SP, Bérubé D, Gagnon MF, Spier S. Reduced interferon-γ production in infants with bronchiolitis and asthma. *Am J Respir Crit Care Med* 1999;**159**:1417–22.

96. Johnston SL, Bardin PG, Pattemore PK. Viruses as precipitants of asthma symptoms III. Rhinoviruses: molecular biology and prospects for future intervention. *Clin Exp Allergy* 1993;**23**:237–46.

97. Grigg J, Riedler J, Robertson CF. Bronchoalveolar lavage fluid cellularity and soluble intercellular adhesion molecule-1 in children with colds. *Pediatr Pulmonol* 1999;**28**:109–16.

98. Smyth RL, Fletcher JN, Thomas HM, Hart CA. Immunological responses to respiratory syncytial virus infection in infancy. *Arch Dis Child* 1997;**76**: 210–14.

99. Øymar K, Bjerknes R. Differential patterns of circulating adhesion molecules in children with bronchial asthma and acute bronchiolitis. *Pediatr Allergy Immunol* 1998;**9**:73–9.

100. Fishaut M, Tubergen D, McIntosh K. Cellular response to respiratory viruses with particular reference to children with disorders of cell-mediated immunity. *J Pediatr* 1980;**96**:179–86.

101. Fernald GW, Almond JR, Henderson FW. Cellular and humoral immunity in recurrent respiratory syncytial virus infections. *Pediatr Res* 1983;**17**:753–8.

102. Isaacs D, Bangham CRM, McMichael AJ. Cell-mediated cytotoxic response to respiratory syncytial virus in infants with bronchiolitis. *Lancet* 1987;**ii**:769–71.

103. Chiba Y, Higashidate Y, Suga K, Honjo K, Tsutsumi H, Ogra PL. Development of cell-mediated cytotoxic immunity to respiratory syncytial virus in human infants following naturally acquired infection. *J Med Virol* 1989;**28**:133–9.

104. Groothuis JR, Simoes EA, Levin MJ, *et al*. Prophylactic administration of respiratory syncytial virus immune globulin to high-risk infants and young children.

The Respiratory Syncytial Virus Immune Globulin Study Group. *New Engl J Med* 1993;**329**:1524–30.

105. Wenzel SE, Gibbs R, Lehr M, Park N, Simoes EAF. Asthma related clinical and physiologic outcomes in high risk children 5–9 years after prophylaxis with RSV IgIV. *Am J Respir Crit Care Med* 2000;**161**:A898.

106. Simoes EA. Respiratory syncytial virus infection. *Lancet* 1999;**354**:847–52.

107. Murphy BR, Graham BS, Prince GA, Walsh EE, Chanock RM, Karzon DT, Wright PF. Serum and nasal-wash immunoglobulin G and A antibody response of infants and children to respiratory syncytial virus F and G glycoproteins following primary infection. *J Clin Micro* 1986;**23**:1009–14.

108. Walzl G, Tafuro S, Moss PA, Openshaw PJM, Hussell T. Influenza virus lung infection protects from respiratory syncytial virus-induced immunopathology. *J Exp Med* 2000;**191**:1317–26.

109. Murphy BR, Alling DW, Snyder MH, *et al.* Effect of age and pre-existing antibody on serum antibody response of infants and children to the F and G glycoproteins during respiratory syncytial virus infection. *J Clin Micro* 1986;**24**:894–8.

110. Nadal D, Ogra PL. Development of local immunity: role in mechanisms of protection against or pathogenesis of respiratory syncytial viral infections. *Lung* 1990;**168**(Suppl):379–87.

111. Kaul TN, Faden H, Ogra PL. Effect of respiratory syncytial virus and virus-antibody complexes on the oxidative metabolism of human neutrophils. *Infect Immunity* 1981;**32**:649–54.

112. Groothuis JR. Treatment and prevention of severe respiratory syncytial virus infection in young children. *Curr Opin Infect Dis* 1995;**8**:206–8.

113. Glezen WP, Paredes A, Allison JE, Taber LH, Frank AL. Risk of respiratory syncytial virus infection for infants from low-income families in relationship to age, sex, ethnic group, and maternal antibody level. *J Pediatr* 1981;**98**:708–15.

114. Yodfat Y, Silvian I. A prospective study of acute respiratory tract infections among children in a kibbutz: The role of secretory IgA and serum immunoglobulins. *J Infect Dis* 1977;**136**:26–30.

115. Balfour-Lynn IM, Valman HB, Silverman M, Webster ADB. Nasal IgA response in wheezy infants. *Arch Dis Child* 1993;**68**:472–6.

116. Stark JM, Busse WW. Respiratory virus infection and airway hyperreactivity in children. *Pediatr Allergy Immunol* 1991;**2**:95–110.

117. Welliver RC, Kaul TN, Sun M, Ogra PL. Defective regulation of immune responses in respiratory syncytial virus infection. *J Immunol* 1984; **133**:1925–30.

118. Openshaw PJM. Immunity and immunopathology to respiratory syncytial virus: the mouse model. *Am J Respir Crit Care Med* 1995;**152**:S59–62.

119. Dudas RA, Karron RA. Respiratory syncytial virus vaccines. *Clin Microbiol Rev* 1998;**11**:430–9.

120. Crowe JEJ. Immune responses of infants to infection with respiratory viruses and live attenuated respiratory virus candidate vaccines. *Vaccine* 1998; **16**:1423–32.

121. Groothuis JR, King SJ, Hogerman DA, Paradiso PR, Simoes EA. Safety and immunogenicity of a purified F protein respiratory syncytial virus (PFP-2) vaccine in seropositive children with bronchopulmonary dysplasia. *J Infect Dis* 1998;**177**:467–9.

122. Piedra PA, Grace S, Jewell A, Spinelli S, Hogerman DA, Malinoski F, Hiatt PW. Sequential annual administration of purified fusion protein vaccine against respiratory syncytial virus in children with cystic fibrosis. *Pediatr Infect Dis J* 1998;**17**:217–24.

123. Englund J, Glezen WP, Piedra PA. Maternal immunization against viral disease. *Vaccine* 1998; **16**:1456–63.

124. Simoes EA, Sondheimer HM, Top FH J, Meissner HC, Welliver RC, Kramer AA, Groothuis JR. Respiratory syncytial virus immune globulin for prophylaxis against respiratory syncytial virus disease in infants and children with congenital heart disease. *J Pediatr* 1998;**133**:492–9.

125. The Impact-RSV Study Group. Palivizumab, a humanized respiratory syncytial virus monoclonal antibody, reduces hospitalization from respiratory syncytial virus infection in high-risk infants. *Pediatrics* 1998;**102**:531–7.

126. Crowe JEJ, Gilmour PS, Murphy BR, Chanock RM, Duan L, Pomerantz RJ, Pilkington GR. Isolation of a second recombinant human respiratory syncytial virus monoclonal antibody fragment Fab RSVF2-5) that exhibits therapeutic efficacy in vivo. *J Infect Dis* 1998;**177**:1073–6.

127. O'Shea TM, Sevick MA, Givner LB. Costs and benefits of respiratory syncytial virus immunoglobulin to prevent hospitalization for lower respiratory tract illness in very low birth weight infants. *Pediatr Infect Dis J* 1998;**17**:587–93.

128. Silverman M, Wilson NM. Wheezing phenotypes in childhood. *Thorax* 1997;**52**:936–7.

7c

Gastroesophageal reflux

ISI DAB AND ANNE MALFROOT

INTRODUCTION

For several years gastroesophageal reflux belonged exclusively to the domain of gastroenterologists, because it was believed to cause oesophageal injury only, with different degrees of oesophagitis which could cause growth retardation, haematemesis, iron deficiency, pain and oesophageal stenosis. The first report relating gastroesophageal reflux to a respiratory complication came in 1946 when Mendelson[1] observed that the aspiration of gastric contents into the respiratory tract caused asthma. Three decades later Mansfield[2] demonstrated that pulmonary aspiration is not a prerequisite: abnormally low pH values in the oesophagus can also trigger bronchospasm in some subjects. This finding prompted pulmonologists, especially paediatric pulmonologists, to show an increased interest in gastroesophageal reflux and to suspect it whenever patients without underlying infections or allergy experienced unexplained chronic or relapsing respiratory problems, or chronic cough.

Definition

One should not mistake belching or possetting (the regurgitation of a small amount of curdled milk, soon after a feed) for gastroesophageal reflux. The term belching is restricted to harmless events, which may be observed in up to 38% of healthy newborns.[3] Gastroesophageal reflux is an abnormal event, which is often though not always harmful. Reflux and belching have some characteristics in common and are characterized by intermittent retrograde movements of the gastric contents into the oesophagus and occasionally into the pharynx or mouth.

Gastroesophageal reflux can be defined functionally by measuring the frequency and the intensity of the reflux, which in healthy subjects should not exceed a certain threshold. Regurgitations and reflux episodes are thus specified by quantitative characteristics, because although they form a continuum, the exact dividing line between them remains ill-defined. It is not always possible to separate the children who are diseased from those who are not.

Relationship between gastroesophageal reflux and respiratory disease

Theoretically, whenever gastroesophageal reflux and respiratory disease are present together, only three possibilities exist: either the co-existence is purely coincidental without any causal relationship, or reflux is a complication of the respiratory disorder, or the gastroesophageal reflux is the primary disorder and induces respiratory symptoms.

The most frequently studied relationship is that between asthma and gastroesophageal reflux. Studies started originally in adults,[2,4,5] before several investigators embarked upon studying asthmatic children without allergy.[6–13] Most authors, except Moote[4] and Ekström,[5] have shown that asthma was secondary to reflux and not the reverse and that the management of gastroesophageal reflux decreased the asthma attacks, whereas the symptomatic treatment of asthma attacks did not decrease the number or the severity of reflux episodes. More recently Palombini et al.[14] demonstrated that in adults chronic non-productive cough could be caused by gastroesophageal reflux disease. Even in infants and preschool children suffering from cystic fibrosis, gastroesophageal reflux is unexpectedly frequent and it always precedes respiratory complications, especially wheeze and spasmodic cough, which are improved by antireflux therapy.[15] Lung infection has also been considered a possible complication of gastroesophageal reflux, in both children and adults.[16,17] Such infections were, however, believed to be associated with either chronic,[18] or massive airway aspiration of gastric contents.[1,17,19–21] It has more recently been shown that infantile apnoea also can be due to gastroesophageal reflux.[22]

Gastroesophageal reflux can remain asymptomatic for many years, which means that it may not cause any problem; it is then called silent gastroesophageal reflux. Some children will suffer exclusively from oesophagitis, others from asthma only, while very occasionally children will suffer from both respiratory and intestinal complications.

DIAGNOSIS

Clinical clues

Although recurrent vomiting or possetting (especially during sleep) may provide a clue in infants, and symptoms of oesophagitis later in childhood, there are often no gastrointestinal clues to the presence of gastroesophageal reflux.

In infants and children gastroesophageal reflux should be considered at any age when asthma cannot be explained by allergy, infection or other conditions, especially in intractable asthma. Several authors have shown gastroesophageal reflux[6,11,13] to be responsible for symptoms in some 50–60% of such cases of asthma. The asthma associated with gastroesophageal reflux is not characteristic and cannot be differentiated from any other aetiology. It may be particularly unresponsive to usual therapy.[23]

Not every patient needs investigation. Where there are powerful clinical clues (or even a strong suspicion), especially in an older child, a therapeutic trial of anti-reflux therapy may be used (see below).

Investigations

Originally a *barium swallow* was used to demonstrate presence of gastroesophageal reflux. Now most clinicians use x-ray investigations to demonstrate only anatomical abnormalities.[24,25] Gastroenterologists quantified and standardized reflux thoroughly in adults[26] using pH electrodes left for about 24 hours in the lower third of the oesophagus. The same method has been applied to children.[27,28] Other teams have used radiolabelled tracers (scintigraphy) to demonstrate gastroesophageal reflux.[28–30] Manometry of the oesophagus is not used for diagnostic purposes but rather as a research tool to understand the mechanism of the reflux and occasionally to monitor the effect of drugs in oesophageal function.[25,31,32]

pH monitoring and scintiscan remain the best investigations to demonstrate reflux. In order to save time, reflux scintigraphy can be combined with pH monitoring on the same day. If this cannot be done (for practical reasons), and if one investigation remains negative, the other needs to be added. Only if both techniques yield a negative result can the occurrence of reflux be excluded; pH tracings and reflux scintigraphy are quite reproducible[33] and the risk of missing reflux is thus negligible. Reflux documented with a pH electrode is called acid reflux, while reflux documented exclusively by abnormal reflux scintigram, if the pH tracing remains normal, is called non-acid reflux. That non-acid reflux might also be harmful was previously suspected.[11–12] Ninety per cent of unexplained asthma with significant gastroesophageal reflux is due to acid reflux and the remaining 10% to non-acid reflux.[9]

pH tracings are obtained with a glass electrode at the tip of a narrow catheter, inserted through the nose, down to the lower third of the oesophagus. The correct position can be checked by chest x-ray. The external part of the probe is connected to a recorder with a 24-hour memory (Figure 7c.1). Oesophageal pH is continuously monitored whatever the position of the patient, over prolonged

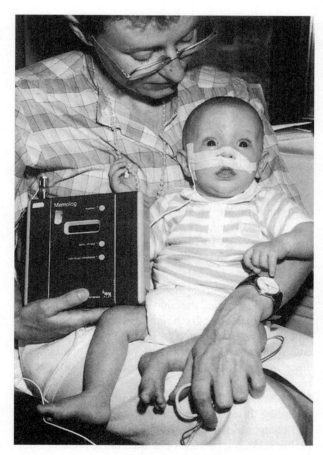

Figure 7c.1 *A baby undergoing pH monitoring in the arms of his mother. The pH probe is inserted through the nose and connected to a 24 h capacity recorder (Memolog). At the end of the measurement period, the Memolog is connected to a computer in order to plot and calculate the degree of reflux (Figure 7c.2).*

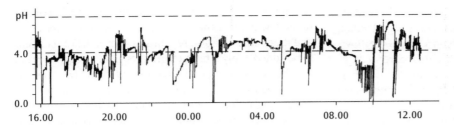

Figure 7c.2 *This is a very abnormal 20 h pH tracing. The lower dashed horizontal line separates the normal oesophageal pH zone (above pH 4) from the abnormal zone. Several prolonged episodes can be seen.*

Table 7c.1 *Definition of the four gastroesophageal reflux variables. These are measured with a pH electrode over a period of about 20–24 hours*

1 *Reflux index*: the ratio of the sum of the durations of all reflux episodes to the entire observation period (%)
2 *The longest reflux duration observed*: (minutes)
3 *The total number of reflux episodes lasting at least 5 minutes* during the entire observation period (expressed per hour)
4 *The total number of reflux episodes observed* during the entire observation period (expressed per hour)

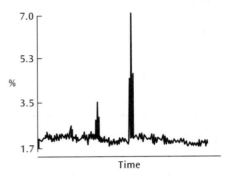

Figure 7c.3 *The duration (x axis) and intensity (y axis) of reflux episodes recorded by the scintigraphic method.*

periods of time. The normal pH of the oesophagus is equal to or higher than 5 and one considers events with a pH of 4 or below to represent acid gastric reflux into the oesophagus (Figure 7c.2). If the contents of the stomach are buffered by food such as milk, reflux will not be detectable by the pH electrode.

Table 7c.1 defines the four variables of acid reflux. Up to 15 months of age, the standards of Vandenplas are used[28] for the normal mean values and for the upper limits of normality. Children older than 15 months have the same standards as adults and for them the standards of de Meester apply.[26] If one of these four variables exceeds its upper limit, the presence of gastroesophageal reflux is unequivocal. In general, more than one variable is abnormal, the most sensitive variables being the reflux index and the longest reflux, followed by the number of reflux episodes lasting more than 5 minutes.

For the *scintigraphic method* the stomach needs to be empty at the start and the child is given a milk feed labelled with a radioisotope of technetium, the amount of the isotope being proportional to the subject's weight. The scintillation camera detects reflux independently of pH (Plate 10). Since the gastric radioactivity decreases in time as the tracer leaves the stomach, the observation period cannot be prolonged for more than one hour, during which the oesophageal radioactivity is recorded every 20 seconds and compared with the remaining gastric radioactivity. Reflux scintigraphy yields one qualitative piece of information, the image (Plate 10) and two important quantitative measurements, the duration of the reflux episode and their magnitude expressed by the intensity of the radioactivity (Figure 7c.3). During the recording the patient needs to remain immobile and in a recumbent position. Reflux scintigraphy is considered a method of choice for the observation of postprandial non-acid reflux,[9,11,30] but is available in very few centres.

In community practice, diagnostic facilities are lacking or they might be too expensive for the patients. In that case, one can start with a *therapeutic trial* (see below). It has however several pitfalls. Firstly, we know that therapeutic response can be delayed up to 3–4 weeks. Secondly, gastroesophageal reflux might be present and responsible for the respiratory disease, though unresponsive to therapy. This can occur when reflux is due to an anatomical abnormality, for example hiatus hernia which requires surgical correction. On the other hand, as is typical for chronic diseases requiring prolonged therapy, even if there is a response to the therapeutic trial, after a while compliance may decrease. In all these cases, we strongly recommend transferring the patient to a team correctly equipped for either confirming the diagnosis of reflux or, if the latter is not present finding another aetiology for the respiratory symptoms.

Natural history

The frequency of belching and possetting decrease with age.[3] Gastroesophageal reflux is more frequently observed in infancy and in early childhood and presumable the disease itself has a tendency to disappear in many infants.[34] A study in cystic fibrosis patients afflicted with gastroesophageal reflux tends to support this hypothesis.[15] The same seems to be true of asthmatic patients with gastroesophageal reflux, though these patients have been less systematically investigated for prolonged periods of time. These observations clearly argue against hasty surgery.

Nevertheless there remain a number of adults with chronic respiratory problems, characterized by either chronic non-productive cough or asthma or both, suffering from gastroesophageal reflux disease and studies in them are ongoing. McGreavy et al.[35] investigated 43 non-smoking adults with chronic non-productive cough (mean duration: 67 months) as the sole respiratory symptom. In eight of them, gastroesophageal reflux was the sole cause of their complaints, whereas no aetiology at all could be found in eight other patients. Palombini et al.[14] investigating thoroughly 78 non-smoking adults with chronic cough demonstrated that the latter was due to multiple causes in 62% of them, gastroesophageal reflux being the third most frequent reason (41%) either as a single aetiology or in combination with asthma and postnasal drip. Only specific antireflux therapy could help these patients. The association between reflux and chronic cough (without wheeze) probably also applies to children.

POSSIBLE MECHANISMS INVOLVED IN ASTHMA ATTACKS

Classic lung function is usually normal between asthma attacks and the occasional bronchial obstruction shows a good response to bronchodilator therapy.

We studied *histamine sensitivity* in most of our patients older than 5 years before the start of antireflux therapy and the challenge was repeated after at least one symptom-free year. At the start, as well as one-year later histamine challenges were positive and neither the threshold nor the intensity of the response to histamine changed (personal data). The acid and non-acid refluxers reacted comparably to the inhalation of histamine. An explanation might be that gastroesophageal reflux will only cause asthma in those children who already have underlying bronchial hyperresponsiveness, which can increase transitorily during reflux. In children with nocturnal gastroesophageal reflux Wilson et al.[8] observed an increase in histamine sensitivity induced by oesophageal acidification. Gastroesophageal reflux is then simply a trigger and the level of host responsiveness to this trigger can be controlled by antireflux therapy, or if it disappears naturally, symptoms seem to vanish despite persisting bronchial hyperreactivity.

The importance of host responsiveness has also been pointed by Hampton et al.[12] who found no relationship between the amount of gastroesophageal reflux and the degree of respiratory dysfunction. They concluded that predisposing factors such as bronchial hyperresponsiveness could determine the importance of the respiratory symptoms. Mansfield[2] believed that oesophageal acidity was responsible for a vagal reflex inducing asthma attacks. Other explanations, however, are needed for non-acid reflux because these too can prompt asthma in non-allergic children.[9,12] Some believe that the relation between non-acid reflux and asthma can only be explained by microaspiration[20] of gastric contents into the respiratory tract and others are convinced that asthma results from a vagal reflex induced by oesophageal dilatation during reflux episodes.[2]

The *microaspiration* theory is not easy to verify. Late recordings of lung radioactivity after scintigraphy are very insensitive. Gastric radioactivity continuously declines during the study and even if microaspirations did occur, the small quantity reaching the lungs would be dispersed and the radioactivity would be close to background activity and hence undetectable. It has been suggested that aspiration of gastric contents might produce lipid inclusions in macrophages and that the quantity of lipid-laden macrophages and the number of inclusions in each macrophage could be a marker of microaspiration. Many have investigated this thoroughly in adults[17,36] and in children,[18–21] but conflicting results suggest that this test is neither sensitive nor specific. The mechanisms which cause asthma in non-acid gastroesophageal reflux are still poorly understood.

Many authors are now convinced that *abnormal oesophageal motility* may explain why non-acid reflux may also be harmful. Fouad et al.[36] studied the pathophysiology of the oesophagus in 98 adults with chronic respiratory disorders and abnormal oesophageal pH-metry. Their respiratory patients often showed statistically more ineffective oesophageal motility than those with exclusively oesophagitis. These abnormalities were seen most frequently with chronic cough followed by asthma and by laryngitis. Orenstein[37] considered that in infancy the motility factors of the oesophagus are more important than the acid secretion. Prokinetic pharmacotherapy seems more efficacious than the acid suppression. This contrasts with the efficacy of pharmacotherapy inhibiting gastric acid secretion or directed against acid in case of oesophagitis.

TREATMENT OF GASTROESOPHAGEAL REFLUX

Medical therapy

Medical treatment has two components: non-drug therapy (diet or position therapy or a combination of both) or drug therapy.

Different *body positions* have been advocated for use in infants. These are rarely successful. *Diet* can help and in some infants adding solids, rather than only liquids can decrease reflux.

Inhibitors of the acid secretion and antacid therapy with alginates (such as gaviscon) and histamine H_2 receptor antagonists may occasionally be helpful though this is not the rule.[38] In non-acid reflux, however, these medications are certainly ineffective.

Since with respiratory complications, motility factors might have a more important role, *prokinetic pharmacotherapy* should be the first choice.[38] Of the prokinetic drugs, cisapride was the most effective and has been extensively used in the treatment of paediatric gastrointestinal motility disorders.[38–43] It stimulates gastrointestinal motor function through indirect cholinergic mechanisms at the level of the myenteric plexus. It differs from existing motility-enhancing drugs by not presenting dopamine receptor-blocking properties or direct cholinergic receptor stimulating properties at therapeutic doses, avoiding the associated side effects. It increases reduced lower oesophageal sphincter tonus and oesophageal clearance. It also improves gastric emptying and the peristalsis in the small intestine and colon, thereby preventing stasis and reflux. The activity lasts for about 6 hours and therefore the drug needs to be taken four times a day before the meals on empty stomach, each dose consisting of 0.2 mg/kg. A total daily dose of 0.8 mg/kg should not be exceeded in infants. Minor transient side effects at the start of the treatment include diarrhoea, abdominal cramps and occasionally vomiting. These can be avoided in sensitive children by starting lower doses and increasing them progressively to the therapeutic level. Cisapride also interacts with medications which inhibit the cytochrome P450 oxydase such as macrolides and imidazole antifungals. It was shown that the cytochrome P450 is responsible for the biotransformation and excretion of cisapride and that very young and immature infants are at greatest risk for accumulation of cisapride plasma concentrations.[44] Moreover, reports of cardiac adverse effects have raised the issue of its safety in prematures and infants so that cisapride is no longer licensed in several countries. Cisapride can prolong the QT interval by blocking the rapid component of the delayed rectifying K+ current in the myocardium.[44,45] A Cochrane Review[46] reported a significant reduction in reflux index, but no symptomatic benefit, publication bias and no greater effect than carobel plug Gaviscon. Because of its effect on Q-T intervals, the drug has been withdrawn. Nevertheless, the authors believe, according to the European Medical Statement,[44] that total restriction should not be applied and that cisapride might be prescribed to paediatric patients who are healthy except for their gastrointestinal motility disorder, provided that a correct dosage schedule is used that no interacting drugs are given and that it is avoided in infants younger than 3 months, prematures and infants with electrolyte disturbances. In such patients ECG monitoring before initiation of therapy and after 3 days of treatment should be done.

If the respiratory symptoms do not improve during therapy, one has to ascertain whether reflux is controlled by repeating during therapy all previously abnormal examinations. If reflux is under control, one can conclude that the reflux is not the main aetiological factor for the respiratory problems. If, on the other hand, none of the therapies has any influence on reflux, anatomical abnormalities for example incompetent cardia or a sliding hernia, might be responsible for the gastroesophageal reflux. Radiological and endoscopic investigations should then be performed, with a view to surgical correction.

If the therapy decreases both the reflux and the asthma attacks, we recommend the treatment to be continued for about one year before being withdrawn and check then whether respiratory symptoms recur. After treatment interruption, only those investigations which were previously abnormal need to be repeated, if indicated. In some patients the antireflux therapy will need to be continued for several years.

Surgery

Although conservative medical therapy remains the first choice, in some patients with severe asthma, reflux persists despite medical therapy. These patients might benefit from a fundoplication.[7,47] Anatomical abnormalities also need surgical repair if medical therapy fails. In the authors' personal experience, surgical therapy is rarely needed but if clearly indicated, yields excellent results.[7,9,11,47]

Normally one should try to postpone surgery, whenever possible, until after the age of 18 months as reflux may decrease with age. This holds also for incompetent cardia and sliding hernia.[3]

REFERENCES

1. Mendelson CL. The aspiration of stomach contents into the lungs during obstetric anaesthesia. *Am J Obstet Gynecol* 1946;**52**:191.
2. Mansfield LE, Stein MR. Gastroesophageal reflux and asthma. Demonstration of a possible reflex mechanism. *Am Rev Respir Dis* 1978;**117**:72.
3. Grysboski J. Infant gastroesophageal reflux. Management implications. *J Clin Gastroenterol* 1979;**1**:153–4.
4. Moote DW, Lloyd DA, McCourtie DR, Welss GA. Increase in gastroesophageal reflux during metacholine-induced bronchospasm. *J Allergy Clin Immunol* 1986;**78**:619–23.
5. Ekström T, Tibbling L. Gastroesophageal reflux and triggering of bronchial asthma: a negative report. *Eur J Respir Dis* 1987;**71**:177–80.
6. Euler AR, Byrne WJ, Ament ME, *et al.* Recurrent pulmonary disease in children: a complication of gastroesophageal reflux. *Pediatrics* 1979;**63**:47–51.
7. Jollye SG, Herbst JJ, Johnson DF, Matlak ME, Books LS. Surgery in children with gastroesophageal reflux and respiratory problems. *J Pediatr* 1980;**96**:194–8.
8. Wilson NM, Charette L, Thomson AH, Silverman M. Gastro-oesophageal reflux and childhood asthma: the acid test. *Thorax* 1985;**40**:592–7.
9. Malfroot A, Giocoli M, Dab I. Respiratory complications of gastroesophageal reflux in children: asthma versus recurrent infections. In: AG Little, MK Ferguson, DB Skinner, eds. *Disease of the Oesophagus, Vol II: Benign Diseases.* Futura Publishing, New York 1990, pp. 127–37.

10. Malfroot A, Vandenplas Y, Dab I. Relationship between gastroesophageal reflux and chronic bronchopulmonary disease in infants and children. *Clin Respir Physiol* 1986;**22**(S8):995.

11. Malfroot A, Vandenplas Y, Verlinden M, Piepsz A, Dab I. Gastroesophageal reflux and unexplained chronic respiratory disease in infants and children. *Pediat Pulmonol* 1987;**3**:208–13.

12. Hampton FJ, MacFayden UM, Beardsmore CS, Simpson H. Gastroesophageal reflux and respiratory function in infants with respiratory symptoms. *Arch Dis Child* 1991;**66**:848–53.

13. Hoyoux CL, Forget P, Lambrechts L, Geubelle F. Chronic bronchopulmonary disease and gastroesophageal reflux in children. *Pediatr Pulmonol* 1985;**1**:149–53.

14. Palombini BC, Villanova CA, Araujo E, *et al.* A pathogenic triad in chronic cough: asthma, postnasal drip syndrome, and gastroesophageal reflux disease. *Chest* 1999;**116**:279–84.

15. Malfroot A, Dab I. New insights on gastroesophageal reflux in cystic fibrosis by longitudinal follow-up. *Arch Dis Child* 1991;**66**:1339–45.

16. Berquist WE, Rachelefsky GS, Kadden M, *et al.* Gastroesophageal reflux-associated recurrent pneumonia and chronic asthma in children. *Pediatrics* 1981;**68**:29–35.

17. Corwin RW, Irwin RI. The lipid-laden alveolar macrophage as a marker of aspiration in parenchymal lung disease. *Am Rev Respir Dis* 1985;**132**:576–81.

18. Ahrens P, Noll C, Kitz R, Willigens P, Zielen S, Hofmann D. Lipid-laden alveolar macrophages (LLAM): a useful marker of silent aspiration in children. *Pediatr Pulmonol* 1999;**28**:79–82.

19. Moran JR, Block SM, Lyerey AD, *et al.* Lipid laden alveolar macrophage and lactose assay as markers of aspiration in neonates with lung disease. *J Pediatr* 1988;**112**:643–9.

20. Nickerson BG. A test for recurrent aspiration in children. *Pediatr Pulmonol* 1987;**3**:65–6.

21. Colombo JL, Hallberg TK. Recurrent aspiration in children: lipid-laden alveolar macrophage quantitation. *Pediatr Pulmonol* 1987;**3**:86–9.

22. Orenstein SR. Update on gastroesophageal reflux and respiratory disease in children. *Can J Gastroenterol* 2000;**14**:131–5.

23. Behar J, Biancani P, Sheahan DG. Evaluation of esophageal tests in the diagnosis of reflux esophagitis. *Gastroenterology* 1976;**71**:9–15.

24. Wu WC. Ancillary tests in the diagnosis of gastroesophageal reflux. *Gastroenterol Clin North Am* 1990;**19**:671–82.

25. De Meester TR, Johnson LF, Joseph GJ, *et al.* Patterns of gastroesophageal reflux in health and disease. *Ann Surg* 1976;**184**:459–70.

26. Euler AR, Amen MOE. Detection of gastroesophageal reflux in the pediatric-age patient by oesophageal intraluminal pH probe measurements. *Pediatrics* 1977;**60**:65–8.

27. Vandenplas Y, Sacré-Smits L. Continuous 24 hours esophageal pH monitoring in 283 asymptomatic infants (0 to 15 months old). *J Pediatr Gastroenterol Nutr* 1987;**6**:220–4.

28. Fisher RS, Malmud LS, Roberts GS, Lobis IE. Gastroesophageal scintiscanning to detect and quantitate reflux. *Gastroenterology* 1976;**70**: 301–8.

29. Piepsz A, Georges L, Perlmutter N, Rodesch P, Cadranel S. Gastroesophageal scintiscanning in children. *Pediatr Radiol* 1981;**11**:71–4.

30. Mahony MJ, Migliavacca M, Spitz L, Milla PJ. Motor disorders of the oesophagus in gastro-oesophageal reflux. *Arch Dis Child* 1988;**63**:1333–8.

31. Cuchiara S, Santamaria F, Andreotti MR, *et al.* Mechanisms of gastro-oesophageal reflux in cystic fibrosis. *Arch Dis Child* 1991;**66**:617–22.

32. Vandenplas Y, Helven R, Goyvaerts H, Sacré L. Reproducibility of gastro-oesophageal pH monitoring in infant and children. *Gut* 1990;**31**:374–7.

33. Carré IJ. Disorders of the oropharynx and oesophagus. In: CM Anderson, V Burke, eds. *Pediatric Gastroenterology.* Blackwell Scientific Publications, Oxford, 1975, pp. 33–76.

34. McGreavy LP, Heany LG, Lawson JT, *et al.* Evaluation and outcome of patients with chronic non-productive cough using a comprehensive diagnostic protocol. *Thorax* 1998; **53**:738–43.

35. Johnston WW, Frable WJ. *Diagnostic Respiratory Cytopathology.* Masson Publishing, New York, 1979, pp. 75–8.

36. Fouad YM, Katz PO, Hattleback JG, Castell DO. Ineffective esophageal motility: the most common motility abnormality in patients with GERD-associated respiratory symptoms. *Am J Gastroenterol* 1999; **94**:1464–7.

37. Orenstein SR, Izadnia F, Khan S. Gastroesophageal reflux disease in children. *Gastroenterol Clin North Am* 1999;**28**:947–69.

38. Cucchiara S, Staiano A, Capozzi C, *et al.* Cisapride for gastro-oesophageal reflux and peptic oesophagitis. *Arch Dis Child* 1987;**62**:454–7.

39. Cucchiara S, Staiano A, Bocciero A, *et al.* Effect of cisapride on parameters of oesophageal motility and on the prolonged intra-oesophageal pH test in infants and gastro-oesophageal reflux. *Gut* 1990; **31**:21–35.

40. Saey ZN, Forget PP, Geubelle F. Effect of cisapride on gastroesophageal reflux in children with chronic bronchopulmonary disease. A double blind cross-over pH monitoring study. *Pediatr Pulmonol* 1987;**3**:8–12.

41. Saey ZN, Forget PP. Effect of cisapride on gastroesophageal pH-monitoring in children with reflux associated bronchopulmonary disease. *J Pediatr Gastroenterol Nutr* 1989;**8**:327–32.

42. McCallum RW. Gastric emptying in gastroesophageal reflux and the therapeutic role of prokinetic agents. *Gastroenterol Clin North Am* 1990;**19**:551–64.

43. Vandenplas Y. Clinical use of cisapride and its risk-benefit in paediatric patients. *Eur J Gastroenterol Hepatol* 1998;**10**:871–81.

44. Vandenplas Y, Belli DC, Benatar A, *et al*. A Medical Position Statement of the European Society of Paediatric Gastroenterology, Hepatology and Nutrition. The role of cisapride in the treatment of pediatric gastroesophageal reflux. *JPGN* 1999;**28**:518–28.

45. Lewin MB, Bryant RM, Fenrich AL, Grifka RG. Cisapride-induced long QT interval. *J Pediatr* 1996;**128**:279–81.

46. Augood C, McLennan S, Gilbert R, Logan S. Cisapride treatment for gastrooesophageal reflux in children (Cochrane Review). Cochrane Library Issue 3. Oxford: Update software 2000.

47. Ahrens P, Heller K, Beyer P, *et al*. Antireflux surgery in children suffering from reflux-associated respiratory diseases. *Pediatr Pulmonol* 1999; **28**(2):89–93.

Food intolerance

NICOLA WILSON

INTRODUCTION

The role of adverse reactions to food as a trigger of asthma is controversial. Certain dietary items have a known potential to affect airway function and indeed are perceived by many children and parents to exacerbate asthma.[1,2] Yet folklore concerning the relationship between diet and symptoms abounds and many cases of alleged food intolerance cannot be substantiated by double-blind challenge[3] or elimination diets.[4]

In this chapter, some information about the perceived prevalence of food and drink-related asthma will be presented. An appraisal of different diagnostic approaches to identify reactions to ingested proteins and intolerance to other ingested substances that can affect the airways will be provided. The mechanisms of food intolerance in asthmatic children will be mentioned. Finally, food and drink-related symptoms will be considered in the clinical context of childhood asthma.

Epidemiologists have demonstrated an association between regional variations in nutritional habits in the population and differences in asthma prevalence,[5,6] so-called 'ecological' evidence. This and other nutritional aspects of the epidemiology of asthma, such as the effects of diets rich in fish oils and antioxidants, are discussed further in Chapter 2.

CLINICAL EVIDENCE AND PREVALENCE OF FOOD INTOLERANCE IN ASTHMA

There is very little information about the true prevalence of food-related asthma in either children or adults. Self-completed questionnaires which enquire about the perceived relationship between diet and symptoms, provide an estimate of the reported prevalence, reflecting current cultural fads and fashions, the powers of observation of subjects, and true symptomatology. In answer to a general question about diet and symptoms, Anderson and colleagues[7] reported that 6% of 8 to 10-year-olds gave food as a precipitating factor in asthma. In a survey of 177 children attending hospital clinics in London, the result of a combination of postal and personal questionnaires, suggested that 67% of Caucasian and 87% of children of South Asian ethnic origin considered at least one item of their diet exacerbated their symptoms.[1] If reactions to orange squash and fizzy drinks, ice and oil were excluded, 28% of the non-Asian and 66% of the Asian children considered one or more of the remaining items affected their symptoms, nuts being the most frequently incriminated. This and other studies[8] suggest that food is commonly considered to be a factor in asthma symptoms. In contrast, challenge under controlled conditions elicits food-induced asthma only in a small minority of adults and children.[3]

Ingested allergens

An allergic response to ingested protein often includes wheezing even in those in whom it has not been recognized.[9–14] In a recent large study of 544 children with known food allergy, 8.6% had respiratory symptoms induced as their main manifestation of a response to controlled challenge.[12] This occurred rarely in those under 3 years and was particularly marked with peanuts. When children with asthma were considered respiratory symptoms occurred in 5.6% of 140 children following double-blind challenge,[10] but it was seen as an isolated symptom in only one child.[13] In another study of children with suspected food allergy and respiratory symptoms, 67/168 (40%) exhibited wheezing as part of their response. Only in five (3%) was it the only symptom.[11] In a French study of 300 patients with asthma including children, 8.3% of subjects reported food allergy.[14] However, following blinded challenge, asthma occurred in only 2.3% and was the sole symptom in 1.3%. When 10 adults, who reported that their asthma was precipitated by dairy products, were challenged no clear adverse response was detected.[15]

So, although asthma does occur as a response to challenge in subjects with known food allergy, it is rarely the sole manifestation of an adverse response in those with ongoing asthma. Furthermore, food allergy is very rarely, if ever, the sole cause of asthma. Children who are affected tend to be highly atopic and react to more than one substance.[12–14] The most frequently incriminated dietary allergens are peanuts, eggs, cow's milk but a wide range of foods can produce a reaction.[11] Unusual substances include figs,[16] natural honey and camomile tea.[17]

Food additives

It has been estimated that in Western industrialized countries, each person eats about 2.5–5 kg of additives a year.[18] In most of the population this does no harm but ingestion of sulphites, particularly in solution, can trigger asthma in some subjects.[19,20] Other substances such as tartrazine, benzoates, nitrates and monosodium glutamate have also been shown to exacerbate asthma in a few individuals.[21–24,25] If only a minority of individuals react then it is not surprising that challenge tests or excluding a particular dietary substance has no overall effect in unselected populations of asthmatic subjects.

METABISULPHITE AND SULPHUR DIOXIDE

Sulphur dioxide and sodium metabisulphite are widely used as preservatives and anti-oxidants which may be added as a gas or stored as metabisulphite added to acidic food and drink. They are usually harmless in recommended concentrations but asthmatics may be sensitive even in high dilutions. Although artificial colourings have been removed from many proprietary drinks metabisulphite remains as a preservative. Between 11% and 35% of children give a history of exacerbation of asthma after soft drinks.[1,23]

When patients in an uncontrolled study with a history of soft drink-induced asthma were challenged with metabisulphite in the concentrations found in proprietary drinks, 14 out of 30 responded by rapid falls in FEV_1.[23] In a further study of asthmatic children, 19/29 (66%) responded to an acidified oral solution but not to metabisulphite capsules.[26] Children may be at greater risk than

adults, as they consume large quantities of soft drinks. Of particular danger are the kind that need diluting, as preservatives can then inadvertently be given in high concentrations. At least one child has suffered a very severe attack of asthma shortly after being given a concentrated orange drink inadequately diluted by a sibling (personal observation). When a group of adults with reported food-induced asthma were challenged with a range of additives, a reaction to metabisulphite was the most frequently found.[25] However, in adults with severe asthma known to respond to ingested metabisulphite capsules, wheezing was only infrequently induced by challenge with a wide variety of foods treated with sulphites as for normal consumption.[27] Also, avoidance of acetyl salicylic acid and metabisulphite had no overall benefit in a group of childhood asthmatics although a few individuals were considered to benefit.[26] All the same, rare life-threatening asthma has been reported.[19,25,27]

ARTIFICIAL COLOURINGS AND OTHER PRESERVATIVES

These have had a bad press in the past decade but many children perceived by their parents to be intolerant have been found to be unaffected by controlled single or multiple challenges.[28,29] Nonetheless, individual subjects including atopic children have been shown to develop asthma following ingestion of tartrazine[21,28] and sodium benzoate.[21,23,28] It is not clear how frequent a problem it is in childhood asthma but in a group of asthmatic children tartrazine and benzoate avoidance did not result in improvement of asthma symptoms.[28] In a population of adults with severe asthma, reactions to a number of different azo and non-azo dyes were only found in two out of 45 subjects.[22] In contrast, in the same study, aspirin intolerance was seen in 20 out of 45. However, carmine dye has been reported to cause a severe reaction in a number of individuals with asthma.[30] Nitrite and nitrate salts are commonly used preservatives and have been reported to induce asthma in adults,[25] and a case of anaphylaxis has been reported in a 22-year-old following nitrate challenge.[31] An assessment of nitrate-induced reactions in children with asthma is not available.

ASPIRIN AND ACETYLACETIC ACID

Aspirin-induced asthma, particularly associated with nasal polyps, is usually considered a feature of adults with non-atopic asthma. The data in children are conflicting, perhaps due to variations in populations selected for assessment. In one study 14 out of 50 (28%) children without a history of aspirin intolerance responded to controlled challenge.[32] Girls with severe atopic asthma were particularly affected. In the other study seven out of 56 (13%) had a positive challenge but the intolerance was already suspected.[33] None of the 56 children studied showed intolerance to tartrazine. In a further group of asthmatic children, no intolerance

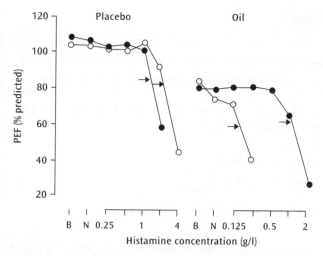

Figure 7d.1 *Effect on the dose–response curve to inhaled histamine of challenge with oil in an individual child of South Asian (Indian) ethnic origin, tested on two separate days. B: baseline; N: normal saline. Arrows indicate PC_{20}. (From ref. 39 with permission.)*

to aspirin was detected.[34] Other cyclo-oxygenase inhibitors may cross-react with aspirin in sensitive subjects.[35]

MISCELLANEOUS CHEMICALS

Food cooked in oil has been shown to exacerbate asthma in some children and adults originating from the Indian subcontinent (South Asian)[1] (Figure 7d.1). This confirms the claim of a number of such children that fried foods, particularly French fries (chips), worsen their asthma.[1] Some chemical in reheated oil may be responsible but the mechanism is not known. This raises the possibility that other chemical properties of food could affect airway function.

PHYSICAL AGENTS

Ingested substances may not only contain allergenic proteins and chemicals, but also have other physical properties which can affect airway function. Following the claim, particularly by children whose ethnic origin is the Indian subcontinent,[1] that cold and fizzy drinks with a low pH exacerbate asthma, challenge with ice and dilute HCl (pH 3.1) has been shown to exacerbate asthma in selected individuals[36–39] (Figure 7d.2). The mechanism is not altogether clear but probably results from oesophageal stimulation.[37] The danger to a susceptible person of eating ice cream has been highlighted.[40]

MECHANISMS (TABLE 7d.1)

An adverse response to food can be divided into several categories (Figure 7d.3).

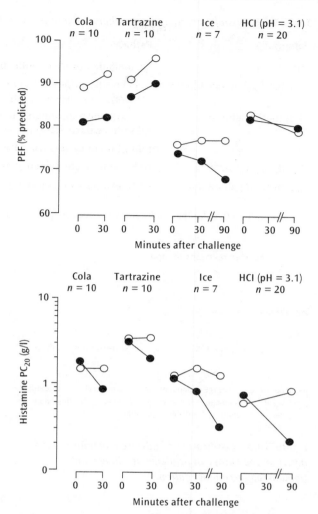

Figure 7d.2 *The effect on peak flow and histamine PC_{20} of challenge with cola and, tartrazine, ice and dilute hydrochloric acid (closed circles) and control agents (open circles) in groups of children with a positive history. (From ref. 39 with permission.)*

Immune mediated

The best characterized are those which involve the production of *food-specific IgE*. The process of sensitization to ingested allergens is discussed in Chapters 4c and 7a. After the food allergen has crossed the gastrointestinal mucosal barrier, the IgE antibodies on the various cell types within the target organ bind with the food allergen causing release of a number of mediators, including histamine, prostaglandins, leukotrienes, tryptase and thromboxane A2.[47] This results in symptoms of immediate hypersensitivity. Late responses have not been objectively demonstrated.[3]

Possible *non-IgE mediated immune processes* include specific food immunoglobulins other than IgE,[48] food immune complexes[49] and cell mediated immunity[49] have been suggested. The relevance of these processes to an allergic response to asthma is controversial,[50] except perhaps that associated with cow's milk intolerance.[48,49]

Table 7d.1 *Possible mechanisms in asthma induced by ingested substances*

Stimulus	Pathway
Allergen	IgE mediated process; milk an exception, since no particular antibody consistently found[41]
Inhaled SO_2/metabisulphite	Not certain; proposed action via parasympathetic or non-cholinergic excitatory neural pathways[42] or enzyme inhibition;[43]
Oral metabisulphite*	IgE mechanism postulated but if exists, rare; non-immunological release of mediators and sulphite oxidase deficiency other possibilities[19,20]
Aspirin	Inhibition of cyclo-oxygenase pathway
Azo dyes, benzoate*	Unknown, except evidence of IgE to carmine dye[44]
Monosodium glutamate*	Unknown; possible peripheral neurociliary effect[24]

*An aspirin-like effect for these substances has been suggested, via thromboxane β_2 inhibition.[45]

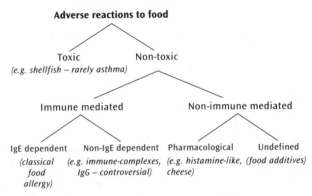

Figure 7d.3 *Classification of adverse reactions to food based on the European Academy of Allergy and Immunology recommendation.*[46]

Non-immune mediated

The mechanism by which most non-immune mediated processes effect the lung are largely unknown (Table 7d.1). It is thought that most cases of sulphite sensitivity result from inhalation of SO_2 released when a solution of metabisulphite is consumed.[19] This may simply be a non-specific response similar in nature to enhanced histamine or methacholine responsiveness, because inhaled metabisulphite hyperresponsiveness is found in most asthmatic subjects.[42] SO_2 release is enhanced by acidification[19] and it has been suggested that carbonated drinks may yield their SO_2 more rapidly than still drinks when the pressure is lowered prior to consumption.[23]

CLINICAL ASSESSMENT

Presentation and clinical features

Ingested substances can undoubtedly exacerbate asthma in some children through IgE-mediated pathways, chemical reactions or physical stimulation (Table 7d.1). The extent of the problem is not known. To complicate matters,

the magnitude of the response in a susceptible individual may depend not only upon the amount ingested,[11] but also on the state of the airways at the time of consumption, in a similar manner to the magnitude of airway response to other environmental stimuli. This makes estimates of the prevalence difficult and confounds challenge procedures. The reporting of severe asthma immediately following ingestion of a particular substance, especially if associated with other allergic manifestations, does not give rise to a diagnostic problem and confirmation is frequently unnecessary, particularly if the substance is not a basic dietary constituent. Peanuts are a good example of this situation.

BRONCHIAL RESPONSIVENESS

The adverse response to an ingested substance is often reported as an increase in the response to other triggers of asthma such as exercise.[1,39] This raises the possibility that the deleterious effect on the airways may not always be manifest as airway narrowing but as an increase in bronchial responsiveness.[39,51] This phenomenon has been demonstrated in a number of studies of children using a histamine challenge test to measure bronchial responsiveness before and after oral challenge with physical and chemical agents as well as allergens[1,36–39] (Figures 7d.1, 7d.2, 7d.4). In many cases, the increase in bronchial responsiveness occurred without change in baseline lung function. In this situation the adverse response would not have been detected in the laboratory without a test of bronchial responsiveness. An example of a child challenged with peanuts on two days is shown in Figure 7d.4. On one day measurements of peak flow alone were used to assess the response and on the other histamine responsiveness was assessed before and after oral challenge. A positive response was seen only when bronchial responsiveness was measured, thus confirming the spontaneous claim of many children.[1,39] This approach has also been validated in adults.[25,52]

ETHNIC DIFFERENCES

A survey of hospital-based children with asthma highlighted a significant difference in the reporting of

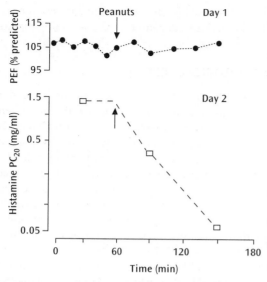

Figure 7d.4 *Comparison of two methods of assessing peanut challenge in the same child. Following the same challenge with peanuts there was no change in PEF on day 1, but a marked fall in PC_{20} (i.e. increase in responsiveness) on day 2.*

Table 7d.2 *Cross-reactions between food and inhalant or contact allergy[55,57–9]*

Inhaled/contact agent	Fruit group or other agent
Ragweed	Watermelon, melon, banana, gourd family
Birch	Apple, pear, peach, hazelnut,* carrot, potato, celery,* fennel
Grass	Tomato, melon, watermelon, kiwi, latex
Hazel	Hazelnut
Mugwort	Celery
Dermatophagiodes pteronyssinus	Crustacians, molluscs (e.g. snail),* peanuts, garlic, tomato, onion, egg, port, variety of fruits
Latex	Avocado,* banana,* chestnut,* variety of fruits

* Potential to cause anaphylaxis.

diet-induced asthma between children of South Asian and non-Asian origin, with many South Asian children incriminating cola drinks, ice and fried foods, especially French fries.[1] The difference was not explained by a greater severity of asthma in the children of Asian origin, as in fact they were using less medication. One possibility is that cultural beliefs account for this difference,[53] although it has been shown that these substances can affect lung function under controlled conditions in selected South Asian subjects[36–39] (Figures 7d.1, 7d.2, 7d.4).

REPORTED TIMING OF ONSET OF FOOD-INDUCED ASTHMA

When a pulmonary response does develop, the peak asthmatic response usually occurs within minutes if it is part of an anaphylactic response, or up to 2 hours after food challenge or ingestion.[9,10,12–14,54] In a survey of the reported timing of asthma induced by ingested substances, the onset of symptoms varied between a few minutes and more than 24 hours.[1] In 36% of the children symptoms returned or were first noticed during the subsequent night. This pattern occurred both following classic allergens such as milk, nuts and eggs and physical stimuli such as fizzy drinks and ice. Though a common complaint, this dual response has not been confirmed objectively. Indeed, in one study in which the children were followed for 24 hours after challenge, no delayed responses were detected.[3]

CROSS REACTIVITY BETWEEN ALLERGENS AND UNRELATED FRESH FRUIT AND VEGETABLES

The association between pollinosis and reactions to unrelated fresh fruit and vegetables has been recognized

for many years and is best described as the 'pollen-food allergy syndrome'[55–57] (Table 7d.2). It can be caused by cross-reacting, specific IgE antibodies to pollens and a variety of fruit and vegetables.[55] Many of the reactions can be explained by the presence of cytoskeletal proteins (profilins) which are present in several different pollen species.[56] They are also present in many plants, so may act as pan allergens. The symptoms occur a few minutes after local contact with the offending fruit or vegetable, with resulting oropharyngeal itching, tingling and lip swelling. If ingestion occurs despite local symptoms more severe local and systemic reactions may occur. In one series, 92/706 (13%) experienced glottic oedema and 15 (2.1%) anaphylaxis.[57]

A similar association between an allergen and a reaction to fresh fruit and vegetables is seen in those allergic to *Dermataphagoides pteronyssinus*[58] or latex[59] (Table 7d.2).

NATURAL HISTORY

Children tend to grow out of food allergies[60] so rechallenge at intervals may be necessary, especially if the substance is a basic dietary ingredient such as milk. Although it used to be said that cow's milk protein intolerance was a condition of the first few years of life, it is now recognized that this persists in some children, particularly those with multiple allergies or a delayed response,[61] or an early IgE response.[49] Allergy to peanuts and fish is usually lifelong.[62] Symptoms of food allergy change with age, with atopic dermatitis occurring in younger children and respiratory disorders, anaphylaxis and oral syndromes increasing as children get older.[63] It should be noted that a dangerously increased reaction may occur after the substance has been excluded for a period of time.

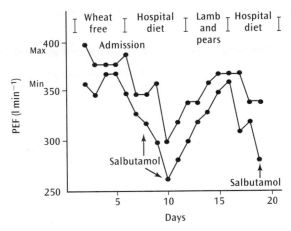

Figure 7d.5 *Twice daily peak flow readings during a diet containing wheat and its subsequent exclusion, in a woman with multiple skin tests to food. (From ref. 75 with permission.)*

Investigation and interpretation

WHEN TO INVESTIGATE

Many more patients attribute a reaction to food as a cause for their symptoms than can be objectively demonstrated.[3] So unless the substance is nutritionally unimportant, the history unequivocal or a severe reaction reported, this history needs confirmation by a formal challenge in controlled conditions or by an indisputable improvement when the substance is eliminated from the diet[64] (Figure 7d.5). This is particularly true for chronic disease, such as asthma, when the association is difficult to detect.

DOUBLE-BLIND FOOD CHALLENGE (DBFC)[65,66]

If possible, the food needs disguising, as a positive response is sometimes seen under open conditions but not when the challenge is blinded. It may be possible to do this with the use of freeze-dried food contained in capsules.[64] In asthma, a positive response is shown by a significantly greater fall in lung function after ingestion of the active ingredient than a placebo preparation. It is however difficult to demonstrate a reaction occurring more than a few hours after ingestion because of the spontaneous variation in lung function that occurs with time, especially in severe asthma.

There are other drawbacks to this test as a diagnostic procedure, particularly if a test of bronchial responsiveness is not included (see above). Repeated 'doses' may be needed or, as with other triggers of asthma, the response may depend on or be enhanced by the presence of additional stimuli. Also, asthma is a very variable condition and any adverse response will depend on the underlying degree of bronchial responsiveness at the time of challenge. A multiple challenge protocol given over an extended period may overcome this to some extent but is not without its own problems.[28] In addition, the response may be attenuated by prophylactic medication, the need for which could, theoretically, depend on the continuing ingestion of the substance.

IMMUNOLOGICAL TESTS

There have been many appraisals of the use of skin and RAST tests as indicators of clinically significant IgE sensitization to specific food proteins.[54,67–69,71] Immediate reactions, confirmed in the laboratory, are usually associated with positive tests. However, a positive IgE response has a low positive predictive value for a positive challenge result, as many subjects with a significant specific IgE do not react clinically. On the other hand, a negative RAST or skin test virtually excludes an IgE mediated response.[63] Some diagnostic success has been claimed for leukocyte histamine release and RAST in the detection of hidden sensitivity.[69] Children who outgrow food allergy often retain positive skin tests to food and there are many atopic children with positive skin tests, particularly to wheat, who are asymptomatic.[72] Proven delayed asthmatic responses to ingested proteins such as milk have been shown to be associated with negative skin tests.[70] The role of immunological markers in diagnosing asthma associated with food allergy is therefore limited.

ELIMINATION DIETS

This is the only method available to diagnose hidden food-induced asthma. Either a few commonly ingested foods can be eliminated or alternatively a 'few foods' diet instituted.[73] The diagnosis of food intolerance using an elimination diet requires improvement after exclusion of the item in question and deterioration after reintroduction (Figure 7d.5). Day-to-day variation in the severity of asthma, particularly with exacerbations associated with viral infections, usually makes this a cumbersome process in asthmatic children. Unless there are clues to possible culprits, multiple food eliminations are necessary. This is very difficult to enforce and can be nutritionally detrimental unless carefully supervised.[62]

HIDDEN FOOD-INDUCED ASTHMA

An allergic reaction is nearly always well-recognized by parents. Nonetheless, the possibility of an unrecognized adverse response as a cause of continuing symptoms may remain, particularly with parents. In addition, there are several reports of greatly improved asthma in adults and older children following elimination of various food substances[72,74,75] (Figure 7d.5). Asthma induced by an adverse response to an ingested substance is less likely to be recognized if wheeze is the only symptom, without other pointers such as vomiting or eczema, or if the onset were more than 2 hours after ingestion. However, reported features suggesting hidden food-allergic asthma include multisystem involvement and a highly atopic background including positive or negative skin-prick tests to food allergens.[10,74] The only way to diagnose hidden food-induced asthma is with the institution of a carefully conducted elimination diet. It should be remembered that, in the vast majority of patients, effective asthma treatment is much simpler than the problems of diagnostic and therapeutic elimination diets. Such diagnostic diets need expert supervision, are not always easy to interpret and can result in malnutrition.[62] This makes treating asthma, with its multiple precipitating factors, a more sensible option than looking for the very rare case of hidden food allergy.

MANAGEMENT

BREAST-FEEDING

The place of dietary exclusion in infants and lactating mothers in the prevention of allergic disease has been hotly debated for over 50 years.[76–78] Breast-feeding appears to confer protection against lower respiratory illness in developing countries but the evidence for this in industrialized areas is conflicting.[79,80] Confusion may arise firstly, because of the failure to control for confounding factors, such as maternal smoking, the fact that the maternal diet can sensitize breast-fed babies and because infants from highly atopic families are more likely to breastfeed. Secondly, breast-feeding provides long-term protection against infections, including virus associated wheeze.[81] Two studies suggest a probable reduction in virus-associated wheeze in breast-fed infants. One showed that in breast-fed infants, wheezing was reduced in atopic children for the first 2 years of life but this protection lasted until 7 years in non-atopic children.[82] In the other, breast-feeding conferred protection against transient early wheeze, but was a risk factor for asthma.[80] The conflicting findings on the effect of breast-feeding and asthma may arise from the fact that virus infections precipitate wheeze and asthma on the one hand, but on the other, early infections protect against allergic disease (See Chapter 2.)

Breast-fed children of atopic mothers may be at greater risk of asthma.[83]

Therapy

Broadly speaking, consideration of food or drink-induced asthma can be divided clinically into four categories:

1 *Intermittent mild asthma occasionally triggered by ingested substances.* Common triggers of this type of event include peanuts, shellfish and ice or cola drinks (Figures 7d.2 and 7d.4) in South Asian children. Avoidance is the best policy but occasional indiscretions can be treated with bronchodilators. The role of leukotriene receptor antagonists (LTRAs) in aspirin-sensitive asthma has been demonstrated in adults.[82a]

2 *Children requiring prophylactic (preventer) treatment for asthma.* When the level of asthma control is good, apart from exacerbations by viral infections, screening for hidden food or drink intolerance is unjustified. It is probably worth attempting to avoid cola drinks and ice in South Asian children and concentrated proprietary drinks (containing metabisulphite) in most children, as well as any other recognized offenders, such as nuts. Like other environmental triggers, most potential adverse responses to food will be prevented or reduced by prophylactic treatment with inhaled corticosteroids. Institution of an additive-free diet is unnecessary and is not in any case recommended for children, although aspirin can usually be avoided.

3 *Severe asthma requiring high-dose inhaled or oral corticosteroids.* Pets and other aeroallergens are much more likely to be responsible for continuing symptoms than food. In highly motivated subjects with multisystem allergic manifestations, with or without positive skin-prick tests to food, an elimination diet to screen for hidden food – or drink-induced asthma may be worth considering after all other possibilities have been excluded, in those who continue to have troublesome symptoms. Case reports, particularly of adults, have demonstrated dramatic improvements in a few individuals after removal of a particular dietary substance. There is no general appraisal of such a procedure in children, probably because assessment is so difficult. Exclusion diets are very demanding on children and their families; the use of oral cromoglycate may be an easier option.[13]

4 *Wheezing in infancy.* Breast-feeding should be encouraged to reduce wheezing in the first few years of life in non-atopic families.[83] Further studies are necessary to evaluate the part played by milk and soya intolerance in chronic infant wheezing. The dramatic improvement that often occurs in episodic viral wheeze between 2 and 4 years must be borne in mind when assessing the benefit of dietary manipulation.

ANAPHYLAXIS

Although rare as its sole manifestation, quite severe asthma may be one of the manifestations of anaphylaxis. There are usually warning symptoms (oral tingling or tongue swelling, generalized itching, nausea and vomiting) as well as extra-pulmonary signs (systemic, circulatory effects, upper airway obstruction, facial swelling, urticaria and abdominal cramps). Management of airway obstruction should take place alongside standard therapy with adrenaline (epinephrine) and antihistamine. Adrenaline administered by inhalation from a metered dose inhaler, may have bronchodilator as well as systemic effects.

An exclusion diet is mandatory and an epinephrine self-injection kit should be available at all times, at school and elsewhere.

REFERENCES

1. Wilson NM. Food related asthma: a difference between two ethnic groups. *Arch Dis Child* 1985;**60**:861–5.

2. Dawson KP, Ford R, Mogridge N. Childhood asthma: what do parents add or avoid in their children's diets? *NZ Med J* 1990;**103**:239–40.

3. May CD. Objective clinical and laboratory studies of immediate reactions to foods in asthmatic children. *J Allergy Clin Immunol* 1976;**58**:500–15.

4. Van Metre TE, Anderson AD, Bennard JH. A controlled study of the effects on manifestations of chronic asthma of a rigid elimination diet based on Rowe's cereal free diet 1.2.3. *J Allergy* 1968;**41**:196–204.

5. Fogarty A, Britton J. The role of diet in the aetiology of asthma. *Clin Exp Allergy* 2000;**30**:615–27.

6. Weiss ST. Diet as a risk factor for asthma. *Ciba Found Symp* 1997;**206**:244–57.

7. Anderson HR, Palmer JC, Brailey P, *et al*. *A community survey of asthma and wheezing illness in 8–10 year old children.* Report to South West Thames Regional Health Authority, London, 1981.

8. Woods RK, Abramson M, Raven JM, Walters EH. Reported food intolerance and respiratory symptoms in young adults. *Eur J Respir Med* 1998;**11**:151–5.

9. Lessof MH, Wraith DG, Merritt TG, *et al*. Food allergy and intolerance in 100 patients. Local and systemic effects. *Q J Med* 1980;**193**:239–71.

10. Minford AMB, Macdonald A, Littlewood JM. Food intolerance and food allergy in children: a review of 68 cases. *Arch Dis Child* 1982;**57**:742–7.

11. Bock SA. Respiratory reactions induced by food challenges in children with pulmonary disease. *Pediatr Allergy Immunol* 2000;**3**:188–94.

12. Rance F, Kanny G, Dutau G, Moneret-Vautrin DA. Food hypersensitivity in children: clinical aspects and distribution of allergens. *Pediatr Allergy Immunol* 1999;**10**:33–8.

13. November E., de Martino M, Viernci A. Foods and respiratory allergy. *J Allergy Clin Immunol* 1988;**81**:1059–65.

14. Onorato J, Merland N, Terral B, Michel FB, Bousquet J. Placebo-controlled double-blind food challenge in asthma. *J Allergy Clin Immunol* 1986;**78**:1139–46.

15. Woods RK, Weiner JM, Abramson M, Thien F, Walters EH. Do dairy products induce bronchoconstriction in adults with asthma? *J Allergy Clin Immunol* 1998;**101**:45–50.

16. Dechamp C, Bessot JC, Pauli G, Deviller P. First report of anaphylactic reaction after fig (*Ficus carica*) ingestion. *Allergy* 1995:**50**:514–16.

17. Florido-Lopez JF, Gonzalez DP, Saenz-de-San PB, Perez MC, Arias-de-Saavedra JM, Marin-Pozo JF. Allergy to natural honeys and camomile tea. *Int Arch Allergy Immunol* 1995;**108**:170–4.

18. Lessof M. Adverse reactions to food additives. *J Roy Coll Phys* 1987;**21**:237–40.

19. Bush RK, Taylor SL, Busse W. A critical evaluation of trials in reactions to sulphites. *J Allergy Clin Immunol* 1986;**75**:197–201.

20. Simon RA. Sulphite sensitivity. *Ann Allergy* 1986; **56**:281–8.

21. Hariparsad H, Wilson N, Dixon C, *et al*. Oral tartrazine challenge in childhood asthma: effect on bronchial reactivity. *Clin Allergy* 1984;**14**:81–5.

22. Weber RW, Hoffman M, Raine DA, *et al*. Incidence of bronchoconstriction due to aspirin, azo dyes, preservatives in a population of perennial asthmatics. *J Allergy Clin Immunol* 1979;**64**:32–7.

23. Freedman BJ. Asthma induced by sulphur dioxide, benzoate and tartrazine in orange drinks. *Clin Allergy* 1977;**7**:407–15.

24. Allen DH, Delohery J, Baker G. Monosodium glutamate-induced asthma. *J Allergy Clin Immunol* 1987;**80**:530–7.

25. Hodge L, Yan KY, Loblay RL. Assessment of food chemical intolerance in adult asthmatic subjects. *Thorax* 1996;**51**:805–9.

26. Towns SJ, Mellis CM. Role of acetyl salicylic acid and sodium metabisulphite in chronic childhood asthma. *Pediatrics* 1984;**73**:631–7.

27. Taylor SL, Bush RK, Selner JC, *et al*. Sensitivity to sulphited foods among sulphite sensitive subjects with asthma. *J Allergy Clin Immunol* 1988;**81**:1159–67.

28. Taulo SM, Broder I. Tartrazine and benzoate challenge and dietary avoidance in chronic asthma. *Clin Allergy* 1982;**12**:303–12.

29. Wilson NM, Scott A. A double blind assessment of additive intolerance in children using a 12 day challenge period at home. *Clin Exp Allergy* 1989; **19**:267–72.

30. Kagi MK, Wuthrich B, Johansson SG. Campari-Orange anaphylaxis due to carmine allergy letter. *Lancet* 1994;**344**:60–1.

31. Hawkins CA, Katelaris CH. Nitrate anaphylaxis. *Ann Allergy Asthma Immunol* 2000;**85**:74–6.

32. Rachelefsky GS, Coalson A, Siega SC, *et al*. Aspirin intolerance in chronic childhood asthma: detected by oral challenge. *Pediatrics* 1975;**56**:443–8.

33. Vedanthan PK, Mearn MM, Bell TD, *et al*. Aspirin and tartrazine oral challenge: incidence of adverse response in chronic childhood asthma. *J Allergy Clin Immunol* 1977;**60**:8–13.

34. Schuhl JF, Pereira JG. Oral acetyl salicylic acid (aspirin) challenge in asthmatic children. *Clin Allergy* 1979; **9**:83–8.

35. Szczeklik A. Adverse reactions to aspirin and nonsteroidal anti-inflammatory drugs. *Ann Allergy* 1987;**59**:113–18.

36. Wilson NM, Dixon C, Silverman M. Increased bronchial responsiveness caused by ingestion of ice. *Eur Respir J* 1985;**66**:25–30.

37. Wilson NM, Choudry N, Silverman M. Role of the oesophagus in asthma induced by the ingestion of ice and acid. *Thorax* 1987;**42**:506–10.

38. Wilson NM, Vickers H, Silverman M. Objective test for food sensitivity in asthmatic children: increased bronchial reactivity after cola drinks. *Br Med J* 1982;**284**:1226–8.

39. Wilson NM. Diet-related asthma in children. *Paediatr Respir Med* 1993;**1**:14–20.

40. Oppenheimer JJ, Bock SA. The ice cream parlour challenge could be a killer. *J Allergy Clin Immunol* 1998;**102**:325–6.

41. Tainio VM, Savilahti E. Value of immunologic tests in cow's milk. *Allergy* 1990;**45**:189–96.

42. Nichol GM, Nix A, Chung KF, *et al.* Characterisation of bronchoconstrictor response to sodium metabisulphite aerosol in atopic subjects with and without asthma. *Thorax* 1989;**44**:1009–14.

43. Simon RA. Sulphite sensitivity. *Ann Allergy* 1986; **56**:281–8.

44. DiCello MC, Myc A, Baker-JR J, Baldwin JL. Anaphylaxis after ingestion of carmine coloured foods: two case reports and a review of the literature. *Allergy Asthma Proc* 1999;**20**:377–82.

45. Williams WR, Pawlowicz A, Davies BH. Aspirin-like effects of selected food additives and industrial sensitizing agents. *Clin Exp Allergy* **19**:533–7.

46. Ortolani C, Vighi G. Definition of adverse reactions to food. *Allergy* 1995;**50**(20 Suppl):8–13.

47. Ohtsuka T, Matsumaru S, Uchida K, *et al.* Pathogenic role of thromboxane A2 in immediate food hypersensitivity reactions in children. *Ann Allergy Asthma Immunol* 1996;**77**:55–9.

48. Duchen K, Einarsson R, Grodzinsky E, Hattevig G, Bjorksten B. Development of IgG1 and IgG4 antibodies against beta-lactoglobulin and ovalbumin in healthy and atopic children. *Ann Allergy Asthma Immunol* 1997;**78**:363–8.

49. Host A. Cow's milk protein allergy and intolerance in infancy. Some clinical, epidemiological and immunological aspects. *Pediatr Allergy Immunol* 1994;**5**:1–36.

50. Barnes RM. IgG and IgA antibodies to dietary antigens in food allergy and intolerance. *Clin Exp Allergy* 1995;**25**(Suppl 1):7–9.

51. Wilson NM, Silverman M. Diagnosis of food sensitivity in asthma. *J Royal Soc Med* 1985;**78**(Suppl 5):11–15.

52. James J, Eigenmann PA, Eggleston PA, Sampson HA. Airway reactivity changes in asthmatic patients undergoing blinded food challenges. *Am J Respir Crit Care Med* 1996;**153**:597–603.

53. De San Lazaro C. Food related asthma: a difference between two ethnic groups. *Arch Dis Child* 1986; **1**:97 (letter).

54. Yazicioglu M, Baspinar I, Ones U, Pala O, Kiziler U. Egg and milk allergy in asthmatic children: assessment by immulite allergy food panel, skin prick tests and double-blind placebo-controlled food challenges. *Allergol Immunopathol Madr* 1999;**27**:287–93.

55. Kelso JM. Pollen-food allergy. *Clin Exp Allergy* 2000;**30**:905–7.

56. Valenta R, Duchene M, Ebner C, *et al.* Profilins constitute a novel family of functional plant pan-allergens. *J Exp Med* 1992;**175**:377–85.

57. Ortolani C, Pastorello EA, Farioli L, *et al.* IgE-mediated allergy from vegetable allergens. *Ann Allergy* 1993; **71**:470–6.

58. Pajno GB, Morabito L, Barberio G. Allergy to house dust mite and snails: a model of cross-reaction between food and inhalant allergens with a clinical impact. *Pediatr Pulmonol* (Suppl) 1999;**18**:163–4.

59. Frankland AW. Food reactions in pollen and latex allergic patients editorial. *Clin Exp Allergy* 1995; **25**:580–1.

60. Host A, Jacobsen HP, Halken S, Holmenlund D. The natural history of cow's milk protein allergy/intolerance. *Eur J Clin Nutr* 1995; **49**(Suppl 1):S13–18.

61. Iacono G, Cavataio F, Montalto G, Soresi M, Notarbartolo A, Carroccio A. Persistent cow's milk protein intolerance in infants: the changing faces of the same disease. *Clin Exp Allergy* 1998;**28**:817–23.

62. David TJ, Waddington E, Stanton RH. Nutritional hazards of elimination diets in children with atopic eczema. *Arch Dis Child* 1984;**59**:323–5.

63. Bock SA, Atkins FM. Patterns of food hypersensitivity during 16 years of double-blind placebo-controlled challenges. *J Pediatr* 1990;**117**:561–7.

64. Lessof MH. The diagnosis of food intolerance. *Clin Exp Allergy* 1995;**25**(Suppl 1):14–15.

65. Bock SA, Sampson HA, Atkins FM, *et al.* Double-blind, placebo controlled food challenge (DBPCFC) as an office procedure; a manual. *J Allergy Clin Immunol* 1998;**82**:986–97.

66. Sicherer SH. Food allergy: when and how to perform oral food challenges. *Pediatr Allergy Immunol* 1999;**10**:226–34.

67. Wraith DG, Merritt S, Roth A, *et al.* Recognition of food-allergic patients and their allergens by RAST technique and clinical investigation. *Clin Allergy* 1979;**9**:25–36.

68. Galant S, Bullock J, Frick OL. An immunological approach to the diagnosis of food sensitivity. *Clin Allergy* 1973;**3**:363–72.

69. Bock SA, Lee WY, Remigo L, Holst A, May CD. Appraisal of skin tests with food extracts for diagnosis of food sensitivity. *Clin Allergy* 1978;**8**:559–64.

70. Wraith DG. Asthma and rhinitis. *Clin Immunol Allergy* 1982;**2**:101–12.

71. Adler BR, Assadullahi J, Warner JA, Warner JO. Evaluation of multiple food specific IgE antibody test

compared to parental perception, allergy skin test and RAST. *Clin Exp Allergy* 1991;**21**:683–8.

72. Bock SA. The natural history of food sensitivity. *J Allergy Clin Immunol* 1982;**69**:173–7.

73. Carter C. Dietary treatment of food allergy and intolerance. *Clin Exp Allergy* 1995;**25**(Suppl 1):34–42.

74. Hoj L, Ostenballe O, Bundgaard A, *et al.* A double blind controlled trial of elemental diet in severe perennial asthma. *Allergy* 1981; **36**:257–62.

75. Williams AJ, Church SE, Finn R. An unsuspected case of wheat-induced asthma. *Thorax* 1987;**42**:205–6.

76. Kramer MS. Does breast feeding help protect against atopic disease? Biology, methodology and a golden jubilee of controversy. *J Pediatr* 1988;**112**:181–90.

77. Golding J, Emmett PM, Rogers IS. Eczema, asthma and allergy. *Early Hum Dev* 1997;**49**(Suppl):S121–30.

78. Oddy WH, Holt PG, Sly PD, *et al.* Association between breast feeding and asthma in 6 year old children: findings of a prospective birth cohort study. *Br Med J* 1999;**319**:815–19.

79. Wright AL, Holberg CJ, Martinez FD, *et al.* Breast-feeding and lower respiratory tract illness in the first year of life. *Br Med J* 1989; **299**:946–9.

80. Rusconi F, Galassi C, Corbo GM, *et al.* Risk factors for early, persistent, and late-onset wheezing in young children. SIDRIA Collaborative Group. *Am J Respir Crit Care Med.* 1999;**160**:1617–22.

81. Hanson LA. Human milk and host defence: immediate and long-term effects. *Acta Paediatr* (Suppl) 1999;**88**:42–6.

82. Burt ML, Limb ES, Maguire MJ, *et al.* Infant feeding, wheezing and allergy: a prospective study. *Arch Dis Child* 1993;**68**:724–8.

82a. Dahlen SE, Malmstron K, Nizankowska E, *et al.* Improvement of aspirin-intolerant asthma by monteleakast, a leukotriene antogonist: a randomized, double-blind placebo controlled trial. *Am J Respir Crit Care Med* 2002;**16**:9–14.

83. Wright AL, Holberg CJ, Taussing LM, Martinez FD. Factors influencing the relation of infant feeding to asthma and recurrent wheeze in childhood. *Thorax* 2001;**56**:192–7.

7e

Passive smoking

JONATHAN M COURIEL

INTRODUCTION

It is almost 30 years since the first studies showed that adult tobacco smoking damages the health of children. In 1974, Colley showed the frequency of pneumonia and bronchitis in infants was related to the parents' smoking habits: if neither parent smoked the annual incidence was 7.8%, if one smoked it was 11.4%, and if both parents smoked it was 17.6%.[1] In the same year, Harlap and Davies showed a dose–response relationship between maternal smoking and hospital admissions for pneumonia or bronchitis in the first year of life: the admission rate for infants of mothers who smoked was 28% higher than that of the infants of non-smokers.[2] Surprisingly, primary care contacts for children with asthma do not appear to be greater for those with reported passive smoke exposure or with greater urinary cortinine levels.[3]

Since these landmark papers, there have been over 3500 publications on the effects of passive smoking on the health of children. From this mass of information, a consistent picture has gradually emerged. It is now clear that passive smoking is an important and potentially avoidable cause of illness and death in children. Awareness of the effects of passive (involuntary) smoking has been increased by several reports[2–5] and by a series of systematic reviews.[6–15] The evidence supports a causal relationship between children's exposure to cigarette smoke, both postnatally, and *in utero* if the mother smokes during pregnancy, and many different adverse outcomes. Although the respiratory tract is the main site of impact, other systems are also affected (Table 7e.1). For example, parental smoking is now the most important avoidable cause of the sudden infant death syndrome in industrialized countries.[16]

The main effects of passive smoking on the respiratory health of children are summarized in Table 7e.2. Overall, the odds ratios for a wide range of respiratory symptoms and illnesses are between 1.2 and 1.6 if either parent smokes. Some effects, such as lower respiratory tract infections, are greater in the first two years of life than in older children,[6,15] but others persist throughout childhood. For many outcomes, there is a dose–response relationship, with higher rates if both rather than only one parent smokes, or with higher daily consumption of cigarettes. Maternal smoking has a greater effect than paternal smoking. Current evidence suggests that this reflects

Table 7e.1 *Main effects of parental smoking on children*

Fetus
- intrauterine growth retardation
- increased spontaneous abortions (miscarriages)
- increased perinatal mortality
- increased premature delivery
- impaired lung development

Infant
- increased sudden infant death syndrome
- increased lower respiratory tract infections
- increased hospital admissions
- abnormal lung function

Child
- increase of all respiratory symptoms
- increased asthma
- increased acute and chronic middle ear disease
- decreased airway function

Adult
- increased risk of malignancies
- increased likelihood of active smoking
- ? precursor of chronic obstructive pulmonary disease

Table 7e.2 *Summary of effects of parental smoking on respiratory health of children (From Cook & Strachan[14])*

Outcome	Either parent OR (95% CI)	Mother OR (95% CI)
Lower respiratory illness, 0–2 yrs		
All studies	1.57 (1.42–1.74)	1.72 (1.55–1.91)
Community studies of wheeze	1.55 (1.16–2.08)	2.08 (1.59–2.71)
Hospital admissions for LRI	1.71 (1.21–2.40)	1.53 (1.25–1.86)
Prevalence rates, age 5–16 yrs		
Wheeze	1.24 (1.17–1.31)	1.28 (1.19–1.38)
Cough	1.40 (1.27–1.53)	1.40 (1.20–1.64)
Breathlessness	1.31 (1.08–1.59)	
Asthma (cross-sectional studies)	1.21 (1.10–1.34)	1.36 (1.20–1.55)
Asthma (case–control studies)	1.37 (1.15–1.64)	
Bronchial reactivity		1.29 (1.10–1.50)
Skin prick positivity		0.87 (0.64–1.24)
Incidence of asthma		
Under age 6		1.31 (1.22–1.41)
Over age 6		1.13 (1.04–1.22)

OR: odds ratio; CI: confidence intervals; LRI: lower respiratory illness.

antenatal exposure of the fetus to tobacco toxins, such as nicotine or carbon monoxide, which cross the placenta, but postnatal exposure to environmental tobacco smoke (ETS) is also important.

This chapter will focus on the relationship between parental smoking and asthma and other wheezing disorders in children. Before doing so, we need to consider the nature of ETS.

THE COMPOSITION AND MEASUREMENT OF ENVIRONMENTAL TOBACCO SMOKE

The scale of the problem

Tobacco smoke is the commonest and most important indoor pollutant to which children are exposed. They are particularly vulnerable, as their rapidly developing lungs are structurally and immunologically immature. As children spend most of their early life in the presence of their parents, those with parents who smoke have prolonged exposure to ETS. In Britain, 3.7 million children aged less than ten live with at least one adult who smokes: in 11% of homes only the mother smokes, in 19% the father smokes, and in a further 20% of homes both parents smoke (Figure 7e.1).[17] Although the proportion of children exposed to ETS has fallen slightly in the last decade, almost half the children in the UK are still smoking passively.[18]

The composition of ETS

Tobacco smoke enters the environment in two ways. *Mainstream smoke* is the complex aerosol of over 3500 chemicals inhaled by the smoker, filtered by the lungs and then exhaled. *Sidestream smoke* enters the environment

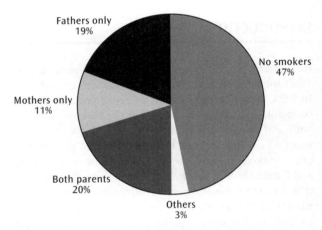

Figure 7e.1 *Passive exposure to tobacco smoke in 5 to 7-year-olds. (From ref. 17.)*

directly from the burning tip of a cigarette: it accounts for 85% of ETS. Both contain toxins such as carbon monoxide, ammonia, formaldehyde, oxides of nitrogen, nicotine and hydrogen cyanide, and over 40 proven carcinogens including benzo-[a]pyrene, 2-naphthylamine, benzene and nitrosamines. Many constituents are in higher concentrations in sidestream than in mainstream smoke. How much of these toxins an individual inhales passively depends on the type and number of cigarettes smoked, the proximity to the smoker, the size and the ventilation of the room, and the length of exposure.[19]

Measuring exposure to environmental tobacco smoke

Early studies of passive smoking relied on a history of whether one or both parents smoked or of the number of cigarettes they consumed daily. Recent studies have quantified exposure by measuring levels of biochemical markers of tobacco smoke. *Cotinine*, the principal metabolite of nicotine, is the most sensitive (97%) and specific (99%) indicator of smoking. It can be measured in serum, saliva, urine, hair and meconium. It has a median half-life in children of 27–28 hours.[20] Cotinine levels correlate closely with air nicotine levels within the home[21] and with questionnaires on smoking habits of parents.[22] Parental self-reporting is less reliable if children suffer from chronic chest illness: Kohler showed 30–60% underreporting by the parents of children with asthma or cystic fibrosis when compared with urinary cotinine levels.[23] Significant levels of cotinine occur in children from non-smoking households,[18] as children inhale ETS from sources other than their parents. Cotinine levels are influenced by the number of smokers in the home, and by social class, type of accommodation, day of the week and season.[17] Urinary cotinine levels measured in the first weeks of life are higher in infants of smoking mothers than in the infants of non-smokers. Levels are five times higher in the breast-fed than the bottle-fed infants of smokers, indicating that nicotine and cotinine are excreted in breast milk as well as being inhaled.[24]

Cotinine measurements give a useful measure of recent ETS exposure, but do not tell us about the duration of exposure or about the intake of other components of tobacco smoke which may be more important than nicotine. Nevertheless, Jarvis estimated that the nicotine dose received by children whose parents smoke is equivalent to the children actively smoking 60–150 cigarettes a year.[25]

ENVIRONMENTAL TOBACCO SMOKE, ASTHMA AND WHEEZING

Epidemiological evidence

Until recently, it was difficult to compare or collate the many hundred studies of the relationship between parental smoking and asthma and other wheezing disorders in childhood. Prospective, case–control and cross-sectional study designs have been used, from both community and hospital-based populations, often with different, poorly defined outcome measures. The degree to which important confounding variables such as socio-economic status, prematurity, atopy and family size have been controlled for, has varied greatly. It has been difficult to separate the effects of intrauterine exposure from postnatal passive smoking, as 90% of women who smoke in pregnancy are still smoking 5 years later.

Our understanding of these complex issues has been aided greatly by a comprehensive series of systematic quantitative reviews by Strachan and Cook published recently in *Thorax*,[6–14] by a recent review by Le Souëf,[56] and by studies of lung function in infants.

Wheezing and non-wheezing lower respiratory illness

In their first review, Strachan and Cook assessed the evidence relating parental smoking to acute lower respiratory illnesses (LRIs) in the first 3 years of life.[6] The results of the 24 community-based and 17 hospital studies they identified were broadly consistent, with a pooled odds ratio for LRI of 1.57 (95% CI 1.42–1.74) if either parent smoked and 1.72 (1.55–1.92) if only the mother smoked. The contribution of postnatal as well as antenatal exposure was confirmed by a significant association even if the mother did not smoke.

Fifteen studies focused on LRIs in which the child wheezed. All but one found an increased risk associated with parental smoking: maternal smoking was more important than paternal. Analysis of case–control studies of RSV infection also found a significant effect. The authors concluded there is a causal relationship between parental smoking and LRI in early childhood.

Prevalence of asthma and other respiratory symptoms

In later reviews, they examined the relationship between parental smoking and the prevalence of asthma and other respiratory symptoms in school-age children (5–16 years)[6,11] (Table 7e.2). Once again, paternal and maternal smoking were both significant, but the mother's smoking had a greater effect. Despite variations in methodology and outcome measures in the 60 studies they analysed, a consistent pattern emerged. In the 25 studies containing quantitative data specifically on asthma, all but two showed an odds ratio of greater than one, but in many the confidence limits included unity. The pooled odds ratio was 1.21 (1.10–1.34) for asthma. For wheeze, it was 1.24 (1.17–1.31) if either parent smoked. In some studies, heavy smoking by the mother (more than 15–20 cigarettes a day), was associated with far higher odds ratios, re-emphasizing that the 'dose' of ETS is important.

Similar sized effects were present for cough, phlegm and breathlessness.[8] Again there was a high degree of consistency amongst the studies and the effects were robust to adjustment for a wide range of confounding variables.

Analysis of 51 longitudinal and case–control studies of childhood asthma showed maternal smoking increased the risk of wheezing illness.[11] The effect was stronger up to the age of 6 years (pooled OR 1.31) than in older children (1.13). Children whose mothers smoked were more likely to lose their symptoms in the early years, particularly if they had no evidence of atopy. However, several indicators of asthma severity, including symptom scores, attack frequency, and use of asthma medication, were positively related to ETS exposure.

Strachan and Cook suggest the explanation for this apparent paradox may be that tobacco smoke is a co-factor provoking wheezing attacks in susceptible individuals rather than a cause of the underlying asthmatic tendency. In other words, ETS provokes exacerbations rather than inducing or initiating asthma. By contrast, the authors of the California Environmental Protection Agency review of ETS found 'compelling evidence' that ETS contributes to both the induction and exacerbation of asthma.[4]

Exacerbations

It is perhaps surprising that several studies have found no evidence that passive smoking increases the risk of hospital admission for acute asthma in children. For example, Reese found no association between urinary cotinine levels and asthma admissions, in contrast to the positive correlation with admissions for bronchiolitis they reported.[26] Ehrlich showed a correlation between recent passive smoking, as assessed by questionnaire and urinary cotinine, and a diagnosis of asthma, but no association with acute exacerbations.[27] He suggested that passive smoking increases hyperreactivity rather than causing bronchospasm. By contrast, Chilmonczyk found higher urinary cotinine levels in children with asthma were associated with a higher incidence of acute exacerbations.[28]

EFFECTS OF PARENTAL SMOKING ON LUNG FUNCTION

Our understanding of how adult smoking causes respiratory symptoms in children has been aided by elegant physiological studies of lung function in children, particularly in infants.

Airway function in school-children

Passive smoking has a statistically significant but small effect on spirometry values in children. In an analysis of 21 surveys of school-children, the mean reduction in FEV_1 associated with parental smoking was only 1.4% (95% CI 1.0–1.9%). There were greater reductions in more sensitive indices of airway function, such as maximal mid-expiratory (mean reduction 5.0%) and end-expiratory flow rates (mean 4.3%).[13] Maternal smoking was more important than paternal smoking. The size of the effect was related to the level of exposure to ETS. Analysis of these data, and the results of a recent large multicentre study from California,[29] suggests antenatal rather than current exposure to ETS is the key factor.

Studies of the relationship between parental smoking and bronchial hyperreactivity or hyperresponsiveness have produced confusing and conflicting findings.[12] Some studies have shown a significant association with current ETS exposure[30] but others have not. This may reflect differences in the study populations, the challenge

test employed, or other methodological issues. By contrast, five studies of circadian changes in peak expiratory flow have shown greater diurnal variation in children exposed to ETS than controls.[12]

Airway function in infants

Recent physiological studies in infants support the concept that antenatal exposure to tobacco toxins has a prolonged effect on the growth and function of the lungs.[31,32] Hanrahan and Tager showed that maternal smoking in pregnancy results in an increased incidence of wheezing illness in infancy and reduced forced expiratory flow rates at functional residual capacity (VmaxFRC) (mean 74.3 vs 150.4 ml/s/cm in infants of smokers vs infants of non-smokers: $p = 0.0007$)[33,34] (see also Chapter 4b). They found a strong negative correlation between VmaxFRC and the urinary cotinine levels measured during pregnancy. Further measurements in this cohort at 18 months of age showed persistent reductions in both FRC and VmaxFRC in the offspring of smoking mothers, particularly in girls.[35] The authors suggest smoking in pregnancy impairs fetal airway development and alters the elastic properties of the lung.

The Perth group has shown several abnormalities of lung function in infants enrolled into a prospective, community-based cohort. Preliminary analysis suggested that parental smoking contributed to the development of bronchial hyperresponsiveness, as assessed by histamine challenge, in the first weeks of life.[36] In that paper, VmaxFRC was not lower in the infants of smokers. In a later report, the time to peak expiratory flow as a proportion of expiratory time was significantly lower in 461 newborn infants whose mothers smoked more than 10 cigarettes a day, suggesting airway dysfunction.[37] In the most recent analyses of the full cohort, Young reported that maternal smoking during pregnancy was associated with significantly lower values of VmaxFRC in both boys and girls, when compared with the infants of non-smokers.[38,39] This effect persisted throughout the first year of life: paternal smoking had no detectable effect. There was no effect on neonatal bronchial responsiveness.[39]

Data from other studies in the UK, America and Norway broadly support these findings.[12,14,32] Milner showed reduced static compliance and conductance in the infants of smoking mothers, with some differences between girls and boys, but no effect on expiratory flow.[40] In the Tuscon cohort of infants, Martinez et al. have shown diminished respiratory conductance and lower maximal expiratory flows in the early months, before any respiratory infections, in those infants who subsequently wheezed.[41–43]

Both the Tuscon and the Perth longitudinal cohort studies have shown that reduced lung function early in life both precedes and predicts a greater risk of wheezing with viral infections, including classical RSV bronchiolitis. Although many of these children stop having recurrent episodes of wheeze in early childhood ('transient early wheezers')[42,43] they continue to show evidence of reduced lung function in a pattern which suggests they have smaller pulmonary airways than the children of non-smokers. This may be a precursor of chronic obstructive airways disease in adult life.[31]

The physiological evidence that intrauterine exposure to tobacco toxins impairs normal lung growth and development is supported by morphometric and histological studies in both humans and experimental animals. Abnormal bronchial and alveolar anatomy, decreased lung volume, weight and nucleic acid content, and reduced parenchymal elastic tissues and decreased attachment of airways to lung parenchyma, have all been associated with exposure of the fetus to tobacco products.[38,44,45,57] Some of these effects may be hormonally mediated. Nicotine and carbon monoxide can both reduce uterine blood flow and fetal oxygen delivery.[45] Maternal smoking also reduces fetal breathing movements, an important part of normal lung development.

Maternal smoking in pregnancy is the most important, potentially avoidable cause of abnormal airway function in early childhood.

Other possible mechanisms

As well as impairing lung development, there are several other pathways by which passive smoking could influence asthma and other wheezing conditions (Figure 7e.2).

There is a controversial relationship between viral (upper) and respiratory tract infections and associated wheezing low respiratory tract illness, in early childhood, and later childhood asthma (see Chapter 2). As passive smoking increases both the frequency and severity of such infections, this may have an important influence on asthma and other wheezing illnesses.

In the past, it was suggested that exposure to ETS altered some aspects of the immune response, such as IgE production, thereby increasing the risk of allergic sensitisation and atopic illnesses.[46] However, a systematic review failed to identify a consistent relationship between passive smoking and serum IgE levels, skin-prick test responses, or atopic conditions such as eczema or allergic rhinitis.[10]

THE POTENTIAL FOR INTERVENTION

All of those involved in the care of children have a responsibility to inform parents of the hazards of smoking and to help them to quit. Many clinicians believe such discussions rarely make a difference, but very few studies have assessed this. One randomized controlled trial confirmed that simply telling the parents of asthmatic children that smoking was harmful to their children had no effect on their smoking or the cotinine levels in the children.[47] But in another RCT, a series of counselling sessions was effective in reducing children's exposure to ETS.[48]

There is now convincing evidence that several strategies increase the proportion of adult smokers who quit.[45,49,50] We now have practical guidelines for smoking cessation from the British Thoracic Society (Table 7e.3).[51] *Smoking cessation interventions* are behavioural (counselling, education), pharmacological (nicotine replacement therapy, bupropion), or a combination of the two.[45] Population-based interventions, such as health warnings on cigarette packets, self-help leaflets, or public education campaigns, often have little impact. For example, despite a sustained campaign to discourage young people in the UK from smoking, the proportion of 11 to 15-year-olds who smoke regularly has risen progressively since 1986.[45]

Individual counselling of smokers is more effective. A systematic review of 31 randomized controlled trials involving over 26 000 adult smokers showed that brief advice about stopping smoking had a significant, if small, effect on cessation rates 6 months later.[49] More intensive advice produced only a slightly greater benefit. Group therapy may be more cost-effective.

Nicotine replacement therapy (NRT) with chewing gum, transdermal patches, sublingual tablets or inhalation increases quit rates 1.5 to 2-fold, and about 20% of those given NRT with counselling remain non-smokers a year

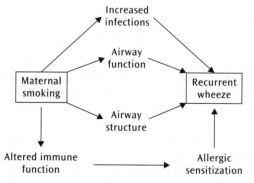

Figure 7e.2 *Possible mechanisms for effects of maternal smoking on recurrent wheeze.*

Table 7e.3 *Principles of effective smoking cessation (Based on the British Thoracic Society guidelines[51])*

- Assess the smoking status of patients (parents) at every opportunity
- Advise all smokers to stop
- Assist all those interested in doing so
- Refer to specialist cessation service if necessary
- Recommend smokers who want to stop to use nicotine replacement therapy or bupropion (not pregnant women)
- Provide accurate information and advice on treatment
- Pregnant women should be given firm and clear advice to stop smoking during pregnancy

later.[52] *Bupropion* is a new pharmacological treatment for smokers. Developed as an anti-depressant, its mechanism of action in smoking cessation is unclear.[52] In one of several controlled trials, the rates of quitting one year after a seven week course of oral bupropion 100–300 mg daily were 20–23%, compared with 12% in those given placebo.[53] Bupropion is more effective and cheaper than NRT, but there may be benefits in using both together.[54]

About 25–30% of women in the UK smoke in pregnancy and there has been no decrease in this figure in the last 8 years.[45] Given what we now know about the effects of smoking on the fetus, is it not logical to target women smokers presenting for *antenatal care*? Smoking cessation in pregnancy is effective, resulting in a reduction in the proportion of women smoking of 6–8%.[51,55] It is recommended that such counselling should be used routinely.[51] Unfortunately, nicotine replacement therapy and bupropion are contraindicated during pregnancy in the UK, although they are probably safer than smoking.

CONCLUSIONS

Environmental tobacco smoke is an important, and potentially avoidable, cause of wheeze and other respiratory symptoms in children. There is increasing evidence that antenatal exposure of the fetus to tobacco toxins in mothers who smoke, impairs lung development and leads to abnormal airway function in their offspring as infants, older children, and conceivably as adults. Additional postnatal exposure to smoking by either parent adds to these effects.

We can debate whether passive smoking simply exacerbates symptoms or whether it also induces childhood asthma. This is a somewhat semantic argument. What is now irrefutable is that ETS exposure increases the risk of a child developing recurrent wheeze, cough and breathlessness, whatever diagnostic label we may choose to describe this symptom complex. However, there is some evidence that parents who smoke are less likely to bring these symptomatic children to the attention of doctors.[3]

What direction should future research in this field take? New epidemiological or physiological studies are unlikely to increase greatly our understanding of the effects of passive smoking. Observational studies of passive smoking are numbered in their thousands, but there has been only a handful of studies of interventions to reduce ETS exposure in children. The challenge now is to design and assess strategies that reduce children's exposure.[58] We should implement what is already known about smoking cessation more effectively and more enthusiastically. At a time of intense interest in the primary or secondary prevention of asthma, reducing the burden that passive smoking imposes on children is a challenge we can no longer reasonably ignore.

REFERENCES

1. Colley JRT, Holland WW, Corkhill RT. Influence of passive smoking and parental phlegm on pneumonia and bronchitis in early childhood. *Lancet* 1974;**ii**:1031–4.
2. Harlap S, Davies AM. Infant admissions to hospital and maternal smoking. *Lancet* 1974;**i**:529–32.
3. Crombie IK, Wright A, Irvine L, Clark RA, Slane PW. Does passive smoking increase the frequency of health service contacts in children with asthma? *Thorax* 2001;**56**:9–12.
4. Dunn A, Zeise L, eds. Health effects of exposure to environmental tobacco smoke. *California Environmental Protection Agency*, 1997.
5. Couriel JM. Passive smoking and the health of children. *Thorax* 1994;**49**:731–4.
6. Strachan DP, Cook DG. Health effects of passive smoking. 1. Parental smoking and lower respiratory illness in infancy and early childhood. *Thorax* 1997;**52**:905–14.
7. Anderson HR, Cook DG. Health effects of passive smoking. 2. Passive smoking and sudden infant death syndrome. Review of the epidemiological evidence. *Thorax* 1997;**52**:1003–9.
8. Cook DG, Strachan DP. Health effects of passive smoking. 3. Parental smoking and respiratory symptoms in schoolchildren. *Thorax* 1997;**52**:1081–94.
9. Strachan DP, Cook DG. Health effects of passive smoking. 4. Parental smoking, middle ear disease and adenotonsillectomy in children. *Thorax* 1998;**53**:50–6.
10. Strachan DP, Cook DG. Health effects of passive smoking. 5. Parental smoking and allergic sensitisation in children. *Thorax* 1998;**53**:117–23.
11. Strachan DP, Cook DG. Health effects of passive smoking. 6. Parental smoking and childhood asthma: longitudinal and case-control studies. *Thorax* 1998;**53**:204–12.
12. Cook DG, Strachan DP. Health effects of passive smoking. 7. Parental smoking, bronchial reactivity and peak flow variability in children. *Thorax* 1998;**53**:295–301.
13. Cook DG, Strachan DP, Carey IM. Health effects of passive smoking. 9. Parental smoking and spirometric indices in children. *Thorax* 1998;**53**:884–93.
14. Cook DG, Strachan DP. Summary of effects of parental smoking on the respiratory health of children and implications for research. *Thorax* 1999;**54**:357–66.
15. Li JSM, Peat JK, Xuan W, Berry G. Meta-analysis on the association between ETS exposure and the prevalence of lower respiratory tract infection in early childhood. *Pediatr Pulmonol* 1999;**27**:5–13.
16. Blair PS, Fleming PJ, Bensley D, *et al*. Smoking and the sudden infant death syndrome: results from 1993–5 case–control study for confidential inquiry into

stillbirths and deaths in infancy. *Br Med J* 1996;**313**:195–8.

17. Cook DG, Whincup PH, Jarvis MJ, Strachan DP, Papacosta O, Bryant A. Passive exposure to tobacco smoke in children aged 5–7 years: individual, family and community factors. *Br Med J* 1994;**308**:384–9.

18. Jarvis MJ, Goddard E, Higgins V, Feyerabend C, Bryant A, Cook DG. Children's exposure to passive smoking in England since the 1980s: cotinine evidence from population surveys. *Br Med J* 2000;**321**:343–5.

19. Fielding JE, Phenow KJ. Health effects of involuntary smoking. *N Engl J Med* 1988;**319**:1452–60.

20. Leong JW, Dore ND, Shelley K, Holt EJ, *et al.* The elimination half-life of urinary cotinine in children of tobacco smoking mothers. *Pulm Pharmacol Ther* 1998;**11**:287–90.

21. Henderson FW, Reid HF, Morris R, *et al.* Home air nicotine levels and urinary cotinine excretion in preschool children. *Am Rev Respir Dis* 1989;**140**:197–201.

22. Cook DG, Whincup PH, Papacosta O, Strachan DP, Jarvis MJ, Bryant A. Relation of passive smoking as assessed by salivary cotinine concentrations and questionnaire to spirometric indices in children. *Thorax* 1993;**48**:14–20.

23. Kohler E, Sollich V, Schuster R, Thal W. Passive smoke exposure in children with respiratory tract disease. *Hum Exp Toxicol* 1999;**18**:212–17.

24. Becker AB, Mnafreda J, Fergusson AC, *et al.* Breast-feeding and environmental tobacco smoke exposure. *Arch Pediatr Adolesc Med* 1999; **153**:689–91.

25. Jarvis MJ, McNeill AD, Russell MAH, West RJ, Bryant A, Feyerabend C. Passive smoking in adolescents: one-year stability of exposure in the home. *Lancet* 1987;**i**:1324–5.

26. Reese AC, James IR, Landau LI, Lesouef PN. Relationship between urinary cotinine level and diagnosis in children admitted to hospital. *Am Rev Respir Dis* 1992;**146**:66–70.

27. Ehrlich R, Kattan M, Godbold J, Saltzberg DS, Grimm KT, Landrigan PJ, Liliefield DE. Childhood asthma and passive smoking: urinary cotinine as a biomarker of exposure. *Am Rev Respir Dis* 1992;**145**:594–9.

28. Chilmonczyk BA, Salmun LM, Megathlin KN, *et al.* Association between exposure to environmental tobacco smoke and exacerbations of asthma in children. *N Engl J Med* 1993;**328**:1665–9.

29. Gilliland FD, Berhane K, McConnell R, Gauderman WJ, Vora H, Rappaport EB, Avol E, Peter JM. Maternal smoking during pregnancy, ETS exposure and childhood lung function. *Thorax* 2000;**55**:271–6.

30. Murray AB, Morrison BJ. The effect of cigarette smoke from the mother on bronchial hyperresponsiveness and severity of symptoms in children with asthma. *J Allergy Clin Immunol* 1986;**77**:575–81.

31. Silverman M. Out of the mouths and babes and sucklings: lessons from early childhood asthma. *Thorax* 1993;**48**:1200–4.

32. Morgan WJ, Martinez FD. Maternal smoking and infant lung function. *Am J Respir Crit Care Med* 1998;**158**:689–90.

33. Hanrahan JP, Tager IB, Segal MR, *et al.* The effect of maternal smoking during pregnancy on early infant lung function. *Am Rev Respir Dis* 1992;**145**:1129–35.

34. Tager IB, Hanrahan JP, Tosteson TD, Castile RG, Brown RW, Weiss ST, Speizer FE. Lung function, pre- and postnatal smoke exposure and wheezing in the first year of life. *Am Rev Respir Dis* 1993;**147**:811–17.

35. Tager IB, Ngo L, Hanrahan JP. Maternal smoking during pregnancy. Effects on lung function during the first 18 months of life. *Am J Respir Crit Care Med* 1995;**152**:977–83.

36. Young S, Le Souef PN, Geelhoed GC, Stick SM, Turner KJ, Landau LI. The influence of a family history of asthma and parental smoking on airway responsiveness in early infancy. *N Engl J Med* 1991;**324**:1168–73.

37. Stick SM, Burton PR, Gurrin L, Sly PD, LeSouef PN. Effects of maternal smoking during pregnancy and a family history of asthma on respiratory function in newborn infants. *Lancet* 1996;**348**:1060–4.

38. Young S, Sherrill DL, Arnott J, Diepeveen D, LeSouef PN, Landau LI. Parental factors affecting lung function during the first year of life. *Pediatr Pulmonol* 2000;**29**:3331–40.

39. Young S, Arnott J, O'Keefe PT, LeSouef PN, Landau LI. The association between early life lung function and wheezing during the first two years of life. *Eur Respir J* 2000;**15**:151–7.

40. Milner AD, Marsh MJ, Ingram DM, Fox GF, Susiva C. Effects of smoking in pregnancy on neonatal lung function. *Arch Dis Child Fetal Neonat Ed* 1999;**80**:F8–14.

41. Martinez FD, Antognoni G, Macri F, *et al.* Parental smoking enhances bronchial responsiveness in nine-year old children. *Am Rev Respir Dis* 1988;**138**: 518–23.

42. Martinez FD, Morgan WJ, Wright AL, Holberg C, Taussig LM, the Group Health Medical Associates. Initial airway function is a risk factor for recurrent wheezing respiratory illnesses during the first three years of life. *Am Rev Respir Dis* 1991;**143**:312–16.

43. Stein RT, Holberg CJ, Sherrill D, Wright AL, Morgan WJ, Taussig L, Martinez FD. Influence of parental smoking on respiratory symptoms during the first decade of life: the Tuscon Children's Respiratory Study. *Am J Epidemiol* 1999;**149**:1030–7.

44. Moessinger AC. Mothers who smoke and the lungs of their offspring. *Ann NY Acad Sci* 1989;**562**:101–4.

45. Royal College of Physicians. *Nicotine Addiction in Britain.* RCP, London, 2000.

46. Kjellman NIM. Effect of parental smoking on IgE levels in children. *Lancet* 1981;**i**:993.

47. Irvine L, Crombie IK, Clark RA, Slone PW, Feyerabend C, Goodman KE, Cater IJ. Advising parents of asthmatic children on smoking: randomised controlled trial. *Br Med J* 1999;**318**:1456–9.

48. Hovell MF, Zakarian JM, Matt GE, Hofstetter CR, Bernert JT, Pirkle J. Effect of counselling mothers on their children's exposure to ETS: randomised controlled trial. *Br Med J* 2000;**321**:337–42.

49. Silagy C. Physician advice for smoking cessation (*Cochrane Review*). Cochrane Library, Issue 2, 2000, Oxford, Software Update.

50. Campbell IA. Smoking cessation. *Thorax* 2000; **55**(Suppl 1):S28–31.

51. Raw M, McNeill A, West RJ. Smoking cessation guidelines for health care professionals. *Thorax* 1998;**53**(Suppl 5, Pt 1):S1–19.

52. Britton J, Jarvis M. Bupropion: a new treatment for smokers. *Br Med J* 2000;**321**:65–6.

53. Hurt RD, Sachs DL, Glover ED, *et al*. A comparison of sustained-release bupropion and placebo for smoking cessation. *N Engl J Med* 1997;**337**:1195–1202.

54. Jorenby DE, Leischow SJ, Nides MA, *et al*. A controlled trial of sustained release bupropion, a nicotine patch or both for smoking cessation. *N Engl J Med* 1999; **340**:685–91.

55. Lumley J, Oliver S, Waters E. Interventions for promoting smoking cessation during pregnancy (Cochrane Review). *Cochrane Library*, Issue 2, 2000, Oxford, Update Software.

56. Le Souëf PN. Tobacco related lung disease in childhood. *Thorax* 2000;**55**:1063–7.

57. Elliot J, Carroll N, Bosco M, McCrohan M, Robinson P. Increased airway responsiveness and decreased alveolar attachment points following in utero smoke exposure in the guinea pig. *Am J Respir Crit Care Med* 2001;**163**:140–4.

58. Ferrence R, Ashley M. Protecting children from passive smoking. *Br Med J* 2000;**321**:310–11.

8a

Clinical pharmacology and therapeutics

SØREN PEDERSEN AND HANS BISGAARD

INTRODUCTION

An immense amount of information is available about the various drugs and treatments for childhood wheeze and asthma. The information is derived from many sources, including whole-animal studies, *in vitro* studies on tissue and cells from animals and humans, *in vivo* studies in adults, and *in vivo* studies in children. In the following only the main information from studies in humans or on human tissues and cells is presented. Furthermore, in the pharmacokinetic and pharmacodynamic sections data from studies in children are used preferentially (when available). When the results from clinical studies are discussed main emphasis has been based wherever possible on the Cochrane Database of Systematic Reviews. Where Cochrane reviews are unavailable, the evidence is based on peer-reviewed systematic reviews of randomized trials in children with asthma. When no such reviews exist individual double-blind randomized controlled trials are scrutinized for evidence.

The clinical effect and effectiveness of the various groups of drugs used in management has been reviewed. The clinical evidence about a particular treatment or healthcare intervention should ideally address three basic questions: can it work (efficacy), does it work in actual clinical practice (effectiveness), and is it worth it (efficiency).[1] However, at present the majority of our information on childhood asthma treatment is based on efficacy studies. In addition other factors such as asthma severity, the benefits and the risks of each treatment, and the availability of the various forms of asthma treatment should influence the choice of treatment. Cultural preferences and differences in healthcare systems also need to be considered. The final choice of treatment should integrate individual clinical expertise with patient preferences and the best available evidence from systematic, clinically relevant research in children.

β-ADRENERGIC AGENTS

For many years treatment with β-adrenoceptor agonists has been the mainstay of asthma treatment in children. Today these drugs are by far the most effective bronchodilators available and therefore the drug of choice in acute asthma. However, the exact role of β-agonists in the maintenance treatment of asthma is undergoing re-appraisal after the introduction of long-acting inhaled β-agonists.

Pharmacological action

β-agonists act through β-adrenoceptors, which belong to a family of G-protein linked receptors in the cell membrane (Figure 8a.1).[2] β_1 and β_2-receptors have been cloned and their sequences determined. Stimulation of the receptor causes activation of intracellular adenylate cyclase which catalyses the production of cyclic adenosine monophosphate (AMP), which in turn causes bronchodilation. These effects are only observed at relatively high concentrations of β-agonist when maximal relaxation responses have been exceeded. However, much lower concentrations of β-agonists have been shown to open membrane K^+ channels and induce smooth muscle relaxation without

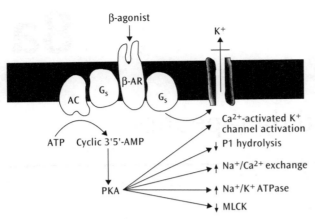

Figure 8a.1 *Molecular mechanisms involved in the bronchodilator response to β-agonists. β-adrenoceptor (β-AR) stimulation activates a stimulatory G-protein (G_s) which may couple directly to a large conductance Ca^{2+}-activated K^+ channel or may activate adenylyl cyclase (AC), leading to an increase in cyclic adenosine monophosphate (AMP). Cyclic AMP activates protein kinase A (PKA), resulting in phosphorylation of various proteins, including K^+ channels, myosin light chain kinase (MLCK) and enzymes involved in phosphoinositide (PI) hydrolysis. ATP: adenosine triphosphate; ATPase: adenosine triphosphatase. (From ref. 2 with permission.)*

Table 8a.1 *Possible modulatory effects of long-acting β₂-agonists on airway inflammation: preclinical observations*

Cell type	Effects
T-lymphocyte	Inhibition of cytokine production
Macrophage/monocyte	Inhibition of mediator and cytokine release
Mast cell	Inhibition of mediator and cytokine release
Eosinophil	Inhibition of oxidative burst, mediator release and cationic protein release
Neutrophil	Inhibition of oxidative burst and mediator release. Inhibition of neutrophil recruitment
Sensory nerves	Inhibition of tachykinin release
Endothelial cells	Decreased permeability
Epithelial cells	Decreased permeability, inhibition of cytokine expression
Fibroblast	Inhibition of adhesion molecules
Smooth muscle cell	Inhibition of proliferation, inhibition of cytokine production

a rise in AMP, suggesting that this direct effect is a more important mechanism of airway smooth muscle response to β-agonists.[2]

The most important effect of β₂-agonists is *bronchodilation*. This action is mainly due to relaxation of airway smooth muscle. However, additional effects may also contribute to their anti-asthma action.

- *Modulation of cholinergic neurotransmission* via prejunctional β₂-receptors on postganglionic nerves.[3] The clinical importance of this is unknown.
- *Inhibition of the release of histamine* from human mast cells. Whether these *in vitro* findings are relevant to *in vivo* use of the drugs is uncertain. However, functional evidence suggests that β-agonists may have an effect on mast cells *in vivo* since inhaled β-agonists have a significantly greater effect on bronchoconstriction induced by indirectly acting (via mast cells) constrictors such as AMP than on bronchoconstriction induced by directly acting constrictors such as histamine and methacholine.[4,5] The possible effects on airway inflammation of long-acting β₂-agonists have recently been summarized (Table 8a.1).[6]
- *Reduction of vascular permeability* in the airways, probably by an action at β₂ adrenoceptors at the level of postcapillary venules.[7] The extent to which physiological doses of β₂-agonists produce this effect is uncertain.[7,8]
- β₂-agonists may significantly *enhance mucociliary clearance* and maintain the functional integrity of the airways.[9]

Adrenoceptor agonists

β-receptors are widely distributed throughout the body in most tissues and cells. β₁-receptors are mainly located in the heart while β₂-receptors are found in the airways, the heart, blood vessels, muscles and inflammatory cells. Stimulation of *α-adrenoceptors* causes constriction of bronchial muscle, peripheral blood vessels and sphincters of the alimentary tract. Furthermore, it causes decreased motility and tone of the alimentary tract and inhibition of lipolysis and insulin secretion. Stimulation of *β₁-adrenoceptors* has a positive chronotropic and inotropic effect on cardiac muscle and stimulates lipolysis. Stimulation of *β₂-adrenoceptors* relaxes smooth muscles in the airways, alimentary tract and peripheral blood vessels, increases tremor in skeletal muscle and stimulates glycogenolysis, glycolysis and insulin secretion. Stimulation of *β₃-adrenoceptors* may produce a number of metabolic effects.

Adrenaline (epinephrine), the first adrenoceptor agonist to be used for asthma, has both α and β activity. Although it is an effective bronchodilator, it has undesirable side effects caused by its α and β₁ actions: anxiety, tremor, hypertension, tachycardia, palpitations and cardiac arrhythmias. As a consequence its use in modern asthma treatment is obsolete. It is sometimes suggested that adrenaline, with its α-adrenoceptor vasoconstricting activity would be better than other drugs at decreasing bronchial oedema because of its constrictor effects on arterioles. However, it also causes venous vasoconstriction and this effect could negate or even overwhelm any beneficial effect on arterial constriction and controlled clinical trials do not demonstrate any advantages over the modern adrenoceptor agonists in relieving airway obstruction in children (other than acute laryngo-tracheo-bronchitis).[10] However, the α stimulating action makes adrenaline the drug of choice for the treatment of anaphylactic shock. *Isoprenaline* has no α activity but an equal activity on β_1 and β_2-receptors. It is rapidly metabolized and has a very short duration of action. Selective β_2-agonists with longer duration of action have been developed and today isoprenaline should not be used for asthma treatment if these drugs are available. At present no purely β_2 specific agonists have been developed. All also show dose-dependent stimulation of β_1-receptors.

SELECTIVITY

Salbutamol, terbutaline and formoterol seem to have the same β_2 selectivity, whereas fenoterol may be somewhat less β_2 selective.[3,6,11] Salmeterol seems to be even more β_2 selective than any of the other β_2-agonists.[6,12] The differences in β_2-selectivity between the various modern β_2-agonists have not been shown to be clinically important in day-to-day treatment.

EFFICACY

Some β_2-agonists (salmeterol and salbutamol) are partial agonists with 60–85% of the efficacy of isoprenaline.[12,13] The clinical relevance of this is not known since in clinical practice there is no evidence that one β-agonist causes a greater maximal effect than another or that one drug diminishes the effect of another. However, studies in acute asthma have not yet been performed to assess this.

POTENCY

Marked differences are seen in potency between the various β-agonists. They are unimportant, however, since lower potency can be compensated for by giving a higher dose of the drug. Differences in dose equivalence between recommended doses of different β-agonists is more important. In this respect salbutamol 200 μg, terbutaline 500 μg, formoterol 6 μg, and salmeterol 50 μg appear to have roughly similar effects on β_2-receptors for each dose from a dry powder inhaler. Fenoterol 200 μg has somewhere between two and four times higher effect on both β_1 and β_2-receptors.[11]

DURATION OF ACTION

After inhalation the duration of action of 'conventional' inhaled β_2-agonists largely depends on dose; the higher the dose the longer the duration of action. Equipotent bronchodilating doses of salbutamol, terbutaline and fenoterol seem to have the same duration of action.

The normal duration of action of a standard dose of a short-acting β_2-agonists (SABA) is 1–5 hours depending upon the outcome parameter. Protection against exercise-induced asthma is briefer than the duration of bronchodilation.[14] Salmeterol and formoterol have both been shown to have significant bronchodilator and protective effects against various challenges for 10 hours or more after a single dose.[6,12,13,15,16] This prolonged action is only seen after inhalation and not after oral or systemic dosing so these drugs are only given by the inhaled route. Both drugs are substantially more lipophilic than other β_2-agonists. This combined with a high receptor affinity seems to be important for the long duration of action. However, in addition salmeterol probably also binds to a specific exo-site domain of the β_2-receptor protein to produce continuous stimulation of the active site of the receptor (Figure 8a.2).

CLINICAL EFFECT

The main action of β-agonists is to inhibit or reverse bronchoconstriction. Pretreatment with a single dose of an inhaled β_2-agonist protects against virtually all bronchoconstrictor stimuli including histamine, methacholine, hyperventilation, cold air, exercise, AMP and allergen. Normally a parallel shift to the right in the dose–response curve is seen so that higher doses of the constrictor are required to produce a certain fall in lung function (Figure 8a.3). However, sometimes the treatment may not only cause a parallel shift in the curve but also change its shape so that the slope becomes steeper and the magnitude of the response is unaffected or increased (Figure 8a.3).[17]

Pharmacokinetics and dynamics

SYSTEMIC ADMINISTRATION

The pharmacokinetics of systemically administered β-agonists have not been studied extensively in children, so it is not known whether important differences exist between the various drugs. However, in general terms about 33% of an oral dose is systemically absorbed in school-children.[18,19] Because of a high first-pass metabolism in the wall of the gastrointestinal tract and in the liver the bioavailability after oral dosing is only about 10–15% when plain tablets are used and about 30% lower after administration of a slow release product. Therefore, somewhat higher doses should be used when therapy is changed from plain to slow release tablets. Concomitant intake of food further reduces gastrointestinal bioavailability by about one third.

Peak plasma drug levels are measured 1–2 h after oral dosing. Most of the absorbed drug is excreted in the urine mainly as unchanged drug or a sulphate conjugate.[19,20] Renal clearance correlates with creatinine clearance and dose reductions should be considered in patients with

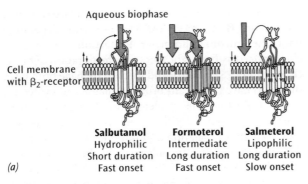

(a)

Smooth muscle cell preparations	
Membrane affinity	Salmeterol > Formoterol
Duration	Salmeterol > Formoterol
Selectivity	Salmeterol > Formoterol
Onset	Formoterol > Salmeterol
Potency	Formoterol > Salmeterol
Efficacy	Formoterol > Salmeterol
Inflammatory cells	
Inhibition of guinea pig eosinophil activation	Formoterol > Salmeterol
Inhibition of human mast cell activation	Formoterol > Salmeterol

(b)

Figure 8a.2 *Pharmacologic differences and similarities between salmeterol and formoterol. (a) The salmeterol molecule consists of the saligenin head of the salbutamol molecule that binds to the active site of the β_2-adrenergic receptor (β_2 AR), coupled to a long alphatic side chain that markedly increases the lipophilicity of the molecule. The molecule is thought to diffuse laterally through the cell membrane to approach the β_2 AR. The side chain then interacts with an auxiliary binding site (exo-site), a group of highly hydrophobic amino acids within the fourth domain of the β_2 AR. Binding to the exo-site prevents dissociation of salmeterol from the β_2 AR and allows the active saligenin head to repeatedly engage at the active site of the receptor. This results in a long duration of the effect, but a slow onset of action. The length of the side chain and the resulting lipophilicity of formoterol is intermediate between salmeterol and salbutamol. This moderate lipophilicity allows formoterol to enter the plasmalemma and to be retained. From this depot, the molecule slowly diffuses to activate the β_2 AR over a prolonged period. Conversely, sufficient drug remains available in the aqueous biophase to allow rapid interaction with the active site of the receptor and hence a rapid response. (b) The most important differences and similarities of salmeterol and formoterol. (From ref. 383.)*

impaired renal function.[21] As for most other drugs the clearance of β-agonists is a little higher in children than in adults.[19,20]

A significant correlation is seen between plasma drug levels and bronchodilating effect after systemic

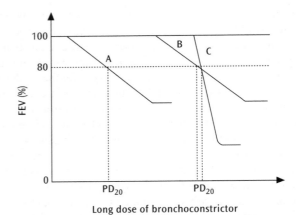

Figure 8a.3 *Three dose–response curves after provocation with a bronchoconstrictor agent: curve A is without any pretreatment; curve B and C after pretreatment with a β_2-agonist. In curve B, a parallel shift in the dose–response curve is seen without any change in the slope of the curve or the magnitude of the response. In C the same degree of protection is seen but the slope is steeper and the maximum fall in lung function is greater. Although the shift to the right of this curve is beneficial, the steepness and the magnitude of the response are potentially dangerous.*

administration of a β-agonist.[22] However, considerable inter-individual variation exists in both plasma level and physiological effect after a given dose.[22] Therefore standard doses are not feasible, and dosing should be individualized by monitoring of the therapeutic response and the occurrence of side effects.[20] A rational approach would be to start at a dose around 0.15 mg/kg/day and then gradually increase the dose until a sufficient clinical effect or systemic side effects are seen. Oral doses of terbutaline around 0.5 mg/kg/day are probably required to produce significant clinical effects.[23] This is higher than the normally recommended dose and emphasizes the importance of individual dose titration.

Continuous treatment with oral β-agonists does not protect effectively against exercise-induced asthma,[23] though it improves symptoms and peak expiratory flow and protects against nocturnal asthma, particulary when slow release products are used.[23,24]

INHALATION

β-agonists should preferably be given by inhalation since this allows bronchodilation to be achieved more rapidly, at a lower dose and with fewer side effects than by either oral or intravenous administration.[25,26] After inhalation a measurable bronchodilator effect is seen within one minute, reaching >90% of maximal within 10 minutes.[27] Inhalers usually deliver rather large doses so one dose results in near maximum bronchodilation when the patient is not suffering from severe airway obstruction.

Furthermore, inhalation offers significant protection against exercise-induced asthma and other challenges[14] which is not seen after systemic administration.[23] Generally quite low doses (25% of the normal dose in the inhaler) produce marked bronchodilation whereas higher doses are required to protect effectively against various challenges. Most of the drug that is deposited in the intrapulmonary airways is systemically absorbed and excreted in the urine, though some may be metabolized locally in the airways. The clinical effects after inhalation correlate with dose and not with plasma level.

Clinical trials of short-acting β₂-agonists

SCHOOL-CHILDREN

Inhaled SABA have repeatedly proved their superiority to other drugs in the treatment of acute episodes of wheeze.[28,29] Furthermore, premedication with such single-dose therapy effectively diminishes exercise-induced asthma.[14]

Continuous treatment with oral SABA does not protect as effectively against exercise-induced asthma as an occasional single dose,[23] though it improves symptoms and peak expiratory flow and protects against nocturnal asthma, particularly when slow release products are used.[23,24] A combination of theophylline and oral SABA has been found to be more effective than either drug used alone,[24] though it is not known whether the combination is preferable to single drug therapy when the drug is used in optimal doses.

PRESCHOOL CHILDREN AND INFANTS

Bronchodilation,[30–32] and bronchoprotection[33,34] from inhaled SABA have been demonstrated with objective measurements in preschool children. Early studies failed to find any bronchodilator response to nebulized SABA in infants, which led to the belief that SABA were ineffective in this age group. A fall in transcutaneous oxygen pressure was interpreted as lack of bronchodilator response, though alternative explanations have been suggested including acidity of the nebulizer solution,[35] and ventilation–perfusion mismatch. Others have reported an increase in transcutaneous oxygen.[36] Placebo-controlled double-blind studies have demonstrated significant bronchodilator effects, protective effects against bronchoconstrictor agents and clinical improvement in infants treated with SABA either alone or in combination with steroids,[37] indicating the presence of functioning β-adrenoceptors. The reason for this discrepancy is not clear. The various studies have differed with respect to dose, device (spacer, nebulizer), baseline lung function, duration of symptoms, method of lung function measurement, and age of subjects. The discrepancy is only seen in studies assessing bronchodilator effects. All studies find a significant protection against bronchoconstriction induced. Thus, it seems that infants

have functional β₂-receptors from birth and that stimulation of these receptors can produce the same effects as in older children. For very young infants with bronchiolitis, the effects are less clear cut (Chapter 9).

ACUTE ASTHMA

The value of *inhaled β₂-agonists* in the treatment of acute asthma in school and preschool children has been demonstrated in several controlled trials.[38–45] Such treatment is superior to treatment with all other bronchodilators. Similarly, subcutaneous, intramuscular or intravenous administration is associated with a significant effect.[22] For the same β₂-agonist the inhaled route is as effective or more effective than other routes of administration, but with fewer side effects. Nebulizers are normally preferred for the delivery though the same results can often be obtained with spacers.[38,39,44,45]

The optimal dose of nebulized β₂-agonist for acute asthma depends upon the nebulizer brand and volume fill and upon the severity of the attack. However, high doses (0.30 mg salbutamol/kg) were better than low doses (0.15 mg/kg) when given at 3-hourly intervals.[43] Furthermore, continuous nebulization of 0.3 mg salbutamol/kg/h produced better results than the same dose nebulized intermittently over 20 minutes every hour.[46] Similarly, a single dose of six puffs terbutaline (1500 µg) from a spacer was less effective than three puffs given twice at 15 minute intervals.[40]

An *intravenous loading dose* of 2 µg/kg terbutaline followed by a continuous infusion of up to 5 µg/kg/h seems to be optimal for the majority of children.[22] The same seems to be the case when salbutamol is used.[47] When systemic administration is combined with high-dose inhaled therapy the systemic doses should probably be reduced. A Cochrane review questioned the role of intravenous β₂-agonists in the management of acute severe asthma.[48] The review concluded that there is no evidence to support the use of IV β₂-agonists in patients with severe acute asthma who are also treated with inhaled β₂-agonists. In these situations β₂-agonists should preferably be given by inhalation. No subgroups were identified in which the IV route should be considered.

Bronchodilators may have a modest, short-term clinical effect in mild to moderate acute infantile bronchiolitis.[49] This is contentious (see Chapter 9).

ADVERSE EFFECTS OF SHORT-ACTING β₂-AGONISTS

The occurrence of side effects is directly proportional to the plasma concentrations of drug and therefore mainly depends on route of administration as well as on selectivity. Skeletal muscle tremor, headache, palpitations and some agitation are the most common complaints when high doses are used. After systemic administration these complaints seem to occur when the top of the bronchodilator dose–response curve is reached.[22] Tolerance to side effects seems to develop easily so that they disappear with continued use of the drug.[50,51]

A small drop in blood pressure and a compensatory increase in pulse rate is seen after systemic use or administration of high doses of inhaled drug. Furthermore, hyperglycaemia, hypokalaemia (which should be monitored) and an increase in free fatty acids are common under these conditions,[51] but disappear with continuous treatment. β_2-agonists reduce the nocturnal secretion of growth hormone.[52] The clinical importance of this is unknown.

Asthma is associated with considerable ventilation–perfusion imbalance. This may result in low PaO_2 and hypoxaemia. β-agonists have two pharmacological actions which may effect PaO_2 in different directions. Firstly, they may decrease PaO_2 by causing pulmonary vasodilation, which increases perfusion of the poorly ventilated areas and thus increases the shunt effect. Secondly, β-agonists will increase cardiac output, decrease peripheral resistance and cause bronchodilation, all of which will increase PaO_2. The net effect on PaO_2 is the balance of these effects. The clinical significance of any β-agonist-induced fall in PaO_2 depends on the initial oxygen tension of the patient. Concomitant use of theophylline may enhance most of the side effects.

Long-acting β-adrenergic agents

PHARMACOKINETICS AND DYNAMICS

The long-acting selective β_2-agonists (LABA) salmeterol and formoterol exert prolonged bronchodilation (>12 hours) as well as prolonged protection against EIB and other challenges. Some children achieve full bronchoprotection for more than 12 hours after a single dose, although considerable heterogeneity in duration and magnitude of response may be seen.[53]

Salmeterol and formoterol differ in many respects (Figure 8a.2).[6] *Salmeterol* is more lipophilic, has a slower onset of action, is only a partial agonist (formoterol is a full agonist), is more β_2-selective and has a somewhat longer duration of action *in vitro* but not *in vivo*. The clinical importance of these differences is not known. Though highly lipophilic there is no evidence of accumulation of drug in the tissues after prolonged use.

Inhaled *formoterol* has a rapid onset of action (3 minutes) and a maximum effect at 30 minutes to 1 hour after inhalation in asthmatic children similar to the effect of the short-acting β_2-agonist, salbutamol.[54,55] Inhaled salmeterol has a relatively slow onset of action with a significant effect reported 10–20 minutes after inhalation of a single dose of salmeterol 50 mg,[56] and comparable to the effect of salbutamol after 30 minutes.[57] Because of its slow onset salmeterol is not recommended for the treatment of acute asthma symptoms including exercise-induced bronchoconstriction or in the treatment of patients with rapidly deteriorating asthma. Patients prescribed salmeterol should have a short-acting β2-agonist available at all times to treat breakthrough symptoms.

The recommended dosage of formoterol for children >6 years is 6 mg (nominal dose) bid, which is probably close to the top of the dose–response curve of formoterol in children with asthma. Individual responses show considerable variation and some patients may benefit from doses above the usual recommended dose. The recommended dosage of salmeterol for children >4 years of age is 50 mg bid, which is probably close to the top of the dose–response curve.

TACHYPHYLAXIS AND TOLERANCE

Tolerance and attenuated response is seen with chronic stimulation with high concentrations of β-agonists in animals and *in vitro*.[58] The protective effect of β-agonists on inhibition of the release of histamine and other mast cell mediators readily shows tachyphylaxis.[59] Bronchoprotection against stimuli which cause bronchoconstriction such as exercise and cold air is reduced when SABA or LABA is given regularly[60] independently of any concurrent steroid treatment (Figure 8a.4). The reduced protection is mainly seen as a reduction in the duration of protection, so if the treatment has been taken shortly before exercise the protection will be close to the maximum achievable. In contrast the bronchodilator response to LABA is relatively resistant to tachyphylaxis.[61] The disparity between tolerance to bronchodilation and bronchoprotection is poorly understood. The clinical significance of this tolerance is not yet clear, but may be at least partially explained by polymorphisms in the β_2-adrenoceptor gene[62] (Chapter 4d).

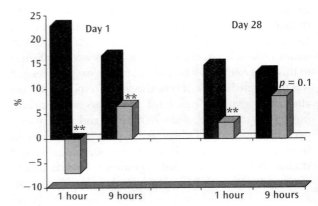

Figure 8a.4 *Protection by salmeterol (▨) against exercise-induced fall in FEV₁ compared with placebo (■). After a single dose, significant protection is seen both 1 and 9 hours after dosing. After the children have been treated with salmeterol 50 μg bid for 4 weeks the protection is attenuated and no longer significant 9 hours after dosing. Notice also the marked reduction in post-exercise fall in FEV₁ after 4 weeks of placebo treatment. (From ref. 60 with permission.)*

Prolonged treatment with systemic β_2-agonists also produces a marked tolerance to the occurrence of side effects such as tremor and headache.[51]

CLINICAL TRIALS

Single-dose therapy effectively diminishes exercise-induced asthma though with a certain heterogeneity of effect.[53] Regular mono-therapy with LABA should be avoided since it does not control the underlying airway inflammation and loss of lung function and increased airway hyper-reactivity has been reported in children with moderate asthma severity receiving mono-therapy with salmeterol for one year (Figure 8a.5).[63]

Regular LABA may be used as add-on to established treatment with ICS (Figure 8a.6). However, the available double-blind randomized controlled trials of such add-on treatment in children with poorly controlled asthma are inconclusive and reported improvements have been much less than for adult patients.[64-66] Most trials find a statistically significant albeit small improvement in lung function. The effect on other outcomes such as symptoms and exacerbations is more variable and often marginal. The reason for this apparent discrepancy between the findings in children and adults is not known. Generally adult patients have had lower lung function and more frequent symptoms and exacerbations during placebo treatment than the children enrolled in the paediatric studies, so there may have been less room for improvement in the paediatric studies. The only add-on study in children which included patients with frequent symptoms and low lung function found the most marked benefit, although still not as much as in the adult studies.

Studies in adults have suggested that the addition of LABA to existing corticosteroid therapy may be more efficient in controlling asthma symptoms and lung function than doubling the dose of inhaled corticosteroid. A similar study in childhood asthma management failed to show any effect of either LABA as add-on or of doubling the dose of ICS. Continuing the lower dose of ICS was equally effective and associated with an improved asthma control and lung function during the treatment period so that the patients at the end of the study period had improved so much spontaneously that they would no longer have been candidates for the study.[67]

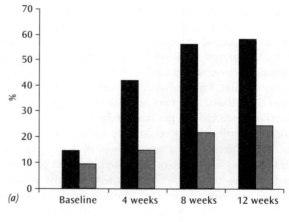

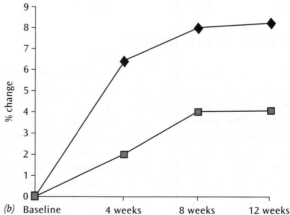

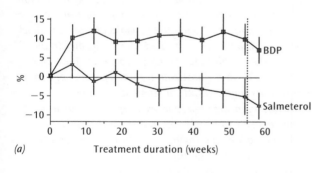

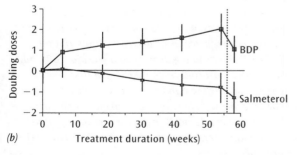

Figure 8a.5 *(a) Changes in FEV$_1$ % predicted (mean, 95% CI) from baseline during treatment of children with asthma, with salmeterol or beclomethasone (BDP). (b) Changes in airway responsiveness (PD$_{20}$) in doubling doses (mean, 95% CI) from baseline during treatment with salmeterol (●) or beclomethasone (■). A significant reduction in FEV$_1$ and a worsening of airway responsiveness was seen during treatment with salmeterol. (From ref. 63 with permission.)*

Figure 8a.6 *(a) Changes in FEV$_1$ from baseline during treatment with salmeterol (♦) or placebo (■) in children whose asthma was uncontrolled during continuous treatment with inhaled corticosteroids. (b) Changes in symptom free days in the same patients. Significant improvements were seen in both parameters. (From ref. 65)*

SIDE EFFECTS

LABA are well-tolerated drugs, even after long-term use, with an adverse effect profile comparable with that of short-acting β_2-agonists.

CORTICOSTEROIDS

Cortisone and hydrocortisone were the first glucocorticosteroids to be used therapeutically. Subsequent structural modifications separated the mineralocorticoid from the metabolic and anti-inflammatory effect. However, so far it has not been possible to remove the metabolic effects and isolate the desired anti-inflammatory properties. Halogenation increases topical potency by increasing receptor affinity but the systemic potency is also increased and biotransformation rate decreased so that the clinical effect/systemic effect ratio is unchanged. [68] When budesonide was designed it was found that structural modifications at positions 16, 17 and 22 could increase anti-inflammatory and topical potency without a corresponding rise in unwanted systemic activity. The various structural changes have led to new molecules with high topical anti-inflammatory potency and low systemic bioavailability and activity. Thus it has been estimated that 1 mg inhaled budesonide per day produces an anti-asthma effect equivalent to approximately 45 mg oral prednisone per day, while the systemic effect is only equivalent to approximately 8 mg prednisone per day. In children the systemic effects of 800 μg budesonide per day are less than the systemic effects of 2.5 mg prednisolone per day.[70–72] For these reasons inhaled steroids are superior to oral steroids for maintenance treatment of childhood asthma. Oral steroids should be reserved for the treatment of acute exercabations.

Pharmacological action[73]

Glucocorticosteroids exert their effects by binding to a single *glucocorticoid receptor* (GR), which is predominantly located in the cytoplasm of the target cells, and only on binding of the glucocorticoid does it move into the nuclear compartment where it produces its effect by regulating the transcription of certain target genes (Figure 8a.7). In this way several aspects of the inflammatory process may be modified through increasing or decreasing gene transcription.

Steroids have *direct inhibitory actions on most of the inflammatory cells* implicated in asthma[74] and on airway microvascular leak induced by inflammatory mediators. Furthermore, inhaled steroids inhibit the increased expression of GM–CSF in airway epithelial cells of asthmatic patients[75] and the increased mucus secretion in the airways. The latter probably by a direct action on submucosal gland cells. Finally, steroids increase the *expression*

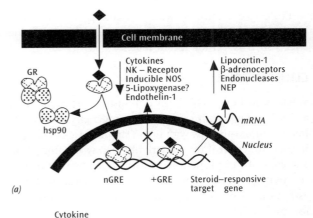

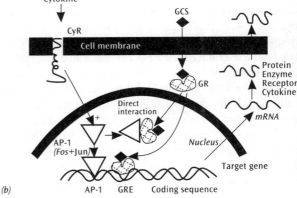

Figure 8a.7 *(a) Molecular mechanism of glucocorticosteroid (GCS) action. GCS binds to a cytosolic glucocorticoid receptor (GR) that is normally bound to two molecules of heat shock protein 90 (hsp 90). The activated GR translocates to the nucleus where it binds to specific glucocorticoid response elements (GRE) in the upstream regulatory region of genes, which either inhibit (nGRE) or stimulate (+GRE) transcription in steroid-responsive target genes (of which many are likely to be relevant in asthma therapy). (b) Interaction between cytokines and glucocorticosteroids (GCS). Cytokines bind to surface receptors (CyR) that lead to activation of transcription factors such as activator protein-1 (AP-1) in the nucleus. Activated AP-1 binds to AP-1 consensus sequences in the upstream regulatory portion of a gene and either increases or decreases transcription. Similarly, GCS binds to a glucocorticoid receptor (GR) that binds to a glucocorticoid response element (GRE) on the same gene and has the opposite effect on transcription, thereby blocking the effect of the cytokine. Furthermore, AP-1 and GR may interact directly via a protein-protein interaction and thereby neutralize each other. (From ref. 384 with permission.)*

of β-receptors, which may increase β-adrenergic bronchodilator responsiveness and reduce the down-regulation of β-receptors that may occur after prolonged β-agonist exposure. As a result of all these actions steroids are very effective in controlling chronic inflammation in asthmatic airways. Several biopsy studies have demonstrated normalization of the numbers of

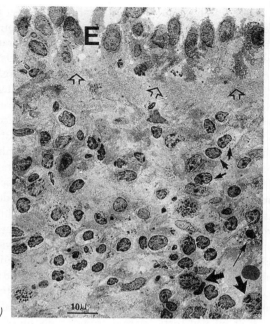

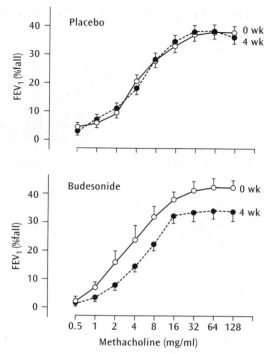

Figure 8a.9 *Mean (±SEM) dose–response curves to inhaled methacholine before (○) and after (●) 4 weeks treatment with placebo (upper panel) and budesonide (lower panel) in two groups of eight subjects with mild asthma. Budesonide not only caused a shift to the right of the dose–response curve but also a reduction in the magnitude of the maximum response. (From ref. 87 with permission.)*

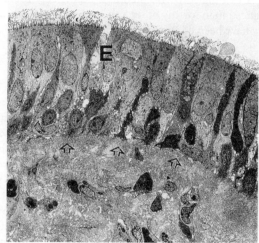

Figure 8a.8 *(a) Electron microscopic picture of a section of a biopsy specimen obtained from airway of a patient with extrinsic asthma of 9 months duration. Patient has a highly damaged airway epithelium (E). Deeper in lamina propria, beneath basement membrane (thick arrows), an intense inflammatory reaction can be observed. Different types of inflammatory cells, eosinophils, lymphocytes, and plasma cells reflect chronic inflammation. Mast cells (thin black arrows) are highly degranulated; bar, 10. (b) Airway of same patient after 3 months of inhaled budesonide treatment. Normal airway epithelium (E) with ciliated and goblet cells is restored on basement membrane (thick black arrows) and inflammatory cells have disappeared. Picture is comparable to that obtained in normal airways (from ref. 385 with permission).*

Inhaled steroids *reduce airway responsiveness* to both direct and indirect stimuli.[76] Single doses reduce the late response and continuous treatment reduce early and late responses to allergen and the subsequent delayed increase in BHR.[77] Chronic treatment reduces airway responsiveness to inhaled histamine and methacholine,[77–80] the bronchoconstriction elicited by metabisulphite and bradykinin (which may act via neural mechanisms), and hyperosmolar, hyperventilation and exercise challenges (which may act via mast cells).[81–86] These effects are probably a result of the reduction in the underlying inflammation, but the component of increased airway responsiveness caused by structural changes in the airway ('remodelling') seems to be irreversible by steroids. Unlike all other drugs steroids not only shift the dose–response curve to spasmogens to the right, but also limit the maximum narrowing in response to the spasmogen[87] (Figure 8a.9).

Pharmacodynamics

Dose–response studies are important to determine the clinically relevant doses of inhaled corticosteroid to use in trials in various patient groups.

Over the last 5 years a number of well conducted *dose–response studies or dose titration studies* have been

eosinophils, macrophages, mast cells, and lymphocytes, restoration of the disrupted epithelium and normalization of the ciliated-to-goblet cell ratio after inhaled steroid treatment (Figure 8a.8).

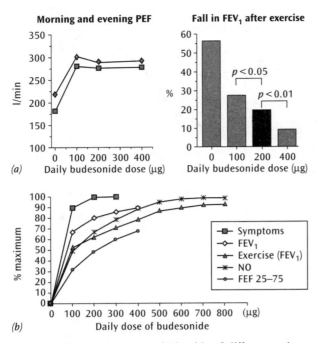

Figure 8a.10 *Dose–response relationship of different asthma outcomes in children treated with budesonide delivered by a metered dose inhaler with a spacer. (a) Measured increase in morning and evening peak expiratory flow and fall in FEV$_1$ after exercise in children with moderate and severe asthma. (From ref. 89.) (b) Dose–response curves constructed upon the basis of dose–response studies in children with moderate asthma. The shape of the dose–response curves for normalization of the chronic inflammatory changes in the airways or for maintaining normal growth of lung function are not known. (From ref. 229.)*

carried out in children with mild, moderate and severe asthma.[88–92] All studies demonstrate marked and rapid clinical improvements and changes in symptoms, and lung function at very low daily doses around 100 µg (Figure 8a.10). Further improvement with increasing doses is rather small, often taking a four-fold increase in dose to produce further statistically significant (but clinically trivial) effects. In patients with mild disease low doses have also been found to normalize the exhaled NO concentration (eNO) and to offer full protection against exercise-induced asthma,[92,93] whereas children with more severe asthma may require four weeks treatment with a daily dose of budesonide of 400 µg from a pMDI with a spacer to achieve a maximum protection against exercise-induced asthma. Low doses are clinically effective, such that even very large, well-conducted studies normally fail to show any statistically significant or clinically relevant additional effect on symptoms and lung function when the dose is increased beyond 100 µg per day. The marked effect of low doses may be even more pronounced in children with mild disease, but at present no studies have used daily doses <100 µg in this category.

These findings and several clinical trials suggest that the vast majority of school-children will achieve optimal symptom control, maximum effect on peak expiratory flow, and marked and clinically significant effects on other outcome parameters at daily doses of <400 µg/day of inhaled steroids. However, the dose of inhaled steroid required to produce the maximum clinical effect seems to depend upon several factors, including the outcome measure studied, the duration of administration of the inhaled steroid, the severity of the disease, the drug/ inhaler combination used, the age of the patient and the duration of asthma when treatment is initiated. As a consequence, each patient may have her/his own individual dose–response curve, which also depends on the main clinical problem (and therefore outcome) in that particular patient. This emphasizes the importance of regular, individual tailoring of the dose. If this is done the majority of patients will be optimally controlled on daily doses of inhaled corticosteroid <400 µg. Moreover, a large number of studies have found that, in children, the beneficial effects of low doses of inhaled corticosteroid are normally more pronounced than for any other anti-asthma drug with which they have been compared.[63,79,93–101]

Pharmacokinetics

The systemically available inhaled corticosteroid derives from two sources (Figure 8a.11) (Table 8a.2): the majority of steroid deposited in the intrapulmonary airways is absorbed systemically, since the available steroids are only metabolized in the liver and not in the airways; the inhaled drug that is deposited in the oropharynx is swallowed and absorbed from the gastrointestinal tract. The extent to which the latter occurs depends upon the inhaled corticosteroid used and the amount of drug deposited in the oropharynx, the latter mainly determined by the inhaler device. The degree of first-pass metabolism in children differs markedly between the various corticosteroids (from 50–99%). Drugs with high first-pass metabolism will have low systemic availability after absorption from the gastrointestinal tract. The contribution of oro-pharyngeal deposition to systemic effect is important in children, because children deposit a much higher proportion of the inhaled dose in the oropharynx than adults.[102–104] On the other hand, children metabolize budesonide about 40% faster than adults.[104,105] The pharmacokinetics of other inhaled corticosteroids have not been studied in children.

Clinical trials

SCHOOL-CHILDREN

Several controlled trials have established that inhaled steroids are highly effective in children irrespective of asthma severity.[63,76–79,92–99,101,106–116] Continuous treatment controls asthma symptoms, reduces the frequency of acute

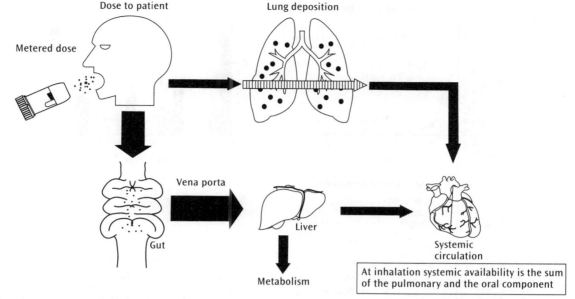

Figure 8a.11 *The fate of inhaled corticosteroids. The amount of an inhaled corticosteroid reaching the systemic circulation is the sum of the pulmonary and orally bioavailable fractions. The fraction deposited in the mouth will be swallowed, and the systemic availability will be determined by absorption from the gastrointestinal tract and degree of first-pass metabolism. The fraction deposited in the intrapulmonary airways is likely to be more or less completely absorbed in active form to the systemic circulation, as there is no evidence for metabolic inactivation of any currently available inhaled corticosteroid in airway tissue. The systemic concentration will be reduced by continuous re-circulation and inactivation of the drug by the liver.*

Table 8a.2 *Basic pharmacokinetic parameters of inhaled corticosteroids which have been studied in children. Children metabolize budesonide and fluticasone propionate faster than adults. There are not sufficient data to assess whether this is also the case for beclomethasone*

Inhaled steroid	T1/2 (h)	MRT (h)	Vss (l/kg)	CL (l/min)	Oral availability (%)
Beclomethasone	2.7	2.8	1.7	0.90	50
Budesonide	3.5	2.1	2.2	0.91	10
Fluticasone	7.5	4.1	4.3	0.87	<2

The half life and clearance of beclomethasone cannot be compared to those of budesonide and fluticasone since the sampling period in the beclomethasone study was shorter and the assay less sensitive. Vss – volume of distribution at steady state, CL – clearance, MRT – mean residence time, T1/2 – half life.

exacerbations and the number of hospital admissions, improves quality of life, lung functions and bronchial responsiveness, reduces exercise-induced bronchoconstriction, eNO and sputum eosinophils[97] both in hospital patients and in primary care. Symptom control and improvements in peak expiratory flow rate occur rapidly (1–2 weeks) at low doses around 100 μg per day in children with moderate and severe asthma, whereas longer treatment (1–3 months) or sometimes somewhat higher doses (around 400 μg/day) is required to achieve maximum effect on bronchial responsiveness as assessed by an exercise challenge test. When steroid treatment is

discontinued there is usually a deterioration of the asthma control and bronchial responsiveness to pretreatment level within weeks to months, though in some patients the effect is maintained much longer.[117]

As for other asthma drugs most studies with inhaled corticosteroids have been of rather short duration. However, three long-term studies (two years or longer) with inhaled budesonide have added interesting information on the beneficial clinical effects and risk of side effects associated with long-term continuous use.[79,98,101] All studies found marked reductions in exacerbations and visits to the emergency room and improvements in lung function, morning and evening peak flow, symptoms, use of rescue β₂-agonists and bronchial hyperresponsiveness in children treated with budesonide (Figure 8a.12). The differences were maintained throughout the study periods in two of the studies whereas the difference from placebo diminished with time in the third study so that the effect on post-bronchodilator FEV_1 was no longer significant after 4 years of treatment.[101] A small reduction in FEV_1 with time was seen in children who did not receive budesonide in two of the studies.[79,98] Furthermore, in one study the effect on lung function was significantly greater when budesonide was started early (within 2 years) after asthma was diagnosed (Figure 8a.13).[98]

PRESCHOOL CHILDREN

Oral steroids have been reported effective in the treatment of *acute exacerbations of recurrent wheezing* in

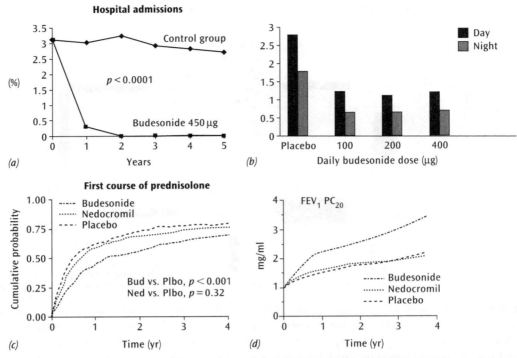

Figure 8a.12 *Clinical effects of budesonide inhaled from a Turbuhaler. (a) Hospital admissions with acute severe asthma. The control group received all kinds of asthma medication except inhaled corticosteroids. (From ref. 98.) (b) Effect on day and night symptoms measured on a scale of 0 to 5. (From ref. 182.) (c) Effect on exacerbations requiring prednisolone. The probability of receiving prednisolone was significantly lower in children treated with budesonide than in children treated with nedocromil sodium or placebo. (From ref. 101.) (d) Effect of budesonide 400 µg per day on bronchial hyperresponsiveness. Budesonide had a significantly greater effect than nedocromil sodium and placebo. (From ref. 101.)*

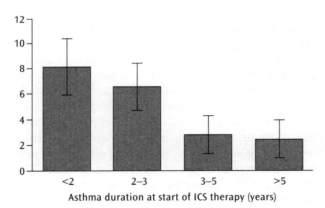

Figure 8a.13 *Influence of asthma duration at the start of inhaled budesonide on the mean annual increase in FEV$_1$ after initiation of budesonide treatment. Children who started treatment sooner had a more rapid and attained significantly better lung function than children who did not receive budesonide treatment until some years after the onset of asthma symptoms. (From ref. 98.)*

children from the age of 2 months in some double-blind randomized controlled trials,[37,118] though not in others.[119] Budesonide (BUD) and fluticasone (FP) administered from pMDI and spacer devices have benefited young asthmatic children of 0–3 years in six double blind randomized controlled trials[120–125] comprising a total of 469 young children; as well as in a study of slightly older children.[126] Nebulized beclomethasone (BDP) suspension from jet-nebulizer has failed to show convincing effects, probably due to inefficient nebulization of this particular steroid preparation.[127] Nebulized BUD from jet-nebulizer has shown significant steroid sparing effect[128] as well as improvement of other health outcomes in large parallel double-blind randomized controlled trials of children of ½–8 years[129,130].

Subsets of young children may not benefit from the treatment. Generally, young asthmatic children do not become symptom-free. ICS typically reduce the number of asthma exacerbations by half,[123,124] but do not completely prevent exacerbations. Whether this is due to insufficient adherence, too low doses (or inefficient delivery systems) or subsets of wheezers unresponsive to treatment is the important focus of future studies.

The variable nature of recurrent wheeze in young children and the strong seasonality partly explain the difficulty in performing clinical trials and the difficulty in clinical practice. Often patients are given preventer therapy or included in a trial during periods of exacerbation, typically during winter season. Simple regression towards the mean is exaggerated in such children by the strong seasonality and variable course of the disease. This is very clearly reflected in the pronounced improvement during placebo treatment in most trials.

Corticosteroids 259

A dose–response relation on exacerbation rate was documented from daily dose of 100 µg vs. 200 µg of fluticasone propionate delivered from pMDI and spacer.[124] Since only two dose-steps were applied the plateau of the dose–response relation was not defined. Accordingly, the doses chosen are at the steep part of the dose–response relation, but higher doses may be required to obtain a full effect. Comparison of 0.25 mg, 0.5 mg and 1.0 mg nebulized budesonide once daily and twice daily[130] showed significant improvement over placebo treatment but failed to indicate a dose–response effect. Another study suggested a dose-effect from 0.25 to 1.0 mg nebulized budesonide bid.[131] Individual dose-finding studies have been performed with nebulized budesonide.[132] Marked individual variations were seen and the conclusion of both studies was that the dose of nebulized budesonide must be individualized.

Lung function and BHR have been reported as primary endpoints in six small double-blind randomized controlled trials of ICS in young *chronically wheezy children*. BDP nebulized suspension was used in two trials though this is a comparatively inefficient steroid regime (vide supra).

BDP pMDI from spacer have been applied in two physiological studies in infants with recurrent wheeze. Infants with a history of persistent wheezing were treated in a placebo-controlled, parallel double-blind randomized controlled trial with a daily dose of 400 µg of BDP pMDI via spacer with face-mask. Forced flow at FRC (rapid thoraco-abdominal compression technique) was used to measured BHR to histamine.[133] BHR improved significantly in the active treatment group, though symptoms did not improve. Lung function (whole body plethysmograph estimates of thoracic gas volume and airway conductance) improved in a controlled trial of 29 infants of 2–25 months with recurrent wheezing.[120]

The effect of BUD pMDI via a metal spacer has been studied in a double-blind randomized controlled trial in 38 young asthmatics aged 2–5 years.[134] Symptoms improved significantly, with exacerbation rate as the best discriminator between active and placebo treatment; bronchial hyperresponsiveness improved significantly as measured by the cold, dry air hyperventilation method, but not by methacholine challenge.

In summary, the available evidence suggests that symptoms, lung function and BHR in young chronically wheezy children are improved by ICS. A rise in exhaled NO subsequent to dose reduction of ICS has been reported in young asthmatic children of 2–5 years, indirectly suggesting an anti-inflammatory effect. None of the available studies on ICS in young children have reported on the effect on blood eosinophils or markers.

Acute viral bronchiolitis (usually caused by respiratory syncytial virus) in previously healthy young infants is unresponsive to steroid treatment. Double-blind randomized controlled trials have found no short- or long-term clinical benefits from the administration of systemic[135–137] or inhaled steroids,[138–141] though some short-term improvements have been reported.[37,142]

Viral episodic symptoms in young children without regular symptoms may benefit marginally from ICS. Intermittent high-dose ICS administered for 1–2 weeks in association with virus induced wheeze reduced the severity of the symptoms.[143,144] The differences between placebo and inhaled steroids were statistically significant though generally small and inhaled corticosteroids did not reduce the need for oral steroids or frequency of hospitalization. One small study reported no effect from regular steroid ICS treatment on viral induced wheeze attacks. The small clinical benefit may not justify ICS treatment in this subset of wheezy children. Accordingly it was the conclusion of a Cochrane review, that episodic high-dose inhaled corticosteroids provide a partially effective strategy for the treatment of mild episodic viral wheeze of childhood, but there is no current evidence to favour maintenance low-dose inhaled corticosteroids in the prevention and management of episodic mild viral induced wheeze.[145]

In conclusion, ICS are clearly effective in young children with regular symptoms as reflected in health-outcomes, lung function measurements and measurements of inflammatory markers. Steroids have no effect on the isolated acute attack of wheeze in a previously healthy young infant (bronchiolitis). However, ICS are effective in viral exacerbation in young children with a history of chronic symptoms. ICS also have little effect on viral induced episodic symptoms in children without chronic symptoms.

ACUTE ASTHMA

The beneficial effects of systemic steroids in the management of acute severe asthma has been shown in several controlled trials in *all age groups except infants* and the value of such therapy has only rarely been questioned. Thus a Cochrane analysis found that use of corticosteroids within 1 hour of presentation to an emergency department significantly reduced the need for hospital admission in patients with acute asthma. Benefits appeared greatest in patients with more severe asthma, and those not currently receiving steroids. Children appeared to respond well to oral steroids.[146]

The optimal doses of steroid and route of administration have not been carefully evaluated, so the recommendations for this condition are rather empirical and based upon personal experience and the dose regimens used in studies evaluating the treatment. Undoubtedly, oral prednisolone is sufficient in the majority of children, especially when used early during the exacerbation[146,147] when it has been shown to reduce the severity of virus induced exacerbations and hospital admissions. In some patients intravenous hydrocortisone or methylprednisolone may be preferable. Theoretically, methylprednisolone is preferable to hydrocortisone because of its lesser mineralocorticoid effect and better penetration into the lung tissue.[148] Very high doses of steroids are probably not necessary and may cause hypokalaemia, fluid retention and an acute myopathy. A recent Cochrane analysis in mainly adult patients concluded that no differences in effect were identified among different doses of corticosteroids in acute asthma requiring hospital admission. Low-dose corticosteroids (80 mg/day or less of methylprednisolone or 400 mg/day or less of hydrocortisone) appeared to be adequate in the initial management of these adult patients. Higher doses did not appear to offer a therapeutic advantage.

The normally recommended steroid doses for acute asthma are: prednisolone – loading dose 0.5–1 mg/kg, followed by 1 mg/kg/24 h; methylprednisolone – loading dose 1 mg/kg, followed by 0.5 mg/kg every 6 h.

Systemic dexamethasone or oral prednisolone were of little benefit *in infants* with acute wheeze in two studies but of significant benefit in another.[37] Therefore, further studies are needed in this age group.

High doses of *inhaled* corticosteroids are sometimes recommended for the treatment of exacerbations. However, at present there are no studies to support this except for a recent study which did find a significant additional effect of nebulized budesonide in acute wheeze in children up to 18 months of age.[37] It seems, however, that if given early to children with asthma provoked by viral upper respiratory tract infection such treatment can reduce the severity of asthma attacks but probably not the incidence of hospital admissions.[143,149] A recent Cochrane review on this topic concluded that early use of inhaled steroids during the acute attack reduced admission rates in patients with acute asthma.[146] It was unclear if there also was a benefit of ICS when used in addition to systemic corticosteroids. Similarly, there was insufficient evidence that ICS alone is as effective as systemic steroids.

Systemic effects and clinically important adverse effects

Often no distinction is made between a measurable systemic effect and a clinically relevant adverse effect of an inhaled corticosteroid. This may lead to unwarranted and unnecessary fear among physicians and patients. All inhaled corticosteroids are systemically absorbed to some extent. Whether the absorbed drug leads to a measurable systemic effect depends upon the amount of drug that is absorbed, the potency and pharmacokinetics of the drug and the sensitivity of the method used for measuring the systemic effect. Most doses will be measurable in one or more systemic effect models. However, more often than not, these measurable effects merely reflect small changes within the normal range of the normal biological feedback system and may be without clinical relevance. There are several examples in children of detectable systemic effects of asthma drugs the clinical relevance of which must be questioned. This does not just apply to the effects of inhaled corticosteroid therapy. For example, sodium cromoglycate treatment has been found to have a significant effect on urinary excretion of growth hormone (GH)[150] and markers of bone metabolism,[151] and

treatment with inhaled β_2-agonists has been found to adversely affect the secretion of GH.[52,152] Although statistically significant, these findings are probably not clinically relevant though, as yet, there have been no thorough clinical studies to assess this.

The vast majority of studies evaluating the risk of systemic effects have been in children older than 5 years. Our knowledge about the dose levels at which measurable systemic effects of inhaled corticosteroids are seen in short-term controlled studies in patients with mild disease is quite good. Though the clinical relevance of the finding in such studies may be questioned it can probably be assumed that doses of an inhaled corticosteroid which are not associated with any measurable systemic effects in sensitive laboratory test systems are also clinically safe (Figure 8a.14).

Clinically relevant adverse effects should be studied in controlled, long-term clinical trials, using clinically relevant doses in groups of patients with a disease severity and age similar to the groups in which the drugs would normally be prescribed. Such studies require large numbers of patients and are difficult to conduct.

BONES

In children the rate of bone modelling or turnover is much higher than in adults. Furthermore, in adults the skeletal mass is decreasing over time, while in children it is increasing over time until peak bone mass/density is reached in early adulthood. The increase in bone mass is not a constant process but varies with age and season of the year.

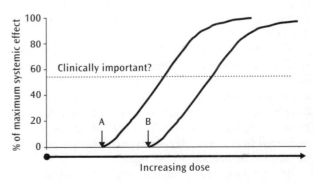

Figure 8a.14 *Dose–response curves for systemic effects of two inhaled corticosteroids or inhaler devices; A being more potent than B. For a given drug or inhaler there will always be a dose below which no effect can be detected. Then there will be a dose range within which the effects are measurable (depending on the outcome studied). Within a certain dose range there will be a linear (or log linear) relationship between the magnitude of the effect and dose of drug. We have very good knowledge of the doses of various corticosteroids at which a systemic effect can be detected. The clinical relevance of a detectable systemic effect is not well defined either in its magnitude or duration.*

The *skeletal modelling*/turnover rate and the retention of calcium is highest during spring and summer and during infancy and adolescence. Normally, most of the skeletal mass will be accumulated by late adolescence. Just as adult height in relation to predicted adult height is the most important outcome measure of growth in children, so fracture or maximal peak bone mass/density is probably the most clinically relevant outcome measure for assessing the influence of steroids on bones in children. In addition to nutrition (including calcium intake), heredity (both parents), endocrine factors (sexual development), poor asthma control and physical activity appear to have profound effects on peak bone mass formation.[153–158] Some chronic diseases have also been reported to be associated with reduced peak bone mass in children.[159] The finding that delayed puberty in itself is associated with a significantly lower peak bone mass/density[159,160] is particularly important in the clinical management of children with asthma since this condition is seen in many children with asthma and atopy, independent of treatment. Obviously, these confounding factors must be considered when the effects of steroids on bone metabolism are assessed. Finally, children show a remarkably ability to repair steroid induced bone loss. Children <3 years with Synacthen-induced compression fractures of the spine had normal x-rays of the spine 5–10 years later.[161] Such remodelling and repair is not seen in adults.

The effect of exogenous steroids on bone can be evaluated by measurement of *biochemical markers* of bone metabolism (bone formation and degradation), bone mineral density (BMD) or frequency of fractures. Several studies have assessed markers of bone resorption and formation. They all found that only high daily doses of inhaled steroids (800 μg may have a detectable effect on some markers in children, suggesting a reduction in both bone formation and degradation at this dose. Daily doses of 400 μg or less had no effect in any of the studies.[151,162–170] All these studies were short term and involved patients with mild disease. So, no adverse effects on markers of bone formation and degradation have been reported at standard paediatric doses of inhaled corticosteroids, whereas high doses may cause significant changes, which suggest a reduced bone turnover rate. The clinical importance of this has yet to be elucidated.

Bone densitometry has been applied to assess the bone mineral density in children receiving inhaled corticosteroids in two long-term trials. The findings have been consistent. A long-term, prospective study found that total body bone mineral density (BMD) of children treated with 3–6 years of continuous inhaled budesonide at an average daily dose of around 500 μg was not different from the BMD of 112 children with asthma, who had never received inhaled or oral steroids (Figure 8a.15).[171] Furthermore, bone density did not correlate with years of treatment or current or accumulated dose. These findings were corroborated in a prospective, randomized, double-blind study on 1000 children, which compared the changes in BMD over four years in three groups of children with mild asthma. No differences were found in increases in BMD between the group which received inhaled budesonide at a daily dose around 400 μg, and the groups of children treated with nedocromil or placebo.[101] Several cross-sectional studies and prospective, longitudinal studies on much smaller groups of children treated for shorter periods of time with inhaled steroids have reported similar results.[170,172–174]

In summary, long-term treatment with inhaled corticosteroids at an average daily dose of 400 μg is not associated with an increased risk of osteoporosis or fracture in children. Standard paediatric doses are not associated with any changes in biochemical markers of bone formation or degradation, whereas low doses of prednisolone (2.5–5 mg/day) and high doses of inhaled corticosteroids adversely affect some of these markers. Further controlled prospective studies are needed to assess the effect of long-term treatment on peak bone mass/density.

ADRENAL SUPPRESSION

Adrenal suppression is the most extensively studied systemic effect of inhaled corticosteroids. However, any effect rarely appears to be clinically important, as no cases of adrenal crisis have been reported in adults using only inhaled corticosteroids while only a few such cases have been reported in children.[175–177]

No significant effects on *urinary cortisol excretion* have been reported with doses up to 400 μg/day budesonide pMDI plus spacer[89,126,164,178–180] and 200 μg/day budesonide Turbuhaler.[181] In contrast, 200 μg/day and 400 μg/day fluticasone propionate Diskhaler, and 400 μg/day budesonide Turbuhaler seemed to reduce urinary cortisol excretion.[181,182] A significant effect on urinary

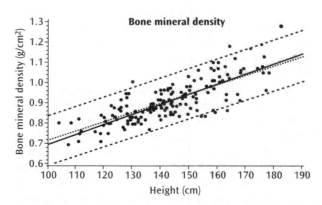

Figure 8a.15 *Individual bone mineral density as a function of height and age in 157 asthmatic children treated continuously for 3–6 years with the inhaled corticosteroid budesonide at a mean daily dose of 504 μg. For comparison the 95% prediction interval and mean regression lines from measurements in 111 children with asthma, who had never received continuous treatment with exogenous steroids are given. (From ref. 171.)*

cortisol excretion by 300–400 µg/day BDP has been found in some studies,[163,183–185] but not others.[152,186–189] Cortisol excretion was still within the normal range in all the studies which reported a significant effect.

Among studies in which *plasma cortisol* was measured at frequent intervals during night-time or over a 24 h period, 400–1000 µg/day BDP pMDI was associated with a significant reduction in the normal physiological secretion of cortisol.[185,190–192] Similar findings have been reported for budesonide pMDI with large volume plastic spacer when plasma cortisol was measured at frequent intervals during night-time. Overnight urinary cortisol excretion was also affected, whereas no effects were seen on *ACTH or growth hormone values*.[185] In contrast, preschool children treated with daily doses of 200–300 µg budesonide for 3–5 years showed normal adrenal function as assessed by frequent plasma cortisol measurements over 24 h.[193] Finally, a daily dose of 200 µg fluticasone propionate and 800 µg budesonide did not affect plasma cortisol profile over a 24 h period, or the increase in plasma cortisol increase after ACTH stimulation.[194] Both had significantly less effect than 2.5–7.5 mg prednisolone per day.

Most studies assessing long-term treatment with BDP or BUD in doses of up to 400 µg/day have found no suppression of the *HPA-axis response to stimulation*.[187,195,196] One study evaluating high-dose therapy with these drugs found a reduced response in some children,[197] and another found abnormal insulin tolerance test in a group of 16 children, nine of whom had also received oral steroids in the past, as compared with a group of normal non-asthmatic children. The results of that study were challenged[198] with regard to the timing of the tests and the fact that the control group were non-asthmatics. None of the children in these studies had any clinical symptoms of adrenal insufficiency, although isolated examples have been described in clinical practice.[177]

Improvements in HPA-axis function have been repeatedly shown in glucocorticoid-dependent patients when their oral steroid dose is reduced following the introduction of inhaled corticosteroids.[199,200] However, the effect of chronic administration of oral steroids may continue for a long time after reduction of the oral dose.

Summary. Though differences exist between the various inhaled corticosteroids and inhalation devices, treatment with low doses (<400 µg/day) of inhaled corticosteroids is not normally associated with any significant suppression of the HPA-axis in children. With higher doses, small changes can be detected with sensitive methods. The clinical relevance of these findings needs further study.

LUNG DEVELOPMENT

Systemic steroids given to rats during the first two post-natal weeks have been shown to impair normal alveolar development.[201] Fears have sometimes been raised that inhaled corticosteroids may have similar effects in young children.[202] However, there are no data to substantiate these fears and marked differences exist in lung development between baby rats and young children. Thus, if inhaled corticosteroids have a definite positive clinical effect in a young child, concerns about possible adverse effects upon lung growth should not be a reason to withhold the treatment.[203]

CATARACTS

Atopic patients, particularly patients with atopic eczema, may have a higher occurrence of cataracts than non-atopic subjects.[204] Four recent studies have evaluated the risk of posterior subcapsular cataracts in more than 800 children receiving long-term treatment with inhaled corticosteroids. The conclusions were that continuous treatment with inhaled corticosteroids is not associated with an increased occurrence of cataract development in children.[205–207] These findings corroborate those reported in previously published studies of smaller groups of less well-characterized children and of adolescent patients treated for shorter periods of time with inhaled glucocorticosteroids.[208–211] These data suggest that long-term treatment with inhaled corticosteroids in the doses required to control mild and moderate asthma is unlikely to cause cataract formation.

CENTRAL NERVOUS SYSTEM EFFECTS

For inhaled corticosteroids, the published evidence concerning CNS effects is limited to isolated case reports in a total of nine patients (three adults and six children).[212–214] The manifestations have been hyperactive behaviour, aggressiveness, insomnia, uninhibited behaviour and impaired concentration. All returned to normal after discontinuation of the inhaled corticosteroid.

OROPHARYNGEAL EFFECTS

Oral candidiasis is seldom a problem in children treated with inhaled or systemic steroids. The occurrence seems to be related to concomitant use of antibiotics, dose, and dose. Spacers seem to reduce the incidence.[215–217] Mouth-rinsing has not been reported to be beneficial. The condition is easily treated and rarely necessitates withdrawal of the treatment.

Increased level of *dental erosion* has been reported in asthmatic children.[218–220] The exact reason is not known. Increased frequency of mouth-breathing and a marked lowering of pH in saliva after inhalation of certain drugs such as β_2-agonists have been suggested.[221,222] The findings had been reported before inhaled corticosteroids were used in children and at present there are no studies to suggest that they contribute to this problem.

Hoarseness has been reported in adults treated with high doses of inhaled corticosteroids. Few studies have assessed its occurrence in children. One study found that three to six years' treatment of 178 children with inhaled budesonide at an average daily dose of about 500 µg was not associated with an increased occurrence of hoarseness or other noticeable voice changes.[368] Hoarseness is reversible after withdrawal of treatment, but unlike thrush, it tends to recur when the treatment is reintroduced. Spacers do not appear to protect against dysphonia.

OTHER SIDE EFFECTS

There is no evidence of an increase in infections, including tuberculosis, of the lower respiratory tract after chronic use of inhaled steroids. Although thinning of the skin around the mouth may occur in young children treated with nebulized corticosteroids through a face-mask, there is no evidence for a similar process in the airways. Bruising is not increased by inhaled corticosteroid use in children.

Growth effects of corticosteroids

GENERAL CONSIDERATIONS

The relationships between childhood asthma, corticosteroids therapy, and growth are thoroughly reviewed in Chapter 15, along with the published evidence. They will be summarized here (Table 8a.3).

Many chronic diseases of childhood have been shown to adversely affect the normal growth pattern of a child. The most commonly observed effect of asthma on growth is a reduction in growth rate, which is most often seen towards the end of the first decade of life. This reduced growth rate continues into the mid-teens and is associated with *a delay in the onset of puberty*. The pre-pubertal deceleration of growth velocity resembles growth retardation. However, the delay in pubertal growth is also associated with a delay in skeletal maturation so that the bone age of the child corresponds to the height. Ultimately, there is no decreased adult height, although it is reached at a later than normal age. This difference in growth pattern seems to be unrelated to the use of inhaled corticosteroids, and may affect non-asthmatic atopic children too (Chapter 15).

Poorly controlled asthma may itself adversely affect growth. Thus, height standard deviation scores before effective treatment with inhaled corticosteroids were found to correlate significantly with lung function and degree of asthma control and severe asthma may adversely affect final adult height. The exact mechanisms by which severe or poorly controlled asthma adversely affects growth are unclear, but there may be similarities with the factors operating in poor socio-economic conditions. These issues must be considered when assessing the possible effects of corticosteroid therapy on growth.

The disease and level of lung function may affect the *systemic availability of inhaled corticosteroid*. Several

Table 8a.3 *Summary of effects of inhaled corticosteroids on statural growth*

Short and intermediate effects
- No controlled studies have reported any statistically or clinically significant adverse effect on growth with daily doses of 100–200 µg of inhaled corticosteroid.
- Growth retardation may be seen with all inhaled corticosteroids when a sufficiently high dose is administered without any dose adjustment for disease severity.
- Growth suppression in both short- and intermediate-term studies is dose dependent.
- Important differences seem to exist between the growth retarding effects of different inhaled corticosteroids (and their respective delivery devices).
- Different age groups seem to differ in susceptibility to the growth retarding effects of inhaled corticosteroids; children aged 4–10 years being more susceptible than pubertal children.
- The growth retarding effect of inhaled corticosteroid treatment seems to be more marked at the beginning of the treatment and in some way becomes attenuated with continued treatment.

Adult height attained
- Uncontrolled or severe asthma seems to adversely affect growth and attained adult height.
- Corticosteroid-induced changes in growth rate during the first one or two years of treatment do not affect adult height.
- Children with asthma treated with inhaled corticosteroids have consistently been found to attain normal final adult height.

studies have suggested that the systemic bioavailability and systemic effects of an inhaled drug are more pronounced in patients with mild asthma than in patients with more severe disease,[223–226] probably due to differences in deposition pattern caused by a smaller airway diameter in more severe disease or possibly due to the differential effects of airway inflammation in absorption. This means that children with mild disease are more likely to experience adverse growth effects of a given dose of inhaled corticosteroid than children with more severe disease.

Short-term growth studies

Knemometry (the accurate measurement of the length of the lower leg, from knee to heel) can be used to measure changes in short-term linear growth over periods as short as 4 weeks. This measurement may be a valuable adjunct/alternative to traditional growth studies since knemometry allows very controlled designs. All children participating in placebo-controlled, double-blind knemometry studies assessing the effects of inhaled corticosteroids on lower leg growth have been mild asthmatics that have not required continuous treatment with inhaled corticosteroids.

The findings in these studies can be summarized as follows: the short-term effect of inhaled corticosteroids on lower leg growth rate is dose-dependent. Generally, low doses (200 μg per day or lower) are not associated with detectable effects, but higher doses are. Moreover, the growth inhibition dose–response curves seem to differ between the various inhaled corticosteroids, BDP having greater effects than other corticosteroids.

As a marker of long-term linear growth, knemometry studies still need further assessment since steroid-induced changes in short-term in lower leg growth rate explain virtually nothing of the variation in annual statural height velocity. This means that knemometry exaggerates the growth stunting effects of exogenous steroids. On the other hand, we believe that if an exogenous steroid has no adverse effect on lower leg growth in a properly performed knemometry study, it is unlikely that such treatment will be associated with any growth suppression during long-term treatment. This assumption is supported by the finding that so far none of three well powered growth studies have found any adverse effects on statural growth of doses of inhaled corticosteroid, which in well designed knemometry studies had no effect on lower leg growth rate.

INTERMEDIATE-TERM STATURAL GROWTH STUDIES

Over the years the influence of inhaled corticosteroids on growth of asthmatic children have been studied extensively. There have been flaws in the designs of most studies. Several have been retrospective or uncontrolled. Others have been conducted under artificial conditions, which are very different from the day-to-day treatment situation. This makes it difficult for the clinician to draw unequivocal conclusions about their clinical relevance. A brief summary of the findings and the conclusions is given below. A large number of intermediate-term studies have evaluated the effect of inhaled corticosteroids on statural growth. None of these studies, comprising more than 3500 children treated for mean periods of 1–13 years found any adverse effect upon growth. A metanalysis of 21 studies representing 810 patients to some extent corroborated the findings in these studies.[227] Significant but small reduction in attained height was found in children receiving oral steroids whereas children treated with inhaled steroids attained normal height. Furthermore, there was no statistical evidence of an association between inhaled steroid therapy and growth impairment at higher doses or during extended therapy.

A follow-up of a cohort of 3347 children with asthma treated in primary care settings corroborated these findings. The vast majority of children had normal growth rates. Only children receiving daily doses of inhaled corticosteroids ≥400 μg showed growth impairment. However, this effect on growth was smaller than the effect of poor socio-economic status or severe asthma.[228] This study illustrates how important it is to account for confounders in growth studies.

Prospective controlled growth studies using parallel group designs have been conducted in recent years. The results differ between the three main agents: beclomethasone dipropionate (BDP), budesonide (BUD) and fluticasone propionate (FP).

Beclomethasone dipropionate caused significant growth retardation in children with mild asthma treated continuously for 9–12 months with a fixed daily dose of beclomethasone ≥400 μg.[229] This dose is markedly higher than the dose normally required to control mild asthma. A dry powder inhaler or a pMDI was used for the administration of BDP in all studies. These devices deposit a large amount of drug in the oropharynx, which is extensively absorbed (50%) into the systemic circulation through the gastrointestinal tract resulting in a subsequent increase in systemic effect. The growth retarding effect in these studies would have been smaller if a spacer device and dose titration had been used. The effects may be transient.[100,230] The magnitude of the growth reduction in these trials has been rather consistent at 1.5 cm per year of treatment.[231]

In a prospective observational study of *inhaled budesonide*, high doses (>400 μg/day) were associated with poor control and with lower growth rates.[98] Other studies have given inconsistent results, but the biggest (around 1000 patients aged 5 to 12 years) and longest randomized, controlled growth study conducted so far found that growth over 4.3 years during treatment with 400 μg BUD per day by Turbuhaler was significantly lower (around 1 cm over 4 years) than in the two other groups.[101] The difference between the three groups was only significant during the first year of treatment. The growth rate during the last 3 years of the study was similar in the three groups and at the end of the study bone age, projected final height and Tanner stage were similar to those in the placebo group. The authors concluded that extrapolation from one-year growth studies to projected loss in subsequent years is not appropriate.

Fluticasone propionate in daily doses of 100 and 200 μg had no effect on growth.[232] The effect of *other inhaled corticosteroids* upon growth has not been thoroughly assessed though a retrospective study did not find any adverse effects upon growth during one year's treatment with triamcinolone.[233]

Though no formal dose–response studies have been conducted these data suggest that the effect of inhaled corticosteroids on statural growth in short-term studies is dose dependent.[67]

Comparison of the effect of different inhaled corticosteroids on growth: The annual growth rate of prepubertal children was higher during treatment with FP 400 μg/day (4.99 cm/year) than with 400 μg BDP per day (4.09 cm/ year)[234] (Table 15.1, Chapter 15). In other studies treatment with BUD 800 μg per day adversely affected growth significantly more than treatment with FP 400 µg/day (a supposedly clinically equivalent dose),[235] and BDP 400 µg per day had a significantly greater influence on growth than FP 200 µg per day.[236] The differences in growth rate between the various treatments may be caused by differences in dose, differences between the drugs or both.

Long-term studies and studies on final adult height: Most physicians consider attained adult height the most important growth outcome and the seminal question with regard to effects on growth is whether slowing in short-term growth rates leads ultimately to a diminished adult height. Several prospective long-term studies on attained adult height have been conducted.

Retrospective studies have shown that in the era prior to the introduction of inhaled corticosteroids, asthma itself was associated with a reduction in adult height attained.[237] Several studies compared measured adult heights of corticosteroid treated children with their target adult heights. All reported no effect of corticosteroid treatment on final adult height, although some noted an adverse effect of severe asthma.[238–240]

Prospective observation studies: In two of the most influential studies, Balfour-Lynn[241,242] found no difference in overall growth rate between children who received inhaled BDP and those who did not. Predicted height was estimated from bone age measurement in children, and not from parental height. These findings were corroborated by a 14-year prospective study of children treated with inhaled budesonide for several years in doses tailored to disease severity.[243] Long-term treatment with inhaled budesonide did not adversely affect adult height (Figure 8a.16) whereas poorly controlled asthma did (Figure 8a.17). Furthermore, slowing in growth rate during the first year of budesonide treatment was not helpful in predicting adult height. These conclusions agree with the findings of the largest randomized growth study conducted so far.[101]

PRESCHOOL CHILDREN

Some aspects of the assessment of safety are unique to preschool children, including the rapid growth velocity and somewhat different metabolism. Therefore the safety findings in school-children or adults cannot uncritically be extrapolated to young children. Growth in the first 2–3 years of life is mainly influenced by factors similar to those controlling fetal growth, and the growth from age 3 mainly by endocrine factors.

Short-term growth measurements by knemometry show dose-related effects of budesonide by pMDI and spacer in toddlers 1–2 years of age with mild recurrent wheezing. A daily dose of 200 µg of budesonide pMDI from spacer may be safe treatment in 1–2-year-old toddlers.

Intermediate growth studies have not been reported specifically for toddlers, but nebulized budesonide ranged from 0.5 to 1.0 mg caused a statistically significant decrease

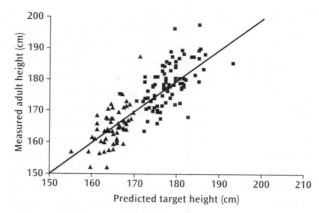

Figure 8a.16 *Measured adult height in relation to target adult height in 142 children treated with inhaled budesonide for 3–13 years.* ▲: *females;* ■: *males. The black line is the line of identity. (From ref. 243.)*

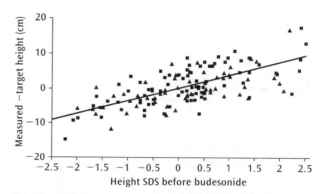

Figure 8a.17 *Correlation between height standard deviation score before budesonide treatment and the difference between measured and target adult height. The correlation was highly significant ($p < 0.001$) so that children who were short for age (had a low height standard deviation score) before treatment with budesonide tended to end up shorter than expected, whereas children who were tall before treatment with budesonide tended to end up taller than expected. The dose of inhaled budesonide and the duration of treatment before adult height was attained did not influence adult height.* ▲: *females;* ■: *males. Height SDS – height standard deviation score. (From ref. 243.)*

in growth velocity of −0.8 cm/year compared with the controls.[244]

Long-term observations of 3–5 years have not shown growth impairment during treatment with 200–300 µg budesonide per day from a pMDI with a spacer, but there are no controlled studies in preschool children.

IS THERE VARIATION IN INDIVIDUAL SENSITIVITY TO STEROIDS?

Case reports suggest that individual children may be particularly sensitive to the growth retarding effects of exogenous corticosteroids. When such reports are evaluated it must be remembered that growth is a complex process that may be affected by a host of factors including disease severity, social and psychological factors, nutrition, body composition, age, puberty, genetic factors and treatment.

Healthy children show spontaneous fluctuations in growth velocity, often with seasonal variations, most children growing faster in the summer. In some children fluctuations are not purely seasonal, but cycles of growth may span two or more years. This leads to a very poor correlation between the growth velocity in one year and that in the next year. These variations in combination with the standard error of the height measurement, which for trained observers is around 0.2–0.3 cm, and unusual growth patterns seen in many asthmatic children, independently of the use of inhaled corticosteroids, mean that case reports of apparently reduced growth in association with an asthma treatment should be interpreted with caution.

There is no evidence of subgroups of children who are more susceptible to the effects of long-term treatment with inhaled corticosteroids.

Summary

Inhaled steroids have been used for the treatment of asthma in children for 30 years. During this time, a substantial number of studies have been performed evaluating the safety and efficacy of this therapy. Inhaled corticosteroids have been found to have a marked benefit on both immediate and long-term outcome of asthma. In patients with mild and moderate asthma, low daily doses of around 100–200 μg/day of inhaled steroid produce a clinical effect that, in most trials, is better than the effect of any other treatment to which it has been compared. No adverse effects on growth have been associated with treatment in this dose range and idiosyncratic adverse reactions are rare. Higher doses of inhaled corticosteroids can reduce growth rate during the first years of treatment, particularly in patients with mild disease. Potentially, suppression of the adolescent growth spurt could have long-lasting effects. However, attained adult height is not adversely affected even if such doses are used for several years. It seems that these children will be somewhat shorter than their peers for some years. This risk will also be there if the asthmatic condition is not sufficiently controlled, but in contrast to the growth retardation caused by high-dose inhaled corticosteroids, the growth inhibition caused by uncontrolled disease may also adversely affect adult height.

Since the occurrence of measurable systemic effects and risk of clinical side effects increases with dose, the lowest dose which controls the disease should always be used. Furthermore, inhaler–steroid combinations with a high clinical efficacy/systemic effect ratio should be used. If a child is not sufficiently controlled on a low dose of inhaled steroid it might be better to add another drug to the low-dose inhaled steroid treatment rather than to increase the steroid dose. Further studies are needed to resolve this question. The answer may be different for each individual steroid–device combination.

LEUKOTRIENE MODIFIERS

Cysteinyl leukotrienes, synthesized *de novo* from cell membrane phospholipids, are proinflammatory mediators that play a major role in the pathophysiology of asthma.[245–247] These mediators are potent bronchoconstrictors and cause vasodilation, increased microvascular permeability, exudation of macromolecules, and oedema. Cysteinyl leukotrienes also have chemoattractant properties for eosinophils and reduce ciliary motility. In addition, these mediators are potent secretagogues (Figure 8a.18). Asthmatic patients demonstrate increased production of cysteinyl leukotrienes during naturally occurring asthma and acute asthma attacks as well as after allergen and exercise challenge. These observations suggest that the cysteinyl leukotrienes represent a novel therapeutic target and that leukotriene blockade may operate additively with corticosteroid therapy in asthma.

The leukotriene receptor antagonists (LTRA) montelukast, zafirlukast, and pranlukast inhibit bronchoconstriction in asthmatic patients undergoing allergen, exercise, cold air, or aspirin challenge.[248,249] Montelukast attenuates the hallmarks of asthmatic inflammation, including eosinophilia in the airway mucosa and peripheral blood.[250–252] Moreover, exhaled NO concentrations decrease during montelukast treatment in children in contrast to adults.[253]

Pharmacokinetics and pharmacodynamics

The onset of action of LTRA is within few hours to days, but not rapid enough to make them useful as rescue medication. They are all administered orally. Intravenous preparations may be made available for trial in acute severe asthma in the future.

At present three Cys-LTRA are available for the treatment of asthma in children. *Zafirlukast*, an orally available Cys-LTRA approved for treatment of asthma in children 7 years and older in some countries, is administered twice daily. Dose-ranging studies have not been performed in children. As a consequence the optimal dose in children is uncertain. There is up to a 40% reduction in bioavailability when zafirlukast is taken with food.[254] Zafirlukast is metabolized by the liver, and hepatic cytochrome P450 is inhibited by therapeutic concentrations of zafirlukast. Therefore, there is a risk of drug interactions, and transient elevations of liver enzymes have been reported. *Pranlukast* is available on few markets and further introduction has been postponed because of suspected liver toxicity.

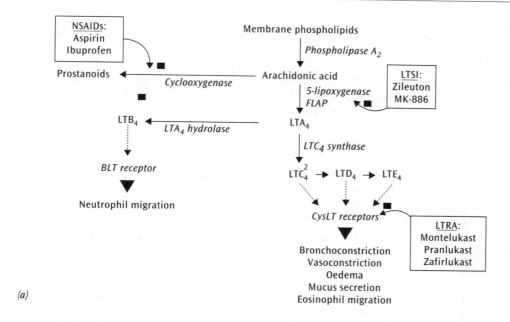

(a)

Potential sites and effects of cysteinyl leukotrienes relevant to a pathophysiological role in asthma

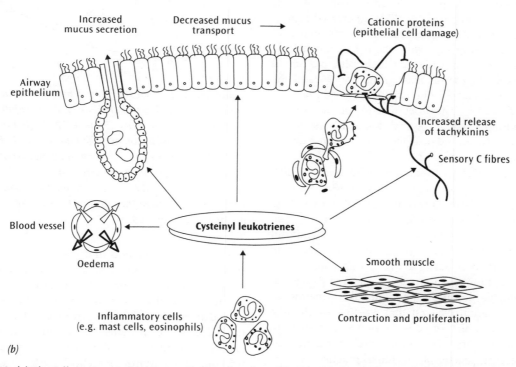

(b)

Figure 8a.18 *(a) The 5-lipozygenase pathway and sites of action of leukotriene modifier drugs. (From ref. 386.) (b) Possible modulatory effects of leukotriene receptor antagonists on airway inflammation. (Adapted from ref. 387.)*

Montelukast is an oral Cys-LTRA administered once daily.[255] In some countries the drug has been approved for the treatment of asthma in children 2 years and older. There is no difference in systemic bioavailability in young and elderly patients, and food does not have a clinically important influence on the systemical bioavailability of the drug. Therapeutic concentrations of montelukast do not inhibit the cytochrome P450 isoenzymes. Dose-ranging studies have not been performed in children. Instead, the paediatric dosage has been chosen as the dosage yielding a pharmacokinetic profile (single-dose area under the plasma concentration-time curve) in children comparable to that achieved with the 10-mg tablet in adults.[252]

Clinical trials

SCHOOL-CHILDREN

Zafirlukast has been shown to be modestly effective in moderate to severe asthmatics of 12 years and older.[256–258] The studies failed to define a plateau at the highest dose used, indicating that higher doses might be more effective. This is however prevented by the risk of side effects. The therapeutic effects of zafirlukast have been reported in one paediatric double-blind randomized controlled trial of asthmatic children from 6 to 14 years of age.[259] Treatment with zafirlukast provided 20–30% protection against exercise-induced bronchoconstriction 4 hours after dosing. Montelukast provided a similar reduction in maximum percentage fall in FEV_1 at approximately 20 hours after dosing.[260]

Montelukast has been compared with placebo in 336 children aged 6 to 15 years with moderate to severe asthma (Mean FEV_1 72% predicted; 2–3 daily doses of β_2-agonist; 1–2 nocturnal awakenings per week) (Figure 8a.19).[261] Approximately one third of the children were maintained on inhaled steroids during the study at a constant dose. The primary outcome variable, FEV_1, increased significantly by a mean of 8% from baseline, compared with 4% in the placebo group, while the use of inhaled β_2-agonists was significantly reduced. Eighty-five per cent of the patients in the montelukast group and 96% of the patients in the placebo group experienced asthma exacerbations ($p < 0.05$). The onset of action of montelukast occurred within 1 day of the first dose, with maximum effect after a few days, and no evidence of tolerance during the 8-week treatment period.

Adding montelukast to children with a mean FEV_1 of 78% predicted, and a reversibility of 18.1% after a β_2-agonist, whose asthma was not controlled on 400 µg budesonide per day was studied in 279 children,[262] and resulted in a small improvement in FEV_1, significant increases in morning and evening PEF, a decrease in asthma exacerbation days (15.9% during placebo and 12.2% during montelukast) and a decreased β_2-agonist use (0.3 puffs/day lower during montelukast treatment). Clinical observations suggest that 30–40% of children with moderate asthma respond to montelukast therapy. Since the benefits are seen within a week, a trial in individual subjects is practicable in clinical practice.

The clinical effect of leukotriene antagonists has rarely been compared with the effect of other drugs in children. In one study the protective effect against exercise-induced bronchoconstriction of montelukast 10 mg per day was found to be significantly less than than that of budesonide 400 µg/day (Figure 8a.19).[263]

PRESCHOOL CHILDREN

Montelukast was studied in 689 in preschool children, who had asthma symptoms and used beta-agonists 6 days/week.[264] Compared with placebo there were

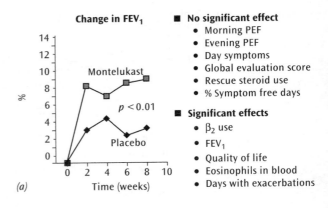

(a)

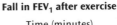

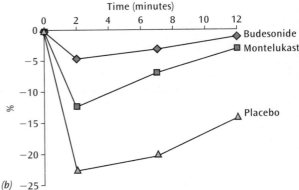

(b)

Figure 8a.19 *(a) Clinical effects of montelukast in a large double-blind, parallel group study on children with moderate asthma severity. (From ref. 261.) (b) Protective effect of montelukast on exercise-induced fall in FEV_1. Compared with placebo treatment montelukast offered a significant attenuation of exercise-induced fall in lung function. However, the effect of montelukast was significantly less than the effect of budesonide 400 µg per day. (From ref. 263.)*

significant improvements in day and night-time asthma symptoms, percentage of days without asthma and the need for beta-agonist or oral corticosteroids. The effect was independent of concomitant use of inhaled corticosteroid or cromolyn therapy. Caregiver global evaluations, the percentage of patients experiencing asthma attacks, and improvements in quality-of-life scores were not significantly different from placebo.

Cold-air hyperventilation was found to cause a 17% increase in airway resistance after pretreatment with montelukast compared with 47% after placebo pretreatment, a significant difference.[265]

In conclusion, the leukotriene receptor antagonist montelukast has significant clinical effects when used alone or in addition to inhaled corticosteroids, in children over 2 years old. Its place as a first-line preventer in mild asthma, in place of low-dose inhaled corticosteroids, has yet to be fully established. There are individual differences in response which could, in part, be explained by genetic polymorphisms in the promoter gene for 5-lypoxygenase (ALOX5).[62] This could be the basis for a screening test.

SODIUM CROMOGLYCATE AND NEDOCROMIL

Pharmacological action

The exact mechanisms of action of sodium cromoglycate (SCG) and the related cromone nedocromil sodium are not fully understood, although these non-steroidal anti-inflammatory medications partly inhibit IgE-mediated mediator release from human mast cells in a dose-dependent way, and they have a cell-selective and mediator-selective suppressive effect on other inflammatory cells (macrophages, eosinophils, monocytes). There is some evidence that these medications inhibit a chloride channel on target cells.[266]

In asthmatic patients cromones inhibit *allergen induced bronchospasm*, both immediate and delayed responses.[267–269] Furthermore, in the laboratory single doses of SCG and nedocromil given just prior to a *challenge* have shown protective effect against airway obstruction induced by exercise,[270–278] hypertonic saline, and hyperventilation.[279] The effect of continuous treatment on these challenges has not been thoroughly studied except for exercise where long-term continuous treatment with SCG does not offer any significant protection against exercise-induced bronchoconstriction unless given just prior to the exercise. Most controlled studies have found that continuous treatment with SCG does not affect the non-specific bronchial hyperreactivity to histamine or methacholine in patients with asthma,[280] though some have found an effect. In one study, 16 mg nedocromil sodium daily for periods of 12–16 weeks decreased histamine responsiveness significantly compared to placebo. However, no effect was seen on the responsiveness to fog.[281] In contrast 4 years' treatment of 300 children with nedocromil sodium 8 mg/day did not significantly decrease bronchial responsiveness to methacholine compared to placebo.[101] Other studies have also failed to show any effect on methacholine or histamine hyperresponsiveness.

Neither SCG nor nedocromil has been shown to affect the *chronic inflammatory changes* or epithelial disruption seen in the airways of asthmatic patients. However, in several studies *in vitro* and *in vivo* anti-inflammatory effects have been found.[282–285] The exact clinical importance of these findings remains unknown since the magnitude of the clinical benefit reported in the majority of controlled clinical trials is modest compared with the reported effect on various inflammatory mediators and challenges in laboratory studies. Thus nedocromil sodium does not reduce exhaled nitric oxide in children.[93,286]

Pharmacokinetics and dynamics

No pharmacokinetic studies are available on children so all information comes from adult studies.[287,288] Both SCG and nedocromil have to be inhaled to be effective. The drug deposited in the intrapulmonary airways is extensively absorbed and becomes systemically bioavailable.[289] The absorbed drug is not metabolized but mainly excreted in the urine and bile with a half life of around 1.5 hours (nedocromil). The part of the inhaled dose deposited in the oropharynx is swallowed and not absorbed. Since no double-blind, placebo-controlled clinical dose–response trials have been performed in children the optimal daily doses of SCG and nedocromil in the day-to-day management are not known.

Clinical trials

SCHOOL-CHILDREN

It is generally assumed that *SCG* is only beneficial in a proportion of children and that the drug has a more marked effect in children with mild disease. Although several placebo-controlled clinical trials have found SCG to reduce asthma symptoms in school-children, to improve lung functions and decrease the need for concomitant bronchodilators,[290,291] the drug appears to be ineffective in infants and preschool children. A meta-analysis of 22 controlled clinical trials concluded that continuous treatment with SCG in children had not been shown to be significantly better than placebo (Figure 8a.20).[292] The interpretation of the evidence is thought by some to be seriously flawed by merging data from school-children and preschool children (see below).

Nedocromil has been reported to improve symptoms (by 50%), lung function and reduce the use of β$_2$-agonists

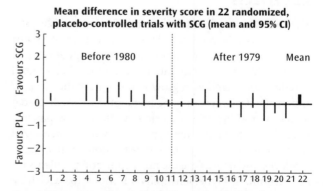

Mean difference in severity score in 22 randomized, placebo-controlled trials with SCG (mean and 95% CI)

Figure 8a.20 *Meta-analysis of placebo-controlled clinical trials with sodium cromoglycate in children. Overall no significant clinical effect was seen. Trials conducted before 1980 (mainly in school-children) were more often in favour of SCG, while after 1997 (almost all in preschool children and infants) there was no benefit. The funnel plots suggested publication bias; small studies with negative or equal outcomes were lacking. (From ref. 292.)*

when given in a daily dose of 16 mg.[293] A systematic review concluded that nedocromil given prior to an exercise test reduces the severity and duration of exercise-induced bronchoconstriction.[294] A combination of nedocromil and salbutamol might provide better protection against exercise-induced bronchoconstriction than salbutamol alone.[272] In contrast, a well powered long-term, placebo-controlled trial only found a significant albeit small effect of nedocromil 8 mg per day on exacerbations (but not other outcomes) as compared with placebo (Figure 8a.12).[101] Nedocromil was markedly less clinically effective than budesonide 400 μg per day.

Treatment with SCG is normally less effective than treatment with inhaled corticosteroids[97] with respect to symptoms, lung function, exercise-induced asthma and bronchial responsiveness.

Cromones do not have a role in the management of acute asthma attacks at any age.

PRESCHOOL CHILDREN

The clinical documentation on sodium cromoglycate in preschool children is very sparse, and there are no reports on nedocromil. The available double-blind randomized controlled trials are conflicting with several unable to demonstrate any effect of nebulized SCG in a dose of 20 mg 3–4 times daily on health outcomes or lung function while other studies have indicated a significant effect of the same magnitude as theophylline. A recent double-blind randomized controlled trial using a pMDI with a spacer for the administration of SCG also failed to show any benefits of SCG over placebo. Indeed, the children in the SCG group experienced more troublesome cough and and perioral skin irritation than the children in the placebo group.[295] Overall, in preschool children there is probably no clinical effect (Figure 8a.20).

SIDE EFFECTS

The risk of systemic side effects of the cromones has not been extensively reported. However, neither SCG nor nedocromil appear to have important systemic side effects. Sodium cromoglycate treatment has been found to reduce the excretion of growth hormone in the urine,[150] and to affect markers of bone metabolism. Cough, throat irritation and bronchoconstriction affect a few patients treated with SCG and the hypotonicity of the nebulized solution may cause bronchoconstriction. A bad taste, headache and nausea are the most common problems for nedocromil.[293] Hypersensitivity reactions to SCG have been reported but are probably extremely rare.

XANTHINES (THEOPHYLLINE)

Theophylline has been used in asthma treatment since the early 1920s. For many decades the use of this drug rested a great deal on clinical impressions and an evolving therapeutic tradition. At the beginning of the 1970s the clinical scientific documentation of theophylline was not advanced and its role in therapy was questioned (particularly in Europe). During the period 1970–1990 slow release theophylline preparations and reliable theophylline assays have increased the use of this drug in asthma therapy and it is the still a frequently prescribed oral agent used for maintenance therapy in many countries.

Chemically theophylline is a dimethylated xanthine that is similar in structure to the common dietary xanthines caffeine and theobromine. Over the years the molecule has been substituted at various positions with subsequent modifications in effects. Although these changes have provided interesting new information about the possible modes of action, they have not yet resulted in new xanthine molecules which are available in the day-to-day treatment.

Caffeine has been used in the management of asthma and has weak bronchodilator effects.[296] It may be important to warn patients to avoid tea and coffee for two hours before attending for lung function tests!

Pharmacological action

A large number of subcellular mechanisms including adenosine antagonism, phosphodiesterase inhibition, release of catecholamines, interactions with G-proteins, 5′-nucleotidase inhibition, prostaglandin antagonism and effects on calcium metabolism have been proposed for theophylline.[297] However, the exact anti-asthmatic mechanism still remains unknown (Table 8a.4).

Of the effects listed in Table 8a.4, some are probably without any important clinical relevance. Recently, it has been argued that the clinical effect of theophylline may reflect anti-inflammatory properties more than smooth muscle relaxation.[298] *In vitro* the drug reduces the activity of basophils, macrophages, mast cells, platelets, lymphocytes and polymorpho-nuclear leukocytes.[298–300] At therapeutic levels theophylline produces a slight reduction of immediate response in asthmatics challenged with

Table 8a.4 *Therapeutic effects of theophylline*

- Bronchial smooth muscle relaxation: related to phosphodiesterase inhibition and is mainly seen at high concentrations (>55 μmol/l)
- Increase in mucociliary clearance
- Inhibition of release of mediators
- Suppression of vascular permeability
- Improved contractility of fatigued diaphragm[374]
- Central stimulation of ventilation[375]
- Anti-inflammatory effects:[376] due to an unknown mechanism; may occur at low concentrations (25–55 μmol/l) and influence chronic asthmatic airway inflammation[221,377]

allergen. In addition, it markedly inhibits the late response occurring after several hours. The effect on vascular permeability seen in patients with allergic rhinitis[7] may be important in preventing this late reaction. Theophylline also significantly inhibits the late reaction followed by toluene diisocyanate challenge.[301,302] However, it does not affect the subsequent increase in bronchial responsiveness or inhibit allergen induced increase in airway responsiveness to methacholine.[298,303] Furthermore, several weeks of treatment does not change the bronchial responsiveness of asthmatics in comparison to the marked attenuation achieved with inhaled steroids over the same period.[304] Finally, there is no clinical evidence that continuous theophylline treatment modifies the chronic inflammation or epithelial disruption in the asthmatic airways, though one study suggested that theophylline treatment may reduce the number of eosinophils in the airway mucosa.[305]

Theophylline has a weak acute protective effect on histamine and methacholine responsiveness in patients with mild asthma and also some effect on exercise-induced bronchospasm.[306,307] Furthermore, the drug also attenuates the bronchial response to provocation with distilled water. There is, however, no evidence of any important effect on non-specific bronchial hyperresponsiveness in patients with severe asthma.[304]

Pharmacokinetics and dynamics

Dose–response studies with theophylline in a limited number of patients have mainly assessed bronchodilator effects[308] and protective effect against exercise-induced asthma.[306] A therapeutic range of 55–110 mmol/l has been defined upon the basis of such studies. Significantly better clinical results have been demonstrated in children with plasma theophylline levels around 75 mmol/l than in children with levels around 35 mmol/l. However, many children have been shown to obtain significant clinical results and some bronchodilation at lower plasma levels.[309,310] Furthermore, the other actions of theophylline such as its anti-inflammatory properties may not require such high concentrations. Thus, after so many years there is still considerable difference in opinion regarding the optimum plasma levels for a child with asthma. It seems rational to individualize the dose upon the basis of the clinical effect, and to use plasma levels to prevent toxic effects.

The pharmacokinetics of theophylline in children have been thoroughly described in an excellent review.[311] Ninety per cent of a theophylline dose is eliminated by metabolic degradation in the liver and around 10% is renally excreted. Generally children metabolize theophylline much more rapidly than adults, and in the child population the elimination rate also varies with age so that young children have a much higher clearance than older children. The normally recommended theophylline

doses for maintenance therapy in different age groups have been:

<1 year: (0.3)*(age in weeks)	+8 mg/kg/24 h
1 to 9 years:	24 mg/kg/24 h
9 to 12 years:	20 mg/kg/24 h
12 to 16 years:	18 mg/kg/24 h
Over 16 years:	10 mg/kg/24 h

These dose recommendations are based upon lean body weight and they aim at plasma theophylline levels between 55 and 110 mmol/l, which, as mentioned earlier, may be too high. It is appropriate to aim for a level of 55 mmol/l for the best ratio of benefit to risk. Within each age group the inter-individual variations in theophylline half life may be up to 10-fold and in addition other drugs including β_2-agonists (increase clearance so that higher doses are required) and viral infections (reduce clearance) may also affect the metabolism. Therefore, theophylline dose must always be individualized and if high doses are used plasma theophylline levels must be measured. When dose adjustments are made upon the basis of serum theophylline determinations it is important to remember that theophylline often shows dose dependent kinetics so that on average the per cent change in serum concentration is about 50% greater than the per cent change in dose.

Gastrointestinal absorption from plain tablets is complete and almost as rapid as from a solution. The absorption may be somewhat slower but not less complete when the tablets are taken with food. Because children metabolize theophylline very rapidly frequent dosing (4–6 times per day) is required when plain tablets are used for continuous treatment. Slow release products are preferable for maintenance therapy, since this administration allows twice daily dosing in most children. However, concomitant intake of food may change the absorption characteristics of many slow release theophylline products in an unpredictable way. Reduced absorption, dose dumping and marked variations in absorption profiles may be seen.[312] This complicates safe, effective treatment. As the food effect is quite unpredictable only slow release products which have been shown to be well-absorbed in combination with food should be used for maintenance treatment. In this respect it is important to evaluate both mean and individual absorption profiles. The variation in absorption seems to be more pronounced in schoolchildren than adults. Slow release theophylline products with reliable absorption profiles and complete bioavailability also with food have been developed.[313]

Clinical trials

SCHOOL-CHILDREN

The vast majority of theophylline studies in children have only assessed the drug's pharmacokinetic properties and not its clinical effect. However, studies have found that theophylline is significantly better than placebo in

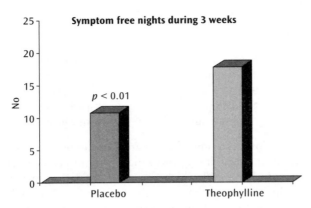

Figure 8a.21 *Clinical effect of treatment with slow release theophylline on nocturnal asthma in children with moderate to severe asthma. The study was a double-blind, randomized, crossover study in children who during run-in had nocturnal asthma at least twice a week. (From ref. 310.)*

controlling symptoms and improving lung function even at doses below the normally recommended therapeutic range.[309,310] Furthermore, a single dose of 15 mg/kg of slow release theophylline taken before bedtime is effective against nocturnal asthma (Figure 8a.21).[310] Continuous treatment offers some protective effect against exercise-induced asthma,[306] though this effect is far less than the effect of an inhaled β_2-agonist or continuous treatment with inhaled corticosteroids. Though definite beneficial effects have been demonstrated, continuous theophylline treatment was found ineffective in preventing asthma deterioration induced by viral infections.[314]

Theophylline treatment is normally far less effective than low doses of inhaled corticosteroids.[96,106] On the other hand theophylline has been found to improve asthma control and reduce the maintenance steroid dose in children with severe asthma treated with inhaled or oral steroids.

Theophylline and oral β_2-agonists seem to have an additive effect.[24] However, it remains unclear whether the combination has any clear advantages compared with either drug used alone.

INFANTS AND PRESCHOOL CHILDREN

The majority of studies in *preschool children* have only evaluated theophylline pharmacokinetics and not clinical effects. Thus, although there are clear indications that theophylline treatment offers some beneficial clinical effects and also some bronchodilation in these age groups, further double-blind studies are needed to assess the optimal dose and place of theophylline relative to other treatments in young children. The effect of continuous theophylline treatment has not been assessed in double-blind controlled studies in *infants with wheeze*.

ACUTE ASTHMA

Xanthine derivates (aminophylline or theophylline) have been used for many years in the treatment of acute severe

asthma in children (Chapter 12). The number of controlled studies assessing the acute effect is relatively sparse. However, it has been shown that a bolus dose of theophylline causes significant increases in lung function in school-children with wheeze.[315] Only one controlled trial has supported its use in hospitalized children with severe asthma. However, that study did not use aggressive therapy with inhaled β_2-agonists. No formal dose–response studies have been conducted in children with acute wheeze, but the bronchodilating effect seems to some extent to correlate with the plasma theophylline level. Therefore, it is normally recommended that the therapeutic strategy in such situations is to aim at plasma levels between 55 and 110 µmol/l. This can be achieved in all age groups by giving an intravenous bolus of 6 mg/kg lean body weight over 5 minutes to a child who has not received any theophylline for 12 hours prior to the treatment (volume of distribution = 0.5 l/kg) and then continue with theophylline infusion rates as mentioned for oral therapy. If the child is already receiving treatment with theophylline additional theophylline therapy should only be given under the guidance of plasma theophylline monitoring.

Although acute bronchodilating effects have been demonstrated by theophylline its role in the modern management of acute asthma is still controversial and two meta-analyses have come to different conclusions. One meta-analysis of 13 double-blind controlled studies on the treatment of acute asthma in children and adults concluded that there was no clinical benefit of adding theophylline to treatment with steroids and sympathomimetics.[316] In contrast a Cochrane meta-analysis of seven trials[317] concluded that addition of intravenous aminophylline should be considered early in the treatment of children hospitalized with acute severe asthma and who have a suboptimal response to the initial inhaled bronchodilator therapy. Although the improvement was sustained for 24 hours, there was no apparent reduction in length of hospital stay or number of inhaled β_2-agonists nebulizations. It was also found that treatment with aminophylline was associated with an increased risk of vomiting.

Side effects

In recent years the use of theophylline has been somewhat controversial since the incidence of side effects has continued unabated. The drug has a narrow therapeutic window and potentially lethal side effects when overdosed.[318,319] Deaths have been reported in studies with theophylline.[320] The most common side effects are anorexia, nausea, vomiting and headache.[318,319,321] These symptoms are quite common especially when initiating theophylline therapy and are often the practical dose-limiting side effects in maintenance therapy. Mild central nervous stimulation, palpitations, tachycardia, arrhythmias, sleep disturbance, abdominal pain, diarrhoea and, rarely, gastric bleeding may also occur. In maintenance therapy, initial dosage should be low to avoid side effects, which seem to occur much more frequently if the initial dose is high. Some patients do not tolerate theophylline at all no matter which precautions are taken.

The most serious toxicity is the risk of seizures, which have been associated with a mortality rate as high as 50%. However, seizures appear to be rare at serum levels less than 220 mmol/l. In theophylline-induced seizures higher than normal doses of benzodiazepines should be used as theophylline antagonizes the effect of benzodiazepines on GABA receptors in the brain. If modern kinetic principles are used seizures should not occur.

Theophylline has been reported to induce changes in mood and personality and impairment of school performance in children.[322] However, subsequent studies have not reproduced these findings[323] and it seems that these problems are not a widespread general problem associated with the treatment but rather a phenomenon that may occur at an unknown frequency in single individuals.

ANTICHOLINERGIC AGENTS

Anticholinergic alkaloids such as atropine exist in many plants and have been used in herbal remedies for centuries. The natural agents produced unpleasant side effects which limited their use. These problems have now been overcome by the development of synthetic anticholinergics that are much less prone to produce side effects and therefore potentially more useful clinically.

Clinical pharmacology

The clinical pharmacology of atropine and its synthetic relatives has been described in thorough reviews.[324] Anticholinergic alkaloids act on muscarinic receptors in the human airways interfering with the cholinergic sympathetic nervous system's control of airway calibre. Several subtypes of receptors have been recognized pharmacologically. M_1-receptors are partly responsible for vagal nerve transmission in ganglia. M_2-receptors are located pre-synaptic on postganglionic vagal nerves where they are stimulated by acetylcholine secreted in the synaptic cleft (negative feedback). M_3-receptors are located on bronchial smooth muscle and submucosal glands. All anticholinergic drugs available for clinical use act on prejunctional and smooth muscle muscarinic receptors with equal effect. As a consequence, they both increase ACh release and block its effect on the muscles. In animals low doses of ipratropium bromide may actually increase vagally mediated bronchoconstriction and it has been suggested that the paradoxical bronchoconstriction which is occasionally seen with inhaled anticholinergics may be due to this effect. Further information about this will be available when drugs that are selective for the muscarinic receptors on airways smooth muscle (M_3-antagonists) have been developed.

Anticholinergic drugs inhibit cholinergic smooth muscle contraction and reduce the release of secretion from submucosal glands. The first action is clinically most important so anticholinergics should be considered mainly as bronchodilators.

In laboratory studies anticholinergics provide partial protection against bronchoconstriction induced by stimuli such as exercise,[325] hyperventilation,[326] inhalation of cold and dry air[327] and non-specific dust. The effects are smaller than the effect of an inhaled β_2-agonist though the addition of ipratropium bromide may prolong the duration of the protection of the β_2-agonist.

Continuous treatment does not influence non-specific bronchial hyperreactivity and anticholinergic agents have not been shown to influence the chronic inflammation and epithelium disruption in the asthmatic airways.

Pharmacokinetics and dynamics

No pharmacokinetic studies are available in children so all information is derived from studies in adults. Virtually all pharmacodynamic data in children refer to one drug: *ipratropium bromide*. The dose ranging studies in schoolchildren have all used a nebulizer for the delivery so the optimal dose is only known for this administration. It would be expected that the optimal dose from a metered dose inhaler would be lower. Various studies have found that increasing the dose above 250 μg adds no extra benefit in protection against exercise-induced asthma,[325] cold air hyperventilation or in bronchodilation.[328] The same dose (250 μg) has also been used in most studies on preschool children. No formal dose–response studies have been performed in infants but a dose of 25 μg/kg has produced beneficial effects in one study.[329] The optimal dose frequency remains unknown.

Clinical trials

SCHOOL-CHILDREN

Significant bronchodilation and improvement of symptoms have been shown in some studies in school-children after both single dose and regular therapy.[328] However, in another study treatment with 250 μg ipratropium bromide three times daily did not diminish symptoms, diurnal variation in airway calibre or bronchodilator responsiveness. The response to ipratropium bromide seems to be quite variable and always less than the response after inhalation of a β_2-agonist. Furthermore, there is no benefit from adding the drug to regular β_2-agonist treatment in the day-to-day management.[330] These findings indicate that these drugs have no or a very limited role in the day-to-day management of asthma in school-children.

INFANTS AND PRESCHOOL CHILDREN

In *preschool children* bronchodilation is seen after single dose inhalation of ipratropium bromide. The effect in these studies being similar to the effect of 5 mg nebulized salbutamol. However, in one study regular treatment (ipratropium bromide 250 μg three times a day) was no better than placebo in the day-to-day management. Paradoxical bronchoconstriction has been described following the use of this agent in young children. Up to 40% of *infants* studied between acute attacks have been reported to improve their lung functions after inhalation of 250 μg ipratropium bromide from a nebulizer in an open study.[331] A Cochrane review concluded that there is not enough evidence to support the uncritical use of anti-cholinergic agents for wheezing infants, although patients using it at home were able to identify some benefits.[332]

ACUTE ASTHMA

Anticholinergics result in less bronchodilation than inhaled β_2-agonists and administrated alone these drugs have no role in the management of acute severe asthma in school-children.[333] However, controlled studies have found that the combination of a β_2-agonist and an anti-cholinergic agent produces somewhat better results than either drug used alone[333–335] without an increase in side effects. Though statistically highly significant, the advantages of the combination therapy were small in most studies. This may be the reason why other studies failed to find any benefit of such combined therapy. A meta-analysis in children concluded that: the addition of ipratropium bromide to a β_2-agonist produces statistically better improvement in FEV_1 and (probably) a reduction in the need for hospital admission[336] (Figure 8a.22). Another independent systematic review reached the same conclusions.[337] As it may cause deterioration in PEF in severely asthmatic children, ipratropium bromide should not be used universally for acute childhood asthma until further research determines the clinical significance of these spirometric changes.[338]

SIDE EFFECTS

Paradoxical bronchoconstriction after inhalation and dryness of the mouth may be a problem in some patients.[339,340]

Lung function

Trial	Treatment group		Control group		Standardized mean difference (95% CI)	Weight (%)	Standardized mean difference (95% CI)
	No	Mean (SD)	No	Mean (SD)			
Single dose protocol							
Change in spirometry							
No glucocorticoids							
Schuh *et al.* 1995	39	22.10 (15.30)	41	15.00 (13.80)		65	
Subtotal							−0.48 (−0.93 to 0.04)
Glucocorticoid use variable							
Beck *et al.* 1985	13	20.40 (19.50)	12	4.10 (6.20)		18	
Phanichyakam *et al.* 1990	10	36.40 (36.00)	10	22.00 (38.30)		17	
Subtotal							−0.74 (−1.35 to −0.12)
Total						100	−0.57 (−0.93 to −0.21)
Multiple dose protocol							
Change in spirometry							
Glucocorticoids							
Qureshi *et al.* 1997	45	33.60 (11.30)	45	24.10 (14.60)		45	
Subtotal							−0.72 (−1.15 to −0.29)
No glucocorticoids							
Schuh *et al.* 1995	39	23.44 (20.60)	38	13.20 (13.30)		39	
Watson *et al.* 1988	16	89.30 (13.20)	16	80.00 (14.00)		16	
Subtotal							−0.61 (−0.99 to −0.22)
Total						100	−0.66 (−0.95 to −0.37)

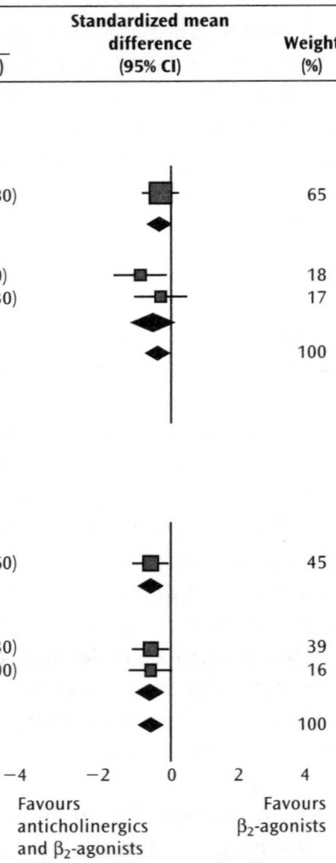

−4   −2   0   2   4

Favours anticholinergics and β_2-agonists   Favours β_2-agonists

Figure 8a.22 *Meta-analysis of placebo-controlled clinical trials with anti-cholinergics used as add-on therapy to inhaled β_2-agonists in children with acute wheeze concluded that the addition of ipratropium bromide to a β_2-agonist offers a statistically significant improvement in percentage predicted FEV_1 but no clinical benefit. (From ref. 336.)*

Some of these incidents seemed to be due to benzalkonium chloride which has now been removed from the nebulizer solution. Otherwise no important side effects are associated with treatment with inhaled ipratropium bromide.

OTHER AGENTS

Antihistamines

Given the importance of mast-cell activation and histamine release in allergic disorders in general, there ought to be a role for antihistamines (H_1 receptor antagonists) in the management of asthma.[341] There is evidence from studies in adults for effects in exercise-induced asthma.[342] There may be additional effects in moderately severe asthma in conjunction with leukotriene receptor antagonists. One large prospective study of cetirizine[343] has shown marginal effects, preventing the development of asthma in a small subset of children at risk (see Chapter 14). Except for *ketotifen*, however, there are little data in children.

KETOTIFEN

Ketotifen is an orally active benzocyclo-heptathiophine derivate, which is widely used in the treatment of asthma in many parts of the world, especially in children. Yet its role in the management of childhood asthma is increasingly being questioned.

The most clearcut *action of ketotifen* in humans is histamine H_1 receptor antagonism. Thus histamine-induced skin weal and bronchoconstriction are potently blocked by the drug.[344] Ketotifen can abrogate the development of tachyphylaxis of β-adrenergic receptor that occurs after continuous exposure to high doses of β-agonists.[345] The diminished β_2-receptor density and responsiveness seen in lymphocytes of asthmatic patients is increased to values within the normal range by ketotifen treatment.[346,347]

Ketotifen does not affect non-specific bronchial hyper-reactivity as assessed by methacholine provocation even after high-dose treatment for 12 weeks[348] and the effect against exercise-induced asthma is inconsistent.[346,349,350] The drug seems to have an effect against allergen provocation which is compatible with an H_1 blocking effect, i.e. some attenuation of the early response but no effect upon the late-phase reaction or the subsequent increase in non-specific bronchial reactivity.[344] It has not been shown to influence the chronic inflammation or epithelial disruption seen in the airways of asthmatic patients.

No *pharmacokinetic* trials have been conducted in children and no dose–response studies are available, so the optimal dose of the drug is not known. Most clinical studies have used the same dose, 1 mg twice daily, irrespective of the age or the size of the patient. In very young children younger than 1 year, 0.1 mg/kg has normally been used.[351,352]

Some *double-blind placebo-controlled clinical trials* have found that ketotifen treatment improves symptoms significantly and reduces concomitant use of theophylline and β_2-agonists in children assessed to have mild and moderate asthma.[353–355] In one of the studies a significant effect on lung function was also seen.[354] Other studies have failed to show convincing therapeutic effects.[348,356]

The results from controlled clinical trials in *preschool children* have been conflicting. Four controlled, double-blind studies involving a total of 227 children did not find any significant effect of ketotifen[357–360] whereas similar studies on 33 and 107 children found that ketotifen improved symptoms and reduced the use of rescue β_2-agonists.[348,361,362] As in older children, the magnitude of the effect has not been properly assessed by comparisons with other drugs in controlled trials. Ketotifen was found to be equieffective with SCG in a double-blind trial which was not placebo-controlled and therefore not capable of demonstrating a clinical effect (especially as SCG is probably ineffective in this group!). In a similarly designed trial ketotifen was found somewhat less effective than theophylline.[363]

It has been suggested that one year's prophylactic continuous ketotifen treatment of children with atopic dermatitis (but no wheeze) reduces the number of wheezing episodes during the treatment period,[364] suggesting that the treatment prevents or delays the onset of asthma in these children. No account was taken of important confounding factors. A large study of cetirizine, set up to replicate these observations, failed to do so.[342] No double-blind placebo-controlled trials have been performed in infants. Ketotifen has not been shown to be of any value in the treatment of acute asthma attacks.

Side effects include: drowsiness, dry mouth, and abnormal weight gain.[351,359,360] The frequency of these events is not known. No studies have assessed the implication of the sedative effect on intellectual performance.

Other agents

Several *immunosuppressive/modulating* agents have been shown to have an anti-asthma effect, including low-dose methotrexate, oral gold, cyclosporin, and intravenous γ-globulins.[365–367] Recent case reports suggest cyclosporin may sometimes be of benefit to children with difficult asthma. Its renal side effects demand careful monitoring.[368] Placebo-controlled trials in children are lacking, but generally these therapies have side effects that may be more troublesome than those of oral steroids and therefore they are indicated only as an additional therapy to reduce the requirement for oral steroids and not as additional therapy to inhaled steroids. Several other drugs including azathioprine, dapsone, and hydroxychloroquine have not been found to be beneficial.

Treatments which are used specifically in *acute severe asthma*, such as magnesium sulphate, heliox, an dintravenous theophylline, are discussed in Chapter 12.

Table 8a.5 *New drugs for asthma*

Cytokine blocking agents
  Anti-IL-5 monoclonal antibody[378]
  Soluble IL-4 receptor[379]
Immunomodulatory agents
  Anti-IgE (omalizumab)[380]
  Anti-chemokines and receptors
  T-cell targetting [381]
Blockers of mediator release or action
  COX-2 inhibitors[382]

Drug interactions are rarely a problem in childhood asthma, but must be borne in mind when antibiotic or anticonvulsant therapies are used concomitantly,[369] especially with theophylline.

Macrolide antibiotics have weak anti-inflammatory effects which may be of marginal benefit in severe asthma.[370]

New treatments in development

Several new lines of therapy are being developed, mostly aimed at specific inflammatory targets (Table 8a.5). Their use in children will await clinical trials in adults. So far, the effect of anti-cytokines has been disappointing, but that of the anti-IgE monoclonal antibody omalizumab is encouraging. It binds to the FCe RI binding site of the circulating IgE molecule, so that IgE is no longer capable of binding to receptors and is cleared without inducing any adverse effects. Serum IgE levels fall to very low levels. In adolescents and adults, there are significant beneficial effects in moderate-severe asthma, on a wide range of inflammatory, physiological, and clinical outcomes, of repeated intravenous or subcutaneous injections over periods of several months.[371-373] Concomitant allergies also improve. However, because it is expensive and requires parental administration, its use is likely to be restricted to severe or therapy-resistant atopic asthma. New opportunities will continue to present themselves.[388,389]

REFERENCES

1. Haynes B. Can it work? Does it work? Is it worth it? The testing of health care interventions is evolving. *Br Med J* 1999;**319**:652–3.
2. Barnes PJ. Beta-adrenoceptors on smooth muscle, nerves and inflammatory cells. *Life Sci* 1993;**52**:2101–9.
3. Rhoden KJ, Barnes PJ. Inhibition of cholinergic neurotransmission in human airways by beta-2-adrenoceptors. *J Appl Physiol* 1988;**65**:700–5.
4. O'Connor BJ, Ridge SM, Barnes PJ, Fuller RW. Comparative effect of terbutaline on mast cell and neurally mediated bronchoconstriction in asthma. *Thorax* 1991;**46**:745.
5. Phillips GD, Finnerty JT, Holgate S. Comparative protective effect of inhaled β2-agonist salbutamol (albuterol) on bronchoconstriction provoked by histamine, methacholine, and adenosine 5-monophosphate in asthma. *J Allergy Clin Immunol* 1990;**85**:755–62.
6. Kips JC, Pauwels RA. Long-acting inhaled β2-agonist therapy in asthma. *Am J Respir Crit Care Med* 2001;**164**:923–32.
7. Persson CGA. Role of plasma exudation in asthmatic airways. *Lancet* 1986;**2**:1126–9.
8. Chung KF, Rogers DF, Barnes PJ, Evans TW. The role of increased airway microvascular permeability and plasma exudation in asthma. *Eur Respir J* 1990;**3**:329–37.
9. Pavia D, Agnew JE, Sutton PP, *et al*. Effect of terbutaline administered from metered dose inhaler (2 mg) and subcutaneously (0.25 mg) on tracheobronchial clearance in mild asthma. *Br J Dis Chest* 1987;**81**:361–70.
10. Kornberg AE, Zuckerman S, Welliver JR, Mezzadri F, Aquino N. Effect of injected long-acting epinephrine in addition to aerosolized albuterol in the treatment of acute asthma in children. *Pediatr Emerg Care* 1991;**7**:1–3.
11. Wong CS, Pavord ID, Williams J, Britton J, Tattersfield A. Bronchodilator, cardiovascular, and hypokalaemic effects of fenoterol, salbutamol, and terbutaline in asthma. *Lancet* 1990;**336**:1396–9.
12. Brogden RN, Faulds D. Salmeterol xinafoate. A review of its pharmacological properties and therapeutic potential in reversible obstructive airways disease. *Drugs* 1991;**42**:895–912.
13. Jack D. A way of looking at agonism and antagonism: lessons from salbutamol, salmeterol and other beta-adrenoceptor agonists. *Br J Clin Pharmacol* 1991;**31**:501–14.
14. Henriksen JM, Agertoft L, Pedersen S. Protective effect and duration of action of inhaled formoterol and salbutamol on exercise-induced asthma in children. *J Allergy Clin Immunol* 1992;**89**:1176–82.
15. Green CP, Price J. Prevention of exercise-induced asthma by inhaled salmeterol xinafoate. *Arch Dis Child* 1992;**67**:1014–17.
16. Verberne AA, Hop WC, Bos AB, Kerrebijn K. Effect of a single dose of inhaled salmeterol on baseline airway caliber and methacholine-induced airway obstruction in asthmatic children. *J Allergy Clin Immunol* 1993;**91**:127–34.
17. Bel EH, Zwinderman AH, Timmers MC, Dijkman JH, Sterk PJ. The effect of beta-adrenergic bronchodilator on maximal airway narrowing to bronchoconstrictor stimuli in asthma and chronic obstructive pulmonary disease. *Thorax* 1991;**46**:9–14.
18. Fuglsang G, Hertz B, Holm EB, Borgström L. Absolute bioavailability of terbutaline from af CR-granulate in

asthmatic children. *Biopharm Drug Dispos* 1990;
11:85–90.

19. Hultquist C, Lindberg C, Nyberg L, Kjellman B,
Wettrell G. Pharmacokinetics of intravenous
terbutaline in asthmatic children. *Dev Pharmacol
Ther* 1989;**13**:11–20.

20. Morgan DJ. Clinical pharmacokinetics of beta-agonists.
Clin Pharmacokinet 1990;**18**:270–94.

21. Hochhaus G, Mollmann H. Pharmacokinetic/
pharmacodynamic characteristics of the beta-2-agonists
terbutaline, salbutamol and fenoterol. *Int J Clin
Pharmacol Ther Toxicol* 1992;**30**:342–62.

22. Fuglsang G, Pedersen S, Borgström L. Dose–response
relationships of intravenously administered
terbutaline in children with asthma. *J Pediatr*
1989;**114**:315–20.

23. Fuglsang G, Hertz B, Holm B. No protection by oral
terbutaline against exercise-induced asthma in
children: a dose response study. *Eur Respir J*
1993;**6**:527–30.

24. Chow OK, Fung KP. Slow-release terbutaline and
theophylline for the long-term therapy of children with
asthma: a Latin square and factorial study of drug
effects and interactions. *Pediatrics* 1989;**84**:119–25.

25. Thiringer G, Svedmyr N. Comparison of infused and
inhaled terbutaline in patients with asthma. *Scand
J Respir Dis* 1976;**57**:17–24.

26. Williams SJ, Winner SJ, Clark TJH. Comparison of
inhaled and intravenous terbutaline in acute severe
asthma. *Thorax* 1981;**36**:629–31.

27. Pedersen S. Inhaler use in children with asthma.
Danish Med Bull 1987;**34**:234–49.

28. Pedersen S. Aerosol treatment of bronchoconstriction
in children, with or without a tube spacer. *New Engl
J Med* 1983;**308**:1328–30.

29. Pedersen S. Treatment of acute bronchoconstriction
in children with use of a tube spacer aerosol and
a dry powder inhaler. *Allergy* 1985;**40**:300–4.

30. Kraemer R, Frey U, Sommer CW, Russi E. Short term
effect of albuterol, delivered via a new auxiliary
device, in wheezy infants. *Am Rev Respir Dis*
1991;**144**:347–51.

31. Nussbaum E, Eyzaguirre M, Galant S. Dose–response
relationship of inhaled metaproterenol sulfate in
preschool children with mild asthma. *Pediatrics*
1990;**85**:1072–5.

32. Conner WT, Dolovich M, Frame RA, Newhouse MT.
Reliable salbutamol administration in 6 to 36 month
old children by means of a metered dose inhaler and
aerochamber with mask. *Pediatr Pulmonol* 1989;
6:263–7.

33. Prendiville A, Green S, Silverman M. Airway
responsiveness in wheezy infants: evidence for
functional beta adrenergic receptors. *Thorax*
1987;**42**:100–4.

34. O'Callaghan C, Milner AD, Swarbrick A. Nebulised
salbutamol does have a protective effect on airways in
children under one year old. *Arch Dis Child*
1988;**63**:479–83.

35. Seidenberg J, Mir Y, Von der Hardt H. Hypoxaemia
after nebulized salbutamol in wheezy infants: the
importance of aerosol acidity. *Arch Dis Child*
1991;**66**:672–5.

36. Holmgren D, Sixt R. Transcutaneous and arterial blood
gas monitoring during acute asthmatic symptoms in
older children. *Pediatr Pulmonol* 1992;**14**:80–4.

37. Daugbjerg P, Brenøe E, Forchammer H, *et al.*
A comparison between nebulized terbutaline,
nebulized corticosteroid and systemic corticosteroid
for acuta wheezing in children up to 18 months of age.
Acta Paediatr 1993;**82**:547–51.

38. Pendergast J, Hopkins J, Timms B, Van Asperen PP.
Comparative efficacy of terbutaline administered by
Nebuhaler and by nebulizer in young children with
acute asthma. *Med J Aust* 1989;**151**:406–8.

39. Fuglsang G, Pedersen S. Comparison of a new
multidose powder inhaler with a pressurized aerosol
in children with asthma. *Pediatr Pulmonol* 1989;
7:112–15.

40. Phanichyakarn P, Kraisarin C, Sasisakulporn C,
Kittikool J. A comparison of different intervals of
administration of inhaled terbutaline in children with
acute asthma. *Asian Pac J Allergy Immunol* 1992;**10**:
89–94.

41. Kelly HW, McWilliams B, Katz R, Murphy S. Safety
of frequent high dose nebulized terbutaline in
children with acute severe asthma. *Ann Allergy* 1990;
64: 229–33.

42. Portnoy J, Aggarwal J. Continuous terbutaline
nebulization for the treatment of severe exacerbations
of asthma in children. *Ann Allergy* 1988;**60**:368–71.

43. Schuh S, Reider MJ, Canny G, Pender E, Forbes T,
Tan YK, Bailey D, Levison H. Nebulized albuterol in
acute childhood asthma: comparison of two doses.
Pediatrics 1990;**86**:509–13.

44. Scalabrin DM, Naspitz CK. Efficacy and side effects of
salbutamol in acute asthma in children: comparison
of oral route and two different nebulizer systems.
J Asthma 1993;**30**:51–9.

45. Lowenthal D, Kattan M. Facemasks versus
mouthpieces for aerosol treatment of asthmatic
children. *Pediatr Pulmonol* 1992;**14**:192–6.

46. Papo MC, Frank J, Thompson AE. A prospective,
randomized study of continuous versus intermittent
nebulized albuterol for severe status asthmaticus in
children. *Crit Care Med* 1993;**21**:1479–86.

47. Bohn D, Kalloghlian A, Jenkins J, Edmunds J, Barker G.
Intravenous salbutamol in the treatment of status
asthmaticus in children. *Crit Care Med* 1984;
12:892–6.

48. Travers A, Jones AP, Kelly K, Barker SJ, Camargo CA,
Rowe BH. Intravenous β2-agonists for acute asthma in
the emergency department (Cochrane Review).
Cochrane Database Syst Rev **2**:CD002988, 2001.

49. Kellner JD, Ohlsson A, Gadomski AM, Wang EE. Efficacy of bronchodilator therapy in bronchiolitis. A meta-analysis. *Arch Pediatr Adolesc Med* 1996; **150**:1166–72.

50. Bengtsson B, Fagerström PO. Extrapulmonary effects of terbutaline during prolonged administration. *Clin Pharmacol Ther* 1982;**31**:726–32.

51. Larsson S, Svedmyr N, Thiringer G. Lack of bronchial beta adrenoceptor resistance in asthmatic patients during long term treatment with terbutaline. *J Allergy Clin Immunol* 1977;**59**:93–100.

52. Ghigo E, Valetto MR, Gaggero L, *et al.* Therapeutic doses of salbutamol inhibit the somatotropic responsiveness to growth hormone-releasing hormone in asthmatic children. *J Endocrin Invest* 1993;**16**:271–5.

53. Bisgaard H. Long-acting beta(2)-agonists in management of childhood asthma: A critical review of the literature. *Pediatr Pulmonol* 2000;**29**:221–34.

54. von Berg A, Berdel D. Formoterol and salbutamol metered aerosols: comparison of a new and an established beta-2-agonist for their bronchodilating efficacy in the treatment of childhood bronchial asthma. *Pediatr Pulmonol* 1989;**7**:89–93.

55. Graff-Lonnevig V, Browaldh L. Twelve hours' bronchodilating effect of inhaled formoterol in children with asthma: a double-blind cross-over study versus salbutamol. *Clin Exp Allergy* 1990;**20**:429–32.

56. Barbato A, Cracco A, Tormena F, Novello A, Jr. The first 20 minutes after a single dose of inhaled salmeterol in asthmatic children. *Allergy* 1995;**50**:506–10.

57. Simons FE, Soni NR, Watson WT, Becker AB. Bronchodilator and bronchoprotective effects of salmeterol in young patients with asthma [see comments]. *J Allergy Clin Immunol* 1992;**90**:840–6.

58. Brodde O-E, Brinkmann M, Schemuth R, O'Hara N, Daul A. Terbutaline induced desensitization of humal lymphocyte β_2-adrenoceptors. *J Clin Invest* 1985; **76**:1096–101.

59. O'Connor BJ, Aikman SL, Barnes RJ. Tolerance to the non-bronchodilator effects of inhaled beta-2-agonists in asthma. *New Engl J Med* 1992;**237**:1204–8.

60. Simons FE, Gerstner TV, Cheang MS. Tolerance to the bronchoprotective effect of salmeterol in adolescents with exercise-induced asthma using concurrent inhaled glucocorticoid treatment. *Pediatrics* 1997;**99**:655–9.

61. O'Connor BJ, Aikman SL, Barnes RJ. Tolerance to the non-bronchodilator effects of inhaled beta-2-agonists in asthma. *New Engl J Med* 1992;**237**:1204–8.

62. Nanavaty U, Goldstein AD, Levine SJ. Polymorphisms in candidate asthma genes. *Am J Med Sci* 2001; **321**:11–16.

63. Verberne AA, Frost C, Roorda RJ, van der Laag H, Kerrebijn K. One year treatment with salmeterol, compared with beclomethasone in children with asthma. *Am J Respir Crit Care Med* 1997;**156**:688–95.

64. Meijer GG, Postma DS, Mulder P, van Aalderen WM. Long-term circadian effects of salmeterol in asthmatic children treated with inhaled corticosteroids. *Am J Respir Crit Care Med* 1995;**152**:1887–92.

65. Russell G, Williams DA, Weller P, Price JF. Salmeterol xinafoate in children on high dose inhaled steroids. *Ann Allergy Asthma Immunol* 1995;**75**:423–8.

66. Zarkovic J, Gotz MH, Holgate ST, Taak NK. Effect of long-term regular salmeterol treatment in children with moderate asthma. *Clin Drug Invest* 1998; **15**:169–75.

67. Verberne AA, Frost C, Duiverman EJ, Grol MH, Kerrebijn KF. Addition of salmeterol versus doubling the dose of beclomethasone in children with asthma. *Am J Respir Crit Care Med* 1998;**158**:213–19.

68. Brattsand R. Development of glucocorticosteroids with lung selectivity. In: FE Hargreave, JC Hogg, JL Malo, JH Toogood, eds. *Glucocorticoids and Mechanisms of Asthma*. Exerpta Medica, Amsterdam, 1989, pp. 17–39.

69. Toogood JH, Baskerville J, Jennings B, Lefcoe NM, Johansson SÅ. Bioequivalent doses of budesonide and prednisone in moderate and severe asthma. *J Allergy Clin Immunol* 1989;**84**:688–700.

70. Wolthers O, Pedersen S. Controlled study of linear growth in asthmatic children during treatment with inhaled glucocorticoids. *Pediatrics* 1992; **89**:839–42.

71. Wolthers O, Pedersen S. Short term linear growth in asthmatic children during treatment with prednisolone. *Br Med J* 1990;**301**:145–8.

72. Wolthers O, Pedersen S. Growth of asthmatic children during treatment with budesonide: a double blind trial [see comments]. *Br Med J* 1991;**303**:163–5.

73. Barnes PJ, Pedersen S, Busse W. Efficacy and safety of inhaled corticosteroids: New developments. *Am J Respir Crit Care Med* 1998;**157**:1–53.

74. Schleimer RP. Effects of glucocorticoids on inflammatory cells relevant to their therapeutic application in asthma. *Am Rev Respir Dis* 1990; **141**:59–69.

75. Sousa AR, Poston RN, Lane SJ, Narhosteen JA, Lee TH. Detection of GM–CSF in asthmatic bronchial epithelium and decrease by inhaled corticosteroids. *Am Rev Respir Dis* 1993;**147**:1557–61.

76. Barnes PJ. Effect of corticosteroids on airway hyperresponsiveness. *Am Rev Respir Dis* 1990;**141**:70–6.

77. deBaets FM, Goetyn M, Kerrebijn K. The effect of two months of treatment with inhaled budesonide on bronchial responsiveness to histamine and house-dust mite antigen in asthmatic children. *Am Rev Respir Dis* 1990;**142**:581–6.

78. Kerrebijn K, van Essen-Zandvliet E, Neijens HL. Effect of long-term treatment with inhaled corticosteroids and beta-agonists on bronchial responsiveness in asthmatic children. *J Allergy Clin Immunol* 1987;**79**:653–9.

79. van Essen-Zandvliet E, Hughes MD, Waalkens HJ, Duiverman E, Pocock SJ, Kerrebijn K. Effects of 22 months of treatment with inhaled corticosteroids and/or beta-2-agonists on lung function, airway responsiveness and symptoms in children with asthma. *Am Rev Respir Dis* 1992;**146**:547–54.

80. Østergaard P, Pedersen S. The effect of inhaled disodium cromoglycate and budesonide on bronchial responsiveness to histamine and exercise in asthmatic children: a clinical comparison. In: S Godfrey, ed. *Glucocorticosteroids in Childhood Asthma*. Excerpta Medica, Amsterdam, 1987, pp. 55–65.

81. Henriksen JM. Effect of inhalation of corticosteroids on exercise-induced asthma: Randomised double blind cross-over study of budesonide in asthmatic children. *Br Med J* 1985;**291**:248–9.

82. Groot CAR, Lammers J-WJ, Molema J, Festen J, van Herwaarden CL. Effect of inhaled beclomethasone and nedocromil sodium on bronchial hyperresponsiveness to histamine and distilled water. *Eur Respir J* 1992;**5**:1075–82.

83. O'Connor BJ, Rigde SM, Barnes PJ, Fuller RW. Greater effect of inhaled budesonide on adenosine 5-monophosphate-induced than on metabisulfite-induced bronchoconstriction in asthma. *Am Rev Respir Dis* 1992;**146**:560–4.

84. Vanthenen AS, Knox A, Wisniewski A, Tattersfield A. Effect of inhaled budesonide on bronchial reactivity to histamine exercise and eucapnic dry air hyperventilation in patients with asthma. *Thorax* 1991;**46**:811–16.

85. Fuller RW, Choudry NB, Eriksson G. Actions of budesonide on asthmatic airway hyperresponsiveness. Effects on directly and indirectly acting bronchoconstrictors. *Chest* 1991;**100**:670–4.

86. Rodwell LT, Anderson SD, Seale JP. Inhaled steroids modify bronchial responses to hyperosmolar saline. *Eur Respir J* 1992;**5**:953–62.

87. Bel EH, Timmers MC, Zwinderman AH, Dijkman JH, Sterk PJ. The effect of inhaled corticosteroids on the maximal degree of airway narrowing to methacholine. *Am Rev Respir Dis* 1991; **143**:109–13.

88. Agertoft L, Pedersen S. A randomized, double-blind dose reduction study to compare the minimal effective dose of budesonide Turbuhaler and fluticasone propionate Diskhaler. *J Allergy Clin Immunol* 1997;**99**:773–80.

89. Pedersen S, Hansen OR. Budesonide treatment of moderate and severe asthma in children. A dose response study. *J Allergy Clin Immunol* 1995;**1**:29–33.

90. Katz Y, Lebas FX, Medley HV, Robson R. Fluticasone propionate 50 mg bid versus 100 mg bid in the treatment of children with persistent asthma. *Clin Ther* 1998;**20**:424–37.

91. Shapiro G, Bronsky EA, LaForce CF, Mendelson L, Pearlman D, Schwartz RH, Szefler SJ. Dose-related efficacy of budesonide administered via a dry powder inhaler in the treatment of children with moderate to severe persistent asthma. *J Pediatr* 1998;**132**:976–82.

92. Jonasson G, Carlsen KH, Blomqvist P. Clinical efficacy of low-dose inhaled budesonide once or twice daily in children with mild asthma not previously treated with steroids. *Eur Respir J* 1998;**12**:1099–104.

93. Agertoft L, Friberg M, Pedersen S. One year treatment of mild asthma in children with budesonide or nedocromil. *J Allergy Clin Immunol* 2000;**105**:260s.

94. Youngchaiyud P, Permpikul C, Suthamsmai T, Wong E. A double-blind comparison of inhaled budesonide, a long-acting theophylline and their combination in the treatment of nocturnal asthma. *Allergy* 1995;**50**:28–33.

95. Price J, Russell G, Hindmarsh P, Weller P, Heaf D, Williams J. Growth during one of treatment with fluticasone propionate or sodium cromoglycate in children with asthma. *Pediatr Pulmonol* 1997;**24**:178–86.

96. Tinkelman DG, Reed CE, Nelson HS, Offord KP. Aerosol beclomethasone dipropionate compared with theophylline as primary treatment of chronic, mild to moderately severe asthma in children [see comments]. *Pediatrics* 1993;**92**:64–77.

97. Price J, Weller P. Comparison of fluticasone propionate and sodium cromoglycate for the treatment of childhood asthma. *Respir Med* 1995;**89**:363–8.

98. Agertoft L, Pedersen S. Effects of long term treatment with an inhaled corticosteroid on growth and pulmonary function in asthmatic children. *Respir Med* 1994;**88**:373–81.

99. Edmunds AT, Goldberg RS, Duper B, Devichand P, Follows RM. A comparison of budesonide 800 micrograms and 400 micrograms via Turbohaler with disodium cromoglycate via Spinhaler for asthma prophylaxis in children. *Br J Clin Res* 1994;**5**:11–23.

100. Simons FE. A comparison of beclomethasone, salmeterol, and placebo in children with asthma. *New Engl J Med* 1997;**337**:1659–65.

101. Long-term effects of budesonide or nedocromil in children with asthma. The Childhood Asthma Management Program Research Group [see comments]. *New Engl J Med* 2000;**340**:1054–63.

102. Anhøj J, Thorsson L, Bisgaard H. Lung deposition of inhaled drugs increases with age. *Am J Respir Crit Care Med* 2000;**162**:1819–22.

103. Zar HJ, Weinberg EG, Binns HJ, Gallie F, Mann MD. Lung deposition of aerosol – a comparison of different spacers. *Arch Dis Child* 2000;**82**:495–8.

104. Agertoft L, Andersen A, Weibull E, Pedersen S. Systemic availability and pharmacokinetics of

nebulized budesonide in pre-school children with asthma. *Arch Dis Child* 1999;**80**:241–7.

105. Pedersen S, Steffensen G, Ekman I, Tönnesson M, Borgå O. Pharmacokinetics of budesonide in children with asthma. *Eur J Clin Pharmacol* 1987;**31**:579–82.

106. Meltzer EO, Orgel HA, Ellis E, Eigen H, Hemstreet MP. Long-term comparison of three combinations of albuterol, theophylline, and beclomethasone in children with chronic asthma. *J Allergy Clin Immunol* 1992;**90**:2–11.

107. Benoist MR, Brouard JJ, Rufin P, Waernessyckle S, de Blic J, Paupe J, Scheinmann P. Dissociation of symptom scores and bronchial hyperreactivity: study in asthmatic children on long-term treatment with inhaled beclomethasone dipropionate. *Pediatr Pulmonol* 1992;**13**:71–7.

108. Gustafsson P, Tsanakas J, Gold M, Primhak R, Radford M, Gillies E. Comparison of the efficacy and safety of inhaled fluticasone propionate 200 micrograms/day with beclomethasone dipropionate 400 micrograms/day in mild and moderate asthma. *Arch Dis Child* 1993;**69**:206–11.

109. Hofstra WB, Neijens HJ, Duiverman EJ, Kouwenberg JM, Mulder PG, Kuethe MC, Sterk PJ. Dose–responses over time to inhaled fluticasone propionate treatment of exercise- and methacholine-induced bronchoconstriction in children with asthma. *Pediatr Pulmonol* 2000;**29**:415–23.

110. Boner A, Piacentini G, Bonizzato C, Dattoli V, Sette L. Effect of inhaled beclomethasone dipropionate on bronchial hyperreactivity in asthmatic children during maximal allergen exposure. *Pediatr Pulmonol* 1991;**10**:2–5.

111. De Baets FM, Goeteyn M, Kerrebijn K. The effect of two months of treatment with inhaled budesonide on bronchial responsiveness to histamine and house-dust mite antigen in asthmatic children. *Am Rev Respir Dis* 1990;**142**:581–6.

112. Eseverri JL, Botey J, Marin AM. Budesonide: treatment of bronchial asthma during childhood. *Allergy Immunol* 1995;**27**:129–35.

113. Ribeiro LB. Budesonide: safety and efficacy aspects of its long-term use in children. *Pediatr Allergy Immunol* 1993;**4**:73–8.

114. MacKenzie CA, Weinberg EG, Tabachnik E, Taylor M, Havnen J, Crescenzi K. A placebo-controlled trial of fluticasone propionate in asthmatic children. *Eur J Pediatr* 1993;**152**:856–60.

115. Perera BJ. Efficacy and cost effectiveness of inhaled steroid in asthma in a developing country. *Arch Dis Child* 1995;**72**:312–16.

116. Connett G, Lenney W, McConchie SM. The cost effectiveness of budesonide in severe asthmatics aged one to three years. *Br J Med Econ* 1993;**6**:127–34.

117. Waalkens HJ, van Essen-Zandvliet E, Hughes MD, *et al.* Cessation of long-term treatment with inhaled

corticosteroid (budesonide) in children with asthma results in deterioration. *Am Rev Respir Dis* 1993;**148**:1252–7.

118. Tal A, Levy N, Bearman JE. Methylprednisolone therapy for acute asthma in infants and toddlers: a controlled clinical trial. *Pediatrics* 1990; **86**:350–6.

119. Webb MSC, Henry RL, Milner AD. Oral corticosteroids for wheezing attacks under 18 months. *Arch Dis Child* 1983;**61**:15–19.

120. Bisgaard H, Munck SL, Nielsen JP, Petersen W, Ohlsson SV. Inhaled budesonide for treatment of recurrent wheezing in early childhood. *Lancet* 1990;**336**:649–51.

121. Noble V, Ruggins NR, Everard ML, Milner AD. Inhaled budesonide via a modified Nebuhaler for chronic wheezing in infants. *Arch Dis Child* 1992;**67**:285–8.

122. Connett G, Warde C, Wooler E, Lenney W. Use of budesonide in severe asthmatics aged 1–3 years. *Arch Dis Child* 1993;**69**:351–5.

123. de Blic J, Delacourt C, Le Bourgeois M, Mahut B, Ostinelli J, Caswell C, Scheinmann P. Efficacy of nebulized budesonide in treatment of severe infantile asthma: a double-blind study. *J Allergy Clin Immunol* 1996;**98**:14–20.

124. Bisgaard H, Gillies J, Groenewald M, Maden C. The effect of inhaled fluticasone propionate in the treatment of young asthmatic children: a dose comparison study. *Am J Respir Crit Care Med* 1999;**160**:126–31.

125. de Benedictis FM, Martinati LC, Solinas LF, Tuteri G, Boner AL. Nebulized flunisolide in infants and young children with asthma: a pilot study. *Pediatr Pulmonol* 1995;**21**:310–15.

126. Gleeson JG, Price J. Controlled trial of budesonide given by the nebuhaler in preschool children with asthma. *Br Med J* 1988;**297**:163–6.

127. O'Callaghan C. Particle size of beclomethasone dipropionate produced by 2 nebulisers and spacers. *Thorax* 1990;**45**:109–11.

128. Ilangovan P, Pedersen S, Godfrey S, Nikander K, Noviski N, Warner J. Treatment of severe steroid dependent preschool asthma with nebulised budesonide suspension. *Arch Dis Child* 1993; **68**:356–9.

129. Shapiro G, Mendelson L, Kraemer MJ, Cruz-Rivera M, Walton-Bowen K, Smith JA. Efficacy and safety of budesonide inhalation suspension (Pulmicort Respules) in young children with inhaled steroid-dependent, persistent asthma. *J Allergy Clin Immunol* 1998;**102**:789–96.

130. Kemp JP, Skoner DP, Szefler SJ, Walton-Bowen K, Cruz-Rivera M, Smith JA. Once-daily budesonide inhalation suspension for the treatment of persistent asthma in infants and young children. *Ann Allergy Asthma Immunol* 1999;**83**:231–9.

131. Vik R, Jorgenson J, Agertoft L, Pedersen S. Dose – titration of nebulized budesonide in young children. *Ped Pulmonol* 1997;**23**:270–7

132. Wennergren G, Nordvall SL, Hedin G, Möller C, Wille S, Åsbrink Nilsson E. Nebulized budesonide for the treatment of moderate to severe asthma in infants and toddlers. *Acta Paediatr* 1996;**85**:183–9.

133. Stick SM, Burton PR, Clough J, Cox M, LeSouef P, Sly P. The effects of inhaled beclomethasone dipropionate on lung function and histamine responsiveness in recurrently wheezy infants. *Arch Dis Child* 1995;**73**:327–32.

134. Nielsen KG, Bisgaard H. The effect of inhaled budesonide on symptoms, lung function, and cold air and methacholine responsiveness in 2- to 5-year-old asthmatic children. *Am J Respir Crit Care Med* 2000;**162**:1500–6.

135. Sung L, Osmond MH, Klassen TP. Randomized, controlled trial of inhaled budesonide as an adjunct to oral prednisone in acute asthma [see comments]. *Acad Emerg Med* 1998;**5**:209–13.

136. Roosevelt G, Sheehan K, Grupp-Phelan J, Tanz RR, Listernick R. Dexamethasone in bronchiolitis: a randomized controlled trial. *Lancet* 1996;**348**:292–5.

137. De Boeck K, Van der AN, Van Lierder S, Corbeel L, Eeckels R. Respiratory syncytial virus bronchiolitis: a double-blind dexamethasone efficacy study. *J Pediatr* 1997;**131**:919–21.

138. Richter H, Seddon P. Early nebulized budesonide in the treatment of bronchiolitis and the prevention of postbronchiolitic wheezing. *J Pediatr* 1998;**132**:849–53.

139. Fox GF, Everard ML, Marsh MJ, Milner AD. Randomised controlled trial of budesonide for the prevention of post-bronchiolitis wheezing. *Arch Dis Child* 1999;**80**:343–7.

140. Cade A, Brownlee KG, Conway SP, *et al.* Randomised placebo-controlled trial of nebulised corticosteroids in acute respiratory syncytial viral bronchiolitis. *Arch Dis Child* 2000;**82**:126–30.

141. Wong JY, Moon S, Beardsmore C, O'Callaghan C, Simpson H. No objective benefit from steroids inhaled via a spacer in infants recovering from bronchiolitis. *Eur Respir J* 2000;**15**:388–94.

142. van Woensel JB, Wolfs TF, van Aalderen WM, Brand PL, Kimpen JL. Randomised double blind placebo-controlled trial of prednisolone in children admitted to hospital with respiratory syncytial virus bronchiolitis. *Thorax* 1997;**52**:634–7.

143. Wilson NM, Silverman M. Treatment of acute, episodic asthma in preschool children using intermittent high dose inhaled steroids at home. *Arch Dis Child* 1990;**65**:407–10.

144. Svedmyr J, Nyberg E, Asbrink-Nilsson E, Hedlin G. Intermittent treatment with inhaled steroids for deterioration of asthma due to upper respiratory tract infections. *Acta Paediatr* 1995;**84**:884–8.

145. McKean M, Ducharme F. Inhaled steroids for episodic viral wheeze of childhood (*Cochrane Review*). Cochrane Database. Update Software, Oxford, 2000.

146. Edmonds ML, Camargo CA, Pollack CV, Rowe BH. Early use of inhaled corticosteroids in the emergency department treatment of acute asthma (*Cochrane Review*). Cochrane Database. Update Software, Oxford, 2001.

147. Brunette MG, Lands L, Thibodeau LP. Childhood asthma: prevention of attacks with short-term corticosteroid treatment of upper respiratory tract infection. *Pediatrics* 1988;**81**:624–9.

148. Vichyanond P, Irvin CG, Larsen G, Szefler S, Hill M. Penetration of corticosteroids into the lung: Evidence for a difference between methylprednisolone and prednisolone. *J Allergy Clin Immunol* 1989;**84**:867–73.

149. Connett G, Lenney W. Prevention of viral-induced asthma attacks using inhaled budesonide. *Arch Dis Child* 1993;**68**:85–7.

150. Soferman R, Sapir N, Spirer Z, Golander A. Effects of inhaled steroids and inhaled cromolyn sodium on urinary growth hormone excretion in asthmatic children. *Pediatr Pulmonol* 1998;**26**:339–43.

151. Martinati LC, Sette L, Chiocca E, Zaninotto M, Plebani M, Boner A. Effect of beclomethasone dipropionate nasal aerosol on serum markers of bone metabolism in children with seasonal allergic rhinitis. *Clin Exp Allergy* 1993;**23**:986–91.

152. Zeitlin S, Wood P, Evans A, Radford M. Overnight urine growth hormone, cortisol and adenosine-3′ 5′-cyclic monophosphate excretion in children with chronic asthma treated with inhaled beclomethasone dipropionate. *Respir Med* 1993;**87**:445–8.

153. Johnston CC, Miller JZ, Slemenda CW, *et al.* Calcium supplementation and increases in bone mineral density in children. *New Engl J Med* 1992;**327**:82–7.

154. Kröger H, Kotaniemi A, Vainio P, Alhava E. Bone densitometry of the spine and femur in children by dual-energy x-ray absorptiometry. *Bone and Mineral* 1992;**17**:75–85.

155. Slemenda CW, Miller JZ, Hui SL, Reister TK, Johnston CC, Jr. Role of physical activity in the development of skeletal mass in children. *J Bone Miner Res* 1991;**6**:1227–33.

156. Michaelsson K, Holmberg L, Mallmin H, Wolk A, Bergstrom R, Ljunghall S. Diet, bone mass, and osteocalcin: a cross-sectional study. *Calcif Tissue Int* 1995;**57**:86–93.

157. Glastre C, Braillon P, David L, Cochat P, Meunier P, Delmas P. Measurement of bone mineral content of the lumbar spine by dual energy X-ray absorptiometry in normal children: correlations with growth parameters. *J Clin Endocrinol Metab* 1990;**70**:1330–3.

158. Gordon CL, Halton JM, Atkinson SA, Webber CE. The contributions of growth and puberty to

peak bone mass. *Growth Develop Aging* 1991; **55**:257–62.

159. Albanese A, Stanhope R, Reed A, Haugen M, Pachman LM, Langman CB. Investigation of delayed puberty abnormalities in serum osteocalcin values in children with chronic rheumatic diseases. *Clin Endocrinol* 1990;**116**:574–80.

160. Finkelstein JS, Klibanski A, Neer RM. A longitudinal evaluation of bone mineral density in adult men with histories of delayed puberty. *J Clin Endocrinol Metab* 1996;**81**:1152–5.

161. Hansen OR, Nøkkentved K. Adverse effects in children treated with ACTH in infantile spasm. *Ugeskr Læger* 1989;**151**:2194–5.

162. Wolthers O, Juul A, Hansen M, Müller J, Pedersen S. The insulin-like growth factor axis and collagen turnover in asthmatic children treated with inhaled budesonide. *Acta Paediatr* 1995;**84**:393–7.

163. Wolthers O, Pedersen S. Short-term growth during treatment with inhaled fluticasone propionate and beclomethasone diproprionate. *Arch Dis Child* 1993;**68**:673–6.

164. Pedersen S. *Safety of Inhaled Glucocorticosteroids*. Excerpta Medica, Amsterdam, 1989, pp. 40–51.

165. Wolthers O, Juel Riis B, Pedersen S. Bone turnover in asthmatic children treated with oral prednisolone or inhaled budesonide. *Pediatr Pulmonol* 1993; **16**:341–6.

166. Wolthers O, Juul A, Hansen M, Müller J, Pedersen S. Growth factors and collagen markers in asthmatic children treated with inhaled budesonide. *Eur Respir J* 1993;**6**(Suppl 17):261.

167. Sorva R, Turpeinen M, Juntunen-Backman K, Karonen SL, Sorva A. Effects of inhaled budesonide on serum markers of bone metabolism in children with asthma. *J Allergy Clin Immunol* 1992;**90**:808–15.

168. Birkebaek NH, Esberg G, Andersen K, Wolthers O, Hassager C. Bone and collagen turnover during treatment with inhaled dry powder budesonide and beclomethasone dipropionate. *Arch Dis Child* 1995;**73**:524–7.

169. Wolthers O, Juul A, Hansen M, Müller J, Pedersen S. The insulin-like growth factor axis and collagen turnover during prednisolone treatment. *Arch Dis Child* 1994;**71**:409–13.

170. König P, Hillman L, Cervantes C, Levine C, Maloney C, Douglass B, Johnson L, Allen S. Bone metabolism in children with asthma treated with inhaled beclomethasone dipropionate. *J Pediatr* 1993;**122**:219–26.

171. Agertoft L, Pedersen S. Bone mineral density in children with asthma receiving long-term treatment with inhaled budesonide. *Am J Respir Crit Care Med* 1998;**157**:1–6.

172. Hopp RJ, Degan JA, Phelan J, Lappe J, Gallagher GC. Cross sectional study of bone density in asthmatic children. *Pediatr Pulmonol* 1995;**20**:189–92.

173. Kinberg K, Hopp RJ, Biven RE, Gallagher JC. Bone mineral density in normal and asthmatic children. *J Allergy Clin Immunol* 1994;**94**:490–7.

174. Boot AM, Verberne AA, Wildeboer G, de Jongste JC, De Muinck Keizer SM. Bone mineral density of prepubertal asthmatic children during long-term treatment with inhaled corticosteroids. *Horm Res* 1995;**44**:86.

175. Santolicandro A, Di Mauro M, Storti S, Buzzigoli G, Morelli C, Borgström L, Giuntini C. Lung deposition of budesonide inhaled through Turbuhaler in asthmatic patients before and after bronchodilation. *Am J Respir Crit Care Med* 1994;**149**:220.

176. Wong J, Black P. Acute adrenal insufficiency associated with high dose inhaled steroids. *Br Med J* 1992;**304**:1415.

177. Todd G, Dunlop K, McNaboe J, Ryan MF, Carson D, Shields MD. Growth and adrenal suppression in asthmatic children treated with high-dose fluticasone propionate. *Lancet* 1996;**348**:27–9.

178. Varsano I, Volovitz B, Malik H, Amir Y. Safety of 1 year of treatment with budesonide in young children with asthma. *J Allergy Clin Immunol* 1990;**85**:914–20.

179. Bisgaard H, Damkjær Nielsen M, *et al*. Adrenal function in children with bronchial asthma treated with beclomethasone dipropionate or budesonide. *J Allergy Clin Immunol* 1988;**81**:1088–95.

180. Wolthers O, Pedersen S. Measures of systemic activity of inhaled glucocorticosteroids in children: a comparison of urine cortisol excretion and knemometry. *Respir Med* 1995;**89**:347–9.

181. Agertoft L, Pedersen S. Short-term knemometry and urine cortisol excretion in children treated with fluticasone propionate and budesonide: a dose response study. *Eur Respir J* 1997;**7**:1507–12.

182. Pedersen S. Comparative study designs and what they show. *Respir Med* 2000;**94**(Suppl D):S40–3.

183. Chang CC, Tam AY. Suppression of adrenal function in children on inhaled steroids. *J Pediatr Child Health* 1991;**27**:232–4.

184. Wolthers O, Hansen M, Juul A, Nielsen HK, Pedersen S. Knemometry, urine cortisol excretion and measures of the insulin-like growth factor axis and collagen turnover in the assessment of systemic activity of inhaled corticosteroids. *Pediatr Res* 1997;**41**:44–50.

185. Nicolaizik WH, Marchant JL, Preece MA, Warner J. Endocrine and lung function in asthmatic children on inhaled corticosteroids. *Am J Respir Crit Care Med* 1994;**150**:624–8.

186. Feigang B, Asthford DR. Adrenal corticol function after long-term beclometasone aerosol therapy in early childhood. *Ann Allergy* 1990;**64**:342–6.

187. Goldstein DE, König P. Effect of inhaled beclometasone dipropionate on hypothalamic-pituitary–adrenal axis function in children with asthma. *Pediatrics* 1983;**72**:60–4.

188. Doull IJ, Donovan SJ, Wood P, Holgate S. Bloodspot cortisol in mild asthma: the effect of inhaled corticosteroids. *Arch Dis Child* 1995;**72**:321–4.

189. Katsunuma T, Akasawa A, Iikura Y. Adrenal function of children with bronchial asthma treated with beclomethasone dipropionate. *Ann Allergy* 1992; **69**:529–32.

190. Phillip M, Aviram M, Leiberman E, *et al*. Integrated plasma cortisol concentration in children with asthma receiving long-term inhaled corticosteroids. *Pediatr Pulmonol* 1992;**12**:84–9.

191. Law CM, Honour JW, Merchant JL, *et al*. Nocturnal adrenal supression in asthmatic children taking inhaled beclomethasone dipropionate. *Lancet* 1986;**i**:942–4.

192. Tabachnik E, Zadik Z. Diurnal cortisol secretion during therapy with inhaled beclomethasone dipropionate in children with asthma. *J Pediatr* 1991;**118**:294–7.

193. Volovitz B, Amir J, Malik H, Kauschansky A, Varsano I. Growth and pituitary–adrenal function in children with severe asthma treated with inhaled budesonide. *New Engl J Med* 1993;**329**:1703–33.

194. Hoffmann-Streb A, L'Allemand D, Niggemann B, Buttner P, Wahn U. Adrenocortical function in children with bronchial asthma under fluticasone treatment. *Monatsschr Kinderheilkd* 1993;**141**:508–12.

195. Prahl P, Jensen T, Bjerregaard-Andersen H. Adrenocortical function in children on high-dose steroid aerosol therapy. Results of serum cortisol, ACTH stimulation test and 24 hour urinary free cortisol excretion. *Allergy* 1987;**42**:541–4.

196. Ribeiro LB. Budesonide: safety and efficacy aspects of its long-term use in children. *Pediatr Allergy Immunol* 1993;**4**:73–8.

197. Ninan T, Reid I, Carter P, Smail P, Russell G. Effects of high doses of inhaled corticosteroids on adrenal function in children with severe persistent asthma. *Thorax* 1993;**48**:599–602.

198. König P, Goldstein DE. Adrenal function after beclomethasone inhalation therapy. *J Pediatr* 1982;**101**:646–7.

199. Laursen J, Wynn V, James V. The adrenocortical response to insulin-induced hypoglycaemia. *J Clin Endocrinol Metab* 1963;**27**:183–9.

200. Tarlo SM, Broder I, Davies GM, Leznoff A, Mintz S, Corey PN. Six-month double-blind, controlled trial of high dose, concentrated beclomethasone dipropionate in the treatment of severe chronic asthma. *Chest* 1988;**93**:998–1002.

201. Burri P, Hislop A. Outcomes – Structural considerations. *Eur Respir Rev* 1998;**12**:59–65.

202. Warner JO. The down-side of early intervention with inhaled corticosteroids. *Clin Exp Allergy* 1997; **27**:999–1001.

203. Pedersen S. Early use of inhaled steroids in children with asthma. *Clin Exp Allergy* 1997;**27**:995–9.

204. Massarano AA, Hollis S, Devlin J, David TJ. Growth in atopic eczema. *Arch Dis Child* 1993;**68**:677–9.

205. Simons FE, Persaud MP, Gillespie CA, Cheang M, Shuckett EP. Absence of posterior subcapsular cataracts in young patients treated with inhaled glucocorticoids. *Lancet* 1993;**342**:776–8.

206. Abuekteish F, Kirkpatrick JN, Russell G. Posterior subcapsular cataract and inhaled corticosteroid therapy. *Thorax* 1995;**50**:674–6.

207. Agertoft L, Pedersen S. Posterior subcapsular cataracts, bruises and hoarseness in children with asthma receiving long-term treatment with inhaled budesonide. *Eur Respir J* 1998;**12/1**:130–5.

208. Toogood JH, Markov A, Baskerville J, Dyson C. Association of ocular cataracts with inhaled and oral steroid therapy during long-term treatment of asthma. *J Allergy Clin Immunol* 1993;**91**:571–9.

209. Sevel D, Weinberg EG, van Niekerk CH. Lenticular complications of long-term steroid therapy in children with asthma and eczema. *J Allergy* 1977; **60**:215–17.

210. Agertoft L, Pedersen S. Bone density in children during long-term treatment with budesonide. *Eur Respir J* 1993;**6**:261S.

211. Nassif E, Weinberger M, Sherman B, Brown K. Extrapulmonary effects of maintenance corticosteroids therapy with alternate-day prednisone and inhaled beclomethasone in children with chronic asthma. *J Allergy Clin Immunol* 1987;**80**:518–29.

212. Phelan MC. Beclomethasone mania. *Br J Psychiatr* 1989;**155**:871–2.

213. Meyboom RHB. Budesonide and psychic side-effects. *Ann Intern Med* 1988;**109**(8):683.

214. Lewis LD, Cochrane GM. Psychosis in a child inhaling budesonide. *Lancet* 1983;**ii**:634.

215. Selroos O, Backman R, Forsen KO, Löfroos AB, Niemistö M, Pietinalho A, Äikäs C, Riska H. Local side-effects during 4-year treatment with inhaled corticosteroids – a comparison between pressurized metered-dose inhalers and Turbuhaler. *Allergy* 1994;**49**:888–90.

216. Müns G, Bergmann KC. Local and systemic side effects of inhalatory corticosteroids – what has been confirmed? *Pneumologie* 1993;**47**:201–8.

217. Settipane GA, Kalliel JN, Klein DE. Rechallenge of patients who developed oral candidiasis or hoarseness with beclomethasone dipropionate. *N Engl Reg Allergy Proc* 1987;**8**:95–7.

218. Shaw L, al Dlaigan YH, Smith A. Childhood asthma and dental erosion. *ASDC J Dent Child* 2000;**67**:102–6.

219. McDerra EJ, Pollard MA, Curzon ME. The dental status of asthmatic British school children. *Pediatr Dent* 1998;**20**:281–7.

220. Kankaala TM, Virtanen JI, Larmas MA. Timing of first fillings in the primary dentition and permanent first molars of asthmatic children. *Acta Odontol Scand* 1998;**56**:20–4.

221. O'Sullivan EA, Curzon MEJ. Drug treatments for asthma may cause erosive tooth damage. *Br Med J* 1998;**317**:820.

222. Kargul B, Tanboga I, Ergeneli S, Karakoc F, Dagli E. Inhaler medicament effects on saliva and plaque pH in asthmatic children. *J Clin Pediatr Dent* 1998; **22**:137–40.

223. Weiner P, Berar-Yanay N, Davidovich A, Magadle R. Nocturnal cortisol secretion in asthmatic patients after inhalation of fluticasone propionate. *Chest* 1999;**116**:931–4.

224. Lipworth BJ, Clark DJ. Effects of airway calibre on lung delivery of nebulised salbutamol. *Thorax* 1997; **52**:1036–9.

225. Falcoz C, Mackie AE, Moss J, *et al.* Pharmacokinetics of fluticasone propionate inhaled from the Diskhaler (r) and the Diskus(r) after repeat doses in healthy subjects and asthmatic patients. *J Allergy Clin Immunol* 1997;**99**:S505.

226. Saari M, Vidgren MT, Koskinen MO, Turjanmaa VM, Waldrep C, Nieminen MM. Regional lung deposition and clearance of 99mTc-labeled beclomethasone-DLPC liposomes in mild and severe asthma. *Chest* 1998;**113**:1573–9.

227. Allen D, Mullen M, Mullen B. A meta-analysis of the effect of oral and inhaled corticosteroids on growth. *J Allergy Clin Immunol* 1994;**93**:967–76.

228. McCowan C, Neville RG, Thomas GE, *et al.* Effect of asthma and its treatment on growth: four year follow up of cohort of children from general practices in Tayside, Scotland. *Br Med J* 1998;**316**:668–72.

229. Pedersen S. Efficacy and safety of inhaled corticosteroids in children. In: R. Schleimer, W Busse, P O'Byrne, eds. *Topical Glucocorticoids in Asthma – Mechanisms and Clinical Actions.* Marcel Dekker, New York, 1996, pp. 551–60.

230. Doull IJ, Freezer NJ, Holgate S. Growth of prepubertal children with mild asthma treated with inhaled beclomethasone dipropionate. *Am J Respir Crit Care Med* 1995;**151**:1715–19.

231. Sharek PJ, Bergman DA. Beclomethasone for asthma in children: effects on linear growth (*Cochrane Review*). Cochrane Database. Update Software, Oxford, 2000.

232. Allen D, Bronsky E, LaForce C, Nathan RA, Tinkelman DG, Vandewalker ML, König P. Growth in asthmatic children treated with inhaled fluticasone propionate. *J Pediatr* 1998;**132**:472–7.

233. Brown DCP, Savacool AM, Letizia CM. A retrospective review of the effects of one year of triamcinolone acetonide aerosol treatment of the growth patterns of asthmatic children. *Ann Allergy* 1989;**63**:47–51.

234. de Benedictis FM, Medley HV, Williams L. Long-term study to compare safety and efficacy of fluticasone propionate (FP) with beclomethasone dipropionate (BDP) in asthmatic children. *Eur Respir J* 1998; **12**:142s.

235. Ferguson AC, Spier S, Manjra A, Versteegh FG, Mark S, Zhang P. Efficacy and safety of high-dose inhaled steroids in children with asthma: a comparison of fluticasone propionate with budesonide. *J Pediatr* 1999;**134**:422–7.

236. Rao R, Gregson RK, Jones AC, Miles EA, Campbell MJ, Warner JO. Systemic effects of inhaled corticosteroids on growth and bone turnover in childhood asthma: a comparison of fluticasone with beclomethasone. *Eur Respir J* 1999;**13**:87–94.

237. Norjavaara E, Gerhardsson de Verdier M, Lindmark B. Reduced height in Swedish men with asthma at the age of conscription for military service. *J Pediatr* 2000;**137**:25–9.

238. Silverstein MD, Yunginger JW, Reed CE, Petterson T, Zimmerman D, Li JT, O'Fallon WM. Attained adult height after childhood asthma: effect of glucocorticoid therapy. *J Allergy Clin Immunol* 1997;**99**:466–74.

239. Inoue T, Doi S, Takamatsu I, Murayama N, Kameda M, Toyoshima K. Effect of long-term treatment with inhaled beclomethasone dipropionate on growth of asthmatic children. *J Asthma* 1999;**36**:159–64.

240. Van Bever HP, Desager KN, Lijssens N, Weyler JJ, Du Caju MV. Does treatment of asthmatic children with inhaled corticosteroids affect their adult height? *Pediatr Pulmonol* 1999;**27**:369–75.

241. Balfour-Lynn L. Effect of asthma on growth and puberty. *Pediatrician* 1987;**14**:237–41.

242. Balfour-Lynn L. Growth and childhood asthma. *Arch Dis Child* 1986;**61**:1049–55.

243. Agertoft L, Pedersen S. Effect of long-term treatment with inhaled budesonide on adult height in children with asthma. *N Engl J Med* 2000;**343**:1064–9.

244. Skoner DP, Szefler SJ, Welch M, Walton-Bowen K, Cruz-Rivera M, Smith JA. Longitudinal growth in infants and young children treated with budesonide inhalation suspension for persistent asthma. *J Allergy Clin Immunol* 2000;**105**:259–68.

245. Lewis RA, Austen KF, Soberman RJ. Leukotrienes and other products of the 5-lipoxygenase pathway. Biochemistry and relation to pathobiology in human diseases. *New Engl J Med* 1990;**323**:645–55.

246. Bisgaard H. Role of leukotrienes in asthma pathophysiology. *Pediatr Pulmonol* 2000;**30**:166–76.

247. Bisgaard H. Pathophysiology of the cysteinyl leukotrienes and effects of leukotriene receptor antagonists in asthma. *Allergy* 2000; **56**(Suppl 66):7–11.

248. Holgate ST, Bradding P, Sampson AP. Leukotriene antagonists and synthesis inhibitors: new directions

in asthma therapy. *J Allergy Clin Immunol* 1996;**98**:1–13.

249. Calhoun WJ. Summary of clinical trials with zafirlukast. *Am J Respir Crit Care Med* 1998;**157**:S238–45.

250. Calhoun WJ, Lavins BJ, Minkwitz MC, Evans R, Gleich GJ, Cohn J. Effect of zafirlukast (Accolate) on cellular mediators of inflammation: bronchoalveolar lavage fluid findings after segmental antigen challenge. *Am J Respir Crit Care Med* 1998;**157**:1381–9.

251. Pizzichini E, Leff JA, Reiss TF, Hendeles L, Boulet LP, Wei LX, Efthimiadis AE, Zhang J, Hargreave FE. Montelukast reduces airway eosinophilic inflammation in asthma: a randomized, controlled trial. *Eur Respir J* 1999;**14**:12–18.

252. Knorr B, Larson P, Nguyen HH, *et al*. Montelukast dose selection in 6- to 14-year-olds: comparison of single-dose pharmacokinetics in children and adults. *J Clin Pharmacol* 1999;**39**:786–93.

253. Bisgaard H, Loland L, Oj JA. NO in exhaled air of asthmatic children is reduced by the leukotriene receptor antagonist montelukast. *Am J Respir Crit Care Med* 1999;**160**:1227–31.

254. Wong SL, Kearns GL, Kemp JP, Drajesk J, Chang M, Locke CS, Dube LM, Awni WM. Pharmacokinetics of a novel 5-lipoxygenase inhibitor (ABT-761) in pediatric patients with asthma. *Eur J Clin Pharmacol* 1998; **54**:715–19.

255. Jones TR, Labelle M, Belley M, *et al*. Pharmacology of montelukast sodium (Singulair), a potent and selective leukotriene D4 receptor antagonist. *Can J Physiol Pharmacol* 1995;**73**:191–201.

256. Spector SL, Smith LJ, Glass M. Effects of 6 weeks of therapy with oral doses of ICI 204,219, a leukotriene D4 receptor antagonist, in subjects with bronchial asthma. ACCOLATE Asthma Trialists Group. *Am J Respir Crit Care Med* 1994;**150**:618–23.

257. Fish JE, Kemp JP, Lockey RF, Glass M, Hanby LA, Bonuccelli CM. Zafirlukast for symptomatic mild-to-moderate asthma: a 13-week multicenter study. The Zafirlukast Trialists Group. *Clin Ther* 1997;**19**:675–90.

258. Nathan RA, Bernstein JA, Bielory L, *et al*. Zafirlukast improves asthma symptoms and quality of life in patients with moderate reversible airflow obstruction. *J Allergy Clin Immunol* 1998; **102**:935–42.

259. Pearlman DS, Ostrom NK, Bronsky EA, Bonuccelli CM, Hanby LA. The leukotriene D4-receptor antagonist zafirlukast attenuates exercise-induced bronchoconstriction in children. *J Pediatr* 1999; **134**:273–9.

260. Villaran C, O'Neill SJ, Helbling A, *et al*. Montelukast versus salmeterol in patients with asthma and exercise-induced bronchosconstriction. *J Allergy Clin Immunol* 1999;**104**:547–53.

261. Knorr B, Matz J, Bernstein JA, Nguyen H, Seidenberg BC, Reiss TF, Becker A. Montelukast for chronic asthma in 6- to 14-year-old children: a randomized, double-blind trial. Pediatric Montelukast Study Group. *JAMA* 1998;**279**:1181–6.

262. Simons FE, Villa JR, Lee BW, *et al*. Montelukast added to budesonide in children with persistent asthma: a randomized, double-blind, crossover study. *J Pediatr* 2001;**138**:694–8.

263. Vidal C, Fernandez-Ovide E, Pineiro J, Nunez R, Gonzalez-Quintela A. Comparison of montelukast versus budesonide in the treatment of exercise-induced bronchoconstriction. *Ann Allergy Asthma Immunol* 2001;**86**:655–8.

264. Knorr B, Franchi LM, Bisgaard H, *et al*. Montelukast, a leukotriene receptor antagonist, for the treatment of persistent asthma in children aged 2 to 5 years. *Pediatrics* 2001;**108**:E48.

265. Bisgaard H, Nielsen KG. Bronchoprotection with a leukotriene receptor antagonist in asthmatic preschool children. *Am J Respir Crit Care Med* 2000;**162**:187–90.

266. Norris AA. Pharmacology of sodium cromoglycate. *Clin Exp Allergy* 1996;**26**(Suppl 4):5–7.

267. Pelikan Z, Knottnerus I. Inhibition of the late asthmatic response by nedocromil sodium administered more than two hours after allergen challenge. *J Allergy Clin Immunol* 1993;**92**:19–28.

268. Cockcroft D, Murdock KY. Comparative effects of inhaled salbutamol, sodium cromoglycate, and beclomethasone dipropionate on allergen induced early asthmatic responses, late asthmatic responses and increased bronchial responsiveness to histamine. *J Allergy Clin Immunol* 1987;**79**:734–40.

269. Mattoli S, Foresi A, Corbo GM, Valente S, Ciappi G. Effects of two doses of cromolyn on allergen-induced late asthmatic response and increased responsiveness. *J Allergy Clin Immunol* 1987;**79**:747–54.

270. Kelly KD, Spooner CH, Rowe BH. Nedocromil sodium versus sodium cromoglycate in treatment of exercise-induced bronchoconstriction: a systematic review. *Eur Respir J* 2001;**17**:39–45.

271. Spooner C, Rowe BH, Saunders LD. Nedocromil sodium in the treatment of exercise-induced asthma: a meta-analysis. *Eur Respir J* 2000;**16**:30–7.

272. de Benedictis FM, Tuteri G, Pazzelli P, Solinas LF, Niccoli A, Parente C. Combination drug therapy for the prevention of exercise-induced bronchoconstriction in children. *Ann Allergy Asthma Immunol* **80**:352–6.

273. Obata T, Matsuda S, Akasawa A, Iikura Y. Preventive effect and duration of action of disodium cromoglycate and procaterol on exercise-induced asthma in asthmatic children. *Ann Allergy* 1993;**70**:123–6.

274. Boner A, Antolini I, Andreoli A, De Stefano G, Sette L. Comparison of the effects of inhaled calcium

antagonist verapamil, sodium cromoglycate and ipratropium bromide on exercise-induced bronchoconstriction in children with asthma. *Eur J Pediatr* 1987;**146**:408–11.

275. Boner A, Vallone G, Bennati D. Nedocromil sodium in exercise-induced bronchoconstriction in children. *Ann Allergy* 198;**62**:38–41.

276. Henriksen JM. Effect of nedocromil sodium non exercise-induced bronchoconstriction in children. *Allergy* 1988;**43**:449–53.

277. Chudry N, Correa F, Silverman M. Nedocromil sodium and exercise-induced asthma. *Arch Dis Child* 1987;**62**:412–14.

278. Ben-Dow I, Bar-Yishay E, Godfrey S. Heterogeneity in the response of asthmatic patients to pre-exercise treatment with cromolyn sodium. *Am Rev Respir Dis* 1983;**127**:113–16.

279. Latimer KM, O'Byrne P, Morris M, Roberts R, Hargreave F. Bronchoconstriction stimulated by airway cooling. Better protection with combined inhalation of terbutaline sulphate and cromolyn sodium than with either alone. *Am Rev Respir Dis* 1983;**128**:440–3.

280. Baki A, Karaguzel G. Short-term effects of budesonide, nedocromil sodium and salmeterol on bronchial hyperresponsiveness in childhood asthma. *Acta Paediatr Jpn* 1998;**40**:247–51.

281. Bel EH, Timmers MC, Hermans J, Dijkman JH, Sterk PJ. The long-term effects of nedocromil sodium and beclomethasone dipropionate on bronchial responsiveness to methacholine in nonatopic asthmatic subjects. *Am Rev Respir Dis* 1990;**141**:21–8.

282. Diaz P, Galleguillos FR, Gonzalez MC, Pantin CF, Kay AB. Bronchoalveolar lavage in asthma: the effect of disodium cromoglycate (cromolyn) on leukocyte counts immunoglobulins, and complement. *J Allergy Clin Immunol* 1984;**74**:41–8.

283. Devalia JL, Rusznak C, Abdelaziz MM, Davies RJ. Nedocromil sodium and airway inflammation in vivo and in vitro. *J Allergy Clin Immunol* 1996;**98**:S51–7.

284. Stelmach I, Jerzynska J, Brzozowska A, Kuna P. Double-blind, randomized, placebo-controlled trial of effect of nedocromil sodium on clinical and inflammatory parameters of asthma in children allergic to dust mite. *Allergy* 2001; **56**:518–24.

285. Corin RE. Nedocromil sodium: a review of the evidence for a dual mechanism of action. *Clin Exp Allergy* 2000;**30**:461–8.

286. Carra S, Gagliardi L, Zanconato S, Scollo M, Azzolin N, Zacchello F, Baraldi E. Budesonide but not nedocromil sodium reduces exhaled nitric oxide levels in asthmatic children. *Respir Med* 2001;**95**:734–9.

287. Brogden N, Sorkin EM. Nedocromil sodium. An updated review on its pharmacological properties and therapeutic efficacy in asthma. *Drugs* 1993;**45**:693–715.

288. Walker SR, Evans ME, Richards AJ, Paterson JW. The fate of [^{14}C]disodium cromoglycate in man. *J Pharm Pharmacol* 1972;**24**:525–31.

289. Aswania OA, Corlett SA, Chrystyn H. Determination of the relative bioavailability of nedocromil sodium to the lung following inhalation using urinary excretion. *Eur J Clin Pharmacol* 1998;**54**:475–8.

290. Selcow J, Mendelson L, Rosen JP. Clinical benefits of cromolyn sodium aerosol (MDI) in the treatment of asthma in children. *Ann Allergy* 1989;**62**:195–9.

291. Eigen H, Reid JJ, Dahl R, *et al.* Evaluation of the addition of cromolyn sodium to bronchodilator maintenence therapy in the long-term management of asthma. *J Allergy Clin Immunol* 1987;**80**:612–21.

292. Tasche MJ, Ujen JH, Bernsen RM, van der Wouden JC. Inhaled disodium cromoglycate as maintenance therapy in children with asthma: a systematic review. *Thorax* 2000;**55**:913–20.

293. Armenio L, Baldini G, Bardare M, *et al.* Double blind, placebo-controlled study of nedocromil sodium in asthma. *Arch Dis Child* 1993;**68**:193–7.

294. Kelly KD, Spooner CH, Rowe BH. Nedocromil sodium versus sodium cromoglycate in treatment of exercise-induced bronchoconstriction: a systematic review. *Eur Respir J* 2001;**17**:39–45.

295. Tasche MJ, van der Wouden JC, Uijen JH, Ponsioen BP, Bernsen RM, van Suijlekom-Smit LW, de Jongste JC. Randomised placebo-controlled trial of inhaled sodium cromoglycate in 1–4-year-old children with moderate asthma. *Lancet* 1997; **350**:1060–4.

296. Bara AI, Barley EA. Caffeine for asthma. *Cochrane Database Syst Rev*. Oxford, Update Software, 2000.

297. Persson CGA, Pauwels R. Pharmacology of anti-asthma xanthines. In: CP Page, PJ Barnes, eds. *Pharmacology of Asthma*. Springer-Verlag, Berlin Heidelberg, 1991, pp. 207–25.

298. Ward AJM, McKenniff M, Evans JM, Page C, Costello J. Theophylline – an immunomodulatory role in asthma? *Am Rev Respir Dis* 1993;**147**:518–23.

299. Lahat N, Nir E, Horenstein L, Colin AA. Effect of theophylline on the proportion and function of T-suppressor cells in asthmatic children. *Allergy* 1985;**40**:453–7.

300. Shohat B, Volovitz B, Varsano I. Induction of suppressor T cells in asthmatic children by theophylline treatment. *Clin Allergy* 1983;**13**:487–93.

301. Mapp C, Boschetto P, Dal Vecchio L, Crescioli S, De Marzo N, Paleari D, Fabbri L. Protective effect of antiasthma drugs on late asthmatic reactions and increased airway responsiveness induces by toluene diisocyanate in sensitized subjects. *Am Rev Respir Dis* 1987;**136**:1403–7.

302. Fabbri L, Maestrelli P, Mapp S, Mapp C. Bronchial hyperreactivity: mechanisms and physiologic

evaluation. Airway inflammation during late asthmatic reactions induced by toluene diisocyanate. *Am Rev Respir Dis* 1991;**143**:37–8.

303. Cockroft D, Murdock KY, Gore BP, O'Byrne P, Manning P. Theophylline does not inhibit allergen-induced increase in airway responsiveness to metacholine. *J Allergy Clin Immunol* 1989;**83**:913–20.

304. Dutoid J, Salome CM, Woolcock A. Inhaled corticosteroids reduce the severity of bronchial hyperresponsiveness in asthma but oral theophyllin does not. *Am Rev Respir Dis* 1987; **136**:1174–8.

305. Sullivan P, Bekir S, Jaffar Z, Page C, Jeffery P, Costello J. Anti-inflammatory effects of low-dose oral theophylline in atopic asthma. *Lancet* 1994; **343**:1006–8.

306. Magnussen H, Reuss G, Jörres R. Methylxanthines inhibit exercise-induced bronchoconstriction at low serum theophylline concentration and in a dose-dependent fashion. *J Allergy Clin Immunol* 1988; **81**:531–7.

307. Phillips MJ, *et al*. The effect of slow-release aminophylline on exercise – induced asthma. *Brit J Dis Chest* 1981;**75**:181–9.

308. Mitenko PA, Ogilvie RI. Rational intravenous doses of theophylline. *New Engl J Med* 1973;**289**:600–3.

309. Bierman C, Pierson W, Shapiro G, Furukawa CT. Is a uniform round-the-clock theophylline blood level necessary for optimal asthma therapy in the adolescent patient? *Am J Med* **85**:17–20.

310. Pedersen S. Treatment of nocturnal asthma in children with a single dose of sustained release theophylline taken after supper. *Clin Allergy* 1985;**15**:79–85.

311. Hendeles L, Iafrate R, Weinberger M. A clinical and pharmacokinetic basis for the selection and use of slow release theophylline products. *Clin Pharmacokinet* 1984;**9**:95–135.

312. Pedersen S. Effects of food on the absorption of theophylline in children. *J Allergy Clin Immunol* 1986;**78**:704–9.

313. Pedersen S, Steffensen G. Absorption characteristics of a once-a-day slow release theophylline preparation in children with asthma. *J Pediatr* 1987;**110**:953–9.

314. Wilson N, Silverman M. Controlled trial of slow release aminophylline in childhood asthma: are shortterm trials valid? *Br Med J* 1982;**284**:863–6.

315. Ishizaki T, Minegishi A, Morishita M, Odajima Y, Kanagawa S, Nagai T, Yamaguchi M. Plasma catecholamine concentrations during a 72-hours aminophylline infusion in children with acute asthma. *J Allergy Clin Immunol* 1988;**82**:146–54.

316. Littenberg B. Aminophyllin treatment in severe, acute asthma. *JAMA* 1988;**259**:1678–84.

317. Mitra A, Bassler D, Ducharme FM. Intravenous aminophylline for acute severe asthma in children

over 2 years using inhaled bronchodilators (*Cochrane Review*). Cochrane Database. Update Software, Oxford, 2001.

318. Barker D. Theophylline toxicity in children. *J Pediatr* 1986;**109**:538–42.

319. Hendeles L, Weinberger M, Szefler S, Ellis E. Safety and efficacy of theophylline in children with asthma. *J Pediatr* 1992;**120**:177–83.

320. Tsiu SJ, Self TH, Burns R. Theophylline toxicity: update. *Ann Allergy* 1990;**64**:241–57.

321. Ellis EF. Theophylline toxicity. *J Allergy Clin Immunol* 1985;**76**:297–301.

322. Furukawa CT, Duhamel T, Weimer L, Shapiro CG, Pierson W, Bierman W. Cognitive and behavioural findings in children taking theophylline. *J Allergy Clin Immunol* 1988;**81**:83–5.

323. Lindgren S, Lokshin B, Stromquist A, Weinberger M, Nassif E, McCubbin M, Frasher R. Does asthma or treatment with theophylline limit children's academic performance? *New Engl J Med* 1992; **327**:926–30.

324. Gross NJ, Skorodin MS. Anticholinergic, antimuscarinic bronchodilators. *Am Rev Respir Dis* 1984;**129**:853–70.

325. Boner A, Vallone G, De Stefano G. Effect of inhaled ipratropium bromide on methacholine and exercise provocation in asthmatic children. *Pediatr Pulmonol* 1989;**6**:81–5.

326. Wilson N, Barnes PJ, Vickers H, Silverman M. Hyperventilation-induced asthma: evidence for two mechanisms. *Thorax* 1982;**37**:657–62.

327. Heaton RW, Henderson AF, Gray BJ, Costello J. The bronchial response to cold air challenge: evidence for different mechanisms in normal and asthmatic subjects. *Thorax* 1983;**38**:506–11.

328. Determination of dose–response relationship for nebulised ipratropium bromide in asthmatic children. *J Pediatr* 1984;**105**:1002–5.

329. Wilkie RA, Bryan MH. Effect of bronchodilators on airway resistance in ventilator-dependent neonates with chronic lung disease. *J Pediatr* 1984;**11**:278–82.

330. Greenough A, Yuksel B, Everett L, Price J. Inhaled ipratropium bromide and terbutaline in asthmatic children. *Respir Med* 1993;**87**:111–14.

331. Prendiville A, Green S, Silverman M. Ipratropium bromide and airways function in wheezy infants. *Arch Dis Child* 1987;**62**:397–400.

332. Everard ML, Bara A, Kurian M. Anti-cholinergic drugs for wheeze in children under the age of two years. *Cochrane Database Syst Rev* CD001279, 2000.

333. Watson WT, Becker AB, Simons FE. Comparison of ipratropium solution, fenoterol solution and their combination administered by nebuliser and face mask to children with acute asthma. *J Allergy Clin Immunol* 1988;**82**:1012–18.

334. Beck R, Robertson C, Galdes-Sebaldt M, Levison H. Combined salbutamol and ipratropium bromide by

inhalation in the treatment of severe acute asthma. *J Pediatr* 1985;**107**:605–8.

335. Phanichyakarn P, Kraisarin C, Sasisakulporn C. Comparison of inhaled terbutaline and inhaled terbutaline plus ipratropium bromide in acute asthmatic children. *Asian Pac J Allergy Immunol* 1990;**8**:45–58.

336. Plotnick LH, Ducharme FM. Should inhaled anticholinergics be added to beta₂ agonists for treating acute childhood and adolescent asthma? A systematic review. *Br Med J* 1998;**317**:971–7.

337. Aaron SD. The use of ipratropium bromide for the management of acute exacerbation in adults and children: a systematic review. *J Asthma* 2001; **38**:521–30.

338. Osmond MH, Klassen TP. Efficacy of ipratropium bromide in acute childhood asthma: a meta-analysis. *Acad Emerg Med* 1995;**2**:651–6.

339. Beasley CR, Rafferty P, Holgate S. Bronchoconstrictor properties of preservatives in ipratropium bromide (Atrovent) nebuliser solution. *Br Med J* 1987; **294**:1197–8.

340. Mann JS, Howarth PH, Holgate S. Bronchoconstriction induced by ipratropium bromide in asthma: relation to hypotonicity. *Br Med J* 1984;**289**:469.

341. Holgate ST, Finnerty JP. Antihistamines in asthma. *J Allergy Clin Immunol* 1989;**83**:537–47.

342. Finnerty JP, Holgate ST. The contribution of histamine release and vagal reflexes alone and in combination to exercise-induced asthma. *Eur Respir J* 1993;**6**:1132–7.

343. Warner JO. A double-blinded, randomized, placebo-controlled trial of cetirizine in preventing the onset of asthma in children with atopic dermatitis: 18 months' treatment and 18 months' post-treatment follow-up. *J Allergy Clin Immunol* 2001;**108**:929–37.

344. Tamura G, Meu S, Takishima T. Protective effect of ketotifen on allergen-induced bronchoconstriction and skin weal. *Clin Allergy* 1989;**16**:535–41.

345. Brodde O, Brinkmann M, Schemuth R, O'Hara N, Daul A. Terbutaline induced desensitization of human lymphocyte b₂ adrenoceptors. *J Clin Invest* 1985;**76**:1096–101.

346. Reinhardt D, Ludwig J, Braun D, Kusenback G, Griese M. Effects of the antiallergic drug ketotifen on bronchial resistance and beta-adrenoceptor density of lymphocytes in children with exercise-induced asthma. *Dev Pharmacol Ther* 1988;**11**:180–8.

347. Brodde O, Howe U, Egerszegi S, Konietzko N, Michel MC. Effect of prednisolone and ketotifen on β₂-adrenoceptors in asthmatic patients receiving β₂-bronchodilators. *Eur J Clin Pharmacol* 1988; **34**:145–50.

348. Graff-Lonnevig V, Hedlin G. The effect of ketotifen on bronchial hyperreactivity in childhood asthma. *J Allergy Clin Immunol* 1985;**76**:59–63.

349. Kennedy JD, Hashan R, Clay MJD, Jones RS. Comparison of the action of disodium cromoglycate and ketotifen on exercise-induced bronchoconstriction in childhood asthma. *Br Med J* 1980;**2**:1458–60.

350. Lilja G, Graff-Lonnevig V, Bevegard S. Comparison of the protective effect of ketotifen and disodium cromoglycate on exercise-induced asthma in asthmatic boys. *Allergy* 1993;**38**:31–5.

351. El-Hefny A. Treatment of wheezy infants and children with ketotifen. *Pharmacotherapeutica* 1983;**3**:388–92.

352. El-Hefny A, El Beshlawy A, Nour S, Said M. Ketotifen in the treatment of infants and young children with wheezy bronchitis and bronchial asthma. *J Int Med Res* 1986;**14**:267–73.

353. Broberger U, Graff-Lonnevig V, Lilja G, Rylander E. Ketotifen in pollen-induced asthma: a double-blind placebo-controlled study. *Clin Allergy* 1986; **16**:119–27.

354. Rackham A, Brown CA, Chandra RK, *et al*. A Candadian multicenter study with Zaditen (ketotifen) in the treatment of bronchial asthma in children aged 5 to 17 years. *J Allergy Clin Immunol* 1989;**84**:286–96.

355. Mylona-Karayanni C, Hadziargurou D, *et al*. Effect of ketotifen on childhood asthma: a double blind study. *J Asthma* 1990;**27**:87–93.

356. Tinkelman DG, Webb CS, Vanderpol GE, *et al*. The use of ketotifen in the prophylaxis of season allergic asthma. *Ann Allergy* 1986;**56**:213–17.

357. White MP, MacDonald TH, Garg RA. Ketotifen in the young asthmatic – a double blind placebo-controlled trial. *J Int Med Res* 1988;**16**:107–13.

358. Loftus BG, Price JF. Long-term, placebo-controlled, trial of ketotifen in the management of preschool children with asthma. *J All Clin Immunol* 1987; **79**:350–5.

359. Volovitz B, Vasano I, Cumella JC, Jaber L. Efficacy and safety of ketotifen in young children with asthma. *J Allergy Clin Immunol* 1988; **81**:526–30.

360. Van Asperen PP, McKay KO, Mellis CM, *et al*. A multicentre randomized placebo-controlled double-blind study on the efficacy of ketotifen in infants with chronic cough or wheeze. *J Pediatr Child Health* 1992;**28**:442–6.

361. Vasano L, Volovitz B, Soferman R, *et al*. Multicenter study with ketotifen (Zatiden) oral drop solution in the treatment of wheezy children aged 6 months to 3 years. *Pediatr Allergy Immunol* 1993;**4**:45–50.

362. Neijens HJ, Knol K. Oral prophylactic treatment in wheezy infants. *Immunol Allergy Pract* 1988; **10**:17–23.

363. Stratton D, Carswell F, Hughes AO, Fysh WJ, Robinson P. Double-blind comparisons of slow release theophylline, ketotifen and placebo for

prophylaxis of asthma in young children. *Br J Dis Chest* 1984;**78**:163–7.

364. Iikura Y, Naspitz CK, Mihura H, *et al*. Prevention of asthma by ketotifen in infants with atopic dermatitis. *Ann Allergy* 1992;**68**:233–6.

365. Shiner RJ, Nunn AJ, Chung KF, Geddes DM. Randomized double blind placebo-controlled trial methotrexate in steroid-dependent asthma. *Lancet* 1990;**336**:137–40.

366. Nierop G, Gijzel WP, Bel EH, Zwinderman AH, Dijkman JH. Auranifin in the treatment of steroid dependent asthma: a double blind study. *Thorax* 1992;**47**:349–54.

367. Alexander AG, Barnes NC, Kay AB. Trial of cyclosporin in corticosteroid-dependent asthma. *Lancet* 1992;**339**:324–8.

368. Coren ME, Rosenthal M, Bush A. The use of cyclosporin in corticosteroid dependent asthma. *Arch Dis Child* 1997;**77**:522–3.

369. Snell NJC. Drug interactions with anti-asthma medication. *Respir Med* 1994;**88**:83–8.

370. Jaffe A, Bush A. Anti-inflammatory effects of macrolides in lung disease. *Ped Pulmonol* 2001; **31**:464–73.

371. Soler M, Matz J, Townley R, Buhl R, O'Brien J, Fox H, Thirlwell J, Gupta N, Della Cioppa G. The anti-IgE antibody omalizumab reduces exacerbations and steroid requirement in allergic asthmatics. *Eur Respir J* 2001;**18**:254–61.

372. Busse W, Corren J, Lanier BQ, McAlary M, Fowler-Taylor A, Cioppa GD, van As A, Gupta N. Omalizumab, anti-IgE recombinant humanized monoclonal antibody, for the treatment of severe allergic asthma. *J Allergy Clin Immunol* 2001; **108**:184–90.

373. Milgrom H, Berger W, Nayak A, Gupta N, Pollard S, McAlary M, Taylor AF, Rohane P. Treatment of childhood asthma with anti-immunoglobulin antibody (omalizumab). *Pediatrics* 2001;**108**:E36.

374. Howell S, Roussos C. Isoproterenol and aminophylline improve contractility of fatigued canine diaphragm. *Am Rev Respir Dis* 1984; **129**:118–24.

375. Hedner J, Hedner T, Wessberg P, *et al*. Central respiratory effects of adenosine analogues, theophylline and enprofylline. In: KE Andersson, CGA Persson, eds. *Anti-asthma Xanthines and Adenosine*. Exerpta Medica, Amsterdam, 1985, pp. 467–71.

376. Barnes PJ, Pauwels RA. Theophylline in the management of asthma: time for reappraisal? *Eur Respir J* 1994;**7**:579–91.

377. Kidney J, Dominguez M, Taylor PM, Rose M, Chung KF, Barnes PJ. Immunomodulation by theophylline in asthma. Demonstration by withdrawal of therapy. *Am J Respir Crit Care Med* 1995;**151**:1907–14.

378. Leckie MJ, Ten BA, Khan J, *et al*. Effects of an interleukin-5 blocking monoclonal antibody on eosinophils, airway hyperresponsiveness, and the late asthmatic response. *Lancet* 2000;**356**:2144–8.

379. Borish LC, Nelson HS, Corren J, *et al*. Efficacy of soluble IL-4 receptor for the treatment of adults with asthma. *J Allergy Clin Immunol* 2001; **107**:963–70.

380. Supplement: Targeting IgE in treatment of asthma. *Am J Respir Crit Care Med* 2001;**164**(8) Pt 2.

381. Stirling RG, Chung KF. New immunological approaches and cytokine targets in asthma and allergy. *Eur Respir J* 2000;**16**:1158–74.

382. Pang L. COX-2 expression in asthmatic airways: the story so far. *Thorax* 2001;**56**:335–6.

383. Anderson GP. Formoterol: pharmacology, molecular basis of agonism, and mechanism of long duration of a highly potent and selective beta 2-adrenoceptor agonist bronchodilator. *Life Sci* 1993;**52**:2145–60.

384. Barnes PJ, Pedersen S. Efficacy and safety of inhaled corticosteroids in asthma. *Am Rev Dis* 1993; **148**:1–26.

385. Laitinen LA, Laitinen A, Haahtela T. A comparative study of the effects of an inhaled corticosteroid, budesonide, and of a beta-2-agonist, terbutaline, on airway inflammation in newly diagnosed asthma. *J Allergy Clin Immunol* 1992;**90**:32–42.

386. Sampson AP. Leukotriene generation. *Clin Exp Allergy Rev* 2001;**1**:196–201.

387. Hay DW, Torphy TJ, Undem BJ. Cysteinyl leukotrienes in asthma: old mediators up to new tricks. *Trends Pharmacol Sci* 1995;**16**:304–9.

388. Holgate ST. Allergic disorders. *Brit Med J* 2000;**320**:231–4.

389. Frossard N, Barnes PJ (eds). Mediators of asthma: new opportunities for treatment. *Eur. Resp. Rev.* 2000;**10(73)**.

Aerosols and other devices

SØREN PEDERSEN AND CHRIS O'CALLAGHAN

INTRODUCTION

When inhaled therapy is used the therapeutic dose is small compared with other routes of administration and consequently the incidence of side effects is normally lower. This is of special importance in the case of treatment with corticosteroids when long-term systemic administration is associated with serious systemic side effects whereas effective inhaled therapy is normally quite safe (Chapter 8a). Compared with oral administration, the delivery of a drug directly to the airways by inhalation has a more rapid onset of action, which is advantageous when bronchodilators are used to treat acute attacks of bronchoconstriction. Furthermore, inhalation of a β_2-agonist offers highly effective protection against exercise-induced asthma, whereas oral administration of high doses of the same drug has no or only a marginal protective effect against this condition. Finally, some agents such as sodium cromoglycate (SCG) and nedocromil are effective only when given by inhalation. For these reasons inhaled therapy has now become accepted as the mainstay of treatment of childhood asthma.

The effect of inhaled therapy seems to depend upon the amount of aerosol reaching the bronchial tree and perhaps also upon its distribution within the airways. However, the distribution of receptor sites in the bronchi is not known in detail and there may be differences between various groups of drugs. Therefore the optimal distribution of aerosol particles within the bronchial tree has not yet been decided. Some studies suggest that a rapid redistribution of drug in the airways may take place after the initial deposition. If this is the case the distribution pattern may not be so important.

Four different inhalation systems constitute the cornerstones of inhalation therapy in children with asthma:

1 conventional metered dose inhalers (MDI);
2 MDI with a spacer attached, with or without a face-mask;
3 dry powder inhalers (DPI);
4 nebulizers (with mouthpiece or face-mask).

They differ with respect to construction, aerosol cloud generation, optimal inhalation technique and ease of use. This may be confusing for paediatricians prescribing inhalation therapy to children and over the years many investigators have reported high frequencies of incorrect inhaler use as a direct cause of treatment failure in asthmatic children. Accurate knowledge about the nature and magnitude of the problems children experience with inhalation therapy and the age groups that can normally use the various inhalation devices correctly is a precondition for effective asthma treatment. Therefore, the principles and construction of the most widely used inhalers and their advantages, disadvantages and limitations will be discussed in some detail with special attention to some of the more important issues:

• Efficiency: which inhaler most consistently delivers the highest fraction of delivered dose to the intrapulmonary airways in each age group during optimal use?
• Acceptability: which inhaler is the most simple to use for each age group?

- Safety: which inhaler has the best clinical effect for a given systemic effect in day-to-day use?

The topic of aerosol therapy in childhood has recently been reviewed.[1,2]

METHODS OF INHALER ASSESSMENT

When information on an inhaler is assessed it is important to consider how the information was derived since inhalers can be evaluated in many different ways.[2]

In vitro measurements

The quality of the generated aerosol is assessed by *in vitro* measurement of the metered dose, the dose retained in the inhaler, the delivered dose and the size distribution of the particles in the aerosol cloud. Particle size and distribution may be measured by a laser diffraction device or by entrapment in a multi-stage impactor. It is important to realize that the dose reaching the intrapulmonary airways is normally substantially lower than both the metered and the delivered dose.

Radioactive deposition studies

Under standardized conditions these measure the deposition pattern of radioactive labelled particles of drug. Most deposition studies use particles with aerodynamic properties as similar to those of drug particles as possible, labelled with radionuclides such as ^{99m}Tc because direct labelling of drugs with γ-emitting radionuclides is difficult. This renders direct correlation between effect and pulmonary deposition difficult. Furthermore, it may also be hard to predict the actual amount of drug delivered to the bronchi because the amount depends not only upon the number but also upon the size of the particles deposited, the dose of drug in a 3 μm particle being nine times higher than that contained in three 1 μm particles. Ipratropium bromide is the only drug with which actual drug labelling has been achieved with ^{77}Br. However, even in this case the active drug and the radioactive label may dissociate in the lungs, which complicates the interpretation of the results.

In recent studies the radiolabel ^{99m}Tc was not chemically bound to the active drug but only acted as a marker for the active drug component in the formulation; thus the label was *associated* to the active drug. This makes it critical that the particle size patterns are the same for the active drug and the radiolabel. Finally, the active drug can be labelled by coprecipitation with ^{99m}Tc, resulting in a mixture of unlabelled and labelled active drug and free radioactive particles. Also with this technique, it is important to ensure that the particle size patterns are the same for the active drug and the radiolabel.

The various labelling techniques may give somewhat different results and clinical conclusions based upon comparisons of results obtained with different techniques should not be made.

Pharmacokinetic studies[3–5]

These assess deposition pattern and the local/systemic effect ratio of the drug. This is achieved by measuring the systemic availability of drug after oral and intravenous administration and after inhalation when the gastrointestinal absorption is blocked, for example by charcoal. When this is blocked, the systemic bioavailability depends exclusively on intact drug absorbed via the lungs. If the drug is not metabolized locally in the lung and the systemic absorption of drug from the airways is 100% then the systemic bioavailability will equal pulmonary deposition. Normally there is a reasonable correlation between the findings in pharmacokinetic studies and the results obtained in deposition studies.

Filter studies[6–8]

The amount of drug delivered to the patient can be measured during inhalation by inserting a filter, which will collect all drug particles larger than the pore size between the inhaler orifice and the mouth of the patient. When the particle size distribution of the aerosol cloud is known, estimates of the amount of drug in respirable particles can be made. As for the other methods, clinical conclusions based upon the results of filter studies should be made with caution.

Clinical effect studies

Laboratory studies, performed under standardized conditions, measure the bronchodilator response or protective effect against various challenges and sometimes systemic effects, often after a single dose of the drug. *Clinical trials* of the day-to-day treatment of patients measure the clinical effect, systemic side effects and ease of inhaler use.

The various methods are complementary since they provide somewhat different information. At present, we do not know the clinical implications of the small but statistically significant differences between devices obtained under standardized laboratory conditions. These may not always reflect the clinical results achieved by patients on a daily basis (effectiveness) when ease of use may be more important in encouraging compliance with therapy.

At present few radioactive label studies or pharmacokinetic studies and filter studies have been performed in children. Due to differences in airway calibre and the anatomy of the upper airways between children and adults, the inspiratory air flow dynamics of children may be quite different from that of adults; therefore conclusions from adult deposition studies should not merely be extrapolated to children. Furthermore, results obtained in school-children may not be valid in infants or very young children. These reservations should be remembered when the various inhalers are discussed. Furthermore, few studies evaluate repeatability of the technique. Often marked variations are seen between patients but little is known about the variation in the individual patient, which may be clinically very important.

PHARMACODYNAMICS

When the effects of various inhalation techniques or inhaler devices are evaluated it is important to consider the quantitative relationships between the dose and the effect of the drug used. There is no single characteristic relationship between drug effect and drug dosage, but in most cases a sigmoid dose–response curve is obtained when the measured effect is plotted against the logarithm of the dose. This means that differences between treatments or inhaler devices are more likely to become apparent when doses of drug are used that ensure the patient is at the beginning of the more or less linear, central portion of the dose–effect curve (Figure 8b.1). If the dose is too high and the clinical response reaches the 'plateau' phase, important differences may be missed. Furthermore, differences between small quantities of drug are more readily detected if the dose–response curve is rather steep. Differences in effect between various inhalers can be compensated for by increasing the dose. However, this is not feasible when inhaled corticosteroids are used because higher doses are more likely to cause unwanted side effects as no inhaler delivers all the drug to the intrapulmonary airways.

General aspects of particle deposition (Figure 8b.2)

The larger the particles of an aerosol and the higher the velocity, the greater the central deposition in the oropharynx, larynx and large conducting airways in adult patients. The optimal size of a particle to reach the periphery of the tracheobronchial tree in children is not known, but in general intrapulmonary deposition of an aerosol in adults is greatest for particles between 2 and 5 μm in diameter. Most particles greater than 8 μm in diameter will impact above the level of the larynx in adults. Particles less than 1 μm in diameter may not be deposited at all. The importance of particle size on the effectiveness of inhaled therapy has been confirmed in some adult studies.

Some therapeutic aerosols are hygroscopic, which means that the inhaled particles may absorb water within the humid environment of the respiratory tract, subsequently enlarging in size, so that their aerodynamic behaviour is difficult to predict. The clinical relevance of this is not known. Studies with terbutaline, which is hygroscopic, and budesonide, which is not, found that total and regional lung deposition was similar for the two drugs, suggesting that it is not important for the deposition pattern.[2]

The four most widely used inhaler systems will be discussed below. Apart from deposition studies, only studies performed in children will be mentioned. No two inhalers are alike. Therefore, conclusions from one inhaler should not be applied to other inhalers of the same class or a different class of inhalers. The terminology of aerosols is important and definitions are provided in Table 8b.1.

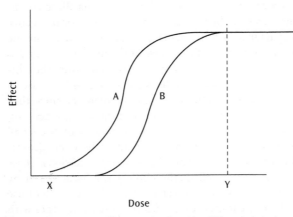

Figure 8b.1 *Dose–effect curves for two different inhalers. Inhaler **A** is more effective than **B**. This difference in effect will only become apparent if doses in the range X–Y are studied. At higher doses, the inhalers seem equally effective because both inhalers have produced maximum effect.*

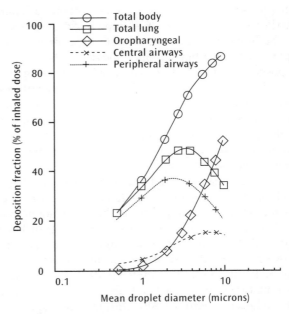

Figure 8b.2 *Effect of particle size on deposition in the airway. (From ref. 98.)*

Table 8b.1 *Aerosols: some definitions (from ref. 2)*

An aerosol: a two phase system made up of a gaseous continuous phase, usually air, and a discontinuous phase of individual liquid or solid particles.

Mass median diameter (MMD): the diameter of a particle such that half the mass of the aerosol is contained in smaller diameter particles, and half in larger.

Mass median aerodynamic diameter (MMAD): the diameter of a sphere of unit density that has the same aerodynamic properties as a particle of median mass from the aerosol.

Geometric standard deviation (GSD): a dimensionless number which gives an indication of the spread of sizes of particles that make up the aerosol. An aerosol with a GSD of 1 is made up of particles of uniform size.

Heterodisperse aerosol: the aerosol is made up of particles of many different sizes. The GSD is >1.2.

Monodisperse aerosol: the aerosol particles are uniform size (or very nearly uniform). The GSD is <1.2.

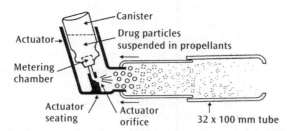

Figure 8b.3 *Metered dose inhaler with a spacer attached. A variety of spacer designs exist. Their main function is to remove large particles and to ensure that the aerosol particles have a lower velocity when they reach the patient.*

PRESSURIZED METERED DOSE INHALERS (pMDIs)

In pMDIs the active drug is dispersed as fine powder particles throughout the propellant kept at a high pressure (about 400 kPa) in an aluminium canister (Figure 8b.3). The particles are very small (MMAD about 3 μm), have a high surface energy and therefore tend to agglomerate. This tendency is reduced by the addition of a surfactant which normally consists of a non-volatile liquid which is soluble in the propellant.[9,10]

The patient actuates a dose from the aerosol by pressing down the canister in the actuator seating. This releases a metered volume of drug, propellants and surfactant through the actuator orifice into the air (Figure 8b.3). The dose is released in less than 0.1s. Just after the release the droplets are rather large (MMAD about 40 μm) and have a high velocity of about 30 m/s. As they travel through the air they are markedly decelerated by the air resistance and their size is reduced due to evaporation of the propellants (velocity about 12 m/s and MMAD about 12 μm 10 m from the actuator orifice). Thus, up to a certain point, the further the droplets travel the lower is their velocity and the smaller their size.[10]

Pressurized aerosols contain multiple doses of the drug and do not have to be reloaded before each inhalation. The canister should be shaken before treatment to ensure proper filling of the metering chamber with a homogenous mixture of the content. If the aerosol is cold due to storage in a refrigerator or in a school bag during winter the dose emitted may decrease as the vapour pressure of the propellants becomes too low to produce an adequate dose and to generate sufficiently small drug particles.

CFC free metered dose inhalers

Chlorofluorocarbons (CFCs) have been shown to damage the earth's ozone layer[11] and their use will become illegal for most purposes over the next few years.[12] Pharmaceutical manufacturers have redesigned their metered dose inhalers using new hydrofluoroalkalane (HFA) propellants. Various formulations have now been released including a non-CFC formulation of salbutamol, beclomethasone dipropionate and fluticasone.

Some of the new drugs have been formulated to have equivalent particle size and drug output to their CFC containing precursors. It cannot be assumed that CFC and the replacement HFA inhalers are equivalent in all situations. For example, the delivered dose of a new HFA salbutamol inhaler from spacer devices is markedly different to the existing CFC formulations.[13] CFC free beclomethasone (3M and Baker Norton) emits drug in very much smaller particles (approximately one micron in size) than the CFC preparation. This results in a much greater lung deposition of a given dose and systemic bioavailability. In the case of beclomethasone dipropionate marketed by 3M, the dose of drug prescribed should be half of that of a conventional metered dose inhaler of this drug.

It is important that the results obtained in adult studies are not extrapolated to young children, particularly those under the age of 5 years where small particles may bypass the nose in significant quantities enhancing lung delivery and subsequent systemic absorption.

The dose released by new CFC free metered dose inhalers tends to be unaffected by storage orientation at ambient temperature and the reproducibility[14] has been improved on the non-CFC metered dose inhaler.[15] The aerosol produced from some HFA formulations is less dense and warmer than that from CFC containing metered dose inhalers. Patients should be reassured that this does not mean the inhaler is not working appropriately.

Inhalation technique

The results from various depositon studies with metered dose inhalers vary, but generally about 80% of the dose from a conventional pMDI lodges in the oropharynx. Of the remaining 20%, 10% is retained in the inhaler and 10% is deposited in the intrapulmonary airways.[2,10] There may be some differences between the various pMDI brands. The mode of inhalation influences the pulmonary deposition of particles from a pMDI. Very slow inhalations (about 30 l/min) followed by a breath-holding pause of 10s after the inhalation have been found to enhance pulmonary deposition as compared with fast inhalations (about 90 l/min) with and without a breath-holding pause.[3,10] Actuating the aerosol 4 cm from the wide open mouth has been suggested to increase pulmonary deposition when compared with actuations with the lips closed around the mouthpiece of the inhaler; however, the results from studies evaluating this have been inconsistent.[10]

Other laboratory studies

The MDI has served as a gold standard for comparison with other inhalers and some of the laboratory studies performed with this device will be discussed in the sections about the other inhalers.

Dose–response studies and single dose studies in school-children have found that a terbutaline pMDI has the same or a lower effect than a pMDI and large volume spacer when both devices are used correctly.[16] Furthermore, a pharmacokinetic study suggested that the intrabronchial deposition of budesonide was somewhat lower after inhalation from a pMDI than after inhalation from a pMDI and large volume spacer. The total area under the serum drug concentration vs time curve (reflecting the bioavailability) was the same for the two devices because the pMDI was associated with a higher gastrointestinal absorption of drug. So even if the spacer produced higher lung deposition the systemic effects of the two inhalers were the same.[5] This indicates that the clinical/systemic effect ratio is lower for budesonide pMDI than for the pMDI and large volume spacer. Similar comparisons have not been performed in children between pMDIs and other devices.

Clinical studies – ease of use

Virtually all children's difficulties with the MDI are related to the high velocity of the aerosol particles (3 m/s) leaving the orifice: problems with coordination of actuation and inhalation, stopping inhalation when the cold aerosol particles reach the soft palate (cold Freon effect), actuation of the aerosol into the mouth followed by inhalation through the nose, and rapid inhalation.[10,17] All these mistakes are associated with a reduced clinical effect. As a consequence more than 50% of children receiving inhalation therapy with a pMDI alone gain less clinical benefit from the prescribed medication[17] when compared with pMDI and spacer or dry powder inhalers.

Therefore, all prescriptions of a pMDI should be accompanied by repeated, thorough tuition of correct inhaler use followed by a demonstration of inhalation technique by the child. Conventional pMDIs cannot normally be recommended for children if alternative devices are available.

When is a pressurized metered dose inhaler empty?

There is currently no way, apart from counting individual actuations, to know when a metered dose inhaler is empty. Counters for metered dose inhalers should be a standard requirement. It has been claimed that the pMDIs float on water when they have delivered their licensed number of doses and it has been suggested that they should be replaced at this time.[18] Ogren clearly demonstrated that this is a very misleading technique.[19]

Breath actuated metered dose inhalers

Breath activated pMDIs incorporate a mechanism that, when activated during inhalation, triggers the metered dose inhaler to fire. In theory, this should reduce tuition time and the need for the patient or parent to coordinate metered dose inhaler actuation with inhalation. Young patients may stop breathing due to the cold Freon effect when the metered dose inhaler is actuated or have a suboptimal inspiration.[20] Use of these devices for the delivery of salbutamol should be restricted to children older than 6–7 years and adults. Here, children can be taught a correct inhalation technique with breath actuated inhalers within 2–3 minutes and then use them during episodes of acute wheeze,[21–23] when they are very effective, or before physical exercise.

Evaluation of their efficacy in children under 5 years of age is limited to eight children in one study.[24] The selection of this group was biased as all children included had to be able to perform reliable peak flows. Only half of the children studied had evidence of bronchodilation following inhalation of β_2-agonist and one child was not able to trigger the device. We are unaware of any trials that have been performed on the use of inhaled steroids from these devices in children or adults. Oral deposition using these devices is still very high, and will be minimized by the use of the conventional metered dose inhaler and spacer instead.

Breath activated pMDIs may be used with a short open tube spacer (Optimizer). Although this may be expected to reduce extra thoracic drug deposition, there are no published evaluations of this.

Intelligent metered dose inhalers such as the Smartmist (Aradigm Corp, California, USA) have been developed to deliver a drug bolus at a pre-programmed point during inhalation, defined by both flow and volume. Although they can also store data on patient use and lung function, costs currently limit their use.[25]

Metered dose inhalers with extended mouthpieces

The Spacehaler (Evans Medical Limited, Leatherhead, UK) has an actuator that is designed to reduce the velocity of the aerosol cloud emerging from the inhaler. This should reduce the impaction of the aerosol in the oropharynx and thus the amount of non-respirable drug delivered to the patient.[26] Although the device appears to be as effective in the delivery of salbutamol to adults as a metered dose inhaler given via a large volume spacer, there are no published studies of this device used by children or for the delivery of steroids.[27]

An open tube spacer known as the Syncroner (Fisons PLC, Loughbrough), is 10 cm long and, if inhalation is not coordinated with actuation of the metered dose inhaler, an aerosol cloud can be seen to escape from the open top of the spacer. It is thought this provides visual feedback for the patient of their poor technique and it was designed primarily as a training aid. In an adult lung deposition study, it has been shown to reduce oropharyngeal deposition of sodium cromoglycate compared to the metered dose inhaler.[28] However, the Syncroner does not function as a holding chamber and good coordination is essential for its use. This precludes its use in young children.

SPACERS

Various devices may be attached to the mouthpiece of a conventional pressurized aerosol to ensure that the aerosol particles have a slower velocity and a small particle size due to evaporation of the propellant within the device, before they reach the patient. This is a theoretical advantage.

The popularity of spacer devices is reflected by their recommended use in Table 8b.2. However, there is a plethora of different spacers available and the emitted dose from different spacers may vary up to 400%, depending on the spacer, the drug, the tidal volume of the patient and their technique. [29]

There are two main types of spacer devices, holding chambers and extension devices.

Extension devices

Such devices increase the distance the aerosolized drug has to travel before the patient inhales. They allow the aerosol to slow and propellants to evaporate and large particles to be trapped within the spacer. Such spacers do not have a one-way valve and coordination is still required for optimal drug delivery. These devices are, therefore, not suitable for young children and may be inappropriate for the many patients of any age who have difficulty in coordination. They should not be used in children under the age of 5 years.

Holding chambers

For the rest of this section, these will be referred to as spacers. They provide a reservoir of drug from which the patient breathes. Holding chambers have the properties of extension devices, but reduce the need for coordination between inhaler actuation and patient inhalation.

If the pressure drop required to open and close the valve is insufficient, the expiration may partly go through the spacer, expelling some of the aerosol, or air entrainment may occur through the side hole or through leaks between the lips and the mouthpiece or the face and the face-mask.[7] This will lead to a reduction in the inhaled dose. Furthermore, a substantial amount of drug may be lost through the valve when the aerosol is fired into a straight tube spacer if the valve is not tight.[8]

Inhalation technique

Slow inhalations improve the effect when a straight extension tube spacer is used in children, whereas breath-holding, tilting of the head during inhalation or inhalation from functional residual capacity instead of residual volume does not influence the effect.[10,30] Quiet tidal breathing results in an optimal effect when a large volume spacer is used.[31]

All spacers reduce the oropharyngeal deposition of drug substantially (by about 50%).[32] As a result the occurrence of oropharyngeal candidiasis is reduced when corticosteroids are used. The amount of drug retained in the inhaler is increased markedly by all spacers (most by the low volume spacers) and hence the dose to the patient is reduced. Yet the dose delivered to the intrapulmonary airways is often the same or higher than that from a pMDI,[9,32] though not all spacers have been thoroughly studied in this respect.

No more than one dose should be fired into the spacer at a time when a large volume spacer is used, otherwise the inhaled dose is reduced.[33] Actuation of more than one puff at a time into low volume spacers is also not recommended.[13]

Static charge

The output of respirable particles from a plastic spacer may be markedly improved by use of an antistatic lining in the spacer.[33]

Static charge accumulates on the walls of many plastic and polycarbonate spacers. These can very rapidly attract the charged particles produced when the metered dose inhaler is actuated. Highly charged spacers deliver less drug than those where the static charge has been reduced by an antistatic lining.[34] Washing polycarbonate spacers with a detergent negates the effect of static charge with some drugs.[35]

In order to overcome the problems with spacer static, a metal spacer (Nebuchamber) has been developed. This is a 280 ml stainless steel device and produces a larger output of both large and small particles than do other spacers. As there is no electrostatic attraction to the spacer walls, there is much less need for the patient to inhale immediately after metered dose inhaler actuation, because particles remain suspended for longer.[36]

Other laboratory studies

One study indicated that there may be important differences between the effect of various spacer devices. The Aerochamber produced less bronchodilation in school-children than the Inspirease or Aerosol Bag.[37] This agrees with the findings in another study measuring the dose of budesonide delivered to children younger than two years after inhalation from a large volume spacer (Nebuhaler) and two low volume spacers (Aerochamber and a Babyspacer).[8] The dose after Aerochamber treatment was significantly lower (about 40%) than the dose delivered from the other spacers. This indicates that the volume of the spacer is not the critical issue in these age groups. The reason for the finding seemed to be that children hyperventilated markedly when a tightly fitting face-mask was placed around their mouth and nose.[8] An in vitro study has found that only at low tidal volumes (around 25 ml) was a low volume spacer like the Aerochamber more efficient at drug delivery;[38] at tidal volumes (around 150 ml) drug delivery was more efficient from the Nebuhaler. Finally, an in vitro study of a circuit designed to administer a pMDI to mechanically ventilated neonates found that the Aerochamber deposited more drug on a filter than did the Aerovent spacer.[39]

Other studies in school-children have compared the pMDI with the Volumatic and the Siriraj spacer[40] or the pMDI and Aerochamber with a pMDI alone[41] and did not find any significant differences in effect between the spacers or between the spacers and the correctly used pMDI.

Assessed by filter studies, drug delivery to preschool children can be markedly improved by attaching a face-mask to the mouthpiece of a large volume spacer, presumably because the face-mask reduces the occurrence of air leakage between the mouthpiece and the lips during the inhalation.[7] The face-mask in this study created a tight seal with the face, but is not the one currently commerically used with this device. The inhalation technique of preschool children, with a large volume spacer and face-mask was not as good as the inhalation technique of older children. As a result, a 2-year-old child had to use a 50% higher dose than a 14-year-old child to get the same amount of drug on the filter.[7] Such age-dependent difference in delivered dose was not seen in children between one and seven years when a low volume spacer (Baby-spacer)

was used.[7] This finding calls for more in vivo studies in different age groups of children to assess the optimal spacer volume.

Infants who cry during administration receive a lower dose.[42,43] Using an antistatic spacer increases the dose and decreases variability.[44]

Clinical studies – ease of use

All spacers reduce the risk of the cold Freon effect and the occurrence of coordination problems. Therefore, spacers are easier to use than a pMDI[10] and some produce a better clinical effect, particularly if they have a valve system. Virtually all school-children can learn to use these devices and to use them effectively during attacks of acute bronchoconstriction when they are as effective as nebulizers.[45,46]

It is also possible to train most preschool children to use valved spacers with face-mask for prophylactic administration of all appropriate anti-asthma medication. Their clinical value has been demonstrated in many clinical trials in all age groups. At present a pMDI and spacer is probably the system of choice in preschool children.[47,48] Problems may occur with opening and closure of the valve of some spacers. This may be reduced by tilting the spacer inhaler upwards during inhalations so that the valve opens by gravity.[47]

Generally spacers have a very favourable clinical/systemic effect ratio, though this has only been studied in school-children not using a face-mask. Most young children breathe through their nose, which serves as an efficient filter of larger particles and may therefore cause considerably reduced drug deposition in the lung.[49,50] So nose breathing may reduce the clinical/systemic effect ratio since many drugs are well-absorbed from the nasal mucosa. However, a spacer retains the large particles, which contain the highest amount of drug, so the importance of nasal breathing may be less.

No formal clinical comparisons between the various spacers have been performed in children.

The main problem with spacers is that they are bulky and difficult to carry about so they are more suitable for prophylactic treatment given at home morning and evening.

Due to their many advantages, new spacer systems are launched every year. Though deceptively similar in appearance, there may be marked differences in the amount of drug retained in them. Therefore, uncritical use of any new spacer device is not recommended until its value has been documented in controlled trials.

DRY POWDER INHALERS

In dry powder inhalers (DPI) the drug is provided as a finely milled powder in individual blisters or gelatin capsules or in a reservoir chamber. Each blister or capsule contains only a single dose so it has to be replaced before each treatment. Often the active drug is mixed with a carrier substance such as lactose or micronized glucose so that the material in the capsules consists of fine drug particles in large aggregates (diameter of about 60 μm), either alone or in combination with the carrier particles. Most of the particles from dry powder inhalers are too large to penetrate into the lungs. However, the turbulent airstream created in the inhaler during inhalation causes the aggregates to break up into particles sufficiently small to be carried into the lower airways. Thus the effective use of powder inhalers is dependent upon a certain minimum amount of energy imparted from the patient's inhalation to create the correct particle size of the drug. Up to a certain point, increases in flow will increase the number of particles within the 'respirable range' and therefore the clinical effect of a dose.[10,51]

The storage of dry powder at high humidity (or exhalation into the device) may cause the drug to go into solution or cause agglomerates to form which are not easily dispersed into fine particles during inhalation.

The devices

INDIVIDUAL DOSE DEVICES

In the *Spinhaler* the gelatine capsule is placed in the middle of a rotor. During inhalation vibration frequencies and the wings of a spinning rotor draw out and disaggregate the dry powder from the capsule. Even with an optimal inhalation technique around 25% of the nominal dose is retained in the capsule and only 6–12% is deposited in the intrapulmonary airways.[51–53]

The *Rotahaler* also uses gelatine capsules. After the capsule is broken a coarse net causes turbulence during the inhalation. This disintegrates the small drug particles from the large lactose particles, which are used as a carrier substance. Intrabronchial deposition with the Rotahaler varies from 6–11% in different studies when an optimal inhalation technique is used. Oropharyngeal deposition is around 80%.[54,55,56]

In the *Diskhaler* active drug and lactose are kept in the airtight aluminium blister that is pierced before inhalation. The Diskhaler also uses a coarse net to disintegrate the particles. Intrabronchial deposition was found to be around 11% in two studies.[57,58] In one the deposition of a Diskhaler was only half the intrabronchial deposition when a pMDI was administered via a Volumatic.[57]

The *Turbuhaler (Turbohaler)* has a powder reservoir, which contains doses of pure drug without any additives. The dose is metered by a dosing disk just prior to inhalation. During inhalation the aggregated drug particles are drawn through spiral formed channels in the mouthpiece. The turbulence generated in these channels disaggregates the large particles. Intrabronchial deposition with this inhaler varies from 17–32% in various studies; 20–25% is retained in the inhaler and around 50% is deposited in the oropharynx. The intrabronchial deposition after Turbuhaler use has been found to be twice the deposition of a correctly used pMDI.[3,56,59]

The *Accuhaler (Diskus)* is a dry powder device that contains 60 individual doses on a foil strip. A dose counter is included. The device is of lower resistance than a Turbohaler and has been designed to deliver a similar dose to that received from a metered dose inhaler of similar nominal strength. It is taking over from the Diskhaler.

Comparative studies of the Turbohaler and the Accuhaler are inconsistent and confined to adults and older children.[60,61] *In vitro* studies suggest the Accuhaler is more consistent in the dose delivered at different flows, although it has a reduced fine particle mass and emits more large particles than the Turbohaler.

MULTIDOSE DEVICES

The *Clickhaler* is a generic dry powder device designed to look similar to a metered dose inhaler, even mimicking the press down action of a metered dose inhaler to load a unit dose for inhalation. The device gives similar results to properly used metered dose inhalers and has a dose counter and warning near the end of its 200 doses. It locks when these are completed, making it impossible for the patient to inadvertently try to administer medication from an empty device.

Dry powder spacer: to overcome the requirement of the patient to use their inhalation to aerosolize the drug, a power assisted dry powder inhaler has been developed which uses a mechanical piston of compressed air to force the powder into a spacer from which it may be inhaled. A modification to the Turbohaler that involves the mechanical actuation of the aerosol into a non-electrostatic spacer has been described. The half life for the dry powder is 82 seconds within this device. It has yet to be marketed.[62]

Inhalation technique

Fast inhalations enhance the effect of dry powder inhalers in children, whereas breathholding, tilting of the head during inhalation or inhalation from functional residual capacity instead of residual volume have no influence.[10,51] The number of respirable particles and the clinical effect may decrease with decreasing inspiratory flow rates. The inhalation effort and the inhalation flow rate needed to generate a therapeutic aerosol vary between different DPIs. Therefore, results obtained with one inhaler cannot be used to characterize another. At present no correctly performed comparisons between the various DPIs have been done so that the clinical importance of these differences is not known. They are most likely to be important in preschool children, who may not be able to generate such high inspiratory flows and therefore benefit less than older children from dry powder inhaler treatment.[10,63,64] Until further studies are available DPIs should be reserved for children older than 5 years.

Other laboratory studies

Pharmacokinetic studies and filter studies in school-children suggest that the intrabronchial deposition is twice as high after Turbuhaler treatment as after treatment with a pMDI and large volume spacer.[4,5] In accordance with this, the terbutaline Turbuhaler was more effective than a pMDI in preventing exercise-induced asthma in school-children.[65] Furthermore, the Turbuhaler produced better bronchodilation than a Rotahaler in children with exercise-induced asthma[66] and it was assessed as being somewhat more effective than the Rotahaler in 3–5-year-old children in an open, controlled trial.[67] The findings in other studies have been at variance with these results.[41,68,69] However, not all of these studies ensured that the comparison took place with doses on the steep part of the dose–response curve (Figure 8b.1) and therefore many are unsuitable for detecting differences between the various inhalers. The same problem applies to other laboratory comparisons between DPIs and between DPIs and other inhalers. Therefore, no firm conclusions about equi-effective doses from the various inhalers can be based upon these results.

Clinical studies

Effectiveness in day-to-day use may depend more on ease of use than on arcane laboratory experiments. DPIs are breath-actuated, thereby reducing or eliminating the coordination problems which are seen with the pMDI.[10] For many years dry powder inhalers have been single dose inhalers and therefore less convenient but easier to use than the MDI. Some children have difficulties with correct loading and splitting of the capsules when using the single dose inhalers, particularly during episodes of acute wheeze.[10,70] The newer multiple dose powder inhalers are easier to use and more convenient and so are preferred to the single dose inhalers (and possibly MDIs) by school-children.

The main problem with multidose DPIs is to train the child not to exhale through the inhaler before inhaling, since that will blow the dose out of the inhaler or cause it to clog. The Turbuhaler should be loaded in the upright position otherwise the metered dose will be reduced when the powder reservoir is less than half full.

Clinical studies have indicated that there is not a molar dose equipotency between DPI and pMDI. The Rotahaler is somewhat less effective than the MDI,[71] whereas the Turbuhaler is twice as effective as a MDI plus Nebuhaler.[72,73] These findings agree with various deposition studies and emphasize the importance of not applying

conclusions from one inhaler to other inhalers of the same class.

NEBULIZERS

Jet-nebulizers

In a jet-nebulizer, air or oxygen from an electric compressor or compressed gas supply passes through a narrow orifice, known as a venturi. At the venturi, the velocity of the gas increases and hence the pressure falls. Liquid from a reservoir is sucked up a tube and expelled in the form of fine 'ligaments' that collapse into droplets due to the surface tension (Figure 8b.4). Only about 0.5% of this primary droplet mass (comprising the smallest droplets) leaves the nebulizer directly; the remaining 99.5% impacts on baffles within the nebulizer or on the internal walls,[74] returns to the reservoir and is nebulized again. Thus the nebulizer produces a spray continuously over a treatment period of several minutes.

A variety of designs of jet-nebulizers exist. Some have no baffle, others possess baffles in varying sizes and shapes and some have concentric air and liquid feeds which are intended to minimize blockage by drug residue and a flat liquid pick-up plate which enables the nebulizer to be tilted by up to 90°. The baffle design has a critical effect upon nebulizer output characteristics, in particular upon droplet size distribution.

During nebulization a fall in temperature of the nebulizer and its contents is seen, being typically 10–15°C at a

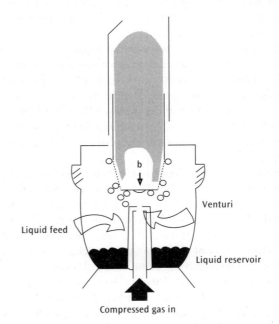

Figure 8b.4 *Operation of a jet-nebulizer. Compressed gas passes through a narrow venturi where negative pressure is created. Liquid is drawn up a feed tube and is fragmented into droplets. Large droplets impact on baffles (b), while smaller droplets are carried away in the inhaled airstream.*

compressed gas flow rate of 8 1/min because the diluent evaporates during nebulization. As a consequence of solvent evaporation, the drug concentration remaining in the nebulizer increases steadily during nebulization.[75] Paradoxical deterioration of infants' lung function from a nebulized β_2-agonist has been reported, possibly due to an increased tonicity of the aerosol during the selective evaporation of solvent during nebulization or due to preservatives.[76–78]

It is not possible to deliver all the fluid as aerosol since some is trapped as a dead or residual volume within the nebulizer, even after nebulization to dryness (when no more spray is produced). Thus an initial volume fill of 4 ml might typically leave a dead volume of 1 ml, but it would be a mistake to think that three-quarters of the drug has been nebulized. If the drug concentration in the reservoir has doubled (as often occurs) then only 50% of the drug has been nebulized. Output from nebulizers is sometimes assessed by weighing the nebulizer before and after nebulization, but this is misleading because it does not take into account the increase in drug concentration within the nebulizer. It is better to wash out the nebulizer after use and assay the amount of drug washed out and subtract this from the amount of drug initially placed in the nebulizer.

Drug output will vary according to the type of nebulizer, variation in dead volume and the volume of fluid initially placed in the nebulizer. Nebulizers work more efficiently (deliver more drug) when higher volume fills are used. To give an example, it may be possible to release only 40% of the dose with a 2 ml fill, and up to 60% with a 4 ml fill.[79]

Modified jet-nebulizers

To reduce the inefficiency of conventional jet-nebulizers, a new breed of jet-nebulizers have emerged over the last few years. They are discussed below briefly in order of their introduction to the market.

OPEN VENT NEBULIZERS

As gas under high pressure expands through the small opening within the nebulizer (the venturi) it expands rapidly creating a negative pressure that sucks aerosol up which is then atomized. The Sidestream nebulizer (Medicaid, UK) incorporates an extra vent that allows air to be drawn through the nebulizer as a result of the negative pressure generated. The additional airflow pushes out more small particles in a given time, reducing nebulization time considerably. Blockage of the vent would allow the nebulizer to release a similar amount of drug but over a much longer time. The main advantage of such systems is that nebulization occurs within half of the usual time. However, because of the high flow of aerosol laden air from the device, the dose received by young children may be surprisingly low due to their lower respiratory tidal flow and volume.

BREATH ENHANCED, OPEN VENT NEBULIZERS (MEDICAID VENTSTREAM, PARI LC PLUS, LC STAR)

These nebulizers also have an extra vent that is protected by a one-way valve. The valve opens only during inspiration. On exhalation, the valve closes and expired air passes out of the device through a separate expiratory port. The amount of drug inhaled on inspiration is increased as the additional airflow generated from the patient's inspiration pulls through more small particles increasing the nebulizer output and again reduces nebulization time. The amount of drug inspired may be doubled but nebulization time is not reduced as much as a simple open vent device.

INTELLIGENT DOSIMETRIC NEBULIZER

The Halo-lite is classed as an intelligent nebulizer that monitors the breathing pattern of the patient continuously. Once the patient has inhaled on three occasions from the device, pulses of aerosol are generated during a specific part of early inspiration only. The constant monitoring allows the device to adapt to the patient's breathing pattern if it changes during the nebulization period. A major advantage of the device is that the dose prescribed may be pre-set and once the patient has inhaled this dose, feedback is given in terms of a beep to the patient. A compliance chip was incorporated in the device used in clinical trials that allowed the time, date and the amount of drug inhaled to be documented. Other devices incorporating flow controllers which release boluses of aerosol early in inspiration are also being developed.

Aerosol characteristics

Most nebulized aerosols are heterodisperse, that is, the droplets in the spray cover a wide range of sizes (Figure 8b.5). MMAD varies with type of nebulizer, drug and gas flow rate through the nebulizer.[80] Normally an increase in air flow is associated with a decrease in MMAD. Information about droplet size provided by manufacturers of nebulizers is often sparse and sometimes misleading. It is common practice for manufacturers' data to quote the number of particles smaller than a given size, for instance, to say that 80% of the droplets are smaller than 5 μm diameter. Since the mass of drug contained in any droplet is proportional to the cube of its radius a single 10 μm droplet will contain the same amount of drug as 1000 1 μm droplets. Hence it is likely that most of the droplet mass will be contained in the 20% of droplets larger than 5 μm in diameter! It is therefore essential to quote droplet sizes from nebulizers in terms of mass or volume distribution if they are to have any meaning. Finally, the output characteristics of the nebulizer may change during ageing.

Nebulization time depends upon the type of nebulizer, the gas flow rate and the volume fill, as well as the

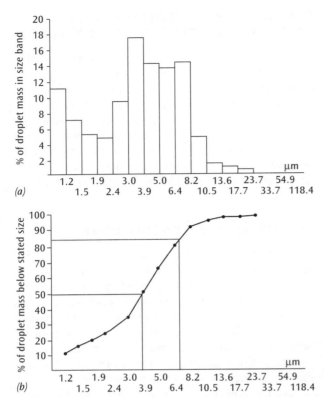

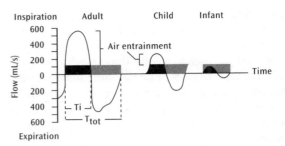

Figure 8b.6 *Air entrainment during tidal breathing from a jet-nebulizer. Inspiratory and expiratory flow patterns are shown. Inspiratory flow exceeds the gas flow through the nebulizer (dark grey blocks) in adults and children, so that the aerosol is diluted by entrained air. Infants may inhale undiluted aerosol. Except for breath-activated or sidestream nebulizers, aerosol is wasted during expiration (light grey blocks). (From ref. 84.)*

Figure 8b.5 *Nebulized droplet size distribution from a jet-nebulizer using a Malvern Instruments series 2600 laser analyzer (Malvern, UK). (a) Percentage of droplet mass contained within each of 15 size bands on a logarithmic scale; (b) cumulative mass distribution. The MMD (50% point on the cumulative distribution) is 3.8 μm diameter; 66% of the aerosol mass is contained in droplets smaller than 5 μm diameter. The GSD (ratio of 84% to 50% points) is 1.8. (From ref. 99.)*

temperature and type of solution. Normally nebulization time should not exceed ten minutes.

Ultrasonic nebulizers

Ultrasonic nebulizers use a piezoelectric crystal vibrating at a high frequency to generate a fountain of liquid in the nebulizer chamber. They operate silently and often produce droplets with a higher MMAD than jet-nebulizers.[75,81,82] Furthermore, they cannot be used for suspensions since they only nebulize the fluid and not the drug. They may not be able to make a spray from some viscous drug solutions and they may cause damage to some drugs.[82] For these reasons ultrasonic nebulizers are not at present as widely used as jet-nebulizers and they will not be discussed in detail.

Inhalation technique

No controlled studies have been done in children on the optimal inhalation technique from nebulizers. However,

quiet tidal breathing is normally recommended because it produces optimal results in adults.[83]

A Spira jet-nebulizer delivered a median of 11% of the nominal dose to the inspiratory filter of children aged 6 months increasing to 14% at 8 years.[7] Approximately 20% of the nominal dose was found on the filter at the expiratory side. This fraction would have been lost as aerosol into the surrounding air. Approximately 68% of the nominal dose was retained in the jet-nebulizer after nebulizing to emptiness. The inhaled dose showed only a weak correlation to age or height of the child. These findings substantiate previous reports suggesting that after 6 months of age the quantity of aerosol inspired from a jet-nebulizer is largely independent of age, since inspiratory flow exceeds jet-nebulized flow during all or part of inspiration[84] (Figure 8b.6). Children aged 1–2 years hyperventilate when a face-mask is applied to their face, permitting air entrainment to take place in these age groups.[8] The distribution of oropharyngeal and intrabronchial deposition is not known.

Suction through the jet-nebulizer, which may occur when there are no holes in the face-mask or mouthpiece, may draw relatively large droplets, which would otherwise fall back into the jet-nebulizer reservoir into the inhaled airstream.[85]

Inhalation through a face-mask 2–3 cm from the face reduces the drug delivery by approximately 50% in school-children with a corresponding increase in release of aerosol to the environment. *In vitro* studies have reported an 85% reduction in the inhaled dose of respirable particles when the face-mask was moved 2 cm from the inspiratory orifice.[39] The clinical effect appears to be the same in school-children whether the inhalation takes place through a mouthpiece or a face-mask.[86]

Other laboratory studies

Simply varying the choice of compressor, jet-nebulizer and size of volume fill has been shown to vary the mass of drug in respirable particles over a ten-fold range.[87] Therefore, ideally each nebulizer/drug combination should be characterized separately. This is very rarely done. Due to this enormous variation it is not meaningful to discuss comparisons with other inhalers in general. However, generally nebulizers are far less efficient (per mg drug) than other inhalation systems in school-children, so higher doses are required to achieve the same clinical effect.[46,88] This difference in delivery seems to be more pronounced for steroids[21] than for β_2-agonists because fewer respirable particles are generated from a steroid suspension.

The pMDI and spacer combination is atleast effective for the administration of β_2-agonists in acute severe asthma as a nebulizer.[89]

Ease of use

Little coordination is required from the patient if continuous nebulization through a face-mask with holes is used. Therefore nebulizers are simple to use. However, compared with other devices nebulizers are expensive, bulky, inconvenient, time-consuming, inefficient delivery systems and with our present knowledge their use for daily treatment should be limited to children who cannot be trained to use another device or for drugs which cannot be delivered by any other inhaler system. In clinical practice this means some children younger than 3–4 years and handicapped older children. In our clinics it is rare for any child to take a nebulizer home.

In spite of all the problems with nebulized therapy nebulizers are still used in the treatment of acute severe asthma in all age groups even if the same results can be obtained with other inhalation systems in school-children.[22,45,46,86,89] In the acute situation it is an advantage that oxygen can be administered through the nebulizer at the same time as the β_2-agonist.

Remarkably few controlled nebulizer studies of day-to-day treatment have been performed. Therefore, our knowledge about optimal dose requirement and nebulizer system for young children is rather limited. At present nebulized therapy to young children has to be based on a few clinical studies and empirical experience. They have clearly demonstrated that nebulizers can be used for effective prophylactic therapy and β_2-agonist administration in children of all ages.[23,90]

The optimal method and frequency of cleaning a nebulizer is not known. Some manufacturers provide instructions. Normally it is recommended to rinse the nebulizer (plus face-mask or mouthpiece) in hot water after each nebulization. In addition, the nebulizer and tubing should be washed in hot soapy water twice weekly and rinsed and disinfected once a week in a mixture of one cup of hot water plus two tablespoons of vinegar. This should be followed by drying by blowing air through the system. Some nebulizers are supplied with needles to unblock the feeding tubes, but generally these should not be used because they may damage the nozzles. Finally the air inlet filter should be changed at regular intervals, depending upon the environment in which the nebulizer is being used.

Though spacers, powder inhalers and nebulizers are apparently easy to use, careful and repeated tuition is required every time one of these inhalers is prescribed otherwise the therapeutic result may not be satisfactory.

CLINICAL – SYSTEMIC EFFECT RATIO

The systemic effect of an inhaled drug depends upon the amount of drug deposited in the intrapulmonary airways and the amount absorbed from the gastrointestinal tract (Figure 8a.11). The clinical effect only depends upon the intrapulmonary deposition. Therefore, a clinically very effective inhaler will also be expected to have a higher systemic effect. In contrast the contribution of the orally deposited drug to the systemic effect is higher for an inhaler with a low intrapulmonary and high oral drug deposition. So, when an inhaler is studied it is important to evaluate both the effect and side effect profile so that an effect-side effect ratio can be defined. This has been done thoroughly for the Turbohaler and for corticosteroids.

Most studies evaluating the use of inhaled corticosteroids have only compared the systemic effect of an identical dose of a corticosteroid delivered from two different inhalers without considering the question of clinically equieffective doses of the two inhalers studied. In such studies it has been shown that beclomethasone delivered via a large volume spacer (Volumatic) has less systemic activity than the same dose delivered from a MDI or a Diskhaler.[91,92,93] Since the Volumatic seems to be at least as effective as these inhalers the clinical-systemic effect ratio for the Volumatic is probably better than the ratio for these inhalers. Furthermore, budesonide from a Nebuhaler has the same systemic effect as budesonide from a MDI and less systemic effect than budesonide from a Turbuhaler.[94,95] However, the Turbuhaler is twice as effective as these inhalers. So the higher systemic effect of the Turbuhaler is mainly due to a higher intrabronchial deposition and hence the clinical-systemic effect ratio is the same for this inhaler and the Nebuhaler.

We have no knowledge about the clinical/systemic effect ratio for the various nebulizer systems. However, nose breathing would be expected to filter off the large particles, which are likely to be absorbed and cause systemic effects without adding to the clinical effect. Jet-nebulizers with spacer-like reservoirs, which filter out large particles, are likely to improve the therapeutic ratio.

In summary, spacer systems have advantages over other devices for delivering inhaled steroids though this has only been studied in school-children not using a face-mask. Most young children breathe through the nose, which serves as an efficient filter to separate most larger particles and therefore may cause considerable drug deposition in the nose and reduced deposition in the lung.[49,50] Nose breathing may reduce the clinical-systemic effect ratio since many drugs are well-absorbed from the nasal mucosa. Furthermore, recent findings with the dry powder inhaler Turbuhaler show that the clinical-systemic effect ratio of this inhaler is quite similar to that of a spacer without a face-mask and the low oral bioavailability of fluticasone probably also reduces the importance of a spacer for this drug. The difference in clinical-systemic effect ratio between the various inhalers is most important when high doses of inhaled corticosteroids are used.

ADHERENCE TO THERAPY

Adherence to asthma medications is poor.[96] Under-use of prescribed medications occurs approximately 50% of the time. There is no evidence that compliance is improved by changing to a different inhaler device, be it small or unobtrusive even though such devices are often marketed on the basis that they are more acceptable to the patient and they will, therefore, be used more. With improvement in technology, there is increasing likelihood in drug delivery devices that can both monitor and prompt patient use.

Implementation of evidence-based pMDI and spacer therapy for acute severe asthma in place of jet-nebulizers takes a great deal of effort and persistence.[97] Thus it is not only patients whose motivation wavers, but health professionals too!

INHALER STRATEGY

Children up to 5 years can use a spacer with a valve system and a face-mask for the delivery of all drugs. If the child cannot be taught correct use of a spacer, a nebulizer should be prescribed (Table 8b.2).

Children over 5 years can be prescribed a multiple dose powder inhaler (if not available, a single dose DPI) or a breath-actuated pMDI for β2-agonists or SCG and a large volume spacer for the administration of inhaled corticosteroids. If these alternatives are not available a conventional DPI or MDI can be used in these age groups provided that careful tuition is given. Fluticasone dipropionate may be given by DPI or spacer pMDI.

Nebulizers are mainly used for severe acute attacks of asthma if children refuse to use a spacer.

With this approach children can be taught effective inhaler use with a minimum of instructional time by the doctor, nurse or therapist, whoever has the necessary skills and patience to succeed. Finally, it must be remembered always to consider the child's wishes since prescription of

Table 8b.2 *The choice of inhalation device (assumes all devices used optimally) (from ref. 2)*

Age (years)	First choice	Second choice	Comments
0–2	MDI + spacer and face-mask	Nebulizer	Avoid 'open vent' nebulizers
3–6	MDI + spacer	Nebulizer	Very few children at this age can use DPIs adequately
6–12 (bronchodilators)	MDI + spacer or breath-actuated MDIs or DPI	–	If using DPI or breath-actuated MDI, also prescribe MDI + spacer for acute exacerbations
6–12 (steroids)	MDI + spacer or Turbohaler or FP DPI	Other DPI or breath-actuated MDI	May need to adjust dose if switching between inhalers Advise mouth rinsing or gargling
12+ (bronchodilators)	DPI or breath-actuated MDI	–	
12+ (steroids)	MDI + spacer or Turbohaler or FP DPI	Other DPI or breath-actuated MDI	May need to adjust dose if switching between inhalers Advise mouth rinsing or gargling
Acute asthma (all **ages**; bronchodilators)	MDI + spacer	Nebulizer	Ensure appropriate dosing Nebulize for a set period of time Provide written instructions

MDI: metered dose inhaler; DPI: dry powder inhaler Fluticasone Propionate.

an inhaler which the physician likes but the child does not is likely to reduce compliance.

AIMS OF FUTURE DEVELOPMENTS

It is obvious that the ideal 'wonderhaler' which can be used by all patients and for all drugs has not yet been developed. The aim of future inhaler development must be to develop a convenient, easy to use, breath actuated, Freon-free, effort-independent multiple dose inhaler, which filters off all larger particles and delivers a reproducible fraction of the dose to the patient in the form of slowly moving respirable particles. Ideally, it should contain a data logger so that, dose by dose, compliance can be recorded. For young children a valve system and a face-mask which prevents nasal inhalation would be ideal. Until such an inhaler has been developed, a more complicated inhaler strategy has to be followed.

REFERENCES

1. Bisgaard H, O'Callaghan C, Smaldone GC, eds. Drug delivery to the lung. In: *Lung Biology in Health and Disease*, vol. 162. Marcel Dekker, New York, 2002.
2. Barry P. Administering treatment – inhaled therapy. In: M Silverman, C O'Callaghan, eds. *Practical Paediatric Respiratory Medicine*. Arnold, London, 2001.
3. Borgstrom L. Methodological studies on lung deposition. Evaluation of inhalation devices and absorption mechanisms. *Acta Univ Upsal* 1993;1–51.
4. Pedersen S, Stefferisen G, Ohlsson SV. The influence of orally-deposited budesonide on the systemic availability of budesonide after inhalation from a Turbuhaler. *Eur J Clin Pharmacol* 1993;**36**:211–14.
5. Pedersen S, Steffensen G, Ekman I, Tonnesson M, Borgaa O. Pharmacokinetics of budesonide in children with asthma. *Eur J Clin Pharmacol* 1987;**31**:579–82.
6. Lodrup Carlsen KC, Nikander K, Carlsen KH. How much nebulized budesonide reaches infants and toddlers? *Arch Dis Child* 1992;**67**:1077–9.
7. Bisgaard H. Aerosol treatment of young children. *Eur Respir Rev* 1994;**4**:15–20.
8. Agertoft L, Pedersen S. Influence of spacer device on drug delivery to young children with asthma. *Arch Dis Child* 1994;**71**:217–20.
9. Moren F. Drug deposition of pressurized inhalation aerosols. I. Influence of actuator tube design. *Int J Pharmacol* 1978;**1**:205–12.
10. Pedersen S. Inhaler use in children with asthma. *Danish Med Bull* 1987;**34**:234–49.
11. Coldiron BM. Thinning of the ozone layer: facts and consequences. *J Am Acad Dermatol* 1992;**27**(5 Pt 1): 653–62.

12. Partridge M, Woodcock A. Metered dose inhalers free of chlorofluorocarbons. *Br Med J* 1995;**310**: 684–5.
13. Barry PW, O'Callaghan C. *In vitro* comparison of the amount of salbutamol available for inhalation from different formulations used with different spacer devices. *Eur Respir J* 1997;**10**:1345–8.
14. June D, Carlson S, Ross D. The effect of temperature on drug delivery characteristics of chloroflurocarbon (CFC) and hydrofluoroalkane (HFA) metered dose inhalers. *Respir Drug Delivery* 1996;**5**:133–44.
15. Everard ML, Devadason SG, Summers QA, Le Souef PN. Factors affecting total and respirable dose delivered by a salbutamol metered dose inhaler. *Thorax* 1995; **50**:746–9.
16. Fuglsang G, Pedersen S. Cumulative dose response relationship of terbutaline delivered by three different inhalers. *Allergy* 1988;**43**:348–52.
17. Pedersen S, Frost L, Arnfred T. Errors in inhalation technique and efficacy of inhaler use in asthmatic children. *Allergy* 1986;**41**:118–24.
18. Williams DJ, Williams AC, Kruchek DG. Problems in assessing contents of metered dose inhalers. *Br Med J* 1993;**307**:771–2.
19. Ogren RA, Baldwin JL, Simon RA. How patients determine when to replace the metered dose inhalers. *Ann Allergy Asthma Immunol* 1995;**75**: 485–9.
20. Pedersen S, Frost L, Arnfred T. Problems in inhalation technique and efficiency in inhaler use in asthmatic children. *Allergy* 1986;**41**:118–24.
21. O'Callaghan C. Particle size of beclomethasone dipropionate produced by 2 nebulizers and spacers. *Thorax* 1990;**45**:109–11.
22. Scalabrin DM, Naspitz CK. Efficacy and side effects of salbutamol in acute asthma in children: comparison of oral route and two different nebulizer systems. *J Asthma* 1993;**30**:51–9.
23. Ilangovan P, Pedersen S, Godfrey S, *et al.* Treatment of severe steroid dependent preschool asthma with nebulised budesonide suspension. *Arch Dis Child* 1993;**68**:356–9.
24. Ruggins NR, Milner AD, Swarbrick A. An assessment of a new breath actuated inhaler device in acutely wheezy children. *Arch Dis Child* 1993;**68**:477–80.
25. Gonda I, Schuster JA, Rubasmen RN, Lloyd P, Cipolla D, Farr SJ. Inhalation delivery systems with compliance and disease management capabilities. *J Controlled Release* 1998;**53**:269–74.
26. Newman SP, Clark SW. Bronchodilator delivery from Gentlehaler, a new low-velocity pressurised aerosol inhaler. *Chest* 1993;**103**:1442–6.
27. Gunawardena KA, Sohal T, Jones JI, Upchurch FC, Crompton GK. The spacehaler for delivery of salbutamol: a comparison with the standard metered-dose inhaler plus volumatic spacer device. *Respir Med* 1997;**91**:311–16.

28. Newman SP, Clarke AR, Talee N, Clarke SW. Pressurised aerosol deposition in the human lung with and without an open spacer device. *Thorax* 1989;**44**:706–10.

29. O'Callaghan C, Barry PW. Spacer devices in the treatment of asthma. *Br Med J* 1997;**314**:1061–2.

30. Pedersen S. Optimal use of tube spacer aerosols in asthmatic children. *Clin Allergy* 1985;**15**:473–8.

31. Gleeson JG, Price JF. Nebuhaler technique. *Br J Dis Chest* 1988;**82**:172–4.

32. Newman SP, Moren F, Pavia D, Little F, Clarke SW. Deposition of pressurized suspension aerosols inhaled through extension devices. *Am Rev Respir Dis* 1981;**124**:317–20.

33. O'Callaghan C, Lynch J, Cant M, Robertson C. Improvement in sodium cromoglycate delivery from a spacer device by use of an antistatic lining, immediate inhalation, and avoiding multiple actuations of drug. *Thorax* 1993;**48**:603–6.

34. O'Callaghan C, Linch J, Cant M, Robertson C. Improvement in drug delivery from spacers devices by use of an antistatic lining. *Thorax* 1993;**48**:603–86.

35. Wildhaber JH, Devadason SG, Hayden MJ, James R, Duffy AP, Fox RA, Sumners QA, Le Souef PN. Electrostatic charge on a plastic spacer device influences the delivery of Salbutamol. *Eur Respir J* 1996;**9**:1943–6.

36. Bisgaard H. A metal aerosol holding chamber device for young children with asthma. *Eur Respir J* 1995;**8**:856–60.

37. Lee H, Evans HE. Evaluation of inhalation aids of metered dose inhalers in asthmatic children. *Chest* 1987;**91**:366–9.

38. Everard ML, Clark AR, Milner AD. Drug delivery from holding chambers with attached face-mask. *Arch Dis Child* 1992;**67**:580–5.

39. Amon S, Grigg J, Nikander K, Silverman M. Delivery of micronized budesonide suspension by metered dose inhaler and jet nebulizer into a neonatal ventilator circuit. *Pediatr Pulmonol* 1992;**13**:172–5.

40. Vichyanond P, Chokephaibulkit K, Kerdsomnuig S, Visitsuntom N, Tuchinda M. Clinical evaluation of the 'Siriraj spacer' in asthmatic Thai children. *Ann Allergy* 1992;**69**:433–8.

41. Rachelefsky GS, Rohr AS, Wo J, *et al*. Use of a tube spacer to improve the efficacy of a metered-dose inhaler in asthmatic children. *Am J Dis Child* 1986;**140**:1191–3.

42. Tal A, Golan H, Grauer N, Aviram M, Albin D, Quastel MR. Deposition pattern of radiolabelled salbutamol inhaled from a metered-dose inhaler by means of a spacer with mask in young children with airway obstruction. *J Ped* 1996;**128**:479–84.

43. Iles R, Lister P, Edmunds AT. Crying significantly reduces absorption of aerosolised drug in infants. *Arch Dis Child* 1999;**81**:163–5.

44. Janssens HM, Heijnen EM, de Jong VM, Hop WC, Holland WP, de Jongste JC, Tiddens HA. Aerosol delivery from spacers in wheezy infants: a daily life study. *Eur Respir J* 2000;**16**:850–6.

45. Fuglsang G, Pedersen S. Comparison of a new multidose powder inhaler with a pressurized aerosol in children with asthma. *Pediatr Pulmonol* 1989;**7**:112–15.

46. Pendergast J, Hopkins J, Timms B, van Asperen PP. Comparative efficacy of terbutaline administered by Nebuhaler and by nebulizer in young children with acute asthma. *Med J Aust* 1989;**151**:406–8.

47. Noble V, Ruggins NR, Everard ML, Milner AD. Inhaled budesonide via a modified Nebuhaler for chronic wheezing in infants. *Arch Dis Child* 1992;**67**:285–8.

48. Bisgaard H, Munck SL, Nielsen JP, Petersen W, Ohlsson SV. Inhaled budesonide for treatment of recurrent wheezing in early childhood. *Lancet* 1990;**336**:649–51.

49. Bisgaard H, Mygind N. Nasal allergy. In: MH Lessof, TH Lee, DM Keremy, eds. *Allergy. An International Textbook*. Wiley, Chichester, 1987, pp. 531–52.

50. Everard ML, Hardy JG, Milner AD. Comparison of nebulised aerosol deposition in the lungs of healthy adults following oral and nasal inhalation. *Thorax* 1993;**48**:1045–6.

51. Richards R, Dickson CR, Renwick AG, Lewis RA, Holgate ST. Absorption and disposition kinetics of cromolyn sodium and the influence of inhalation technique. *J Pharmacol Exp Ther* 1987;**241**:1028–32.

52. Auty RM, Brown K, Neale MG, Snashall PD. Respiratory tract deposition of sodium cromoglycate is highly dependent upon technique of inhalation using the Spinhaler. *Br J Dis Chest* 1987;**81**:371–80.

53. Vidgren M, Karkkainen A, Karjalainen P, Paronen P, Nuutinen J. Effect of powder inhaler design on drug deposition in the respiratory tract. *Int J Pharm* 1988;**42**:211–16.

54. Vidgren M, Paronen P, Vidgren P, Vainio P, Nuutinin J. *In vivo* evaluation of the new multiple dose powder inhaler and the Rotahaler using, the gamma scintigraphy. *Acta Pharm Nord* 1990;**1**:3–10.

55. Roberts CM, Biddiscombe M, Fogarty P, Spiro SG. Lung deposition of dry powder salbutamol delivered by Rotahaler in subjects with chronic airflow obstruction. *Eur Respir J* 1990;**3**(Suppl 10):94.

56. Zainudin BMZ, Biddiscombe M, Tolfree SEJ, Short M, Spiro SG. Comparison of bronchodilator responses and deposition patterns of salbutamol inhaled from a pressurised metered dose inhaler, as a dry powder, and as nebulised solution. *Thorax* 1990;**45**:469–73.

57. Melchior EA. Lung deposition of salbutamol. *Thorax* 1993;**48**:506–11.

58. Biddiscombe M, Marriott RJ, Melchior R, *et al*. The preparation and evaluation of pressurized

metered dose and dry powder inhalers containing 99 mTc labelled salbutamol. *J Aer Med* 1991; **4**(Suppl 1):9.

59. Newman SP, Moren F, Trofast E, Talaee N, Clarke SW. Deposition and clinical efficacy of terbutaline sulphate from Turbuhaler, a new multi-dose powder inhaler. *Eur Respir J* 1989;**2**:247–52.

60. Schlaeppi M, Edwards K, Fuller RW, Sharma R. Patient perception on the Diskus inhaler: a comparison with the Turbohaler inhaler. *Br J Clin Pract* 1996;**50**:14–19.

61. Venebles TL, Addlestone MB, Smithers AJ, Blagden MD, West D, Gooding T, Carr EP, Follows RMA. A comparison of the efficacy and patient acceptability of once daily Budesonide via a Turbohaler and twice daily Fluticasone Propionate Diskhaler at an equal daily dose of 400 micrograms in adult asthmatics. *Br J Clin Res* 1996; 7:15–32.

62. Bisgaard H. Automatic actuation of a dry powder inhaler into a non-electrostatic spacer. *Am Rev Respir Crit Care Med* 1998;**157**:518–21.

63. Pedersen S, Hansen OR, Fuglsang G. Influence of inspiratory flow rate upon the effect of a Turbuhaler. *Arch Dis Child* 1990;**65**:308–10.

64. Bisgaard H, Pedersen S, Nikander K. Use of budesonide Turbuhaler in young children suspected of asthma. *Eur Respir J* 1994;**7**:740–2.

65. Arborelius MJ, Svenonius E, Wiberg R, Stahl E. A comparison of terbutaline inhaled by Turbuhaler and by a chlorofluorocarbon (CFC) inhaler in children with exercise-induced asthma. *Allergy* 1994;**49**:408–12.

66. Pedersen S. Effect of terbutaline sulphate Turbuhaler in children with exercise induced bronchoconstriction. In: SP Newman, F Moren, GK Crompton, eds. *A New Concept in Inhalation Therapy*. Medicom, London, 1987, pp.166–72.

67. Seddon PC, Heaf DP. How well do children use dry powder inhalers? *Thorax* 1990;**45**:818.

68. Boggard JM, Slingerland R, Verbraak AF. Dose–effect relationship of terbutaline using a multi-dose powder inhalation system (Turbuhaler) and salbutamol administered by powder inhalation (Rotahaler) in asthmatics. *Pharmatherapeutica* 1989;**5**:400–6.

69. Rufin P, Benoist MR, de Blic J, Braunstein G, Scheinmann P. Terbutaline powder in asthma exacerbations. *Arch Dis Child* 1991;**66**:1465–6.

70. Pedersen S. Treatment of acute bronchoconstriction in children with use of a tube spacer aerosol and a dry powder inhaler. *Allergy* 1985;**40**:300–4.

71. Bisgaard H, Andersen JB, Bach-Mortensen N, *et al.* A clinical comparison of aerosol and powder administration of beclomethasone dipropionate in childhood asthma. *Allergy* 1984;**39**:365–9.

72. Agertoft L, Pedersen S. The importance of delivery system for the effect of budesonide. *Arch Dis Child* 1993;**69**:130–3.

73. Agertoft LA, Pedersen S. Effects of long-term treatment with an inhaled corticosteroid on growth and pulmonary function in asthmatic children. *Respir Med* 1994;**88**:327–81.

74. Mercer TT. Production of therapeutic aerosols: principles and techniques. *Chest* 1981;**80**(Suppl): 813–18.

75. Wood JA, Wilson RSE, Bray J. Changes in salbutamol concentration in the reservoir solution of a jet nebulizer. *Br J Dis Chest* 1986;**80**:164–9.

76. Schoni MH, Kraemer R. Osmolality changes in nebulizer solutions. *Eur Respir J* 1989;**2**:887–92.

77. O'Callaghan C, Milner AD, Swarbrick A. Paradoxical deterioration in lung function after nebulised salbutamol in wheezy infants. *Lancet* 1986;**ii**:1424–5.

78. O'Callaghan C, Milner AD, Swarbrick A. Paradoxical bronchoconstriction in wheezing infants after nebulised preservative free iso-osmolar ipratropium bromide. *Br Med J* 1989;**299**:1433–4.

79. Clay MM, Pavia D, Newman SP, Lennard-Jones TR, Clarke SW. Assessment of jet nebulizers for lung aerosol therapy. *Lancet* 1983;**2**:592–4.

80. Newman SP, Pellow PGD, Clarke SW. Droplet size distributions of nebulised aerosols for inhalation therapy. *Clin Phys Physiol Meas* 1986;**7**:139–46.

81. Matthys H, Kohler D. Pulmonary deposition of aerosols by different mechanical devices. *Respiration* 1985;**48**:269–76.

82. Sterk PJ, Plomp A, van der Vate JF, Quanjer PH. Physical properties of aerosols produced by several jet and ultrasonic nebulizers. *Bull Eur Physiopathol Bl Respir* 1984;**20**:65–72.

83. Ryan G, Dolovich MB, Obminski G, *et al.* Standardisation of inhalation provocation tests: influence of nebulizer output, particle size and method of inhalation. *J Allergy Clin Immunol* 1981; **67**:156–61.

84. Collis GG, Cole CH, Le Souef PN. Dilution of nebulised aerosols by air entrainment in children. *Lancet* 1990;**336**:341–3.

85. Mercer TT, Goddard RF, Flores RL. Effect of auxiliary air flow on the output characteristics of compressed-air nebulizers. *Ann Allergy* 1969;**27**:211–17.

86. Lowenthal D, Kattan M. Facemasks versus mouthpieces for aerosol treatment of asthmatic children. *Pediatr Pulmonol* 1992;**14**:192–6.

87. Newman SP, Pellow PGD, Clay MM, Clarke SW. Evaluation of jet nebulizers for use with gentamycin solution. *Thorax* 1985;**40**:671–6.

88. Blackhall MI, O'Donnell SR. A dose–response study of inhaled terbutaline administered via nebuhaler or nebulizer to asthmatic children. *Eur J Respir Dis* 1987; **71**:96–101.

89. Adams N, Cates CJ, Bestall J. Holding chambers versus nebulizers for inhaled steroids in chronic asthma. *Cochrane Review* 2001: *The Cochrane Library Issue 4*. Oxford. Update Software.

90. Wilson NM, Silverman M. Treatment of acute episodic asthma in preschool children using intermittent high dose inhaled steroids at home. *Arch Dis Child* 1990;**65**:407–10.

91. Farrer M, Francis AJ, Pearce SJ. Morning serum cortisol concentrations after 2 mg inhaled beclomethasone dipropionate in normal subjects: effect of a 750 ml spacing device. *Thorax* 1990; **46**:891–4.

92. Brown PH, Blundell G, Greening AP, Crompton GK. Do large volume spacer devices reduce the systemic effects of high dose inhaled corticosteroids? *Thorax* 1990;**45**:736–9.

93. Pedersen S. Safety aspects of cortico-steroids in children. *Eur Respir Rev* 1994;**4**:33–43.

94. Selroos O, Halme M. Effect of a volumatic spacer and mouth-rinsing on systemic absorption of inhaled corticosteroids from a metered dose inhaler and a dry powder inhaler. *Thorax* 1991; **46**:891–4.

95. Pedersen S, Hansen OR. Treatment of asthmatic children with budesonide from a Turbuhaler and a MDI with a Nebuhaler. *35th Nordic Congress of Pneumonology*, 1990, p. 35.

96. Coutts JA, Gibson NA, Paton JY. Measuring compliance with inhaled medication in asthma. *Arch Dis Child* 1992;**67**:332–3.

97. Powell CVE, Maskell GR, Marks MK, South M, Robertson CF, Lenney W. Successful implementation of spacer treatment guideline for acute asthma. *Arch Dis Child* 2001;**84**:142–6.

98. Rudolph G, Kobrich R, Stahlofen W. Modelling and algebraic formulation of regional aerosol deposition in man. *J Aerosol Sci* 1990;**21**:S306–406.

99. Newman SP, Pellow PG, Clarke SW. Droplet size distributions of nebulized aerosols for inhalation therapy. *Clin Phys Physiol Meas* 1986;**7**:139–46.

9

Wheezing disorders in infants and young children

MICHAEL SILVERMAN

THE NATURE OF WHEEZING IN EARLY CHILDHOOD

A brief history of wheeze

Attitudes to infant wheezing disorders have come full circle over the last 40 years. While the techniques which led paediatricians[1] and family doctors[2] in the 1960s to recognize that infant wheezing disorders differed in important ways from childhood asthma can be criticized, their conclusions were very perceptive. In particular, these observers noticed that wheezing in the youngest children was episodic, associated with upper respiratory tract infection and that the overwhelming majority of wheezy infants, including some who had been admitted to hospital many times, out-grew their disease so that by school age they were unlikely to exhibit the features of asthma (Figure 9.1). Recent studies of birth cohorts collected from a whole population and from groups at high risk of developing atopic asthma have confirmed some of these observations (Chapter 3).

A different message was promulgated in the 1970s and 1980s. Alarm at the apparent epidemic of childhood asthma and awareness that under-diagnosis and under-treatment of asthma could lead to excess morbidity and mortality, along with the ready availability of all the main therapeutic agents which are in use today, caused paediatricians to abandon vague descriptive terms such as 'wheezy bronchitis' in favour of the apparently more precise and prescriptive term 'asthma' for all ages, although terminology for those under one year remained contentious.

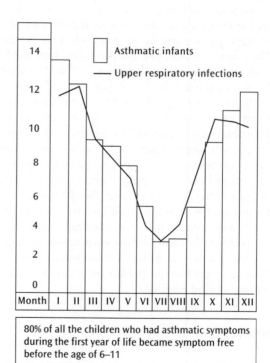

80% of all the children who had asthmatic symptoms during the first year of life became symptom free before the age of 6–11

Figure 9.1 *Concordance of community reporting of upper respiratory infections and admissions to one hospital with acute severe asthma in the first year of life. (From ref. 1 with permission.)*

By this means, it was hoped that appropriate therapy, including bronchodilators and prophylactic anti-asthma agents, would be prescribed for young wheezy children in place of the ineffectual antibiotics and antitussives which

Table 9.1 *Major differences between the risk factors for wheezing lower respiratory illness in infants and for asthma in school*

Risk factors*	Episodic viral wheeze in infants	Atopic asthma in schoolchildren
Tobacco smoke exposure		
In utero	+++	?
Childhood	++	++
Virus infection	++++	++
Atopy	−	+++
Aeroallergen exposure	−	+++
Infant formula feeding	+	−**
Low birth weight	+	+

*The risk factors for the aetiology of wheezing disease or asthma may not be the same as the trigger factors for the manifestation of symptoms. **In infants of allergic mothers.

had been customary. Up to a point, this clinically driven paradigm was valuable. It certainly raised awareness of asthma and abated the shift away from the inappropriate use of antibiotics for young wheezy children. But by lumping all wheezers under a single diagnostic label, diagnostic, therapeutic and prognostic subgroups lay hidden.

In the last 15 years, it has become clear that early wheezing disorders, particularly in the first 2–3 years of life, should be considered as largely independent of later childhood asthma (Table 9.1 and Chapter 3). The evidence includes the characteristic infant patterns of episodic wheeze, the viral aetiology of wheeze in the youngest age groups, recent evidence demonstrating the absence of chronic inflammation in episodic viral wheeze, the overwhelmingly non-atopic nature of infant wheezing, the generally poor response of wheezing infants to therapeutic agents and the lack of progression to atopic childhood asthma in the majority of cases. By opening up the debate again, we are no longer in danger of throwing out the wheezy baby with the bath water. Instead, it would be wise to admit that the term 'asthma' encompasses a range of disorders, and to qualify the term with descriptors in order later to target therapy, predict prognosis and conduct focused clinical research.[3]

Terminology

Wheeze is a symptom, not a diagnosis (Chapter 6a). The use of the term leads to a problem-orientated rather than a diagnosis-led approach to management which affects all aspects of care, including the identification of contributory factors, clinical evaluation, therapeutic measures and determination of outcome. The range of names applied to the commonest group of wheezing infants and toddlers is wide: wheezy bronchitis, wheezy baby syndrome, wheezing LRI (lower respiratory illness), wheeze-associated respiratory illness, recurrent bronchiolitis, infantile asthma

or simply asthma. As the term 'wheezy bronchitis' implies, in addition to wheeze, cough is an important symptom. The thorny question of the existence of 'cough-variant asthma' is considered in Chapter 6a. Even the term 'wheeze' is ill-defined, and may be mis-interpreted by parents (Chapter 6a). Other types of noisy breathing such as rattly or bubbly noises (called 'ruttles' in the English Midlands) which emanate from the large airways or pharynx, and even stridor, are sometimes mistakenly labelled wheeze by parents and sometimes by health professionals too.[4]

Despite using the deliberately vague term 'wheezy child', the label 'asthma' still has a place in management, if only to simplify discussion with the parents of wheezy children. However, it should be used only as a general term. Arguments concerning the number of episodes of wheeze required to justify the label of asthma are reminiscent of medieval debate: how many angels can sit on the point of a needle?

The relationship between *acute infantile bronchiolitis* and wheezing disorders in infancy is not entirely clear: bronchiolitis is part of the spectrum of wheezing, albeit at one extreme, and not a 'cause' of recurrent wheezing LRI (see below). The term 'recurrent bronchiolitis' is confusing and therefore unhelpful and should be dropped. Even the term 'bronchiolitis' is used differently in North America where it is applied to episodes of wheeze, whether isolated or recurrent, in the first 2 years of life. In Europe, it applies to the first episode of infantile lower respiratory wheezing illness, generally caused by RSV, in infants of less than 6–8 months old.

Disease patterns

As is the case for other age groups, disease patterns can be broken into three types (Figure 1.2, Chapter 1).

1 Most wheezy young children simply have *episodic attacks of wheeze* and cough associated with evidence of viral upper respiratory infection, punctuated by symptom-free intervals of variable duration. At one extreme, some children have a single episode, either a mild attack lasting from 2–3 days, often with their first RSV infection or a severe but isolated attack of acute bronchiolitis; at the other extreme, monthly admissions to hospital may be precipitated by each passing cold.

2 A less common pattern of illness consists not only of acute episodic wheeze and cough with virus infection, but also includes *interval* symptoms between episodes, brought on by laughter or crying or at night, for instance.

3 The least frequent pattern in the community (although common in hospital outpatient practice) is the young child with *persistent wheeze* who even at his or her best appears to be functioning suboptimally. If well-adapted, fat and content, the term

'happy wheezer' is sometimes applied; however this is an inappropriate term which may encourage therapeutic nihilism. In addition, in such a child, symptoms may vary from day to day and acute episodes may complicate viral respiratory infections. Without lung function tests, the degree of persistent airway obstruction from which such children suffer can only be guessed.

Whereas for school-children disease patterns can be constructed from a combination of lung function (domiciliary PEF monitoring) and symptom diaries, for infants only the latter are available, supplemented by careful history taking to fill the gaps and to establish the severity of symptoms. These patterns of disease are of major importance in management for several reasons:

- as is the case for asthmatic school-children, evaluation of control is based on day-to-day symptoms, which thus determine the level of 'preventer' therapy;
- the therapy of acute episodes may differ from the management of interval symptoms, so that acute episodes need to be identified and their severity gauged;
- the outcome for children with purely episodic symptoms may be better than for those with interval symptoms, although this is disputed.

Acute viral bronchiolitis deserves special mention as a distinctive acute lower respiratory illness characteristically due to infection with the respiratory syncytial virus (RSV). In its hospitalized form it has a peak incidence at the age of about 3 months, much earlier than the onset of most wheezing disorders. Although the main symptom is cough rather than wheeze and the main physical signs are hyperinflation, intercostal and subcostal recession and crackles rather than rhonchi, the relevance of acute bronchiolitis to wheezing disorders is that the majority of infants (up to 90% in some studies) subsequently suffer recurrent, episodic viral wheeze during early childhood (Chapter 7b). Whether RSV causes lung 'damage', leading to recurrent wheeze, or whether RSV merely picks out infants at a particularly early age who are susceptible to recurrent wheezy LRI (or both) is not entirely clear (Chapter 3).[5] Recent research showing that premorbid lung function is abnormal in infants who develop bronchiolitis, supports the latter.[6] The fact that RSV is also responsible for much wheezing illness in slightly older infants and has an excellent long-term prognosis supports the latter hypothesis. Atopy, as normally defined, certainly has little role in acute bronchiolitis.

Acute bronchiolitis does nevertheless present particular problems because of the scale of the illness (1–2% of all infants in the UK require admission to hospital), the age and size of victims, the relatively frequent occurrence of severe respiratory failure needing high dependency or intensive care in up to 5% of hospital cases, the poor response to treatment and the predilection of children with other disorders (such as chronic lung disease of prematurity, congenital heart disease or cystic fibrosis) to be over-represented in hospitalized populations.

OTHER CAUSES OF WHEEZE

The respiratory system has a limited range of pathological and physiological responses. The range of symptoms and signs is even more limited. It is not surprising that a large number of conditions which affect airflow in the lower respiratory tract can cause wheeze (Table 9.2). In population terms, most of these are very rare (Figure 9.2) and in clinical terms many are obvious. (See also Chapters 6a and 13a.) But it is important to consider that some of these conditions may contribute to symptoms in children who are independently predisposed to wheeze – gastroesophageal reflux is an example (Chapter 7c); clues to differential diagnosis should always be sought and acted upon (Table 9.3); the presence of wheezing in one of these alternative conditions may in any case demand the same management as simple recurrent wheeze – chronic lung disease of prematurity (Chapter 13b) and cystic fibrosis (Chapter 13a) are examples.

The range of investigations which might be invoked to examine all the possible diagnoses is huge. In practice, the only 'routine' investigation of value is the chest radiograph. All others should be selected as appropriate.

Table 9.2 *Differential diagnosis of chronic or recurrent wheezing in infancy*

Developmental anomalies
 Tracheoesophageal fistula and related disorders
 Bronchomalacia (localized or generalized)
 Stove-pipe or rat-tail trachea
 Airway compression syndromes
 - vascular ring
 - anomalous origin of R. subclavian artery
 - bronchial or pericardial cyst
 Congenital heart disease (L–R shunting)
 Granulomata or polyps
Host defence defect
 Cystic fibrosis
 Ciliary dyskinesia
 Defects of immunity
 - severe combined immune deficiency
 - combined IgA and IgG_2 deficiency
Postviral syndromes
 Obliterative bronchiolitis
 Airway stricture or granuloma or lymphadenitis
Recurrent aspiration
 Gastroesophageal reflux
 Disorders of swallowing
 Neuromuscular disease
 Mechanical disorders
Perinatal disorders
 Chronic lung disease of prematurity
 Congenital infection

Paediatricians should have a low threshold for sweat testing, and CF genotyping, even in the presence of population screening for cystic fibrosis. The role of investigations for gastroesophageal reflux has been reviewed in Chapter 7c and other investigations are discussed below.

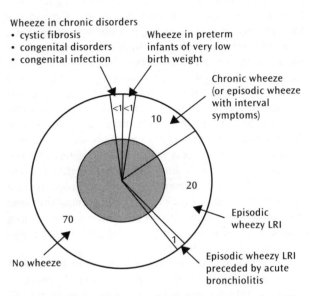

Figure 9.2 *Likely frequency of wheezing disorders in a UK population of infants. Figures are percentages. The central hatched area represents the random distribution of the atopic genotype (at about 30%) across all groups.*

EPIDEMIOLOGY

Natural history and risk factors

Assuming that they are causally related to wheeze, important factors for clinical management are those which are amenable to modification (Table 9.1). The feeding regime will have been decided by the time most infants develop wheezing. Similarly, it will be too late to avoid smoking in pregnancy! Household smoking is the only remediable factor and should be addressed (Chapter 7e). If parents cannot quit smoking, they should at least avoid smoking in the dwelling. Virus infections, the main precipitants of acute episodes (Chapter 7b), are more common in children from large families, with parents who have asthma and who attend day care. Where mother is a smoker, the risk of viral infections in day care may be the lesser of the two evils. These risk factors are reviewed in Chapters 2 and 3. Paradoxically, some risk factors for early wheeze (absence of breast-feeding and exposure to more viral infections) are protective against later allergic asthma,[7] although data on breast-feeding are disputed.[8] It is probable that risk factors for asthma and wheeze differ in high-risk and low-risk populations.[9]

Prospective studies of cohorts of newborn children have provided more reliable information on the natural history and prognosis of wheeze in young children (Chapter 3), but there are insufficient longitudinal data to be certain about the long-term outcome for individual wheezy infants.

Table 9.3

Clinical clue	Possible diagnosis
Perinatal and family history	
Symptoms present from birth; perinatal lung problem	Developmental anomaly; perinatal infection; CF; CLD; ciliary dyskinesia
Neonatal conjunctivitis	Chlamydial infection
Family history of unusual chest disease	CF; developmental anomaly
Severe upper respiratory tract disease	Defect of host defence
Recurrent febrile illnesses	Infective cause (host defence defect)
Symptoms and signs	
Persistent cough without wheeze	Recurrent aspiration; perinatal infection
Excessive vomiting	Recurrent aspiration
Feeding difficulty or symptoms during feeding	Developmental anomaly; recurrent aspiration
Abnormal voice or cry	Neurodevelopmental anomaly
Focal physical signs in the chest	Focal developmental disease; postviral syndrome
Crackles in the absence of acute infection	Pulmonary oedema or fibrosis; host defence defect
Inspiratory stridor as well as wheeze	Major central airway or laryngeal disorder
Failure to thrive	CF; host defence defect; gastroesophageal reflux
Unusual skin rashes (i.e. other than eczema)	Granulomatous or storage disorder
Investigations	
Focal or persistent radiological signs	Developmental disorder; post-infective disorder; recurrent aspirations; inhaled foreign body
Pattern of 'airway closure' or expiratory obstruction during lung function measurement	Bronchomalacia; central airway disease

CF: cystic fibrosis; CLD: chronic lung disease of prematurity.

For the majority of infants in the population, including those who present initially with bronchiolitis, symptoms are largely confined to the preschool years; by middle childhood except for those who develop atopic childhood asthma, most children become symptom-free (Figure 9.3). Persistent mild bronchial hyperresponsiveness may be a temporary feature of ex-bronchiolitics and indeed hospital-based cohorts of wheezy infants may also be different from population-based groups in the greater contribution of atopy and likelihood of later disease. Such differences could explain much of the controversy regarding prognosis when viewed from the different perspectives of hospital and community. Hospital-recruited populations are more likely to suffer long-term wheeze as are those children who have more attacks in their preschool years.[10] In the latter study, 33% of children who had four or more attacks by the age of four were still wheezy at ten. One large prospective population study in the USA has reported that a family history of either atopy or asthma is a risk factor for any lower respiratory illness in very young infants, while wheezing in patients (but not atopy) was a risk factor for doctor diagnosed asthma by 18 months.[11]

Prognostic factors for individual preschool wheezy children, gleaned from several studies, are given in Table 9.4. Even the best combination of predictions of later asthma in young recurrently wheezy children are of low sensitivity.[12] Inflammatory markers related to esinophil activation, have been shown to be of prognostic significance in some studies[13,14] but not others.[15,16] They may simply be markers of atopy, a well known association of

asthma! These conflicting studies were based on small numbers. If large numbers are needed to demonstrate prediction, then the tests will be too insensitive for clinical application.

In late adolescence and early adult life, follow-up studies of birth cohorts suggest that those who had LRI in the first 2 years are more prone to productive early morning cough and have a significant but small reduction in lung function[17] and enhancement of BHR.

There may be very long-term consequences to apparently benign wheezing infantile LRI. Recent evidence links premorbid lung function to the risk of early childhood wheezing and later asthma,[18–21] suggesting intrauterine risk factors, of which maternal cigarette smoking is one

Table 9.4 *Factors which indicate increased risk of later asthma, in young children with wheeze (from several sources)*

Risk factor	Size of effect
Parental asthma	+++
Personal eczema	+++
Wheeze without colds	++
Several episodes of wheeze	++
Older age at onset of wheeze	++
Allergic rhinitis	+
Eosinophilia (>95% CI)	+
Raised EPX or ECP	+
Serum soluble IL-2R level	+
Cockroach allergen load	+
Prematurity	+

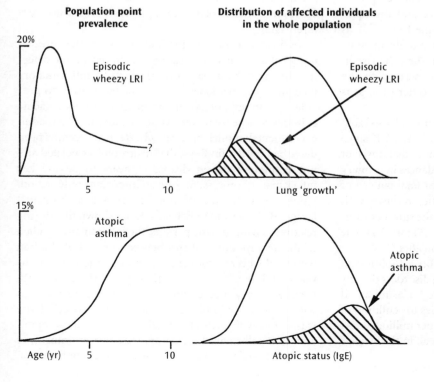

Figure 9.3 *The graphs indicate the changing prevalence of recurrent wheezy lower respiratory illness (LRI) and atopic asthma in childhood. The two distribution curves suggest the major recognizable factors which determine the distribution of affected individuals. For episodic wheezing LRI, an additional 'viral factor' is needed; for atopic asthma, perhaps bronchial responsiveness in response to aeroallergen sensitization is a necessary factor.*

example. Other data link size at birth and the presence of LRI in infancy with reduced lung function and excess mortality from chronic obstructive pulmonary disease (COPD) in late adult life.[22] These observations raise the intriguing possibility that fetal lung maldevelopment predisposes both to LRI in infancy and COPD later in life.[22]

Prevalence

The prevalence of wheezing disorders is difficult to establish, since there is no clear dividing line between health and disease. However, the recorded cumulative prevalence over the first years of life varies between 25–60% for different populations depending on definition.[23–27] The prevalence of viral respiratory tract infection[28] and the influence of smoking and social contacts are important variables.[29,30]

Currently in the UK preschool children account for about 80% of admissions to hospital for childhood asthma and wheezing disorders and about half of asthma admissions at all ages. These disorders account for 25% of all acute admissions of children to hospital and this figure may increase to 50% during RSV epidemics when acute bronchiolitis looms large. In Sweden, most of the recent increase in hospital admissions for obstructive airway disease in all age groups was due to the under-fives and this was not explained by RSV bronchiolitis in the under-ones.[31] In contrast, the distribution of wheezing disorders in the community reveals quite a different distribution (Figure 9.2), with mild episodic wheeze being the most common variety. It would appear from the results of a UK cohort study, that the reported prevalence of both episodic/transient wheeze and multiple/persistent wheeze has increased during the 1990s.[27] If, as is believed, the former pattern occurs mainly in non-atopic and the latter in atopic children, then the rise in preschool wheezing cannot simply be ascribed to the increase in allergic sensitization. Some other process is at work.

Recent trends suggest that the 'epidemic' of wheezing in preschool children may have peaked in the UK since 1990–93, admissions to hospital with a diagnosis of asthma or related conditions[32] and attendances in primary care[33] have declined nationwide. The seasonal pattern of presentation in primary care in the UK ties in closely with the school year, showing a major peak as the summer vacation ends and viral infections proliferate (Figure 9.4). The peak for hospital admissions follows soon after.[34]

With the exception of acute viral bronchiolitis and bronchopulmonary dysplasia, wheezing disorders of early life are very rarely fatal. The death rate for asthma and related conditions for England and Wales for children of all ages, has fallen from about 4.5 to 2.5 per million at risk per year, over the last 15 years, with a peak in the teenage years.

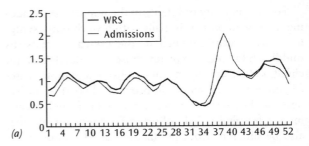

(a)

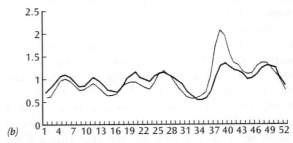

(b)

Figure 9.4 *Weekly seasonal indices of general practice episodes and hospital admissions by age group plotted as 3-week moving averages. (a) 0–4 years; (b) 5–14 years. WRS weekly return service. (From ref. 34.)*

MECHANISMS

Physiopathology

Until recently the pathological basis for airway disease in infancy and young children was known only from fatal cases of acute bronchiolitis and chronic lung disease of prematurity. Neither situation is representative of the common patterns of wheezing disease, which are very rarely fatal.

Indirect, non-invasive methods which use the nose as a model of acute airway disease or which rely on the detection of the stable breakdown products of inflammatory mediators and cytokines in the urine have begun to provide data to support an inflammatory process in acute episodes of wheeze in very young children.[35,36] An adult experimental model of viral wheeze has recently been described.[37,38] Its findings, that neutrophil-associated and not eosinophil driven disease, appears to be the key inflammatory process, may be an important observation. Using the technique of non-bronchoscopic bronchial lavage (BAL), a team in Belfast, UK has shown that during relatively asymptomatic periods, the inflammatory milieu of the airways differentiates between preschool children with viral wheeze, atopic non-asthmatic and atopic asthmatic children.[39] In a bronchoscopic BAL study of 20 wheezy, mostly atopic children (mean age 15 months) with 'episodes' or 'prolonged' wheeze, excessive cellularity was found with increases in all cell types.[40] Eosinophils and mast cell derived mediators were not prominent, in contrast to older asthmatics. This is further confirmation of the separate phenotypes which comprise preschool wheezing disease.

Methods of studying airway inflammation in young children have recently been reviewed.[41] As yet, they do not contribute to clinical management (Chapter 6d). Most indirect methods of studying eosinophilic airway inflammation from blood markers simply relate to atopic status,[16,42] but some markers may relate more specifically to viral wheeze.[43]

The nature of viral susceptibility is unknown or even whether children with wheezy LRI have more viral illness than other children. There is weak evidence for a familial aggregation of lower respiratory symptoms,[44] but not of increased bronchial responsiveness[20,45,46] or of atopy.[47] Risk factors for transient wheeze differ from those for persistent disease.[48] Knowledge of the specific virus involved may allow appropriate immunization therapy to be considered in the future.

That acute episodes are predominantly viral in aetiology is not in doubt (Chapter 7b). Other organisms also contribute. Using molecular techniques *Chlamydia pneumoniae* (about 5% of cases) and *Mycoplasma pneumoniae* (less than 5%) have been reported.[49,50] Bacterial secondary infections are probably very uncommon, but there are no reliable data.

Pulmonary physiology

The developmental basis for infant wheeze and the physiological abnormalities in wheezy infants has been described earlier (Chapters 3 and 5). Much knowledge has been gained by *airway function tests* but the demanding nature of such measurements means that there are no tests which can easily be applied in the routine management of infants. New techniques based simply on tidal flow–volume curves recorded during natural sleep have been shown to have diagnostic value[51] in infants with noisy breathing (Figure 9.5). A number of more demanding methods have been used in research in this age group (Chapter 5). Some techniques were analagous to those used in older subjects, and may thus be more easily interpreted and more useful in longitudinal studies.[52]

The issue of *bronchial hyperresponsiveness* and its role in preschool wheeze and asthma is contentious. Two prospective studies have shown that female infants with levels of airway responsiveness in the first few weeks of life had the greatest risk of infantile wheeze[19,20] suggesting the importance of fetal developmental or genetic determinants of BHR and wheeze. However, later in infancy, there was no difference in bronchial responsiveness between those with and without LRI[20,45,46] possibly because of the interaction of many postnatal environmental factors. One group has found neonatal bronchial responsiveness to be a risk factor for asthma (but not BHR) later in childhood.[21] Less invasive techniques for measuring BHR in infants may permit a better evaluation of their role in the clinical management of wheezy infants.[53,54]

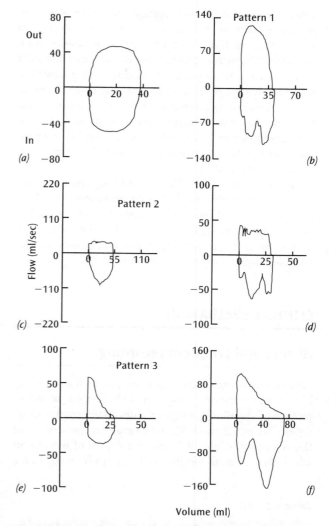

Figure 9.5 *Tidal breathing flow–volume loop patterns. (a) Normal pattern: round-shaped inspiratory (in) and expiratory (out) limbs. (b) Pattern 1: irregular fluctuations of the inspiratory flow (inspiratory fluttering), with normal expiratory shape (associated with laryngomalacia). (c) Pattern 2: flattening of the expiratory limb of the loop with a normal (or variably flattened) inspiratory shape (associated with an airway obstruction between the glottis and mainstem bronchi). (d) Association between expiratory flattening (Pattern 2) and inspiratory fluttering (Pattern 1) in a child with laryngomalacia and primary tracheomalacia. (e) Pattern 3: early expiratory peak flow followed by reduced flow rates at lower volumes, with normal inspiration (associated with reactive airway disease). (f) Association between peripheral airflow limitation (Pattern 3) and inspiratory fluttering (Pattern 1) in a child with laryngomalacia and asthma. (From ref. 51)*

Disturbances of *gas exchange* are invariable in wheezy infants. The ready availability of oximetry has taught us that moderate hypoxaemia (SaO_2 85–92%) is common in acute severe episodes (Chapter 6b). This puts infants at risk of acute severe hypoxaemia if, for instance, against a background of moderate hypoxaemia they develop additional episodes of obstructive apnoea during sleep. This is a significant risk, especially in young infants. Additional factors, such as chronic lung disease of prematurity (Chapter 13b) or congenital heart disease (e.g. ventricular septal defect), put infants at great risk since exacerbation of pre-existing pulmonary hypertension can lead to right-to-left shunt or exaggerated intrapulmonary ventilation/perfusion imbalance with acute, severe hypoxaemia. Sedation of wheezy infants for investigations may exacerbate hypoxaemia.[55]

In severe *respiratory failure*, ventilatory compensation for hypoxaemia becomes impaired with consequent CO_2 retention. Arterial blood gas estimations are needed in critical cases, although in general, other clinical features decide the need for intensive care or mechanical ventilation (see assessment of severity below).

CLINICAL EVALUATION

History and symptom recording

Careful recording of the perinatal, personal and family history allows the doctor or nurse to build up a subjective picture of the illness, to glean clues to alternative diagnoses (Tables 9.2 and 9.3), and to evaluate the severity of the symptoms (Table 9.5) and the degree of disruption which they cause to family life. The steps involved in the

evaluation of an infant are outlined in Figure 9.6 and in detail in Figure 1.4 (Chapter 1).

Severity can be defined in various ways (Table 9.5). The severity before starting treatment gives a guide to the appropriate starting level for therapy. Adequate control is defined as the abolition of symptoms by therapy or their amelioration to a level which renders them trivial.

Questions should be directed in such a way that the pattern of acute and chronic symptoms emerges (Chapter 1, Figure 1.2). Particular attention should be paid to perinatal factors (Chapter 13b), gastrointestinal symptoms (Chapter 7c), cigarette smoke exposure (Chapter 7e) and the timing of symptoms in relation to the introduction of a weaning diet (Chapter 7d). Inhalant allergens may be important triggers and should not be overlooked.

In order to evaluate the cardinal symptoms of wheeze and cough (Chapter 6a) attention should be paid to sleep disturbance, disruption of feeding, the relationship to non-specific provoking factors such as laughter, exercise or smoke or to specific factors such as viral respiratory tract infections. In my experience, the report of wheeze provoked by laughter (tickle-induced asthma), crying or exercise implies airway hyperresponsiveness and should have the same implications for diagnosis and management as a report of exercise-induced asthma in an older child. There are many features which suggest alternative diagnoses (Table 9.3). Two of the most important clues to important alternative diagnoses are: the presence of persistent 'moist' cough (apart from colds), which suggests chronic infection, and wheeze of very sudden onset,

Table 9.5

Severity or control	Pattern of illness		
	Steady state-reversible	Steady state-irreversible	Acute episode
Mild (good control)	Intermittent mild symptoms (wheeze, dry cough) which do not limit any normal activity by day or night	Unremitting symptoms (wheeze, dry cough) which rarely disturb the child, by day or night	Symptoms worse than steady state, with limitation of active play, and some sleep disruption, but not of feeding or sedentary activities; may respond to β_2-agonist
Moderate	Intermittent symptoms including breathlessness, which limit vigorous activity but not feeding or sedentary activities and rarely disturb sleep	Unremitting symptoms with breathlessness, which limit vigorous activities and disturb sleep several times each week	Symptoms worse than steady-state, with unwillingness to play, misery and frequent sleep disruption; may respond to β_2-agonist
Severe (poor control)	Intermittent symptoms which affect all but sedentary activities on most days, with sleep disruption on most nights	Unremitting symptoms which limit all but sedentary activities, and wake the child every night	Will not feed or play actively; too breathless to lie down; brief or no response to β_2-agonist
Life-threatening		Unremitting breathlessness with misery, difficulty feeding, talking or playing; frequent nightly sleep disruption	Too breathless to feed, talk or play; frightened, cyanosed; no response to β_2-agonist

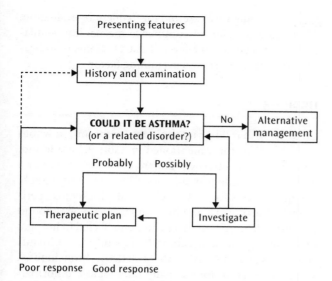

Figure 9.6 *The bare bones of diagnosis. The diagnosis is always provisional in very young children. The algorithm is presented more fully in Figure 1.4, Chapter 1.*

Table 9.6 *Features of a severe acute episode in infancy*

Unable to settle, sleep, or lie down
Unable to feed or drink
Agitated, restless, frightened
Cyanosis*, $SaO_2 < 90\%$
Tachypnoea (>60–70) with use of accessory muscles of breathing
Tachycardia (>150)

*Suggests life-threatening airway obstruction.

which may be the only clue to the presence of an inhaled foreign body.

The older the child, the more informative is the assessment of response to prior therapy, especially inhaled β_2-agonists and inhaled or oral corticosteroids (assuming an adequate delivery device and adequate compliance). Neither is especially effective in young infants, so failure of response does not have the same diagnostic implications as in older children and adults.

Symptom recording systems such as diary cards for school-children with asthma are appropriate for infants. The accuracy of such systems and the statistical treatment of symptom 'scores' have not been adequately determined (Chapter 6a). There are no criteria for defining or quantifying acute episodes and no 'objective' lung function measurements to back up symptom reporting. The work of Clough and colleagues on the definition of acute episodes in older children may be applicable to infants,[56] but it is of interest that even this group uses subjective methods to define episodes in their own research![57]

The evaluation of the severity of acute severe episodes in infants demands different questions. The features which suggest a severe attack requiring management in hospital are listed in Table 9.6. Scoring systems for acute bronchiolitis and other acute episodes have been devised but never fully evaluated for interobserver bias or statistically justified (Chapter 6a). Nevertheless, they do provide a simple means to detect trends and have been used, in default of objective measures, in therapeutic trials.[58]

Physical examination

A remarkable variety of physical features is found in wheezy babies: thin or fat; happy or miserable when wheezy; atopic features such as eczema or none; hyperinflated chest or small, possibly hypoplastic thoracic cage; crackles during acute episodes or simply wheezes. Their significance is not always obvious. Physical signs are important in the identification of alternative diagnoses and in the assessment of severity (Tables 9.3 and 9.6) as well as in the ongoing management of acute episodes. A completely normal examination does not preclude significant morbidity, especially if the disease is episodic in nature.

Examining *wheezy toddlers* may be a challenge to the inexperienced. In general, however, there are no particular features which do not apply to older children (Chapter 6a). Again, except in an acute episode, most children have no abnormal residual signs. The presence of abnormalities between episodes is thus of great importance, implying chronic (poorly controlled) inflammation or some other underlying structural or functional abnormality (Table 9.2).

A common clinical problem is posed by the presence of 'transmitted', 'rattly' or 'noisy' breath sounds (euphonically called 'ruttles' in the English East Midlands[4]). The quality and amplitude of breath sounds seem to convey little useful information and in fact one often wonders whether the stethoscope is not a redundant instrument, retained simply as a badge of office. Features such as hyperinflation, recession or the use of accessory muscles are better guides to severity. Asymmetrical breath sounds, persistent crackles and a persistent wet cough are important clues to alternative diagnoses.

Investigations

LUNG FUNCTION MEASUREMENTS

Measurements of lung mechanics and bronchial responsiveness have played an important part in research into the mechanisms, epidemiology and therapeutics of wheezing disorders. Most methods are technically demanding, and in infants, usually require a face-mask for tidal flow and volume measurements, and sedation.[59] Techniques based on non-invasive monitoring of the motion of the chest wall and abdomen during tidal breathing have been developed, and could be useful in monitoring. Methods of monitoring based on breath-sound analysis promise to be useful for monitoring children in hospital or at home. New methods of signal processing may allow patterns of tidal breathing to be analysed on a continuous basis in the near future, to monitor children at home or in hospital in order to detect changes in breathing pattern which indicate changes in airway obstruction. Details of infant lung function techniques are provided in Chapter 6b.

Of the range of techniques available for measuring airway function in awake preschool children, the following are currently practicable, but all require the use of a mouthpiece:

- *spirometry*, success is variable,[60,61] although with incentive training, 80% success is reported.[62]
- *interrupter methods* for measuring resistance (Rint), based on tidal breathing methods, which have been used to demonstrate bronchodilator responsiveness for diagnostic or therapeutic purposes in toddlers.[63,64]
- *plethysmography* with the infant seated on parent's knee, to provide an index of specific airway resistance (sRaw).[65]
- *impedance* methods for measuring airway resistance and reactance to which, like the interrupter technique, are very sensitive to upper airway distortion.[65]

Disturbed gas exchange is a feature of acute wheezing episodes and bronchiolitis. Clinical observations suggest that infants who enter an acute episode with pre-existing problems such as chronic lung disease of prematurity may quickly exhaust their ability to maintain alveolar ventilation and ventilation/perfusion matching in the lung and thus develop more severe hypoxaemia than those who are free of disease between attacks. Oximetry is the appropriate technique to detect hypoxaemia and to monitor the response to oxygen therapy and bronchodilators. Nebulized β_2-agonist bronchodilators may worsen hypoxaemia but this does not seem to happen with β_2-agonists given by MDI and spacer or with ipratropium bromide or adrenaline. Transcutaneous PO_2 and PCO_2 devices are useful for trend monitoring or for detecting significant change after interventions, but their absolute accuracy is poor and they have been superseded by oximetry in clinical practice.

For critical or deteriorating acute severe episodes or bronchiolitis, direct *arterial puncture* is occasionally useful. It should be achievable so quickly in a sleeping infant that the sample is in the syringe before the steady state is disturbed by crying. Otherwise, thorough analgesia should be used, starting with a local anaesthetic skin patch and followed by local anaesthetic infiltration around the radial artery (no adrenaline (epinephrine) should be used in the local anaesthetic). The key measurement is the arterial PCO_2 since hypoxaemia is likely to have been treated with oxygen therapy and is in any case detectable by oximetry. $PaCO_2$ values of 6–8 kPa suggest early respiratory failure and such infants should be nursed in a high dependency area; values over 8 kPa in conjunction with signs of exhaustion and a rising inspired oxygen concentration indicate the need for intensive care and for frequent re-evaluation. Although a decision to commence mechanical ventilation is not made on the level of $PaCO_2$ alone, blood gas analysis is an important determining factor.

Imaging

Children with mild or intermittent symptoms, in whom none of the features mentioned in Table 9.3 are found, need no further investigation. Troublesome wheeze or a first acute episode demands a simple chest radiograph. Abnormalities such as bronchial wall thickening, peribronchial shadowing and hyperinflation are often found in chest radiographs of older children referred to hospital for the management of asthma.[66] In a study of 101 infants (median age 9 months) with 'obstructive bronchiolitis', Wennergren *et al.* found many radiological abnormalities including perihilar infiltrates (19%), peripheral infiltrates (32%) and atelectasis (3%).[67] Radiological changes were not useful predictions of outcome; 70% of the children were symptom free at the age of 10 years.[68] Unexpected diagnoses can occasionally be made simply as a result of chest radiograph (Chapter 6a). Children who have features listed in Table 9.3 will all need a plain chest radiograph as a minimum.

A repeat chest radiograph is not needed for subsequent episodes unless clinical features suggest major segmental collapse or consolidation or an air leak. Specialized imaging under sedation or anaesthesia (CT, MRI, angiography and ventilation/perfusion radioisotope scanning) is performed rarely in order to follow up clues to alternative diagnoses (Table 9.3 and Chapter 6a).

Host defence and allergy

Sweat testing should be performed if there is a family history of cystic fibrosis or if there are clinical features compatible with the disease, such as a failure to thrive, malabsorption syndrome, meconium ileus equivalent or troublesome chest disease. The latter may include persistent or moist cough, repeated febrile LRI and unusually delayed recovery from acute viral bronchiolitis. With the recognition of new gene polymorphisms, the old certainties of an 'all or none' approach to the diagnosis of cystic fibrosis have weakened.

Allergy tests to identify either a general atopic predisposition (serum IgE level) or specific sensitization (by skin-prick testing or specific IgE test) are increasingly useful in children beyond the first year. Apart from the rare response to food allergens, the long-term significance of which is often unclear, skin testing is generally negative in infants, even those who are subsequently shown to have been sensitized.[69] A positive skin test to inhalant allergens has low sensitivity but high specificity for allergic disease in a wheezy infant. The immunological process which takes place during the 'silent phase' between early aeroallergen sensitization and the subsequent onset of clinical disease is a topic of much research (Chapter 7a). Atopy plays a significant role in only a minority of wheezy infants, even those with atopic parents, but an increasing role in older wheezers, as discussed earlier.

The value of *other tests* of immune function such as total serum immunoglobulin levels and IgG subclasses is dubious. The reference range is very wide in healthy infants (Appendix). Without evidence of transient neonatal respiratory distress followed by troublesome ENT infections, tests for ciliary dyskinesia are probably unwarranted.[70]

Other investigations

Claims that *bronchoscopy* reveals many unsuspected abnormalities may be the result of over-enthusiasm by the bronchoscopist! Bronchoscopy is clearly indicated for some problems.[71,72] A study of 30 wheezy infants under 18 months who were poorly responsive to β_2-agonists, reported 40% segmental trachomalacia (over 50% under 6 months of age) mainly due to extrinsic compression.[73] The fact that the prevalence fell with increasing age raises questions about the relevance of the findings, and whether dynamic narrowing was mistakenly reported as trachomalacia. A similar rate of anomaly has been reported in infants with chronic cough.[74] At the moment, this sort of investigation is still in the realms of research, but gleaning as much information as possible from each clinically justified bronchoscopic procedure is imperative.[40]

The relationship between cause and effect in *gastroesophageal reflux* and wheeze is often unclear and the interpretation of relevant investigations is rarely straightforward (Chapter 7c). *Microbiological studies* provide little therapeutic information but do help in the management of a clinical service by permitting isolation and cohort nursing of potentially infectious acutely wheezy children and by giving warning of the onset of an impending epidemic (of RSV infection, for instance). Certain adenoviral subtypes may lead to obliterative bronchiolitis; bronchiectasis or airway granuloma formation, especially but not exclusively in malnourished children, or those with concurrent viral infections (measles and *Herpes simplex*, for example).[75] It is important to diagnose such infections for prognostic reasons. It is doubtful whether awareness of chlamydial, mycoplasma or bacterial pathogens in the airways of uncomplicated wheezy young children alters management or prognosis.

Reaching a diagnosis

In infants and very young children, to a greater extent than for older children, reaching a diagnosis of asthma (or one of its phenotypes) is simply one stage in an interative process (Figure 1.4, Chapter 1). The central question 'Could it be asthma?' implies the provisional nature of the diagnosis. It should be addressed at every point

of contact between the child and family and a health professional.

As implied above, the reasons for this cautious approach in infants and young children are many: the frequency and importance of alternative diagnosis; the weak relationship to markers of allergy; lack of physiological measurement tools; the poor response to 'standard' anti-asthma therapy; the rapidly changing prognosis. Nevertheless, at the end of the period of clinical evaluation, the child's parent(s) need(s) to be told a diagnosis and given a management plan!

THERAPEUTIC MEASURES

General aspects of management

The aims of management are to abolish or minimize symptoms with the minimum disturbance to the child and family. Good management depends on mutual respect and understanding between the families of young children and health professionals. More than at any other age, care in the community by community paediatric nurses, health visitors and public health doctors supplements the work of family doctors, paediatricians and hospital staff. The tangible outcome of medical consultation should be a guided self-management plan for the family, built on information and advice, which takes into account the extent to which the family can cope with self-management decisions, and which is based as far as possible on published evidence.

A number of international and national consensus statements dealing with adult and childhood asthma have been published, but only one deals purely with childhood asthma and has considered the management of infants and young children in any detail.[76] It must be acknowledged that the evidence base for management in early childhood is slim.

Avoiding trigger factors

Cigarette smoke is probably the major avoidable factor, although it is possible that many of its damaging effects takes place during fetal life (Chapter 7e). Apart from *viral infection* against which active and passive immunization are now possible for certain viruses (RSV and influenza A, for example), there are few other important triggers. Overcrowding day care and the presence of several older siblings may increase the risk of viral infection, as does day care.[77,78] Paradoxically, the increased risk of wheezing in the first years of life translates into a reduced risk of asthma at school age. *Indoor air pollution* may aggravate the risk of wheeze.[56] *Breast-feeding* probably reduces the risk of wheezing LRI, whatever its disputed value in relation to atopic disease (Chapter 2),[9,26,79] the major effect occurring in the first two years.

Primary *allergen avoidance* measures in general are contentious and there is an emerging realization that the effects of exposure (or avoidance) during pregnancy or early infancy may have different risks and benefits to children at high risk (i.e. for atopic or asthmatic families) and to those at low risk. Recent evidence suggests that primary avoidance of dust mite before birth and during the first year reduces the prevalence of chronic and severe wheeze (but not virus-induced episodes) in infants of atopic parents.[80]

Atopic asthma may begin in infancy. A strong family history and active eczema are pointers. Tertiary intervention by reduction of sources of aero-allergens such as house-dust mites and cats may be worthwhile if there is supporting evidence from the history (such as wheezing after visiting grandma and her cats) and positive tests for allergic sensitization. The house-dust mite content of infants' bedding is minimal except for fleece bedding in New Zealand, although the mite may even thrive on the surface of impermeable mattress coverings. The main source of aerial Der pI is natural wool carpeting in humid, centrally heated houses (especially those with furry pets). Measures to reduce house-dust mite levels are reviewed in Chapter 14.

The evidence to support an alteration in *feeding practices* for infants or young children with wheezing illnesses. However, where there is a clear history of the onset of wheeze with weaning from breast to bottle milk or with the introduction of specific foodstuffs such as egg, especially with the supporting evidence of food-sensitive eczema, a trial of a dietician-supervised elimination diet is worthwhile. Wheeze is very rarely the sole manifestation of allergy to cow's milk. Soya-based infant formula should not be used as a substitute for cow's milk formula, since sensitization to soya is common in cow's milk-sensitive infants[81] and its use does not reduce the risk of wheezing in the infants of atopic families.[82] Trial periods of 4–6 weeks should be allowed on low-allergy formula, with phased reintroduction if no benefit occurs. With clear benefit, supervised reintroduction should be postponed until the child is 2 years old.

Pet ownership is a controversial issue, some cross-sectional studies seeming to show a protective effect against allergy, of cat ownership. However, prospective studies clearly show that cat ownership leads to sensitization.[80, 83] Once sensitization has occurred, avoiding the ever-present cat antigen Fel d I is almost impossible.

Education

The aim of part of every consultation should be to provide information about the nature of the illness and its management, according to the parents' wants and needs; but information by itself is unlikely to improve their child's health. Training is required in the skills needed to monitor the disease, to fill in record cards and to administer medication. Although advice is often accepted better when provided by a trained nurse or other health professional rather than by a doctor, its quality may be less good (Chapter 18). The value of guided self-management programs in improving healthcare in preschool children has not been proved by randomized trial. In fact, a recent two-centre UK trial of a structured discharge programme for 200 preschool children attending an Emergency Department or admitted to a Children's Ward (incorporating parental training, a guided self-management plan, written information and follow-up session reinforcement) failed to show any effect on subsequent morbidity or caregiver quality of life over any part of the subsequent 12 months.[84] The contrast with the outcome of similar research in older children is striking and suggests either that current management guidelines are inappropriate for the (mainly) episodic pattern of preschool wheezing disease, or that our 'educational' techniques are not appropriate.

Anybody who deals with the parents of sick children must appreciate their anxiety. This may lead to questions which the doctor may consider irrelevant, but which should be patiently tackled with the help of published literature. The most frequent question concerns *prognosis*. Explaining that the frequency and severity of acute episodes in infancy tend to decline with age and do not necessarily carry a poor long-term prognosis can be very reassuring (Table 9.4 and Chapter 3).

Drug therapy: review of therapeutic trials

GENERAL CONSIDERATIONS

In the era of evidence-based medicine (EBM), the double-blind randomized controlled trial (RCT) is master and the systematic review (with or without meta-analysis) is king. But clinical trials are usually designed to show efficacy; effectiveness in clinical practice is always much less, partly because motivation and therefore adherence falls and partly because RCTs are usually performed on small, highly selected groups of subjects, whereas their results are often generalized indiscriminately. Systematic review has the aura of extreme objectivity, but in practice, it too can be subject to bias, as illustrated by the conflicting outcomes of two reviews of the evidence relating to house-dust mite avoidance.[85,86] Nevertheless, RCTs are the essential starting point for rational prescribing.

Many variables demand consideration in any review of clinical trials of asthma. In young children, some of these are particularly important (Table 9.7) in determining the validity and generalizability of clinical trials. Symptom pattern (episodes or chronic symptoms) has already been emphasized, but is rarely taken into account in clinical trials. A large proportion of all published trials concern the short-term, physiological outcome of single doses of bronchodilators administered by jet-nebulizer. While this sort of study may be important, for instance in dose-ranging investigations, as technical studies or as a preliminary to

Table 9.7 *Therapeutic trials in wheezy infants – important variables to note*

Target population
Hospital or domiciliary
Acute episodes or intercurrent symptoms
Age

Drug administration
Dose and form of agent
Device for administration
Route of administration

Trial design
Randomized controlled trial or other format
Size of study and statistical power

Outcome measures
Physiological or clinical, short- or long-term
Toxicity

a full clinical trial, the results cannot be generalized to most clinical situations. Very few studies have been carried out at home.

The influence of devices used for the administration of aerosols on the dose delivered to the lungs of infants has only recently been explored (Chapter 8b). Metered dose inhalers (MDI) can be used with a spacer and integral face-mask from the neonatal period. Small volume spacers, close application of the face-mask, single activations and minimal residence time are all important in increasing efficiency of drug delivery.[87] Infants who fight the application of a face-mask, a problem which increases with age, may peacefully accept their therapy while asleep. Crying reduces drug availability.[88] Although nebulized therapy is widely used, we find it less acceptable for most young children and subject to many technical difficulties, both for freely breathing and for intubated subjects. A systematic review and two trials in infants have demonstrated slight superiority for MDI spacer over jet-nebulizer for bronchodilator therapy,[89–91] although for both, the dose delivered to the lungs is very small (<1–2%), lower in younger subjects[92] and very variable.[93]

Age is an important determinant of the response to treatment. Animal studies have shown major developmental changes in the structure of the airways[94,95] an in the distribution of receptors[96] during postnatal maturation as well as in the relative dimensions of the various structures.[97] These and other factors will have differential effects with age on such important effects as smooth muscle contractility,[98] airway collapsibility with bronchodilators[67] and aerosol distribution.[100] One other major age-related factor which limits pulmonary deposition of aerosol is the nose which acts as a natural filter.[101]

Bronchodilators

A review of *short-acting β₂-agonists* in infant wheeze in 1984 concluded that while clinicians recognized a clinical response in some patients, former clinical trials had shown little benefit.[102] The efficacy of these drugs increases with increasing age. Since then, many more studies have been performed, but the message is the same. It is possible to draw a number of conclusions.

1 A single dose of nebulized albuterol (salbutamol) in infants with acute wheeze or bronchiolitis or after recovery commonly leads to a transient worsening of hypoxaemia[103–107] and no change or even a diminution in forced expiratory flows by the squeeze technique[108–110] in contrast to the passive deflation method.[111] Airway resistance as measured plethysmographically during quiet breathing in a convalescent or recovery phase either changes little[108,110,112] or seems to improve.[113,114] A novel transfer impedance method showed significant (25%) reduction in airway resistance.[112]

2 The transient adverse effects of nebulized β₂ agonists may be in part due to the pH of the aerosol and to other additives.[104,115] Another explanation is that the airway effects of β₂-agonists simply alter the compliance (floppiness) of the airway wall rendering it more likely to narrow during expiration, without sufficient compensatory increase in airway calibre, in the youngest children. β₂-agonist-induced pulmonary vasodilation then causes (transient) worsening of V/Q imbalance. MDI/spacer administration of β₂-agonists appears to be less troublesome and possibly clinically more effective[90,113] than nebulizer, and is the method of choice.[89]

3 There is no evidence for an overall beneficial clinical effect of nebulized β₂-agonists in acute severe episodes in infancy or acute bronchiolitis,[114–118] although some infants may seem to respond. A systematic review suggested marginal benefits in recurrent episodes in (presumably older) children in the first 2 years of life.[119]

4 Regular short-acting inhaled β₂-agonist therapy is no better than placebo in infants with chronic wheeze.[120]

5 Nevertheless, β₂-agonists do seem to protect against bronchial challenge[121–123] and to hasten recovery from challenge in infants,[124] suggesting that there are effective β₂-receptors in infant airway smooth muscle. Lack of a β₂ response in acute episodes implies that the mechanisms of airway obstruction during natural acute episodes and during artificially induced airway obstruction differ. Failure of β₂-agonists to cause bronchodilation, despite their protective role in challenge, is in direct contrast to the situation of β₂-agonist 'tolerance' induced in adults by excessive β₂-agonist use. Thus, the situation in infants is not equivalent to 'tolerance' in older subjects. It is possible that acute viral episodes, the commonest form of asthma in young children, lead to transient down-regulation of β₂-receptors on airway smooth muscle,[125] hence reducing the efficacy of β₂-agonists in acute episodes of wheeze or asthma (at all ages[126]).

6 The likelihood of a clinical response to β_2-agonists increases with age.[127,128] This may be explained partly by the greater dose delivered to larger children by some (but not all) devices.[129,130]

In contrast to β_2-agonists, *adrenaline* (epinephrine) has benefits on clinical scores, oxygenation and lung function.[117,131,132] Its use deserves further clinical evaluation in acute severe episodes, where an adrenergic effect may serve to reduce submucosal swelling of vascular origin. Whether repeated administration could lead to rebound mucosal oedema has not been ascertained.

Long-acting β_2-agonists are commonly added to low-dose inhaled corticosteroids in managing poorly controlled asthma in young children, despite almost total lack of clinical trial data in this age group. One bronchoprotection study of salmeterol delivered by MDI and spacer to preschool children showed significant effects on methacholine induced bronchoconstriction, of single 50 and 100 μg doses, after a 1 hour interval.[133] Duration of protection is unknown. Recent concerns about the development of β_2-tolerance with chronic use, should engender caution[134] (Chapter 8a).

There is a perception that the *antimuscarinic, anticholinergic bronchodilator* ipratropium bromide is more effective in wheezy infants than β_2-agonists, but a recent systematic review[135] did not support its 'uncritical' use in children under 2 years. Another recommended it as add-on therapy to β_2-agonists for severe asthma attacks in children of school age.[136] Single dose physiological studies have also proved disappointing.[137,138] The complexity of the muscarinic receptor system[139] raises the possibility of developmental changes which could be exploited by increased selectivity of receptor subtype agonists or antagonists.

Corticosteroids

Very few of the variables listed in Table 9.7 have been adequately addressed in clinical trials of corticosteroid therapy in infants and young children. Some statements can be made and practical conclusions drawn (Table 9.8).

1 Clinical trials over a 30-year period have failed to demonstrate any benefit from oral or inhaled corticosteroids in acute viral bronchiolitis.[140–149] A meta-analysis would be helpful.

2 Short course oral or inhaled (high-dose) corticosteroids have trivial or no effects on acute wheeze in infancy,[150–153] but one trial has shown an effect of dexamethasone.[154] A single i.m. dose of dexamethasone may be as effective (or ineffective) as a 5-day course of prednisolone.[155]

3 Double-blind studies have shown benefit from regular inhaled corticosteroids as preventer therapy for chronic wheeze in infants and toddlers when administered by MDI/spacer[156–160] or nebulizer.[161–166]

4 Regular inhaled corticosteroids are of no benefit in purely episodic viral wheeze at any age.[167]

The apparent paradox of the lack of effect of corticosteroid prophylaxis in acute episodes in the absence of interval symptoms, contrasting with their beneficial effects on both acute and interval symptoms in those with chronic (relapsing) asthma requires explanation. A hypothetical explanation is provided in Figure 9.7.

There are data showing medium-term safety of inhaled steroid therapy in infants and young children.[168–169] One study raised concern about effects on linear growth.[159] One particular aspect of long-term inhaled steroid therapy which has not been addressed adequately is the potential to inhibit the active process of alveolization which takes place over the first postnatal year (Chapter 4a). Doses administered to infants and toddlers tend to be high, in part to compensate for deposition in the nose by nasal filtration of droplets. If nasal deposition leads to absorption, the potential for systemic effects, as well as local effects in the nose, will be proportionately greater in infants, at an age when the rate of body growth is maximal.

Other agents

A recent systematic review[170] showed that *cromoglycate* (cromolyn sodium) is ineffective in preschool children despite an apparently protective effect against acute challenge with nebulized distilled water.[171] Similarly, *theophylline* has never been shown to work in infants with bronchiolitis[172] or acutely wheezy preschool children as emergency therapy.[173] A meta-analysis reported no

Table 9.8 *The efficacy of corticosteroid therapy in wheezy infants and preschool children*

| Therapy | Acute viral bronchiolitis | Episodic viral wheeze | Chronic wheeze | |
			Episodic	Interval symptoms
Acute therapy:				
Inhaled	0	±	?	−
Oral	0	?	?	−
Chronic therapy	0*	0	+	++

*For several weeks after the acute illness.

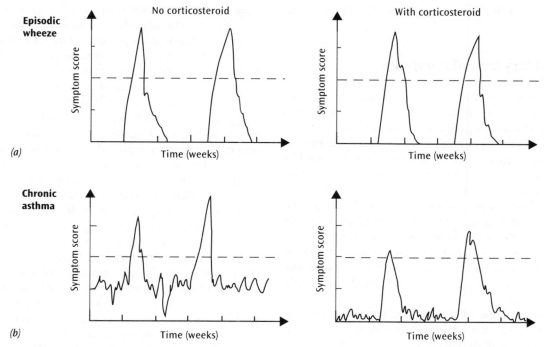

Figure 9.7 *Possible explanation for the apparent paradox that inhaled corticosteroid preventer therapy (a) appears to have little or no effect on acute attacks of purely episodic viral wheeze (without interval symptoms), but (b) ameliorates episodes in children with chronic asthma (with interval symptoms as well as acute epidsodes), by reducing the variable baseline of interval symptoms.*

significant benefit in older children.[174] The resurgence of interest in its low-dose, anti-inflammatory actions suggests the need for its re-examination as oral therapy in young children with chronic symptoms. Antiviral agents such as *ribavirin* have a marginal role in the management of acute RSV bronchiolitis in the compromised infant.[175] There is little, if any evidence of long-term benefit.[175,176]

Antibiotic therapy has not been subjected to clinical trial in infantile wheezers, possibly because of the slender evidence that bacterial infection is relevant.[177] 'Atypical' infections such as *Chlamydia pneumoniae* or *Mycoplasma pneumoniae* may be more common than suspected, warranting a trial of a macrolide antibiotic if clinically indicated.

Leukotriene receptor antagonists (LTRAs) have a potential role to play in acute viral wheeze (Chapter 8a) and in young children with exercise-induced exacerbations of chronic asthma.[178] Clinical trials in the preschool age group are beginning to demonstrate efficacy.[76,178,179]

Physical forms of therapy

Chest physiotherapy (physical therapy) has no role in acute bronchiolitis or wheezy preschool children and in our experience, causes deterioration in clinical status and in oxygenation in infants with acute severe airway obstruction.[180] Respiratory support for acute bronchiolitis by

means of positive airway pressure[181] or mechanical ventilation[182] is discussed in Chapter 12.

Drug therapy: clinical management

OVERALL STRATEGY

Management schemes will be based on the recognition of three components to the pattern of asthma (Chapter 1, Figure 1.2): day-to-day symptoms such as nocturnal, laughter- or exercise-induced cough and wheeze; acute episodes generally associated with viral infection; and persistently suboptimal function, indicated by unremitting symptoms poorly responsive to therapy.

Guided self-management

The flexibility to vary doses of preventer agents and to start additional therapy for exacerbations, within written and agreed limits, is the essence of guided self-management. Alterations in the level of therapy must be decided on symptoms alone in preschool children; useful lung function monitoring is impossible. The basis for written plans may be pre-printed material such as the Children's Asthma Card developed by the UK National Asthma Campaign, or simply a blank piece of paper, filled in by parent and health professional to produce an agreed plan. Although guided self-management seems entirely reasonable, it has yet to be proved effective in this age group.[84]

Domiciliary (ambulatory) care

The *stepwise hierarchy* of drug administration for day-to-day use is similar in many respects to that employed for older children (Figure 9.8). Oral bronchodilator therapy should be used only in the mildest intermittent cases in infancy. Aerosol therapy is given where tolerated by MDI/spacer and, for under-twos, face-mask and, if not, by jet-nebulizer and face-mask (Chapter 8b, Table 8b.2).

The doses employed for infants and young children have never been adequately standardized and seem by adult standards to be excessive (Table 9.8). This is partly because the agents are less effective in infancy, mainly because the delivery devices are less efficient and possibly because of the very effective nasal filter, as discussed above.

At one extreme of therapy, for infants with stable, non-life threatening symptoms, one must question the possible long-term risks of dubious short-term symptomatic gains. In many cases it is prudent to advise parents that the symptoms are preferable, when all alternative avenues of management have been explored.

Most wheezy infants have only *acute episodes* with few or no intervening symptoms. The evidence that any therapy helps the very youngest infants is poor, as reviewed above. With increasing age and with recurrent episodes,[119] β_2-agonist treatment becomes more effective. Self-management plans should indicate the amount and frequency of bronchodilator therapy which may be administered at home. It is wise to administer an initial nebulized dose of a β_2-agonist under supervised conditions to ensure that hypoxaemia is not exacerbated.[103-107] Hypoxaemia does not seem to be a problem with metered dose inhaler/spacer administration. The only significant risk of short-term high-dose β_2-agonists, is the possibility of arrhythmias in the presence of hypoxia. There is no rationale for paediatricians' preference for ipratropium bromide for wheezy infants.[135] Clear instructions must be given to contact medical help if before a second (or subsequent) dose of bronchodilator is due, symptoms relapse or deteriorate further. Oral prednisolone should be started at the first sign of coryzal symptoms if a consequent severe attack is predicted on previous experience or at the first sign of significant lower respiratory tract symptoms, but it has to be said that evidence of efficacy from controlled clinical trials in infants is not available. There is no evidence to support the use of acute high-dose topical corticosteroid therapy in this age group.[167]

The question is frequently raised as to whether regular *preventer therapy* with inhaled corticosteroids can reduce the frequency or severity of acute viral LRI. (There is no evidence at all to support the use of cromoglycate.) The effect of long-term preventer therapy seems to differ between those children who only suffer from episodic viral wheeze, without interval symptoms, in whom there is no evidence for efficacy[167] and those who have chronic interval symptoms as well as episodes in whom inhaled corticosteroids are effective (see above). Trials conducted in the latter group generally show benefit both in symptoms and in the frequency or severity of acute episodes. Direct comparison between MDI/spacer and nebulizer therapy has not been carried out in this age group, but evidence for older age groups suggests that MDI/spacer is at least as effective as a nebulizer.

Children who receive more than occasional bronchodilator therapy should be reviewed at least 3-monthly, for several reasons.

1 Opportunity should be made to reinforce advice, to review the technique of drug administration and

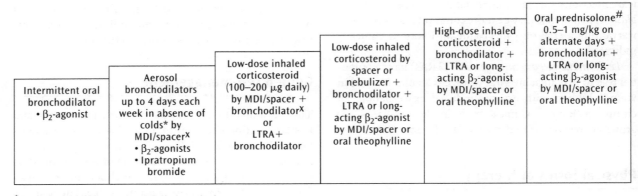

* or 4–6 times daily for short periods during episodes
x or by nebulizer if spacer unacceptable
the lowest dose possible as a supplement to high-dose topical corticosteroids can be tried once control has been achieved.
LTRA: leukotriene receptor antagonist (Montelukast)

Figure 9.8 *Stepwise hierarchy of drug therapy for chronic symptoms in infants and young children. Only the first three steps may be managed without specialist advice.*

to ensure that parental assessment of the child's condition is appropriate.

2 The pattern of disease evolves rapidly early in childhood so doses of drugs may need to be adjusted up or down; with increasing age, preventer therapy is more likely to become effective and its introduction considered.

3 Growth monitoring is mandatory for any children given corticosteroid preparations; other complications which should be sought include oral candidiasis and facial cutaneous thinning for those receiving inhaled corticosteroids by jet-nebulizer and face-masks. Monitoring is especially important for children who also receive topical steroid therapy for other conditions, such as rhinitis or eczema.

4 The earlier the onset of symptoms, the more one should question the diagnosis (Chapter 1, Figure 1.4)!

Any infant who requires inhaled steroid therapy or who has moderate or severe wheezing disease and any toddler on more than low-dose therapy, should be referred to a paediatrician for management. Any child on high-dose steroids or with severe chronic or episodic symptoms should be under the care of a specialist in paediatric respiratory medicine. Indications for acute referral to hospital are given in Table 9.6. Before and during transfer, nebulized bronchodilators and oxygen should be given.

Acute severe episodes in hospital

Any infant or preschool child referred to hospital with acute airway obstruction should be managed from the time of arrival by members of the paediatric team. Triage procedures in the accident and emergency department should assign a high priority, especially to infants. Oximetry should be carried out and oxygen therapy administered if the SaO_2 is below 90% in air. After initial evaluation, bronchodilator treatment should be initiated in the emergency department if the child is in a critical state, before transfer to another part of the hospital. Children with mild symptoms may be held in an observation area, pending discharge home, while most will be admitted to a children's ward (Figure 9.9) for monitoring and treatment. Those with critical signs (Table 9.6) should be managed in a high dependency area with access to full resuscitation facilities and blood gas analysis.

General aspects of care include oxygen therapy for significant hypoxia ($SaO_2 < 90\%$), by headbox (for infants) or fine nasal (if the nose is not blocked) or nasopharyngeal low-flow cannula. If the child is too breathless to feed or drink, intravenous fluid therapy should be administered at usual maintenance levels, taking care to detect the syndrome of inappropriate ADH secretion in severely obstructed young infants, especially those with acute viral bronchiolitis, by daily weighing and serum sodium estimation. Nasogastric tube feeding should in general be avoided for breathless infants, since by increasing the nasal airway resistance with a catheter, respiratory difficulties may be worsened. This is a matter for clinical judgement. Heart rate monitoring, oximetry and a symptom score chart, if used, should be instituted. Infants whose clinical state is exacerbated by crying can benefit from a hypnotic dose of chloral hydrate. This requires experienced judgement and careful monitoring, and if either is not available it should be avoided.

Specific drug therapy is controversial. In particular, evidence for the efficacy of bronchodilator therapy is poor in the youngest infants and there is good evidence that nebulized β_2-agonists may cause worsening of hypoxaemia with little relief of airway obstruction whereas nebulized adrenaline may be less likely to have adverse effects.[132] Ipratropium bromide has been considered to provide benefit in acute episodic wheeze in infants although objective evidence is lacking.[135] None of these has convincingly been shown to be of short or long-term benefit in acute infantile bronchiolitis. Clinical experience suggests that all are increasingly likely to be effective in older infants and toddlers. Trial doses of β_2-agonist and of ipratropium bromide should be given and repeated as necessary if effective. Tachycardia and tremor result from β_2-agonist overdosage, and serum potassium should be monitored daily for children in high dependency or intensive care units.

Corticosteroids have no role in the management of acute infantile bronchiolitis. For older infants and toddlers, oral or intravenous corticosteroids should be given as for acute severe asthma in older children (Table 9.9 and Chapters 10 and 11). High-dose inhaled steroids appear to be ineffective in established acute severe infantile wheeze, although there are no trial data. Any response to oral corticosteroid therapy should be followed up by oral prednisolone 1–2 mg/kg daily given for 2–3 days after discharge from hospital, together with any bronchodilator which has proved to be effective. The latter should be administered by MDI with a small volume spacer and face-mask, such as the Aerochamber (Trudell) Babyhaler (GSK) or Nebuchamber (AZ) for infants, or a large volume spacer for toddlers.

Other forms of therapy which may be considered include ribavirin for severe RSV bronchiolitis in infants at risk (chronic lung disease of prematurity and congenital heart disease). The complexities of administration and its marginal benefits, cost and teratogenic potential are the main arguments against its use.[175]

About 5% of young children admitted to hospital with an acute severe episode develop sufficiently severe respiratory failure to warrant admission to an *intensive care unit*, but very few need mechanical ventilation. Mechanical ventilation is more likely for smaller, younger infants, those who were born prematurely, and those with a second underlying diagnosis. The duration of mechanical ventilation is likely to be longer if there are infiltrations on the chest radiograph, if there is a family history of atopy and if sedation has been used.[182] Criteria for instituting mechanical ventilation vary widely (Chapter 12).

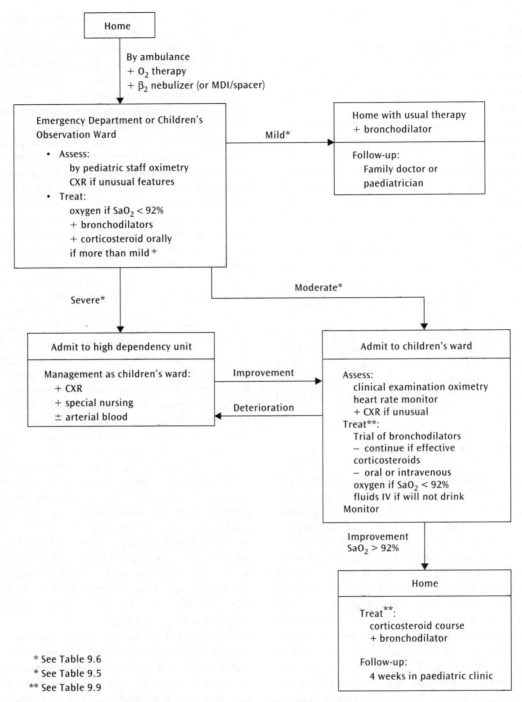

Figure 9.9 *Flow chart for secondary care for acute severe attack in infant or young child.*

Follow-up arrangements at discharge are important. It is generally easier to review the events surrounding the admission in the calm of a consulting room. Potential causal factors can be sought. Delays in self-referral or in medical referral for the acute attack can be identified and a plan set up to obviate such problems in the future. The need for regular or emergency therapy, a guided self-management plan and revision of inhaler use can all be examined.

OUTLOOK

Prognosis

As discussed earlier, the long-term outlook for many wheezy preschool children is excellent. At one extreme, some will experience monthly severe attacks requiring hospital inpatient management for the first 2 years of life.

Table 9.9 *Drug doses for infants and young children*

| | Domiciliary (ambulatory) care | | Secondary care for acute severe episodes (excluding acute infantile bronchiolitis) |
	Therapy for day-to-day (steady state) symptoms	Therapy of acute episodes	
Bronchodilators			
β_2-agonist	100–500 µg up to 4 times daily by pMDI + spacer	Up to 1 mg by pMDI + spacer or 2.5–5 mg by jet nebulizer 3–4 hourly as needed	2.5–5 mg by jet-nebulizer (or IV therapy) as frequently as needed, if responsive
Ipratropium bromide	40–240 µg up to 4 times daily by pMDI + spacer	120–240 µg by pMDI + spacer or 250 µg by jet nebulizer 6 hourly	250 µg by jet-nebulizer 4–6 hourly if responsive
Long-acting β_2-agonist	Usual childhood dose by pMDI + spacer 12 hourly	–	–
LTRA	Montelukast 4 mg orally at bedtime	–	–
Theophylline	(see Chapter 8a)	–	Not recommended
Corticosteroids*	50 µg–400 µg by pMDI + spacer or up to 2 mg by jet-nebulizer (see Figure 9.8) 12 hourly	Prednisolone 1–2 mg/kg daily for 1–3 days	Prednisolone 1–2 mg/kg daily or hydrocortisone sodium succinate 4 mg/kg IV and 1 mg/kg/h by IV infusion

PMDI: metered dose inhaler (with spacer and face-mask); LTRA: long-acting leukotriene antagonist (currently for children over 2 years old).
*Inhaled doses in 'BDP equivalent' doses.

Just as parental despair and medical disillusion begin to set in, spontaneous improvement usually occurs, with a strong likelihood of a healthy and symptom-free middle childhood (Chapter 3). There is no satisfactory prognostic formula; prognostic features are summarized in Table 9.4. Many studies have confirmed the obvious: that atopy is a risk factor for later asthma.[12,183–188] The hypothesis that children with purely episodic wheeze (usually non-atopic) may have a better prognosis than children with intercurrent symptoms (normally atopic) (Figure 9.3) discussed above, has been confirmed by recent work.[187] Early anti-inflammatory treatment of young children with severe, acute wheeze does not appear to alter the medium-term prognosis.[183] Whether early intervention in children at high risk of later asthma (those with atopy of a strong family history) can alter the natural history, has yet to be established (Chapter 14).

There is no reason to believe that infants whose wheezing career starts with acute bronchiolitis are likely to behave any differently from other episodic, viral wheezers. The weight of evidence is that recurrent wheeze after an episode of RSV-induced lower respiratory illness in infancy, is transient and is not associated with persistence of wheeze or allergy by late childhood.[189] For hospitalized cases of acute infantile bronchiolitis, the prognosis may be different.[63] As discussed above,[140–149] corticosteroid therapy for acute infantile bronchiolitis has no long-term prognostic benefits.[190] Other viruses may damage the lungs, leading to obliterative bronchiolitis[75,191] or chronic idiopathic post-infective bronchiolitis.[192]

The mortality rate for disorders encompassed by the umbrella term 'asthma' has decreased in the 0–4 age group in the UK, despite evidence of an increase in the prevalence of these disorders. Most deaths from acute severe episodes occur in infants compromised by congenital heart disease or underlying pulmonary diseases such as cystic fibrosis and chronic lung disease of prematurity.

Changing attitudes

In contrast to the research effort in the field of (atopic) asthma, viral wheeze and bronchiolitis attract meagre support. The research field is wide open, since we know little of the genetics, biomechanisms, potential drug targets or social and economic impact of these prevalent disorders.

But the therapeutic nihilism of a few years ago is being gradually modified by clinical trials based on more than single-dose physiological studies in convalescent or mildly affected infants. Improved inhalation devices have recently been developed after many years of neglect. Advances in our ability to treat viral infection, the most important trigger factor in this age group, are taking place. RSV vaccine will drastically reduce the incidence of acute bronchiolitis, while agents which can block rhinovirus adherence to respiratory epithelium will, if effective, modify most of the rest of acute wheezing LRI in infants. Better understanding of the causes and mechanisms involved in viral wheeze will require new investigative techniques.[41] These will go a long way towards the development of targeted or preventative programmes, aimed at therapies relieving suffering and preventing long-term disease.[193]

REFERENCES

1. Selander P. Asthmatic symptoms in the first year of life. *Acta Paediatr* 1960;**49**:265–9.
2. Fry J. 'Acute wheezy chests'. Clinical patterns and natural history. *Br Med J* 1961;**1**:227–32.
3. Silverman M, Wilson NM. Asthma: time for a change of name? *Arch Dis Child* 1997;**77**:62–4.
4. Elphick HE, Sherlock P, Foxall G, Simpson EJ, Shiell NA, Primhak RA, Everard ML. Survey of respiratory sounds in children. *Arch Dis Child* 2001;**84**:35–9.
5. Supplement: The link between respiratory syncytial virus and reactive airway disease. *Am J Respir Crit Care Med* 2001;**162**(2):XX–XX.
6. Turner SW, Yolung S, Landan LI, LeSouef PN. Reduced lung function both before bronchiolitis and at eleven. *Arch Dis Child* 2002; in press.
7. Rusconi F, Galassi C, Corbo GM, Forastiere F, Biggeri A, Ciccone G, Renzoni E. Risk factors for early, persistent, and late-onset wheezing in young children. SIDRIA Collaborative Group. *Am J Respir Crit Care Med* 1999;**160**:1617–22.
8. Oddy WH, Holt PG, Sly PD, Read AW, Landau LI, Stanley FJ, Kendall GE, Burton PR. Association between breast feeding and asthma in 6 year old children: findings of a prospective birth cohort study. *Br Med J* 1999;**319**:815–19.
9. Wright AL, Holberg CJ, Taussig LM, Martinez FD. Factors influencing the relation of infant feeding to asthma and recurrent wheeze in childhood. *Thorax* 2001;**56**:192–7.
10. Park EJ, Golding J, Carswell F, Stewart-Brown S. Preschool wheezing and prognosis at 10. *Arch Dis Child* 1986;**61**:642–6.
11. Bosken CH, Hunt WC, Lambert WC, Samet JM. A parental history of asthma is a risk factor for wheezing and non-wheezing respiratory illness in infants younger than 8 months of age. *Am J Respir Crit Care Med* 2000;**161**:1810–15.
12. Castro-Rodriguez JA, Holberg CJ, Wright AL, Martinez FD. A clinical index to define risk of asthma in young children with recurrent wheezing. *Am J Respir Crit Care Med* 2000;**162**:1403–6.
13. Koller DY, Wojnarowski C, Herkner KR, Weinlander G, Raderer M, Eichler I, Frischer T. High levels of eosinophil cationic protein in wheezing infants predict the development of asthma. *J Allergy Clin Immunol* 1997;**99**:752–6.
14. Reijonen TMM, Korppi M, Kleemola M, Savainen K, Kuikka L, Mononen I, Remes K. Nasopharyngeal eosinophil cationic protein in bronchiolitis: relation to viral findings and subsequent wheezing. *Pediatr Pulmonol* 1997;**24**:35–41.
15. Oymar K, Bjerknes R. Is serum eosinophil cationic protein in bronchiolitis a predictor of asthma? *Pediatr Allergy Immunol* 1998;**9**:204–7.
16. Sigurs N, Bjarnason R, Sigurbergsson F. Eosinophil cationic protein in nasal secretion and in serum and myeloperoxidase in serum in respiratory syncytial virus bronchiolitis: relation to asthma and atopy. *Acta Pediatr* 1994;**83**:1151–5.
17. Strachan DP. Do chesty children become chesty adults? *Arch Dis Child* 1990;**65**:161–6.
18. Martinez FD, Morgan WJ, Wright AL, et al. Initial airway function is a risk factor for recurrent wheezing respiratory illness during the first 3 years of life. *Am Rev Respir Dis* 1991;**143**:312–16.
19. Clarke JR, Salmon B, Silverman M. Bronchial responsiveness in the neonatal period as a risk factor for recurrent lower respiratory illness in infancy. *Am J Respir Crit Care Med* 1995;**151**:1434–40.
20. Young S, Arnott J, O'Keeffe PT, Le Souef PN, Landau LI. The association between early life lung function and wheezing during the first 2 years of life. *Eur Respir J* 2000;**15**:151–7.
21. Palmer LJ, Rye PJ, Gibson NA, Burton PR, Landau LI, Le Souef PN. Airway responsiveness in early infancy predicts asthma, lung function, and respiratory symptoms by school age. *Am J Respir Crit Care Med* 2001;**163**:37–42.
22. Barker DJ. A new model for the origins of chronic disease. *Med Health Care Philos* 2001;**4**:31–4.
23. Wright AL, Taussig LM, Ray CG, et al. The Tucson children's respiratory study. II Lower respiratory tract illness in the first years of life. *Am J Epidemiol* 1989;**129**:1232–46.
24. Taylor B, Wadsworth J. Maternal smoking during pregnancy and lower respiratory tract illness in early life. *Arch Dis Child* 1987;**62**:786–91.
25. Tager IB, Hanrahan JP, Tosteson TD, et al. Lung function, pre- and postnatal smoke exposure, and wheezing in the first years of life. *Am Rev Respir Dis* 1993;**147**:811–17.
26. Haby MM, Peat JK, Marks GB, Woolcock AJ, Leeder SR. Asthma in preschool children: prevalence and risk factors. *Thorax* 2001;**56**;589–95.
27. Kuehni CE, Davis A, Brooke AM, Silverman M. Are all preschool wheezing disorders in very young (preschool) children increasing in prevalence? *Lancet* 2001;**357**:1821–5.
28. Isaacs D. Cold comfort for the catarrhal child. *Arch Dis Child* 1990;**65**:1295–6.
29. Wright AL, Holberg C, Martinez FD, Taussig LM. Relationship of parental smoking to wheezing and non-wheezing lower respiratory tract illness in infancy. *J Paediatr* 1991;**118**:207–14.
30. Lux AL, Henderson AJ, Pocock SJ and the Aspal Team. Wheeze associated with pre-natal tobacco smoke

exposure: a prospective longitudinal study. *Arch Dis Child* 2000;**83**:307–12.

31. Wickman M, Farahmand BY, Persson PG, Pershagen G. Hospitalization for lower respiratory disease during 20 years among under 5 year old children in Stockholm County: a population based survey. *Eur Respir J* 1998;**11**:366–70.

32. Lung and Asthma Information Agency; http://www.sghms.ac.uk/depts/laia.htm

33. Fleming DM, Sunderland R, Cross K, Ross AM. Declining incidence of episodes of asthma: a study of trends in new episodes presenting to general practitioners in the period 1989–98. *Thorax* 2000; **55**:657–61.

34. Fleming DM, Cross KW, Sunderland R, Ross AM. Comparison of the seasonal patterns of asthma identified in general practitioner episodes, hospital admissions, and deaths. *Thorax* 2000; **55**:662–5.

35. Balfour-Lynn L, Valman B, Silverman M, Webster AD. Nasal IgA response in wheezy infants. *Arch Dis Child* 1993;**68**:472–6.

36. Balfour-Lynn LM, Valman HB, Wellings R, *et al.* Tumour necrosis factor-a and leukotriene E4 production in wheezy infants. *Clin Exp Allergy* 1993;**24**:121–6.

37. McKean MC, Leech M, Lambert PC, Hewitt C, Myint S, Silverman M. A model of viral wheeze in nonasthmatic adults: symptoms and physiology. *Eur Respir J* 2001;**18**:23–32.

38. McKean MC, Leech M, Lambert PC, Hewitt C, Myint S, Silverman M. An adult model of viral wheeze: inflammation in the upper and lower respiratory tracts. *Clin Exp Allergy* 2002; in press.

39. Stevenson EC, Turner G, Heaney GG, Schock BC, Taylor R, Gallagher T, Ennis M, Shields MD. Bronchoalveolar lavage findings suggest two different forms of childhood asthma. *Clin Exp Allergy* 1997;**9**:1027–35.

40. Krawiec ME, Westcott JY, Chu HW, Balzar S, Trudeau JB, Schwartz LB, Wenzel SE. Persistent wheezing in very young children is associated with lower respiratory inflammation. *Am J Respir Crit Care Med* 2001;**163**:1338–43.

41. Silverman M, Pedersen S, Grigg J, eds. Measurement of airway inflammation in children. *Am J Respir Crit Care Med* 2000;**162**:(Suppl).

42. Shields MD, Brown V, Stevenson EC, Fitch PS, Schock BC, Turner G, Taylor R, Ennis M. Serum eosinophilic cationic protein and blood eosinophil counts for the prediction of the presence of airways inflammation in children with wheezing. *Clin Exp Allergy* 1999;**10**:1382–9.

43. Marguet C, Dean TP, Warner JO. Soluble intercellular adhesion molecule-1 (sICAM-1) and interferon-gamma in bronchoalveolar lavage fluid from children with airway diseases. *Am J Respir Crit Care Med* 2000; **162**:1016–22.

44. Camilli AE, Holberg CJ, Wright AL, *et al.* Parental childhood respiratory illness and respiratory illness in their infants. *Pediatr Pulmonol* 1993;**16**:275–80.

45. Stick SM, Arnolt J, Turner DJ, Young S, Landau LI, LeSouef PN. Bronchial responsiveness and lung function in recurrently wheezy infants. *Am Rev Respir Dis* 1991;**114**:1012–15.

46. Clarke JR, Reese A, Silverman M. Bronchial responsiveness and lung function in infants with lower respiratory tract illness over the first 6 months of life. *Arch Dis Child* 1992;**67**:1454–8.

47. Halonen M, Stern D, Taussig LM, *et al.* The predictive relationship between serum IgE levels at birth and subsequent incidences of lower respiratory tract illness and eczema in infants. *Am Rev Respir Dis* 1992;**146**:866–70.

48. Halonen M, Stern DA, Lohman C, Wright AL, Brown MA, Martinez FD. Two subphenotypes of childhood asthma that differ in maternal and paternal influences on asthma risk. *Am J Respir Crit Care Med* 1999;**160**:564–70.

49. Freymouth F, Vabret A, Brouard J, Toutain F, Verdon R, Petitjean J, Gouarin S, Duhamel JF, Guillois B. Detection of viral, Chlamydia pneumoniae and Mycoplasma pneumoniae infections in exacerbations of asthma in children. *J Clin Virol* 1999;**3**:131–9.

50. Zarm HJ, Van Dyk A, Yeats JK, Hanslo D. Chlamydia trachomatis lower respiratory tract infection in infants. *Ann Trop Paediatr* 1999;**1**:9–13.

51. Filippone M, Narne S, Pettenazzo A, Zaccello F, Baraldi E. Functional approach to infants and young children with noisy breathing. *Am J Respir Crit Care Med* 2000;**162**:1795–800.

52. Castile R, Filbrun D, Flucke R, Franklin W, McCoy K. Adult-type pulmonary function tests in infants without respiratory disease. *Pediatr Pulmon* 2000;**30**:215–17.

53. Frey U, Jackson AC, Silverman M. Differences in airway wall compliance as a possible mechanism for wheezing disorders in infants. *Eur Respir J* 1998; **12**:136–42.

54. Springer C, Godfrey S, Picard E, Uwyyed K, Rotschild M, Hananya S, Noviski N, Avital A. Efficacy and safety of methacholine bronchial challenge performed by ouscultation in young asthmatic children. *Am J Respir Crit Care Med* 2000;**162**:857–60.

55. Mallol J, Sly PD. Effect of chloral hydrate on arterial and oxygen saturation in wheezy infants. *Pediatr Pulmonol* 1988;**5**:96–9.

56. Clough J, Sly PD. Association between lower respiratory tract symptoms and falls in peak expiratory flow in children. *Eur Respir J* 1995; **8**:718–22.

57. Linaker CH, Coggan D, Holgate ST, Clough J, Josephs L, Chauhan AJ, Inskip HM. Personal exposure to nitrogen dioxide and risk of airflow obstruction in asthmatic children with upper respiratory infection. *Thorax* 2000;**55**:930–3.

58. Sanchez I, Koster J, Powell RE, Wolstein R, Chernick V. Effect of racemic epinephrine and salbutamol on clinical score and pulmonary mechanics in infants with bronchiolitis. *J Pediatr* 1993;**122**:145–51.

59. Standards for infant respiratory function testing: ERS/ATS Task Force. Series published in *Eur Respir J* 2000–2001, Volumes 16–17.

60. Kanengiser S, Dozer AJ. Forced expiratory manoeuvres in children aged 3–5 years. *Pediatr Pulmonol* 1994; **18**:144–9.

61. Eigen H, Bieler H, Grant D, Christoph K, Terrill D, Heilman DK, Ambrosius WT, Tepper RS. Spirometric pulmonary function in healthy preschool children. *Am J Respir Crit Care Med* 2001;**163**:619–23.

62. Vilozni D, Barker M, Jellouschek H, Heimann G, Blau H. An interactive computer-animated system (SpiroGame) facilitates spirometry in preschool children. *Am J Respir Crit Care Med* 2001;**164**: 2200–5.

63. McKenzie SA, Bridge PD, Healy MJR. Airway resistance and atopy in preschool children with wheeze and cough. *Eur Respir J* 2000;**15**:833–8.

64. Merkus PJ, Mijnsbergen JY, Hop WC, de Jongste JC. Interrupter resistance in preschool children: measurement characteristics and reference values. *Am J Respir Crit Care Med* 2001;**163**:1350–5.

65. Klug B, Bisgaard H. Specific airway resistance, interrupter resistance, and respiratory impedance in healthy children aged 2–7 years. *Pediatr Pulmonol* 1998;**25**:322–31.

66. Faure C. Imaging of the lower respiratory tract. *Curr Opin Ped* 1991;**3**:12–20.

67. Wennergren G, Hansson S, Enstrom I, *et al.* Characteristics and prognosis of hospital-treated obstructive bronchitis in children aged less than 2 years. *Acta Paediatr* 1992;**81**:40–5.

68. Wennergren G, Amark M, Amark K, Oskarsdottir S, Sten G, Redfors S. Wheezing bronchitis reinvestigated at the age of 10 years. *Acta Paediatr* 1997;**86**:351–5.

69. Van Asperen PP, Kemp AS. The natural history of IgE sensitization and atopic disease in early childhood. *Acta Paediatr* 1989;**78**:239–45.

70. Bush A, Cole P, Hariri M, Mackay I, Phillips G, O'Callaghan C, Wilson R, Warner JO. Primary ciliary dyskinesia: diagnosis and standards of care. *Eur Respir J* 1998;**12**:982–8.

71. De Blic J, Scheinmann P. Fibreoptic bronchoscopy in infants. *Arch Dis Child* 1992;**67**:159–61.

72. Wood RE. Flexible bronchoscopy in infants. *Int Anesth Clin* 1992;**30**:125–32.

73. Schellhase DE, Fawcett DD, Schutze GE, Lensing SY, Tryka AF. Clinical utility of flexible bronchoscopy and bronchoalveolar lavage in young children with recurrent wheezing. *J Pediatr* 1998;**132**:312–18.

74. Holinger LD, Sanders AD. Chronic cough in infants and children: an update. *Laryngoscope* 1991; **101**:596–605.

75. Chang AB, Masel JP, Masters B. Post-infectious bronchiolitis obliterans: clinical, radiological and pulmonary function sequelae. *Pediatr Radiol* 1998; **1**:23–9.

76. Warner JO, Naspitz CK. Third international pediatric consensus statement on the management of childhood asthma. International Pediatric Asthma Consensus Group. *Pediatr Pulmonol* 1998;**25**:1–17.

77. Celedon JC, Litonjua AA, Weiss ST, Gold DR. Day care attendance in the first year of life and illnesses of the upper and lower respiratory tract in children with a familial history of atopy. *Pediatrics* 1999; **104**:495–500.

78. Ball TM, Castro-Rodriguez JA, Griffith KA, Holberg CJ, Martinez FD, Wright AL. Siblings, day-care attendance, and the risk of asthma and wheezing during childhood. *N Engl J Med* 2000;**343**:538–43.

79. Wright AL, Holberg CJ, Taussig LM, Martinez FD. Factors influencing the relation of infant feeding to asthma and recurrent wheeze in childhood. *Thorax* 2001;**56**:192–7.

80. Custovic A, Simpson BM, Kissen P, Woodcock A, for NAC Manchester Asthma + Allergy Group. Effect of environmental manipulation in pregnancy and early life on respiratory symptoms and atopy during the first year of life: a randomised trial. *Lancet* 2001; **358**:188–93.

81. Garson JZ, Maningas CS. Cows milk allergy: prevalence and manifestations in an unselected series of newborns. *Paediatr Scand* 1973;**234**(Suppl):1–21.

82. Burr ML, Limb ES, Maguire MJ, Amarah L, Eldridge BA, Layzell JC, Merrett TG. Infant feeding, wheezing and allergy: a prospective study. *Arch Dis Child* 1993;**68**:724–8.

83. Wahn U, Lau S, Bergmann R, Kulig M, Forster J, Bergmann K, Bauer CP, Guggenmoos-Holzmann I. Indoor allergen exposure is a risk factor for sensitization during the first three years of life. *J Allergy Clin Immunol* 1997;**99**:763–9.

84. Stevens CA, Wesseldine LJ, Couriel JM, Dyer AJ, Osman LM, Silverman M. Parental education and guided self-management of asthma and wheezing in the preschool child: a randomised controlled trial. *Thorax* 2002;**57**:39–44.

85. Gotzsche PC, Hammarquist C, Burr M. House dust mite control measures for asthma: (Cochrane Review) Cochrane Database Syst. Rev 2001:2.

86. Custovic A, Simpson A, Chapman MD, Woodcock A. Allergen avoidance in the treatment of asthma and atopic disorders. *Thorax* 1998;**53**:63–72.

87. Barry P. Administering treatment – inhaled therapy. In: M Silverman, C O'Callaghan, eds. *Practical Paediatric Respiratory Medicine*. Arnold, London, 2001.

88. Iles R, Lister P, Edmunds AT. Crying significantly reduces absorption of aerosolised drug in infants. *Arch Dis Child* 1999;**81**:163–5.

89. Cates CJ, Rowe BH. Holding chambers versus nebulizers for β-agonist treatment of acute asthma (*Cochrane Review*). The Cochrane Library, 4, 2000. Update Software, Oxford.

90. Rubilar L, Castro-Rodriguez JA, Girardi G. Randomized trial of salbutamol via metered-dose inhaler with spacer versus nebulizer for acute wheezing in children less than 2 years of age. *Pediatr Pulmonol* 2000;**29**:264–9.

91. Ploin D, Chapuis FR, Stamm D, Robert J, David L, Chatelain PG, Dutau G, Floret D. High-dose albuterol by metered-dose inhaler plus a spacer device versus nebulization in preschool children with recurrent wheezing: a double-blind, randomized equivalence trial. *Pediatrics* 2000;**106**:311–17.

92. Salmon B, Wilson NM, Silverman M. How much aerosol reaches the lungs of wheezy infants and toddlers? *Arch Dis Child* 1990;**64**:401–3.

93. Janssens HM, Devadason SG, Hop WC, LeSouef PN, De Jongste JC, Tiddens HA. Variability of aerosol delivery via spacer devices in young asthmatic children in daily life. *Eur Respir J* 1999;**13**:787–91.

94. Penn RB, Wolfson MR, Shaffer TH. Development differences in tracheal cartilage mechanics. *Pediatr Res* 1989;**26**:429–33.

95. Panitch HP, Deoras KS, Wolfson MR, Shaffer TH. Maturational changes in airway smooth muscle structure-function relationships. *Pediatr Res* 1992;**31**:151–6.

96. Schell DN, Durham D, Murphree SS, Muntz KH, Shawl PW. Ontogeny of beta-adrenergic receptors in pulmonary arterial smooth muscle, bronchial smooth muscle and alveolar lining cells in the rat. *Am J Respir Cell Mol Biol* 1992;**7**:317–24.

97. Griscom NT, Whol MBB. Dimensions of the growing trachea related to body height. Length, anteroposterior and transverse diameters, cross-sectional area, and volume in subjects younger than 20 years of age. *Am Rev Respir Dis* 1985; **131**:840–4.

98. Sparrow M, Mitchell HW. Contraction of smooth muscle pig airway tissues from before birth to maturity. *J Appl Physiol* 1990;**68**:468–77.

99. Bhutani VK, Koslo RJ, Shaffer TH. The effect of tracheal smooth muscle tone on neonatal airway collapsibility. *Pediatr Res* 1986;**20**:492–5.

100. Behr P. Inhalation pathways in relation to infants and children. In: GB Gerbo, H Metivier, H Smith, eds. *Age Related Factors in Radionuclide Metabolism and Dosimetry*. Martinus Nighoff, Dordrecht, 1987, pp. 67–78.

101. Everard ML, Hardy JG, Milner AD. Comparison of nebulized aerosol deposition in the lungs of healthy adults following oral and nasal inhalation. *Thorax* 1993;**48**:1045–6.

102. Silverman M. Bronchodilators for wheezy infants? *Arch Dis Child* 1984;**59**:84–7.

103. Prendiville A, Rose A, Maxwell DL, Silverman M. Hypoxaemia in wheezy infants after bronchodilator treatment. *Arch Dis Child* 1987;**62**:997–1000.

104. Seidenberg J, Mir Y, con der Hardt H. Hypoxaemia and after nebulized salbutamol in wheezy infants: the importance of aerosol acidity. *Arch Dis Child* 1991;**66**:672–5.

105. Ho L, Collis G, Landau LI, Le Souef PN. Effect of salbutamol on oxygen saturation in bronchiolitis. *Arch Dis Child* 1991;**66**:1061–4.

106. Connett G, Lenney W. Prolonged hypoxaemia after nebulized salbutamol. *Thorax* 1993;**48**:574–5.

107. Alaris AJ, Lewander W, Dehenney P, *et al.* The efficacy of nebulized meta proterenol in wheezing infants and young children. *Am J Dis Child* 1992; **146**:412–18.

108. Prendiville A, Green S, Silverman M. Paradoxical response to nebulized salbutamol in wheezy infants, assessed by partial expiratory flow-volume curves. *Thorax* 1987;**42**:86–91.

109. Sly PD, Lanteri CJ, Raven JM. Do wheezy infants recovering from bronchiolitis respond to inhaled salbutamol? *Pediatr Pulmonol* 1991;**10**:36–9.

110. Hughes DM, Le Souef PN, Landau LI. Effect of salbutamol on respiratory mechanics in bronchiolitis. *Pediatr Res* 1987;**22**:83–6.

111. Mallory GB, Motoyama EK, Koumbourlis AC, Mutich RL, Nakayama DK. Bronchial reactivity in infants in acute respiratory failure with viral bronchiolitis. *Pediatr Pulmonol* 1989;**6**:253–9.

112. Jackson AC, Tennhoff W, Kraemer R, Frey U. Airway and tissue resistance in wheezy infants: effects of albuterol. *Am J Respir Crit Care Med* 1999;**2**:557–63.

113. Kraemer R, Frey U, Sommer DW, Russi E. Short-term effect of albuterol delivered via a new auxiliary device in wheezy infants. *Am Rev Respir Dis* 1991;**144**:347–51.

114. Soto ME, Sly PD, Uren E, Taussig LM, Landau LI. Bronchodilator response during acute viral bronchiolitis in infancy. *Pediatr Pulmonol* 1985; **1**:85–90.

115. O'Callaghan C, Milner AD, Swarbrick A. Paradoxical deterioration in lung function after nebulized salbutamol in wheezy infants. *Lancet* 1986;**ii**:424–5.

116. Bentur L, Canny GJ, Shields MD, *et al.* Controlled trial of nebulized albuterol in children younger than two years of age with acute asthma. *Pediatrics* 1992; **89**:133–7.

117. Sanchez I, Koster J, de Powell RE, Wolstein R, Chernick V. Effect of racemic epinephrine and salbutamol on clinical score and pulmonary mechanics in infants with bronchiolitis. *J Pediatr* 1993;**122**:145–51.

118. Dobson JV, Stephens-Groff SM, McMahon SR, Stemmier MM, Brallier SL, Bay C. The use of albuterol in hospitalized infants with bronchiolitis. *Pediatrics* 1998;**101**:361–8.

119. Kellner JD, Ohlsson A, Gadomski AM, Wang EEL. Bronchodilators for bronchiolitis (*Cochrane Review*). The Cochrane Library, 3, 2000. Update Software, Oxford.

120. Chavasse RJ, Bastian-Lee Y, Richter H, Hilliard T, Seddon P. Inhaled salbutamol for wheezy infants: a randomised controlled trial. *Arch Dis Child* 2000;**82**:370–5.

121. Prendiville A, Green S, Silverman M. Airway responsiveness in wheezy infants: evidence for functional beta-adrenergic receptors. *Thorax* 1987;**42**:100–4.

122. O'Callaghan C, Milner AD, Swarbrick A. Nebulized salbutamol does have a protective effect on airways in children under 1 year old. *Arch Dis Child* 1988; **63**:479–83.

123. Clarke JR, Aston H, Silverman M. Delivery of salbutamol by metered dose inhaler and valved spacer to wheezy infants: effect on bronchial responsiveness. *Arch Dis Child* 1993;**69**:125–9.

124. Henderson AJW, Young S, Stick SM, Landau LI, Le Souef PN. Effect of salbutamol on histamine induced bronchoconstriction in healthy infants. *Thorax* 1993;**48**:317–23.

125. Henry PJ, Rigby PJ, McKenzie JS, Goldie RG. Effect of respiratory tract viral infection on murine airway β adrenoceptor function, distribution and density. *Br J Pharmacol* 1991;**104**:914–21.

126. Reddel H, Ware S, Marks G, Sahme C, Jenkins C, Woolcock A. Differences between asthma exacerbations and poor asthma control. *Lancet* 1999; **353**:364–9.

127. Holmgren D, Bjure J, Engrostrom I, *et al.* Transcutaneous blood gas monitoring during salbutamol inhalation in young children with acute asthmatic symptoms. *Pediatr Pulmonol* 1992; **14**:75–9.

128. Turner DJ, Landau LI, Le Souef PN. The effect of age on bronchodilator responsiveness. *Pediatr Pulmonol* 1993;**15**:98–104.

129. Turpeinen M, Nikander K, Malmberg LP, Pelkonen A. Metered dose inhaler add-on devices: is the inhaled mass of drug dependent on the size of the infant? *J Aerosol Med* 1999;**12**:171–6.

130. Wildhaber JH, Janssens HM, Pierart F, Dore ND, Devadason SG, Le Souef PN. High-percentage lung delivery in children from detergent-treated spacers. *Pediatr Pulmonol* 2000;**29**:389–93.

131. Kristjansson S, Lodrup-Carlsen KC, Wennergren G, Stannegard I-L, Carlsen K-H. Nebulized racemic adrenaline in the treatment of acute bronchiolitis in infants and toddlers. *Arch Dis Child* 1993;**69**: 650–4.

132. Bertrand P, Aranibar H, Castro E, Sanchez I. Efficacy of nebulized epinephrine versus salbutamol in hospitalized infants with bronchiolitis. *Pediatr Pulmonol* 2001;**31**:284–8.

133. Primhak RA, Smith CM, Yong SC, Wach R, Kurian M, Brown R, Efthimiou J. The bronchoprotective effect of inhaled salmeterol in preschool children: a dose-ranging study. *Eur Respir J* 1999;**1**:78–81.

134. Bisgaard H. Long-acting beta(2)-agonists in management of childhood asthma: A critical review of the literature. *Pediatr Pulmonol* 2000;**29**:221–34.

135. Everard ML, Bara A, Kurian M. Anti-cholinergic drugs for wheeze in children under the age of two years (*Cochrane Review*). The Cochrane Library, 2, 2000. Update Software, Oxford.

136. Plotnick LH, Ducharme FM. Combined inhaled anticholinergics and β₂-agonists for initial treatment of acute asthma in children (*Cochrane Review*). The Cochrane Library, 4, 2000. Update Software, Oxford.

137. Henry RL, Milner AD, Stokes GM. Ineffectiveness of ipratropium bromide in acute bronchiolitis. *Arch Dis Child* 1983;**58**:925–6.

138. Prendiville A, Green S, Silverman M. Ipratropium bromide and airways function in wheezy infants. *Arch Dis Child* 1987;**62**:397–400.

139. Barnes PJ. Muscarinic receptor subtypes in airways. *Eur Respir J* 1993;**6**:328–31.

140. Connelly JH, Field CMB, Glasgow JFT, Slattery CM, MacLynn DM. A double blind trial of prednisolone in epidemic bronchiolitis due to respiratory syncytial virus. *Acta Paediatr Scand* 1969;**58**:116–20.

141. Leer JA, Green JL, Heimlich EM, *et al.* Corticosteroid treatment in bronchiolitis: a controlled collaborative study in 297 infants and children. *Am J Dis Child* 1969;**117**:495–503.

142. Springer C, Bar-Yishay E, Uwayyed K, *et al.* Corticosteroids do not affect the clinical or physiological status of infants with bronchiolitis. *Pediatr Pulmonol* 1990;**9**:181–5.

143. Roosevelt G, Sheehan K, Grupp-Phelan J, Tanz RR, Listernick R. Dexamethasone in bronchiolitis: a randomised controlled trial. *Lancet* 1996;**348**:292–5.

144. Klassen TP, Sutcliffe T, Watters LK, Wells GA, Allen UD, Li MM. Dexamethasone in salbutamol-treated inpatients with acute bronchiolitis: a randomized, controlled trial. *J Pediatr* 1997;**130**:191–6.

145. Berger I, Argaman Z, Schwartz SE, Segal E, Kiderman A, Branski D, Kerem E. Efficacy of corticosteroids in acute bronchiolitis: short-term and long-term follow-up. *Pediatr Pulmonol* 1998;**26**:162–6.

146. Richter H, Seddon P. Early nebulized budesonide in the treatment of bronchiolitis and the prevention of postbronchiolitic wheezing. *J Pediatr* 1998; **132**:849–53.

147. Wong JYW, Moon S, Beardsmore C, O'Callaghan C, Simpson H. No objective benefit from steroids inhaled via a spacer in infants recovering from bronchiolitis. *Eur Respir J* 2000;**15**:388–94.

148. Cade A, Brownlee KG, Conway SP, *et al.* A. Randomised placebo controlled trial of

nebulised corticosteroids in acute respiratory syncytial viral bronchiolitis. *Arch Dis Child* 2000;**82**:126–30.

150. Webb MSC, Henry RL, Milner AD. Oral corticosteroids for wheezing attacks under 18 months. *Arch Dis Child* 1986;**61**:15–19.

151. Wilson NM, Silverman M. Treatment of acute, episodic asthma in preschool children using intermittent high dose inhaled steroids at home. *Arch Dis Child* 1990;**65**:407–10.

152. Connett G, Lenney W. Prevention of viral induced asthma attacks using inhaled budesonide. *Arch Dis Child* 1993;**68**:85–7.

153. Svedmyr J, Thunguist P, Asbrink-Nilsson E, Hedlin G. Prophylactic intermittent treatment with inhaled corticosteroids of asthma deterioration due to upper respiratory tract infections in young children. *Acta Paediatr* 1999;**88**:42–7.

154. Tal A, Bavilski C, Yohai D, *et al.* Dexamethasone and salbutamol in the treatment of acute wheezing in infants. *Pediatrics* 1983;**71**:13–18.

155. Gries DM, Moffitt DR, Pulos E, Carter ER. A single dose of intramuscularly administered dexamethasone acetate is as effective as oral prednisolone to treat asthma exacerbations in young children. *J Pediatr* 2000;**136**:298–303.

156. Noble V, Ruggins NR, Everard ML, Milner AD. Inhaled budesonide for chronic wheezing under 18 months of age. *Arch Dis Child* 1992;**67**:285–8.

157. Bisgaard H, Munch BL, Nielsen JP, Petersen W, Ohlsson SV. Inhaled budesonide for treatment of recurrent wheezing in early childhood. *Lancet* 1990;**336**:649–51.

158. Kraemer R, Graf Bigler U, Casaulta Aebischer C, Weder M, Birrer P. Clinical and physiological improvement after inhalation of low-dose beclomethasone dipropionate and salbutamol in wheezy infants. *Respiration* 1997;**64**:342–9.

159. Bisgaard H, Gillies J, Groenewald M, Maden C. The effect of inhaled fluticasone propionate in the treatment of young asthmatic children: a dose comparison study. *Am J Respir Crit Care Med* 1999;**160**:126–31.

160. Chavasse RJ, Bastian-Lee Y, Richter H, Hilliard T, Seddon P. Persistent wheezing in infants with an atopic tendency responds to inhaled fluticasone. *Arch Dis Child* 2001;**85**:143–8.

161. Van Bever HP, Schuddinck L, Wojciechowski M, Stevens WJ. Aerosolized budesonide in asthmatic infants; a double blind study. *Pediatr Pulmonol* 1990;**9**:177–80.

162. Maayan C, Itzhaki T, Bar-Yishay E, *et al.* The functional response of infants with persistent wheezing to nebulized beclomethasone dipropionate. *Pediatr Pulmonol* 1986;**2**:9–14.

163. De Blic J, Delacourt C, le Bourgeois M, *et al.* Efficacy of nebulized budesonide in treatment of severe infantile asthma: a double-blind study. *J Allergy Clin Immunol* 1996;**98**:14–20.

164. Allen ED, Whittaker ER, Ryu G. Six-week trial of nebulized flunisolide nasal spray: efficacy in young children with moderately severe asthma. *Pediatr Pulmonol* 1997;**6**:397–405.

165. Baker JW, Mellon M, Wald J, Welch M, Cruz-Rivera M, Walton-Bowen K. A multiple-dosing, placebo-controlled study of budesonide inhalation suspension given once or twice daily for treatment of persistent asthma in young children and infants. *Pediatrics* 1999;**103**:414–21.

166. Kemp JP, Skoner DP, Szefler SJ, Walton-Bowen K, Cruz-Rivera M, Smith JA. Once-daily budesonide inhalation suspension for the treatment of persistent asthma in infants and young children. *Ann Allergy Asthma Immunol* 1999;**83**:231–9.

167. McKean M, Ducharme F. Inhaled steroids for episodic viral wheeze of childhood (*Cochrane Review*). The Cochrane Library, 4, 2000. Update Software, Oxford.

168. Hedlin G, Svedmyr J, Ryden AC. Systemic effects of a short course of betamethasone compared with high-dose inhaled budesonide in early childhood asthma. *Acta Paediatr* 1999;**88**:48–51.

169. Scott MB, Skoner DP. Short-term safety of budesonide inhalation suspension in infants and young children with persistent asthma. *J Allergy Clin Immunol* 1999;**104**:200–9.

170. Tasche MJ, Uijen JH, Bernsen RM, de Jongste JC, van der Wouden JC. Inhaled disodium cromoglycate (DSCG) as maintenance therapy in children with asthma: a systematic review. *Thorax* 2000;**55**:913–20.

171. O'Callaghan C, Milner AD, Swarbrick A. Nebulized sodium cromoglycate in infancy: airway protection after deterioration. *Arch Dis Child* 1990;**54**:404–6.

172. Brooks LJ, Cropp GJA. Theophylline therapy in bronchiolitis. A retrospective study. *Am J Dis Child* 1981;**135**:934–6.

173. Vieira SE, Lotufo JP, Ejzenberg B, Okay Y. Efficacy of IV aminophylline as a supplemental therapy in moderate broncho-obstructive crisis in infants and preschool children. *Pulm Pharmac Ther* 2000;**13**:189–94.

174. Goodman DC, Littenberg B, O'Connor GT, Brooks JG. Theophylline in acute childhood asthma: a meta-analysis of its efficacy. *Pediatr Pulmonol* 1996;**21**:211–18.

175. McBride JT, McConnochie KM. RSV, recurrent wheezing, and ribavirin. *Pediatr Pulmonol* 1998;**25**:145–6.

176. Rodriguez WJ, Arrobio J, Fink R, Kim HW, Milburn C. Prospective follow-up and pulmonary functions from a placebo-controlled randomized trial of ribavirin therapy in respiratory syncytial virus bronchiolitis. Ribavirin Study Group. *Arch Pediatr Adolesc Med* 1999;**153**:469–74.

177. Korppi M, Leinonen M, Koskela M, Makela P, Launiala K. Bacterial co-infection in children hospitalized with respiratory syncytial virus infections. *Pediatr Infect Dis J* 1989;**8**:687–92.

178. Bisgaard H, Neilsen KG. Bronchoprotection with a leukotriene receptor antagonist in asthmatic preschool children. *Am J Respir Crit Care Med* 2000;**162**:187–90.

179. Knorr B, Franchi LM, Bisgaard H, *et al*. Montelukast, a leukotriene receptor antagonist, for the treatment of persistent asthma in children aged 2 to 5 years. *Pediatrics* 2001;**108**:E48.

180. Webb MS, Martin JA, Cartlidge PH, Ng YK, Wright NA. Chest physiotherapy in acute bronchiolitis. *Arch Dis Child* 1985;**60**:1078–9.

181. Soong WJ, Hwang B, Tang R-B. Continuous positive airway pressure by nasal prongs in bronchiolitis. *Pediatr Pulmonol* 1993;**16**:163–6.

182. Lebel MH, Gauthier M, Lacroix J, Rousseau E, Buthieu M. Respiratory failure and mechanical ventilation in severe bronchiolitis. *Arch Dis Child* 1989;**64**:1431–7.

183. Reijonen TM, Korppi M. One-year follow-up of young children hospitalized for wheezing: the influence of early anti-inflammatory therapy and risk factors for subsequent wheezing and asthma. *Pediatr Pulmonol* 1998;**2**:113–19.

184. Clough JB, Keeping KA, Edwards LC, Freeman WM, Warner JA, Warner JO. Can we predict which wheezy infants will continue to wheeze? *Am J Respir Crit Care Med* 1999;**160**:1473–80.

185. Wever-Hess J, Kouwenberg JM, Duiverman EJ, Hermans J, Wever AM. Prognostic characteristics of asthma diagnosis in early childhood in clinical practice. *Acta Paediatr* 1999;**8**:827–34.

186. Wever-Hess J, Kouwenberg JM, Duiverman EJ, Hermans J, Wever AM. Risk factors for exacerbations and hospital admissions in asthma of early childhood. *Pediatr Pulmonol* 2000;**4**:250–6.

187. Martinez FD, Wright AL, Taussig LM, *et al*. Asthma and wheezing in the first six years of life. *New Engl J Med* 1995;**332**:133–8.

188. Stein RT, Holberg CJ, Morgan WJ, Wright AL, Lombardi E, Taussig L, Martinez FD. Peak flow variability, methacholine responsiveness and atopy as markers for detecting different wheezing phenotypes in childhood. *Thorax* 1997;**52**:946–52.

189. Stein RT, Sherrill D, Morgan WJ, Holberg CJ, Halonen M, Taussig LM, Wright AL, Martinez FD. Respiratory syncytial virus in early life and risk of wheeze and allergy by age 13 years. *Lancet* 1999;**354**:541–5.

190. van Woensel JB, Kimpen JL, Sprikkelman AB, Ouwehand A, van Aalderen WM. Long-term effects of prednisolone in the acute phase of bronchiolitis caused by respiratory syncytial virus. *Pediatr Pulmonol* 2000;**30**:92–6.

191. Hardy KA, Schidlow DV, Zaeri N. Obliterative bronchiolitis in children. *Chest* 1988;**93**:460–6.

192. Hull J, Chow CW, Robertson CF. Chronic idiopathic bronchiolitis of infancy. *Arch Dis Child* 1997; **77**:512–15.

193. Martinez FD. Present and future treatment of asthma in infants and young children. *J Allergy Clin Immunol* 1999;**104**:169–74.

10

The management of asthma in school-children

JOHN F PRICE

INTRODUCTION

Throughout the world the high and increasing prevalence of asthma has stimulated the development of guidelines which set standards and make recommendations for the management of asthma (Table 10.1). The implementation of the Global Initiative for Asthma (GINA) international guidelines[1] was tested recently by a survey of patients, of whom about 750 were children, in seven European countries.[2] Asthma control comparable with the overall aims of the GINA guidelines was seen in only 6% of children surveyed. Nearly 40% had symptoms weekly, 30% experienced significant limitation of activity and 60% had never had any form of lung function test. In this survey 46% of the children reported persistent symptoms ranging from mild to severe (Figure 10.1). All recent national and international guidelines including GINA recommend the use of inhaled steroids in children with persistent symptoms. However of the 46% of children with persistent symptoms less than one third were taking an inhaled steroid. The results of this study clearly indicate that although the management of asthma is well standardized and described in guidelines, their implementation is far from perfect (Chapter 18).

Table 10.1 *Recommendations for asthma control*

- minimal chronic symptoms
- minimal episodes
- no emergency visits
- minimal bronchodilator use
- no limitation of activity
- near normal lung function

Good management of asthma in children depends on accurate diagnosis, careful assessment of severity, recognition of environmental influences and selection of age-appropriate treatment. These principles need to be understood and accepted by the child and family and form the basis of a partnership leading to guided self-management (sometimes referred to as 'home management', to reflect the role of the whole family). Asthma care includes dealing with specific patterns of illness at home and at school and regular review. Most recurrent wheezing in school age children is caused by asthma and the diagnosis can usually be made from a carefully taken history (Chapter 6a). Reversible airway obstruction should be confirmed by lung function testing (Chapter 6b). Historically asthma has carried the stigma of a small thin child who is breathless and ill. Occasionally there is still a reluctance to tell parents that their child has asthma. As long as appropriate explanation and management follow, the child and parents' anxiety is much more

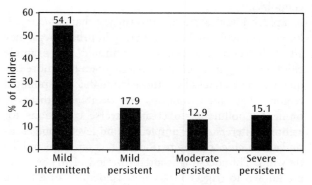

Figure 10.1 *Childhood asthma classified according to frequency and severity of symptoms. (Adapted from ref. 1.)*

likely to be relieved than increased by being told the diagnosis.

ENVIRONMENTAL ISSUES IN MANAGEMENT

There are three main ways in which an adverse environment will affect asthma control: outdoor and indoor air pollution, the presence of allergens to which the child is sensitized and individual or family psychopathology.

Air pollution and smoking

Air pollutants may influence the severity of asthma by a direct irritant action provoking bronchoconstriction, by causing inflammation in the airways and thus increasing bronchial responsiveness or by altering the immune response to environmental allergens.

Many asthmatic children are exposed to high levels of *tobacco smoke at home*.[3] A total of 86% of children exposed to adults who smoke have salivary cotinine concentrations greater than 0.6 ng/ml.[4] Exposure to tobacco smoke *in utero* is associated with raised IgE concentrations in cord blood,[5] reduced lung function,[6] and more wheezing illness in early life.[7] Antenatal clinics have a responsibility to warn pregnant mothers of the dangers of cigarette smoke to their unborn infants and offer help with stopping smoking.[8] Such guidance is of course particularly important in families with a strong history of atopy. There is good evidence that children with asthma have more severe symptoms if their parents smoke.[9] Evidence for an association with increased bronchial reactivity and with increased allergic sensitization have been reviewed[10] (Chapter 7e). Exposure to cigarette smoke provokes asthma attacks and chronic exposure has a cumulative adverse effect on the lung function of asthmatic children.[11] Parental smoking is an important marker of non-attendance at education programs about asthma.[12] Moreover a randomized trial of intervention informing parents about the harmful effects of smoking on their children did not encourage them to stop smoking. Salivary cotinine levels in the children before and one year after the intervention were the primary endpoints.[13]

Epidemiological studies also suggest that *outdoor pollutants*, particularly those occurring in urban areas, may affect the severity of childhood asthma.[14] For example children living in a polluted area of Spain had more frequent asthma attacks than those living in a non-polluted region.[15] Climatic conditions may combine with environmental pollutants to create adverse conditions for asthma sufferers; for example, ground level ozone accumulates in cities during periods of hot sunshine and little wind. Thunderstorms after a period of dry weather are known to trigger local 'mini-epidemics' of asthma. The increased release of mould spores or possibly the fragmentation of pollen grains may be responsible. Part

of the management of asthma is to make families aware of this and to be alert to the possibility of deterioration in symptoms during certain types of weather.

Allergen exposure

In low altitude temperate zones the main environmental allergens are house-dust mite (*Dermatophagoides pteronyssinus*) antigen Der p1 in faecal pellets, cat antigen (Fel d 1) in saliva, and seasonal pollens especially grasses. Other allergens may be important elsewhere (Table 7a.2). It is easy to identify an allergic precipitant of asthma if exposure repeatedly causes acute symptoms. More often however continued exposure causes chronic symptoms. The role of an allergen in the consequent increase in vulnerability to asthma attacks provoked by other factors such as viral infection and exercise is then difficult to discern. Improvement in asthma when children go on holiday without any other change in their management, strongly suggests an allergic trigger at home. If negative, skin-prick tests or measurement of specific IgE antibodies rule out allergic sensitization, but false positives are common. The threshold for carrying out skin testing in children varies widely in different countries. They should certainly be done before embarking on house-dust mite avoidance or recommending removal of pets.

The allergen to which asthmatic children in the UK most commonly become sensitized is the house-dust mite. Unfortunately no particular pattern of symptoms characterizes house-dust mite allergy. Exposure to mite allergens is highest at night but asthma symptoms in children generally tend to be worse at night anyway. House-mite allergy often causes severe nasal symptoms in the early morning and this may be a useful clue. When children sensitized to mite reside at high altitude in the European Alps or in a hospital environment, where mite allergen concentrations are low, symptoms and bronchial responsiveness decrease. Return to the home environment causes rapid relapse.[16] A meta-analysis of the efficacy of house-dust mite avoidance concluded there was marginal benefit.[17] This analysis was subsequently criticized for including trials that succeeded with those which failed to reduce allergen concentrations in the home. Mite reduction in the home is time consuming and re-accumulation of mites occurs rapidly. A trial of mite reduction measures, including removal of carpets in the bedroom, covering mattresses, vacuuming, freezing or removal of soft toys and washing bed linen at 60 degrees, is only worth considering in highly motivated families with children who have good evidence of mite allergy. House construction has a marked influence on mite concentrations. The number of mites is related to temperature and humidity; well-heated and poorly ventilated houses are those most conducive to mite proliferation. In Denmark experimental houses with mechanical ventilation systems contain very low levels of mite antigen.[18] Whether factors relating to mite proliferation will be taken into consideration in future house building remains to be seen. The topic of mite avoidance in the management of childhood asthma has recently been reviewed[19] and is considered in Chapter 14.

Families with an asthmatic child should be encouraged not to acquire pets. Pets should be removed when allergy has been clearly established. Cat allergens are particularly pervasive in Europe. Children with cat sensitivity in a class at school in which more than 18% of the children own cats have worse asthma as a result of school attendance.[20] When cats are removed it may be months before the dander disappears completely from dust in the home.[21] One must be quite sure a household pet really is triggering asthma before advising its removal because the resulting emotional upset could make things worse. When removal of a cat is likely to cause great upset it has been suggested that a weekly wash will reduce levels of cat antigen and this, together with removing carpets, frequent vacuuming and air filtration, may allow the family cat to be retained.[22]

Psychosocial issues

Individual or family psychopathology can influence childhood asthma directly by its association with deteriorating symptoms or indirectly by acting as a barrier to asthma education and adherence to treatment (Chapter 13e). Stressful events in children's lives have been linked with decreased school performance,[23] a requirement for increased doses of steroids[24] and prolonged admissions to hospital.[25] Several mechanisms have been proposed to explain the association between psychopathology and poor asthma control. The pathophysiology and clinical manifestations of asthma depend on complex neural mechanisms and changes in the autonomic nervous system. In depression β-adrenergic hyporesponsiveness has been demonstrated. Certain neuropeptides thought to regulate airway inflammation and responsiveness are released during stress. Alterations in immune responses observed during stress may have implications for the exacerbation of asthma particularly by increasing the risk of respiratory infections.[26] Family support naturally has an important influence on a child's asthma. Many of the psychosocial factors implicated in poor asthma control, including childhood anxiety, depression, non-adherence and family conflict, are dependent on family structure and function. There is some evidence that exposure to violence is associated with deterioration in asthma among inner city children.[27] Acute and chronic stress have different effects.[28]

Psychosocial factors may affect perception of asthma control and can influence attitudes to treatment and self-management adversely. Adherence to prescribed treatment is poorer in children and families with psychological problems although very few studies have examined this specifically in children with asthma. One study however found that the level of family conflict predicted adherence with theophylline treatment.[29] Psychosocial barriers to asthma education include economic status, literacy level and ethnicity. Socio-economic status has a significant effect on patterns of asthma symptoms. A study in the UK has shown that socio-economic status does not influence asthma diagnosis or prescribed treatment, but children in less privileged social classes have more frequent asthma attacks especially at night.[30]

In the past there has been a tendency for polarization of views about the role of psychosocial issues in asthma. Collaborative research between respiratory physicians and psychologists is needed to advance our knowledge in this complex area.

DRUG THERAPY

Guidelines and their implementation

National and international guidelines for the management of childhood asthma have the advantages of promoting good clinical practice and providing a basis for clinic audit. In the past, most have been compiled by consensus, but henceforth will be expected to describe the level of evidence on which recommendations are based. They should not be regarded as inflexible protocols but rather to be adapted according to local circumstances and the needs of individual patients and families. They require regular updating as new drugs and delivery systems become available.

Most guidelines propose a step-wise or algorithmic approach to drug management, choosing a treatment regimen based on the initial assessment of severity. Asthma guidelines generally divide children with asthma into those with intermittent and those with persistent symptoms. A fundamental assumption is that children with persistent symptoms have chronic airway inflammation and therefore require regular anti-inflammatory therapy. For ethical reasons there is little histological evidence to support this assumption in mild persistent asthma in children. Nevertheless, by analogy with the situation in young adults with asthma, the increase in bronchial responsiveness characteristic of children who develop chronic symptoms provides strong indirect evidence for underlying airway inflammation. By convention persistent asthma has been divided into mild, moderate and severe (Figure 10.2). A recent survey[2] using a symptom severity index similar to that applied in Global Initiative for Asthma (GINA) guidelines[1] suggests that intermittent asthma may be slightly more common and persistent asthma a little less common in children than in adults. A suggested scheme for classifying severity and control of acute and chronic (steady-state) symptoms in young children is given in Chapter 9 (Table 9.7) and can easily be adapted for school-children.

Frequency and severity of symptoms	Regular preventive medication
Mild intermittent (Step 1)	None
Mild persistent (Step 2)	Inhaled steroid 100–200 µg/day or Inhaled cromone
	Consider Oral leukotriene receptor antagonist
Moderate persistent (Step 3)	Inhaled steroid 400–800 µg/day or Inhaled steriod 200–400 µg/day plus either Inhaled long acting β-agonist or Oral leukotriene receptor antagonist
Severe persistent (Step 4)	Inhaled steroid up to 1000 µg/day plus Inhaled long acting β-agonist or Oral leukotriene receptor antagonist and/or Oral slow release theophylline (low dose) and/or Inhaled anticholinergic agent
Difficult asthma (Step 5)	As above plus Oral alternate day prednisolone
	Consider Cyclosporin Methotrexate

Figure 10.2 *Symptom severity and drug treatment in school-children.*

Mild intermittent asthma – Step 1

This category includes children who over a period of several months have symptoms of asthma occurring less than once a week and nocturnal asthma no more than twice a month. Spirometry and peak flow variability return to normal between symptomatic episodes. Symptoms rarely interfere with daytime activity or sleep. Children who fall into this category need to have available bronchodilator medication given by inhalation to relieve symptoms. The selective, short-acting β$_2$-adrenergic agonists (albuterol/salbutamol, terbutaline) are the most rapidly effective and safest bronchodilators. In school-children β$_2$-adrenergic agonists should be used in preference to anticholinergic agents such as ipratropium bromide.

Some children experience seasonally troublesome asthma, but for the remainder of the year, have few symptoms. For instance those with symptoms provoked predominantly by viral respiratory infection may have mild symptoms during the summer but more frequent virus-induced episodes in the winter. For such episodes, they may need to take a bronchodilator regularly during and for a week or two after a cold. Treatment with a prophylactic agent should be considered if they have symptoms between viral episodes. However, there is no evidence that school-age children with mild intermittent symptoms provoked only by viral infections benefit from low-dose inhaled steroid treatment.[31] Although there are theoretical reasons for believing leukotriene receptor antagonists may have a place in treating wheezing provoked by viral upper respiratory infections there are as yet no published studies to support their use in children with mild intermittent asthma. Some children who do not normally wheeze with exercise may develop coughing or wheezing during physical activity when they have a cold. A single dose of an inhaled β-adrenergic agonist taken shortly beforehand helps to prevent this.

Conversely, children with seasonal asthma due to pollen allergy may require a step-up during the pollen season, but little more than intermittent bronchodilator therapy (Step 1) at other times.

Mild persistent asthma – Step 2

School-children with persistent asthma are usually atopic or have an atopic family history. Wheezing may be triggered by allergic, physical or emotional factors although viral respiratory infections remain the predominant trigger of acute asthma attacks in school-age children. Spirometry may be close to normal between attacks, but some indices of small-airway obstruction, such as MEF_{25} and MEF_{50} (Chapter 6b) may remain depressed. Persistent asthma is considered mild if the child has symptoms at least once a week but less than daily, occasionally affecting daytime activity and causing sleep disturbance (less than weekly). Bronchodilator medication may be needed on most days. Parents and children may have difficulty remembering the frequency of cough and wheeze. Recording day and night symptoms and morning and evening peak flow on a diary card for a brief period (say 4 weeks) may help in determining the pattern and severity of symptoms, and the need for regular medication. A written record can be helpful in persuading parents and children that regular preventer therapy is necessary.

Some guidelines include 'cough variant asthma' in the category of mild persistent asthma but this is controversial in school-children (Chapter 6a). Cough is undoubtedly a common symptom of asthma but it has been estimated that less than 10% of asthma presents with cough alone.[32,33] In a community setting, isolated cough (in the absence of wheeze) is rarely due to asthma, rarely responds to asthma medications[34] and is quite often over-diagnosed as asthma.[32] However, in a specialist clinic, where a highly selected group of children are seen, children who cough in response to typical asthma triggers, and improve when treated with asthma medications are not uncommonly seen.[35] Bronchoscopic and bronchoalveolar lavage studies have shown that many children with chronic cough have no evidence of eosinophilic airway inflammation.[36–38] Others however will show increasing bronchial reactivity over time, start wheezing and develop the typical clinical picture of asthma.[39] If coughing is troublesome and no other diagnosis is evident a therapeutic trial with anti-inflammatory treatment is justified. The only danger is that ineffectual and potentially harmful medication may be continued long-term. An adequate therapeutic trial should

demonstrate improvement with treatment, deterioration when it is stopped and improvement again when it is restarted. In school-children with chronic cough who can perform lung function, there is little justification for a therapeutic trial of anti-inflammatory treatment without first attempting to document variable airflow obstruction.

There is currently a choice of two types of agent to control airway inflammation in mild persistent asthma, inhaled steroids and cromones. Future studies may show that the leukotriene receptor antagonists (LTRA) also have a place in treating mild persistent asthma in school-children.

INHALED STEROIDS

A systematic review published in 1997 analysed 24 randomized controlled trials of inhaled steroid treatment in children.[40] The mean improvement was 50% for symptoms and 11% of predicted for lung function. There was a mean reduction in bronchodilator use of 37% and a mean decrease in oral steroid use of 28%. Nevertheless the best way to use these highly effective agents in children with asthma is still not entirely clear. There is evidence that it is no better to start with a high dose and wean down than to start low and work up (if necessary)[40a]. Low-dose inhaled steroid therapy (100–200 μg/day) is highly effective in mild persistent asthma.

In recent years concern has been expressed about the safety of inhaled steroids particularly when used to treat relatively mild disease. Local side effects are rare and there is no evidence that inhaled steroid therapy causes cataracts in children. There is some systemic adsorption with all inhaled steroids and this leads to dose-dependent inhibition of the hypothalamic pituitary adrenal feedback loop. Over 160 studies have investigated the impact of inhaled steroids on growth in children but only six of them have been double-blind controlled trials (see also Chapters 8a and 15). Four concluded that beclomethasone dipropionate 400 μg/day was associated with a growth deceleration of just over 1 cm in one year. In one of these studies the children treated had only mild intermittent asthma.[41] Another has been criticized for including pubertal children.[42] In two studies the dose of inhaled steroid would normally have been reduced after 3 months because of the excellent therapeutic response.[43,44] Thus none gave a clinically generalizable result! Despite this effect on medium term growth there is no evidence that long-term treatment with inhaled steroid adversely effects final height.[45,46] The remaining randomized double-blind studies both monitored growth over one year and did not demonstrate growth suppression with fluticasone propionate, which is about twice as potent as beclomethasone but has less systemic bioavailability, in doses of 100 and 200 μg/day.[47,48] Growth in children with mild persistent asthma taking fluticasone propionate 100 μg per day is comparable to that in children taking sodium cromoglycate but asthma control is better.[49] Patients with mild disease appear more vulnerable to the systemic effects of inhaled steroids than those with severe disease; this makes a strong argument for using the lowest possible dose to maintain control. Normally inhaled steroids are given twice daily. There is no therapeutic justification for more frequent dosage and adherence declines with increasing frequency of dosing.[50] Once asthma control has been achieved it can often be maintained with once daily inhaled steroid.[51] Inhaled steroids should not be given to children via unmodified metered dose aerosol inhalers; an efficient powder inhaler (e.g. Turbohaler) or large-volume spacer device should be used (Chapter 8b).

CROMONES

Until recently sodium cromoglycate was recommended as the first line preventive agent for children with mild to moderate asthma. Early studies indicated that if taken regularly it controlled symptoms in about 60% of school-age children with frequent asthma.[52] The aerosol is as effective as the powder in children who are able to use a metered dose aerosol properly and is slightly less likely to cause coughing after inhalation.[53] Sodium cromoglycate is safe with virtually no known side effects even when taken regularly for years. The requirement for cromoglycate to be taken three or preferably four times a day is a serious disadvantage. Comparative studies indicate sodium cromoglycate is less effective than a low dose of inhaled steroid when initiating anti-inflammatory treatment in children with mild persistent asthma.[54] A recent systematic review which analysed[24] randomized controlled trials of sodium cromoglycate concluded there is insufficient evidence that it has a beneficial effect as maintenance treatment in children with asthma[55] although these conclusions hide an important difference between infants (where there is no evidence of benefit) and school-children (where there is evidence of benefit). In many countries (but not Japan, Chapter 17) cromones have been virtually superseded by low-dose inhaled steroids. However the systematic review did not address the question of exercise-induced asthma and single dose studies provide clear evidence that cromones inhibit exercise-induced bronchoconstriction.

Nedrocromil sodium inhibits the activation of a variety of inflammatory cells and is a potent mast cell stabilizer *in vitro*. Few trials have been done in children but it has efficacy in seasonal asthma.[48] Like cromoglycate, it needs to be administered four times a day.

Moderate persistent asthma – Step 3

Moderate persistent asthma in children is characterized by persistent, daily symptoms and nocturnal symptoms at least once a week. Inevitably daily activity (such as exercise) and sleep are affected. Lung function frequently falls below 80% of predicted or best and there is wide peak flow variability. Children also fall into this category if although initially assessed as having mild persistent asthma satisfactory symptom control and near normal

lung function can not be achieved with low doses of inhaled steroid together with intermittent short-acting bronchodilators. When a careful search for remedial environmental triggers and attention to compliance and inhaler technique have failed to result in improvement there are three choices for treatment: increase the dose of inhaled steroid; add a long-acting bronchodilator; or add a leukotriene receptor antagonist (LTRA).

INCREASE THE DOSE OF INHALED STEROID

There have been very few good studies to define the plateau of the dose response curve for inhaled steroids in children. One study has indicated that the top of the dose–response curve for inhaled steroids in children with mild and moderate persistent asthma is not more than 400–800 μg/day.[56] Although most guidelines advise doubling the dose of inhaled steroid during exacerbations of asthma, this recommendation is not supported by a controlled trial.[57] The increasing evidence of systemic effects of inhaled steroids at doses of greater than 400 μg/day, highlights the importance of combining moderate doses of inhaled steroid with other non-steroid compounds that may have a synergistic effect.

ADD A LONG-ACTING β-AGONIST

There are theoretical reasons for regarding the actions of the long-acting β-agonist bronchodilators (LABA) salmeterol and formoterol and inhaled steroids as complementary. For example steroids may potentiate β-receptor synthesis while long-acting β-agonist may prime intracellular steroid receptors. Concerns that treatment with LABA may mask ongoing airway inflammation have not been borne out by airway biopsy studies in adults.[58] We know nothing of the interaction of inhaled steroids and LABA at the cellular level in children. Crucially we must ask whether the theoretical synergistic actions of inhaled steroids and LABA are reflected in clinical practice.

In adults there is substantial evidence that combining an inhaled steroid with a LABA improves symptom control to a greater extent than increasing the dose of inhaled steroid and reduces frequency of exacerbations.[59] In a placebo-controlled study asthma symptoms and lung function improved when a LABA was given to children already taking beclomethasone 400 μg/day.[60] However in another study children derived no benefit from either doubling the dose of inhaled steroid or from adding a LABA.[61] The children who took part in this study had near normal lung function at baseline and it may be there was not sufficient room for improvement to demonstrate an effect. Importantly however the children treated with the higher dose of inhaled steroid (800 μg/day) grew less well than those on combination therapy.

Long-acting β-agonists are potent and prolonged inhibitors of exercise-induced asthma[62] although this inhibitory effect may decline with regular administration.[63] The evidence for declining benefit with regular LABA therapy in children has been reviewed (Chapter 8a) but remains controversial. The incorporation of an inhaled steroid (fluticasone) and a long-acting bronchodilator (salmeterol) in one inhaler device makes the administration of this combination more convenient. The one study so far published testing this product in children shows it is at least as effective as the two agents given separately and is free of side effects.[64]

ADD A LEUKOTRIENE RECEPTOR ANTAGONIST (LTRA)

The cysteinyl leukotrienes are released from a range of inflammatory cells, notably mast cells and eosinophils, and are potent mediators of bronchoconstriction, stimulate mucus secretion and increased vascular permeability. Leukotriene synthesis is one of the few components of the inflammatory cascade that is not affected by corticosteroids and therefore leukotriene inhibition could complement the action of steroids in asthma. Montelukast and zafirlukast interfere with receptor binding of LTC4 and LTD4. Montelukast, a once daily chewable tablet, is effective in children over 2 years. Zafirlukast, a twice daily tablet, has been shown to be effective in children over 12 years. In one multicentre placebo-controlled trial, montelukast was superior to placebo for symptom control, lung function and for all three domains of a quality of life assessment in school-children.[65] Its safety profile was very reassuring with no difference in adverse events between montelukast and placebo. Both montelukast[66] and zafirlukast[67] inhibit exercise-induced asthma: in the case of montelukast this inhibition persists for 24 hours after a dose.

The positioning of LTRA in current treatment guidelines is not clearly established. As yet there are no direct comparisons between LTRA and either low-dose inhaled steroid in children with mild persistent asthma or long-acting β-agonists as add on therapy in children with moderate persistent asthma already receiving inhaled steroids. The sound theoretical basis for a complementary action with inhaled steroids and the results of the large placebo-controlled study justifies their inclusion as one of the choices to combine with an inhaled steroid in children with moderate persistent asthma. Leukotreine receptor antagonists inhibit exercise-induced asthma and unlike long-acting β-agonists there is no indication this effect decays over time[68] so they may be particularly suitable for children with troublesome activity related symptoms. In time the therapeutic role for leukotriene receptor antagonists in mild and severe persistent asthma should become clearer. Common sense dictates that adherence will be better with a once daily tablet than with inhaled treatment taken twice daily, but there is no evidence to confirm or refute this at the moment.

In all of the clinical trials, the rate of onset of clinical and physiological benefit is rapid, the maximum benefit occurring over 1–2 days. This means that in practice, under stable clinical conditions, it should be possible to assess the benefit of introducing LTRA therapy over a 1–2 week period.

Severe persistent asthma – Step 4

Some children have almost continuous day-time and nocturnal symptoms, waking frequently at night and almost invariably coughing and wheezing in the mornings. Such children miss a lot of schooling, school performance may be affected and they are often unable to participate in sporting activities. Despite treatment with an inhaled steroid and either a long-acting β-agonist or a leukotriene receptor antagonist these children also have asthma attacks and may require hospital admissions. They are nearly always atopic and usually have abnormal lung function between attacks. Chest deformity may result from chronic persistent airflow obstruction and lung hyperinflation.

Management of severe childhood asthma is a fine balance between the benefits of controlling symptoms and the inconvenience and adverse effects of therapy. Optimal asthma control and normal lung function may not be achievable without unacceptable imposition on daily life or undesirable side effects from treatment. The dose–response relationship for inhaled steroids is likely to be different from that in mild or moderate asthma with a higher plateau for efficacy and a less steep curve for adverse effects. Thus in children with severe disease doses of up to 1000 μg per day of inhaled steroid may relieve symptoms without impairing growth.

Other options available in addition to high-dose inhaled steroids plus long-acting β-agonists and leukotriene antagonists include oral slow release theophylline and anti-cholinergic agents. Slow-release theophylline in doses that are titrated to give blood levels of 50–100 mmol/l will control asthma in about 60% of children with frequent symptoms, but are relatively ineffective in preventing the wheezing episodes which accompany viral upper respiratory tract infections.[69] One study has shown that the addition of oral slow-release theophylline improves asthma control in children with symptoms despite taking an inhaled steroid.[70] The high frequency of side effects and the narrow therapeutic index are reasons why in many countries the use of oral theophyllines has become restricted to the severe end of the asthma spectrum. There is a clinical impression that some children with severe asthma benefit from treatment with inhaled anti-cholinergic agents, but no controlled studies have been done. They may be worth considering in children experiencing side effects such as tremor or headache when taking both long and short-acting β-agonists.

Difficult asthma – Step 5 and beyond

Most children with correctly diagnosed asthma, who take measures to avoid known provoking factors and who are given appropriate medication will improve. Several

Table 10.2 *Factors which may contribute to difficult asthma (Step 5 and beyond)*

- incorrect diagnosis
- co-morbidity
- unrecognized environmental agents
- psychosocial stress
- non-adherence with therapy (compliance)

possibilities should be considered when children do not or apparently do not respond to treatment (Table 10.2). Firstly the diagnosis may be wrong. Vocal cord dysfunction, a condition in which there is paradoxical adduction of the vocal cords sufficient to cause airflow limitation at the level of the larynx may mimic or co-exist with asthma (Chapter 13a). This condition commonly appears in early adolescence. Gastroesophageal reflux or hyperventilation may similarly mimic or co-exist with asthma. Secondly there may be environmental or psychosocial factors affecting the asthma that have not been recognized. Thirdly the prescribed treatment may not be taken, either by accident or by design.

However, a very small number of school-children, despite good adherence to the treatment regimes described above, continue to experience frequent incapacitating and occasionally life-threatening symptoms. The final step in the asthma guidelines for these children is regular oral corticosteroids. Other options are available for those who do not respond to oral steroids. Before embarking on these options that often carry a high risk of side effects an attempt should be made to document the presence and nature of airway inflammation. There are probably different subgroups of very severe asthma that are distinguished for example by presence or absence of eosinophilia[71] or the level of exhaled nitric oxide.[72] The pathological basis of very severe childhood asthma needs to be better understood if we are to develop a rational basis for its treatment.[73]

ORAL AND NEBULIZED STEROIDS

A survey in the UK of almost 4000 asthmatic children under 16 years of age found only 27 children who were taking regular oral steroids.[74] The use of regular prednisolone involves a balance between its benefits and side effects. Both excessive doses of prednisolone and poorly controlled asthma suppress growth in childhood. It is therefore particularly important to monitor growth in these children. Oral prednisolone suppresses the hypothalamo–pituitary–adrenal axis, but this may be lessened by taking a single dose on alternate days. The drug should never be stopped suddenly and additional doses may be required for patients undergoing surgery. Children on regular oral steroids should not be given live vaccines and are at increased risk of severe chickenpox.

The use of nebulized steroids in very severe steroid-dependent childhood asthma is controversial. In a small open study in adults, 55% were able to reduce their oral steroid intake when treated with nebulized budesonide 2 mg/day.[75] A small reduction in daily prednisolone was also seen in adults with steroid dependent asthma when they were given nebulized fluticasone 4 mg/day.[76] No study of nebulized steroid has been done in school-age children with steroid dependent asthma. If a child can use a spacer device efficiently it seems unlikely that switching to a nebulized steroid will confer additional benefit.

IMMUNOSUPPRESSIVE AGENTS

Cyclosporin inhibits T-lymphocyte activation. Small trials in adults with severe asthma, in which oral cyclosporin has been given for 12 weeks[77] and 36 weeks[78] have shown improvement in lung function, reduction in exacerbations and reduced prednisolone use compared with placebo. No controlled trials have been carried out on children. However there is a case report of its use in five children on regular oral steroids, three of whom experienced a definite benefit.[79] The side effects in adults include hirsutism, paraesthesia, mild hypertension, headaches, and tremor. The only concern in the paediatric reports was hirsutism, which led to one girl stopping its use even though her steroid dose had been profoundly reduced.[79] There is obviously a concern about renal impairment with long-term use, so renal function must be carefully monitored, and cyclosporin blood concentrations maintained at 80–150 mg/l.

Methotrexate is an immunosuppressive and anti-inflammatory agent. Three small open label studies on children have shown steroid doses could be reduced in some of the children while lung function was maintained or improved.[80–82] Doses of methotrexate used were between 7.5 and 17 mg/week for up to 2 years[80,81] and 0.6 mg/kg per week for 3 months.[82] Reported side effects in the children were gastrointestinal upset and transiently raised liver transaminases. Low doses seem to be relatively safe, and its use may be considered in some children with very severe asthma.

PARTNERSHIP IN MANAGEMENT

If asthma management is to be successful a partnership needs to be established between the child, family, primary and secondary healthcare workers and other temporary carers such as schoolteachers. The object of this partnership is to evolve a guided management plan, to enable asthmatic children and their parents to deal with symptoms day-to-day and to feel confident about when to make adjustments themselves and when to call for help. The route to achieving this includes the identification of family anxieties and beliefs about asthma, the provision of appropriate information about asthma and its treatment and an agreed therapeutic approach which is then written down (Table 10.3).

Table 10.3 *Route to a guided self-management plan for families of children with asthma*

- establish frequency, severity and pattern of symptoms
- identify anxieties and beliefs about asthma
- provide information about:
  - nature of asthma
  - how to judge severity
  - principles of prevention and relief medication
- identify and if possible remove triggers
- agree treatment regime
- choose and demonstrate use of inhalers
- advise on use and limitations of peak flow measurement
- write down the management plan on an asthma card

History taking

The history taking should include open questions that help to clarify not only the severity and frequency of symptoms but also underlying anxieties and beliefs about asthma and its treatment. In general during the primary school years parents have a clearer perception of asthma severity than the children themselves. However as children approach adolescence their own perception of their symptoms more closely resembles objective measures than that of their parents.[83] Some parents fear their child will die during an asthma attack, to such an extent that it interferes with their ability to deal rationally with the attack.[84] Other parents underestimate the severity of their child's symptoms.[85] During an acute attack this can lead to delay in starting, emergency treatment[86] and may be a contributory factor in some asthma deaths.[87] Misconceptions about the hazards of asthma medication are common. In one study over a third of parents considered asthma drugs to be addictive or unsafe in the long-term[86] and a questionnaire survey of 13 to 14-year-olds found 60% of them thought asthma medication was addictive.[88]

INFORMATION AND EDUCATION

The goals of any educational program should be to: reinforce the process of shared care between the family and the doctor, improve adherence to medication, increase the family's confidence in making assessments and judgements about symptom severity and help children to be physically active at home and at school. Intelligence, education and the ability to understand information about the nature of asthma bears little relationship to adherence with treatment.[89] Nevertheless the provision of information in an accessible form aids the development of self-management plans. Children and parents should be offered information about the nature of asthma, how to assess severity and the principles of 'preventer and reliever' medication. A wealth of education programs have been developed, along with booklets, audio cassettes and videos. They are useful supplements to but not substitutes for regular personal contact between families and appropriately trained health professionals.

Delivery devices

Most treatment for asthma in school-children is given by inhalation and choice of delivery device with careful instruction in their correct use is central to successful management (Chapter 8b). One of the most common reasons for failure of asthma treatment is inappropriate selection or incorrect use of the inhaler. Most children under the age of 10 years are unable to achieve the coordination needed to use an unmodified metered dose aerosol inhaler and less than 50% of children obtain benefit from these devices because of poor inhalation technique. Breath-actuated metered dose inhalers (Autohaler, Easibreathe) are easier to use but young children tend to close their glottis when the breath-actuated valve opens. The number of children able to use these inhalers declines rapidly under the age of 7 years.[90]

Children become fully aware of their own breathing and recognize the difference between inspiration and expiration by about the age of 3 years. From this age most children can use valved spacers with an integral mouthpiece. By school age children have learnt how to take a full inspiration and most will be able to use breath-actuated powder inhalers. However, low inspiratory flow rates particularly during wheezy episodes limit the use of this type of inhaler in children under 7. Breath-actuated powder inhalers are either single dose (e.g. Spinhaler, Rotahaler) or multi-dose (e.g. Diskhaler, Turbuhaler, Accuhaler).

Peak flow measurement

Some children over the age of 3 and most over the age of 6 can use a peak flow meter. It is the cheapest and most convenient way to measure lung function in children with asthma. In the past it has been the mainstay of home monitoring programs and has often been used as a primary variable in asthma trials. Peak expiratory flow measurement does however have serious limitations. Although PEF is highly reproducible, mini-Wright peak flow meters are non-linear. This results in underestimation at low and high recordings and overestimation in the mid range. It is preferable to relate values to the child's 'best' with a given meter than to relate the value to mean predicted. PEF recordings on diary card records can easily be fabricated and are very unreliable.[91] PEF measurement in outpatient clinics is of little value in establishing severity and pattern of disease. Single measurements of PEF can be compared with the child's and parents' assessment of the severity of their airway obstruction at the time in order to understand better their perception of the severity of the airway obstruction. Regular monitoring of PEF has proved to be less sensitive than symptoms in identifying acute episodes of asthma. In self-management programs, PEF monitoring confers no additional benefit as an adjunct to symptom control.[92]

PEF measurement before and after a bronchodilator can be helpful in making the diagnosis, but spirometry (FEV_1) is more informative (Chapter 6b). Measurements made in the morning and evening over a short period (1–2 weeks) can be useful in determining whether a change in treatment is required or to evaluate the introduction of a new treatment, provided the results are reliable![91] (Figure 10.3). PEF can also be used to guide families during the early stages of an asthma attack. Broadly speaking, a value of less than 70–80% of best indicates the need for

some remedial action (additional bronchodilator); a value of less than 50% which is unrelieved by bronchodilator indicates the need to start a short course of prednisolene (if this is part of the agreed management plan) and to seek medical advice; and a value of less than 25–30% indicates a severe or life threatening attack (Chapter 11).

Asthma cards

Once a management plan has been developed it should be written down. One way to do this is by using asthma cards. The cards need to be robust, clear and didactic and not too wordy (Figure 10.4).

Figure 10.3 *Variation in peak flow recorded morning and evening at home. Mean predicted value: 200 l/min.*

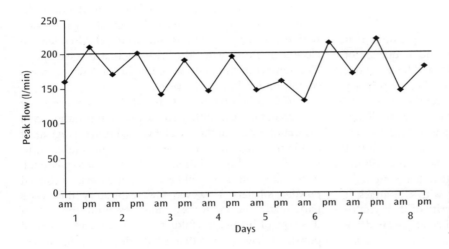

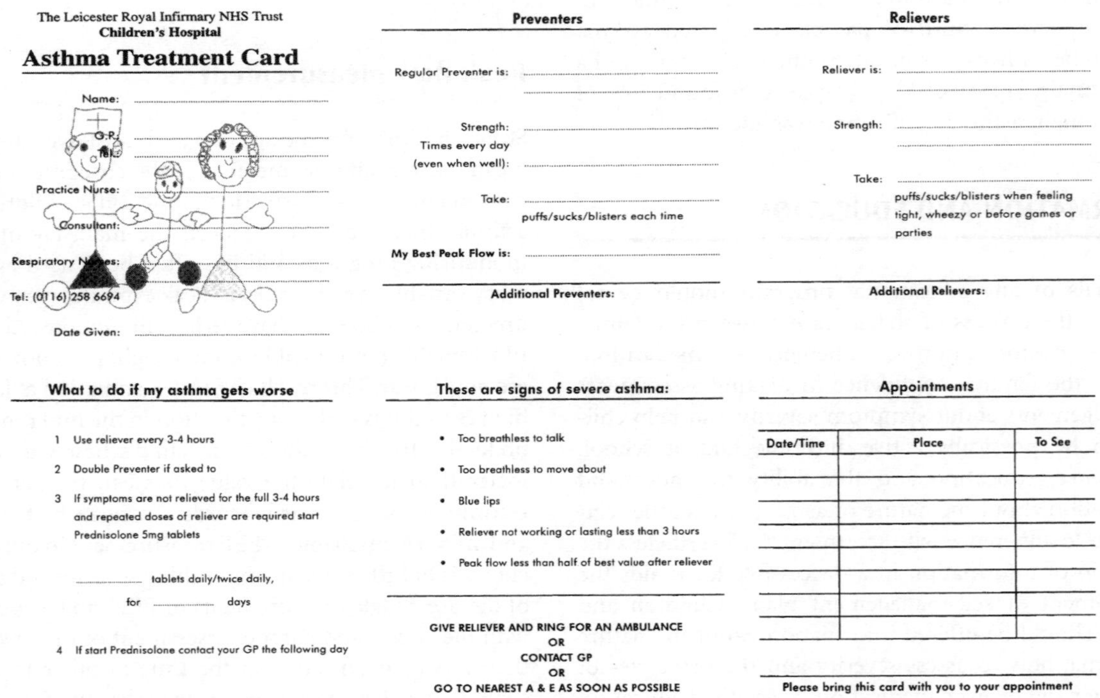

Figure 10.4 *Asthma card for home management.*

The key elements are:

- names and doses of drugs and inhalers;
- a plan of what to do when asthma becomes worse;
- what to do if the child has a severe attack;
- when, whom, and how to call for help.

PATTERNS OF ASTHMA

Nocturnal asthma

A combination of factors relating to circadian rhythms, environment and posture predispose to cough and wheezing at night (Table 10.4). The importance of nocturnal symptoms is highlighted by a questionnaire survey conducted in the UK involving 773 asthmatic children and 248 parents. One third of the children reported waking at least once a week due to asthma and school performance was often affected the following day.[93] A more recent survey of children with asthma in seven European countries showed little has changed; 28% of school-age children reported asthma related sleep disturbance more than once a week.[2] Nocturnal symptoms and particularly nocturnal cough often go unrecognized. In a study of asthmatic children aged 7–14 years nocturnal cough was reported by 66% but was heard by tape recording during the night in 90%.[94]

The term nocturnal asthma is misleading because it implies asthma at night is a separate entity. In fact there is strong evidence that the frequency of nocturnal symptoms reflects overall asthma severity. Overnight oxygen saturation and to a lesser extent, cough are related to the severity of day-time asthma in children recovering from acute attacks.[95] The most common time for asthma deaths to occur is at night or in the early morning and most children who die of asthma have previously had severe nocturnal symptoms.[96,97]

Since nocturnal symptoms reflect overall severity and probably indicate chronic inflammation in the lung airways, it is generally not appropriate to treat nocturnal

asthma simply by giving a bronchodilator at bedtime. Although this may be justified in a child with occasional and transient nocturnal symptoms associated with viral respiratory tract infections, persistent nocturnal cough or wheezing requires regular anti-inflammatory therapy, the dose depending on overall frequency and severity of symptoms. If day-time symptoms improve but nocturnal asthma persists despite moderate doses of inhaled steroid (400 mg/day), consider giving an inhaled long-acting β-agonist at bedtime.[98] Slow-release oral theophylline as a single dose in the evening has also been shown to improve nocturnal symptoms[99] but may disturb sleep and, in younger children, induce enuresis.

If a child has predominantly nocturnal symptoms it is important to consider environmental factors such as cigarette smoke exposure and contact with allergen in the bedroom. The degree of sensitivity to house-dust mite can be assessed by skin-prick testing. This can be helpful to the clinician in deciding whether to advise mite eradication measures in the bedroom and provides a demonstration to the families and an incentive to embark on such measures. Some attention should also be paid to day-time exposure to pets or pollens because nocturnal symptoms may be the result of a late asthmatic response to allergen exposure several hours previously. Gastroesophageal reflux is more common in asthmatic children than in those without asthma. Treatment with ranitidine, however, produces only a modest improvement in asthma symptoms at night.[100] The relevance of diurnal variation in plasma cortisol to nocturnal asthma is not clear because 24-hour infusions of hydrocortisone have failed to prevent the early morning fall in peak flow. On the other hand, oral prednisolone given to asthmatic patients at 15.00 h has been shown to reduce parameters of airway inflammation the following night.[101] The practical implication in children with very severe asthma and frequent nocturnal symptoms who require oral corticosteroid therapy is that perhaps the appropriate time to give the steroid may be mid-afternoon.

Seasonal asthma

The most common cause of seasonal asthma in children is pollen allergy. A relatively small number of grass species account for practically all grass pollen allergy and there is extensive cross-reactivity between them. Pollen asthma usually accompanies pollen hay fever in the early summer. Symptoms of allergic rhinitis may precede the development of asthma by several years, but the peak prevalence for hayfever is in teenage, a few years later than the peak for asthma. Sensitization to tree pollens causes symptoms in the early spring and to ragweed pollen, in North America, in the autumn. Often pollen allergy is one of several trigger factors and perennial asthma becomes worse in the summer months. The diagnosis is usually obvious. It is important to treat the hay fever adequately

Table 10.4 *Factors which may predispose to asthma at night*

Circadian rhythms
Airway responsiveness
Plasma catecholamines
Vagal tone
Non-adrenergic, non-cholinergic airway control
Plasma cortisol
Sleep state

Environment and posture
Allergen exposure (e.g. house-dust mite)
Non-specific irritants (e.g. cigarette smoke)
Gastroesophageal reflux
Mucociliary clearance (slower)

as well as the asthma. Exposure to seasonal pollens can be reduced by keeping windows closed during the day when it is warm and windy and pollen counts are high. Hot and humid conditions and especially thunderstorms can be very troublesome. The efficacy of air conditioners and air filters is not established. In a child with a history of seasonal asthma treatment with an inhaled steroid should be started or the dose increased about 2 weeks before the onset of the pollen season and continued until about two weeks after pollen counts have fallen.

Food-related asthma

Food and drink-related asthma in children may be of more relevance to young infants than older children and their role has been a subject of dispute for many years[102] (Chapter 7d). One survey estimated about 6% of school-age children could identify a food as a precipitating cause.[103] Diagnostic tests for food allergy as a cause for asthma are generally unsatisfactory and the only sure way to confirm food allergy is by elimination and double-blind challenge. This is quite difficult to achieve in children and the results are often inconclusive. The mechanism by which food intolerance predisposes to asthma may be by an effect on bronchial responsiveness.[104] An indirect challenge technique has been described, whereby a change in bronchial responsiveness is determined after ingestion of a suspected food trigger. The correlation between the clinical history and the results of such challenge tests is good so that reliance can be placed on the history alone.[105] In one hospital-based children's asthma clinic, food-induced symptoms were found in over 90% of children of South Asian origin in contrast to about 60% of other (mainly Caucasian) children.[106] The difference was caused by sensitivity to acidic drinks, ice-cold drinks and fried foods, and not to foods that are commonly thought of as 'allergenic'. The onset of symptoms may range from minutes to hours after exposure or may even be delayed to the next day. Often food ingestion alone is insufficient and additional factors, such as a recent cold (URTI) or exercise, are necessary to cause symptoms.

Anaphylactic reactions to foods are sudden, dramatic and sometimes fatal. Nuts, sea foods and eggs are the commonest agents to be incriminated. Acute severe asthma often accompanies anaphylaxis. Adrenaline (epinephrine) 1:1000, 0.01 ml/kg (10 μg/kg) i.m. is the emergency treatment.

Asthma and exercise

THE SIZE OF THE PROBLEM

Perhaps the strongest impact asthma can have on a school-child's well-being and ability to mix with their peers is through restriction of daily activity. Two large UK surveys have documented prevalence rates of exercise-related symptoms in 87%[107] and 80%[93] of asthmatic

children. One of these surveys found that more than 50% of children were at times unable to complete a sports lesson because of asthma. Sports that involve outdoor running were those most affected. Nevertheless 11% of children found swimming provoked symptoms, a sport generally considered to be well-tolerated by asthma sufferers. Many children also found that social play and other outdoor activities such a camping, horse riding and walking in the country were curtailed by their asthma. Asthma may interfere with playground activity and because schoolteachers are sometimes reluctant to allow asthmatic children to join school trips involving camping or walking in the country,[93] they are at risk of being isolated from their peers. Impairment of activity is also a problem in secondary school-children with asthma. This was assessed in students aged 13–14 years attending Australian schools. Asthma limited the activities of 35% of students during the previous 2 weeks, most commonly affecting outdoor sports, running up hills, cycling and swimming.[88]

Although many asthma provoking physical activities take place at school, studies in the UK[108] and Australia[88] have shown that schoolteachers are not well-informed about exercise-induced asthma and its management. Three-quarters of secondary schoolteachers were unable to name a β-agonist as useful treatment during an asthma attack, and only 6% were able to give the correct answer when asked about prevention of exercise-induced asthma.[88] In many schools children are not encouraged to keep their inhalers with them so inevitably management of exercise-induced asthma is not ideal. A child with a cold who is simultaneously exposed to allergen (e.g. during the pollen season) or air pollution (e.g. at the roadside in hot weather) is more vulnerable to exercise-induced asthma.

CHOICES OF TREATMENT

The *short-acting β-adrenergic* agonists salbutamol and terbutaline are potent inhibitors of exercise-induced asthma but the duration of protective effect is less than 4 hours.[109] The value of short-acting β-agonists to treat activity-induced symptoms in school-children is limited where local school regulations prevent children carrying their own inhalers. Children are active throughout the day and it is impractical to keep giving treatment before every period of physical exercise. *Long-acting β2-agonists* afford protection against exercise-induced asthma for at least 9 hours.[62] This prolonged protection is achieved with low inspiratory flow (30 l/min) from a dry powder breath actuated inhaler.[110] Both 25 μg and 50 μg of salmeterol given to children aged 7–14 years almost completely inhibited airway obstruction 1 hour after exercise, but 50 μg afforded better protection after 12 hours.[111] Formoterol has a more rapid onset of bronchodilation than salmeterol and gives greater than 60% inhibition of exercise-induced bronchoconstriction 12 hours following pretreatment.[112] These single dose studies suggest that a long-acting β-agonist given in the morning will offer some protection throughout the day against symptoms provoked by sport and other physical activity. With regular administration the duration of inhibition of exercise-induced asthma by a long-acting β-agonist declines (Chapter 8a). In a randomized, double-blind cross-over study salmeterol 50 μg was given once daily to young adolescents aged 12–16 years with asthma for 28 days. On the first day of treatment there was effective inhibition of bronchoconstriction with salmeterol at 1 and 9 hours. On the 28th day of treatment the protective effect of salmeterol at 1 hour was undiminished, but the protective effect at 9 hours was reduced. Treatment with an inhaled steroid did not prevent this apparent development of tolerance.[63]

Sodium cromoglycate and nedocromil sodium give similar protection against exercise-induced asthma,[113] reducing bronchoconstriction by at least 50%.[114] The duration of protection with both compounds lasts less than 2 hours.[113] Nedocromil sodium has an unpleasant taste and sodium cromoglycate may cause coughing immediately after inhalation. Because β-agonists are bronchodilators as well as protecting against exercise-induced asthma, it has been proposed they should be used before exercise in children with pre-existing airway obstruction. The use of cromones may be more appropriate in children with vulnerability to activity induced symptoms but no airway obstruction before exercise.[115]

Cysteinyl leukotriene release has been implicated as a mechanism in exercise-induced asthma and the *leukotriene receptor antagonists* have an inhibitory effect on EIB.[66–68] An increase in urinary LTE4 has been observed after exercise in adults and in children with severe asthma[116] although neither the pre-exercise level nor the rise in LTE4 after exercise correlate with the degree of exercise-induced bronchoconstriction.[117] The effect of 5 mg montelukast administered once daily on exercise challenge was assessed in 27 children aged between 6–14 years with stable asthma. Six minute treadmill exercise challenges were performed 20–24 hours after the last dose in each trial period. Montelukast significantly reduced the 'area under the curve' (mean difference 60%) and the maximum % fall in FEV_1 (mean difference 8%), but not the time to recovery relative to placebo. There was no correlation between age and the degree of inhibition of EIB and no suggestion that younger children were less well-protected.[66] A further study examined the impact of montelukast on activity-induced symptoms through the use of a quality of life questionnaire during an 8-week treatment period. The 'activity domain' questions showed improvement for montelukast compared with placebo.[65] No controlled studies have been published to describe the impact of long-term treatment with LRAs on exercise-induced asthma in asthmatic children. However studies in adults suggest tolerance and loss of protective effect do not occur.[68]

When deciding on treatment it is important to take into account the whole pattern of illness and not just the wheezing with exercise. Although we do not have histological confirmation, it is likely that the presence of exercise-induced asthma implies persistent underlying airway inflammation and is therefore an indication to start or modify the dose of an inhaled steroid. Regular treatment with inhaled steroids for 1–2 months attenuates airway obstruction following exercise.[56] Some data indicates however that the protective effect of inhaled steroids may decrease over time.[118]

Asthma at school

Asthma remains the most frequent physical cause of school absence in the UK and the amount of school missed is a good measure of asthma morbidity and asthma control.[119] Academic performance is affected by school absence and by tiredness and lack of concentration following disturbed nights. The disadvantageous effects on education continue into adulthood. One study has shown that adults who had asthma in childhood have a higher than average rate of unemployment even if they become asymptomatic.[120] Several studies have revealed misconceptions about asthma among schoolteachers with respect to sporting activity. A commonly held view noted in one survey was that because exercise caused wheezing, exercise was bad for asthma.[109] In fact sports fitness programs, particularly those involving swimming, have been found to reduce exacerbations of asthma and improve school attendance.[121] It is important for teachers to have information about asthma and its relationship to exercise, classroom pets and chemical fumes. School asthma cards such as those produced by the UK National Asthma Campaign help to promote good communication between schoolteachers, nurses, school doctors, general practitioners and hospital paediatricians, but require regular updating. Schools often have special knowledge of family relationships relevant to the child's asthma that is not possessed by the general practitioner or hospital clinic. It is important this information is shared. A written policy regarding the administration of drugs in school is essential and children should have ready access to their inhalers before exercise and when they develop symptoms (Table 10.5). Much anxiety is generated about the participation of asthmatic children in trips and camps away from the school. This can be alleviated by providing written information that can be taken on the trip about routine medication and what to do in the event of an asthma attack.

In the past it was common practice for children with asthma to be sent to special schools, often in the mountains or by the sea. This practice is declining but such schools still perform a valuable function for a small minority of children with very severe asthma, accompanied by special emotional and psychological problems. Children attending school at altitude in a relatively allergen-free environment often show a marked improvement in symptoms and reduction in bronchial responsiveness.

Table 10.5 *Key points for good asthma management in schools*

- information for teachers about recognition and treatment of asthma
- written policy regarding administration of drugs and emergency action plan
- good lines of communication between education and health professionals
- monitoring of potential asthma triggers such as classroom pets and chemical fumes
- written instructions on routine and emergency medication for school trips
- availability of a β_2-agonist inhaler and large volume spacer in the emergency cupboard for use by *any* child in an emergency

Unfortunately asthma symptoms and responsiveness usually recur within a few days or weeks of returning to the home environment.[16]

REGULAR REVIEW AND STEP DOWN

Regular treatment with an anti-inflammatory drug is likely to be needed for years rather than months. Asthma can alter in severity over time and the doses of medication that are needed to maintain optimal asthma control also vary. A child with asthma who is taking regular inhaled steroid treatment needs to be reviewed at least every 6 months and those with severe asthma at least every 3 months. At reviews useful checkpoints are: number and severity of asthma attacks; frequency of daytime and night-time symptoms; use of relief medication; days off school; effect of exercise and other activities; inhaler technique; and understanding of treatment. Growth needs to be monitored in all children with persistent asthma. Height should be measured by a trained observer, using a stadiometer that is calibrated regularly.

Lung function should be assessed at each visit. Spirometry before and after taking a bronchodilator gives more information about overall asthma control than PEF. However PEF recorded at home in the morning and evening during the week or two before attending the clinic may reveal variations which would not be apparent from a single clinic measurement, if reliable.[91] Abnormalities in the maximum expiratory flow–volume (MEFV) curve at low lung volumes that probably reflect small airway obstruction are often seen in children with a relatively normal PEF and FEV_1.[122] However recordings made from the MEFV at low lung volume have relatively poor repeatability[123] and are especially prone to error in young children. Measurement of lung volumes by plethysmography requires considerable cooperation from the child but can be made in most school-age children. Such measurements are generally only available in tertiary centres and are not necessary in routine management. They have

the great advantage of being effort independent and have a place in difficult asthma.

Preventive therapy should be reduced when a child has been virtually asymptomatic and there has been little requirement for bronchodilator treatment for three months and a seasonal exacerbation is not anticipated. If a child is asymptomatic on a minimal dose of inhaled steroid a trial of withdrawal is justified but close supervision is needed. If symptoms recur this will serve both to confirm the asthma has not resolved and demonstrate to parents that regular prophylaxis is still required. Even if withdrawal of preventer therapy is possible, it is likely that remission will be followed, albeit mild and many years later, by relapse.

REFERENCES

1. Global Initiative for Asthma. Global strategy for Asthma Management and Prevention. *NIH Publication No.* 02-3659, 2002.
2. Rabe KF, Vermeire PA, Soriano JB, Maier WC. Clinical management of asthma 1999: the Asthma Insights and Reality in Europe (AIRE) study. *Eur Respir J* 2000;**16**:802–7.
3. Irvine L, Crombie IK, Clark RA, *et al.* What determines levels of passive smoking in children with asthma. *Thorax* 1997;**52**:766–9.
4. Cook DG, Whincup PH, Papacosta O, Strachan DP, Jarvis MJ, Bryant A. Relation of passive smoking as assessed by salivary cotinine concentration and questionnaire to spirometric indices in children. *Thorax* 1993;**48**:14–20.
5. Magnusson CGM. Maternal smoking influences serum IgE and IgD levels and increases risk for subsequent infant allergy. *J Allergy Clin Immunol* 1986;**78**:878–904.
6. Lodrup Carlsen KC, Jaakkola JJ, Nafstad P, Carlsen KH. In utero exposure to cigarette smoking influences lung function at birth. *Eur Respir J* 1997;**10**:1774–9.
7. Martinez FD, Cline M, Burrows B. Increased incidence of asthma in children of smoking mothers. *Pediatrics* 1992;**89**:21.
8. West R, McNeill A, Raw M. Smoking cessation guidelines for health professionals: an update. Health Education Authority. *Thorax* 2000;**55**:987–99.
9. Strachan DP. Parental smoking and childhood asthma: longitudinal and case control studies. *Thorax* 1998;**53**:204–12.
10. Cook DG, Strachan DP. Summary of effects of parental smoking on the respiratory health of children and implications for research. *Thorax* 1999;**54**:357–66.
11. Murray AB, Morrison BJ. Passive smoking by asthmatics: its greater effect on boys than on girls and on older than on younger children. *Pediatrics* 1989;**84**:451–9.

12. Fish L, Wilson SR, Latini DM, Starr NJ. An education program for parents of children with asthma: differences in attendance between smoking and non-smoking parents. *Am J Public Health* 1996;**86**:246–8.

13. Irvine L, Crombie IK, Clark RA, *et al*. Advising parents of asthmatic children on passive smoking: randomised controlled trial. *Br Med J* 1999;**318**:1456–9.

14. Grigg J. The health effects of fossil fuel derived particles. *Arch Dis Child* 2002;**86**:79–83.

15. Berciano FA, Dominguez J, Alvarez FV. Influence of air pollution on extrinsic asthma in childhood. *Ann Allergy* 1989;**5**:201–7.

16. Peroni G, Boner A, Vallone G, Antoline I, Warner JO. Effective allergen avoidance at high altitude reduces allergen-induced bronchial responsiveness. *Am J Respir Crit Care Med* 1994;**149**:1442–6.

17. Gotzsche PC, Hammarquist C, Burr M. House-dust mite control measures for asthma: (Cochrane Review). Cochrane Database Syst Rev. 2000: 2.

18. Harding H, Hansen LG, Korsgaard J, *et al*. House-dust mite allergy and anti mite measures in the indoor environment. *Allergy* 1991;**46**:33–8.

19. Custovic A, Woodcock A. Avoiding environmental triggers. In Silverman M, O'Callaghan CLP, eds. Practical paediatric respiratory medicine. Arnold, London 2001.

20. Almqvist C, Wickman N, Perfetti L, *et al*. Worsening of asthma in children allergic to cats, after indirect exposure to cat at school. *Am J Respir Crit Care Med* 2001;**163**:694–8.

21. Van de Brempt X, Charpin D, Haddi E, daMata P, Vervloet D. Cat removal and Fel d I levels in mattresses. *J Allergy Clin Immunol* 1991;**87**:595–6.

22. De Blay F, Chapman MD, Platts-Mills TAE. Airborne cat allergen (Fel d 1):environmental control with cat in situ. *Am Rev Respir Dis* 1991;**143**:1334–9.

23. Gutstadt LB, Gillette JW, Mrazek DA, *et al*. Determinants of school performance in children with chronic asthma. *Am J Dis Child* 1989;**143**:471–5.

24. Fritz GK, Overholser JC. Patterns of response to childhood asthma. *Psychosom Med* 1989;**51**:347–55.

25. Kaptein AA. Psychological correlates of length of hospitalisation and re-hospitalisation in patients with severe acute asthma. *Soc Sci Med* 1982; **16**:725–9.

26. Wright RJ, Rodriguez M, Cohen S. Review of psychosocial stress and asthma: an integrated biopsychosocial approach. *Thorax* 1998;**53**:1066–74.

27. Wright RJ, Hanrahan JP, Tager I, *et al*. Effect of the exposure to violence on the occurrence and severity of childhood asthma in an inner city population. *Am J Respir Crit Care Med* 1997;**155**:A972.

28. Sandberg S, Paton JY, Ahola S, McCann DC, McGuinness D, Hillary CR, Oja H. The role of acute and chronic stress in asthma attacks in children. *Lancet* 2000;**356**:982–7.

29. Christiaanse ME, Labigne JV, Lerner CV. Psychosocial aspects of compliance in children and adolescents with asthma. *J Develop Behav Pediatr* 1989;**10**:75–80.

30. Strachan DP, Anderson HR, Limb ES, O'Neill A, Wells N. A national survey of asthma prevalence, severity and treatment in Great Britain. *Arch Dis Child* 1994; **70**:174–8.

31. McKean M, Ducharme F. Inhaled steroids for episodic viral wheeze of childhood (*Cochrane Review*). The Cochrane Library, Issue 2, 2001. Oxford.

32. Kelly YJ, Brabin BJ, Milligan PJM, Reif JA, Heaf D, Pearson MG. The clinical significance of cough in the diagnosis of asthma in the community. *Arch Dis Child* 1996;**75**:489–93.

33. Ninan TK, MacDonald L, Russell G. Persistent nocturnal cough in childhood: a population base study. *Arch Dis Child* 1995;**73**:403–7.

34. Chang AB. Isolated cough – probably not asthma? *Arch Dis Child* 1999;**80**:211–13.

35. Cloutier MM, Loughlin GM. Chronic cough in children: a manifestation of airway hyperreactivity. *Pediatrics* 1981;**67**:6–12.

36. Stevenson EC, Turner G, Heaney LG, *et al*. Bronchoalveolar lavage findings suggest two different forms of childhood asthma. *Clin Exp Allergy* 1997; **27**:1027–35.

37. Marguet C, Jouen-Bodes F, Dean TP, Warner JO. Bronchoalveolar cell profiles in children with asthma, infantile wheeze, chronic cough, or cystic fibrosis. *Am J Respir Crit Care Med* 1999;**159**: 1533–40.

38. Krawiec ME, Westcott JY, Chu HW, *et al*. Persistent wheezing in very young children is associated with lower respiratory inflammation. *Am J Respir Crit Care Med* 2001;**163**:699–704.

39. Koh YY, Jeong JY, Park Y, Kim CK. Development of wheezing in patients with cough variant asthma during an increase in airway responsiveness. *Eur Respir J* 1999;**14**:302–8.

40. Calpin C, Macarthur C, Stephens D, Feldman W, Parkin PC. Effectiveness of prophylactic inhaled steroids in childhood asthma: a systematic review of the literature. *J Allergy Clin Immunol* 1997;**100**:452–7.

40a. Visser MJ, Postma DS, Arends LR, deVries DW, Duiverman EJ, Brand PLP. One year treatment with different dosing schedules of fluticason propionate in childhood asthma. *Am J Resp Crit Care Med* 2001;**164**:2073–7.

41. Doull IJM, Freezer NJ, Holgate ST. Growth of prepubertal children with mild asthma treated with inhaled beclomethasone dipropionate. *Am J Respir Crit Care Med* 1995;**151**:1715–19.

42. Tinkelman DG, Reed CE, Nelson HS, *et al*. Aerosol beclomethasone dipropionate compared with theophylline as primary treatment of chronic, mild to moderately severe asthma in children. *Pediatrics* 1993;**92**:64–77.

43. Verberne AAPH, Frost C, Roorda RJ, *et al*. One year's treatment with salmeterol compared with beclomethasone in children with asthma. *Am J Respir Crit Care Med* 1997;**156**:688–95.

44. Simons ER, Canadian Beclomethasone Dipropionate – Salmeterol Xinafoate Study Group. A comparison of beclomethasone, salmeterol and placebo in children with asthma. *N Eng J Med* 1997;**337**:1659–65.

45. Silverstein MD, Yunginger JW, Reed CE, *et al*. Attained adult height after childhood asthma: Effect of glucocorticoid therapy. *J Allergy Clin Immunol* 1997;**99**:466–74.

46. Agertoft L, Pedersen S. Effect of long term treatment with inhaled budesonide on adult height in children with asthma. *N Engl J Med* 2000;**343**:1064–9.

47. Allen DB, Bronsky EA, LaForce CF, *et al*. Growth in asthmatic children treated with fluticasone propionate. *J Pediatr* 1998;**132**:472–7.

48. de Benedictis FM, Teper A, Green RJ, Boner AL, Williams L, Medley HV. Effects of 2 inhaled corticosteroids on growth: results of a randomized controlled trial. *Arch Pediatr Adolesc Med* 2001;**155**:1248–54.

49. Price JF, Russell G, Hindmarsh PC, *et al*. Growth during one year of treatment with fluticasone propionate or sodium cromoglycate in children with asthma. *Pediatr Pulmonol* 1997;**24**:178–86.

50. Coutts JA, Gibson NA, Paton JY. Measuring compliance with inhaled medication in asthma. *Arch Dis Child* 1992;**67**:332–3.

51. Jonasson G, Carlsen K-H, Jonasson C, *et al*. Low dose inhaled budesonide once or twice daily for 27 months in children with mild asthma. *Allergy* 2000;**55**:740–8.

52. Silverman M, Connolly NM, Balfour-Lynn L, Godfrey S. Long term trial of disodium cromoglycate and isoprenaline in children with asthma. *Br Med J* 1972;**3**:378–81.

53. Lozewicz S, Robertson CF, Costello JF, Price JF. Delivery of sodium cromoglycate by pressurised aerosol. *Clin Allergy* 1984;**14**:187–91.

54. Price JF, Weller PH. Comparison of fluticasone propionate and sodium cromoglycate for the treatment of childhood asthma. *Respir Med* 1995;**89**:363–8.

55. Tasche MJA, Uilen JHJM, Bersen RMD, de Jongste JC, van der Wouden JC. Inhaled disodium cromoglycate (DSCG) as maintenance therapy in children with asthma: a systematic review. *Thorax* 2000;**55**:913–20.

56. Pedersen S, Hansen OR. Budesonide treatment of moderate and severe asthma in children: a dose response study. *J Allergy Clin Immunol* 1995;**95**:29–33.

57. Garrett J, Williams S, Wong C, Holdaway D. Treatment of acute asthmatic exacerbation with an increased dose of inhaled steroid. *Arch Dis Child* 1998;**79**:12–17.

58. Li X, Ward C, Thien F, *et al*. An anti-inflammatory effect of salmeterol, a long-acting beta 2 agonist, assessed in airway biopsies and bronchoalveolar lavage in asthma. *Am J Respir Crit Care Med* 1999;**160**:1493–9.

59. Greening AP, Ind PW, Northfield M, Shaw G. Added salmeterol versus higher dose corticosteroid in asthma patients with symptoms on existing inhaled corticosteroid. *Lancet* 1994;**334**:219–24.

60. Russell G, Williams DA, Weller P, Price JF. Salmeterol xinafoate in children on high dose inhaled steroids. *Ann Allergy Asthma Immunol* 1995;**75**:423–8.

61. Verberne AA, Frost C, Duiverman EJ, Grol MH, Kerrebijn KF. Addition of salmeterol versus doubling the dose of beclomethasone in children with asthma. The Dutch Asthma Study Group. *Am J Respir Crit Care Med* 1998;**158**:213–19.

62. Green CP, Price JF. Prevention of exercise-induced asthma by inhaled salmeterol xinafoate. *Arch Dis Child* 1992;**67**:1014–17.

63. Simons FE, Gerstner TV, Cheang MS. Tolerance to the protective effect of salmeterol in adolescents with exercise-induced asthma using concurrent inhaled glucocorticoid treatment. *Pediatrics* 1997;**99**:655–9.

64. Van den Berg NJ, Ossip MS, Hederos CA, *et al*. Salmeterol/fluticasone propionate (50/100 microg) in combination in a Diskus inhaler (Seretide) is effective and safe in children with asthma. *Pediatr Pulmonol* 2000;**30**:97–105.

65. Knorr B, Matz J, Bernstein JA, *et al*. Montelukast for chronic asthma in 6- to 14-year-old children: a randomised, double-blind trial. Pediatric montelukast Study Group. *JAMA* 1998;**279**:1181–6.

66. Kemp JP, Dockhorn RJ, Shapiro GG, *et al*. Montelukast once daily inhibits exercise-induced bronchoconstriction in 6–14 year old children with asthma. *J Pediatr* 1998;**133**:424–8.

67. Pearlman DS, Ostrom NK, Bronsky EA, *et al*. The leukotriene D4-receptor antagonist zafirlukast attenuates exercise-induced bronchoconstriction in children. *J Pediatr* 1999;**134**:273–9.

68. Leff JA, Busse WW, Pearlman D, *et al*. Montelukast, a leukotriene receptor antagonist, for the treatment of mild asthma and exercise-induced bronchoconstriction. *New Eng J Med* 1998;**339**:147–52.

69. Wilson N, Silverman M. Controlled trial of slow release aminophylline in childhood asthma: are short term trials valid? *Br Med J* 1982;**285**:863–6.

70. Nassif EG, Weinberger M, Thompson M, Huntley W. The value of maintenance theophylline in steroid-dependent asthma. *New Engl J Med* 1981;**304**:71–5.

71. Payne DNR, Wilson NM, James A, Hablas H, Agrafioti C, Bush A. Evidence for different subgroups of difficult asthma in children. *Thorax* 2001;**56**:345–50.

72. Pavord ID, Brightling CE, Woltmann G, *et al*. Non-eosinophilic corticosteroid unresponsive asthma. *Lancet* 1999;**353**:2213–14.

73. Payne DNR, McKenzie SA, Stacey S, Misra D, Haxby E, Bush A. Safety and ethics of bronchoscopy and endobronchial biopsy in difficult asthma. *Arch Dis Child* 2001;**84**:422–5.

74. Hoskins G, McCowan C, Neville RG, *et al*. Risk factors and costs associated with an asthma attack. *Thorax* 2000;**55**:19–24.

75. Higenbottam TW, Clark RA, Luksza AR, *et al*. The role of nebulised budesonide in permitting a reduction in the dose of oral steroid in persistent severe asthma. *Eur J Clin Res* 1994;**5**:1–10.

76. Westbroek J, Saarelainen S, Laher M, *et al*. Oral steroid-sparing effect of two doses of nebulised fluticasone propionate and placebo in patients with severe chronic asthma. *Respir Med* 1999;**93**:689–99.

77. Alexander AG, Barnes NC, Kay AB. Trial of cyclosporin in corticosteroid-dependent chronic severe asthma. *Lancet* 1992;**339**:324–8.

78. Lock SH, Kay AB, Barnes NC. Double-blind placebo-controlled study of cyclosporin A as a corticosteroid sparing agent in corticosteroid dependent asthma. *Am J Respir Crit Care Med* 1996;**153**:509–14.

79. Coren ME, Rosenthal M, Bush A. The use of cyclosporin in corticosteroid dependent asthma. *Arch Dis Child* 1997;**77**:522–3.

80. Stempel DA, Lammert J, Mullarkey MF. Use of methotrexate in the treatment of steroid-dependent adolescent asthmatics. *Ann Allergy* 1991;**67**:346–8.

81. Guss S, Portnoy J. Methotrexate treatment of severe asthma in children. *Pediatrics* 1992;**89**:635–9.

82. Sole D, Costa-Carvalho BT, Soares FJ, *et al*. Methotrexate in the treatment of corticodependent asthmatic children. *J Invest Allergol Clin Immunol* 1996;**6**:126–30.

83. Guyatt GH, Juniper EF, Griffith LE, Feeny DH, Ferrie PJ. Children and adult perceptions of childhood asthma. *Pediatrics* 1997;**99**:165–8.

84. Clark NM, Feldman CH, Freudenberg N, *et al*. Developing education for children with asthma through study of self-management behaviour. *Health Educ Q* 1980;**7**:278–96.

85. Deaves DM. An assessment of the value of health education in the prevention of childhood asthma. *J Adv Nursing* 1993;**18**:354–63.

86. Evans D, Mellins RB. Educational programs for children with asthma. *Paediatrician* 1991;**18**:317–23.

87. Cushley MJ, Tattersfield AE. Sudden death in asthma; a discussion paper. *J Roy Soc Med* 1983;**76**:662–6.

88. Gibson PG, Henry RL, Vimpani GV, Halliday J. Asthma knowledge, attitudes, and quality of life in adolescents. *Arch Dis Child* 1995;**73**:321–6.

89. Rand CS, Wise RA. Measuring adherence to asthma medication regimes. *Am J Respir Crit Care Med* 1994;**149**:869–76.

90. Pedersen S, Mortensen S. Use of different inhalation devices in children. *Lung* 1990;**168**(Suppl):90–8.

91. Kamps A, Roorda R, Brand P. Peak flow diaries in childhood asthma are unreliable. *Thorax* 2001;**56**:180–2.

92. Charlton I, Charlton G, Broomfield J, Mullee MA. Evaluation of peak expiratory flow and symptoms only self management plans for control of asthma in general practice. *Br Med J* 1990;**301**:135.

93. Lenney W, Wells NE, O'Neill BA. The burden of paediatric asthma. *Eur Respir Rev* 1994;**4**(18):49–62.

94. Falconer A, Oldman C, Helms P. Poor agreement between reported and recorded nocturnal cough in asthma. *Pediatr Pulmonol* 1993;**15**:209–11.

95. Hoskins EW, Heaton DM, Beardsmore CS, Simpson H. Asthma severity at night during recovery from an acute asthma attack. *Arch Dis Child* 1991;**66**:1204–8.

96. Fletcher HJ, Ibrahim SA, Speight ANP. Survey of asthma deaths in the Northern Region 1970–1985. *Arch Dis Child* 1990;**65**:163–7.

97. Robertson CF, Rubinfield AR, Bowes G. Pediatric asthma deaths in Victoria: the mild are at risk. *Pediatr Pulmonol* 1992;**13**:95–100.

98. Verberne AAPH, Hop WCJ, Bos AB, Kerrebijn KF. Effect of a single dose of inhaled salmeterol on baseline-airway calibre and methacholine-induced airway obstruction in asthmatic children. *J Allergy Clin Immunol* 1993;**91**:127–34.

99. Pedersen S. Treatment of nocturnal asthma in children with a single dose of sustained release theothylline. *Clin Allergy* 1985;**15**:79–85.

100. Gustafsson PM, Kjellman NI, Tibbling L. A trial of ranitidine in asthmatic children and adolescents with and without pathological gastro-oesophageal reflux. *Eur Respir J* 1992;**5**:201–6.

101. Beam WR, Wiener DE, Martin RJ. Timing of prednisolone and alterations of airway inflammation in nocturnal asthma. *Am Rev Respir Dis* 1992;**146**:1524–30.

102. Wilson NM. Food and drink related asthma in children. *Paediatr Respir Med* 1993;**3**:14–20.

103. Anderson HR, Palmer JC, Brailey P, *et al*. A community survey of asthma and wheezing illness in 8–10 year old children. *Report to the South West Thames Regional Health Authority*, London, 1981.

104. Wilson NM, Silverman M. Diagnosis of food sensitivity in childhood asthma. *J Roy Soc Med* 1985;**78**:11–16.

105. Silverman M, Wilson NM. The clinical physiology of food intolerance in asthma. *J Allergy Clin Immunol* 1986;**77**(Suppl):457–62.

106. Wilson NM. Food related asthma: a difference between two ethnic groups. *Arch Dis Child* 1985;**60**:861–5.

107. Coughlin SP. Sport and the asthmatic child: a study of exercise-induced asthma and the resultant handicap. *J Royal Coll Gen Pract* 1988;**38**:253–5.

108. Bevis M, Taylor B. What do schoolteachers know about asthma? *Arch Dis Child* 1990;**65**:622–5.

109. Berkowitz R, Schwartz E, Bukstein D, Grunstein M, Chai H. Albuterol protects against exercise-induced asthma longer than metaproterenol sulfate. *Pediatrics* 1986;**77**:173–8.

110. Nielsen KG, Auk IL, Bojsen K, Ifversen M, Klug B, Bisgaard H. Clinical effect of Discus™ dry powder inhaler at low and high inspiratory flow rates in asthmatic children. *Eur Respir J* 1998;**11**:350–4.

111. de Benedictis FM, Tuteri G, Pazzelli P, Niccoli A, Mezzetti D, Vaccaro R. Salmeterol in exercise-induced bronchoconstriction in asthmatic children: comparison of two doses. *Eur Respir J* 1996;**9**:2099–103.

112. Boner AL, Vallone G, Chiesa M, Spezia E, Fambri L, Sette L. Inhaled formoterol in the prevention of exercise-induced bronchoconstriction in asthmatic children. *Am J Respir Crit Care Med* 1994;**149**:935–9.

113. Morton AR, Ogle SL, Fitch KD. Effects of nedocromil sodium, cromolyn sodium and a placebo in exercise-induced asthma. *Ann Allergy* 1992;**68**:143–8.

114. Comis A, Vallette EA, Sette L, *et al.* Comparison of nedocromil sodium and sodium cromoglycate administered by pressurised aerosol, with and without a spacer device in exercise-induced asthma in children. *Eur Respir J* 1993;**6**:523–6.

115. Anderson SD. Drugs and the control of exercise-induced asthma. *Eur Respir J* 1993;**6**:1090–2.

116. Kikawa Y, Miyanomae T, Inoue Y, *et al.* Urinary leukotriene E4 after exercise challenge in children with asthma. *J Allergy Clin Immunol* 1992;**89**: 1111–19.

117. Reiss TF, Hill JB, Harman E, *et al.* Increased urinary excretion of LTE4 after exercise and attenuation of exercise-induced bronchospasm by montelukast, a cysteinyl leukotriene receptor antagonist. *Thorax* 1997;**52**:1030–5.

118. Freezer NJ, Croasdell H, Doull IJM, Holgate ST. Effect of regular inhaled beclomethasone on exercise and methacholine airway responses in school children with recurrent wheeze. *Eur Respir J* 1995;**8**:488–93.

119. Jones KP, Bain DG, Middleton M, Mullee MA. Correlates of asthma severity in primary care. *Br Med J* 1992;**304**:361–4.

120. Sibbald B, Anderson HR, McGuigan S. Asthma and employment in young adults. *Thorax* 1992;**47**:19–24.

121. Huang SW, Veiga R, Sila U, Reed E, Hines S. The effect of swimming in asthmatic children – participants in a swimming program in the city of Baltimore. *J Asthma* 1989;**26**:117–21.

122. Clough JB, Sly PD. Can peak expiratory flow be used as a predictor of lower respiratory symptoms. *Am Rev Respir Dis* 1993;**147**:267.

123. Lebecque P, Kiakulanda P, Coates AL. Spirometry in the asthmatic child: is FEF25-75 a more sensitive test than FEV_1/FVC? *Pediatr Pulmonol* 1993;**16**:19–22.

11

Asthma in young people

SUSAN M SAWYER

INTRODUCTION

Adolescence is the life stage that refers to the developmental period between childhood and adulthood. According to culture and context, adolescents are commonly known as teenagers, young people or youth.[1] For every young person, it is a time of complex interaction between physical, cognitive, emotional and social development; adolescence is a time of change, a time of challenge and a time of health risk in respect of respiratory health and adolescent well-being.

Ingersoll[2] defines adolescence as 'a period of personal development during which a young person must establish a personal sense of individual identity and feelings of self-worth which include an alteration of his or her body image, adaptation to more mature intellectual abilities, adjustments to society's demands for behavioural maturity, internalizing a personal value system, and preparing for adult roles'. A range of age definitions is used, with 10–24 years being the broadest definition in common use.[3]

Asthma causes a significant burden of disease during adolescence. This is especially due to the range and severity of symptoms, but also from the increasing asthma mortality in adolescence when compared to childhood. Physiological changes associated with puberty play a part (Chapter 15). The dynamic nature of asthma in the teenage years indicates that young people may no longer need the same amount of medication as previously. However, poor adherence may also mean they are taking little of the medication they actually need and previously prescribed aerosol delivery devices may no longer be indicated or appropriately used. These features highlight the critical need for close medical attention during the adolescent years.

ADOLESCENT DEVELOPMENT

Adolescent development is characterized by maturation of physical growth, cognitive development and psychosocial–sexual development.[4] Early adolescence is characterized by the physical changes of puberty with a rapid growth spurt heralding the development of secondary sexual characteristics and the potential of fertility. Adolescent development constitutes far more than simply physical development. The less easily measured changes of cognition and psychosocial development are of particular importance when it comes to maximizing positive outcomes for young people with asthma.

An increased capacity for abstract thought is a feature of adolescence. This is characterized by a maturing ability for complex logical reasoning and the consideration of alternative positions, such as life without asthma or medications. In contrast to the now imaginable (and advertised) ideals of health, beauty and family and societal functioning, the reality of less perfect states is something that young people must come to terms with at this time.

During adolescence, young people move from the position of relative dependence within the family to relative independence. This shift is commonly mediated through external influences, with peer friendships assuming greater importance during the teenage years. Educational, vocational and recreational opportunities are of increasing importance during later adolescence. During these years, the capacity for intimacy matures, as does a coherent sense of sexual identity.

Development in these three domains is neither linear nor synchronous. For example, the level of psychosocial or cognitive development cannot be inferred from the level of physical maturity. Notwithstanding this, health professionals frequently assume congruent development. For example, it is all too easy to approach a physically mature 15-year-old girl with asthma like one might an adult, forgetting that she may be cognitively less mature. We also risk approaching a 15-year-old boy with significant pubertal delay as we would the 13-year-old he looks like. Neither approach facilitates healthy developmental or asthma outcomes.

EPIDEMIOLOGY

Asthma and respiratory allergies are the most common chronic illnesses affecting young people in the developed world.[5] Asthma is also one of the most common reasons for young people to visit primary care practitioners.[6]

Asthma results in substantial morbidity in young people, whether from current wheeze, sleep disturbance, exercise-induced symptoms or associated eczema and allergic rhinitis.[7,8] These symptoms can have a significant impact on educational and recreational participation during adolescence. There is also a significant increase in mortality from asthma during adolescence when compared with the pre-adolescent population.[9]

The increasing prevalence of childhood asthma in many countries raises many questions about the natural history of asthma during and beyond adolescence. As has been addressed elsewhere (Chapter 2), childhood and adolescent years are a time of change in relationship to asthma prevalence, severity and pattern.

The changing prevalence can be crudely seen in the statistic that one in four children, one in seven adolescents and one in 10 adults in Australia has asthma. There is commonly some amelioration in asthma symptoms during adolescence, especially early adolescence, however it is far less common for children to truly 'grow out of asthma' during adolescence. Only 5% of those with persistent symptoms in childhood will become totally wheeze free by early adult life; approximately 15% will suffer from only trivial episodes of wheezing, 25% will have relatively infrequent asthma, and 50% will continue to have significant symptoms in early adult life.[10–12]

The greater proportion of boys with more severe asthma in childhood and early adolescence is a phenomenon not seen in later adolescence and early adult life when the ratio of males to females is the same in those with continuing asthma.[10–12]

THREATS TO RESPIRATORY HEALTH IN ADOLESCENCE

Young people are poorly motivated by future health goals

Health professionals generally aim to achieve the best treatment of the disease. We commonly focus on future health goals and expect this to motivate our patients' current behaviour. However, young people are more influenced by the 'here and now'; their perspective is more commonly focused on achieving the developmental goals of adolescence rather than in improving their lung health for the sake of it, whether now or in the future.

In contrast, young people are often very concerned by particular impacts of asthma on their lives, whether because of reduced sporting participation, school absenteeism or concerns of poor growth. Health professionals, therefore, have significant opportunities to make better asthma management relevant for young people if they can specifically link the goals of asthma management (optimizing lung health) to reducing the particular impacts of asthma for that young person.[13]

A priority of asthma consultations with young people is to identify how asthma affects their life, now. Since young people are less influenced by future perspectives, the task for health professionals is to frame this into concrete goals with immediate or short-term relevance (weeks to months). Examples are to improve sporting participation for the current netball season, or to enable participation in the school camp next month.

Young people may have little understanding of asthma

Many young people have had asthma for as long as they can remember. Given that parents are the common recipients of asthma education, young people themselves can have poor understanding of asthma and its management. Any opportunity to review asthma management with the young person should be grasped. Seeing the young person on their own for at least part of the medical consultation is a particularly helpful strategy to promote greater ownership of asthma by the young person and encourage honest communication about asthma. It is best to respectfully assume they know little.

There is little evidence that improving asthma *knowledge*, of itself, improves asthma outcomes.[14] However, there is evidence for improved asthma outcomes using approaches that are based on exploring the person's understanding and beliefs about asthma, that focus on developing skills for identifying asthma and responding to it, and that include written asthma management plan.[15] This approach allows asthma education to be focused on identified issues of concern for the young person.

Information must be provided at a developmentally and cognitively appropriate level. It must be sufficient to enable them to perform tasks, yet relevant and simple enough to be remembered. Avoid jargon. Repetition is essential, and understanding should be confirmed with specific questioning.

Common among concerns in young people is the belief that they will 'grow out of' asthma. Many are unimpressed, even angry, if their asthma is still problematic as they mature. Other concerns focus on growth which, regardless of asthma, is of major interest to young people. Concerns about inhaled corticosteroids are common and it is important to explore beliefs about steroids. Exercise-induced asthma and the approach to its management are also important to explore, as are barriers to asthma management at school.[16]

Lack of routine is a threat to adherence with medication

The best asthma medication in the world is only effective if it is actually taken, and taken correctly. The issue of adherence (the extent to which a patient follows medical advice) is increasingly being taken seriously as the negative impacts of poor adherence on asthma outcomes are recognized.[17] Risk factors for poor adherence include the nature of illness (chronic or relapsing illnesses are more commonly associated with poor adherence), the complexity of the medical regimen (the more drugs are prescribed with greater dosing frequency, the less likely that any will be taken), and social disadvantage.[18] Adolescents are commonly reported to be very poorly adherent with medication. There is, however, little objective evidence to suggest they are significantly less adherent than adults. Parental nagging around poor adherence with asthma medication is a common issue for young people (and their parents). Paradoxically, it is likely to reduce rather than improve adherence.

Efforts to improve adherence with medication should be a routine aspect of all asthma consultations with young people. Knowledge of adolescent development is an important aspect of adherence promoting strategies. After hearing the parental perspective, seeing the young person alone for part of the consultation is a useful technique that helps avoid young people automatically assuming the doctor will have a natural alliance with the parent. A non-judgmental approach that normalizes poor adherence is a strategy to encourage more honest self-report of less than ideal behaviour. For example, 'Most people I see your age have difficulty taking medication regularly. Tell me, how are things going with you? Are you more likely to forget your morning or evening medication?'

Routine – or the lack of it – is a major determinant of adherence with medication in young people with asthma. Young people commonly have routines for one dose but not the other, resulting in less than optimal adherence.[19]

For example, an evening routine resulting in good adherence may be cleaning their teeth, setting their alarm clock, and then taking their asthma medication. However the lack of routine in the morning may make morning adherence less reliable. Developing routines for taking medication before school can require specific assistance, encouragement and review for many young people.

Improving adherence in order to reduce parental nagging is a useful short-term goal that equally achieves the health professionals' aim of achieving better asthma outcomes. Encouraging the young person to keep a visible diary chart for a short period (e.g. a week) is a technique that can help young people differentiate parental 'reminding' (if there is no tick and the young person is about to go to school or bed) from 'nagging' (if there is a tick). In this way, appropriate parental concern can be harnessed as a positive influence along the way to greater autonomy by young people, instead of the usual interpretation by young people of parental input as unhelpful.

Smoking is a key health-risk behaviour in adolescence

Nicotine addiction is the single largest preventable cause of death and disease in adults. About 90% of adults who smoke commenced smoking during their adolescent years,[20] highlighting that smoking is a child and adolescent health problem.[21,22]

While rates of smoking are gradually declining in most adult populations, there is little evidence of reducing rates of teenage smoking.[23,24] Young people commonly experiment with smoking in middle adolescence, with a significant proportion becoming occasional and regular users over time. The incidence of smoking increases rapidly during the secondary school years, such that nearly 40% of 16-years-olds smoke at least occasionally.[23,25] Rates of smoking in teenage girls are significantly higher than in boys. Boys and girls experiment with smoking at the same rate, but more girls progress to regular smoking than boys.[26]

However, tobacco smoking is equally concerning because of the strength of associations with a range of other health-risk behaviours and conditions, such as regular marijuana use, problem alcohol use, unprotected sexual intercourse and depression.[27,28] In this context, tobacco smoking could be viewed as a beacon of distress.

Tobacco smoking, both active and passive (Chapter 7e), is known to have significantly negative effects on asthma.[29] In this context, it is very concerning that the physical experience of asthma does not seem to influence adolescents with asthma not to smoke. Indeed, a number of studies now highlight that both young people and adults with asthma are as likely – even more likely – to smoke than those without asthma.[30,31] Active smoking is a risk factor for symptomatic asthma in adolescents.[8] Active smoking is also associated, in a dose–response relationship, with lower levels of lung function and reduced rate of lung growth, with some evidence that girls may be more vulnerable than boys.[32]

Preventing adolescents from starting to smoke is critical to reducing the future burden of disease in our community. Advocacy efforts for public policy, public health interventions and school-based measures to reduce access to tobacco for young people in our society are increasingly indicated. As physicians of young people with asthma however, we can also use specific individual strategies that aim to prevent adolescent smoking and promote parental and adolescent smoking cessation[33,34] (Table 11.1).

Brief anti-smoking messages from physicians have a powerful impact on patients.[35] Promoting parental smoking cessation is one strategy to reducing the rate of teenage smokers as children whose parents smoke are twice as likely to become smokers as adolescents.[36]

Table 11.1 *Ten clinical strategies to prevent adolescents from smoking. From Rutishauser* et al.[33]

1 Take a smoking history. This should include details of personal, sibling, peer and parental smoking.
2 Identify other risk factors for initiation of smoking (e.g. low self-esteem, depressive symptoms, problems with weight control) as well as check for smoking-associated risk behaviours such use of marijuana, binge drinking, unprotected sexual intercourse.
3 Education. Highlight short-term rather than long-term smoking effects. For example, smoking causes bad breath, smelly clothes, yellow teeth and costs money.
4 Reinforce non-smoking as a healthy choice in non-smoking preadolescents and adolescents.
5 Anticipate peer pressure. Use rehearsal strategies to help young people feel more confident in refusing cigarettes, such as 'Only idiots smoke', 'I gave it up years ago', 'My doctor tells me I shouldn't smoke'.
6 Encourage parents to quit smoking. Emphasize their positive value as role models in addition to the personal benefits of non-smoking.
7 Identify 'teachable moments' when young people will be more motivated to think about the role of tobacco, such as a hospital admission for asthma, or grandparental illness due to smoking.
8 Encourage the adolescent smoker to think about quitting. Discuss the tobacco industry's manipulation of young peoples' opinions. Discuss smoking cessation options.
9 If the teenager is motivated to quit, set a 'quit date'; identify trigger factors for smoking and discuss strategies to avoid them; suggest substitute activities such as chewing gum; anticipate and discuss management of withdrawal symptoms; suggest increasing exercise or relaxation techniques; spend more time with non-smoking peers; plan how the adolescent can reward their success; review their progress early and often, by telephone or in person.
10 Play an active role in anti-tobacco policy and advocacy, such as supporting public health initiatives.

Smoking status should be identified in all young people. Avoid a lecture on the adverse effects of cigarette smoking on asthma; many young people do not experience (or admit to experiencing) that smoking exacerbates their asthma in the short term. However, asthma should be used as an important reason why they should not smoke. Specifically address myths about smoking and asthma, such as the common belief that marijuana makes asthma better.[37]

Many health professionals feel uncomfortable consulting with young people

Young people with asthma face a range of barriers in obtaining quality healthcare. These barriers include aspects of adolescent development itself, structural barriers, and aspects of health professional training.[1]

A key barrier to young people with asthma obtaining good healthcare is the lack of priority that they give to health in comparison to other competing life demands. This makes them less likely to seek medical care themselves and more dependent on parental encouragement for attendance. Structural barriers include issues of funding. Quality consultations with young people can take time; financial disincentives to longer consultations can reduce the likelihood of young people getting the time they deserve within the medical consultation.[38,39]

A barrier to young people obtaining quality healthcare is the lack of confidence that many health professionals have in consulting with adolescents.[38,39] Health professionals identify lack of training around skills at engaging young people as well as a lack of confidentiality guidelines as particularly problematic.[39]

Reassuringly however, health professionals can improve their skills in working with young people by specific professional development.[40] The HEADSS acronym (Table 11.2) provides a useful framework for taking a psychosocial history in young people.[41] What activities do they enjoy? How might these be affected by asthma? What are their educational and vocational goals? What do they do with their peers? Do most of their peers smoke or not? Do they smoke? What about other health-risk behaviours?

The first three themes within HEADSS provide a good mechanism to build rapport with a young person. Interweaving a routine asthma history with a psychosocial history is equally a technique to identify motivating factors with asthma management and approaches that can be used to improve adherence with medication. Identifying concerns to address in further appointments, such as the need to monitor growth, is a good mechanism to encourage regular review. Skills to explore the key socializing influences on young people (family, peers, school) and to elicit health risk and protective factors are also important if the broader health of the young person is to be managed, not just asthma.

Table 11.2 *An approach to taking a psychosocial history in adolescents. (From Goldenring and Cohen[41])*

HEADSS	Area	Questions
H	Home	Where do you live?
		Who do you live with?
E	Education	Are you at school? What year are you in?
		What are your marks like?
A	Activities	What do you do for fun?
		What do you do with your friends?
D	Drugs	Many young people experiment with alcohol, cigarettes and drugs. Have you ever smoked tobacco?
		What about marijuana?
S	Sexuality	Most young people become more interested in sex at your age. Have you had a sexual relationship with anyone?
S	Depression and suicide	Many people feel down or sad at times. Have you ever thought that life is not worth living?

Explicit articulation of confidentiality guidelines is an important part of all consultations with young people, including asthma consultations. Many young people are unaware of the health professional's duty to maintain confidentiality.[42] Others are fearful their parents or others will find out about specific aspects of the consultation, such as smoking behaviour.[43] Although the young person is part of a family, it should be remembered that they, not their family, are the patient. Medico-legal rights to confidentiality all generally younger than the legal age of majority. Multiple studies now confirm that clarification of confidentiality during consultations with young people significantly improves the likelihood of honest and open communication.[42–44]

Schools are a key setting for young people and their health

The impact of asthma within the education sector is substantial. Equally substantial, given the time that young people spend at school, is the capacity of schools to actively promote positive asthma outcomes.

Asthma is responsible for more school absenteeism than any other single chronic illness[45] although there is wide variation in the reported frequency of school absence due to asthma.[46–48]

Asthma education programs for teachers continue to demonstrate low levels of knowledge about asthma and its management.[48–50] One Australian study identified that almost all teachers had deficiencies in knowledge about reliever medication and the management of exercise-induced asthma (EIA) before an educational intervention. The 2-hour educational intervention achieved significant effects on symptom knowledge, pathophysiology, preventive medication and side effects. However, despite the intervention, only one third of teachers correctly answered questions about reliever medication and

management of EIA.[49] Appropriate management of EIA is particularly important within schools, not only because up to 90% of people with asthma experience it[51,52] but also because of increasing rates of obesity in young people including young people with asthma.

Approaches to teacher asthma education are more likely to be successful if they are part of a school asthma policy. All schools should have an asthma policy which specifically includes background information for teachers about recognizing the symptoms of asthma, written policies regarding the administration of medication (which highlight the appropriateness of young people taking responsibility for their own reliever medication within secondary schools), appropriate strategies to manage EIA, the availability of emergency treatment of asthma at school or on school camps, and the presence of written asthma management plans for all students with asthma. School asthma policies are now available.[53] Teacher training in association with an asthma policy can have significant results. For example, the implementation of one school program that included a School Asthma First Aid Kit, training workshops for school staff and individual Crisis Management Plans for students with asthma doubled the rate of school registrations of students with asthma, and resulted in completion of School Asthma Crisis Plans by 68% of students with asthma.[54]

However, given the prevalence of asthma, it is also appropriate for schools to take more proactive stances in terms of asthma education. There are creative ways of incorporating asthma care within the education curriculum. Lurie *et al.*[55] innovatively incorporated daily student peak flow measurement within a mathematics class as an approach to understanding variation within populations generally, with the added expectation of reducing the stigmatization of asthma, modelling peak flow measurements for students at risk and improving students' interest in personal asthma management. Broader health promotion approaches are also being explored. The use of peer educators within schools in a school-based asthma health promotion program (The Adolescent Asthma Action (Triple A) Program) is an innovative program that has demonstrated substantial benefits in asthma knowledge, quality of life, frequency of asthma attacks and asthma awareness within school communities.[56–58]

OPPORTUNITIES TO PROMOTE RESPIRATORY HEALTH IN ADOLESCENTS

In summary, adolescence is a time of change. It is a time of change as it relates to asthma, whether in terms of its pattern or severity in adolescence. It is equally a time of change as it relates to adolescent development. These changes can result in substantial threats to the health of young people with asthma, whether from infrequent clinic attendance, poor adherence with medication, or smoking.

Yet there are equally substantial opportunities for intervention. Clinicians with an understanding of adolescent development have many opportunities to use this knowledge to promote the health and well-being of young people with asthma. Seeing young people alone for at least part of the consultation, taking a psychosocial history and having an understanding of confidentiality are integral aspects of consultations with young people.

Communication skills that identify how asthma most impacts on a young person are important, as it is this information (rather than achieving 'good asthma control' for the sake of it) that most motivates young people to achieve better asthma control. The clinical challenge is to assist young people develop the skills to better manage their asthma as they mature through adolescence. Too often, asthma becomes a focus of parental nagging or family arguments in adolescence. Rather, the goal of good asthma self-management is for young people to be sufficiently empowered and skilled such that routine asthma care becomes incorporated into their lives.

In this way, it should be the goal of both clinicians and parents that young people feel sufficiently comfortable and able to access medical care that their asthma is regularly reviewed. We should aim for young people to be sufficiently informed about their asthma that they understand the rationale for preventive medication and are reasonably reliable takers of medication. We should aim for young people with asthma to grow up in a smoke free environment. Equally, we should aim for young people to know how and when to seek emergency care if it was required.

As parents know only too well, young people do not develop these skills overnight. Regular medical review by informed and skilled clinicians is a key opportunity to promote better health outcomes for young people with asthma.

REFERENCES

1. Sawyer SM, Bowes G. Adolescence on the health agenda. *Lancet* 1999;**354**(Suppl II):31–4.
2. Ingersoll GM. *Adolescence*, 2nd edn. Prentice-Hall, Englewood Cliffs, NJ, 1989.
3. World Health Organization. *The Health of Young People*. World Health Organization, Geneva, 1993.
4. McAnarney ER, Kreipe RE, Orr DP, Comerci GD. *Textbook of Adolescent Medicine*. WB Saunders, London, 1992.
5. Newacheck PW, McManus MA, Fox HB. Prevalence and impact of chronic illness among adolescents. *Am J Dis Child* 1991;**145**:1367–73.
6. Moon L, Meyer P, Grau J. Australia's youth: their health and well being. Australian Institute of Health and Welfare, Canberra, 1999.
7. Robertson CF, Dalton MF, Peat JK, Haby MM, Bauman A, Kennedy DJ, Landau LI. Asthma and other atopic diseases in Australian children. *Med J Aust* 1998;**168**:434–8.
8. Withers NJ, Low L, Holgate ST, Clough JB. The natural history of respiratory symptoms in a cohort of adolescents. *Am J Respir Crit Care Med* 1998;**158**:352–7.
9. Robertson CF, Rubinfeld AR, Bowes G. Pediatric asthma deaths in Victoria: the mild are at risk. *Pediatr Pulmonol* 1992;**13**:95–1000.
10. Williams H, McNicol KN. Prevalence, natural history and relationship of wheezy bronchitis and asthma in children. An epidemiological study. *Br Med J* 1969;**4**:321–5.
11. Martin AJ, McLennan LA, Landau LI, Phelan PD. The natural history of childhood asthma to adult life. *Br Med J* 1980;**280**:1397–400.
12. Martin AJ, Landau LI, Phelan PD. Asthma from childhood to age 21: the patient and his disease. *Br Med J Clin Res* 1982;**284**:380–2.
13. SM Sawyer. Managing asthma in adolescents. In: RS Walls, CM Jenkins, eds. *Understanding Asthma*. MacLennan and Petty, Australia, 2000, pp. 262–70.
14. Gibson PG, Coughlin J, Wilson AJ, Abramson M, Bauman A, Hensley MJ, Walters EH. Self-management education and regular practitioner review for adults with asthma (*Cochrane Review*). The Cochrane Library, 4, 2000. Oxford, Update Software.
15. Clark NM, Gong M, Schork MA, Evans D, Roloff D, Hurwitz M, Maiman L, Mellins RB. Impact of education for physicians on patient outcomes. *Pediatrics* 1998;**101**:831–6.
16. Sawyer S, Aroni R, Abramson M, Douglass J, Thien F, Stewart K. Adolescents with asthma: a qualitative study of adherence and the impact of families and healthcare professionals. *J Paediatr Child Health* 1999;**35**:A7.

17. National Asthma Campaign. *Asthma Adherence: a Guide for Health Professionals.* Department of Health and Aged Care, Australia, 1999.

18. Sackett DL, Haynes RB. *Compliance with Therapeutic Regimens.* The Johns Hopkins University Press, Baltimore and London, 1976.

19. Sawyer SM, Dakin V. Adherence in adolescents with asthma: comparison of self report with parental report and objective measurement. *Respirology* 2000;**5**:A25.

20. US Department of Health and Human Services. *Preventing Tobacco use Among Young People.* A report of the Surgeon General. Washington, DC, Office of Smoking and Health, 1994.

21. Kessler DA. The Tobacco Settlement. *N Engl J Med* 1997;**337**:1082.

22. Koop CE. The pediatrician's obligation in smoking education. *AJDC* 1985;**139**:973.

23. Hill D. Why we should tackle adult smoking first. *Tobacco Control* 1999;**8**:333–5.

24. US Department of Health and Human Services. *Preventing Tobacco Use Among Young People.* A report of the Surgeon General. Atlanta, Georgia. US Department of Health and Human Services, Public Health Service, Centers for Disease Control and Prevention, National Centre for Chronic Disease Prevention and Health Promotion, Office on Smoking and Health, 1994.

25. Patton GC, Hibbert M, Rosier MJ, Carlin JB, Caust J, Bowes G. Is smoking associated with depression and anxiety in teenagers? *Am J Public Health* 1996; **86**:225–30.

26. Patton GC, Carlin JB, Coffey C, Wolfe R, Hibbert M, Bowes G. The course of early smoking: a population-based cohort study over three years. *Addiction* 1998;**93**:1251–60.

27. Hibbert M, Caust J, Patton G, Rosier M, Bowes G. *The Health of Young People in Victoria. Adolescent Health Survey.* Centre for Adolescent Health, 1996.

28. Zubrick SR, Silburn SR, Gurrin L, Teoh H, Sheperd C, Carlton J, Lawrence D. *Western Australian Child Health Survey: Education, Health and Competence.* Australian Bureau of Statistics and the TVW Telethon Institute for Child Health Research, Perth, WA, 1997.

29. National Health and Medical Research Council. *Effects of Passive Smoking on Health.* Report of the NHMRC working party on the Effects of Passive Smoking on Health. Australian Government Publishing Service, Canberra, 1998.

30. Forero R, Bauman A, Young L, Booth M, Nutbeam D. Asthma, health behaviors, social adjustment, and psychosomatic symptoms in adolescence. *J Asthma* 1996;**33**:157–64.

31. Wakefield M, Ruffin R, Campbell D, Roberts L, Wilson D. Smoking-related beliefs and behaviour among adults with asthma in a representative population sample. *Aust NZ J Med* 1995; **25**:12–17.

32. Gold DR, Wang X, Wypij D, Speizer FE, Ware JH, Dockery D. Effects of cigarette smoking on lung function in adolescent boys and girls. *N Eng J Med* 1996;**335**:931–7.

33. Rutishauser C, Sanci L, Sawyer S. Clinical strategies to reduce teenage smoking. *Aust Paediatr Rev* 1997;**2**:4–5.

34. Ammerman SD. Helping kids kick butts. *Contemp Pediatr* 1998;**15**:64–74.

35. Fiore MC, Bailey WC, Cohen SJ, *et al.* Smoking cessation: quick reference guide for smoking cessation specialists. *Clin Pract Guidelines* No 18.

36. Shean RE, de Klerk NH, Armstrong BK, Walker NR. Seven-year follow-up of a smoking-prevention program for children. *Aust J Publ Health* 1994;**18**:205–8.

37. Sawyer S, Aroni R, Goeman D, Abramson M, Thien F, Douglass J, Stewart K. Smoking in adolescents with asthma: premedication to promote social participation. *Respirology* 2000;**5S**:A24.

38. Veit FC, Sanci LA, Young DY, Bowes G. Adolescent healthcare: perspectives of Victorian general practitioners. *Med J Aust* 1995;**163**:16–18.

39. Veit FC, Sanci LA, Coffey CM, Young DY, Bowes G. Barriers to effective primary healthcare for adolescents. *Med J Aust* 1996;**165**:131–3.

40. Sanci LA, Coffey CM, Veit FC, Carr-Gregg M, Patton GC, Day N, Bowes G. Evaluation of the effectiveness of an educational intervention for general practitioners in adolescent healthcare: randomised controlled trial. *Br Med J* 2000;**320**:224–30.

41. Goldenring JM, Cohen E. Getting into adolescents heads. *Contemp Pediatr* 1988;**15**:75–90.

42. Cheng TL, Savageau JA, Sattler AL, DeWitt TG. Confidentiality in healthcare. A survey of knowledge, perceptions and attitudes among high school students. *JAMA* 1993;**269**:1404–7.

43. Marks A, Malizio J, Hoch J, Brody R, Fisher M. Assessment of health needs and willingness to utilize healthcare resources of adolescents in a suburban population. *J Pediatr* 1983;**102**:456–60.

44. Ford CA, Millstein SG, Halpern-Felsher BL, Irwin CE. Influence of physician confidentiality assurances on adolescents' willingness to disclose information and seek future healthcare. A randomized controlled trial. *JAMA* 1997;**278**:1029–34.

45. Newacheck PW, Taylor WR. Childhood chronic illness: prevalence, severity, impact. *Am J Publ Health* 1992; **82**:364–71.

46. Fowler MG, Davenport MG, Garg R. School functioning of US children with asthma. *Pediatrics* 1992; **90**(6):939–44.

47. Speight ANP, Lee DA, Hey EN. Underdiagnosis and undertreatment of asthma in childhood. *Br Med J* 1983;**286**:1253–6.

48. Fillmore EJ, Jones N, Blankson JM. Achieving treatment goals for schoolchildren with asthma. *Arch Dis Child* 1997;**77**:420–2.

49. Henry RL, Hazell J, Halliday JA. Two hour seminar improves knowledge about childhood asthma in school staff. *J Paediatr Child Health* 1994;**30**:403–5.

50. Bevis M, Taylor B. What do school teachers know about asthma? *Arch Dis Child* 1990;**65**:622–5.

51. Kawabori I, Pierson WE, Conquest LL, Bierman CW. Incidence of exercise-induced asthma in children. *J Allergy Clin Immunol* 1976;**58**:447–55.

52. McFadden ER, Gilbert IA. Exercise-induced asthma. *N Engl J Med* 1994;**330**:1362–7.

53. http://www.asthma.org.au/brochures/school.htm

54. Shah S, Gibson PG, Wachinger S. Recognition and crisis management of asthma in schools. *J Paediatr Child Health* 1994;**30**:312–15.

55. Lurie N, Straub MJ, Goodman N, Bauer EJ. Incorporating asthma education into a traditional school curriculum. *Am J Publ Health* 1998; **88**:822–3.

56. Gibson PG, Shah S, Mamoon HA. Peer-led asthma education for adolescents: impact evaluation. *J Adolesc Health* 1998;**22**:66–72.

57. Shah S. *Adolescent Asthma Action Project 1993–2000* (final report). Commonwealth of Australia, 2001.

58. Shah S, Peat JK, Mazurski EJ, Wang H, Sindhusake D, Bruce C, Henry RL, Gibson PG. Effect of peer led programme for asthma education in adolescents: cluster randomised controlled trial. *Br Med J* 2001; **322**:583–5.

12

The management of acute severe asthma

WARREN LENNEY AND JOHN ALEXANDER

INTRODUCTION

Although the prevalence of childhood asthma continues to rise,[1–3] at last we now have some evidence that acute severe exacerbations may be on the decline. Hospital admissions in the UK have reduced from their peak in the early 1990s by approximately one third[4] with similar findings in Sweden[5] and other European countries. Visits to primary care doctors are less than those previously recorded,[6] the need for admission to paediatric intensive care units is less and the mortality rate is falling.[3]

Contrast this with statements made in the 1980s that 'there seems to be little change in the frequency of acute wheezing episodes over recent years'[7] and that hospital admissions have increased nationally[8] and internationally.[9]

Good management of acute severe asthma remains dependent upon early recognition that control is being lost. The first part of this chapter therefore deals with how to recognize such changes and act accordingly. The increased input into patient education, self-management plans and the development of care pathways may well be beginning to pay dividends. Treatment of acute severe asthma is dealt with in the second part of the chapter. Here, home management and management by the primary care team is separated from that in hospital. The third part of the chapter discusses the management of life-threatening attacks, the role of the paediatric intensive care unit with particular reference to mechanical ventilation and the subsequent aftercare.

The recognition and management of acute severe asthma have not seen major changes over the past 6 years but 'fine tuning' may have resulted in reduced episodes. The burden of paediatric asthma world-wide remains huge, however.[10] Differential costings show clearly that severe asthma requiring hospital admission is a greater burden to the patients, their families and the health services than more mild disease.[11]

THE RECOGNITION OF ACUTE SEVERE ASTHMA

At home

The *features of severe airway obstruction* (Table 12.1) are important, but of much greater value is the ability to recognize early warning signs in the individual patient and thereby to institute early treatment may stave off the progression of symptoms. The majority of severe episodes are triggered by viral infections[12,13] but in some particularly sensitive children, environmental allergens may be important. The development of home management

Table 12.1 *Features of severe airway obstruction*

Symptoms and signs
Inability or difficulty in speech or feeding
Exhaustion, agitation or reduced level of consciousness
Progressive tachycardia and/or tachypnoea
Use of accessory muscles
Poor chest movement and quiet breath sounds

Lung function
PEF <30% expected

Response
Deterioration despite recent use of appropriate rescue medication
Transient (<2 h) or partial response to bronchodilator (e.g. albuterol (salbutamol) 2.5–5 mg by nebulizer)

Experience
Knowledge of progress in previous attacks

programs has been confounded by the relatively poor quality of some programs.[14] A meta-analysis[15] of home management programs suggested they did not seem to reduce morbidity but the authors suggested that programs designed to target patients with clearly defined characteristics might result in benefits. Two discharge planning programs targeted on children admitted to UK hospitals with acute severe asthma have led to impressive reductions in hospital re-admission rates.[16,17]

Prodromal features have been described as early warning signs in individual patients. Parents not infrequently note features such as dark rings developing around their child's eyes, an increasingly pale complexion, a facial twitch or generalized itching.[18] Beer *et al.*[19] stated that each child has his own constant set of prodromal features. They listed a large number of behavioural changes, gastrointestinal symptoms, fever, skin eruptions, itching and toothache and suggested that awareness of them may lead to the early introduction of treatment thereby avoiding or abbreviating some acute episodes. Little attention has been paid to these prodromal symptoms in the development of national[20,21] and international[22,23] guidelines for asthma and perhaps they should be revisited.

Few parents are taught how to measure their child's breathing rate. Increasing tachypnoea is an important and well recognized sign of *deterioration*. It can interfere with appetite and exercise/activity tolerance. As the work of breathing increases the child becomes less active, withdrawn and stops speaking. Parents can be shown how to observe chest wall movements, the use of the accessory muscles and the increased use of the diaphragm. Progression of the above signs may be rapid, over a few hours, or may take place slowly over a period of days. The latter might indicate deteriorating or poorly controlled asthma suggesting the need to alter the dose of preventative medications. The former might suggest it is more beneficial to concentrate on the early intervention with relief bronchodilator treatment. Diurnal variation of PEF is greater when chronic asthma control is poor but does not significantly differ between exacerbations and stable asthma.[24] Increasing diurnal variation of PEF as an objective way of differentiating poor asthma control from an asthma exacerbation may occasionally be useful.

Parents of children over 5 years of age may find *peak flow meters* useful[25] to estimate the severity of the acute exacerbation or monitor response to bronchodilator therapy. However in a recent US study[26] only a small proportion of parents had been given PEF meters and only one out of 220 parents reported using it to monitor the severity of an attack or the response to treatment. This study also showed that in inner-city children previously admitted to hospital with asthma, guidelines for home management of asthma exacerbations were not being followed. A symptom-based approach rather than a reliance on PEF values has also been favoured in other studies,[27,16] since symptoms are more sensitive indicators of deterioration (and recovery) in acute episodes, than PEF (Chapter 6b).

In primary care

INITIAL ASSESSMENT

Most children with asthma are totally managed in primary care, where access to *medical records* can be helpful: Has the child had a recent hospital admission or visits to the emergency department? Have there been exacerbations associated with rapid clinical deterioration? Are the parents able to assess and safely manage their child's asthma symptoms? Are follow-up appointments regularly kept and have prescriptions been collected appropriately? The process of healthcare should be appropriate: when the family is concerned that the child is deteriorating can a consultation be arranged immediately? Has the professional who assesses the child received appropriate training in asthma management?

A full *history* needs to be taken. The time and pattern of onset of the present attack needs to be noted as do the times and dosages of the treatments given. If there have been previous attacks how does the present one compare with them? Is there evidence of rapid deterioration? The features in Table 12.1 can be used as a guide but the following should be noted:

- respiratory rate may not correlate well with severity;[28]
- although cyanosis is a marker of a severe disease it can be difficult to assess clinically;[29]
- peak flow is an insensitive measure during an acute exacerbation;[30]
- parental anxiety may influence the clinical presentation, especially in very young children;
- response to inhaled bronchodilator therapy is vital to assess clinical progress and often determines the need for hospital admission.

A quiet room with comfortable seating is essential as is sufficient time to fully assess the clinical situation. Remember that other conditions can mimic acute severe asthma (e.g. inhaled foreign body, croup, hyperventilation, cystic fibrosis and vocal cord dysfunction) and these conditions need to be ruled out. To assess response to *bronchodilator therapy* it is important to evaluate the child before and after treatment. These assessments should be clearly documented. Peak flow monitoring, before and after treatment may be helpful in children old enough but it cannot be relied upon. Other objective assessments such as oxygen saturation monitoring (SaO_2) should be available in primary care, since there is no other reliable way to detect significant hypoxaemia (i.e. <90% saturation).

Referral to hospital/emergency department

The factors which suggest that a referral to a secondary care facility is necessary for safe and more effective management are:

- short attack with rapid deterioration;
- limited or brief response to bronchodilator therapy;

- drowsiness or altered state of consciousness;
- evidence of dehydration;
- inability of child to drink or talk;
- inability of parents to cope.

The development of care pathways with clearly defined protocols may be helpful in the future management in children with acute severe asthma in primary care settings.

In the emergency department

The availability of professional staff 24 hours a day, together with objective monitoring aids should enable assessment in an emergency department or children's acute assessment unit to be easily accomplished. However, the research literature dealing with emergency management is confusing and often parochial and therefore difficult to transpose from one country to another because of major differences in healthcare and its resources. There are differences of opinion concerning the value of *specific asthma scoring systems* in adults.[31–34] Objective measures of *lung function* such as PEF and FEV_1 have also been unhelpful.[32,35,36] Attempts to develop predictive indices for children requiring hospital admission have been relatively unsuccessful.[35,37,38] A problem in paediatric asthma is the high proportion of admissions in the preschool age group where reliable measurements of lung function cannot be obtained.

Children admitted to hospital can often be cared for elsewhere.[39] This study in the US showed that 70% of the children could have been cared for in alternative settings if oxygen was available there.

In the emergency room does SaO_2 measured by *pulse oximetry* predict the need for hospitalization? Several studies have examined this. Geelhoed et al.[40] showed that an initial SaO_2 of 91% or below was predictive of hospital admission or re-attendance at the emergency department. In another study[41] the same authors showed that the initial SaO_2 was lower in those admitted than in those discharged home from the emergency department. Whilst initial SaO_2 levels have high specificity, low values are insensitive to the need for admission.[42–45]

Admission *per se* is influenced by factors such as the experience of the medical staff, the availability of local medical services and the social circumstances of the family. The above studies do show that an initial high SaO_2 value is a good predictor that the child will not require admission to hospital. In one of the above studies[43] an SaO_2 of less than 91% ten minutes after inhaled bronchodilator therapy was a good discriminator for the need of intravenous therapy.

Does the presence of *pulsus paradoxus* help to define the severity of an asthma attack in children? During an acute severe attack, the swings in pleural pressure widen, the inspiratory (and mean) pleural pressure falls and left ventricular afterload increases. (Left ventricular afterload = aortic pressure − pleural pressure). In addition, increased venous return causes a shift of the intraventricular septum to the left, reducing the end-diastolic volume of the left ventricle. The increased left ventricular afterload produces a fall in systolic blood pressure during inspiration leading to the clinical sign of pulsus paradoxus, measured by sphygmomanometer.[45] A pressure difference of >20 mmHg is considered indicative of moderate to severe airway obstruction and it is said that a detectable pulsus paradoxus indicates the PEF will be 50% or less of predicted.[46] One study[47] suggested that detection of pulsus paradoxus was very useful in children but under-represented children of preschool age. During development of the 1993 UK National Guidelines for Asthma Management[48] the usefulness of pulsus paradoxus was reviewed. The consensus paediatric view was that it was of little clinical benefit. In practice, inflating the sphygmomanometer in a young child may increase distress. Movement artefact makes the reading unreliable so that in a very distressed child the reading may be impossible to obtain. Non-invasive methods of measuring pulsus paradoxus during oximetry may prove useful in measuring and monitoring this controversial sign.[49]

A *clinical scoring system* may be helpful (Table 12.2). Such systems remain unproven as the subjective interpretation of signs of airway obstruction is susceptible to inter-observer variation.[49] It is also known that clinical features correlate poorly with objective measures such as PEF and SaO_2.[27,51] The scoring system shown in Table 12.2 has been used to assess improvement following β_2-agonist therapy over short (20 minute) periods.[50]

Why children attend the emergency department

It is unlikely the same criteria can be applied in all hospitals in relation to hospital admissions policy. In 1997–1998 we undertook a study to discover the reason why children with asthma attended our local emergency department, what assessments were undertaken, what factors decided whether the child should be admitted and what was the subsequent outcome.[50] The reasons for attendance were variable:

- the parents did not want to disturb their general practitioner (50% attended between 18.00 hours and 06.00 hours);
- the parents thought their general practitioner did not know much about asthma;
- the parents assessment was that the attack was severe;
- the general practitioner did not have a nebulizer;
- some patients had no general practitioner and used the emergency department as their primary source of care.

Similar findings have been reported from the USA in inner-city, deprived populations. In one study[52] 51% of the children had 10 or more prior visits to the emergency department, 72% had functional severity scores in the

Table 12.2 *Asthma severity score*

Score	Wheeze	Anxiety	Chest
0	No wheeze/minimal wheeze/ wheezes on deep respiration	Settled/undisturbed	Normal breath/normal chest shape
1	Obvious wheeze all areas	Increased respiratory effort/undisturbed	Detectable hyperinflation
2	Obvious wheeze with detectable tachypnoea	Obvious dyspnoea/not distressed	Obvious hyperinflation
3	Obvious wheeze/moderate tachypnoea	Moderate dyspnoea, fretful/unsettled	Moderate hyperinflation/subcostal and supraclavicular recession
4	Detectable decrease in breath sounds	Moderate dyspnoea, restless/anxious	Moderate hyperinflation/marked intercostal recession
5	Moderate decrease in breath sounds	Distressed. Air hunger	As above plus accessory muscle respiration, maximal inflation
6	Marked decrease in breath sounds	Very distressed, tiring	Marked accessory muscle respiration, maximal inflation

moderate to severe range and only 11% used regular anti-inflammatory medications. No patient had a written self-management plan.

We discovered that assessments in the emergency department were not being carried in accordance with protocols and the decision to admit patients to the paediatric wards was not based on any guidelines. Patients discharged from the emergency department had no clear follow-up arrangements. Following the study we adopted well-defined triage plans,[53] developed care pathways for children with asthma and the follow-up arrangements have been formalized (see Figure 12.1).

Hospital admission

It is not possible to recommend specific indications to admit to hospital because of the world-wide variation in healthcare systems and resources. Local care pathways or their equivalent need to be developed.

A number of factors inform the decision to admit to hospital, or to discharge home, usually after a period of observation:

- triage level;
- limited or brief response to bronchodilator therapy;
- low SaO_2 (<90% in air) especially 10 minutes after bronchodilator therapy;
- local hospital admission policy;
- availability of primary care medical services;
- time of day;
- ability of parent(s) to cope and social circumstances.

MANAGEMENT

At home

Satisfactory regimes for the management of acute severe asthma depend on individualized plans together with

good communication between healthcare professionals and the family. The initial thrust of management is effective bronchodilator therapy, backed up by systematic corticosteroids. Failure to respond to treatment warrants immediate referral to secondary care.

Therapeutic management

Some of the following section also applies to acute severe asthma managed in the emergency room. To avoid repetition, the evidence concerning each agent is summarized here.

SHORT-ACTING β₂-AGONISTS

These are the mainstay of treatment for acute severe asthma, administered in inhaled form using a metered-dose inhaler (MDI) attached to a spacer device or using a nebulizer. There is little to choose between the two most commonly used β₂-agonists salbutamol (albuterol) and terbutaline as their onset of action and duration of effect is very similar. A spacer device increases deposition into the lungs and during an acute attack children find it easier to inhale the medication through the spacer rather than with an MDI alone. In acute severe episodes dry powder devices may be unreliable and are not recommended (Chapter 8b).

Individual β₂-agonist aerosol actuations should be used allowing 20–30 seconds between each actuation. After each actuation the MDI canister should be removed, shaken and replaced to maximize medication output. The dose regimes used in the home setting for children with acute severe asthma have not been well studied, but there is no reason to believe they should be different to those used in the emergency department which have been proven to be both effective and safe. The dose should have been determined by healthcare professionals, agreed with the family, individualized to the patient's needs and recorded in a self-management plan. A suitable starting regime for an acute severe attack would be

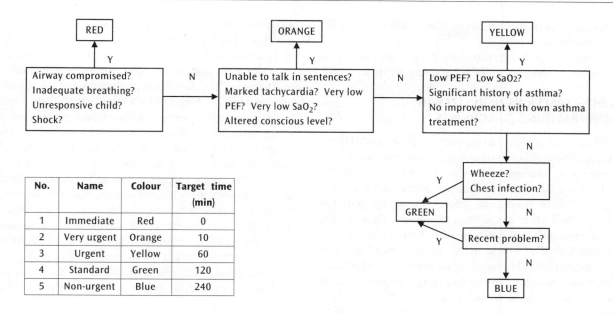

No.	Name	Colour	Target time (min)
1	Immediate	Red	0
2	Very urgent	Orange	10
3	Urgent	Yellow	60
4	Standard	Green	120
5	Non-urgent	Blue	240

Chart notes (Asthma Triage Chart)

This is a presentation-defined flow diagram which is intended for use with patients who present with exacerbations of known asthma. The severity of asthma at presentation varies from life threatening to patients requiring a repeat prescription of inhalers. A number of general discriminators are used, including *Life threat, Conscious level* (in adults and children) and *Oxygen saturation*. Specific discriminators are included to identify those signs and symptoms which point to severe and life-threatening asthma.

Specific discriminators	Explanation
Marked tachycardia	A heart rate over 120 in an adult. In children this needs to be related to the age of child.
Very low SaO$_2$	This is a saturation <95% in O$_2$ therapy or <90% in air.
Very low PEF	This is a PEF of 33% or less of best in predicted PEF.
Low SaO$_2$	This is a saturation of 90–95% in air.
Low PEF	This is a PEF of 50% or less of best or predicted PEF.
Significant history of asthma	A history of brittle asthma or previous life-threatening episodes is significant.
No improvement with own asthma treatment	This history should be available from the patient. A failure to improve with bronchodilator therapy given by the GP or paramedic is equally significant.
Wheeze	This can be audible wheeze or a feeling of wheeze. Remember, very severe airway obstruction is silent (no air can move).

Figure 12.1 *Asthma triage chart. (From ref. 53.)*

up to 1000 μg (10 puffs) of salbutamol (albuterol) or its equivalent carefully assessing the benefit over the next few minutes. If no improvement is seen after 10 minutes the procedure should be repeated. Lack of response following the second treatment warrants immediate contact with a healthcare professional and/or direct access to the emergency department. Doses of β$_2$-agonists can be repeated 2–4 hourly at home but once again the frequency should be agreed and documented in a written treatment plan. The better the child and family understand the response to therapy and the earlier the bronchodilator is started following the onset of symptoms the less likely will be the need to involve others in the child's management.

Long-acting β_2-agonists have no proven role in the emergency management of acute severe asthma.

MDI + SPACER VS NEBULIZER IN ADMINISTERING β_2-AGONISTS

There is clear evidence to support the use of an MDI and spacer combination to treat acute severe asthma in preference to a nebulizer in the emergency department.[54–57] MDI and spacers take less time to administer the medication,[58] have fewer side effects, are more portable, cheaper and easier to use than nebulizers. They are also more efficient[59] and can be used in very young children by attaching a face-mask to the spacer device.[60] It therefore seems rational to recommend such devices for use in the home as well as in the emergency department. An additional benefit is the lack of need for the use of O_2, a gas which is often recommended to drive the nebulizer gas flow to prevent hypoxaemia resulting from ventilation–perfusion mismatch. Hypoxaemia has not been reported using an MDI and spacer.

A small number of children (particularly the very young) seem unable to use an MDI and spacer and in them nebulizers may be the only practical form of therapy.

CORTICOSTEROIDS

Inhaled corticosteroids are unquestionably the cornerstone of chronic asthma treatment in both adults and children. The use of systemic corticosteroids in acute severe asthma, however, has been more controversial. Some earlier studies failed to show benefit, the reasons suggested were: the patients were spontaneously improving thereby minimizing the steroid benefit;[61] the patient numbers were too small[62] or the improvement was masked by the use of large doses of bronchodilators.[63] More recently other studies undertaken in the emergency department have also produced negative results.[64–66] This is strange, given what we know of corticosteroid action in asthma.[67,68]

One of the best early studies to show benefit in adult patients[69] used intravenous methyl prednisolone in the emergency department. When assessed four hours after treatment the number needing hospital admission was considerably reduced. This study was repeated in children using oral prednisolone rather than intravenous methyl prednisolone[70] with very similar results. Both studies were double-blind and controlled, the steroid treatment being given in addition to bronchodilator therapy. Other studies have shown that the addition of steroids in acute severe asthma reduces the need for hospital admission,[71,72] shortens the length of the attack[73–75] and reduces the rate of relapse.[72,76,77]

Intravenous steroids may have an earlier onset of action than oral steroids (1 hour vs 3 hours) but the time to peak clinical effect is very similar so that oral steroids are usually the preferred method of administration.[78,79] Most guidelines on asthma management recommend the early use of oral prednisolone during an acute attack especially in those already receiving inhaled corticosteroid therapy or in those not responding fully to inhaled bronchodilator therapy. The dose of oral prednisolone is usually recommended as 1–2 mg/kg/day as a once daily dose. There is no evidence base for such a dose schedule and a recent study showed no differences between 0.5 mg, 1.0 mg and 2 mg/kg/day prednisolone given during an acute attack.[80] Given the flat dose–response curve of corticosteroids and the possible need for repeated dosings to prevent secondary care management it seems reasonable to recommend the lowest dose schedule early in acute attacks of asthma in children. The severity of each acute attack of asthma will differ and it seems unreasonable, therefore, to stipulate the optimal length of treatment with oral prednisolone. Most guidelines recommend 1–5 days allowing the parent or the child to end the course when a target response is achieved.

Corticosteroids are also available in nebulized preparations. Twice daily nebulized budesonide has been shown to be more effective than once daily dosing in stable asthma.[81] Francis et al. showed that nebulized fluticasone propionate was as effective as once daily oral prednisolone in the treatment of preschool children with an acute exacerbation[82] and a recent study demonstrated nebulized fluticasone was as effective as oral prednisolone in children aged 4–16 years old presenting with an acute exacerbation of asthma.[83]

Controversy about the use of corticosteroids in acute asthma has also occurred because of the apparent difference in response depending on whether the child has atopic asthma or virus-induced wheeze. Although one study showed that the use of oral prednisolone was beneficial when used at the first sign of a runny nose in viral-induced wheeze,[84] it was not controlled and concerns have been raised about the possible effects on short-term linear growth[85] if repeated courses are given. Studies using intermittent high-dose inhaled corticosteroids during virus-induced wheezing or at the onset of upper respiratory symptoms[86,87] only produced modest benefits. The traditional recommendation of doubling the dose of inhaled corticosteroids during an acute wheezing episode has clearly been questioned by another study[88] showing no differences between the active and placebo groups. One of the issues in virus-induced wheeze may be that the cellular response in the airways (as shown in bronchoalveolar lavage studies)[89] is not susceptible to corticosteroid therapy.

Corticosteroid therapy is not without the possibility of side effects. Repeated doses of oral prednisolone have the ability to interfere with short-term and long-term growth. The long-term effects on bone density are unknown. The benefits to very young children (under 2 years old) with asthma are poorly reported and, as with bronchodilators, it is probable that the response is less good. Caution is needed on the frequency, the dosage and the length of the steroid courses in all children. A child who requires four or more oral prednisolone doses within a 12-month period should be referred to a respiratory paediatrician for evaluation of asthma control and subsequent follow-up.

In summary, there is strong evidence in atopic asthma for the early use of oral prednisolone in an acute severe attack. A dose of 0.5 mg/kg/day appears as effective as higher doses. The evidence for the use of corticosteroids in viral-induced wheeze is less clear.

ANTICHOLINERGIC AGENTS

In inhaled form these act by blocking muscarinic para-sympathetic bronchoconstriction in the central and peripheral airways.[90] The only commonly available inhaled anticholinergic agent is ipratropium bromide which, because of its insolubility in lipid, is a safe medication even in high doses. A recent study by Qureshi and colleagues showed that in combination with a β_2-agonist, it reduced hospital admissions in children with severe asthma compared with β_2-agonist therapy alone.[91] In doses of up to 750 μg within an hour, it leads to significant additional bronchodilation.[92] Most consensus statements on the management of acute severe asthma suggest, however, that ipratropium bromide is not a first line therapeutic agent.[93] Two meta-analyses[94,95] indicate that the addition of ipratropium to β_2-agonist therapy improves lung function by 10–12% but it should not be used universally until further research determines the clinical significance of these lung function changes.

METHYLXANTHINES

Some studies have suggested that theophylline provides benefit when added to β_2-agonist therapy[96] and may reduce hospital admission[97] but others have shown no benefit with increased likelihood of side effects.[98–100] For discussion of the use of theophyllines in children admitted to hospital with very severe exacerbations see the relevant section below.

Emergency department

Effective management depends on the use of:

- an initial triage system to determine the severity of the attack and the urgency of pharmacotherapy;
- a management protocol, carefully followed according to the response to therapy;
- an effective, well-tested assessment schedule;
- clear plans on the need for admission to hospital or discharge home;
- a discharge plan including agreed follow-up arrangements.

The most effective way to do this, as already discussed, is by the development of *asthma care-pathways* in each

centre. These pathways will differ according to the provision of the local medical services. The following therapeutic protocols are only a guide as we recognize that local needs will vary.

If the initial *triage* colour is red or orange commence SaO_2 monitoring. Immediate treatment with nebulized salbutamol 5 mg or terbutaline 10 mg is mandatory, driven by oxygen at a flow rate of 7 l/min. Nebulizations should be continuous, intravenous (IV) access must be obtained for fluid replacement, the commencement of IV corticosteroids and IV salbutamol. For further management see in-patient treatment below. This presentation can be classified as critical asthma.

For less critical presentations with an initial triage colour of yellow (or below) the emergency department protocol in Table 12.3 can be used.

Whilst functional severity scores have been developed to assess chronic childhood asthma,[102] probably the best way to assess the severity of the acute attack is the degree and rapidity of response to the above regimes. This is especially true in the preschool age group which accounts for approximately half of the referrals to emergency departments.

Table 12.3 *Emergency department protocol*

1 Take a full history, examine the child, monitor the SaO_2 and commence O_2 if necessary. If the child is well enough or old enough PEF can be measured and evaluated using a standard chart[101] (Figure 12.2). If urgent, give nebulized β_2-agonist without delay and assess simultaneously.
2 Give nebulized bronchodilator or inhaled salbutamol/terbutaline through an MDI and spacer device. (See text.) Various protocols suggest half dosages in children <6 years old. A face-mask can be added to the spacer in very young children. Also give soluble prednisolone 0.5 mg/kg orally to children over 18 months (unless the attack is mild or there is very rapid return to normality).
3 Reassess after 5–10 minutes and repeat the treatment every 20 minutes for the first hour (or give continuous nebulization) as necessary. Reassessments should include SaO_2, a clinical severity assessment and PEF readings if appropriate.
4 A decision to admit or not should be made during the first hour depending on local guidelines and the available medical service. Admission should be mandatory if PEF remains low, SaO_2 remains <92% in air and if the family is unlikely to manage at home.
5 If the decision is to send the child home ensure the child has sufficient bronchodilator therapy and a suitable spacer device (±face-mask). Consider the need to give a short 1–5 day course of soluble prednisolone (0.5 mg/kg/day). Determine the ability of the parent(s) to continue home management.
6 Ensure a clear written management plan is given to the parent(s) and complete the plans for follow-up before discharge home.

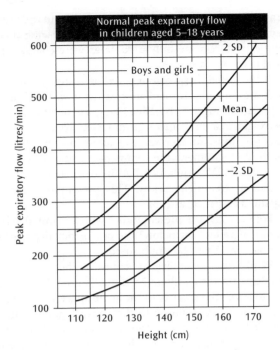

Figure 12.2 *Reference data for peak expiratory flow. (From ref. 101.)*

When discharging patients home from the emergency department there seems agreement that some form of written treatment plan is helpful (Table 12.4). Such a plan should be as simple as possible and include the arrangements for follow-up. The discharge plan will vary with local healthcare facilities.

Hospital management

Children presenting to hospital with severe asthma (triage level of orange or red) should be treated as medical emergencies because of their potential to deteriorate rapidly. In the emergency room, they should be nursed in high dependency areas where frequent observations can be made to assess severity of the attack and the response to treatment.

The aims of treatment are to relieve hypoxia, reverse airflow obstruction, prevent progression of the attack and facilitate early discharge from the emergency department or admissions unit. A number of treatment options are available with variable degrees of supportive evidence and it may be helpful to divide these options into those with reasonably strong supportive evidence and those where the evidence is not conclusive.

Treatment

OXYGEN

Initial assessment of any asthma attack should include pulse oximetry to detect the presence of hypoxia. In an

Table 12.4 *Emergency department discharge plan*

INFORMATION FOR PARENTS

In the emergency department your child has received treatment for an asthma attack. Further treatment is likely to be needed after arrival at home. Your child has been given some inhaled medicine and some medicine to take by mouth.

Inhaled medicine
.... is an inhaled medicine which works quickly to help stop wheezing and ease breathlessness. Use up to .... puffs as you have been shown, using the spacer, every 2–4 hours until your child is back to normal. If the medicine is not working, or does not last for at least 2 hours, bring your child immediately back to the emergency department or phone .... for advice.

Medicine by mouth (Soluble prednisolone 5 mg tablets)
Give .... tablets tomorrow morning, dissolved in a drink.
Give the same dose the next day if your child is not back to normal. There are enough tablets to give up to 4 days treatment if you think it necessary. Give the same dose each day; stop when your child is much better.
If your child normally takes regular inhaled medicine, give this as before.

Follow-up arrangement
A follow-up appointment has been made for
.... on ....(day/date) at
................(time) in ....(hospital/community clinic or surgery).

acute exacerbation, the maldistribution of airway obstruction results in ventilation perfusion mismatch,[104] due to a combination of increased dead space ventilation and intrapulmonary shunting. Both these mechanisms can cause hypoxia which occurs early during an attack and correlates with the severity of the episode.[105] Hypoxia (SaO_2 <92% in air) should be treated with high flow oxygen (8–10 l/min) via face-mask immediately on arrival at the hospital. If there is poor response to treatment with high flow oxygen it is important that other causes of respiratory distress, pneumothorax in particular, are sought.

β₂-AGONISTS

Definitive treatment of bronchospasm is with inhaled short-acting β_2-agonists administered by a metered dose inhaler (MDI) through a spacer device, or in young patients (less than 4 years of age) and those in severe respiratory distress by nebulizer. All short-acting β_2-agonists given in equivalent doses produce equal bronchodilation[106] and the choice will depend on local preference (Table 12.5).

Patients with severe asthma should receive a dose of β_2-agonist immediately after initial assessment, no later than 10 minutes after arrival. The effect of treatment should be apparent within 15 minutes of the first dose.

Table 12.5 *Short-acting β₂-agonists and their doses*

Drug	MDI and spacer	Nebulized dose	Subcutaneous	Intravenous
Salbutamol	6–12 puffs of 100 μg every 3 breaths	2.5–5 mg intermittent 0.5 mg/kg/h continuous	8 μg/kg/dose	15 μg/kg load* 1–5 μg/kg/min infusion
Terbutaline	6–10 puffs of 250 μg every 3 breaths	2–5 mg intermittent 0.5 mg/kg/h continuous	5–10 μg/kg/dose	10 μg/kg load* 1–4 μg/kg/min
Bitolterol	Not studied in acute severe asthma			
Pirbuterol	Not studied in acute severe asthma			

*Omit if inhaled dose has been high.

If there is poor response to the first dose, a repeat dose 20 minutes later is indicated. The optimum dose and interval for the administration of β₂-agonist depends on the severity of the attack and the response to the first dose. Doses given every 20 minutes are more effective than hourly doses[107] and continuous nebulization is more effective than intermittent dosing.[108,109]

β₂-Agonists can be administered intravenously and are effective when there has been a poor response to the first nebulized dose.[110] On the other hand, intravenous administration does not confer any benefit over the nebulized route if effective nebulization occurs.[111] Lack of response to nebulized therapy may occur because the patient generates tidal volumes that are too small to facilitate aerosol delivery to the lungs or because mucosal oedema and mucous plugging contribute to a significant proportion of airway obstruction. Side effects of β₂-agonists include tachycardia, dysrhythmias, hypertension, hypokalaemia, hyperglycaemia and lactic acidosis.

CORTICOSTEROIDS

All patients with an acute exacerbation of asthma should receive steroid treatment as early as possible. The parenteral route does not confer any advantage over the enteral route and should be reserved for the patient who is vomiting or unable to take oral fluids. Discussion of the optimal dose has been covered previously.

ANTICHOLINERGIC AGENTS

Ipratropium bromide (a quarternary derivative of atropine) has been shown to produce benefit when used with β₂-agonists in very severe asthma attacks.[112,92,113] It is thought to act mainly on the larger airways[91] and therefore complements the action of β₂-agonists, which may have a more peripheral action. In a very severe attack, ipratropium bromide (125–250 μg per dose) should be administered with a β₂-agonist every 20 minutes for the first hour and every 4 hours thereafter, by MDI and spacer, or by nebulizer.

FLUID REPLACEMENT

Mild dehydration is common in patients with severe asthma and younger patients may have a significant fluid deficit from a combination of poor intake prior to admission, increased loss through the respiratory tract and faster metabolism.[114] Oral fluid replacement is normally adequate unless the patient is vomiting or in severe respiratory distress. Intravenous fluid replacement should be used judiciously because of the risk of precipitating pulmonary oedema, since the high negative transpulmonary pressure may lead to fluid accumulation around the respiratory bronchiole.[115] Normal saline or 0.45% saline should be the fluid of choice and it is prudent to restrict fluid administration to 70% of daily requirement. There should be a low threshold for the addition of potassium chloride to the fluid as hypokalaemia may accompany the use of β₂-agonists.[111,116,117]

Optional treatment

Despite maximal recommended treatment, a small proportion of patients will continue to deteriorate and a number of additional therapies have been used in an attempt to avoid intubation and mechanical ventilation.

AMINOPHYLLINE

Aminophylline is a xanthine derivative that is postulated to cause bronchodilation by mechanisms which include modulation of intracellular calcium, prostaglandin antagonism, inhibition of phosphodiesterase effects on cyclic AMP and β-adrenergic receptor agonism. It has also been shown to increase diaphragmatic contractility.[118–120] Although in clinical use for over 50 years, there is poor evidence to support its continuing use in mild to moderate asthma as demonstrated in two meta-analyses.[121,122] One study in very severe asthma suggested that the use of intravenous aminophylline reduced the need for intubation and mechanical ventilation.[123] However there was a significantly higher rate of adverse effects in the treated group which was nearly nine times as likely as the placebo group to discontinue treatment because of these effects. Adverse events are closely related to serum concentration of the drug[124] and include irritability, nausea, vomiting and diarrhoea with lower doses and cardiac arrhythmia, hypotension, seizures and cardiac arrest with higher doses. Intravenous aminophylline should therefore only be considered in patients who have not responded to oxygen, nebulized and/or intravenous β_2-agonists, nebulized anticholinergics, corticosteroids and fluid replacement. At this stage, mechanical ventilation is probably the best option. Serum levels should be monitored and may vary as a result of drug interactions. If used at all, this treatment should be carried out in the setting of an intensive care or high dependency unit where close monitoring and rapid reaction to adverse events are available.

MAGNESIUM SULPHATE

There have been anecdotal reports of the use of slow intravenous magnesium sulphate infusion in severe asthma for over 60 years but clinical trials show conflicting evidence of benefit.[125–132] A meta-analysis of seven trials, two in children, showed no significant benefit from the use of magnesium sulphate overall but subgroup analysis suggests possible benefit when used in very severe asthma.[133] It is not clear how magnesium sulphate exerts its therapeutic effect but postulated mechanisms include inhibition of calcium channels through plasma membranes, decreased acetylcholine release at neuromuscular junctions and effects on adenosine triphosphatases. A response is said to occur within minutes and the effect lasts for up to two hours. A wide range of doses has been used and the drug is well tolerated if given by slow intravenous infusion. Side effects are minimal and include flushing and mild sedation. Large doses may cause hypotension and loss of deep tendon reflexes.

HELIOX

Blends of helium and oxygen in ratios of 60:40, 70:30 and 80:20 are less dense than air and are said to reduce resistance to gas flow and thereby reduce the work of breathing, potentially retarding the progression of respiratory failure. It can be delivered by a tight-fitting face-mask or through a ventilator circuit in mechanically ventilated patients. There is conflicting evidence of its value in severe asthma[134–139] and until clinical trials can clearly demonstrate a benefit, few would recommend its use.

Treatment in the intensive care unit

The vast majority of patients with severe asthma respond to emergency room treatment and will either be admitted to a general paediatric ward or discharged home. Patients in status asthmaticus – defined as progressive worsening of an asthma attack and respiratory failure not responding to standard treatment – need admission to an intensive care unit. Early transfer to an intensive care unit is recommended in the following situations.

History of previous attack resulting in ITU admission. Some patients have a pattern of attacks characterized by rapid deterioration in respiratory function during an attack.[125] Close monitoring and intensive treatment may

prevent progression to respiratory failure and mechanical ventilation.

Arterial carbon dioxide tension >6 kPa (45 mmHg) or rising at more than 1.5 kPa/h (10 mmHg). During an acute attack, increased ventilation, driven by hypoxia and by mechanical factors, usually leads to lower than normal values of $PaCO_2$. Although $PaCO_2$ levels do not correlate well with the degree of airway obstruction, levels above normal occur when the FEV_1 is less than 20% predicted.[105]

PEF or FEV_1 <33% predicted. Most children with severe asthma cannot perform pulmonary function tests reliably (the majority of children admitted to hospital are below 6 years old), especially when acutely ill. They are more useful as indicators of response to therapy during recovery.

Arterial oxygen tension less than 8 kPa (60 mmHg) despite oxygen therapy. As discussed above, hypoxia is common during an attack but is usually easily corrected. In the absence of an air leak, persistence of hypoxia suggests gross ventilation perfusion mismatch due to a combination of hyperinflation and segmental atelectasis.

Depressed conscious level. This is usually the end result of persistent hypoxia and exhaustion, occurs late in the course of an attack and may be a prelude to cardiorespiratory arrest.

Metabolic acidosis. May occur in very severe attacks and is thought to be a result of renal bicarbonate loss, tissue hypoxia and the side effects of β_2-agonist treatment. Acidosis together with hypercapnia and hypoxia depresses cardiovascular function and could lead to cardiorespiratory arrest.

Pneumothorax or pneumomediastinum. Although uncommon, should either of these occur, treatment should take place in the intensive care unit.

Basic therapy which was started in the emergency room should be continued unless the patient requires mechanical ventilation immediately. A nasogastric tube should be placed to empty the stomach and the patient should have at least two points of venous access. An indwelling arterial catheter will facilitate continuous monitoring of blood pressure and allow repeated arterial blood gas sampling.

INTUBATION

The need for mechanical ventilation is relatively rare and most paediatric intensive care units will only ventilate a handful of patients each year. Consequently there is a paucity of controlled data on ventilatory strategy in the management of these patients. Practical aspects of intubation and mechanical ventilation have recently been reviewed.[140] The following section is based on a summary of a number of review articles on the management of patients in status asthmaticus.[141–143] The decision to initiate ventilation should be made early rather than late.

Apart from cardiorespiratory arrest, there are no absolute indications for ventilation and the decision to intubate is usually based on a subjective assessment by the clinician that maximal pharmacological treatment has failed to relieve respiratory distress and that respiratory failure is imminent.

Rapid sequence intubation should be carried out by an experienced physician who is aware of the particular dangers of intubating a patient with severe asthma. Instrumentation of the airway can provoke pharyngeal and laryngeal reflexes leading to laryngospasm and pre-treatment with atropine and a local anaesthetic to the hypopharynx is advisable.

Sedation with morphine should be avoided because of the risk of histamine release worsening bronchospasm. The sedative drug of choice is ketamine hydrochloride 1–3 mg/kg, an intravenous anaesthetic that has some bronchodilating properties in addition to sedative and analgesic effects. Ketamine is a dissociative agent and it is advisable to add a benzodiazepine like midazolam or lorazepam to counteract its well-described dysphoric effects. A short-acting muscle relaxant like succinylcholine or rocuronium should be used during intubation.

Oral intubation is easier than nasal intubation and a cuffed endotracheal tube should be used if available. Ventilatory strategies in asthma involve very high gas flows and it is important to choose the largest appropriate endotracheal tube to reduce tube resistance. This has the added benefit of facilitating suctioning of the airway. One of the risks of intubation in severe asthma is cardiovascular instability due to a combination of worsening lung hyperinflation, relative hypovolaemia and sedation, all of which may affect venous return and left ventricular filling pressure. This may require cardiovascular support with fluid boluses and administration of inotropic agents.

VENTILATORY STRATEGY

In the presence of severe airway obstruction, the challenge in ventilating a severe asthmatic is to relieve hypoxia and reduce hypercapnia and respiratory acidosis without causing barotrauma or exacerbating lung hyperinflation. Mechanical ventilation is effective at reducing hypercapnia but its primary role is to provide sorely needed rest to fatigued respiratory muscles while pharmacological agents reverse bronchoconstriction. The over-riding priority therefore is to minimize the risk of iatrogenic lung injury. A number of ventilatory strategies have been put forward but there are no controlled trials that would help to choose between them. In general, volume controlled ventilation is preferred initially with a low respiratory rate (approximately half the normal rate for the child's age) with a short inspiratory time and I:E ratio of 1:3 to 1:6 to facilitate passive expiration and reduce the risk of lung hyperinflation. Tidal volumes of 6–10 ml/kg will limit inspiratory pressure and avoid barotrauma. A lower minute ventilation is feasible with the acceptance of permissive hypercapnia ($PaCO_2$ up to 8 kPa or 60 mmHg) so long as the pH is maintained above 7.2. Positive end-expiratory pressure (PEEP) should be kept low (0–3 cmH$_2$O) to avoid exacerbating lung hyperinflation. As bronchoconstriction improves, PEEP can be increased to aid oxygenation. If there is a large leak around the endotracheal tube or if the inspiratory pressure generated during volume controlled ventilation exceeds 40 cmH$_2$O, pressure control ventilation should be considered. A maximal peak inspiratory pressure of 35–40 cmH$_2$O, PEEP of 0–3 cmH$_2$O and rate of 10–15 breaths per minute would be reasonable initial ventilator settings. When airway obstruction begins to lessen, inspiratory pressures can be reduced and support ventilatory modes like volume support or pressure support can be used to wean the patient off the ventilator.

In addition to assisted ventilation, endotracheal intubation will allow clearance of airway secretions that contribute significantly to airway narrowing. In very severe cases, bronchoscopic lavage has been used to clear secretions in the airway. Instrumentation of the airway may however provoke bronchospasm and pre-treatment with topical anaesthetic is usually needed.

SEDATION

Patients on mechanical ventilation need to be sedated and given a muscle relaxant during the initial phase of ventilation to allow rest and to prevent patient/ventilator asynchrony. Sedation with benzodiazepines (midazolam, lorazepam) and analgesia with ketamine are usually adequate. Ketamine has the theoretical advantage of providing sedation and a small degree of bronchodilation.

Muscle relaxation is best achieved with a continuous infusion of a non-depolarizing agent like vecuronium 2–4 mg/kg/min. Prolonged use of muscle relaxants in the presence of high-dose steroids is occasionally associated with muscle weakness, myopathy and neuropathy. Intermittent discontinuation of muscle relaxation may reduce the likelihood of these complications.

UNUSUAL TREATMENTS

There are anecdotal reports of agents used with some success in ventilated patients resistant to normal treatment. There are no controlled trials using these agents and they may have significant adverse effects. Inhalational anaesthetic agents like halothane and isofluorane have been used with varying success. The effects are said to be immediate and may provide some additional bronchodilation. However, hypotension invariably accompanies the use of anaesthetic agents and will need to be treated with fluid boluses and inotropic support. Nitric oxide has been used with some success in children but data are too scanty to recommend this treatment. Methyl-xanthines, magnesium sulphate and helium are considered earlier.

Discharge plans

When discharging patients from hospital a written treatment plan similar to that recommended in the emergency department is helpful. It should clearly indicate arrangements for follow-up as already discussed. Despite an overall increase in the prevalence of asthma, one study has documented a fall in the number of children needing admission or re-admission for mechanical ventilation, possibly because of greater use of preventer therapy.[153] Children who have had intensive care therapy for asthma are at higher subsequent risk of a fatal attack.

Repeated studies have demonstrated a cluster of features that distinguish children with severe (near-fatal) asthma attacks.[150,154] They include:

- teenage, male sex;
- severe, poorly controlled asthma;
- low compliance with inhaled corticosteroids and excessive reliance on short-acting β_2-agonists;
- recent admission to hospital (or ICU);
- delay in seeking medical help, despite adequate warning signs;
- psychosocial factors in the family.

Identifying such children is only the first step in changing their behaviour (Chapters 11 and 18).

FATAL ASTHMA

Childhood deaths from asthma are infrequent but a significant number should be preventable.[144] The Global Initiative for Asthma (GINA), set a world-wide target to reduce childhood asthma deaths by 50% over the 5 years from 1998. Detailed analysis of childhood asthma mortality rates are plagued by the problems of insufficient data from developing countries and variations in ascertainment elsewhere, making cross-sectional comparisons difficult. Nevertheless, following a period of increasing mortality in the two decades from 1970–1990, there is evidence of a fall in mortality rate at least in the developed countries. Data from England and Wales show an average 6% fall in deaths in the 5–14 year age group from 1983 to 1995.[145] A similar pattern has been reported in Denmark[146] and the United States.[147] Although these are encouraging trends, it has to be recognized that there was a significant increase in mortality prior to this and that the crude mortality rate remains higher than in the early 1970s. Fatal asthma in childhood has recently been reviewed.[148]

The relatively small number of childhood deaths from asthma and variations in reporting between countries, reduces the likelihood of identifying risk factors for fatal asthma in children. There is some consensus that fatal asthma in children is rare in the very young, is usually very rapid (less than 2 hours) in onset, occurs in children who are not under secondary care (and whose asthma

has not been previously recognized as very severe), who are under-treated with inhaled corticosteroids and whose compliance with therapy is poor.[149–153] There is also a small but distinct group of children with asthma that is difficult to control and who have had significant chronic problems including previous mechanical ventilation, admission to an intensive care unit and psychosocial problems.[149,150] Corticosteroid resistance could be a specific additional factor.[155]

Additional factors thought to contribute to fatality in these patients include failure to appreciate the severity of the attack, increased exposure to allergens that precipitate the attack and a blunted response to hypoxia and hypercapnia in chronic poorly controlled patients. It is of note that fatal attacks often appear to be extremely rapid in onset (less than 1 hour in many cases) and, unlike most severe episodes, not preceded by an obvious upper respiratory tract infection. Some occur in apparently mild asthma, raising the possibility of 'pulmonary anaphylaxis'. However, in a large adult series, absence of a self-management plan and failure to use steroids in the attack distinguished fatal from severe asthma.[156] One cannot draw inferences about fatal asthma from 'near-fatal' (i.e. mechanically ventilated) patients.[150]

REFERENCES

1. The International Study of Asthma and Allergies in Childhood (ISAAC) Steering Committee. Worldwide variation in the prevalence of asthma symptoms: The International Study of Asthma and Allergies in Childhood (ISAAC). *Eur Respir J* 1998;**12**:315–35.
2. Ninan TK, Russell G. Respiratory symptoms and atopy in Aberdeen school children: evidence from two surveys 25 years apart. *Br Med J* 1992;**304**:873–5.
3. Vollmer WM, Osborne M, Buist AS. 20 year trends in the prevalence of asthma and chronic airflow obstruction in an HMO. *Am Respir Crit Care Med* 1998;**157**:1079–84.
4. Flemming DM, Sunderland R, Cross AW, *et al.* Declining incidence of episodes of asthma: a study of trends in new episodes presenting to general practitioners in the period 1989–98. *Thorax* 2000;**55**:657–61.
5. Wennergren G, Kristjánnsson S, Strannegård I-L. Decrease in hospitalisation for treatment of childhood asthma with increased use of anti-inflammatory treatment despite an increase in the prevalence of asthma. *J Allergy Clin Immunol* 1996;**97**:742–8.
6. Royal College of General Practitioners – Asthma Group. 1997. *Annual Report.*
7. Anderson HR, Bailey PA, Cooper JS, *et al.* Medical care of asthma and wheezing illness in children: A community survey. *J Epidemiol Comm Health* 1983;**37**:180–6.

8. Storr J, Barrell E, Lenney W. Rising asthma admissions and self referral. *Arch Dis Child* 1988;**63**:774–9.
9. Mitchell EA. International trends in hospital admission rates for asthma. *Arch Dis Child* 1985;**60**:376–8.
10. Lenney W. The Burden of Paediatric Asthma. *Pediatr Pulmonol* (Suppl)1997;**15**:13–16.
11. Toelle BG, Peat JK, Mellis CM, *et al.* The cost of childhood asthma to Australian families. *Ped Pulmonol* 1995;**19**:330–5.
12. Pattemore P, Johnston S, Bardin P, *et al.* Viruses as precipitants of asthma symptoms. I. Epidemiology. *Clin Exp Allergy* 1992;**22**:325–36.
13. Storr J, Lenney W. School holidays and admissions with asthma. *Arch Dis Child* 1989;**64**:103–7.
14. Howland J, Bauchner H, Adair R. The impact of pediatric asthma education on morbidity. Assessing the evidence. *Chest* 1988;**94**:964–9.
15. Bernard-Bonnin AC, Stachenko S, Bonin D, *et al.* Self-management teaching programs and morbidity of paediatric asthma: a meta-analysis. *J Allergy Clin Immunol* 1995;**95**:34–41.
16. Madge P, McColl J, Paton J. Impact of a nurse-led home management training programme in children admitted to hospital with acute asthma: a randomised controlled study. *Thorax* 1997;**52**:223–8.
17. Wesseldine LJ, McCarthy P, Silverman M. Structured discharge procedure for children admitted to hospital with acute asthma: a randomised controlled trial of nursing practice. *Arch Dis Child* 1999;**80**:110–14.
18. David TJ, Wibrew M, Hennessen U. Prodromal itching in childhood asthma. *Lancet* 1984;**ii**:154–5.
19. Beer S, Laver J, Karpuch J. Prodromal features of asthma. *Arch Dis Child* 1987;**62**:345–8.
20. The British Guidelines on Asthma Management. 1995 Review and Position Statement. *Thorax* 1997; **52**(Suppl 1):S1–21.
21. Expert Panel Report 2. *Guidelines for the Diagnosis and Management of Asthma.* National Institutes of Health, Bethesda, MD, 1998.
22. GINA Guidelines. *Global Strategy for Asthma Management and Prevention.* NHLBI, Bethesda MD, NIH Publication Number 02–3659, 2002.
23. Warner JO, Naspitz CK, Cropp GJA. Third international pediatric consensus statement on the management of childhood asthma. *Pediatr Pulmonol* 1998; **25**:1–17.
24. Reddel H, Ware S, Marks G, *et al.* Differences between asthma exacerbations and poor asthma control. *Lancet* 1999;**353**:364–9.
25. Lloyd BW, Ali MH. How useful do parents find home peak flow monitoring for children with asthma? *Br Med J* 1992;**305**:1128–9.
26. Warman KL, Silver EJ, McCourt MP, *et al.* How does home management of asthma exacerbations by parents of inner-city children differ from NHLBI Guideline recommendations? *Pediatrics* 1999; **103**:422–7.
27. Charlton I, Charlton G, Broomfield J, *et al.* Evaluation of peak flow and symptoms on self-management plans for control of asthma in general practice. *Br Med J* 1990;**301**:1355–9.
28. Kesten S, Maleki-Yazdi MR, Sanders BR, *et al.* Respiratory rate during acute asthma. *Chest* 1990; **97**:58–62.
29. Comore JH Jr, Botelho S. The unreliability of cyanosis in the recognition of arterial anoxemia. *Am J Med Sci* 1947;**214**:1–6.
30. Clark NM, Evans D, Mellins RB. Patient use of peak flow monitoring. *Am Rev Respir Dis* 1992;**145**:772–5.
31. Fischl MA, Pitchenik A, Gerdner LB. An index predicting relapse and the need for hospitalisation in patients with acute bronchial asthma. *New Engl J Med* 1981;**305**:783–9.
32. Kelsen SG, Kelsen DP, Fleeger BF, *et al.* Emergency room assessment and treatment of patients with acute asthma: adequacy of conventional approach. *Am J Med* 1978;**64**:622–8.
33. Rose CC, Murphy JG, Schwartz JS. Performance of an index predicting the response of patients with acute bronchial asthma to intensive emergency department treatment. *New Engl J Med* 1984;**310**:573–7.
34. Centor R, Yarbrough B, Wood J. Inability to predict relapse in acute asthma. *New Engl J Med* 1984;**310**: 577–80.
35. Skoner DP, Fischer TJ, Gromley C, *et al.* Paediatric predictive index for hospitalisation in patients with acute asthma. *Ann Emerg Med* 1987;**16**:25–31.
36. Martin TG, Elenbaas RM, Pingleton SH. Failure of peak expiratory flow rate to predict hospital admission in acute asthma. *Ann Emerg Med* 1982;**11**:466–70.
37. Ownby DR, Abarzua J, Anderson JA. Attempting to predict hospital admissions in acute asthma. *Am J Dis Child* 1984;**138**:1062–6.
38. Lulla S, Newcomb RW. Emergency management of asthma in children. *J Pediatr* 1980;**97**:346–50.
39. McConnochie KM, Russo MJ, McBride JT, *et al.* How commonly are children hospitalized for asthma eligible for care in alternative settings? *Arch Pediatr Adolesc Med* 1999;**153**:49–55.
40. Geelhoed GC, Landau LI, Le Souëf PN. Predictive value of oxygen saturation in emergency evaluation of asthmatic children. *Br Med J* 1988;**297**:395–6.
41. Geelhoed GC, Landau LI, Le Souëf PN. Oximetry and peak expiratory flow in assessment of acute childhood asthma. *J Pediatr* 1990;**117**:907–9.
42. Connett GJ, Lenney W. Use of oximetry in acute asthma in childhood. *Pediatr Pulmonol* 1993; **15**:345–9.
43. Wright RO, Santucci KA, Jay GD, *et al.* Evaluation of pre- and post-treatment pulse oximetry in acute childhood asthma. *Acad Emerg Med* 1997;**4**:114–17.
44. Mayefsky JH, L-Shinaway Y. The usefulness of pulse oximetry in evaluating acutely ill asthmatics. *Pediatr Emerg Care* 1992;**8**:262–4.

45. Frey B, Freezer N. Diagnostic value and pathophysiologic basis of pulsus paradox in infants and children with respiratory disease. *Pediatr Pulmonol* 2001;**31**:138–43.

46. Rebuck A, Pengally L. Development of pulsus paradox in the presence of airway obstruction. *New Engl J Med* 1973;**288**:66.

47. Galant SP, Graucy CE, Shaw KC. The value of pulsus paradoxus in assessing the child with status asthmaticus. *Pediatrics* 1978;**61**:46–51.

48. Guidelines on the Management of Asthma. *Thorax* 1993;**48**:(Suppl)S1–24.

49. Frey B, Butt W. Pulse oximetry for assessment of pulsus paradoxus: a clinical study in children. *Intens Care Med* 1998;**24**:242–6.

50. Lenney W, Clayton S. A&E attendances for children with asthma. *Thorax* 1998;**53**:(Suppl 4)A5.

51. Weng TR, Levison H. Pulmonary function in children with asthma at acute attack and symptom-free status. *Am Rev Respir Dis* 1969;**99**:719–23.

52. Farber HJ, Johnson C, Beckerman RC. Young inner-city children visiting the emergency room (ER) for asthma: Risk factors and chronic care behaviors. *J Asthma* 1998;**35**:547–52.

53. Mackway-Jones K, ed. *Emergency Triage, Manchester Triage Group*. BMJ Publishing Group, London, 1997.

54. Cates CJ. Comparison of holding chambers and nebulisers for beta agonists in acute asthma. A systemic review of randomised controlled trials (*Cochrane Review*). Update Software, Cochrane Library, Oxford, 1999.

55. Kerem E, Levison H, Schuh S, et al. Efficacy of albuterol administered by nebuliser versus spacer device in children. *J Pediatr* 1993;**123**:313–17.

56. Chou KJ, Cunningham SJ, Crain EF. Metered-dose inhalers with spacers vs nebulisers for paediatric asthma. *Arch Paediatr Adoles Med* 1995;**149**:201–5.

57. Dewar AL, Stewart A, Cogswell JJ. A randomised controlled trial to assess the relative benefits of large volume spacers and nebulisers to treat acute asthma in hospital. *Arch Dis Child* 1999; **80**:421–3.

58. Anon. Nebulisers in the treatment of asthma. *Drugs Therapeut Bull* 1987;**25**:101–3.

59. Salmon B, Wilson NM, Silverman M. How much aerosol reaches the lungs of wheezy infants and toddlers? *Arch Dis Child* 1990;**65**:401–3.

60. Parkin PC, Saunders NR, Diamond SA, et al. Randomised trial spacer – v – nebuliser for acute asthma. *Arch Dis Child* 1995;**72**:239–40.

61. Harris JB, Weinberger MM, Nassif E, et al. Early intervention with short courses of prednisolone to prevent progression of asthma in ambulatory patients incompletely responsive to bronchodilators. *J Pediatr* 1987;**110**:627–33.

62. McFadden ERT, Kisser R, DeGroot WJ. A controlled study on the effects of a single dose of hydrocortisone on the reduction of acute attacks of asthma. *Am J Med* 1976;**60**:52–9.

63. Kattan M, Gurwitz D, Levison H. Corticosteroids in status asthmaticus. *J Pediatr* 1980;**96**:596–9.

64. Stein LM, Cole RP. Early administration of corticosteroids in emergency room treatment of acute asthma. *Ann Intern Med* 1990;**112**:822–7.

65. Wolfson DH, Nypaver MM, Blaser M, et al. A controlled trial of prednisolone in the early emergency department treatment of acute asthma in children. *Pediatr Emerg Care* 1994;**10**:335–8.

66. Lin RY, Pesola GR, Westfal RE, et al. Early parenteral corticosteroid administration in acute asthma. *Am J Emerg Med* 1997;**15**:621–5.

67. Morris HG. Mechanisms of action and therapeutic role of corticosteroids in asthma. *J Allergy Clin Immunol* 1985;**75**:1–13.

68. Barnes PJ. A new approach to the treatment of asthma. *N Engl J Med* 1989;**321**:1517–27.

69. Littenberg B, Gluck EH. A controlled trial of methylprednisolone in the emergency treatment of acute asthma. *N Engl J Med* 1986;**314**:150–2.

70. Storr J, Barry W, Barrell E, et al. Effect of a single dose of prednisolone in acute childhood asthma. *Lancet* 1987;**i**:879–82.

71. Tal A, Levy N, Bearman JE, et al. Methylprednisolone therapy for acute asthma in infants and toddlers: A controlled clinical trial. *Pediatrics* 1990;**86**:350–6.

72. Rowe BH, Keller JL, Oxman AD. Effectiveness of steroid therapy in acute exacerbations of asthma: A meta-analysis. *Am J Emerg Med* 1992;**10**:301–10.

73. Fanta CH, Rossing TH, McFadden ER. Glucocorticoids in acute asthma: a critical controlled trial. *Am J Med* 1983;**74**:845–51.

74. Shapiro GG, Furukawa CT, Pierson WE, et al. Double-blind evaluation of methylprednisolone versus placebo for acute asthma episodes. *Pediatrics* 1983;**71**:510–14.

75. Younger RE, Gerber PS, Herrod HG, et al. Intravenous methylprednisolone efficacy in status asthmaticus of childhood. *Pediatrics* 1987;**80**:225–30.

76. Fiel SB, Swartz MA, Glanz K, et al. Efficacy of short-term corticosteroid therapy in out-patient treatment of acute bronchial asthma. *Am J Med* 1983;**75**:259–62.

77. Chapman KR, Verbeek PR, White JG, et al. Effect of a short course of prednisolone in the prevention of early relapse after the emergency room treatment of acute asthma. *N Engl J Med* 1991;**324**:788–94.

78. Ellul-Micallef R, Fenech FF. Intravenous prednisolone in chronic bronchial asthma. *Thorax* 1975;**30**:312–15.

79. Ellul-Micallef R, Borthwick RC, McHardy GJ. The time course of response to prednisolone in chronic bronchial asthma. *Clin Sci Mol Med* 1974;**47**:105–17.

80. Langton-Hewer S, Hobbs J, Reid F, et al. Prednisolone in acute childhood asthma: Clinical responses to three dosages. *Respir Med* 1998;**92**:541–6.

81. Baker J, Mellon M, Wald J. A multiple-dosing, placebo-controlled study of budesonide inhalation suspension given once or twice daily for treatment of persistent asthma in young children and infants. *Pediatrics* 1999;**103**:414–21.

82. Francis P, Geelhoed G, Harris MA, *et al*. Effect of nebulised fluticasone propionate1mg twice daily compared with oral prednisolone in pre-school children aged 48 months or less with an acute exacerbation of asthma. *Eur Respir J* 1997;**10**:275S.

83. Manjra AI, Price J, Lenney W, *et al*. Efficacy of nebulized fluticasone propionate compared with oral prednisolone in children with an acute exacerbation of asthma. *Respir Med* 2000;**94**:1206–14.

84. Brunette MG, Lands L, Thibidou LP. Childhood asthma: prevention of attacks with short-term corticosteroid treatment of upper respiratory infection. *Pediatrics* 1988;**81**:624–9.

85. Wolthers OD, Pedersen S. Short-term linear growth in asthmatic children during treatment with prednisolone. *Br Med J* 1990;**301**:145–8.

86. Wilson MN, Silverman M. Treatment of acute, episodic asthma in pre-school children using intermittent high-dose inhaled steroids at home. *Arch Dis Child* 1990;**65**:407–10.

87. Connett G, Lenney W. Prevention of viral-induced asthma attacks using inhaled budesonide. *Arch Dis Child* 1993;**68**:85–7.

88. Garrett J, Williams S, Wong C, *et al*. Treatment of acute asthmatic exacerbations with an increased dose of inhaled steroid. *Arch Dis Child* 1998;**79**:12–17.

89. Stevenson ECG, Turner LG, Heaney BC, *et al*. Bronchoalveolar lavage findings suggest two different forms of childhood asthma. *Clin Exp Allergy* 1997;**27**:1027–35.

90. Gross NJ. Ipratropium bromide. *N Engl J Med* 1988;**319**:486–94.

91. Quershi F, Pestian J, Davis P, *et al*. Effect of nebulised ipratropium on the hospitalisation rates of children with asthma. *N Engl J Med* 1998;**339**:1030–5.

92. Schuh S, Johnson DW, Callahan S, Canny G, Levison H. Efficacy of frequent nebulized ipratropium bromide added to frequent high-dose albuterol therapy in severe childhood asthma. *J Pediatr* 1995;**126**:639–45.

93. Mitchell EA and ad hoc Paediatric Group. Consensus of acute asthma management in children. *NZ Med J* 1992;**105**:353–5.

94. Henry RL. Ipratropium bromide: an added effect? *J Pediatr Child Health* 1990;**26**:124–5.

95. Osmond MH, Klassen TP. Efficacy of ipratropium bromide in acute childhood asthma: A meta-analysis. *Acad Emerg Med* 1995;**2**:651–6.

96. Pierson WE, Bierman CW, Stamm SJ, *et al*. Double-blind trial of aminophylline in status asthmaticus. *Pediatrics* 1971;**48**:642–6.

97. Wrenn K, Slovis CM, Murphy F, *et al*. Aminophylline therapy for acute bronchospastic disease in the emergency room. *Ann Intern Med* 1991;**115**:241–7.

98. Murphy DG, McDermott MF, Rydman RJ, *et al*. Aminophylline in the treatment of acute asthma when beta 2-adrenergics and steroids are provided. *Arch Intern Med* 1993;**153**:1784–8.

99. Appel D, Shim C. Comparative effect of epinephrine and aminophylline in the treatment of asthma. *Lung* 1981;**159**:243–54.

100. Strauss RE, Wertheim DL, Bonagura VR, *et al*. Aminophylline therapy does not improve outcome and increases adverse effects in children hospitalised with acute asthmatic exacerbations. *Pediatrics* 1994;**93**:205–10.

101. Godfrey S, Kamburoff PL, Nairn JR. Spriometry, lung volumes and airway resistance in normal children aged 5–18 years. *Br J Dis Chest* 1970;**64**:15–24.

102. Rosier MJ, Bishop J, Nolan T, *et al*. Measurement of functional severity of asthma in children. *Am J Respir Crit Care Med* 1994;**149**:1434–41.

103. Hogg JC. The pathophysiology of asthma. *Chest* (Suppl)1982;**82**:8S.

104. Ledbetter MK, Bruck E, Farhi LE. Perfusion of the underventilated compartment of the lungs in asthmatic children. *J Clin Invest* 1964;**43**:2333.

105. McFadden ER Jr, Lyons HA. Arterial blood gas tension in asthma. *N Eng J Med* 1968;**278**:1029.

106. Gaddie J, Legge JS, Palmer RNV. Aerosols of salbutamol, terbutaline and isoprenaline/phenylephrine in asthma. *Br J Chest Dis* 1973;**67**:215.

107. Schuh S, Parkin P, Rajan A, *et al*. High versus low-dose frequently administered nebulized albuterol in children with severe, acute asthma. *Pediatrics* 1989;**83**:513.

108. Moler FW, Hurwitz ME, Custer JR. Improvement in clinical asthma score and $PaCO_2$ in children with severe asthma treated with continuously nebulized terbutaline. *J Allergy Clin Immunol* 1988;**81**:1101.

109. Papo MC, Frank J, Thompson AE. A prospective, randomized study of continuous versus intermittent nebulized albuterol for severe status asthmaticus in children. *Crit Care Med* 1993;**21**:1479.

110. Browne GJ, Penna AS, Phung X, Soo M. Randomised trial of intravenous salbutamol in early management of acute severe asthma in children. *Lancet* 1997;**349**:301–5.

111. Salmeron S, Brochard L, Mal H, *et al*. Nebulized versus intravenous albuterol in hypercapnic acute asthma. A multicenter, double-blind, randomized study. *Am J Respir Crit Care Med* 1994;**149**:1466–70.

112. Plotnick LH, Ducharme FM. Combined inhaled anticholinergic agents and beta-2-agonists for initial treatment of acute asthma in children (*Cochrane Review*). The Cochrane Library, Issue 3, 2000. Update Software, Oxford.

113. Zorc JJ, Pusic MV, Ogborn CJ, *et al.* Ipratropium bromide added to asthma treatment in the pediatric emergency department. *Pediatrics* 1999;**103**:748–52.

114. Potter PC, Klein M, Weinberg EG. Hydration in acute severe asthma. *Arch Dis Child* 1991;**66**:216.

115. Stalcup SA, Mellins RB. Mechanical forces producing pulmonary edema and acute asthma. *New Engl J Med* 1977;**297**:592.

116. Hung CH, Chu DM, Wang CL, *et al.* Hypokalemia and salbutamol therapy in asthma. *Pediatr Pulmonol* 1999;**27**:27–31.

117. Singhi SC, Jayashree K, Sarkar B. Hypokalaemia following nebulized salbutamol in children with acute attack of bronchial asthma. *J Paediatr Child Health* 1996;**32**:495–7.

118. Aubier M, DeTroyer A, Sampson M, *et al.* Aminophylline improves diaphragmatic contractility. *NEJM* 1981;**305**:249.

119. Aubier M, Murciano D, Viires N, *et al.* Increased ventilation caused by improved diaphragmatic efficiency during aminophylline infusion. *Am Rev Respir Dis* 1983;**127**:148.

120. Viires N, Aubier M, Murciano D, *et al.* Effects of aminophylline in diaphragmatic fatigue during acute respiratory failure. *Am Rev Respir Dis* 1984; **129**:396.

121. Goodman DC, Littenberg B, O'Connor GT, *et al.* Theophylline in acute childhood asthma: a meta-analysis of its efficacy [see comments]. *Pediatr Pulmonol* 1996;**21**:211–18.

122. Yung M, South M. Randomised controlled trial of aminophylline for severe acute asthma. *Arch Dis Child* 1998;**79**:405–10.

123. Mitra A, Bassler D. Intravenous amniophylline for acute severe asthma in children over two years. *Cochrane Airways Group.* Update Publications, Oxford, 2000.

124. Jacobs MH, Senior RM, Kessler G. Clinical experience with theophylline: relationship between dosage, serum concentration and toxicity. *JAMA* 1976; **235**:1983.

125. Bloch H, Silverman R, Mancherje N, *et al.* Intravenous magnesium sulfate as an adjunct in the treatment of acute asthma. *Chest* 1995;**107**:1576–813.

126. Ciarallo L, Sauer AH, Shannon MW. Intravenous magnesium therapy for moderate to severe pediatric asthma: results of a randomized, placebo-controlled trial [see comments]. *J Pediatr* 1996;**129**:809–14.

127. Corbridge TC, Hall JB. The assessment and management of adults with status asthmaticus. *Am J Respir Crit Care Med* 1995;**151**:1296–316.

128. Devi PR, Kumar L, Singhi SC, *et al.* Intravenous magnesium sulfate in acute severe asthma not responding to conventional therapy. *Indian Pediatr* 1997;**34**:389–976.

129. Green SM, Rothrock SG. Intravenous magnesium for acute asthma: failure to decrease emergency treatment duration or need for hospitalization [see comments]. *Ann Emerg Med* 1992;**21**:260–52.

130. Gurkan F, Haspolat K, Bosnak M, *et al.* Intravenous magnesium sulphate in the management of moderate to severe acute asthmatic children nonresponding to conventional therapy. *Eur J Emerg Med* 1999;**6**:201–55.

131. Skobeloff EM, Spivey WH, McNamara RM, *et al.* Intravenous magnesium sulfate for the treatment of acute asthma in the emergency department [see comments]. *JAMA* 1989;**262**:1210–38.

132. Tiffany B, Berk WA, Todd IK, *et al.* Magnesium bolus or infusion fails to improve expiratory flow in acute asthma exacerbations. *Chest* 1993; **104**:831–44.

133. Rowe BH, Bretzlaff JA, Bourdon C, *et al.* Magnesium sulfate treatment for acute asthmatic exacerbations treated in the emergency department (*Cochrane Reviews*). Cochrane Library, Issue 2. Update Software, Oxford, 1999.

134. Carter ER, Webb CR, Moffitt DR. Evaluation of heliox in children hospitalized with acute severe asthma. A randomized crossover trial. *Chest* 1996;**109**:1256–616.

135. Henderson SO, Acharya P, Kilaghbian T, *et al.* Use of heliox-driven nebulizer therapy in the treatment of acute asthma. *Ann Emerg Med* 1999; **33**:141–63.

136. Kass JE, Terregino CA. The effect of heliox in acute severe asthma: a randomized controlled trial. *Chest* 1999;**116**:296–302.

137. Kudukis TM, Manthous CA, Schmidt GA, *et al.* Inhaled helium-oxygen revisited: effect of inhaled helium-oxygen during the treatment of status asthmaticus in children. *J Pediatr* 1997;**130**:217–45.

138. Manthous CA, Hall JB, Caputo MA, *et al.* Heliox improves pulsus paradoxus and peak expiratory flow in nonintubated patients with severe asthma. *Am J Respir Crit Care Med* 1995;**151**:310–14.

139. Verbeek PR, Chopra A. Heliox does not improve FEV_1 in acute asthma patients. *J Emerg Med* 1998;**16**: 545–84.

140. Silverman M, O'Callaghan CLP, eds. *Practical Paediatric Respiratory Medicine.* See: Chapter 16, D Luyt, Airway management in emergency situations; and Chapter 17, S Nichani, Ventilatory support in the critically ill child. Arnold, London, 2001.

141. DeNicola LK, Monem GF, Gayle MO, *et al.* Treatment of critical status asthmatic in children. *Pediatr Clin N Am* 1994;**41**:1293–324.

142. Halfaer MA, Nichols DG, Rogers MC. Lower airway disease: bronchiolitis and asthma. In: MC Rogers, ed. *Textbook of Pediatric Intensive Care*, 3rd edn. Williams and Wilkins, Baltimore,1996.

143. Downey P, Cox R. Update on the management of status asthmaticus. *Curr Opin Pediatr* 1996;**8**:226–33.

144. Fletcher HJ, Ibrahim SA, Speight N. Survey of asthma deaths in the Northern region, 1970–85. *Arch Dis Child* 1990;**65**:163–7.

145. Campbell MJ, Cogman GR, Holgate ST, *et al.* Age specific trends in asthma mortality in England and Wales, 1983–95: results of an observational study. *Br Med J* 1997;**314**:1439.

146. Jorgensen IM, Bulow S, Jensen VB, *et al.* Asthma mortality in Danish children and young adults, 1973–1994: epidemiology and validity of death certificates. *Eur Respir J* 2000;**15**:844–8.

147. Sly RM. Decreases in asthma mortality in the United States. *Ann Allergy Asthma Immunol* 2000;**85**:121–7.

148. Lemanske RF, Larson GL. Fatal asthma in children. In: AL Sheffer, ed. *Fatal Asthma*. Marcel Dekker, New York, 1998.

149. Robertson CF, Rubinfield AR, Bowes G. Pediatric asthma deaths in Victoria: the mild are at risk. *Pediatr Pulmonol* 1992;**13**:95.

150. Schmitz T, von Kries R, Wjst M, Schuster A. A nationwide survey in Germany on fatal asthma and near-fatal asthma in children: different entities. *Eur Respir J* 2000;**16**:85–849.

151. Turner MO, Noertjojo K, Vedal S, *et al.* Risk factors for near-fatal asthma. A case-control study in hospitalized patients with asthma. *Am J Respir Crit Care Med* 1998;**157**:1804–9.

152. Hannaway PJ. Demographic characteristics of patients experiencing near fatal and fatal asthma: results of a regional survey of 400 asthma specialists. *Ann Allergy Asthma Immunol* 2000;**84**:587–93.

153. Malmstrom K, Kaila M, Korhonen K, Dunder T, Nermes M, Klaukka T, Sarna S, Juntunen-Backman K. Mechanical ventilation in children with severe asthma. *Pediatr Pulmonol* 2001;**31**:405–11

154. Martin AJ, Campbell DA, Gluyas PA, *et al.* Characteristics of near-fatal asthma in childhood. *Pediatr Pulmonol* 1995;**20**:1–8.

155. Warner JO, Nikolaizik WH, Besley CR, Warner JA. A childhood asthma death in a clinical trial: potential indicators of risk. *Eur Respir J* 1998;**11**:229–33.

156. Abramson MJ, Bailey MJ, Couper FJ, Driver JS, Drummer OH, Forbes AB, McNeil JJ, Haydn Walters E; Victorian Asthma Mortality Study Group. Are asthma medications and management related to deaths from asthma? *Am J Respir Crit Care Med* 2001; **163**:12–18.

Unusual syndromes and asthma complicating other disorders

ROBERT DINWIDDIE

INTRODUCTION

A number of conditions other than asthma can result in recurrent wheezing in children. These are principally due to congenital malformations or functional defects which cause disturbed breathing patterns leading to secondary small airway obstruction. Asthma itself is a common disease in childhood and can potentially complicate any other respiratory condition however caused. The major structural and developmental conditions resulting in recurrent wheeze are set out in Table 13a.1.

Table 13a.1 *Structural conditions leading to recurrent wheeze*

Upper airway problems
Pierre Robin sequence
Choanal atresia or stenosis
CHARGE syndrome
Vocal cord paralysis – unilateral or bilateral
   Subglottic or tracheal stenosis

Large airway obstruction
Tracheomalacia/bronchomalacia
Vascular ring; pulmonary artery sling
Enlarged mediastinal glands/bronchogenic cyst

Congenital anomalies of the lungs
Pulmonary agenesis or hypoplasia
Congenital lobar emphysema
Cystic adenomatoid malformation
Lobar sequestration

AIRWAY OBSTRUCTION

Upper airway obstruction

Congenital malformations leading to marked upper airway obstruction can cause recurrent cough and wheeze secondary to aspiration into the lungs during feeding. Infants in particular have difficulty in breathing and sucking adequately at the same time. This leads to failure to thrive and the need to increase nutrition becomes more important. Difficulty in coping with the volume of feed in association with upper airway obstruction results in coughing, spluttering and inhalation of feed into the lower respiratory tract. This situation is exacerbated by the presence of other malformations such as cleft palate or a neurological problem such as bulbar palsy. Examples of these conditions are shown in Table 13a.1.

PIERRE ROBIN SEQUENCE

This condition classically comprises of micrognathia, hypoglossia and cleft palate. Feeding difficulties are seen in almost all cases but can be resolved after the airway obstruction is relieved by the placement of a nasopharyngeal tube.[1] If there is continuing incoordination of swallowing then there is a definite risk of aspiration of respiratory secretions and milk into the lungs. This will result in recurrent episodes of wheeze and areas of patchy consolidation on the chest x-ray. This situation gradually resolves during the first six months of life as the mandible grows forward and the airway obstruction is overcome.

It is very important not to close the palate too early in these children as this often results in recurrence of the upper airway obstruction due to decreased space in the posterior pharyngeal area.

CHARGE ASSOCIATION

Another major condition in which there are often very severe problems in the upper airway, frequently associated with swallowing incoordination and severe gastro-oesophageal reflux, is the CHARGE association.[2,3] These children have multiple anomalies from which the condition derives its name: C, colobomata of the eyes; H, heart disease; A, atresia of the choanae; R, retarded growth and development; G, genital hypoplasia in males; and E, ear deformities. The choanal atresia is usually evident at birth and there is also frequently a major feeding problem due to neurologically determined swallowing incoordination with or without significant gastroesophageal reflux. Many of these children require fundoplication and gastrostomy in order to control the reflux and to facilitate an adequate calorie intake.[3] Those who have the most severe airway problems may need a tracheostomy to allow adequate clearance of liquids, including milk, from the lungs and also from the upper airway. These problems frequently result in acute wheezy episodes with resultant lung infection if they are not adequately controlled. Patients with CHARGE association have lifelong difficulties and need careful long-term supervision.

VOCAL CORD PARALYSIS

Partial or complete paresis of the vocal cords leads to spillover of saliva and milk into the lower respiratory tract and is thus a potent cause of recurrent wheeze in infants. If the cords are paralysed they usually take up a position of mid-abduction. The paralysis can be unilateral or bilateral depending on the underlying aetiology but unilateral is more common. Bilateral palsy is frequent where there is a lesion in the central nervous system (Table 13a.2). Symptoms will include stridor and a weak cry, especially in unilateral paralysis, and airway obstruction with respiratory difficulty, most often seen in those who have bilateral cord palsy.

Diagnosis is by direct inspection under sedation or as the child wakes from anaesthesia. Ultrasound examination

Table 13a.2 *Causes of vocal cord palsy*

Intracranial haemorrhage
Agenesis of cranial nerve nuclei
Encephalocoele
Arnold–Chiari malformation
Hydrocephalus
Trauma from intubation
Paralysis of recurrent laryngeal nerves
Generalized hypotonia

also contributes to the dynamic investigation of this problem. It is important not to splint the vocal cords with the endoscope and to allow the patient to breathe spontaneously so that natural movements of the vocal cords can be observed.

Treatment will depend on the severity of the lesion and the related symptoms of aspiration, recurrent lower respiratory tract infection and wheeze. Unilateral lesions can often be managed conservatively and improve spontaneously with age. Bilateral palsies are much more likely to result in more severe respiratory symptoms and lead to the need for tracheostomy in order to prevent long-term lung damage from recurrent aspiration. Specialized procedures to improve cord function are best left until the patient is fully grown. In extreme cases where recurrent aspiration into the lungs is life-threatening, an epiglottopexy is performed, but this results in permanent loss of voice.

SUBGLOTTIC STENOSIS

This condition is a complication of long-term intubation in the preterm ventilated neonate. It is seen less frequently nowadays as endotracheal tubes which are less traumatic to the airway are used and attention is paid to ensuring that a small leak exists around the tube so that local tissue trauma is minimized. It is also seen as a congenital malformation, probably due to failure of recanalization of the subglottic area in the region of the cricoid cartilage.[4] The congenital form may not be apparent at birth but can come to light during the first few weeks or months of life when an intercurrent infection causes oedema and further narrowing of the area which results in the child having to be intubated for acute airway obstruction.

Symptoms from subglottic stenosis include stridor, which is biphasic, and not infrequently wheezing, particularly during infections such as bronchiolitis. This is secondary to retention of secretions and oedema in the small airways. If stenosis is severe and airflow very limited, the stridor may be almost inaudible. This is an extremely dangerous situation as complete airway obstruction can occur at any time, especially if attempts at intubation provoke further oedema and airway narrowing.

Intra-thoracic airway obstruction

TRACHEAL STENOSIS

Tracheal stenosis can be short segment or long segment. Long segment tracheal stenosis can involve circumferential narrowing caused by the presence of complete tracheal rings throughout all or part of the trachea. In this circumstance there may be insufficient growth post natally thus increasing large airway resistance with time. These children are at special risk during intercurrent infections, especially bronchiolitis, when the work of breathing is increased and the intrinsic airway narrowing is worsened by the accompanying tracheobronchial inflammation which is part of the illness. Some children with tracheal stenosis have either a long narrow trachea (stovepipe trachea) or one which becomes increasingly narrow towards the carina (funnel trachea). One important radiological sign of a narrowed lower trachea is widening of the subcarinal angle. This feature is also seen with a bronchogenic cyst sited just below the carina.

All of these conditions are very difficult to treat especially in the early months of life. Tracheal reconstruction is possible in short segment stenosis, but much more difficult in long segment disease. Various procedures have been tried in a number of children although thus far none has been universally successful. These include the insertion of a Teflon patch or rib graft to enlarge the diameter of the airway, placement of a pericardial patch to open up a segment of the trachea thus increasing its size, and external splinting with various materials or internal stenting.

TRACHEOMALACIA

Tracheomalacia may be localized, usually due to extrinsic compression such as, for example, by a pulmonary artery sling, or in relation to a tracheo-oesophageal fistula with oesophageal atresia. Wheezing is particularly common in this second group of patients, having been reported as a problem in up to 40% of cases on long-term follow-up.[5] Tracheomalacia can also be generalized affecting the trachea throughout most of its length and sometimes spreading into the major bronchi (bronchomalacia). These changes result in stridor and persistent cough. There is often retention of secretions from the lower airways during expiration due to dynamic airway compression and during coughing because of the soft tracheal cartilage. This results in recurrent wheeze, especially during respiratory infections. Radiological imaging of the airway is important to assess the level and degree of involvement. This should include a barium swallow looking for oesophageal indentation by a vessel lying between the oesophagus and trachea.[6] Most children will also require ultrasound and bronchoscopy in order fully to assess the nature and extent of the lesion. Nowadays CT scan can contribute significantly to the localization of the lesion and a dynamic tracheobronchogram may also be particularly useful.[7] Surgical treatment is usually indicated where there is a structural lesion such as a tracheo-oesophageal fistula or a vascular ring. If there is a very short segment of intrinsic tracheomalacia this can also be surgically corrected by resection and anastomosis. Longer segments and particularly those involving the major bronchi are much more difficult to correct although various procedures to splint or enlarge the trachea have been described.

These have only been used in small numbers of cases with limited success. If the disease involves a longer section of the trachea and is causing problems, then an aortopexy can be helpful. This involves moving the aorta forward and stitching it to the back of the sternum, thus splinting the trachea in a more forward and stable position.

When the tracheomalacia is severe and not responsive to conservative treatment, a tracheostomy can be useful in order to splint the airway internally until it has grown large enough to be self-supporting. A very small number of cases require extended periods of positive pressure ventilation during this time and this too is facilitated by the presence of a tracheostomy. The introduction of a tracheal stent has also proved helpful in a number of cases.

VASCULAR ANOMALIES

A number of vascular anomalies occur in the area of the lower trachea which result in tracheal compression and secondary wheezing. These broadly comprise two types (Table 13a.3): vascular rings in which there is complete encirclement of the trachea and oesophagus, such as by a double aortic arch, or a vascular sling where the left pulmonary artery arises anomalously from the right pulmonary artery and takes an aberrant path between the trachea and oesophagus. In a small number of cases there is compression of the anterior wall of the trachea by an anomalous innominate artery arising early from the aorta. This produces direct pressure and is not a true ring constriction as such. Although these lesions often result in stridor secondary to the pressure on the tracheal wall, wheezing is also a common associated feature. This is again due to the fact that airway clearance of secretions is impaired which results in small airway obstruction and tends to prolong resolution of lower respiratory tract infection. Symptoms due to oesophageal compression are uncommon despite the associated vascular compression of the oesophagus itself. Radiological investigation including posteroanterior and lateral chest x-rays, filter view of the large airways, barium swallow and echocardiography.[6] Some cases require CT scan of the chest and occasionally magnetic resonance imaging is necessary to show the anomaly. Angiography is not usually required in straightforward cases but may be necessary where the underlying anatomy is thought to be complex.

Treatment is surgical and involves division of the ring, leaving the major vessel as the aortic supply, or rerouting of the anomalous pulmonary artery.[8] The localized segment of tracheomalacia gradually improves with time once the compression has been removed. The long-term outcome is usually excellent.

Table 13a.3 *Vascular anomalies causing tracheal compression*

Double aortic arch
Right aortic arch with left patent duct arteriosus or
  ligamentum arteriosum
Aberrant right subclavian with patent ductus arteriosus
  or ligamentum arteriosum
Aberrant left pulmonary artery
Anomalous innominate artery

ENLARGED GLANDS OR CYSTS COMPRESSING THE TRACHEA

Enlarged glands in the mediastinum can occur because of non-specific inflammation, tuberculosis (TB) or sarcoidosis. A bronchogenic cyst can also produce an identical picture and should be considered when recurrent wheeze is seen in association with large airway narrowing.[9] If these compress the carina and large airways then retained secretions and associated inflammation distally will result in wheeze. The most specific condition resulting in this problem is TB which is often associated with airway compression leading to overinflation or collapse-consolidation. Treatment consists of identification of the underlying problem and specific drug treatment if available.[10] Surgical intervention is indicated for both diagnostic and therapeutic reasons if the diagnosis cannot be made by other means. If the problem is due to non-specific gland enlargement or a bronchogenic cyst then this approach will result in complete resolution.

DISORDERS OF LUNG DEVELOPMENT

Pulmonary agenesis/hypoplasia

Pulmonary agenesis can sometimes be asymptomatic, only coming to light on an incidental chest x-ray. It is, however, often associated with other tracheobronchial anomalies involving the contralateral lung. The most frequently seen comprise complete tracheal rings and stenosis or malacia of the other main bronchus. There is also an association with pulmonary artery sling which again results in compression of the lower trachea.

All of these anomalies cause marked bronchial narrowing and retention of secretions in the small airways, especially during infections. Vigorous attempts at tracheobronchial suction lead to oedema and further narrowing of a compromised airway. Severe wheeze during acute infection can be life-threatening, especially in the presence of gross hyperinflation. Sometimes external compression of the chest to push the air past the obstruction is the only way to reduce the residual lung volume to more physiological levels. These infants have a poor prognosis and can only survive if the airway can grow sufficiently to overcome the high airway resistance associated with the critically reduced diameter.

Isolated pulmonary hypoplasia can occur without complication and may present as apparent 'unilateral over inflation' of the opposite lung in a wheezy child with asthma. Investigation usually reveals a small lung with a pulmonary artery which is also correspondingly small on ultrasound. Such children do not have major problems and do not develop pulmonary hypertension. Unilateral hypoplasia can also be associated with other congenital malformations such as diaphragmatic hernia where there has been intrauterine compression of the lung. The degree of hypoplasia will depend on the gestation at which compression began and on the size of the lesion. Those with large defects often have major neonatal respiratory problems and require extended periods of ventilation. This, plus the fact that the airways do not develop normally, often results in persistent wheezing in infancy.

A specific condition of hypoplasia affecting the right lung and resulting in wheezing is the 'Scimitar' syndrome.[11] This consists of hypoplasia in association with sequestration of the right lower lobe which is fed by an anomalous arterial supply usually from the descending aorta. The venous system drains to the right atrium or inferior vena cava. This abnormal vein gives a scimitar shaped shadow on the chest x-ray from which the syndrome derives its name. Treatment now consists of embolization of the abnormal arterial supply. The outcome is variable; some children having relatively few problems while others have impaired lung function including significant problems with wheeze. Significant lung damage caused by infection due to the high blood supply may result in bronchiectasis for which the treatment is right lower lobectomy.

Congenital lobar emphysema

This congenital malformation of the lung can present infancy with lobar overinflation leading to adjacent lung compression with small airway obstruction and recurrent wheeze. The symptomatic infant is usually tachypnoeic, hypoxic and distressed. Difficulty in feeding because of the respiratory problem leads to failure to thrive. Milder cases cause few or no symptoms and may be identified incidentally on a chest x-ray. It usually affects the upper lobes or right middle lobe in 95% of cases.[12] Anteroposterior and lateral chest x-rays, ventilation/perfusion lung scan and CT scan of the chest are required for diagnosis. Fourteen per cent have an associated cardiac lesion so this too should be carefully sought. Treatment of symptomatic cases is by surgery to remove the affected lobe if it is nonfunctional. Those cases where the ventilation/perfusion scan does not show major functional impairment or where the other lobes can be seen to be working satisfactorily can be treated conservatively. Where surgery is not undertaken the long-term prognosis is usually good and is associated with improving lung function with time.[13]

CHEST WALL ANOMALIES

The calibre of the small airways is dependent on lung volume which is maintained by a balance between the outward recoil of the chest wall and the inward pull of the elastic tissue within the lung itself. If this balance is disturbed, for example by softening of the ribs or weakness of the intercostal muscles due to neuromuscular disease, then lung volume will fall and small airway

Table 13a.4 *Chest wall problems causing recurrent wheeze*

Rickets
Metabolic bone disease of preterm infant
Spinal muscular atrophy
Myotonic dystrophy
Congenital muscular dystrophy
Myasthenia gravis
Poliomyelitis
Postinfectious polyneuritis (Guillain–Barré syndrome)

calibre will decrease. This results in an increased tendency to wheeze.

If the underlying problem is a generalized neuromuscular condition there may be dysphagia leading to recurrent aspiration of fluid or food into the lungs which may result in wheezing (Table 13a.4). Treatment depends on whether the condition is primary or secondary. If it is primarily inherited and usually fatal such as the severe form of spinal muscular atrophy (Werdnig-Hoffmann disease) then treatment will be symptomatic. If the condition is secondary, for example, to rickets, then appropriate dietary supplementation with vitamin D will result in correction of the underlying defect. The ultimate prognosis therefore depends on the basic problem, its severity and its duration before corrective measures are taken.

ASTHMA UNDERLYING OTHER DISORDERS

Structural and developmental disorders

Children with any of the above problems may well develop asthma in addition. When asthma does complicate these or indeed any other respiratory condition, it is important to recognize its presence and its contribution to the overall symptomatology.

Treatment will be by conventional measures but it must be realized that if there is an underlying structural defect leading to reduced airflow then asthma treatment will only be partially successful in overcoming the problem. There is a danger of over treatment with steroids in an attempt to treat partially irreversible airway obstruction, for example in obliterative bronchiolitis. It is also important to search for other causes of wheezing in the apparently intractable asthmatic since these can complicate the illness and its treatment. An example of this situation would be a child with gastroesophageal reflux in association with underlying asthma (Chapter 7c).

Fortunately many congenital malformations causing persistent symptoms in infancy are nowadays amenable to surgical correction or improve with age as the airways naturally increase in size. Children with these problems who survive the early part of life usually therefore have a relatively good prognosis providing that the underlying problems are recognized and treated appropriately.

Cystic fibrosis

Wheezing is common in patients with cystic fibrosis (CF). It is reported as a problem in approximately 50% of those with the illness.[14] The aetiology in CF is multifactorial and apart from bronchospasm itself, includes factors such as mucous plugging, localized oedema and distortion of airway architecture secondary to bronchial wall thickening and long-term inflammatory damage to small airways. Studies of airway responsiveness in CF have shown that this is variable and that a significant minority may bronchoconstrict due to changes in small airway tone. Many CF patients, however, do benefit from chronic bronchodilator therapy. It is important to demonstrate that the response is indeed beneficial before starting long-term treatment on a regular basis. Atopic asthma itself is probably no more common in CF than in the population at large but in many of these children exercise-induced wheeze can limit normal physical activities. This of course can be blocked in the usual way with the use of beta agonists or cromoglycate inhaled beforehand. Some patients with CF present with RSV bronchiolitis[15] and this too can contribute to recurrent wheeze.

Inhaled steroid therapy to control wheezy symptoms in CF children is very important both in terms of true asthmatic symptoms but also in the inhibition of the major inflammatory response which occurs when the patient is chronically colonized with pathogens such as *Staphylococcus aureus* or *Pseudomonas aeruginosa*.[16] The control of wheeze in the CF patient with advanced disease is one of the most important clinical challenges in this disease although the precise therapeutic role of inhaled steroids in this condition has yet to be determined.[17]

MISCELLANEOUS DISORDERS

Vocal cord dysfunction (VCD)

Vocal cord dysfunction (VCD) is an important cause of wheezing in childhood. It occurs due to paradoxical closure of the vocal cords on inspiration which can result in wheezing virtually indistinguishable from bronchoconstriction in the lower airways typical of asthma. In many cases true asthma also occurs at the same time. Ideally fibreoptic larygnoscopy should be performed to demonstrate the acute closure of the cords during exacerbations of wheeze.

The condition is most commonly seen in mid to late childhood especially in girls. In a number of cases it is a reflection of stress related external influences such as school examinations, family and other emotional disturbances.

Patients with this disorder are often unresponsive to bronchodilator therapy and steroids either inhaled or oral. Between attacks if there is no wheezing auscultation

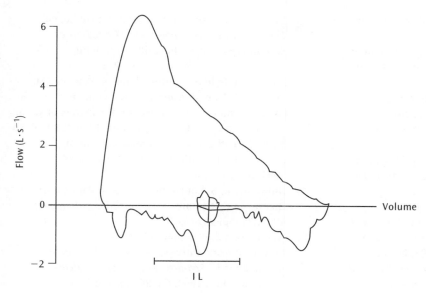

Figure 13.a.1 *Full inspiratory and expiratory maximum flow–volume loop in a girl with vocal cord dysfunction syndrome. The striking intermittent and variable ('saw-tooth') pattern on inspiration was poorly repeatable from blow to blow.*

of the chest is normal. In pure VCD lung function tests may be entirely normal between episodes. During acute attacks, oxygen saturation is normal, but lung function tests can be very revealing. Spirometry should include forced inspiration as well as expiration, revealing variability from blow to blow, with a saw-toothed inspiratory flow–volume curve (Figure 13a.1).

Treatment consists of a thorough evaluation of the patient's lung function, psychological status, ENT review and a critical evaluation of drug therapy for asthma. The treatment is mainly psychological with emotional support although breathing exercises and speech therapy may be helpful in some cases. Unless there is concomitant asthma the drugs which are normally used in this situation should be actively discontinued.[18]

Other forms of dysfunctional breathing may coexist with asthma.[25]

Eosinophilic lung disorders

These represent a number of rare conditions in childhood in which there is chronic pulmonary eosinophilic infiltration. This may be associated with cough, wheezing breathlessness, intermittent pyrexia and failure to thrive. There may be patchy nodular infiltrates throughout the lungs on chest x-ray, although these are not always present.

The condition may be associated with anaemia and increased eosinophils in the peripheral blood count although not in all cases. Lung biopsy is indicated in those with severe disease and demonstrates intra-alveolar and interstitial infiltrates with inflammatory cells including lymphocytes, macrophages and particularly eosinophils.

Treatment is with oral corticosteroids which are effective in the majority of cases. They may however need to be continued for many months for resolution of symptoms. This condition has been associated with nitrofurantoin

therapy and has also been seen in patients with beta-thalassemia major who were receiving desferrioxamine.[19]

Pulmonary eosinophilia can occur in association with parasitic infection, particularly with organisms such as *Toxocara gondii*, *Ascaris lumbriocoides* and *Strongyloides stercoralis*. Toxocara is the most common agent seen in clinical practice in the UK. Treatment is with appropriate anti-parasitic agents for each organism.

Churg–Strauss syndrome is an extremely rare eosinophilic vasculitis which has raised interest recently because of its unmasking during leukotriene receptor antagonist therapy in adults. There are few reports in childhood.[20]

Sickle cell disease

The relationship between asthma and sickle cell disease is controversial. Studies have suggested that bronchodilator responsiveness[21] and airway reactivity (to cold-air challenge)[22] are significantly greater in children with homozygous sickle cell disease than in appropriate controls, although the prevalence of clinical asthma is no more common.[23]

Acute chest syndrome may be accompanied by wheezing and although a trial of inhaled bronchodilator therapy is recommended in this situation, its efficacy is small[24] and has never been subjected to formal clinical trial.

REFERENCES

1. Dinwiddie R. Ear, nose and throat problems. In: R Dinwiddie, ed. *The Diagnosis and Management of Paediatric Respiratory Disease.* Churchill-Livingstone, Edinburgh, 1997, pp. 81–102.
2. Blake KD, Russell-Eggitt IM, Morgan DW, Ratcliffe JM, Wyse RKH. Who's in CHARGE? Multidisciplinary

management of patients with CHARGE association. *Arch Dis Child* 1990;**65**:217–23.

3. Sporik R, Dinwiddie R, Wallis CE. Lung involvement in the multisystem CHARGE association. *Eur Respir J* 1997;**10**:1354–5.

4. Harrier MLL, Irving RM, Gray R. Upper airway disorders. In: A Greenough, NRC Robertson, AD Milner, eds. *Neonatal Respiratory Disorders.* Arnold, London, 1997, pp. 487–502.

5. Chetcuti P, Phelan PD. Respiratory morbidity after repair of oesophageal atresia and tracheoesophageal fistula. *Arch Dis Child* 1993;**68**:167–70.

6. Burch M, Balaji S, Deanfield J, Sullivan ID. Investigation of vascular compression of the trachea: the complementary roles of barium swallow and echocardiography. *Arch Dis Child* 1993;**68**:171–6.

7. Doull IJM, Mok Q, Tasker RC. Tracheobronchomalacia in preterm infants with chronic lung disease. *Arch Dis Child* 1997;**76**:F203–5.

8. Westaby S, Dinwiddie R, Chrispin AR, Stark J. Pulmonary artery sling in identical twins. *Thorac Cardiovasc Surg* 1984;**32**:182–3.

9. Brooks JW, Krummel TM. Tumors of the chest. In: V Chernick, TF Boat, E Kendig, eds. *Disorders of the Respiratory Tract*, 6th edn. Saunders, Philadelphia, 1998, Ch. 45, pp. 754–87.

10. Dinwiddie R. Pulmonary tuberculosis. In: R Dinwiddie, ed. *The Diagnosis and Management of Paediatric Respiratory Disease.* Churchill-Livingstone, Edinburgh, 1997, Ch. 11, pp. 261–71.

11. Partridge JB, Osborne JM, Slaughter RE. Scimitar etcetera, the dysmorphic right lung. *Clin Radiol* 1988;**39**:11–19.

12. Roggin KK, Breuer CK, Carr SR, Hansen K, Kurkchubasche AG, Wesselheoft CW, Tracy TF, Luks FI. The unpredictable character of congenital cystic lung lesions. *J Paediatr Surg* 2000;**35**:801–5.

13. Kennedy CD, Habibi P, Matthew DJ, Gordon I. Lobar emphysema: long term imaging follow up. *Radiology* 1991;**180**:189–93.

14. Dinwiddie R. Cystic fibrosis. In: R Dinwiddie, ed. *The Diagnosis and Management of Paediatric Respiratory Disease.* Churchill-Livingstone, Edinburgh, 1997, Ch. 9, pp. 197–245.

15. Abman SH, Ogle HW, Butler-Simon N, Rumack CM, Accurso FJ. Role of respiratory syncytial virus in early hospitalisations for respiratory distress of young infants with cystic fibrosis. *J Pediatr* 1988;**113**:826–30.

16. Zach MS. Pathogenesis and management of lung disease in cystic fibrosis. *J Roy Soc Med* 1991;**84**(Suppl 18):10–17.

17. Dinwiddie R, Balfour-Lynn IM. Anti-inflammatory therapy in cystic fibrosis. *Pediatr Allergy Immunol* 1997;**7**(Suppl 9):70–3.

18. Wamboldt MZ, Wamboldt FS. Psychiatric aspects of respiratory symptoms. In: LM Taussig, LI Landau, eds. *Pediatric Respiratory Medicine.* Mosby, St Louis, 1999, Ch. 80, pp. 1222–34.

19. Carroll JL, Sterni LM. Eosinophilic lung disorders and hypersensitivity pneumonitis. In: LM Taussig, LI Landau, eds. *Paediatric Respiratory Medicine.* Mosby, London, 1999, Ch. 50, pp. 804–11.

20. Rabusin M, Lepore L, Costaninides F, Bussani R. A child with severe asthma. *Lancet* 1998:**351**:32.

21. Koumbourlis AC, Zar HJ, Hurlet-Jensen A, Goldberg MR. Prevalence and reversibility of lower airway obstruction in children with sickle cell disease. *J Pediatr* 2001;**138**:188–92.

22. Leong MA, Dampier C, Varlotta L, Allen JL. Airway hyperreactivity in children with sickle cell disease. *J Pediatr* 1997;**131**:278–83.

23. Savoy LB, Dy Lim J, Sarnaik SA, Jones DC. Prevalence of atopy in a sickle-cell anemia population. *Ann Allergy* 1988;**61**:129–32.

24. Vichinsky EP, Neumayer LD, Earles AN, *et al.* Causes and outcomes of the acute chest syndrome in sickle cell disease. *N Engl J Med* 2000;**342**: 1855–65.

25. Keeley D, Osman L. Dysfunctional breathing and asthma. *Brit Med J* 2001;**322**:1075–6.

Prematurity and asthma

ANNE MILNER AND ANTHONY MILNER

INTRODUCTION

A small proportion of infants born prematurely and receiving intensive respiratory support are left with extensive obstructive airways disease (bronchopulmonary dysplasia, BPD).[1] There are, however, a much greater number of infants, particularly born at very early gestations, who remain oxygen dependent beyond 28 days after birth (chronic lung disease (CLD)). Infants who have had either BPD or CLD or were simply born at an early gestation have recurrent respiratory symptoms and lung function abnormalities at follow-up which are similar to early childhood asthma. The role of this chapter is to review the information on the incidence of those abnormalities, examine critically possible aetiological factors and assess methods of treatment and prevention.

CLINICAL FEATURES

Symptoms

In the first two to three years of life, preterm infants suffer from both cough and wheeze.[2,3] In the majority of infants these symptoms are not continuous, but can occur on at least 2–3 days per week.[4] The symptoms are often precipitated by infection, aggravated by parental smoking and can temporarily remit either spontaneously or in response to bronchodilator therapy.[2,3,5]

Residual respiratory problems have been frequently reported in preterm infants following discharge from neonatal intensive care.[6–9] A prospective study[4] highlighted that approximately 50% of infants had lower respiratory symptoms in the first year of life. The prevalence does initially decrease with increasing postnatal age, less than half of the infants symptomatic in the first year of life had recurrent problems in the second year,[10] but approximately 33% of VLBW infants continue to wheeze and/or cough throughout their preschool years.[11] At school age prematurely born infants are more likely to have respiratory symptoms than classroom colleagues born at term.[12,13] Although one study[13] found no excess of wheeze in low birth weight children compared with a reference group of school-children, in another, VLBW children at 8–9 years were noted to be more likely to use inhalers, be absent from school or require admission to hospital because of respiratory illness.[14] A recent prospective follow-up study[15] of ninety-six 7-year-old children born preterm and 108 term born controls found that 30% of those with BPD, 24% of those born preterm but without BPD and only 7% of the term control children had recurrent wheezing. In addition, both gestational age and birth weight have been reported to be independent risk factors for wheezy bronchitis.[16]

Lung function abnormalities

Plethysmographic studies performed in the first year of life have demonstrated that infants born preterm, regardless of symptom status, have an elevated airway resistance in comparison to reference ranges from infants born at term.[17,18] The abnormality is particularly marked in preterm infants with recurrent symptoms and is associated with an elevated thoracic gas volume and low functional residual capacity (FRC).[19] This combination of lung function abnormalities suggests gas trapping; in the preterm infants it is reversed by bronchodilator therapy.[20] Despite improvements with age, lung function abnormalities can often be detected in school-aged children and older born of low birth weight and/or prematurely. Children aged 8 years, who following premature birth had required ventilation, were found to have lower values for specific conductance and a greater increase in FEV_1 after salbutamol than non-ventilated children. They had a history of wheezing and recurrent respiratory illnesses; suggesting an increased tendency to reversible airway obstruction.[21] Other studies[15,22] have suggested lung function abnormalities at school age are only present in prematurely born children who had BPD/CLD. In a recent large prospective study,[15] although the mean FVC and FEV_1 results were significantly reduced in 7-year-old children who had had BPD, there were no significant differences in lung function results between those born preterm but without BPD and those born at term. A study of fifteen 10-year-old children who had severe BPD requiring home oxygen therapy for up to 3 years[22] found them to have significantly reduced FEV_1 results compared with both preterm and term control children. The investigators also showed a strong ($r = -0.84$) inverse relationship between the percentage predicted FEV_1 and the duration of supplemental oxygen therapy. A recent report of 11-year-old children of VLBW also implicated oxygen therapy as a major risk factor for reduced FEV_1.[23] Duration of oxygen therapy might be a surrogate for more severe neonatal lung disease. Signs of airflow obstruction affecting small airways can persist up to 15 years of age in children who had had CLD,[24] but others[25] found no significant differences in lung function at a mean of 15.7 years between 164 VLBW infants and controls born at term and matched for gender, parity, place and date of birth. The prevalence of chronic obstructive pulmonary disease in a cohort of 70-year-old men, however, was associated with lower birth weight as well as respiratory illness in infancy.[26]

Hospital admission

The risk of re-admission is increased for all VLBW infants, being ten times greater than for infants born at term, but the CLD infants have double that risk.[10] The primary reason for admission was lower respiratory tract infections, particularly due to RSV. A recent study[15] found that 53% of infants with BPD were re-admitted to hospital in the first 2 years of life, compared with 26% of those born before 32 weeks' gestation but without BPD and 3% of term-born controls. Parental smoking in symptomatic preterm infants has been shown to be associated with a significant longer duration of admission.[4]

Table 13b.1 *Risk factors for respiratory symptoms in children born prematurely*

- Prematurity
- Low birth weight
- Mechanical ventilation
- Respiratory distress syndrome
- Bronchopulmonary dysplasia/chronic lung disease
- Family history of atopy
- Viral infections
- Passive smoking

RISK FACTORS (TABLE 13B.1)

Prematurity

Preterm birth, *per se*, seems an important factor in the development of symptoms and lung function abnormalities. Comparison of two groups of infants living within the same geographic area and of similar socio-economic background, demonstrated that 65% of infants born preterm had respiratory problems in the first year of life, compared with only 33% of those born at term.[4] Infants born preterm, regardless of the need for respiratory support or development of respiratory distress, have lung function abnormalities in the first year of life such as elevated airways resistance when compared with published reference ranges for term infants.[17,27] The data on lung function in later childhood are less consistent. In one study,[21] at approximately 9 years of age, FEV_1 and specific airway conductance were lower in infants born preterm, with or without respiratory distress (RDS), compared with children born at term. There were, however, no differences in lung function at the age of 7 between 53 children born before 32 weeks' gestation who did not develop BPD and 108 term born controls.[15]

Low birth weight (LBW)

Bowman and Yu[28] documented a 48% incidence of wheeze in extremely low birth weight infants which compared unfavourably with an 8% incidence of wheezing in term infants reported in a separate study from Melbourne. At 7 years of age, compared with unselected school-children, LBW infants had significantly reduced FEV_1[29] which was closely associated with low birth weight, but not oxygen treatment, mechanical ventilation or neonatal respiratory illness. Birth weight was a significant predictor of a low FEV_1 in a recent study of VLBW infants.[23]

Artificial ventilation

Abnormalities of airway resistance have been detected at follow-up amongst infants ventilated in the neonatal period, but not in those who received oxygen alone.[17]

Comparison of preterm infants who did and did not require respiratory support[30] demonstrated more symptomatic infants and severe lung function abnormalities in the former group, the difference, however, was only found in infants who required mechanical ventilation and not those who were only oxygen dependent.[30] Those data, however, do not exclude an effect related to the severity of the respiratory distress.

The level of neonatal respiratory support may have a temporary effect on subsequent lung function. We reported[30] differences between groups were present at 6 months of age, but not at 1 year. The evidence for a persisting effect of ventilation on lung function at school age is conflicting. In one study,[31] although airway responsiveness at 7 years in LBW children was twice as common as that found in a random sample of school-children, it was not associated with any perinatal variable including respiratory support.[31] In addition, Chan et al.[32] found reduced lung compliance and increased thoracic volume in very LBW infants examined at 9 years of age, but the abnormalities did not significantly correlate with a requirement for neonatal mechanical ventilation. In a population-based study,[14] however, comparison of 300 VLBW children to 590 controls aged 8–9 years demonstrated that the former had lower FVC and were twice as likely to have signs of obstructive disease and excessive induced bronchospasm. Those abnormalities were associated with prolonged ventilatory support as well as RDS and a requirement for more than 40% supplementary oxygen. In addition, abnormalities of FEV_1, FEV_1/FVC and PEF correlated with days of neonatal ventilatory support at 11 years of age.[33]

Respiratory distress syndrome (RDS)

There is a significant influx of inflammatory cells into the airways of infants with RDS and BPD (see below).[34] Mediator release from neutrophils can increase airway hyperreactivity.[35] At 8–14 years, children who had had RDS had lower FEV_1 and higher resistance than gestational age and gender matched controls without RDS.[36]

Bronchopulmonary dysplasia/chronic lung disease

CLD infants have airway smooth muscle hypertrophy and respond to bronchodilators even while on the NICU. More than 50% of non-selected premature infants were symptomatic in the first year after birth and approximately 33% affected in the second year,[4] but 85% of infants who developed CLD had symptoms in the first 2 years after birth.[37] Oxygen dependency beyond 28 days of life, regardless of the development of BPD, is an important risk factor for chronic respiratory morbidity.[37] The occurrence of symptoms and lung function abnormalities at follow-up being similar in two groups who were both oxygen dependent at least until 28 days after birth, but only one group had BPD as evidenced by classical chest radiograph changes. Problems later in childhood, however, are more severe in those who had radiographic BPD rather than clinical CLD.[38,39]

Family history of atopy

Bertrand et al.[40] demonstrated that both the full-term siblings and mothers of preterm children had a much greater level of airway responsiveness than controls. They suggested that irritability of uterine and airway smooth muscle could act as a common pathway in the aetiology of both premature labour and bronchial hyperresponsiveness in the mothers and their children, both full term and preterm. Evidence of a weak association between maternal asthma and preterm delivery has been repeated elsewhere.[38] Bertrand's study, however, was retrospective and based on only a small number of children and a prospective study[41] did not confirm an increase in maternal asthma, a family history of asthma or airway responsiveness in the mothers of low birth weight children. At follow-up, although prematurely born children with a family history of atopy had a higher airways resistance than those without, this was explained by the lower birth weight of the former group.[42] A requirement for prolonged neonatal respiratory support was demonstrated to be a more significant risk factor than a family history of atopy for recurrent respiratory symptoms throughout the preschool years in children born prematurely.[11] If prematurely born CLD children become symptomatic for the first time at 5 years of age, however, then their symptoms relate to their atopic status rather than their perinatal history.[11] In a national cohort of VLBW children in New Zealand, the main risk factor for a diagnosis of asthma by the age of 7 was a family history of asthma.[42a]

Viral infections

Otherwise healthy prematurely born infants are more likely to acquire RSV infection due to their impaired immunity with reduced transfer of maternal antibodies, and have a more severe illness.[43] Those with CLD are also more likely to suffer serious morbidity, as evidenced by a higher hospitalization rate and longer hospital stay than seen in infants born at term.[44] Risk factors for acquisition of RSV infection include large family size and passive smoking, CLD infants receiving home oxygen therapy are at greatest risk of severe disease.[44] Once admitted to PICU, they often require prolonged ventilatory support due to the additional cardiopulmonary compromise. Some cannot be supported by conventional techniques and represent a high proportion of those who need transfer to extracorporeal membrane oxygenation. Infants born at term who have RSV infection suffer chronic respiratory morbidity, the severity of the initial infection in preterm infants, particularly those with CLD, seems likely to put them at high risk of such an adverse outcome.

Preterm infants with neonatal CLD frequently suffer from acute deteriorations in their respiratory status while remaining on the NICU. Some of the deteriorations are due to viral infections.[45] Follow-up of eight affected infants demonstrated that six had recurrent wheeze and cough at follow-up compared with only two of eight gestational age and gender-matched controls who did not suffer viral infections. In addition, airway resistance was significantly higher and specific conductance significantly lower ($p < 0.05$) in the index cases compared with the controls.[46] These data are similar to findings in infants born at term, in whom viral infections, particularly due to RSV, are associated with an excess of symptoms[47] and abnormal lung function at follow-up[48] (see Chapter 7b).

PATHOPHYSIOLOGY

Following premature birth there is an early inflammatory response,[49] this usually resolves by the end of the first week.[50] Infants who develop CLD are, however, exposed to ongoing insults which results in chronic inflammation and further accumulation of inflammatory cells and mediator production.[49] For example, transforming growth factor β, which increases the degradation of the existing extracellular matrix, is increased in the BAL fluid at 4 days of age in infants who go on to develop CLD.[51] Leukotriene C4, a potent bronchoconstrictor, has been recovered in large quantities in the tracheobronchial effluent of infants who subsequently developed chronic oxygen dependency.[38] At follow-up at approximately 7 months of age, premature infants who had CLD were found to have elevated leukotriene E4 levels in association with elevated TGV, airways resistance and FRC, indicative of obstruction.[52]

THERAPEUTIC MEASURES (TABLE 13B.2)

Acute episodes

NEONATAL PERIOD

A variety of bronchodilators have been administered to preterm infants receiving intensive care. Isoprenaline, salbutamol, isoetharene and ipratropium bromide all

Table 13b.2 *Benefits of anti-asthma therapy*

Reduction in symptom score, active compared to placebo period:

65% by a β-agonist[2]
59% by an anticholinergic agent[3]
49% by sodium cromoglycate[65,66]
37% by inhaled steroids[68]

improve lung function, although the effect rarely persists beyond 60 minutes.[53,54] The improvements include increased specific airway conductance and decreased airways resistance. In a randomized placebo-controlled trial, however, oral salbutamol improved pulmonary resistance after 48 hours of treatment in ventilator dependent preterm infants.[55] Synergism has been noted between ipratropium bromide and salbutomol.[56] Bronchodilator responsiveness is not seen in all infants with CLD; the variability in response seems not to be due to postnatal or postconceptional age,[57] but rather dosage.[58] Administration of 200 μg, but not 100 μg of salbutamol via a metered dose inhaler (MDI) improved lung function in all infants tested.[57] In addition, repeated doses of salbutamol resulted in increased static compliance from as early as the first week after birth, the effect was independent of postnatal age.[59] There are no data, however, to suggest that regular bronchodilator therapy in ventilated infants improves long-term outcome. Sodium cromoglycate administration has been associated with a clinical improvement and reduction in the inspired oxygen concentration and ventilator pressures,[38] but it does not reduce the incidence of CLD.

AT FOLLOW-UP

Nebulized salbutamol[5] or ipratropium bromide[60] can result in acute improvements in lung function, a reduction in airway resistance and an increase in both specific conductance and increase in the FRC:TGV ratio,[60] (Figure 13b.1). The effect appears most pronounced in infants with recurrent respiratory symptoms at follow-up and the worst lung function abnormalities. This positive response occurs even in preterm infants aged only 3 months and is independent of neonatal complications

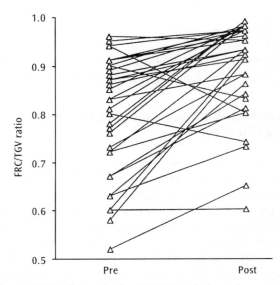

Figure 13b.1 *Change in the FRC:TGV ratio in response to bronchodilator. Individual data are demonstrated by linked data points. (From ref. 60 with permission.)*

or a family history of asthma.[5,60]. As with term infants,[61] nebulized therapy must be administered with caution. In certain infants there is an early paradoxical deterioration in respiratory function, approximately 5 minutes after the nebulization.[62] This may then be followed by an improvement in airways resistance.[62] The deterioration occurs even if a preservative-free solution is used and may be a function of the changing osmolality of the solution as nebulization continues or the relatively low pH of all respiratory solutions. The paradoxical response is unpredictable from the infant's gestational age, postnatal age or baseline lung function.[61,62] It thus seems prudent, if nebulized bronchodilator therapy is to be used, to administer the first dose in hospital where the infant can be closely observed and oxygen can be given. Alternatively, salbutamol can be administered equally as effectively using a metered dose inhaler (MDI) and a spacer device and that method of administration avoids the early paradoxical deterioration.[63]

Nebulized sodium cromoglycate may have some bronchodilator effects in prematurely born patients. In 10 of 18 children studied at 15 months of age specific conductance improved following sodium cromoglycate.[64]

Chronic symptoms

MAINTENANCE THERAPY

Regular bronchodilator therapy given from an inhaler and spacer device can reduce asthma symptoms in preterm infants.[2,3] In several studies, a plastic coffee cup has been used as the spacer device. This has sufficient volume to act as a spacer for preterm infants less than 2 years of age and has the advantages of being light to transport and inexpensive. In both a non-randomized[2] and a randomized study,[3] terbutaline and ipratropium bromide respectively resulted in improvements in lung function and a reduction in symptoms.

PROPHYLAXIS

Although administration of bronchodilators improves symptoms, despite maintenance therapy some infants have residual respiratory problems. In such patients, inhaled sodium cromoglycate may further reduce symptoms and improve lung function with a decrease in bronchodilator usage.[65] Inhaled sodium cromoglycate[66] improves both upper and lower respiratory tract signs; the magnitude of the response does not seem to be related to postnatal or gestational age, nor to the occurrence of neonatal chronic lung disease. Inhaled nedocromil sodium may also have useful prophylactic effects in symptomatic preterm infants.[67]

Inhaled steroids are also useful.[68] Children with a mean age 10.5 months, whose symptoms persisted despite 2 weeks of regular bronchodilator, were randomized to receive 200 mcg of beclomethasone dipropionate twice daily or placebo via an inhaler and spacer, each for 6 weeks. The symptom score was reduced by 37% during the active period and the infants had a mean of 28 bronchodilator-free days when receiving beclomethasone dipropionate compared with 22 days in the placebo period.

Prevention

ANTENATAL PROPHYLAXIS

Antenatal administration of maternal steroids reduces the incidence of RDS, but not CLD. Meta-analysis of randomized trials has demonstrated that administering TRH in combination with corticosteroids offers no additional advantages.[69]

POSTNATAL PROPHYLAXIS

Surfactant

Exogenous surfactant replacement therapy reduces the severity of RDS[70] and may improve lung function at follow-up.[71,72] Abbasi[71] demonstrated administration in the neonatal period of Exosurf rather than placebo resulted in improvements in resistive airflow properties in late infancy. Both airway resistance and specific conductance at 7 months of age were also better in infants treated with Exosurf rather than placebo.[71] High airway resistance at 6 months of age[10] has been previously found to be a sensitive and specific predictor of symptoms such as cough and wheeze persisting into the second year of life, while any dysfunction at 1 year of age appears to track through childhood.[32] These data,[71,72] therefore, suggest that surfactant replacement therapy has the potential to reduce chronic symptoms.

Ventilatory requirements

Randomized trials[73,74] have demonstrated ventilator rates $\geq$60/min (high frequency positive pressure ventilation, HFFPV) compared with $\leq$40/min reduce the incidence of airleak, a risk factor for chronic respiratory morbidity.[10] None of the trials, however, have reported long-term follow-up nor indicated that HFFPV reduces CLD. High frequency oscillation (HFO) does decrease the incidence of CLD, but only if a high volume recruitment strategy and/or exogenous surfactant is used.[75] Pulmonary function follow-up studies have not demonstrated any long-term benefits of HFO over conventional ventilator techniques. Those studies, however, report the outcome of infants exposed during HFO to the inferior low volume strategy, which does not reduce the incidence of CLD.[75]

Corticosteroids

If corticosteroids are administered systemically in the first 2 weeks after birth they reduce both the incidence of CLD and the mortality rate.[77] The exact timing of administration and the effect achieved varies according to which trials are included in the analysis.[77,78] After 3 weeks of age corticosteroids are less efficacious, reducing only the requirement for further systemic courses and facilitating extubation.[79] Administration by the inhaled route has less side effects, but also fewer benefits. Even when administered in the first days after birth only achieving a reduction in the need for systemic therapy and earlier extubation.[80] There are no pulmonary function studies to indicate whether early administration of systemic steroids will impact on the chronic respiratory morbidity associated with premature birth. Data from pre-clinical models suggest that corticosteroids may have an unfavourable effect on long-term lung function. Rats given corticosteroids systemically at a critical period for lung growth, that is in the first days after birth, develop emphysematous lungs.[81]

RSV immunoprophylaxis

Treatment for RSV infection is supportive and thus effective prevention offers the best hope of reducing the chronic respiratory morbidity[47,48] associated with acquisition of this infection. There is no safe and effective vaccine for use in infants. Immunoprophylaxis in randomized trials[82,83] has been demonstrated to reduce hospitalization and PICU admission in preterm infants with and without BPD. Whether such treatment improves long-term outcome remains to be tested. To be cost effective, it seems likely that only infants at high risk of severe RSV infection, that is those who require home oxygen therapy,[84,85] should be selected for immunoprophylaxis. Palivizumab, rather than RSV-IGIV, is the preferred agent,[84] as it is easier to administer (intramuscular injection rather than intravenous infusion), has a better safety profile, does not interfere with vaccines and may be more efficacious, although there are no 'head to head' comparisons of the two therapies.

SUMMARY

There is overwhelming evidence that babies born preterm are more likely than term babies to develop the symptoms of recurrent cough and wheeze which are characteristic of asthma. This tendency can persist for many years. The symptoms are associated with lung function abnormalities which indicate hyperinflation and airways obstruction. Although those needing intensive neonatal respiratory support are more likely to be affected, these changes are also seen in babies born preterm who did not develop neonatal respiratory distress. There is also good evidence that both the symptoms and lung function abnormalities respond, at least partially, to anti-asthma therapy. The nature of the disease in the first year after birth has many features in common with other wheezing disorders of infancy but, unlike later childhood asthma, does not appear to have an atopic basis.

REFERENCES

1. Northway WH, Moss RB, Carlisle KB, et al. Late pulmonary sequelae of bronchopulmonary dysplasia. New Engl J Med 1990;323:1793–9.
2. Yüksel B, Greenough A, Maconochie I. Effective bronchodilator therapy by a simple spacer device for wheezy premature infants in the first two years of life. Arch Dis Child 1990;65:782–5.
3. Yüksel B, Greenough A. Ipratropium bromide for symptomatic preterm infants. Eur J Pediatr 1991;150:854–7.
4. Greenough A, Maconochie I, Yüksel B. Recurrent respiratory symptoms in the first year of life following preterm delivery. J Perinat Med 1990;18:489–94.
5. Yüksel B, Greenough A. Effect of nebulised salbutamol in preterm infants during the first year of life. Eur Respir J 1991;4:1088–91.
6. Sauve RS, Singhal N. Long term morbidity of infants with bronchopulmonary dysplasia. Pediatrics 1985;76:725–33.
7. Andreasson B, Lindstrom M, Mortensson W, Svenningsen NW, Jonson B. Lung function eight years after neonatal ventilation. Arch Dis Child 1989;64:108–13.
8. Riedel F. Long term effects of artificial ventilation in neonates. Acta Paediatr Scand 1987;76:24–32.
9. Smyth JA, Tabachnik E, Duncan WJ, Reilly BJ, Levison H. Pulmonary function and bronchial hyperreactivity in long-term survivors of bronchopulmonary dysplasia. Pediatrics 1981;68:336–40.
10. Yüksel B, Greenough A. Persistence of respiratory symptoms into the second year of life: predictive factors in infants born preterm. Acta Paediatr 1992;81:832–5.
11. Greenough A, Giffin FJ, Yüksel B, Dimitriou G. Respiratory morbidity in young school children born prematurely – chronic lung disease is not a risk factor? Eur J Pediatr 1996;155:823–6.
12. Rona RJ, Gulliford MC, Chinn S. Effects of prematurity and intrauterine growth on respiratory health and lung function in childhood. Br Med J 1993;306:817–20.
13. Chan KN, Elliman A, Bryan E, Silverman M. Respiratory symptoms in children of low birthweight. Arch Dis Child 1989;64:1294.
14. McLeod A, Ross P, Mitchell S, et al. Respiratory health in a total very low birthweight cohort and their classroom controls. Arch Dis Child 1996;74:188–94.
15. Gross SJ, Iannuzzi DM, Kveselis DA, Anbar RD. Effect of preterm birth on pulmonary function at school age: a prospective controlled study. J Pediatr 1998;133:188–92.
16. Alho O, Koivu M, Hartikainen-Sorri AL, Sorri M, Kilkku O, Rantakallio P. Is a child's history of acute otitis media and respiratory infection already

determined in the antenatal and prenatal period? *Internat J Pediatr Otorhinolaryngol* 1990;**19**(2):129–37.

17. Stocks J, Godfrey S. The role of artificial ventilation, oxygen and CPAP in the pathogenesis of lung damage in neonates: assessment by serial measurements of lung function. *Pediatrics* 1976;**75**:352–62.

18. Yüksel B, Greenough A. Lung function in 6–20 month old infants born very preterm but without respiratory problems. *Pediatr Pulmonol* 1992;**14**:214–21.

19. Yüksel B, Greenough A. Relationship of symptoms to lung function abnormalities in preterm infants at follow-up. *Pediatr Pulmonol* 1991;**11**:202–6.

20. Yüksel B, Greenough A. Airway resistance and lung volume before and after bronchodilator therapy in symptomatic preterm infants. *Respir Med* 1994; **88**:281–6.

21. de Kleine MJK, Roos CM, Voorn WJ, Jansen HM, Koppe JG. Lung function 8–18 years after intermittent positive pressure ventilation for hyaline membrane disease. *Thorax* 1990;**45**:941–6.

22. Coates JC, Lands LC, MacNeish CF, Riley SP, Hornby L, Outerbridge EW, Davis GM, Williams RL. Long-term pulmonary sequelae of severe bronchopulmonary dysplasia. *J Pediatr* 1998;**133**:193–200.

23. Kennedy JD, Edward LJ, Bates DJ, Martin AJ, Dip SN, Haslam RR, McPhee AJ, Sturgess RE, Baghurst P. Effects of birthweight and oxygen supplementation on lung function in late childhood in children of very low birthweight. *Paediatr Pulmonol* 2000; **30**:32–40.

24. Koumbourlis AC, Motoyama EK, Mutich RL, Mallory GB, Walczak SA, Fertal K. Longitudinal follow-up of lung function from childhood to adolescence in prematurely born patients with neonatal chronic lung disease. *Pediatr Pulmonol* 1996;**21**:28–34.

25. Matthes JW, Lewis PA, Davies DP, Bethel JA. Birth weight at term and lung function in adolescence: no evidence for a programmed effect. *Arch Dis Child* 1995;**73**:231–4.

26. Barker DJ, Godfrey KM, Fall C, Osmond C, Winter PD, Shaheen SO. Relation of birthweight and childhood respiratory infection to adult lung function and death from chronic obstructive airway disease. *Br Med J* 1991;**303**:671–5.

27. Yüksel B, Greenough A, Green S. Lung function abnormalities at six months of age after neonatal intensive care. *Arch Dis Child* 1991;**66**:472–6.

28. Bowman E, Yu V. Continuing morbidity in extremely low birthweight infants. *Early Hum Develop* 1989; **18**:165–74.

29. Chan KN, Noble-Jamieson CM, Elliman A, Bryan EM, Silverman M. Lung function in children of low birthweight. *Arch Dis Child* 1989;**64**:1284–93.

30. Yüksel B, Greenough A. Neonatal respiratory distress and lung function at follow-up. *Respir Med* 1991; **85**:235–7.

31. Chan KN, Elliman A, Bryan AC, Silverman M. Clinical significance of airway responsiveness in children of low birthweight. *Pediatr Pulmonol* 1989;**7**:251–8.

32. Chan KN, Wong YC, Silverman M. Relationship between lung mechanics and childhood lung function in children of very low birthweight. *Pediatr Pulmonol* 1990;**8**:74–81.

33. Schraeder BD, Czajka C, Kalman DD, McGeady SJ. Respiratory health, lung function and airway responsiveness in school age survivors of very low birthweight. *Clin Pediatr* 1998;**37**:237–45.

34. Merritt TA, Cochrane CG, Holcomb K, *et al.* Elastase and alpha-1 protease inhibitor activity in tracheal aspirates during RDS: the role of inflammation and pathogenesis of bronchopulmonary dysplasia. *J Clin Invest* 1983;**72**:656–66.

35. Motoyama EK, Fort MD, Klesh KW, Mutich R, Guthrie RD. Early onset of airway reactivity in premature infants with bronchopulmonary dysplasia. *Am Rev Respir Dis* 1987;**136**:50–7.

36. Cano A, Payo F. Lung function and airway responsiveness in children and adolescents after hyaline membrane disease: a matched cohort study. *Eur Respir J* 1997;**10**:880–5.

37. Giffin F, Greenough A, Yüksel B. Does the duration of oxygen dependence after birth influence subsequent respiratory morbidity? *Eur J Pediatr* 1994;**153**:34–7.

38. Evans M, Palta M, Sadek M, Weinstein MR, Peters ME. Associations between family history of asthma, bronchopulmonary dysplasia, and childhood asthma in very low birth weight children. *Am J Epidemiol* 1998;**148**:460–6.

39. Demissie K, Breckenridge MB, Rhoads GG. Infant and maternal outcomes in the pregnancies of asthmatic women. *Am J Respir Crit Care Med* 1998;**158**:1091–5.

40. Bertrand JM, Riley SP, Popkin J, Coates AL. The long term pulmonary sequelae of prematurity: the role of familial airway hyperreactivity and the respiratory distress syndrome. *New Engl J Med* 1985;**312**:742–5.

41. Chan KN, Noble-Jamieson CM, Elliman A, Bryan EM, Aber VR, Silverman M. Airway responsiveness in low birthweight children and their mothers. *Arch Dis Child* 1988;**63**:905–10.

42. Giffin F, Greenough A, Yüksel B. Does a family history of atopy influence lung function at follow-up of infants born prematurely? *Acta Paediatr* 1995; **84**:17–21.

42a. Darlow BA, Horwood LJ, Mogridge N. Very low birthweight and asthma by age seven years in a national cohort. *Pediatr Pulmonol* 2000;**30**:291–6.

43. Meert K, Heidemann S, Abella B, Sarnaik A. Does prematurity alter the course of respiratory syncytial virus infection? *Crit Care Med* 1990;**18**:1357–9.

44. Groothuis JR, Gutierrez KM, Lauer BA. Respiratory syncytial virus infection in children with bronchopulmonary dysplasia. *Pediatrics* 1988;**82**:199–203.

45. Yüksel B, Greenough A. Acute deteriorations in neonatal chronic lung disease. *Eur J Pediatrics* 1992;**151**:697–700.

46. Yüksel B, Greenough A. Viral infections acquired on the neonatal unit and lung function of preterm infants at follow-up. *Acta Paediatr* 1994;**83**:117–18.

47. Webb MS, Henry RL, Milner AD, Stokes GM, Swarbrick AS. Continuing respiratory problems three and a half years after acute viral bronchiolitis. *Arch Dis Child* 1985;**60**:1064–7.

48. Stokes GM, Milner AD, Hodges IGC, Groggins RC. Lung function abnormalities after acute bronchiolitis. *J Pediatr* 1981;**98**:871–4.

49. Ozdemir A, Brown MA, Morgan WJ. Markers and mediators of inflammation in neonatal lung disease. *Pediatr Pulmonol* 1997;**23**:292–306.

50. Finkelstein JN, Horowitz S, Sinkin RA, Ryan RM. Cellular and molecular responses to lung injury in relation to induction of tissue repair and fibrosis. *Clin Perinatol* 1992;**19**:603–20.

51. Kotecha S, Wangoo A, Silverman M, Shaw RJ. Increase in the concentration of transforming growth factor beta-I in bronchoalveolar lavage fluid before the development of chronic lung disease of prematurity. *J Pediatr* 1996;**128**:464–9.

52. Cook AJ, Yüksel B, Sampson AP, Greenough A, Price JF. Cysteinyl leukotriene involvement in chronic lung disease in premature infants. *Eur Respir J* 1996;**9**:1907–12.

53. Kao LC, Warburton D, Platzker ACG, Keens TG. Effect of isoproterenol inhalation on airways resistance in chronic bronchopulmonary dysplasia. *Pediatrics* 1984;**73**:509–14.

54. Wilkie RA, Bryan MH. Effect of bronchodilators on airway resistance in ventilator-dependent neonates with chronic lung disease. *J Pediatr* 1987;**111**:278–82.

55. Stefano JL, Bhutani VK, Fox WW. A randomized, placebo-controlled study to evaluate the effects of oral albuterol on pulmonary mechanics in ventilator dependent infants at risk of developing BPD. *Pediatr Pulmonol* 1991;**10**:183–90.

56. Brundage KL, Mohsini KG, Froese AB, Fisher JT. Bronchodilator response to ipratropium bromide in infants with bronchopulmonary dysplasia. *Am Rev Respir Dis* 1990;**142**:1137–42.

57. Kovacs SJ, Fisher JB, Brodsky NL, Hurt H. Use of a beta-agonist in ventilated, very low birth weight babies: a longitudinal evaluation. *Develop Pharmacol Ther* 1990;**15**:61–7.

58. Denjean A, Gulmaraes H, Migdal M, Miramand JL, Dehan M, Gaultier C. Dose-related bronchodilator response to aerosolized salbutamol (albuterol) in ventilator-dependent premature infants. *J Pediatr* 1992;**120**:974–9.

59. Rotschild A, Solimano A, Puterman M, Smyth J, Sharma A, Albersheim S. Increased compliance in response to salbutamol in premature infants with developing bronchopulmonary dysplasia. *J Pediatr* 1989;**15**:984–91.

60. Greenough A, Yüksel B. Variable response to bronchodilator therapy in preterm infants. *Respir Med* 1993;**87**:359–64.

61. O'Callaghan C, Milner AD, Swarbrick A. Paradoxical deterioration in lung function after nebulised salbutamol in wheezy infants. *Lancet* 1986;**ii**:1424–5.

62. Yüksel B, Greenough A. Comparison of the effects on lung function of two methods of bronchodilator administration. *Respir Med* 1994;**88**:229–33.

63. Yüksel B, Greenough A. Bronchodilator effect of nebulized sodium cromoglycate in infants born prematurely. *Eur Respir J* 1993;**6**:387–90.

64. Yüksel B, Greenough A. Nebulized sodium cromoglycate in preterm infants – protection against water challenge-induced bronchoconstriction. *Respir Med* 1993;**87**:37–42.

65. Yüksel B, Greenough A. Inhaled sodium cromoglycate for preterm children with respiratory symptoms at follow-up. *Respir Med* 1992;**86**:131–4.

66. Yüksel B, Greenough A. The effect of sodium cromoglycate on upper/lower respiratory symptoms in preterm infants. *Eur J Pediatr* 1993;**152**:615–18.

67. Yüksel B, Greenough A. Inhaled nedocromil sodium in symptomatic young children born prematurely. *Respir Med* 1996;**90**:467–71.

68. Yüksel B, Greenough A. Randomized trial of inhaled steroids in preterm infants symptomatic at follow-up. *Thorax* 1992;**47**:910–13.

69. Crowther CA, Alfirevic Z, Haslam RR. Prenatal thyrotropin-releasing hormone for preterm birth (*Cochrane Review*). The Cochrane Library, Issue 4. Update Software, Oxford, 1999.

70. Morley CJ, Greenough A, Miller NG, *et al*. Randomised trial of artificial surfactant (ALEC) given at birth to babies from 23–34 weeks gestation. *Early Hum Develop* 1988;**17**:41–54.

71. Abbasi S, Bhutani VK, Gerdes JS. Long term pulmonary consequences of respiratory distress syndrome in preterm infants treated with exogenous surfactant. *J Pediatr* 1993;**122**:446–52.

72. Yüksel B, Greenough A, Gamsu HR. Respiratory function at follow-up after neonatal surfactant replacement therapy. *Respir Med* 1993;**87**:217–21.

73. Oxford Region Controlled Trial of Artificial Ventilation (OCTAVE) Study Group. Multicentre randomised controlled trial of high against low frequency positive pressure ventilation. *Arch Dis Child* 1991;**66**:770–5.

74. Pohlandt F, Saule H, Schröder H, *et al*. Decreased incidence of extra-alveolar air leakage or death prior to air leakage in high versus low rate positive pressure ventilation: results of a randomised seven-centre trial in preterm infants. *Eur J Pediatr* 1992;**151**:904–9.

75. Cools F, Offringa M. Meta-analysis of elective high frequency ventilation in preterm infants with

respiratory distress syndrome. *Arch Dis Child Fetal Neonat Edn* 1999;**80**:F15–20.

76. HIFI Study Group. High frequency oscillatory ventilation compared with conventional mechanical ventilation in the treatment of respiratory failure in preterm infants. *New Engl J Med* 1989;**320**:88–93.

77. Bhuta T, Ohlsson A. Systematic review and meta-analysis of early postnatal dexamethasone for prevention of chronic lung disease. *Arch Dis Child Fetal Neonat Edn* 1998;**79**:F26–33.

78. Arias-Camison JM, Lau J, Cole CH, Frantz ID 3rd. Meta-analysis of dexamethasone therapy started in the first 15 days of life for prevention of chronic lung disease. *Pediatr Pulmonol* 1999;**28**:167–74.

79. Halliday HL, Ehrenkranz RA. Delayed (>3 weeks) postnatal corticosteroids for chronic lung disease in preterm infants (*Cochrane Review*). The Cochrane Library, Issue 1, 2000. Update Software, Oxford.

80. Greenough A. Chronic lung disease of prematurity – prevention by inhaled corticosteroids. *Lancet* 1999;**354**:266–7.

81. Greenough A. Gains and losses from dexamethasone for neonatal chronic lung disease. *Lancet* 1998; **352**:835–6.

82. Wang EEL, Tang NK. Immunoglobulin for preventing respiratory syncitial virus infection (*Cochrane Review*). The Cochrane Library, Issue 3, 2000. Update Software, Oxford.

83. Anonymous. Palivizumab, a humanized respiratory syncytial virus monoclonal antibody, reduces hospitalization from respiratory syncytial virus infection in high-risk infants. The IMpact-RSV Study Group. *Pediatrics* 1998;**102**(3, part 1):531–7.

84. Anonymous. Respiratory syncytial virus immune globulin intravenous: indications for use. American Academy of Pediatrics Committee on Infectious Diseases, Committee on Fetus and Newborn. *Pediatrics* 1997;**99**:645–50.

85. Thomas M, Bedford-Russell A, Sharland M. Hospitalisation for RSV infection in ex-preterm infants – implications for use of RSV immune globulin. *Arch Dis Child* 2000;**83**:122–7.

Psychological factors

PER A GUSTAFSON AND BRYAN LASK

INTRODUCTION

Although much is known about the relationship between biological and psychosocial factors in asthma and about the significance of this relationship in determining the course of the disease, all too often only lip service is paid to this knowledge. The physician will acknowledge that psychosocial factors are relevant but pay only minimal attention to them in practice. In this chapter the research evidence is reviewed, the role of psychosocial factors outlined and an integrated model of treatment is recommended, with a description of the main psychosocial treatments.

MECHANISMS

Psychophysiological mechanisms

Emotional factors have been considered of importance in both the development and the course of asthma. The psychosomatic concept was introduced to explain how psychological factors could induce and influence somatic symptoms. But, as a consequence, it proposes that there is some illness where psychological factors are of no importance, an unlikely situation. Instead the bio-psychosocial model of illness was constructed, where all illness is viewed in biological, psychological and social aspects[1] (Figure 13c.1), and the concept psychosomatic is now used to describe the psychological aspects of that model.

Experimental, epidemiological and clinical observations strongly support the findings that the conditions under which the primary encounter with an antigen takes place influence the immune response for a long time.[2] Neural mechanisms could influence the responses. Inflammatory mediators may activate afferent nerves causing reflex effects on the airway function.[3] Such interactions are mediated through cholinergic or adrenergic mechanisms and neuropeptides, or by a combination. High cortisol levels due to negative stress seem to facilitate the shift

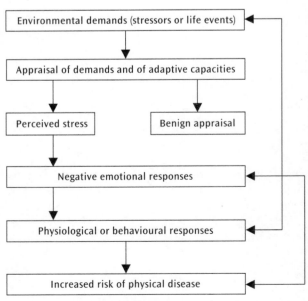

Figure 13c.1 *The bio-psychosocial model of the stress process designed to illustrate the potential integration of the psychological and biological effects of environmental demands. (From ref. 62, after ref. 2.)*

from Th1 to Th2 immunity in allergic subjects.[2] These neuro-humoral mechanisms provide links between psychological and physical aspects of asthma.

It is obvious that the family and the informal social network constitute the most important environment for the child, both from a psychological and social point of view. Dysfunctional family interaction patterns before the onset of illness do not seem to predict the development of wheezing in infants.[4] However, two studies suggest[5,6] that early parental interaction and parenting difficulties may influence the development of asthma so that it seems obvious that a good relationship between parents and child, in which the child can experience challenges without too much stress that could influence the immune system, would be optimal. It is important though to point out that parents do not cause asthma in their children!

Emotional arousal is an everyday event for everyone, children included. Excitement, happiness, anger, sadness, envy, resentment, fear and anxiety are but some of the emotions that children commonly experience. Emotional arousal differs from the other asthma triggers in that it is the only one to be involved in a two-way process. This makes it harder to unravel the complexities of the relationship between emotional arousal and asthma, but this is no excuse for ignoring them. Through the mechanisms described above, any of these feelings may, and in some asthmatic children frequently do, trigger or aggravate episodes of asthma. It is unlikely that they would do so in isolation, although this does happen. More commonly emotional arousal will combine with other triggers such as allergens, pollution, infection or exercise, exerting their effect on the labile bronchus and producing bronchospasm. This phenomenon, among others, explains why asthma attacks can be so unpredictable.

Living conditions

The influence of living conditions on the development of asthma, the social aspect of the bio-psychosocial model, is clearly supported by recent research in the former socialist countries of Eastern Europe where the prevalence of asthma is about 1% compared with 5–8% in the Western countries. The lifestyle, including dietary regimes, the influence on the microbial environment due to crowded houses, ventilation in the apartments, extensive travelling to new environments, stress, etc, in these countries in the beginning of the 1990s was very similar to living conditions in Western Europe some 30–40 years ago, before the dramatic rise in incidence of allergic illness. It is tempting to suggest that one link between social and biological aspects of allergic disease is to be found in differences in the resident intestinal flora of young children, probably due to change in feeding habits, and its effect on the development and priming of the immune system in early childhood,[7] but psychological factors may play a part too.

Course of disease

Although children with asthma differ from others in several psychosocial features, the differences are small and may be secondary to the illness.[61] Nevertheless, psychosocial factors influence the management and the course of the disease. Dysfunctional family interaction patterns and weak social network seem to be risk factors for continuing and more severe allergic illness.[8–11]

DIFFERENT MODELS

The *psychoanalytic model* considers the personality to be of great importance for the development of 'psychosomatic illness'. According to this model, individuals with difficulties in verbalizing their feelings often experience them as body tensions, resulting in 'psychosomatic illness'.[12] Although empirical studies of children with asthma have revealed differences in personality as compared with healthy children, there have been no differences compared with children with other chronic disease, such as congenital heart disease. Thus, personality seems to have been influenced by the disease, not *vice versa*.[13]

Another approach is the *psychophysiologic stress model*, evaluating how everyday life stress as well as severe stressful life events, e.g. death of a close relative, illness in the family etc., influence the course of illness. A number of laboratory experiments have demonstrated the role of psychophysiological mechanisms in the induction of asthma. For example, bronchospasm can be induced by discussion of anxiety-provoking topics[14] or by suggesting that nebulized normal saline is actually an allergen that the subject associates with asthma attacks. Reversal of the bronchospasm can also be induced by inhaled nebulized saline. This process of suggestion can have even more powerful and paradoxical effects. Inhaled bronchodilators and bronchoconstrictors can induce opposite effects to those expected if the subject believes that the bronchodilator is a bronchoconstrictor or vice versa.[15,16] In animals psychological conditioning of the immune system is well established, but the support for such mechanisms in humans is incomplete.[17]

Emotional arousal such as anxiety, sadness, anger or excitement can precipitate bronchospasm by vagal activity.[18] Increased airway responsiveness in asthmatic children is associated with increased autonomic reactivity in other peripheral systems. In asthmatic children with increased autonomic reactivity there is either increased sensitivity to emotional challenge or increased emotional arousal. Also pulmonary function is more sensitive to emotional triggers in asthmatic children, with their relatively greater airway responsiveness, possibly as a result of cholinergic mechanisms. Emotionally determined respiratory behaviours such as laughing and crying can precipitate bronchospasm, probably as a result of hyperventilation.[19]

Another mechanism that may contribute to the interaction is the hypothalamic-limbic midbrain circuit, which plays an important role in response to stress, and can exert influence on the immune system.[20] For a critical research update see Rietveld et al.[21]

Finally, proponents of the *interaction and systems approach* stress the interplay between the individual and family members, other important persons and the total life situation.[10,22–26] Minuchin et al.[27] in their 'psychosomatic family model', proposed a relationship between family interaction patterns with too much closeness (enmeshment), too little flexibility rigidity, diffuse roles and generational boundaries, and 'psychosomatic illness' in the child. Pinkerton[28] found that 86% of hospitalized asthmatic children had parents whose attitude to the asthma tended towards one extreme or the other of the overprotective/denying continuum. However, no uniform characteristics of these families were found, in fact family patterns with too little closeness (disengagement) and to much flexibility (chaotic interaction) were almost as common as the family types proposed by Minuchin.[22,24,29–33] Families may have a primary inherent dysfunction of structure or communications as well as marital discord or substance abuse, or they may experience secondary family dysfunction from environmental stress.

A CONCEPTUAL MODEL

Illness has an *impact on family life*, but family interaction also may influence the predisposition to illness, its onset and course and the adherence to treatment.[22,23] If we consider families at a certain moment of time, some will have dysfunctional interaction patterns. It seems probable that the appearance of severe disease could trigger a psychological crisis in the family and that certain families never reach a functional adaptation to illness.[11] Most parents of children with asthma or other serious diseases react initially with denial and rejection. Some parents never get over that stage; others move to a complementary position of over-protection. With time, parents then achieve an adequate relationship with the child and the illness. Regardless of why the dysfunctional patterns were established, they are of importance for the further development of the family system.

Dysfunctional interaction patterns will reduce problem-solving capacity and diminish the family's capacity to counter stress, and functional patterns *vice versa*. On the other hand illness also has considerable impact on family relations. Dysfunctional patterns can create tension in the family, reduce coping and problem-solving capacity, and thus become risk factors for continuing and more severe illness. In modern treatment of atopic illness information to parents and children about preventive measures and self-management are central. In this situation good problem-solving capacity and coping in the

family become crucial for effective treatment. Social and psychological factors in the environment influence both the child and the family, but worry and concern for the disease and symptoms leading for instance to school absence, also influence psychological well-being and social competence. For example, asthmatic children may develop bronchospasm on some occasions, but not others, when exposed to one of their triggers. Variability in response may to some extent be accounted for by variation in emotional arousal.

It is worth noting that in one study, 80% of parents of asthmatic children considered emotional factors to be important in the aetiology of their attacks.[34] Gustafsson et al.[8] showed the importance of the family for the course of the disease in an ongoing prospective study. It was found that the chance of recovery from atopic illness (wheezing bronchitis and/or eczema) between 1½ and 3 years of age was four times greater in well-functioning families with a good social supportive network (73% recovered), compared with dysfunctional families with a poor social network (18% recovered). Children in families with dysfunctional interaction and a dysfunctional social network had significantly more psychiatric symptoms compared with children in families where both interaction and network were functional. This does not mean that these children have an emotional disturbance, but rather that they are manifesting the close link between emotional arousal and bronchospasm. Socio-economic factors are of importance for children's health, and families of lower socio-economic class seem to take less advantage of preventive paediatric care.[35]

PSYCHOLOGICAL FACTORS ASSOCIATED WITH FATALITIES

A number of specific factors have a significant association with fatal childhood asthma. Fritz and colleagues[36] reviewed the case notes of children who had died from asthma and found consistent themes of childhood depression, emotional triggers for the asthma, denial and a tendency for the families to be unsupportive. Strunk and colleagues[37] found that psychological factors comprised ten of the 14 variables that significantly distinguished children who died from asthma from living matched controls. With adequate treatment asthma in childhood is seldom fatal, thus poor-adherence with treatment regime is a significant risk factor for severe asthma attacks.[38,39] These findings lend further support to the view that psychosocial factors need to be given far more serious consideration than is common practice (Figure 13c.2).

Blunted awareness of severe airway obstruction may be another significant risk factor for severe or fatal asthma, leading to delay in presentation for emergency treatment.[40] Techniques for measuring symptom perception

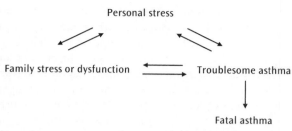

Figure 13c.2 *Interaction of asthma and stress factors.*

in asthma are unsophisticated[41] and the factors which determine the wide individual differences which are seen in children[40] are unresolved and of potential clinical importance.

MANAGEMENT

In modern treatment of allergic illness high demands are put on the patient, and if the patient is a child, on the parents and family life. One is supposed to be an active agent in the treatment, follow lung function with screening tests, learn what precipitate symptoms and how to prevent deterioration. One should learn to foresee attacks and take medicine in advance, ensure good hygiene, avoid allergens (and, as a consequence, avoid much fun, such as riding horses or keeping pets), perhaps even get rid of pets, maintain a diet, etc; in short be a skilled manager of one's treatment. It should be obvious that such an ambitious program demands good capacity for psychological adjustment and problem solving.

Adherence to therapy

The term adherence is used in preference to compliance. The latter terms imply coercion, in contrast to the cooperation that is desirable. Adherence to treatment is something that is all too often assumed to occur without question. If readers question their own experience, it would rapidly become obvious that full adherence is unlikely and that partial adherence is much more likely to be the norm. Degrees of adherence may well vary, both over time and between situations. For example, a child may become less adherent as she gets older or may always take her medication when at home, but not at school or when staying with friends.

There are many reasons for partial-adherence (Chapter 18). Koocher and colleagues[42] have classified partial-adherence in cystic fibrosis, but the principles are applicable to asthma. They describe three main types of partial-adherence.

1 *Inadequate knowledge* implies that lack of information or inadequate understanding of information available is the main contributor.

This faulty process may involve individual characteristics of the physician, child and parent and the manner in which the information is imparted and how frequent such misinformation is.

2 *Psychosocial resistance* includes control struggles with parents and other authority figures. The illness can also induce over-close relations between a parent and the sick child. Cultural and peer group pressures, striving for normality, denial and avoidance and disturbed or chaotic home environment could also be important aspects.

3 *Educated non-adherence* involves conflicts and difficult choices, based on a full understanding of both the reasons for the prescribed regime and the result of not following it. Patients make a quality of life decision in which they may decide that the treatment is worse than the disease.

In childhood asthma any of the above forms of partial-adherence may apply. It should be remembered that in the younger age group parents play a much larger part in determining how much or how frequently medication is taken and very rarely indeed would a parent freely admit to anything other than almost full adherence. In adolescents, on the other hand, the normal drive for self-assertiveness and independence suggests that the patient sometimes should have the opportunity to consultations without the parents. Indeed, it would be wise, when attempting to enquire about adherence, to acknowledge the commonality of partial adherence and then seek information about departure from that norm ('How often do you forget to…?') rather than from the ideal of full adherence.

Attempts to study the extent of the problem are inevitably hampered by the difficulties in getting an accurate picture. However, estimates of satisfactory (*not* complete) adherence vary between10% and 50%.[43] Clinical experience supports these figures.

There are many methods of partial-adherence, apart from the obvious means such as refusal to take medication or straightforward dishonesty. Such techniques include sleight of hand (and mouth) and misuse of inhalers and nebulizers.

To achieve good adherence treatment should be coherent with daily life routines, be based on knowledge of family dynamics, use monitoring and supervision, include self-evaluation, prevent development of symptoms or deterioration of symptoms, including measures to handle anxiety and panic. Unnecessary anxiety and stress should be lifted from the parents, patient and siblings, so that attention can be focused on treatment. Since children and families are different, and have different needs for support and information, it follows that if health professionals have only one way of relating to their patients, most of their clients will be dissatisfied.

Management of partial-adherence is clearly determined to a major extent by the type of problem. Thus there is no standard treatment, but rather it should be individualized.

The three main types of partial adherence require quite different handling. Education will play a major part in the first type, while sensitive exploration of the underlying issues will be in the forefront for the second. Discussion and compromise are likely to be most important in the management of educated non-adherence. Specific treatments are discussed in the next sections.

PSYCHOLOGICAL TREATMENTS

When to refer or intervene

Given the complex interaction between psychosocial and organic factors in the triggering and maintenance of bronchospasm and episodes of asthma, it is logical that management should be comprehensive, taking into account all factors in all cases. However, because of time constraints, lack of resources and sometimes lack of knowledge, detailed attention is commonly paid to psychosocial issues only when these are so complex or severe that they cannot be ignored. A reasonable compromise needs to be found. Paediatricians and general practitioners clearly need to bear in mind psychosocial issues whenever they see a child with asthma. It is important that doctors use their contacts with the family to explain why a psychological assessment is necessary.[44–47] If the psychological consultation can be offered as a conjoint meeting with the doctor and a psychologist at the doctor's outpatient clinic most parents happily accept the suggestion. Psychosocial referral or intervention should be considered whenever there is:[48]

- an obvious psychological trigger for the asthma;
- clear evidence of behavioural or emotional problems;
- family dysfunction or inappropriate handling of the illness;
- concern at school;
- failure of standard treatment;
- significant poor-adherence to treatment;
- life-threatening attacks or attacks requiring intensive care.

The most useful psychosocial interventions include parental counselling, family therapy, behavioural techniques, individual counselling and environmental change. There is no place for psychotropic medication in childhood asthma, unless there is a concurrent psychiatric disorder.

How to introduce a psychological view on illness to the family

A good start is to state that all children can develop symptoms due to emotional arousal, although with varying frequency (about a third experience it sometimes, a few often). The risk of getting an emotionally induced attack is of course influenced by the state of emotional balance of the child. Pharmacological treatment in asthma can cause hyperactivity and bad temper in the child. Disciplining children with chronic illness can be difficult for several reasons: parents can feel guilty if they are firm with a child who suffers from illness; crying or screaming in response to disciplining can precipitate symptoms; much energy is spent on managing the disease and little is left for child-rearing issues. If the parents are overprotective and the siblings also are worried by wheezing attacks the asthmatic child may easily develop a poor, and illness-oriented self-image. The consequent stress for the child may aggravate the asthma, and perpetuate the cycle of ill-health. Some children unconsciously use the illness to get their way and can be perceived as manipulative and controlling.

A certain amount of anxiety, or respect for the disease, is normal while being either not anxious at all or very anxious is dysfunctional.[49] It is rational to take illness seriously and adapt to it, but it is unhelpful to let the disease take over completely, or to take no precautions at all to avoid asthma attacks. To investigate how the family reacts and interacts when they handle the symptoms of the child is often a good way to understand family dynamics and to find out where improvements could be made. Some children have difficulties expressing their needs directly and might find that when they are ill the care and support achieved from their parents also provides emotional satisfaction. For the parent caring can satisfy unspoken emotional needs. Parental self-esteem might be enhanced by being a good caregiver, or difficulties in the relationship between the two parents may be put in the background by focusing on the sick child.

Parental counselling

This should be a *sine qua non* of the management of all childhood illness and should not really be considered as a distinct treatment. Successful parenting involves parents working together as a team, supporting and helping each other in their management of the asthma, sharing the tasks of identifying problems and conflicts and finding ways of resolving these. They need to be consistent between each other and over time. In addition they have to be responsive to the needs of all their children and be available to them at any time. Such tasks are hard enough under normal circumstances but are far harder in the presence of a recurrent and occasionally frightening or even life-threatening illness. Single parents have to do all this without the support of a partner.

The essence of successful parental counselling is the ability to listen and understand, rather than to offer didactic opinions and advice. Rapport is gained by sympathetic listening and empathic acknowledgement. Parental counselling focuses on helping parents to express feelings of anxiety, sadness, resentment and failure, to identify and discuss difficulties and to begin to find possible solutions.

Single parents can also be encouraged to find appropriate support systems. The value of the approach is in its focus on building parental strength and confidence, rather than reinforcing dependency and passivity. It is the emotional counterpart of the physical self-reliance embodied in the concept of guided self-management.

Family therapy

Family therapy appears to be a very useful complement to conventional medical treatment of childhood asthma. A number of studies[9,25,50,51] have shown that family therapy reduces symptoms in asthmatic children. Further, a family counselling program aimed at helping families cope better with their child's asthma and placing a strong emphasis on providing information, new ways of thinking and new behavioural strategies led to increased independence and responsibility for daily healthcare.[52] There have been various descriptions of the application of family therapy in paediatric practice,[44,45,53] as well as specifically in asthma.[9,44,54,55] A systematic review has been carried out.[56]

The main focus in family therapy is neither the symptom nor the child, but the whole family. The rationale is that the family is in the strongest position to help or hinder the asthmatic child. When families are dysfunctional they may, as described in the section on families and family dysfunction, maintain or aggravate the problem. The family therapist attempts to:

- identify the family strengths and weaknesses;
- understand the relationship between the way in which the family functions and the course of the asthma;
- encourage discussion between parents and children about the impact of the illness (and it's management) on quality of life;
- help the family build upon their strengths and resolve any weaknesses.

Issues that are commonly addressed in family therapy include over-involvement and over-protectiveness, denial, fear of fatality, feelings of isolation due to avoidance of allergens, autonomy and independence, including taking responsibility for medication, clear and direct communication, the open expression of feelings and acknowledgement and acceptance of these. Often there is a too tight relationship between one of the parents and the sick child, which could be moderated by engaging the other parent in treatment activities, for instance accompanying the child to physiotherapy. In many cases the sick child needs to develop more autonomy and this can be a joint task for both parents. Work towards more realistic attitudes and hope in the family is important, as well as encouraging activities that have been avoided: in some families this could be soothing and caring, in others encouraging autonomy and adequate demands. Talk about restricted

feelings, anxiety about death, but also about negative feelings towards the sick child.

Behavioural treatments

These are the best evaluated of the psychosocial interventions. Several studies have demonstrated their effectiveness in symptom relief[57] and because they are easily taught, easily learned and economical, they warrant particular attention.

Where anxiety appears to be playing a significant part in asthma attacks, relaxation techniques are particularly helpful. Because the smooth muscle of the bronchus constricts and relaxes in parallel with various voluntary muscle groups, learning to relax the voluntary muscles leads to bronchodilation. Children aged 6 upwards can learn these techniques in just a few minutes. It is best to include the parents in the instruction so that they can supervise the treatment at home. The addition of systematic desensitization as a means of reducing sensitivity to psychological stimuli that trigger bronchospasm enhances the relaxation techniques. A systematic review of relaxation therapy has recently been reported.[63]

Children are taught to identify a stimulus and then, while relaxed, imagine themselves exposed to it. As anxiety and relaxation are incompatible the child gradually overcomes the anxiety, with subsequent reduction in bronchospasm on exposure. It is wise to start with the least worrying of the triggers and when that has been mastered, others can be tackled. Biofeedback equipment can be used to further enhance these techniques and help maintain the child's attention and enthusiasm. A number of centres have devised self-management programs which combine these techniques with training in the identification of attack precipitants and strategies for avoiding them, identifying the prodromal signs of bronchospasm and, more appropriate, the effective use of inhalers.[58,59]

With computer technology becoming so creative, there is considerable scope for developing even more sophisticated methods of integrating relaxation, desensitization and health management biofeedback programs. As a result of a wider Internet use, we will be frequently helping families who are more informed about the clinical issues, and might challenge our recommendations based on information they obtained via the Internet. Interactive, computer mediated, multimedia programs will be available for information of patients and parents.[60]

Individual counselling and psychotherapy

Individual counselling is the equivalent to parental counselling as applied to the child. It focuses on helping the child to express feelings of anxiety, sadness or resentment and identify aspects of life that are stressful or difficult and to begin to find possible solutions.

There is no absolute distinction between this and psychotherapy, although the latter tends to focus more on unconscious processes. The aim is to bring these to the surface, so that they can then be discussed and resolved. For example, many children have deeply suppressed but powerful negative feelings. Unless these can be expressed they remain covert but active, so that the child is in a state of emotional arousal and continuously at risk of bronchospasm.

Counselling is usually a short-term treatment, perhaps eight sessions at 2–3-week intervals. *Psychotherapy* in contrast is likely to last for at least 6 months and often much longer, with weekly meetings. As such it is best reserved for the more intractable cases of childhood asthma. In both instances the medium of communication is any combination of talking, drawing or playing. There have been surprisingly few formal evaluative studies. The only available controlled study showed that asthmatic children treated with short-term individual psychotherapy had a lower relapse rate than did a matched control group who received no psychotherapy.[28]

ENVIRONMENTAL CHANGE

It has long been recognized that some asthmatic children benefit from being separated from their *parents*.[32] This would usually take the form of hospitalization or residential schooling. Clearly it is possible that improvement occurs in response to the child being removed from physical allergens such as house dust, mites and animal fur or pollutants such as cigarette smoke. However, clinical experience indicates that bronchospasm often rapidly returns when parents visit the new environment. Further, Purcell's[32] experiments showed improvement at home for a significant number of children when their parents stayed elsewhere. The concept of 'emotional allergy' is not unreasonable in helping to understand the dramatic differences in a child's physical state when separated from key relatives. Parents and siblings can be just as powerful triggers as the more traditional dust mite or family pet.

Sometimes a *change of school* may also make a considerable difference. There are a number of reasons for considering this as a possibility. The school may be finding it particularly hard to cope with a child who may require hospitalization at any time. Staff anxieties are readily communicated to parents and child. Physical symptoms can lead to peer group problems such as teasing, while frequent absences can result in academic failure and impaired self-image. A change of school may be indicated if the school cannot accommodate and fulfil the child's needs.

Occasionally *residential schooling* may be indicated. This might be considered particularly in cases of intractable asthma, when not infrequently the family environment is playing a major part in the maintenance of the illness. Under such circumstances a trial of family therapy is indicated but should this fail the possibility of residential schooling should certainly be considered, preferably at a school which specializes in children with chronic illness.

CONCLUSIONS

There can no longer be any dispute about the relevance of psychosocial factors in the triggering and maintenance of episodes of asthma. What is now required is for paediatricians, nurses and GPs to pay more attention in practice to current knowledge. When investigating a child with troublesome asthma, using a family and systems perspective can promote understanding and open up possible ways for intervention. Mental health professionals, having convincingly demonstrated the effectiveness of their treatments, need to identify which types of intervention are most suitable for children and families with different psychological characteristics. Child-psychiatric liaison services to paediatrics should be provided. Better problem solving and coping in families of children with asthma may significantly improve the course of the disease. It is possible to live a 'normal' life in spite of chronic illness.

REFERENCES

1. Antonovsky A. *Unraveling the Mystery of Health.* Jossey-Bass, New York, 1987.
2. Herbert TB, Cohen S. Stress and immunity in humans: a meta-analytic review. *Psychosom Med* 1993; **55**:364–79.
3. Barnes PJ. Is asthma a nervous disease? The Parker B. Francis Lectureship. *Chest* 1995;**107**:119–25.
4. Gustafsson PA, Björkstén B, Kjellman N-IM. Family dysfunction in asthma: a prospective study of illness development. *J Pediatr* 1994;**125**:493–8.
5. Askildsen EC, Watten RG, Faleide AO. Are parents of asthmatic children different from other parents? Some follow-up results from the Norwegian PRAD Project. *Psychother Psychosom* 1993;**60**:91–9.
6. Mrazek DA, Klinnert M, Mrazek PJ, *et al.* Prediction of early-onset asthma in genetically at-risk children. *Pediatr Pulmonol* 1999;**27**:85–94.
7. Björkstén B. Environmental influence on the development of childhood immunity. *Nutr Rev* 1998;**56**:106–12.
8. Gustafsson PA, Björkstén B, Kjellman N-IM. Family interaction and supportive social network as salutogenic factors in childhood atopic illness. *Pediatr Allergy Immunol* 2002;**13**:51–57.
9. Liebman R, Minuchin S, Baker L. The use of structural family therapy in the treatment of intractable asthma. *Am J Psychiatr* 1974;**131**:535–40.

10. Onnis L, Tortolani D, Cancrini L. Systemic research on chronicity factors in infantile asthma. *Fam Process* 1986;**25**:107–22.

11. Pinkerton P. Correlating physiologic with psychodynamic data in the study and management of childhood asthma. *J Psychosom Res* 1967;**11**:11–25.

12. Feiguine RJ, Johnson FA. Alexithymia and chronic respiratory disease. A review of current research. *Psychother Psychosom* 1985;**43**:77–89.

13. Hilliard JP, Fritz GK, Lewiston NJ. Goal-setting behavior of asthmatic, diabetic and healthy children. *Child Psychiatr Hum Dev* 1982;**13**:35–47.

14. Dekker E, Pelser H, Green J. Conditioning as a cause of asthmatic attacks. *J Psychosom Res* 1957;**2**:97–104.

15. Kotses H, Rawson JC, Wigal JK, Creer TL. Respiratory airway changes in response to suggestion in normal individuals. *Psychosom Med* 1987;**49**:536–41.

16. Luparello TJ, Leist N, Lourie CH, Sweet P. The interaction of psychologic stimuli and pharmacologic agents on airway reactivity in asthmatic subjects. *Psychosom Med* 1970;**32**:509–13.

17. Cohen N, Moynihan JA, Ader R. Pavlovian conditioning of the immune system. *Int Arch Allergy Immunol* 1994;**105**:101–6.

18. Miller BD, Wood BL. Psychophysiologic reactivity in asthmatic children: a cholinergically mediated confluence of pathways. *J Am Acad Child Adolesc Psychiatr* 1994;**33**:1236–45.

19. Godfrey S. Exercise and hyperventilation induced asthma. In: S Clark, S Godfrey, T Lee, eds. *Asthma.* London: Chapman and Hall, London, 2000.

20. Sandberg S, Paton JY, Ahola S, McCann DC, McGuinness D, Hilary CR, Oja H. The role of acute and chronic stress in asthma in children. *Lancet* 2000;**356**:982–7.

21. Rietveld S, Everaerd W, Creer TL. Stress-induced asthma: a review of research and potential mechanisms. *Clin Exp Allergy* 2000;**30**:1058–66.

22. Campbell TL. Family's impact on health: A critical review. *Fam Syst Med* 1986;**4**:135–329.

23. Dym B. The cybernetics of physical illness. *Fam Proc* 1987;**26**:35–48.

24. Gustafsson PA, Kjellman NI, Ludvigsson J, Cederblad M. Asthma and family interaction. *Arch Dis Child* 1987;**62**:258–63.

25. Lask B, Matthew D. Childhood asthma. A controlled trial of family psychotherapy. *Arch Dis Child* 1979;**54**:116–19.

26. Loader P, Kinston W, Stratford J. Is there a psychosomatogenic family? *J Fam Ther* 1980;**2**:311–26.

27. Minuchin S, Rosman BL. *Psychosomatic Families.* Harvard University Press, Cambridge, MA, 1978.

28. Pinkerton P. Childhood asthma. *Br J Hosp Med* 1971;September:331–8.

29. Baron C, Veilleux P, Lamarre A. The family of the asthmatic child. *Can J Psychiatr* 1992;**37**:12–16.

30. Coyne JC, Anderson BJ. The 'psychosomatic family' reconsidered II: Recalling a defective model and looking ahead. *J Marit Fam Ther* 1989;**15**:139–48.

31. Hermanns J, Florin I, Dietrich M, Rieger C, Hahlweg K. Maternal criticism, mother-child interaction, and bronchial asthma. *J Psychosom Res* 1989;**33**:469–76.

32. Purcell K, Brady K, Chai H, Muser J, Molk L, Gordon N, Means J. The effect on asthma in children of experimental separation from the family. *Psychosom Med* 1969;**31**:144–64.

33. Wirsching M, Stierlin H. *Krankheit und Familie. Konzepte, Forschungsergebnisse, Behandlingsmöglichkeiten.* Klett-Cotta, Stuttgart, 1982.

34. Rees L. The significance of parental attitudes in childhood asthma. *J Psychosom Res* 1963;**7**:181–90.

35. Zeiger RS. Secondary prevention of allergic disease: an adjunct to primary prevention. *Pediatr Allergy Immunol* 1995;**6**:127–38.

36. Fritz GK, Rubinstein S, Lewiston NJ. Psychological factors in fatal childhood asthma. *Am J Orthopsychiatr* 1987;**57**:253–7.

37. Strunk RC, Mrazek DA, Fuhrmann GS, LaBrecque JF. Physiologic and psychological characteristics associated with deaths due to asthma in childhood. A case-controlled study. *JAMA* 1985;**254**:1193–8.

38. Kravis LP. An analysis of fifteen childhood asthma fatalities. *J Allergy Clin Immunol* 1987;**80**:467–72.

39. Molfino NA, Nannini LJ, Rebuck AS, Slutsky AS. The fatality-prone asthmatic patient. Follow-up study after near-fatal attacks. *Chest* 1992;**101**:621–3.

40. Male I, Richter H, Seddon P. Children's perception of breathlessness in acute asthma. *Arch Dis Child* 2000:**83**;325–9.

41. Bonzett R, Dempsey SA, O'Connell DE, Wamboldt MZ. Symptom perception and respiratory sensation in asthma. *Am J Respir Crit Care Med* 2000;**162**:1178–82.

42. Koocher GP, McGrath ML, Gudas LJ. Typologies of nonadherence in cystic fibrosis. *J Dev Behav Pediatr* 1990;**11**:353–8.

43. Hindi-Alexander M. Symptom, perception and compliance. *Acta Paediatr. Latina* 1987;**60**(Suppl 4): 728–34.

44. Godding V, Kruth M, Jamart J. Joint consultation for high-risk asthmatic children and their families, with pediatrician and child psychiatrist as co-therapists: model and evaluation. *Fam Proc* 1997;**36**:265–80.

45. Gustafsson PA, Svedin CG. Cost Effectiveness: Family therapy in a pediatric setting. *Fam Syst Med* 1988;**6**:162–75.

46. Hodas GR, Honig PJ. An approach to psychiatric referrals in pediatric patients. Psychosomatic complaints. *Clin Pediatr (Phila)* 1983;**22**:167–72.

47. Huyse FJ. Consultation/liaison psychiatry: the state of the art and future developments. *Nord J Psychiatr* 1991;**45**:405–22.

48. Lask B. Psychological treatments for childhood asthma. *Arch Dis Child* 1992;**67**:891.

49. Kinsman RA, Dirks JF, Jones NF, Dahlhem NW. Anxiety reduction in asthma: four catches to general application. *Psychosom Med* 1980;**42**: 397–405.

50. Gustafsson PA, Kjellman N-IM, Cederblad M. Family therapy in the treatment of severe childhood asthma. *J Psychosom Res* 1986;**30**:369–74.

51. Rathner G, Messner K. Bronchial asthma and systematic family therapy: treatment concept, initial contact and therapy follow-up. *Pediatr Padol* 1992;**27**:A49–54.

52. Tal D, Gil-Spielberg C, Antonoesky H. Teaching families to cope with childhood asthma. *Fam Syst Med* **8**:135–44.

53. Lask B, Fosson A. *Childhood Illness: The Psychosomatic Approach*. John Wiley, Chichester, 1989.

54. Lask B, Kirk M. Family therapy for childhood asthma. *J Fam Ther* 1979;**1**:33–41.

55. Weinstein AG, Chenkin C, Faust D. Caring for the severely asthmatic child and family. I. The rationale for family systems integrated medical/ psychological treatment. *J Asthma* 1997;**34**:345–52.

56. Panton J, Barley EA. Family therapy for asthma in children (*Cochrane Review*). The Cochrane Library, 4, 2000. Update Software, Oxford.

57. Lehrer PM, Sargunaraj D, Hochron S. Psychological approaches to the treatment of asthma. *J Consult Clin Psychol* 1992;**60**:639–43.

58. Clark NM, Feldman CH, Evans D, Levison MJ, Wasilewski Y, Mellins RB. The impact of health education on frequency and cost of health care use by low income children with asthma. *J Allergy Clin Immunol* 1986;**78**:108–15.

59. Vazquez MI, Buceta JM. Effectiveness of self-management programmes and relaxation training in the treatment of bronchial asthma: relationships with trait anxiety and emotional attack triggers. *J Psychosom Res* 1993;**37**:71–81.

60. Long N. The future of technology in mental health services for children. *Clin Child Psychol Psychiatr* 2000;**5**:165–8.

61. Wjst M, Roell G, Dold S, *et al.* Psychosocial characteristics of asthma. *J Clin Epidemiol* 1996;**49**:461–6.

62. Wright RJ, Rodriquez M, Cohen S. Review of psychosocial stress and asthma: an integrated biopsychosocial approach. *Thorax* 1998;**53**:1066–74.

63. Huntly A, White AR, Ernst E. Relaxation therapies for asthma: a systematic review. *Thorax* 2002;**57**:127–31.

14

Preventing asthma

JOHN O WARNER AND JILL A WARNER

INTRODUCTION

The natural course of asthma appears to be unaffected by any therapeutic strategy hitherto available for the control of the disease. Under such circumstances, attention must focus on the opportunities for prevention of a disease which is chronic, life-long, and incurable, even though it can be very effectively controlled.

The levels of prevention may be considered along the same lines as for tuberculosis. There are, therefore, three separate components to the strategy (Table 14.1). *Primary prophylaxis* is introduced before there is any evidence of sensitization to factors that might be subsequently associated with the disease. As there is increasing evidence that allergic sensitization is a very common precursor to the development of asthma, much primary prophylaxis is focused on prevention of allergic sensitization in very

early life. *Secondary prophylaxis* is employed after primary sensitization to allergen has occurred but before there is any evidence of asthma. This is usually apparent in the first few months of life. Once individuals already manifest atopic disease such as eczema or allergic rhinitis but not yet asthma, the intervention is *tertiary prophylaxis*. Such intervention tends to focus on the first few years of life and includes pharmacotherapeutic interventions as well as immune modulation and environmental control. Once there is already evidence of both sensitization and asthma, intervention primarily involves appropriate allergen avoidance, which may be introduced at any stage in the disease process. However, taking the precedent of occupational asthma, the earlier it is introduced, the better the likely outcomes.[1]

A prerequisite for establishing any form of prevention is having reliable markers to predict progression of

Table 14.1 *Strategies for the prevention of asthma*

	Stage	Targets	Potential modalities
Primary prophylaxis	Before allergic sensitization	Fetus and newborn	Improved maternal health and nutrition No maternal smoking
Secondary prophylaxis	After sensitization but before disease	First months of life	Immune modulation Allergen avoidance
Tertiary prophylaxis	Sensitization and allergic disease but not asthma	Atopic eczema Allergic rhinitis Gastrointestinal food allergy	Pharmacotherapy Allergen immunotherapy Allergen avoidance
Therapy (non-pharmacological)	Established asthma	As early as possible after the onset of asthma	Allergen immunotherapy Allergen avoidance

disease. None have yet been identified which will predict asthma with high sensitivity and specificity. Therefore, a balance must be achieved between the rigours and the side effects of the intervention and the likelihood of preventing disease. The lower the probability that the disease will occur, the less justification there is for any intervention, unless it is non-invasive and without undue cost both socially and financially. However, much research has focused on the development of an index employing various risk factors present in the first years of life to predict with a high likelihood the development of asthma.[2–4]

PRIMARY PROPHYLAXIS

Time course of allergic sensitization

Many studies have now shown that the neonate is capable of mounting a significant immune response to environmental allergens.[5–7] Indeed virtually all neonates, both from atopic and non-atopic families, have T-cell responsiveness to inhalant and ingestant allergens.[8] It has been possible to demonstrate that specific allergen induced responses can occur from as early as 22 weeks of gestation.[9] For sensitization to have occurred, there must have been both allergen exposure via the mother and the presence of mature antigen presenting cells and T-lymphocytes in the fetus. That this is the case is not in doubt. Indeed, it has been clearly shown that the fetus is perfectly able to mount an antigen specific IgE response from as early as 11 weeks gestation, though primarily in the liver and subsequently lung and spleen, and only later in pregnancy from circulating cells.[10,11]

By virtue of the materno–placental–fetal interaction, there is a tendency for all immune responses in infancy to be allergy (Th2 lymphocyte) biased. Thus cytokines, predominantly manufactured by the placenta including IL-4, -10 and -13, will down-regulate maternal Th1 responses to foeto-paternal antigens and, therefore, protect the pregnancy. Those cytokines will also have an impact on the fetus.[12] It is, therefore, not surprising that there is a universal bias towards Th2 responsiveness in the neonate.[13] It is also not surprising that relatively minor perturbations of immune response between the mother, the placenta and

the fetus will alter the probability that a newborn will develop allergic disease and asthma by further biasing the immune response one way or the other. Many factors are involved, including the timing and dose of allergen exposure, the presence or absence of maternal atopy, atopic disease and whether or not the mother is also a smoker or has been exposed to particular microbial organisms at various stages during pregnancy (Table 14.2).

Timing of exposure

One study has identified that birch and timothy grass pollen exposure via the pregnant mother only produces T-cell sensitization of the fetus if this occurs during the first 6 months of a pregnancy. Exposure later in pregnancy appears to either result in immune suppression or tolerance.[14] We have some limited evidence that allergen can be transported across the amnion and is detectable in amniotic fluid.[15] Such allergen will be available to be swallowed by the fetus and could sensitize via the fetal gut. Later in pregnancy, allergen can be transported across the placenta complexed with IgG. Indeed, there may well be a concentrating effect as there is active transport of IgG from mother to fetus.[15–17] A number of studies have suggested that IgG allergen specific antibody might have a role in modulating the fetal immune response to allergen and perhaps even suppressing the development of allergy. This is certainly apparent from animal studies.[18] Furthermore, a high cord blood IgG antibody to cat dander and the major allergen of birch pollen has been associated with less atopic symptoms in children during the first 8 years of life, with an inverse relationship between cat IgE antibodies in children and their levels of cat IgG antibodies at birth.[19] Clearly IgG antibody levels in the cord blood reflect those of maternal IgG which, in turn, is a reflection of maternal allergen exposure. It, therefore, follows that if a mother is exposed to high levels of allergen, this will increase her IgG antibody level which, in turn, might confer some protection. One study of children of mothers who have undergone rye grass immunotherapy during pregnancy and consequently had high IgG antibody levels compared with children born to rye grass allergic mothers who were not treated with immunotherapy showed fewer positive skin tests to rye grass 3–12 years later in the offspring.[20]

Table 14.2 *Maternal factors potentially influencing primary allergic sensitization and asthma*

Maternal factor	Influence	Potential outcome on infant
Timing of allergen exposure in gestation	2nd trimester	Allergic sensitization
	3rd trimester	Tolerance
Maternal health and allergen exposure	Atopic → High IgG	Promotes sensitization
	High allergen → High IgE	Promotes tolerance
Good maternal nutrition	Rapid fetal growth	Higher risk of allergy and asthma
Maternal smoking	No effect on sensitization	Higher risk of wheezing

All these data fit together into a concept of dose and timing of allergen exposure in pregnancy as being critical. Early exposure during the second trimester of pregnancy, even to low doses, could produce sensitization via the fetal gut. Later in pregnancy, particularly if allergen exposure is high and maternal IgG antibody levels are consequently high, protection is more likely to occur. These data provide the first indication that antenatal immune modulation might reduce the frequency of sensitization. It also casts considerable doubt over the wisdom of making any recommendations on allergen avoidance during pregnancy in high-risk families. There is the potential that incomplete allergen avoidance might actually be more harmful than a sustained high dose exposure. Thus until more studies have been conducted, it would perhaps be better not to make any recommendations. Furthermore if this also involves food allergen avoidance, then there are intrinsic dangers in compromising nutrition during pregnancy which might also have an adverse effect on outcomes.[21]

Maternal health and nutrition

There is clearly an increased risk of asthma in the offspring of atopic mothers compared with atopic fathers, at least in early life and this effect is found even when the influence of under-reporting of atopy in fathers by mothers is taken into account.[22] The mechanism by which this occurs remains to be established. It could be a consequence of genetic priming but is far more likely to be due to the intra-uterine environment created by the atopic rather than the non-atopic mother. We have evidence that there are higher levels of IL-10 in the amniotic fluid of atopic than non-atopic mothers and also higher IgE levels.[12] The presence of IgE in the amniotic fluid which can be swallowed together with allergen can enhance allergic sensitization by a phenomenon known as IgE antigen focusing. Indeed, we have proposed that this phenomenon will facilitate sensitization of the fetus to maternal helminth and thereby protect the newborn from the obligate exposure to mothers' parasites.[23] Certainly newborn infants of helminth-infected mothers have specific Th2 biased immune responses to helminth antigen and IgE antibodies to these antigens.[11] It is possible that the molecular configuration of proteins in sensitizing allergens have counterparts in parasites leading to stimulation of the same immune response.

The implication from the above observation is that the higher the maternal IgE, the greater the probability of enhanced allergic sensitization in the second trimester of pregnancy. Treatments which could reduce levels might, therefore, be considered as potentially of benefit in primary prophylaxis. It would be of interest to consider whether the monoclonal IgE currently being developed for the treatment of asthma might have a role in this respect. Trials will be awaited.

Later in pregnancy, fetal growth and nutrition may have an impact on the risks of sensitization. There has

been an association demonstrated between large head circumference at birth and levels of total IgE at birth[24] and childhood[25] and even in adulthood.[26] There is even an association between asthma and particularly severe symptomatic asthma and large head circumference at birth.[25] It has been proposed that these observations are a consequence of a rapid fetal growth trajectory programmed in early pregnancy because of a good nutrient supply which cannot always be sustained later in pregnancy. This paradoxically means that problems of nutrition occur in the rapidly growing fetus later in pregnancy in relation to mothers who are well-nourished at conception. What component of the diet leads to a problem in later pregnancy remains to be established, if indeed the link is causal, and clinical trials of dietary supplementation will be of considerable interest.

The main focus on nutrients and allergy has been on polyunsaturated fatty acids. Diets rich in linolenic acid promote allergic responses.[24] It is well-established that fish oil supplementation decreases the production of pro-inflammatory mediators.[27] However, the effects on asthma are often modest or non-existent.[28] Whether there might be a greater impact if this intervention is employed early in pregnancy, remains to be established. Trials are currently in progress to investigate this hypothesis. Studies will also need to focus on anti-oxidants and the effects that they might have on the early development of asthma. It has been proposed that low fresh fruit and vegetable intake might have an impact on the severity of asthma rather than its prevalence.[29] Abnormal nutrient delivery may, however, also have an effect on lung growth and development. Thus subtle deficiencies of vitamin A can affect airway branching and lung epithelial cell differentiation.[30] There are also effects on surfactant protein production which, in turn, could affect airway host defence producing a greater probability of inflammation and an epithelial cell defect.[31] Collectively, the two latter phenomena are the key immuno-histopathological changes that occur in asthma. There is, therefore, a potential for a wide range of nutrients to have an impact on not only allergic sensitization but also airway development and many will need to be examined as part of a primary asthma prevention strategy.

Tobacco smoke

The health effects of parental smoking on the respiratory health of children has been extensively reviewed.[32] There are independent contributions of pre- and postnatal smoking.[33] Studies have shown clearly that lung function of newborns of smoking and non-smoking mothers differ significantly.[34,35] Furthermore, the infants of smoking mothers are four times more likely to have developed wheezing illnesses in the first year of life.[35] This suggests that at least one of the effects of antenatal smoking is on airway development. However, there is little evidence on meta-analysis that maternal smoking during pregnancy has any effect on allergic sensitization.[36] Nevertheless, the data are so secure in relation to lung growth that the single most important recommendation to make in primary prophylaxis against wheezing illnesses is avoiding pregnancy smoking.

SECONDARY PROPHYLAXIS

The main focus of secondary prophylaxis has been on allergen avoidance and most trials have been done in relation to ingestants with little information on inhalants. However, most recent attention has been directed to the so-called hygiene hypothesis and the potential that there might be intervention strategies which will switch the neonate's Th2 allergic biased immune response postnatally. Even when such strategies are introduced in the first days of life, they are now considered as secondary prophylaxis, because of evidence of T-cell allergen sensitization at birth.[5-9]

Allergen avoidance

There is a general consensus that postnatal allergen avoidance involving primarily breast-feeding has been associated with a reduced prevalence or delayed onset of food allergy and atopic dermatitis in the first 2 years of life, but the majority of studies have shown no protective effects on later airway disease.[37,38] One study has shown a sustained effect of breast-feeding with a subsequent significant effect on asthma.[39] It is difficult to reconcile these differences, though the latter study was initiated some 15 years earlier than most subsequent studies which have failed to show an effect on asthma or even an adverse effect in children from high risk families.[39a] It remains to be seen whether more attention to aeroallergen avoidance immediately postnatally will have any impact on airway disease. However, the Isle of Wight study[37] did attempt to combine dietary manipulation with house-dust mite avoidance and there was still no effect on asthma prevalence at 4 years of age. Certainly more studies are required.

The hygiene hypothesis (Table 14.3 and Chapter 2)

The hygiene hypothesis suggests that the major factor enhancing down-regulation of the weak Th2 allergy-promoting immune response at birth is exposure to environmental microbial antigens. This was first suggested in 1989 when an inverse relationship was found between birth order in families and the prevalence of hay fever. It was proposed that infections in early infancy brought home by older siblings modified the risk of allergy.[40] More recent data substantiate this observation and also show that day care attendance in the first 6 months of life reduces the subsequent prevalence of wheezing illnesses, raised serum IgE and skin test reactivity to any allergen.[41] It is proposed that early infection, whether by viruses or bacteria, will tend to stimulate Th1 immune responsiveness which, if it occurs early enough postnatally, will switch off the weak Th2 biased response of all newborn babies to allergens.[42]

Several other studies support the hygiene hypothesis. In Japan, strong tuberculin responsiveness reflecting a good Th1 response was associated with a significantly reduced odds ratio for asthma and raised IgE levels[43] and an international observational study related increasing regional notification rates for tuberculosis with decreasing regional prevalence of wheezing illnesses.[44] Similarly in Sweden, tuberculin responsiveness was inversely related to atopy in children provided BCG was given in early life but had no effect if the BCG was given in adolescence.[45] In contrast, one study of high-risk children showed no effect on atopy of BCG in early infancy.[46] An intervention trial administering BCG in the neonatal period would establish whether this has any impact on later atopic disease.

Similar inverse relationships have been shown between atopy and prior early life exposure to respiratory tract infections,[47] measles[48] and either helicobacter, hepatitis A or toxoplasma.[49] These observations are in keeping with those found in the day care study.[41] It might also explain the lower prevalence of atopy in children born into traditional farming families who have been observed to have a different microbial flora in the gut.[50-52] Indeed, it has

Table 14.3 *Some evidence in support of the hygiene hypothesis*

Evidence	Effect	Refs
Increasing birth order	Decreasing hay fever and asthma	40, 41
Day care attendance in first 6 months	Decreased atopy and asthma	41
Tuberculin responsiveness and early life BCG	Inversely related to asthma and raised IgE prevalence	43, 44, 45
Early infections – measles, Toxoplasma, Hepatitis A, Helicobacter	Less atopy	48, 49
Farmers' children	Less atopy, hay fever, and asthma	51, 52
Early antibiotic usage	Increased atopy and asthma	54, 55
Anthroposophic lifestyle	Less atopy	56

been suggested that the most important normal influence in reducing atopic disease is the development of satisfactory intestinal microbial flora.[53]

The first prospective controlled intervention study which addresses the hygiene hypothesis in relation to the prevention of atopic disease has now been published.[53a] The use of a probiotic (lactobacillus GG) prenatally to mothers from 'atopic families' and postnatally to the infants up to 6 months of age resulted in half the cumulative prevalence of atopic eczema by 2 years of age compared with the placebo group. However, this study did not demonstrate any differences in allergic sensitization based on skin tests or IgE antibody measurements and the children were too young to assess whether it had any impact on asthma or allergic rhinitis.

Additional components of an affluent community which might also impact on the hygiene hypothesis are the excessive early use of antibiotics, which has again been suggested to increase prevalence of atopy.[54,55] A suggestion that even early immunizations by reducing early infections also are associated with a higher risk of atopy[54] has not been confirmed by other studies.[55a] If verified, it could explain the lower prevalences of atopy in children of families with an anthroposophic lifestyle which includes an avoidance of immunizations and also, indeed, much other medical treatment.[56] However, these observations must not be taken to indicate that immunizations should be avoided but merely that an attempt should be made to identify which components of active infection might be distilled out to utilize in some form of immune modulation program to reduce prevalence of atopy whilst, at the same time, continuing with immunizations to prevent infection.

A number of groups have begun to develop Th1 immunoadjuvants, taking the form of either DNA vaccines or extracts of particular organisms such as killed listeria which have a particularly potent effect on the Th1 immune response.[57–60] All approaches would potentially restore a cytokine imbalance related to response to allergen that has commonly been demonstrated at birth. There are, however, intrinsic risks in an excessive promotion of a Th1 response at the expense of a Th2 response. The risks of Th1-mediated immune disorders such as insulin dependent diabetes mellitus, or inflammatory bowel disease may increase. In the developing world, where helminth infections are common, IgE-dependent host defences may be rendered less effective.

TERTIARY PROPHYLAXIS

Allergen immunotherapy

Whilst still a contentious approach to the treatment of allergic disease, it is clear from meta-analyses that allergen immunotherapy can reduce asthma symptoms compared with placebo.[61] It has clearly been demonstrated that this form of therapy orchestrates an immunological switch of allergen induced cytokine profiles from Th2 to Th1 pattern.[62,63] This could, therefore, be seen as another potential early intervention strategy. Hitherto, little evidence is available on early use. However, one non-randomized study in 6-year-old asthmatic children demonstrated that specific immunotherapy reduced the development of new allergen sensitizations over a 3-year follow-up period.[64] This has been confirmed for house-dust mite immunotherapy.[64a] A trial is currently being conducted in Europe known as the Preventive Allergy Treatment study (PAT) which has generated a few preliminary results. After 3 years of pollen immunotherapy with pure seasonal allergic rhinitis, fewer children have subsequently developed asthma than in an untreated parallel control group.[65] This approach may, therefore, have some value as secondary prophylaxis, but has never been consistently employed in any children under 5 years of age. Prospects for allergen immunotherapy have recently been reviewed.[115]

Pharmacotherapy

Three studies have investigated the use of *antihistamines* in the prevention of asthma in children. One employed ketotifen or placebo in a double-blind randomized trial conducted over a 1-year period in 121 infants with atopic eczema.[66] This showed that the active treatment significantly reduced the prevalence of asthma. However, the beneficial effect was only observed in those with a raised total IgE at recruitment. A second much larger study in similar infants compared cetirizine with placebo. This study also demonstrated a significant reduction in the prevalence of asthma over an 18-month period of active treatment compared with placebo, but only in those with evidence of house-dust mite or grass pollen sensitivity which constituted 20% of the total population.[67] A third study used ketotifen in infants with a family history of allergy and a raised total IgE level. This intervention also significantly reduced the subsequent prevalence of wheezing illnesses.[68]

The mechanism of action by which antihistamines, such as ketotifen or cetirizine, might have an effect in preventing the development of asthma in already sensitized children is clearly important to identify. One proposition is that antihistamine may prevent allergen induced up-regulation of adhesion molecules such as ICAM-1 and VCAM-1 which in turn will, therefore, inhibit eosinophil trafficking into allergen provoked tissues such as the airway.[69] It will clearly be of considerable interest to investigate other pharmacotherapeutic interventions that might have similar effects in inhibiting eosinophil trafficking. One candidate in this respect would be *leukotriene receptor antagonists*.[70]

NON-PHARMACOLOGICAL THERAPY (Table 14.4)

Pollutant avoidance

It is important to identify non-allergenic triggers which might be avoided for the benefit of children with established asthma. A number of studies have shown that exposure to environmental tobacco smoke (ETS) has deleterious effects on asthma control. Indeed, the Institute of Medicine in the USA reviewed associations between ETS and respiratory illnesses. They found a clear causal relationship between ETS exposure and exacerbations of asthma in preschool children with an estimated 30% increased frequency of symptoms.[71] One study showed a significant effect of maternal smoking on bronchial hyperresponsiveness and severity of symptoms in children with asthma.[72] The same authors were able to show that if the mothers stopped smoking, there was a decrease in asthma severity in their children compared with those whose mothers who continued to smoke.[73] This provides the one piece of evidence that removal of ETS will result in improvement.

There is evidence from epidemiological studies that respiratory symptoms occur more frequently in homes employing unusual forms of heating as well as those where there is significant exposure to ETS.[74] Other surveys have suggested increased risks of respiratory symptoms in children resident in homes using gas cookers. A meta-analysis estimated that the odds of respiratory illness was 20% higher in such children.[75] However, evidence in support of this is not very consistent and recent studies with large numbers of subjects would probably negate the previously positive association on meta-analysis.[74,76] Thus other than avoidance of ETS, it is difficult on the basis of evidence to make any recommendation about other forms of modification of home environment in relation to gaseous pollutants.

A major review through the Department of Health in the UK into associations between outdoor air pollution and asthma came to the conclusion that there was little or no association between the regional distribution of asthma and that of air pollution. There was no convincing evidence that asthma was more common in high pollution urban areas compared with rural areas. However, it was accepted that day-to-day fluctuations in air pollution levels would have a small effect on lung function which, particularly in individuals with severe asthma, may produce exacerbation or need for increased medication. It was also accepted that short-term fluctuations in levels of outdoor air pollutants could be responsible for changes in hospital admissions and accident and emergency attendances for asthma. However overall the effects, if any, were considered to be small and relatively unimportant by comparison with other factors such as infections and allergens,[77] although a role of air pollution in the inception (i.e. incidence) of asthma cannot be ruled out.

Aero-allergen avoidance

In occupational asthma, the more rapid the removal from allergen exposure, the more favourable the outcome. Occupational asthma can resolve completely after the occupational allergen exposure ceases, if avoidance is introduced soon after the onset of symptoms. By analogy, the earlier allergen avoidance is introduced in an atopic

Table 14.4 *Non-pharmacological approaches to asthma treatment*

Factor	Strategy	Problems
Environmental tobacco smoke avoidance	No smoking in house Monitor urinary cotinine	Ubiquitous Poor parental adherence
House-dust mite avoidance	Bedding barrier systems Ventilation/dehumidification	Disputed efficacy
Animal allergens (particularly cat and dog) avoidance	Remove pets from home or regular pet washing	Ubiquitous Poor adherence Little evidence base
Pollens and moulds avoidance	Filters in homes Hoods	Impractical
Food avoidance	Dietary adjustment	Rarely necessary for asthma alone Nutritional and psychosocial consequences
Pollutant avoidance	Filters and ventilation systems in homes	Relevance and importance in asthma disputed
Reduce allergen sensitivity	Allergen immunotherapy Anti-IgE	Risk/benefits and cost/benefits compared to pharmacotherapy unfavourable

asthmatic, the greater the potential benefit. After prolonged exposure, the asthmatic process may well become so well established that avoidance will have no effect.

Severity of asthma symptoms can be related to increased exposure to relevant allergens.[78] Indeed, studies have also been able to show that allergen exposure is a risk for acute asthma and emergency room visits.[79] The implication of such observations is that reduction of exposure would reduce asthma severity and thereby recourse to medical services. However, evidence for the latter is a little more difficult to access, predominantly because allergen avoidance techniques have been far from perfect. Nevertheless, there are sufficient studies to support the assertion that allergen avoidance should be an integral part of asthma management strategies.

House-dust mites

The World Health Organization has endorsed the concept that house-dust mite allergy is a universal problem in association with asthma.[80] However, a recent meta-analysis of controlled house-dust mite avoidance trials suggested that this approach was of marginal benefit in the treatment of asthma.[81] However, this meta-analysis was based on single interventions and included some that did not even reduce house mite levels with others that may well be effective. Others have commented that the meta-analysis was unsatisfactory in its conclusion.[82] Indeed, an independent systematic review of essentially the same data sets came to the conclusion that house-dust mite avoidance is effective in asthma.[83] Better and longer trials are required before firm recommendations can be given.

Recently, one of us reviewed all controlled studies that have attempted house mite avoidance and came to the conclusion that a number of strategies were clearly efficacious (Table 14.5). These included encasing of bedding, removal of carpets and soft furnishings, and the use of high efficiency vacuum cleaners. Rather less effect was identified from the use of acaracides and insufficient studies are being conducted on the use of dehumidification systems.[84] Perhaps the most compelling evidence that house-dust mite avoidance will be effective comes from studies at *high altitude* where mite levels are very low indeed. Children with mite sensitivity taken to high altitude have dramatic reductions in symptoms, requirements for pharmacotherapy, bronchial hyperresponsiveness and both total IgE and dust mite specific IgE levels. This occurs within 3 months of avoidance and there is furthermore even a reduction in hyperresponsiveness induced by a house mite challenge.[85] However, the problem is rapid relapse after return to a home environment with high mite exposure. This should encourage further controlled trials using combined strategies which may have a far greater chance of being efficacious.

The use of *bedding encasings* has achieved the most consistent beneficial results, both in reducing mite allergen and improving symptoms.[86–88] However, these studies did not employ encasings alone but variously added effective vacuuming and the use of acaracides. It is clear that in order to achieve adequate reduction in mite levels, it is important to cover all components of the bedding, namely the mattress, pillow and duvet.[89]

Effective *vacuuming* may reduce mite levels, particularly if they are of high efficiency and contain appropriate filters. However, it is rather more difficult to demonstrate clinical efficacy.[90] Indeed, a recent study remarkably showed that a high efficiency vacuum cleaner can indeed improve clinical symptoms in house mite sensitive asthmatics. However, the effect appeared to relate to reductions in cat rather than house mite allergen and only occurred in the individuals who were also cat allergic.[91] While the use of acaracides can be shown to reduce house mite allergen levels, clinical efficacy is rather more difficult to demonstrate.[86,92] Other strategies that have been investigated in trials include *dehumidification* and the use of mechanical ventilation systems.[93] While this latter British study failed to show any effect either on mite allergen levels or symptoms, studies using mechanical ventilation systems in other countries, where perhaps it is possible to reduce humidity more easily, have been more successful.[94] Even in the UK, this approach may achieve efficacy if combined with additional measures such as high efficiency vacuuming.[95] *Other techniques*, such as high temperature washing, freezing with liquid nitrogen, the use of electric blanket and exposure to direct sunlight have all been shown to reduce mite levels but hitherto none has proved to have efficacy in clinical trials.[84]

Thus in summary, effective dust mite control requires a combination of bedding encasings, removal of carpets,

Table 14.5 *House-dust mite avoidance strategies*

	Reduction in allergen	Clinical efficacy
Barrier bedding covers	Yes	Effective
Acaricides/denaturants	Yes	Minimal effect
High performance vacuum cleaners	Yes	Too few trials
Dehumidifiers/ventilation systems	Results vary depending on geographical location	
Filtration systems	Small effect	Inadequate trials
Ionizers	Small effect	None
Freezing toys and bedding	Yes	No trials

the use of high efficiency vacuum cleaners and perhaps attempts at reducing humidity either by dehumidification or effective ventilation.

Animal allergen

Domestic pets are a significant source of allergens. The principle culprits are cats and dogs which often have the freedom to roam the whole domestic environment, including bedrooms, and spread their allergen generously throughout. Most allergen is on particles of very small size which are able to remain airborne for long periods and to spread way beyond the original source. Thus both cat and dog allergens are widely distributed in public places, presumably either airborne or carried on the clothing of pet owners.[96] Indeed in environments where house-dust mite is relatively less prevalent, such as Northern Sweden, the presence of cat and dog allergen has been implicated as the major allergic stimulus to contribute to the development and aggravation of asthma in such environments.[97] Cat allergen can be detected in air samples from most if not all homes, even those which have not contained a cat.[98] It is, therefore, not surprising that cat and dog allergy is very common in asthmatic children in many diverse environments, being second only to house-dust mite in terms of frequency of sensitization in the UK, but occurring even in environments where house-dust mite does not exist.[99] Exposure also occurs in schools and it has been shown that children of pet owning families will transport sufficient allergen on their clothing to have an adverse effect on bronchial responsiveness and symptoms in allergic asthmatic children in the same classroom.[100,101a] This makes control of cat or dog allergen exposure extremely difficult. Furthermore, there are no good published controlled studies demonstrating clinical benefits from appropriate environmental modification in cat or dog allergic asthmatic children. One might assume that removal of an animal from the home will lead to clinical improvement. However, allergen levels remain high for years after removal.[101,102] Reduction in allergen levels may only be sufficient if additional measures such as efficient vacuuming are carried out.[91] Furthermore, changing bedding or the use of impermeable encasements may also be important as allergen can also be detected in mattresses for years after an animal has been removed.[103]

It has been suggested that reductions might be achieved in allergen levels even with the animal remaining in the home. As the allergen is not the dander but comes from saliva and sebaceous secretions, regular washing of cats together with efficient vacuum cleaning, removal of furnishings and air filtration, can achieve significant reductions. However, the study describing this effect did not measure clinical outcomes.[104] Only one published trial has convincingly shown that reduction of cat allergen exposure in cat allergic individuals can lead to clinical improvement and this occurred in a study which did not have this outcome as its primary objective. The study had initially been designed to attempt to demonstrate an effect in reduction of house mite levels based on the use of high efficiency vacuum cleaners.[91] More research is required to justify the common recommendation about cat and dog avoidance in allergic individuals.

Other allergens

In some environments world-wide, cockroach allergy is common occurring particularly in inner city deprived populations.[105] In such populations, cockroach exposure in cockroach-sensitive children is considered to have a major impact on morbidity in terms of hospitalizations, missed days from schooling and sleepless nights.[106] There is no evidence that attempts at extermination of the cockroach have much effect on cockroach allergen levels and there are no published studies on clinical outcomes.

Mould allergens

A vast range of different mould species can be found both in the indoor and outdoor environment. Indoors, *Aspergillus* and *Penicillium* species predominate. They tend to be found in damp homes with condensation problems. However, the frequency of sensitivity to mould allergens is relatively low and in many environments where there are high mould counts in household dust, there are also high levels of house-dust mite allergen. Thus attempts at mould removal have not been a major focus for intervention but reduction of humidity could be of benefit in relation to both house mite and mould levels.

Outdoor allergens

The major outdoor allergens in temperate climates are grass and tree pollens, while in more arid environments, mould spores such as *Alternaria* predominate.[107,108] Although impossible to avoid completely, it has been suggested that exposure might be reduced by keeping windows and doors closed while the pollen and/or mould counts are high. However, evidence of efficacy is lacking and perhaps the only guidance that can be offered is to intensify pharmacotherapy on a basis of predicted pollen and mould spore counts.

Food allergy

As indicated in the chapter on allergy, food allergy is a rare phenomenon in children with isolated asthma. However where food allergy has been demonstrated convincingly by double-blind placebo controlled challenge, it is necessary to impose an avoidance diet.[109] Such avoidance is particularly imperative in children who have reported acute anaphylactic type reactions to food where the association with asthma confers a higher risk of future fatal reactions.[110]

There is a common public perception that food additives are a cause of asthma exacerbation. However, it is extremely difficult to substantiate such claims and where double-blind placebo controlled challenges have been conducted, it has been rare to substantiate the patients' perceptions.[111]

Preventing infective exacerbations

Most severe exacerbations of asthma and of wheeze in young children are triggered by viral infection (Chapter 7b). Prospects for prevention are huge, but largely unrealized. Influenza vaccination is recommended, and does not exacerbate existing asthma.[112] Active immunization against RSV infection in infancy is likely to be available soon, but current passive techniques have limited benefits.[113]

SUMMARY

Prevention of asthma by environmental modification remains an attractive hypothetical approach to both the prevention and management of asthma. Many parents now demand explanations for the cause of their child's asthma and will not be satisfied with merely administering pharmacotherapy without being empowered to attempt to control their child's disease by environmental modification. Unfortunately, however, reduction of the exposure to key allergens such as house-dust mite, the allergens of cat and dog and indeed outdoor allergens is either very difficult or impossible. Evidence that avoidance has any impact on clinical outcomes in childhood asthma is scanty or non-existent. However given the public demand for such approaches, it is incumbent on paediatricians to conduct more trials utilising more recent insights into potential effective allergen reduction measures. At present, perhaps the only confident recommendation for avoidance that can be made from an evidence base is that of pregnancy and postnatal environmental tobacco smoke exposure.

Recent insights into the early life origins of asthma may well, however, identify other therapeutic approaches which will have effects in preventing the onset of disease.

REFERENCES

1. Paggiaro PL, Vagaggini B, Bacci E, *et al*. Prognosis of occupational asthma. *Europ Respir J* 1994;**7**:761–7.
2. Castro-Rodriguez JA, Holberg CJ, Wright AL, Martinez FD. A clinical index to define risk of asthma in young children with recurrent wheezing. *Am J Respir Crit Care Med* 2000;**162**:1403–6.
3. Warner JO, Warner JA, Clough JB, *et al*. Markers of allergy and inflammation. *Pediatr Allergy Immunol* 1998;**9**(Suppl 11):53–7.
4. Clough JB, Keeping KA, Edwards LC, *et al*. Can we predict which wheezy infants will continue to wheeze? *Am J Respir Crit Care Med* 1999;**160**: 1473–80.
5. Warner JA, Miles EA, Jones AC, *et al*. Is deficiency of interferon-gamma production by allergen triggered cord blood cells a predictor of atopic eczema? *Clin Exp Allergy* 1994;**24**:423–30.
6. Prescott SL, Macaubas C, Holt BJ, *et al*. Transplacental priming of the human immune system to environmental allergens: universal skewing of initial T cell responses towards the Th-2 cytokine profile. *J Immunol* 1998;**160**: 4730–7.
7. Kondo N, Cubiyashi Y, Shinoda S, *et al*. Cord blood lymphocyte responses to food antigens for the prediction of allergic disease. *Arch Dis Child* 1992;**67**:1003–7.
8. Upham JW, Holt BJ, Baron-Hoy MJ, *et al*. Inhalant allergen specific T cell reactivity is detectable in close to 100% of atopic and normal individuals: Covert responses are unmasked by serum free medium. *Clin Exp Allergy* 1995;**25**:634–42.
9. Jones CA, Miles EA, Warner JO, *et al*. Foetal peripheral blood mononuclear cell proliferative responses to mitogenic and allergenic stimulae during gestation. *Pediatr Allergy Immunol* 1996;**7**:109–16.
10. Miller DL, Hirvonen T, Gitlin D. Synthesis of IgE by the human conceptus. *J Allergy Clin Immunol* 1973;**52**:182–8.
11. King CL, Malhotra I, Mungai B, *et al*. B cell sensitization to helminthic infection develops *in utero* in humans. *J Immunol* 1998;**160**:3578–84.
12. Jones CA, Holloway JA, Warner JO. Does atopic disease start in foetal life. *Allergy* 2000;**55**:2–10.
13. Prescott SL, Macaubas C, Smallacombe T, *et al*. Development of allergen specific T cell memory in atopic and normal children. *Lancet* 1999; **353**:196–200.
14. Van Duren-Schmidt K, Pichler J, Ebner C, *et al*. Prenatal contact with inhalant allergens. *Pediatr Res* 1997;**41**:128–31.
15. Holloway JA, Warner JO, Vance GHS, Diaper ND, Warner JA, Jones CA. Two pathways of allergen passage to the human foetus with potential to initiate allergic priming. *Lancet* 2000;**356**:1900–2.
16. Malek A, Sager R, Schneider H. Transport of proteins across the human placenta. *Am J Reprod Immunol* 1998;**40**:347–51.
17. Casas R, Bjorksten B. Detection of fel d 1-IgG immune complexes in the cord blood and sera from allergic and non allergic mothers. *Pediatr Allergy Immunol* 2001;**12**:59–64.
18. Jarrett EEE, Hall E. IgE suppression by maternal IgG. *Immunology* 1983;**48**:49–58.

19. Jenmalm MC, Bjorksten B. Cord blood levels of immunoglobulin G subclass antibodies to food and inhalant allergens in relation to maternal atopy and the development of atopic disease during the first 8 years of life. *Clin Exp Allergy* 2000;**30**:34–40.

20. Glovsky MM, Ghekiere L, Rejzek E. Effect of maternal immunotherapy on immediate skin test reactivity, specific rye IgG and IgE antibody and total IgE of the children. *Ann Allergy* 1991;**67**:21–4.

21. Falth-Magnusson K, Oman H, Kjellman N-IM. Development of atopic disease in babies whose mothers were on exclusion diet during pregnancy – a randomised study. *J Allergy Clin Immunol* 1987;**80**:868–75.

22. Bergmann RL, Edenharter G, Bergmann K, *et al.* Predictability of early atopy by cord blood IgE and parental history. *Clin Exp Allergy* 1997;**27**:752–60.

23. Jones CA, Warner JA, Warner JO. Foetal swallowing of IgE letter. *Lancet* 1998;**351**:1859.

24. Langley-Evans S. Foetal programming of immune function and respiratory disease editorial; comment. *Clin Exp Allergy* 1997;**27**:1377–9.

25. Gregory A, Doull I, Pearce N, *et al.* The relationship between anthropometric measurements at birth: asthma and atopy in childhood. *Clin Exp Allergy* 1999;**29**:330–3.

26. Godfrey KM, Barker DJ, Osmond C. Disproportionate foetal growth and raised IgE concentration in adult life see comments. *Clin Exp Allergy* 1994;**24**:641–8.

27. Arm JP, Horton CE, Spur BW, Mencia-Huerta JM, Lee TH. The effects of dietary supplementation with fish oil lipids on the airways response to inhaled allergen in bronchial asthma. *Am Rev Respir Dis* 1989;**139**:1395–400.

28. Hodge L, Salome CM, Hughes JM, *et al.* Effect of dietary intake of omega-3 and omega-6 fatty acids on severity of asthma in children. *Eur Respir J* 1998;**11**:361–5.

29. Butland BK, Strachan DP, Anderson HR. Fresh fruit intake and asthma symptoms in young British adults: confounding or effect modification by smoking? *Eur Respir J* 1999;**13**:744–50.

30. Cardoso WV, Williams MC, Mitsialis SA, Joyce-Brady M, Rishi AK, Brody JS. Retinoic acid induces changes in the pattern of airway branching and alters epithelial cell differentiation in the developing lung *in vitro*. *Am J Respir Cell Mol Biol* 1995;**12**:464–76.

31. Chailley-Heu B, Chelly N, Lelievre-Pegorier M, Barlier-Mur AM, Merlet-Benichou C, Bourbon JR. Mild vitamin A deficiency delays foetal lung maturation in the rat. *Am J Respir Cell Mol Biol* 1999;**21**:89–96.

32. Cook DG, Strachan DP. Health effects of passive smoking–10: Summary of effects of parental smoking on the respiratory health of children and implications for research. *Thorax* 1999;**54**:357–66.

33. Institute for Environment and Health 2002 (in press).

34. Martinez FD, Wright AL, Taussig LM, Holberg CJ, Halonen M, Morgan WJ. Asthma and wheezing in the first six years of life. The Group Health Medical Associates. *N Engl J Med* 1995;**332**:133–8.

35. Dezateux C, Stocks J, Dundas I, Fletcher ME. Impaired airway function and wheezing in infancy: the influence of maternal smoking and a genetic predisposition to asthma. *Am J Respir Crit Care Med* 1999;**159**:403–10.

36. Strachan DP, Cook DG. Health effects of passive smoking. Parental smoking and childhood asthma: longitudinal and case-control studies. *Thorax* 1998;**53**:204–12.

37. Hide DW, Matthews S, Tariq S, Arshad SH. Allergen avoidance in infancy and allergy at 4 years of age. *Allergy* 1996;**51**:89–93.

38. Zeiger RS, Heller S, Mellon MH, Halsey JF, Hamburger RN, Sampson HA. Genetic and environmental factors affecting the development of atopy through age 4 in children of atopic parents: a prospective randomized study of food allergen avoidance. *Pediatr Allergy Immunol* 1992;**3**:110–27.

39. Saarinen UM, Kajosaari M. Breastfeeding as prophylaxis against atopic disease: prospective follow-up study until 17 years old. *Lancet* 1995;**346**:1065–9.

39a. Wright AL, Holberg CJ, Taussig LM, Martinez FD. Factors influencing the relation of infant feeding to asthma and recurrent wheeze in childhood. *Thorax* 2001;**56**:192–7.

40. Strachan DP. Hay fever, hygiene, and house-hold size. *Br Med J* 1989;**299**:1259–60.

41. Ball TM, Castro-Rodriguez JA, Griffith KA, *et al.* Siblings, day-care attendance, and the risk of asthma and wheezing during childhood. *N Engl J Med* 2000;**343**:538–43.

42. Folkerts G, Walzl G, Openshaw PJM. Do childhood infections teach the immune system not to be allergic? *Immunol Today* 2000;**21**:118–20.

43. Shirakawa T, Enomota T, Shimazu S, *et al.* The inverse association between tuberculin responses and atopic disorder. *Science* 1997;**775**:77–9.

44. Von Mutius E, Pearce N, Beasley R, *et al.* International patterns of tuberculosis and the prevalence of symptoms of asthma, rhinitis and eczema. *Thorax* 2000;**55**:440–53.

45. Strannegard IL, Larsson LO, Wennergren G, *et al.* Prevalence of allergy in children in relation to prior BCG vaccination and infection with atypical micobacteria. *Allergy* 1998;**3**:240–54.

46. Alm JS, Lilja G, Pershagen G, Scheynius A. Early BCG vaccination and development of atopy. *Lancet* 1997;**350**:400–3.

47. Martinez FD, Stern DA, Wright AL, *et al.* Association of non-wheezing low respiratory tract illnesses in early life with persistent diminished serum IgE levels. *Thorax* 1995;**50**:67–72.

48. Shaheen SO, Aaby P, Hall AJ, Barker DJ, Heyes CB, Shiell AW, *et al.* Measles and atopy in Guinea-Bissau. *Lancet* 1996;**347**:1792–6.

49. Matricardi PM, Rosmini F, Ferigno L, *et al.* Exposure to food borne and oro-fecal microbes vs. airborne viruses in relation to atopy and allergic asthma: epidemiological study. *Br Med J* 2000;**320**:412–16.

50. Bjorksten B, Naaber P, Sepp E, Mikelsaar M. The intestinal microflora in allergic Estonian and Swedish 2-year old children. *Clin Exp Allergy* 1999;**29**:342–6.

51. Von Ehrenstein OS, Von Mutius E, Illi S, Baumann L, Bohm O, Von Kries R. Reduced risk of hay fever and asthma among children of farmers. *Clin Exp Allergy* 2000;**30**:187–93.

52. Riedler J, Eder W, Oberfeld G, Schreuer M. Austrian children living on a farm have less hay fever, asthma and allergic sensitization. *Clin Exp Allergy* 2000;**30**:194–200.

53. Holt PG, Sly PD, Bjorksten B. Atopy versus infectious diseases in childhood; a question of balance. *Pediatr Allergy Immunol* 1997;**8**:53–8.

53a. Kalliomaki M, Salminen S, Arvilommi H, Kero P, Koskinen P, Isolauri E. Probiotics in primary prevention of atopic disease: a randomised placebo-controlled trial. *Lancet* 2001;**357**: 1076–9.

54. Farooqi IS, Hopkin JM. Early childhood atopy and infection and atopic disorder. *Thorax* 1998;**53**:927–32.

55. Drostre JHJ, Wieringa MH, Weyler JJ, *et al.* Does the use of antibiotics in early childhood increase the risk of asthma in allergic disease? *Clin Exp Allergy* 2000; **30**:1547–53.

55a. Wickens K, Crane J, Kemp T, *et al.* A case–control study of risk factors for asthma in New Zealand children. *Aust NZ J Public Health* 2001;**25**:44–9.

56. Alm JS, Schwartz J, Lilja G, *et al.* Atopy in children of families with an anthroposophic lifestyle. *Lancet* 1999;**353**:1485–8.

57. Holt PG. Immuno-prophylaxis of atopy: light at the end of the tunnel? *Immunol Today* 1994;**15**:484–9.

58. Umetsu DT, DeKruyff RH. Th1 and Th2 CD4+cells in human allergic diseases. *J Allergy Clin Immunol* 1997;**100**:1–6.

59. Kline JN. Effects of CpG DNA on Th1/Th2 balance in asthma. *Curr Top Microbiol Immunol* 2000;**247**: 211–25.

60. Metzger WJ, Nyce JW. Oligonucleotide therapy of allergic asthma. *J Allergy Clin Immunol* 1999;**104**:260–6.

61. Abramson MJ, Puy RM, Weiner JM. Allergen immunotherapy for asthma (Cochrane Review). In: The Cochrane library, 4. Oxford: Update Software, 2001.

62. Varney VA, Hamid QA, Gaga M, *et al.* Influence of grass pollen immunotherapy on cellular infiltration and cytokine mRNA expression during allergen induced late phase cutaneous responses. *J Clin Invest* 1993;**92**:644–51.

63. Durham SR, Walker SM, Varga E-M, *et al.* Long term clinical efficacy of grass pollen immunotherapy. *New Engl J Med* 1999;**341**:468–75.

64. Des-Roches A, Paradis L, Menardo J-L, *et al.* Immunotherapy with a standardised *Dermatophagoides pteronyssinus* extract VI specific immunotherapy prevents the onset of new sensitizations in children. *J Allergy Clin Immunol* 1997;**99**:450–3.

64a. Panjo GP, Barberio G, DeLuca FR, Morabito L, Parmiani S. Prevention of new sensitisation in asthmatic children mono sensitised to house-dust mite by specific immunotherapy. *Clin Exp All* 2001;**31**:1392–7.

65. Möler C, Dreborg S, Ferdousi HA, *et al.* Pollen immunotherapy reduces the development of asthma in children with seasonal rhinoconjunctivitis (the PAT-study). *J Allergy Clin Immunol* 2002;**109**:251–256.

66. Iikura Y, Naspitz CK, Mikawa H, *et al.* Prevention of asthma by ketotifen in infants with atopic dermatitis. *Ann Allergy* 1992;**68**:233–6.

67. ETAC Study Group. Allergic factors associated with the development of asthma and the influence of cetirizine in a double blind, randomised, placebo controlled trial: first results of ETAC. *Pediatr Allergy Immunol* 1998;**9**:116–24.

68. Bustos GJ, Bustos D, Bustos GJ, Romero O. Prevention of asthma with ketotifen in pre-asthmatic children; a 3-year old follow-up study. *Clin Exp Allergy* 1995;**25**:568–73.

69. Ciprandi G, Passalacqua G, Canonica GW. Effect of H1 antihistamines on adhesion molecules: a possible rationale for long term treatment. *Clin Exp Allergy* 1999;**29**(Suppl 3):49–53.

70. Pizzichini E, Leff JA, Reiss TF, *et al.* Montelukast reduces airway eosinophilic inflammation in asthma: a randomised controlled trial. *Eur Respir J* 1999; **14**:12–18.

71. Institute of Medicine. Exposure to indoor tobacco smoke. In: *Clearing the Air: Asthma and Indoor Exposures.* Committee on the Assessment of Asthma in Indoor Air, Washington, DC National Academy Press, 2000, pp. 263–97.

72. Murray AB, Morrison BJ. The effects of cigarette smoke from the mother on bronchial responsiveness and severity of symptoms in children with asthma. *J Allergy Clin Immunol* 1986;**77**:575–81.

73. Murray AB, Morrison BJ. The decrease in severity of asthma in children of parents who smoke since the parents have been exposing them to less cigarette smoke. *J Allergy Clin Immunol* 1993; **91**:102–11.

74. Burr ML, Anderson HR, Austin JB, *et al.* Respiratory symptoms and home environment in children: a national survey. *Thorax* 1999;**54**:27–32.

75. Hasselbad V, Eddy DM, Kotchmar DJ. Synthesis of environmental evidence: nitrogen dioxide epidemiology studies. *J Air Waste Manage Soc* 1992;**42**:662–71.

76. Strachan DP, Carey IM. Home environment and severe asthma in adolescence: a population base control study. *Br Med J* 1995;**311**:1053–6.

77. Committee on the Medical Effects of Air Pollutants (Department of Health Asthma and Outdoor Air Pollution). HMSO, London, 1995, pp. 1–195.

78. Woodcock A, Custovic A. Role of the indoor environment in determining the severity of asthma. *Thorax* 1998;**53**(Suppl 2):S47–51.

79. Call RS, Smith TF, Morris E, *et al*. Risk factors for asthma in inner city children. *J Pediatr* 1992; **121**:862–6.

80. Platts-Mills TA, Thomas WR, Aalberse RC, *et al*. Dust mite allergens and asthma. Report of the 2nd International Workshop. *J Allergy Clin Immunol* 1992;**89**:1046–60.

81. Gotzsche PC, Hammarquist C, Burr M. House-dust mite control measures for asthma. (Cochrane Review) Cochrane Database Syst. Rev 2001;**2**.

82. Strachan DP. House-dust mite allergen avoidance in asthma. Benefits unproved but not yet excluded (editorial). *Br Med J* 1998;**317**:1096–7.

83. Custovic A, Simpson A, Chapman MD, Woodcock A. Allergen avoidance in the treatment of asthma and atopic disorders. *Thorax* 1998;**53**:63–72.

84. Warner JA. Controlling indoor allergens. *Pediatr Allergy Immunol* 2000;**11**:208–19.

85. Peroni DG, Boner AL, Vallone G, *et al*. Effective allergen avoidance at high altitude reduced allergen induced bronchial hyperresponsiveness. *Am J Respir Crit Care Med* 1994;**149**:1442–6.

86. Ehnert B, Lau-Schadendorf S, Veber A, *et al*. Reducing domestic exposure to dust mite allergen reduces bronchial hyperreactivity in sensitive children with asthma. *J Allergy Clin Immunol* 1992;**90**:135–8.

87. Murray AB, Ferguson AC. Dust-free bedrooms in the treatment of asthmatic children with house-dust or house-dust mite allergy: a controlled trial. *Pediatrics* 1983;**71**:418–22.

88. Sarsfield JK, Gowland G, Toy R, Norman ALE. Mite sensitive asthma in childhood. Trial of avoidance measures. *Arch Dis Child* 1974;**49**:716–21.

89. Frederick JM, Warner JO, Jessop WJ, *et al*. The effect of a bed covering system on children with house-dust mite sensitive asthma. *Europ Respir J* 1997;**10**:361–6.

90. Hegarty JM, Rouhbakhsh S, Warner JA, Warner JO. A comparison of the effect of conventional and filter vacuum cleaners on airborne house-dust mite allergen. *Respir Med* 1995;**89**:279–84.

91. Popplewell EJ, Innes VA, Lloyd-Hughes S, *et al*. The effect of high efficiency and standard vacuum cleaners on mite, cat and dog allergen levels and

clinical progress. *Pediatr Allergy Immunol* 2000; **11**:142–8.

92. Closterman SGM, Schermer TRJ, Bijl-Hofland ID, *et al*. Effects of house-dust mite avoidance measures on Der p 1 concentrations and clinical condition of mild adult house-dust mite allergic asthmatic patients using no inhaled steroids. *Clin Exp Allergy* 1999; **29**:1336–46.

93. Niven R, Fletcher AM, Pickering AC, *et al*. Attempting to control mite allergens with mechanical ventilation and dehumidification in British homes. *J Allergy Clin Immunol* 1999;**103**:756–62.

94. Harving H, Hansen LG, Korsgaard J, *et al*. House-dust mite allergy and anti-mite measures in the indoor environment. *Allergy* 1991;**46**:33–8.

95. Warner JA, Frederick JM, Bryant TN, *et al*. Mechanical ventilation and high efficiency vacuum cleaning: a combined strategy of mite and mite allergen reduction in the control of mite sensitive allergy. *J Allergy Clin Immunol* 2000;**105**:75–82.

96. Custovic A, Green R, Taggart SCO, *et al*. Domestic allergens in public places. II:dog (Can f 1) and cockroach (Bla g 2) allergens in dust and mite, cat, dog and cockroach allergens in the air in public buildings. *Clin Exp Allergy* 1996;**26**:1246–52.

97. Munir AKM, Bjorksten B, Einarsson R, *et al*. Cat (Fel d 1), dog (Can f 1) and cockroach allergens in homes of asthmatic children from 3 climatic zones in Sweden. *Allergy* 1994;**49**:508–16.

98. Bollinger ME, Eggleston PA, Wood RA. Cat antigen in homes with and without cats may induce allergic symptoms. *J Allergy Clin Immunol* 1996; **97**:907–14.

99. Ingram JM, Sporik R, Rose G, *et al*. Quantitative assessment of exposure to dog (Can f 1) and cat (Fel d 1) allergens: relationship to sensitization and asthma among children living in Los Alamos, New Mexico. *J Allergy Clin Immunol* 1995;**96**: 449–56.

100. Lonnkvist K, Hallden D, Dahlen SE, *et al*. Markers of inflammation and bronchial reactivity in children with asthma exposed to animal dander in school dust. *Pediatr Allergy Immunol* 1999;**10**:45–52.

101. Egmar A-C, Emenius G, Almqvist C, Wickman M. Cat and dog allergen in mattresses and textile covered floors of homes which do or do not have pets either in the past or currently. *Pediatr Allergy Immunol* 1998;**9**:31–5.

101a. Almquist C, Wickman M, Perfetti L, Berglind N, Renstrom A, Hedren M, Larsson K, Hedlin G, Malmberg P. Worsening of asthma in children allergic to cats, after indirect exposure to cat at school. *Am J Respir Crit Care Med* 2001;**163**:694–8.

102. Wood RA, Chapman MD, Adkinson NF, *et al*. The effect of cat removal on allergen content in household dust samples. *J Allergy Clin Immunol* 1989;**83**:730–4.

103. Van der Brempt X, Charpin D, Haddi E, *et al.* Cat removal and Fel d 1 levels in mattresses. *J Allergy Clin Immunol* 1991;**87**:595–6.

104. de Blay F, Chapman MD, Platts-Mills TA. Airborne cat allergen (Fel d 1): environmental control with cat *in situ. Am Rev Respir Dis* 1991;**143**:1334–9.

105. Sarpong SB, Hamilton RG, Eggleston PA, Adkinson NF. Socio-economic status and race as risk factors for cockroach allergen exposure and sensitization in children with asthma. *J Allergy Clin Immunol* 1996;**97**:1393–401.

106. Rosenstreich DL, Eggleston P, Kattan M, *et al.* The role of cockroach allergy and exposure to cockroach allergen in causing morbidity among inner city children with asthma. *New Engl J Med* 1997; **336**:1356–63.

107. Peat JK, Tovey E, Mellis CM, *et al.* Importance of house-dust mite and alternaria allergens in childhood asthma: an epidemiological study in two climatic regions of Australia. *Clin Exp Allergy* 1993;**23**:812–20.

108. Halonen M, Stern D, Wright AL, *et al.* Alternaria as a major allergen for asthma in children raised in a desert environment. *Am J Respir Crit Care Med* 1997;**155**:1356–61.

109. Onorato J, Merland N, Terral C, *et al.* Placebo controlled double blind food challenge in asthma. *J Allergy Clin Immunol* 1986;**78**:1139–46.

110. Sampson HA, Mendelson L, Rosen JP. Fatal and near fatal food induced anaphylaxis in children. *New Engl J Med* 1992;**327**:380–4.

111. Young E, Patel S, Stoneham M, *et al.* The prevalence of reaction to food additives in a survey population. *J Roy Coll Phys* 1987;**21**:241–7.

112. Kramarz P, DeStefano F, Gargiullo PM, *et al.* Does influenza vaccination exacerbate asthma? Analysis of a large cohort of children with asthma. Vaccine Safety Datalink Team. *Arch Fam Med* 2000;**9**:617–23.

113. Wong EEL, Tark NK. Immunoglobulin for preventing respiratory syncitial virus infection. Cochrane Airways Group. *Cochrane Library*. Update Publications, Oxford, 2000.

114. Fearby S, Frew AJ. Hunting the magic bullet in immunotherapy: new forms of old treatment or something completely different? *Clin Exp Allergy* 2001;**31**:969–74.

15

Growth and puberty in asthma

GEORGE RUSSELL AND MUSTAFA OSMAN

INTRODUCTION

If the asthma has come on young, he (the asthmatic) is generally below the average height (Salter[1]).

Although they produced no evidence to support this assertion, classical writers such as Salter were in no doubt that childhood asthma was an important cause of stunting of growth. Cohen *et al.*[2] are generally credited with first drawing attention to the importance of anthropometry in recording the progress of allergic children, and later[3] presented data which confirmed the association between uncontrolled allergy and poor growth (and the converse).[3,4] Although it has been widely accepted that asthma has an adverse effect on growth, the literature has contained surprisingly few accounts of the growth of asthmatic children, and even less by way of explanation for growth impairment. Inevitably, interpretation of the literature is bedevilled by problems related on the one hand to the definition of asthma and the assessment of its severity, and on the other to the collection and interpretation of the data on growth. More recently, a further source of confusion has been the effect on growth of systemic and inhaled corticosteroid therapy.

ASSESSMENT OF GROWTH

The assessment of growth is an integral part of paediatric practice. Growth may be assessed in terms of either attained height or height velocity.

Attained height

Attained height summates all the previous growth. Growth is a dynamic process, and a single measurement is therefore of limited value. Attained height, measured using an accurate stadiometer, must be related to age and sex on an appropriate chart, sometimes known as a 'distance' or 'growth' chart. The result is expressed either as a centile, or as a standard deviation score (SDS or z-score), the deviation from the mean in units of standard deviation. Attained adult height summates the effects of all influences on childhood growth.

Height velocity

Height velocity describes growth over a given time-period as an annual increment in height. Change in height is small over short intervals, so the total period studied should be as long as possible. Ideally, several measurements should be made over the period, and growth rate calculated by regression. Again, the results can be expressed as either a centile or an SDS. Height velocity is at its maximum during infancy, following which it declines gradually throughout childhood to reach its lowest childhood level during the pre-pubertal nadir (Figure 15.3). Following the pubertal growth spurt, growth declines gradually, but may take several years to come to a complete stop.

Knemometry

Knemometry was introduced to overcome some of the problems in assessing height velocity over short periods.[5,6]

This technique allows extremely precise measurements to be made of the distance between the heel and the knee, allowing the assessment of lower leg growth over periods of only a few days. Short-term changes cannot be extrapolated to the long-term. Knemometry is useful in allowing the systemic (metabolic) effects of corticosteroids to be detected, rather than as a true measure of growth. Unfortunately, knemometry involves the use of complex, expensive and bulky apparatus, and although valuable research has been performed using it, it has been little used in routine clinical practice.

Measurements of childhood growth, particularly in individuals rather than populations, must be interpreted in the light of four constitutional factors that influence growth: *parental height*; *intrauterine and perinatal influences*; *maturational influences* (usually measured in terms of bone age or pubertal status: children in whom pubertal development is relatively delayed undergo considerable catch-up growth when puberty eventually occurs); *pathological influences* (such as those which directly affect growth and those chronic diseases, including asthma, which may do so indirectly).

EFFECTS OF ASTHMA ON GROWTH

Population-based studies

Several population-based studies have included data on the association between asthma and short stature. Both the Oxford Child Health Survey[7] and the Thousand Family Study in Newcastle upon Tyne[8] demonstrated an association between respiratory symptoms and poor growth. At a time when asthma was generally under-diagnosed, many of these children are likely to have had asthma. However, respiratory symptoms were also related to adverse social circumstances, which in turn have a well-recognized impact on growth, and it would be wise not to over-interpret these data. In Aberdeen[9] and in Melbourne[10] both height and weight were affected adversely by increasing severity of asthmatic symptoms. In Melbourne, Gillam *et al.*[10] found that growth impairment was most marked in children in whom barrel chest testified to the severity of their asthma. However, by 21 years of age, all groups in this study, including children selected because they had unusually severe asthma, had heights in the same range as controls.[11]

Although asthma does not appear to be a common cause of *severe* growth failure,[12,13] Rona and Florey[14] in a later community-based study confirmed that asthma (but not non-specific respiratory symptoms) adversely affected growth independently of social and biological factors assessed. In contrast, the 1958 British Birth Cohort Study[15] failed to find an ill-effect of childhood asthma on growth, perhaps because community studies contain only a small proportion of children with severe asthma. Other recent community-based studies[16–19] have also failed to demonstrate any effect of asthma on growth, except in severe cases in which the effects of asthma are difficult to separate from the potential effects of inhaled corticosteroids used in its management.

It is essential therefore to examine studies from hospital-based clinics, in which severe cases of asthma are more likely to be represented, with particular emphasis on reports that antedate the introduction of effective anti-inflammatory and bronchodilator treatment.

Hospital-based studies

Several workers examined the effects of new corticosteroid therapy on the growth of asthmatic children,[20–27] and in so doing, measured children before corticosteroids were started. Their heights were appreciably lower than predicted (Figure 15.1). More recent studies[28,29] (Figure 15.2) have supported these findings.

Several of these authors also demonstrated retarded bone maturation in association with severe asthma.[23,30]

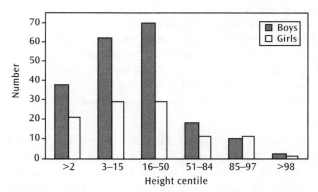

Figure 15.1 *Distribution of height centiles in children studied by Falliers[20] prior to 1961 at the Jewish National Home for Asthmatic Children, a residential hospital-school for children with intractable asthma in Denver, Colorado, USA. Equal numbers of children should lie above and below the 50th centile.*

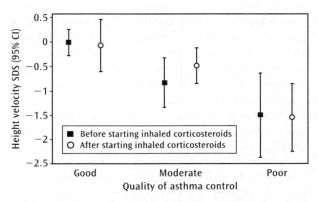

Figure 15.2 *Height velocity SDS in 58 pre-pubertal children studied before and after starting inhaled corticosteroids.[28]*

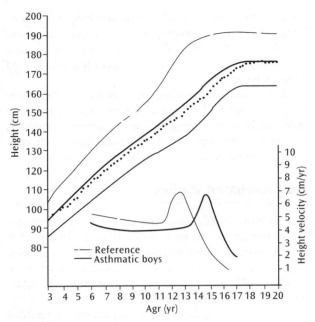

Figure 15.3 *Growth of 531 asthmatic boys based on 1754 mixed longitudinal measurements. The upper graph represents height for age in the reference population, on which is superimposed a dotted line representing the heights of the asthmatic children. The lower graph compares the height velocity and the timing of the pubertal growth spurt in the asthmatic boys with the reference population. Figure modified by Preece et al.[198] from Hauspie et al.[31] (reproduced with permission).*

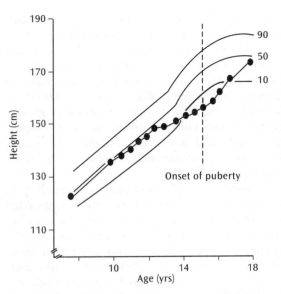

Figure 15.4 *Height record on a Tanner and Whitehouse growth development chart (10th, 50th and 90th centile lines) for a child with mild chronic perennial asthma, virtually symptom-free by 11 years of age, illustrating: (1) the established centile pattern from 7.7 to 12.3 years; (2) the physiological deceleration of growth velocity pattern of delayed puberty; (3) the delayed puberty growth spurt, resulting in a child regaining his original height centile. The broken line represents the onset of puberty. (From ref. 199 with permission.)*

Particularly important evidence comes from a group of children institutionalized for severe asthma[31] (Figure 15.3), who had clear evidence of retardation of height, bone age and pubertal development. Children with delayed puberty typically continue to grow for longer than other children, so that by the time bone maturation finally occurs, normal adult stature has been achieved (Figures 15.4 and 15.5). In Hauspie's study,[31] this was exactly what happened; in subjects followed through to the age of 19 years, adult height was normal.

Snyder[23] related height centile to asthma severity assessed by the frequency of attacks and demonstrated a preponderance of small children in the group with the most frequent attacks. A similar effect is seen in Figure 15.2.[28] Indirect support for an association between asthma severity and impaired growth comes from a few anecdotal reports in which effective asthma treatment has been followed by accelerated or 'catch-up' growth.[32–35]

There has not however been universal agreement that severe asthma is associated with impaired growth. Spock[36] found no impairment of growth in patients who had not received corticosteroids, although in common with other studies,[2,9,37] he found that asthmatic children tended to be relatively underweight. There was however a tendency for Spock's patients to achieve a greater height centile after puberty than at the beginning of the study, a finding that

Crowley[38] has interpreted as a tendency for childhood growth to be retarded, with compensatory catch-up growth during puberty. In a study from Nigeria,[39] socio-economic factors were thought to be more important than asthma in explaining growth impairment, although children with severe asthma were, on average, lighter in weight and shorter in stature than those with mild or moderate disease. Similar conclusions have been reported in a Scottish population survey.[18]

Adult height following asthma

The great majority of reports that have examined adult height following childhood asthma have found normal[11,31,36] or even greater than predicted adult height.[26] However, in a large cohort of 17-year-old Israeli military recruits, Shohat et al.[40] demonstrated statistically significant growth retardation in severe asthmatics, although the actual differences between the various groups were small, and unlikely to be of clinical importance (Figure 15.5). Paradoxically, in this study the subjects with mild or moderate asthma were taller and heavier than controls, a finding that remains unexplained. The findings in this study must however be interpreted with some caution, as full adult height has not necessarily been attained by the age of 17 years, particularly in asthmatics in whom the adolescent growth spurt is commonly delayed.[31] Even

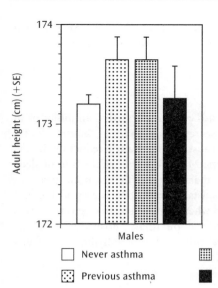
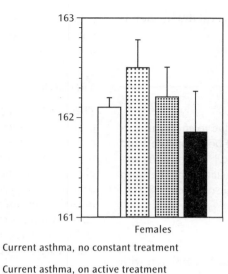

Figure 15.5 *Heights of 54 051 male and 38 102 female Israeli military recruits studied by Shohat et al.[40] Although some of these differences attain statistical significance by virtue of the large numbers studied, it should be noted that the actual differences are extremely small, and that the subjects were only 17 years of age, when full adult height would not have been attained by all subjects.*

Legend for chart:
- Never asthma
- Previous asthma
- Current asthma, no constant treatment
- Current asthma, on active treatment

temporary short stature and lack of sexual development may lead to emotional and social difficulties that may persist after normal height and full sexual maturation are attained.[41]

Summary of evidence relating asthma to growth

Although the quality of some of the evidence relating asthma to growth is less than satisfactory by modern standards, its volume is considerable and suggests that:

- In contrast to milder disease, severe asthma, in the pre-corticosteroid era, was frequently associated with delayed growth during childhood.
- Asthma is associated with delayed puberty and bone maturation, and therefore relative short stature in early teenage, with little or no effect on adult stature.
- The adverse effects of severe asthma were particularly marked in reports prior to the introduction of 'modern' asthma therapy.

MECHANISMS BY WHICH ASTHMA AFFECTS GROWTH AND MATURATION

Allergy

Cohen *et al.*[2] believed that growth retardation was an integral part of the atopic state, presenting case reports involving children with eczema and hay fever as well as asthma. Support for this view has appeared in more recent publications, in which growth impairment has been associated with eczema, particularly with extensive skin involvement,[42–44] the growth pattern being similar to that seen in asthma, with delayed bone maturation[45] resulting

eventually in normal adult height.[46] Upper respiratory tract allergy has also been implicated in growth retardation,[47] although this study did not distinguish clearly between upper and lower respiratory tract allergy.

Endocrine factors

PUBERTAL DELAY

Pubertal delay has been fully documented in only two studies in asthmatic children.[48,49] Delayed radiological bone maturation, presumably secondary to delayed endocrine development, has however been reported widely.[20,23,31,50–52] As in any other group of children with delayed pubertal development, short stature in childhood is balanced by a relatively long period of pre-pubertal growth (Figure 15.4). Although the subsequent pubertal growth spurt is often subnormal, satisfactory adult height is usually attained.

HYPOTHALAMO–PITUITARY DYSFUNCTION

The underlying mechanism has not been elucidated, although hypoxia has been shown to cause hypothalamo–pituitary dysfunction.[53] Pituitary gonadotrophins are depressed in asthmatic adolescents compared with matched controls, associated with depressed levels of testosterone in boys, and oestrogen and progesterone in girls.[54] One study showed that asthmatic children have an exaggerated growth hormone response to exercise,[55] although this has been disputed.[56–58] In two studies the effects on growth were confined to boys.[26,59]

ADRENAL DYSFUNCTION

There is evidence of reduced urinary excretion of the adrenal androgen dehydroepiandrosterone in asthmatic children, whether or not they are on corticosteroid therapy.[60] This could certainly result in maturational delay. Further evidence of adrenocortical dysfunction is an impaired cortisol response to exercise.[61]

Undernutrition

ENERGY IMBALANCE

Growth failure in asthma could be due to energy imbalance resulting from a combination of poor appetite[24] and increased resting energy expenditure.[62,63] However, several studies have failed to show any relationship between energy intake and growth in asthmatic children,[63–66] suggesting that this is not a major factor.

ZINC DEFICIENCY

Zinc deficiency has been demonstrated in children with asthma[67] and eczema,[68,69] although the findings for asthma are not consistent.[70,71] Moreover, zinc deficiency has been postulated as a factor causing bronchial hyperreactivity,[72] so any association between asthma, growth and zinc deficiency is difficult to interpret.

ANTIOXIDANT DEFICIENCY

It has been suggested that dietary antioxidant deficiency might be responsible for the widely observed increase in the prevalence of asthma.[72,73] There are certainly plausible biochemical and epidemiological reasons why this might be so,[74,75] and vitamin C can prevent exercise-induced bronchospasm in some patients.[76]

OTHER DEFICIENCIES

Collipp[77] described *pyridoxine deficiency* in asthmatic children, with a favourable response to treatment, although these findings have not been replicated by other workers.[78,79] Perturbations of pyridoxine metabolism in asthma were probably due to theophylline therapy.[80,81]

At present, there is insufficient evidence to advise the widespread use of dietary supplements to promote growth in asthmatic children, although there is an increasingly strong case for dietary intervention to prevent the development of asthma.[75]

Non-corticosteroid asthma therapy

β_2-AGONISTS

The transient inhibition of growth hormone secretion following the intravenous injection of terbutaline in children is unlikely to be responsible for any clinically relevant inhibition of growth.[82] In adults, the growth hormone response to exercise was blunted following 400 µg salbutamol (albuterol) and abolished following broxaterol.[83] In children, Lanes et al.[84] showed an early but unsustained reduction in both stimulated and spontaneous growth hormone secretion during salbutamol treatment. This

evidence of an interaction between β_2-agonists and growth hormone has not been established as the cause of growth inhibition.

XANTHINES

Theophylline has also been implicated as an inhibitor of growth hormone secretion. In children, Baum[85] found that theophylline caused a significant reduction in the median values of the 24-hour profile, of the 8-hour sleep phase and of the maximal growth hormone peak. In contrast to β_2-agonists, theophylline was available and indeed widely used when some of the most severe growth failure was reported,[20–22] but there is no evidence that the endocrine changes induced by theophylline are of any clinical significance.

CROMONES

Cromoglycate is said to have a beneficial effect on growth,[32] a finding that may be related to the increased growth hormone excretion that occurs during its use.[86]

Oral corticosteroids

EARLY STUDIES

Growth retardation is a well-recognized component of Cushing's syndrome when it occurs in children, and its successful management is followed by catch-up growth.[87] It is therefore hardly surprising that, when corticosteroids were introduced to medical practice, growth retardation soon emerged as an important side effect.[88] Many children had evidence of growth suppression before starting steroids and their administration had little additional effect. Attempts to preserve growth using ACTH injections[90,91] produced unpredictable hyperadrenalism, without affecting adult height.[92] Growth was largely preserved when oral corticosteroids were given on alternate days,[93] and this has almost completely superseded the use of ACTH.

RECENT STUDIES

Using knemometry, Wolthers and Pedersen have shown that *prednisolone in daily doses* as low as 2.5 mg and 5 mg inhibits short-term growth,[94] suggesting that at daily doses likely to be effective in asthma, growth retardation would be inevitable.

Alternate day therapy does not however provide complete protection against the effects of corticosteroids on growth, although it may be difficult to separate the effects of therapy from those of the underlying disease.[25] In one study, children who received prednisone in doses of <15 mg every other day had acceleration of growth, whereas children who received larger doses had further suppression of growth.[26] Much of the growth retardation in asthma appears to be due to the disease itself, but is accelerated by steroid therapy, in proportion to the duration and dosage of daily steroid treatment.[27]

Corticosteroid therapy also delays skeletal maturation. Bone age is delayed more than height-for-age in asthmatic children on oral prednis(ol)one,[95] with slow and variable catch-up after discontinuing treatment.

There is insufficient evidence to identify a 'safe' dose of oral corticosteroid; both continuous and intermittent treatment have been associated with growth retardation. As with all potentially toxic drugs, corticosteroids should be given in as low a dose as possible, for as short a time as possible, and as infrequently as possible. It is as important to step down treatment when the patient is doing well as to step up when he is doing badly. Restraint in the use of corticosteroids is balanced by the undoubted benefits they have brought to the management of both acute and chronic asthma (Chapter 8a).

Inhaled corticosteroid therapy – beclomethasone dipropionate and budesonide

It was hoped that the effects of corticosteroids on growth could be avoided by using tiny doses of topically active corticosteroids by inhalation. Initial trials of inhaled corticosteroid therapy in children demonstrated dramatic improvements in asthma control,[96,97] with no adverse effect on growth.[33,98–100]

Nevertheless, there were observational reports of growth impairment of pre-pubertal children on inhaled corticosteroids[101] and misleading reports of growth retardation around puberty which made no allowance for the delayed pubertal growth spurt that is characteristic of the asthmatic child.[102] Nevertheless, these findings stimulated numerous further studies of childhood growth on inhaled corticosteroids, mostly with reassuring results.[103–106] Indeed, in our own study (Figure 15.2), we were in no doubt that poor asthma control was the major determinant of poor growth.[28,107] Reviewing the literature in 1994, Allen[108] concluded that there was no statistical evidence that beclomethasone dipropionate therapy was associated with growth impairment, regardless of dose, duration of therapy or severity of asthma. This may have been over-optimistic.

STUDIES USING KNEMOMETRY (SHORT-TERM BONE GROWTH)

Knemometry provided the first convincing evidence that inhaled corticosteroids had a dose-related effect on growth. Budesonide in doses up to 400 μg per day had no significant effect, whereas a daily dose of 800 μg slowed lower leg growth[109–112] (Figure 15.6). A reduced dose of budesonide (from 400 μg to 200 μg daily), achieved by adding formoterol to the regimen, was followed by significantly enhanced lower leg growth.[113] Interestingly, budesonide given in a once-daily dose of 800 μg had less

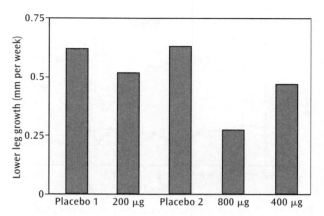

Figure 15.6 *Lower leg growth in children receiving various doses of budesonide in a double-blind study.[109] Only the effect of 800 μg was statistically significant.*

effect on lower leg growth than when the daily dose was divided in two.[114] Budesonide given by nebulizer to very young children in a daily dose of 1–4 mg did not influence growth.[115] In contrast, beclomethasone dipropionate slowed lower leg growth in a daily dose of 400 μg,[116,117] suggesting that its systemic effects were more marked than those of budesonide. Studies using knemometry to assess growth suggest therefore that budesonide might offer some advantages over beclomethasone dipropionate.

The results of studies based on knemometry must be viewed with some caution, since measurements made over extremely short periods cannot be extrapolated to the longer term. In some children lower leg growth apparently slowed to an extent that would have resulted in severe stunting of growth, a finding that has not been seen even in individuals who have received inhaled corticosteroids for most of their childhood years.

STUDIES USING STADIOMETRY (STATURAL GROWTH)

Several studies have now shown clear evidence of growth suppression on inhaled corticosteroids. There have been four randomized controlled trials in which growth has been measured in children receiving beclomethasone dipropionate 400 μg per day.[118–121] These therapeutic trials can be criticized because of the inclusion of children up to 14[120] or 16[118,121] years of age, when puberty might be a confounding variable, or because the indication for treatment was unconventional.[119] It is however difficult to escape the conclusion that the effect on growth was genuine, a view supported by a recent systematic review of the effects of beclomethasone dipropionate on growth,[122] which concluded that beclomethasone dipropionate suppresses height velocity by an average of 1.51 cm per year (95% CI −1.15, −1.87).

Further evidence that inhaled corticosteroids have an inhibitory effect on growth comes from two observational

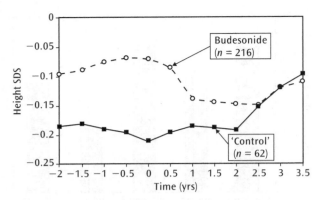

Figure 15.7 *Height standard deviation score in children followed before and after starting budesonide, compared with children who were not given inhaled corticosteroids. Budesonide was started at year 0. (From Agertoft and Pedersen.[106])*

studies. In one, the slowing was independent of dose, was accentuated in the more severe asthmatics, and was most marked during the first year of treatment.[29] When inhaled corticosteroid treatment was discontinued there was evidence of catch-up growth.[123]

EFFECT ON ADULT HEIGHT

Several studies have reported that the eventual adult height of individuals who have received corticosteroid therapy during childhood is unaffected.[123–128] Any slowing of growth is transient (Figure 15.7). Delayed pubertal growth is a feature of steroid treated and of untreated children.[127]

There is therefore good reason to advise parents that, whatever short-term effect inhaled corticosteroids may have on their child's growth, there will be no adverse effect on eventual adult height.

Inhaled corticosteroid therapy – fluticasone propionate

Fluticasone propionate has been introduced as a potent anti-inflammatory corticosteroid that undergoes virtually total first pass hepatic metabolism, and is therefore likely to be associated with fewer systemic side effects than the other steroid molecules given by the inhaled route.[129] On a weight-for-weight basis, it is clinically at least twice as effective as budesonide or beclomethasone dipropionate,[130] and this needs to be borne in mind when comparing its effects on growth with those of the other corticosteroids.

STUDIES USING KNEMOMETRY

Fluticasone propionate had no short-term effect on lower leg growth in doses of 200 µg[116,131,132] or 400 µg[131] daily.

Thus it appears to offer advantages over beclomethasone dipropionate, but no difference was found between budesonide 800 µg daily and fluticasone propionate 400 µg daily.[133]

STUDIES USING STADIOMETRY

Fluticasone propionate was introduced at a time when there was considerable interest in the potential systemic side effects of inhaled corticosteroids. Its effects on growth have therefore been included as an end-point in several clinical trials.

Comparisons with placebo or non-steroidal drugs

In a study comparing fluticasone propionate 100 µg per day with cromoglycate 80 mg per day, similar growth rates were achieved on both drugs.[134] Allen et al.[135] compared fluticasone propionate 100 µg or 200 µg with placebo. Sharek and Bergman[122] reviewed their results and concluded that fluticasone propionate 200 µg per day had a modest growth retarding effect of −0.43 cm per year compared with placebo (95% confidence interval− 0.01 cm, − 0.85 cm).

Comparisons with other inhaled corticosteroids

Barnes et al.[136] found reduced growth rates in 32 children whose asthma was well controlled on either beclomethasone dipropionate or budesonide. Sixteen patients were then switched to fluticasone propionate in equipotent doses, with no loss of asthma control, but their height velocity changed from SDS −0.5 to SDS +1.3. In other words, growth rates did not just return to normal, but there was enhanced growth suggesting catch-up.

Other studies have also shown significantly slower growth on beclomethasone dipropionate than on fluticasone propionate.[137,138] In infants, fluticasone propionate given for six months in doses of either 50 µg or 125 µg had no effect on height standard deviation score.[139]

Studies using greater than licensed doses

All of the above studies used standard (i.e. licensed) doses of fluticasone propionate of up to 200 µg per day, and do not necessarily translate into enhanced safety at higher doses.

There was much concern when Todd et al.[140] reported severe growth retardation and adrenal suppression in six children receiving exceptionally high doses of fluticasone propionate. Fitzgerald et al.[141] found no difference in growth rates between 30 children in a blinded crossover comparison of fluticasone propionate 750 µg per day with beclomethasone dipropionate 1500 µg per day. This unusually high dose of beclomethasone dipropionate could reasonably be expected to have an adverse effect on growth, so these results suggest that, at very high doses, the apparent advantages of standard-dose fluticasone propionate are lost. Unfortunately, the study periods were only 12 weeks, too short to allow accurate assessment of height velocity,

Table 15.1 *Growth velocity on inhaled corticosteroids and other anti-asthmatic drugs (Stempel et al.[146])*

Drug	N	Growth velocity (cm/yr)
Beclomethasone dipropionate	435	4.19
Budesonide	166	4.9
Fluticasone propionate	551	5.78
Other drugs	438	5.69

and coinciding with the period when the effects of inhaled corticosteroids on growth are maximal.[142]

Since then, several further studies on the effects of higher doses of fluticasone propionate have been reported. In doses of 400–500 μg per day, growth is normal[143] or better than equipotent doses of budesonide.[144,145]

Stempel *et al.*[146] analysed data from a number of papers describing growth rates in asthmatic children on beclomethasone dipropionate 400 μg per day, budesonide 800 μg per day, fluticasone propionate 100–400 μg per day, and other drugs (placebo, cromoglycate, salmeterol, theophylline). This analysis encountered the usual problems of heterogeneity of pubertal status, inhaled corticosteroid dose, delivery device, comparator non-steroidal drug, asthma severity and patient population. Nevertheless, the annualized growth rates shown in Table 15.1 suggest that fluticasone propionate in doses of up to 400 μg per day (i.e. twice the licensed dose) has no adverse effect on growth.

Conclusion

Although it is interesting to speculate on the possible aetiology of growth retardation in asthma, there is no clear evidence that any specific factors other than the severity of the asthma and corticosteroid therapy are responsible. As severe uncontrolled asthma is rare with modern management, it is unlikely that the mechanism will now be elucidated.

There is however good evidence from controlled and blinded clinical trials that the use of the older inhaled corticosteroids, particularly beclomethasone dipropionate, is associated with a reduction in growth velocity, although other studies have shown that this has little if any effect on eventual adult height. The most likely explanation for these apparently divergent findings is that inhaled corticosteroids have a retardant effect on bone maturation that balances the effect on bone growth, allowing prolongation of pre-pubertal growth so that catch-up occurs. However, growth suppression is most marked during the initial six weeks after starting treatment with beclomethasone dipropionate, with most suppression occurring during the initial 18 weeks, and normal growth thereafter.[142] Clinical trials,

which of necessity are of relatively brief duration, may simply overemphasize the effects of growth retardation in the early weeks of treatment, and translate what is no more than a temporary phenomenon into a prediction of a significant decrement in annual height gain. Further possible explanations include the greater than normal compliance that occurs during clinical trials, and the fact that in trials treatment continues in a fixed dose even after improvement has occurred, and the airways are less inflamed and thus more readily lead to systemic absorption.[147]

The apparent advantages of fluticasone propionate demonstrated in knemometry studies appear to translate into normal, or very nearly normal, growth as assessed by stadiometry when it is given in licensed or moderately high doses, supporting the view that fluticasone propionate has a better therapeutic ratio than the older inhaled corticosteroids.[130] At very high doses, the advantages of fluticasone propionate may be lost.

Whichever inhaled corticosteroid is selected, the minimum effective dose used should be, and delivered by the inhaler device most appropriate for that child. It is also sensible, particularly when using doses greater than those normally recommended, to adopt strategies designed to enhance airway deposition and minimize oropharyngeal deposition of inhaled corticosteroids (Chapter 8b). Such strategies include the use of spacer devices[148] and/or extra-fine aerosol hydrofluoroalkane metered dose inhalers.[149] Although there have been no studies showing that such methods of delivery have any effect on growth, their use can reasonably be expected to minimize systemic absorption. It is also important to remember that the shallow, sigmoid shape of the dose–response curve for inhaled corticosteroids means that it is seldom advisable to use doses far in excess of those licensed for paediatric use[150] (Chapter 8a).

ASTHMA AND PUBERTY

Introduction

It has long been recognized that asthma tends to worsen around the time of menstruation[151] and that hormonal contraceptives may worsen[152] or relieve symptoms.[153] It is therefore important that paediatricians caring for asthmatic adolescents should be aware of the interplay between female sex hormones and airway function. Moreover, important psychological and social changes occur at adolescence, affect both sexes, and impact on asthma management (Chapter 11).

Managing adolescent patients with asthma is a challenge for patients, parents and clinicians, as the disease is potentially life threatening. Asthma mortality at 15–19 years of age is six times that at 5–9 years.[154] In one study, 15 reported childhood asthma fatalities comprised mainly

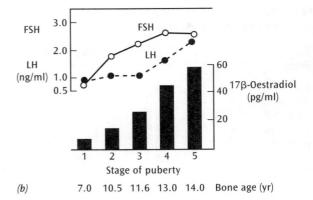

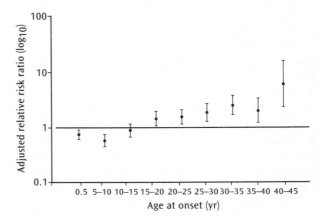

Figure 15.8 *Changes in plasma hormone concentrations in relation to pubertal stage and bone age in (a) males and (b) females. (Reproduced from Ganong,[200] Figure 23.9, p. 383.)*

adolescents, with previous psychiatric consultation in 67% and recorded non-compliance in 40%.[155] In a study of near fatal asthma attacks in children, Martin *et al.*[156] found that over half were adolescents aged 12–15 years.

Parental attitudes are important, though their effects can be unpredictable.[157] Teenagers themselves are often reluctant to take medication for fear of being 'different'. They prefer bronchodilators to prophylactics, and frequently miss doses of regular medication. Compliance may be affected by denial, embarrassment or simply laziness![158]

These findings underline the importance of patient education in this age-group, and the difficulties in ensuring compliance even in the presence of severe asthma (Chapter 18). Involvement of the teenager in management decisions is essential, the presence of friends may foster a positive peer attitude.[159,160]

This chapter will focus on the physical aspects of puberty and their influence on asthma and its management. Social-emotional and educational aspects have been covered elsewhere in the book (Chapters 11, 13c, and 18).

Effects of sex steroids on the lung

BASIC PHYSIOLOGY

High levels of sex steroids *in utero* and soon after birth are necessary for sexual differentiation, and influence the maturation of organs such as the brain and lungs.[161,162] Significant levels are not encountered again until puberty when they are primarily responsible for the acquisition of secondary sexual characteristics. It is clear that even in the earliest stages of puberty sex hormones begin to rise, to peak in adolescence (Figure 15.8).

The ability of sex hormones to modulate immunity is well established[163,164] but has received scant attention from respiratory and allergy specialists. Much of the available evidence comes from the study of autoimmunity, which is more common in females. An immune dimorphism exists with females having higher overall antibody levels.[165] IgE is an exception, and males have higher IgE levels, especially

Figure 15.9 *Data from the European Community Respiratory Health Survey[172] of 18 659 subjects in 16 countries, demonstrating the sex reversal in asthma prevalence at puberty. RR: risk ratio (female/male).*

when young.[166] This difference narrows in the reproductive years but never disappears.[167] Females also have a greater CD4/CD8 ratio.[168] Oestrogen enhances the immune response and androgens are immunosuppressive.[163] There is a biphasic dose response to oestrogen, which promotes a Th1 response at low levels, and a Th2 response at high levels.[165] Progesterone promotes a Th2 response,[169] and both oestrogen and testosterone can cause thymic involution. In pregnancy the high levels of oestrogen and progesterone foster a Th2 environment that prevents fetal rejection, although the precise timing of this Th2 predominance is not known.[170] Sex steroids potentiate the bronchorelaxant effects of catecholamines, and increase prostaglandin synthesis, mucus secretion, β-adrenoceptor density, minute ventilation and smooth muscle contractility.[171]

SEX DIFFERENCES AND THE GENDER SWITCH

Population studies have repeatedly demonstrated a greater male prevalence and incidence of wheeze and asthma in childhood, with a reversal at the time of puberty[172] (Figure 15.9). A more detailed analysis of the gender change in

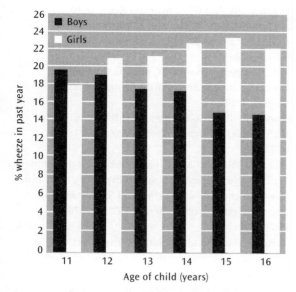

Figure 15.10 *Sex differences in the prevalence of self-reported wheeze in the past year in 27 826 children (based on data of Venn* et al.[173]*).*

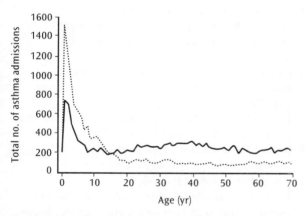

Figure 15.11 *The total number of asthma admissions by age for males (dotted line) and females (solid line) in the USA, demonstrating the male preponderance in childhood, and the female preponderance after puberty (Based on data of Skobeloff* et al.[174]*).*

relation to age (but not to pubertal status) is illustrated in Figure 15.10.[173] A similar sex reversal occurs with asthma-related admissions and lengths of stay in hospital (Figure 15.11).[174] That a similar pattern occurs in hay fever casts doubt on sex differences in airway size and development as the main explanation for this gender switch.[175]

The prevalence of asthma reflects the incidence of the disorder, which in males reaches its peak in the first 5 years of life, declining rapidly thereafter till it reaches a steady state from puberty onwards. In females the incidence decreases slowly from infancy to puberty and then shows a steady rise.[172] Boys tend to experience less severe asthma as they get older, whereas girls are at risk for late onset wheeze, and for persistent and severe symptoms.[176,177]

More boys than girls have atopy and these differences become less apparent later in life[167,178] and may even reverse.[179,180] Sex differences in bronchial reactivity partially explain the excess of asthma in boys,[181,182] although Peat *et al.*[183] found only a small association with sex. In adults, bronchial hyperresponsiveness appears to be more prevalent in women.[184]

MENSTRUAL CYCLE

Although poorly understood, premenstrual asthma is important, and is occasionally associated with respiratory failure[185] and even death. Deterioration during the 10 days before the menses, or during menstruation, affects 30–46% of asthmatic women.[151,171,186–188] Occasionally, this will amount to severe life-threatening exacerbations. It has also been shown that patients with premenstrual asthma tend to have more severe asthma overall.[189]

Even in the absence of symptoms, there may be cyclical changes in peak flow and bronchial responsiveness.[186,190] Tan *et al.*[191] compared asthmatic women with natural cycles with a group on the oral contraceptive pill. During natural cycles, there was a four-fold increase in airway responsiveness to AMP in the luteal phase of the cycle, associated with the rise in oestradiol and progesterone. In the group on the pill, the natural sex steroid levels remained low throughout the month and there was no change in airway responsiveness.

Changes in airway responsiveness between the follicular and luteal phase may explain the worsening of symptoms premenstrually, but there are also immunological changes. IgE values are lower in the periovulatory phase,[192] and sensitivity to skin-prick testing also varies with menstruation, with significant increases in skin reactivity during days 12–16 corresponding to the time of follicular rupture and peak oestrogen levels (Figure 15.12).[193] Skin histamine sensitivity is increased during the early luteal phase.

MANAGEMENT ASPECTS

Paediatricians should be alert to the possibility of cyclical influences. Symptom and peak flow monitoring, along with body temperature measurements, may be helpful in uncovering relationships between asthma control and the menstrual cycle. Possible therapeutic interventions include the avoidance of known trigger factors and increasing conventional treatment at the appropriate point in the cycle. Gonadal suppression, medical or surgical, abolishes premenstrual asthma.[194] The contraceptive pill usually eliminates premenstrual asthma, and is the obvious recommendation in adolescents.[153,195]

In healthy women given oral contraceptives and hormone replacement therapy there may be an increased risk of acquiring asthma related to dose and duration of use.[196] Although pregnancy and its relation to asthma is outwith the scope of this chapter it is worth mentioning that the effect of the contraceptive pill in programming of

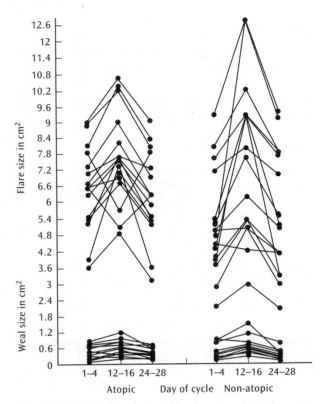

Figure 15.12 *The mean wheal and flare response to histamine prick test in 15 atopic and 15 matched non-atopic females during the menstrual cycle. Observed differences between phases of cycle and between groups are significant. (Based on data from Kalogeromitros et al.[193]).*

the fetal immune system and its relevance to the asthma epidemic remains unexplored.[197]

REFERENCES

1. Salter HH. *On Asthma: its Pathology and Treatment*, 2nd edn. Churchill, London, 1868.
2. Cohen MB, Weller RR, Cohen S. Anthropometry in children. Progress in allergic children as shown by increments in height, weight and maturity. *Am J Dis Child* 1940;**60**:1058–66.
3. Cohen MB, Abram LE. Growth patterns of allergic children. *J Allergy* 1948;**19**:165–71.
4. Welsh JB. The effect of allergic management on the growth and development of allergic children. *J Pediatr* 1951;**38**:571.
5. Hermanussen M, Geiger-Benoit K, Burmeister J, Sippell WG. Knemometry in childhood: accuracy and standardization of a new technique of lower leg length measurement. *Ann Hum Biol* 1988; **15**:1–15.
6. Hermanussen M. Knemometry, a new tool for the investigation of growth. A review. *Eur J Pediatr* 1988;**147**:350–5.
7. Hewitt D, Westropp CK, Acheson RM. Oxford child health survey. Effect of childish ailments on skeletal development. *Br J Prev Soc Med* 1955;**9**:179–86.
8. Miller F, Court S, Walton W, Knox E. *Growing up in Newcastle upon Tyne.* Oxford University Press, London, 1960.
9. Dawson B, Illsley R, Horobin G, Mitchell RG. Survey of childhood asthma in Aberdeen. *Lancet* 1969; **1**:827–30.
10. Gillam GL, McNicol KN, Williams HE. Chest deformity, residual airways obstruction and hyperinflation, and growth in children with asthma. II Significance of chronic chest deformity. *Arch Dis Child* 1970; **45**:789–99.
11. Martin AJ, Landau LI, Phelan PD. The effect on growth of childhood asthma. *Acta Paediatr Scand* 1981;**70**:683–8.
12. Lacey KA, Parkin JM. Causes of short stature. A community study of children in Newcastle upon Tyne. *Lancet* 1974;**i**:42–5.
13. Vimpani GV, Vimpani AF, Farquhar JW. Growth retardation in chronic asthma. *Lancet* 1976;**2**:422.
14. Rona RJ, Florey dV. National study of health and growth: respiratory symptoms and height in primary schoolchildren. *Int J Epidemiol* 1980; **9**:35–43.
15. Power C, Manor O. Asthma, enuresis, and chronic illness: long term impact on height. *Arch Dis Child* 1995;**73**:298–304.
16. Memon IM, Loftus BG. Spectrum of childhood asthma in Galway. *Ir Med J* 1993;**86**:194–5.
17. Neville RG, McCowan C, Thomas G, Crombie IK. Asthma and growth – cause for concern? *Ann Hum Biol* 1996;**23**:323–31.
18. McCowan C, Neville RG, Thomas GE, *et al.* Effect of asthma and its treatment on growth: four year follow up of cohort of children from general practices in Tayside, Scotland. *Br Med J* 1998;**316**:668–72.
19. Norjavaara E, Gerhardsson de Verdier M, Lindmark, B. Asthma and adult registered height during maternity. *Am J Respir Crit Care Med* 2000; **161**:A774.
20. Falliers CJ, Szentivanyi J, McBride M, Bukantz SC. Growth rate of children with intractable asthma. *J Allergy* 1961;**32**:420–34.
21. Norman AP. Steroid treatment in asthma. In: D Gairdner, ed. *Recent Advances in Paediatrics*. Churchill, London, 1965, pp. 294–306.
22. Smith, JM. Long-term steroid treatment in asthmatic children. *Ann Allergy* 1965;**23**:492–6.
23. Snyder RD, Collipp PJ, Greene JS. Growth and ultimate height of children with asthma. *Clin Pediatr* 1967;**6**:389–92.
24. Murray AB, Fraser BM, Hardwick DF, Pirie GE. Chronic asthma and growth failure in children. *Lancet* 1976;**ii**:197–8.

25. Reimer LG, Morris HG, Ellis EF. Growth of asthmatic children during treatment with alternate-day steroids. *J Allergy Clin Immunol* 1975;**55**:224–31.

26. Wittig HJ, McLaughlin ET, Belloit JD. Growth retardation in children with chronic asthma in the absence of prolonged steroid therapy. *Allergol Immunopathol* 1978;**6**:203–8.

27. Chang KC, Miklich DR, Barwise G, Chai H, Miles-Lawrence R. Linear growth of chronic asthmatic children: the effects of the disease and various forms of steroid therapy. *Clin Allergy* 1982;**12**:369–78.

28. Ninan TK, Russell G. Asthma, inhaled corticosteroid treatment, and growth. *Arch Dis Child* 1992;**67**:703–5.

29. Saha MT, Laippala P, Lenko HL. Growth of asthmatic children is slower during than before treatment with inhaled glucocorticoids. *Acta Paediatr* 1997; **86**:138–42.

30. Falliers CJ, Tan LS, Szentivanyi J, Jorgensen JR, Bukantz SC. Childhood asthma and steroid therapy as influences on growth. *Am J Dis Child* 1963; **105**:127–37.

31. Hauspie R, Susanne C, Alexander F. Maturational delay and temporal growth retardation in asthmatic boys. *J Allergy Clin Immunol* 1977;**59**:200–6.

32. Clift AD, Holzel A. Long-term therapy with sodium cromoglycate: effects and side effects. *Ann Allergy* 1978;**41**:313–18.

33. Soderberg-Warner M, Siegel S, Katz R, Rachelefsky, G. Treatment of chronic childhood asthma with beclomethasone dipropionate aerosols (BDA) IV Long-term effects on growth. *J Allergy Clin Immunol* 1979;**64**:164.

34. Smith JM. Prolonged use of disodium cromoglycate in children and young persons – ten years experience. *Schweiz Med Wochenschr* 1980;**110**:183–4.

35. Bacon CJ. Growth retardation in asthmatic children treated with inhaled beclomethasone dipropionate. *Lancet* 1988;**i**:475–6.

36. Spock A. Growth patterns in 200 children with bronchial asthma. *Ann Allergy* 1965;**23**:608–15.

37. Hauspie R, Susanne C, Alexander FA. Mixed longitudinal study of the growth in height and weight in asthmatic children. *Hum Biol* 1976;**48**:271–83.

38. Crowley S. Growth in asthma. *Growth Matters* 1993; **13**:2–4.

39. Aderele WI. Physical growth of Nigerian children with bronchial asthma. *Ann Trop Paediatr* 1981;**1**:107–13.

40. Shohat M, Shohat T, Kedem R, Mimouni M, Danon YL. Childhood asthma and growth outcome. *Arch Dis Child* 1987;**62**:63–5.

41. Albanese A, Stanhope R. Investigation of delayed puberty. *Clin Endocrinol* 1995;**43**:105–10.

42. David TJ. Short stature in children with atopic eczema. *Acta Derm Venereol* (Suppl) 1989;**144**:41–4.

43. Pike MG, Chang CL, Atherton DJ, Carpenter RG, Preece MA. Growth in atopic eczema: a controlled study by questionnaire. *Arch Dis Child* 1989;**64**:1566–9.

44. Massarano AA, Hollis S, Devlin J, David TJ. Growth in atopic eczema. *Arch Dis Child* 1993;**68**:677–9.

45. Patel L, Clayton PE, Addison GM, Price DA, David TJ. Linear growth in prepubertal children with atopic dermatitis. *Arch Dis Child* 1998;**79**:169–72.

46. Patel L, Clayton PE, Jenney ME, Ferguson JE, David TJ. Adult height in patients with childhood onset atopic dermatitis. *Arch Dis Child* 1997;**76**:505–8.

47. Sant'Anna CA, Sole D, Naspitz CK. Short stature in children with respiratory allergy. *Pediatr Allergy Immunol* 1996;**7**:187–92.

48. Hauspie R, Susanne C, Alexander F. Maturational delay and temporal growth retardation in asthmatic boys. *J Allergy Clin Immunol* 1977;**59**:200–6.

49. Balfour-Lynn L. Growth and childhood asthma. *Arch Dis Child* 1986;**61**:1049–55.

50. Ferguson AC, Murray AB, Tze WJ. Short stature and delayed skeletal maturation in children with allergic disease. *J Allergy Clin Immunol* 1982;**69**:461–6.

51. Baum WF, Kloditz E, Bromme W, Bismarck M, Thiemann HH, Weingartner R. Der Einfluss des Asthma bronchiale auf Wachstum und korperliche Entwicklung. *Arztl Jugendkd* 1990;**81**:379–83.

52. Baum WF, Kloditz E, Thiemann HH. Die atopische Skelettretardierung als eine mogliche Ursache fur Kleinwuchs und Brustkorbdeformierung asthmakranker Kinder. *Kinderarztl Prax* 1993; **61**:285–90.

53. Semple PD, Beastall GH, Watson WS, Hume R. Hypothalamic–pituitary dysfunction in respiratory hypoxia. *Thorax* 1981;**36**:605–9.

54. Abdel-Khalek A, Abdel Khalek AA, El-Salahy IM, Abdel-Ghaffar LA. Inter-relationship of adolescence and bronchial asthma. *Eur Respir J* 1999;**14**:178s.

55. Amirav I, Dowdeswell RJ, Plit M, Panz VR, Joffe BI, Seftel HC. Growth hormone response to exercise in asthmatic and normal children. *Eur J Pediatr* 1990;**149**:443–6.

56. Sanders SS, Norman AP. Growth hormone secretion in growth-retarded asthmatic children. *Br Med J* 1969;**3**:25–6.

57. Nigam P, Laungia S, Goyal BM, Dutt B. Growth hormone secretion in growth retarded asthmatic children. *Indian J Pediatr* 1969;**44**:315–19.

58. Morris HG, Jorgensen JR, Jenkins SA. Plasma growth hormone concentration in corticosteroid-treated children. *J Clin Invest* 1968;**47**:427–35.

59. Tinkelman DG, Reed CE, Nelson HS, Offord KP. Aerosol beclomethasone dipropionate compared with theophylline as primary treatment of chronic, mild to moderately severe asthma in children. *Pediatrics* 1993;**92**:64–77.

60. Priftis K, Milner AD, Conway E, Honour JW. Adrenal function in asthma. *Arch Dis Child* 1990;**65**:838–40.

61. Kallenbach JM, Panz V, Girson MS, Joffe BI, Seftel HC. The hormonal response to exercise in asthma. *Eur Respir J* 1990;**3**:171–5.

62. Zeitlin SR, Bond S, Wootton S, Gregson RK, Radford M. Increased resting energy expenditure in childhood asthma: does this contribute towards growth failure? *Arch Dis Child* 1992;**67**:1366–9.

63. Maffeis C, Chiocca E, Zaffanello M, Golinelli M, Pinelli L, Boner AL. Energy intake and energy expenditure in prepubertal males with asthma. *Eur Respir J* 1998;**12**:123–9.

64. Cogswell JJ, El-Bishti MM. Growth retardation in asthma: role of calorie deficiency. *Arch Dis Child* 1982;**57**:473–5.

65. Klein GL, Dungy CI, Galant SP. Growth and the nutritional status of nonsteroid-dependent asthmatic children. *Ann Allergy* 1991;**67**:80–4.

66. Klein G, Duriseti L, Miyamoto S, Wright D, Galant SP. Nutrition and growth in the nonsteroid-dependent asthmatic child. *J Allergy Clin Immunol* 2000;**106**:158–9.

67. el Kholy MS, Gas Allah MA, el Shimi S, el Baz F, el Tayeb H, Abdel-Hamid MS. Zinc and copper status in children with bronchial asthma and atopic dermatitis. *J Egypt Public Health Assoc* 1990;**65**:657–68.

68. David TJ, Wells FE, Sharpe TC, Gibbs AC. Low serum zinc in children with atopic eczema. *Br J Dermatol* 1984;**111**:597–601.

69. David TJ, Wells FE, Sharpe TC, Gibbs AC, Devlin J. Serum levels of trace metals in children with atopic eczema. *Br J Dermatol* 1990;**122**:485–9.

70. Goldey DH, Mansmann HC Jr, Rasmussen AI. Zinc status of asthmatic, prednisone-treated asthmatic, and non-asthmatic children. *J Am Diet Assoc* 1984; **84**:157–63.

71. Di Toro R, Galdo CG, Gialanella G, Miraglia DG, Moro R, Perrone L. Zinc and copper status of allergic children. *Acta Paediatr Scand* 1987;**76**:612–17.

72. Soutar A, Seaton A, Brown K. Bronchial reactivity and dietary antioxidants. *Thorax* 1997;**52**:166–70.

73. Seaton A, Godden DJ, Brown K. Increase in asthma: a more toxic environment or a more susceptible population? *Thorax* 1994;**49**:171–4.

74. Hatch GE. Asthma, inhaled oxidants, and dietary antioxidants. *Am J Clin Nutr* 1995;**61**:625S–630S.

75. Peat JK. Prevention of asthma. *Eur Respir J* 1996;**9**:1545–55.

76. Cohen HA, Neuman I, Nahum H. Blocking effect of vitamin C in exercise-induced asthma. *Arch Pediatr Adolesc Med* 1997;**151**:367–70.

77. Collipp PJ, Chen SY, Sharma RK, Balachandar V, Maddaiah VT. Tryptophane metabolism in bronchial asthma. *Ann Allergy* 1975;**35**:153–8.

78. Hall MA, Thom H, Russell G. Erythrocyte aspartate amino transferase activity in asthmatic and non-asthmatic children and its enhancement by vitamin B_6. *Ann Allergy* 1981;**47**:464–6.

79. Sur S, Camara M, Buchmeier A, Morgan S, Nelson HS. Double-blind trial of pyridoxine (vitamin B_6) in the treatment of steroid-dependent asthma. *Ann Allergy* 1993;**70**:147–52.

80. Delport R, Ubbink JB, Serfontein WJ, Becker PJ, Walters L. Vitamin B6 nutritional status in asthma: the effect of theophylline therapy on plasma pyridoxal-5′-phosphate and pyridoxal levels. *Int J Vitam Nutr Res* 1988;**58**:67–72.

81. Shimizu T, Maeda S, Mochizuki H, Tokuyama K, Morikawa A. Theophylline attenuates circulating vitamin B_6 levels in children with asthma. *Pharmacology* 1994;**49**:392–7.

82. Baum WF, Kloditz E, Schneyer U, Sitka U. Zum Einfluss des Beta-2-Mimetikums Terbutalin auf die Wachstumshormonsekretion prapubertarer asthmakranker Kinder. *Pneumologie* 1997;**51**:513–16.

83. Giustina A, Malerba M, Bresciani E, Desenzani P, Licini M, Zaltieri G, Grassi V. Effect of two beta 2-agonist drugs, salbutamol and broxaterol, on the growth hormone response to exercise in adult patients with asthmatic bronchitis. *J Endocrinol Invest* 1995;**18**:847–52.

84. Lanes R, Duran Z, Aguirre J, Espina L, Alvarez W, Villaroel O, Zdanowicz M. Short- and long-term effect of oral salbutamol on growth hormone secretion in prepubertal asthmatic children. *Metab Clin Exp* 1995;**44**:149–51.

85. Baum WF, Kloditz E, Schneyer U. Hemmung der wachstumshormonsekretion durch theophyllin bei asthmakranken kindern. *Pneumologie* 1996;**50**:238–41.

86. Soferman R, Sapir N, Spirer Z, Golander A. Effects of inhaled corticosteroids and inhaled cromolyn sodium on urinary growth hormone excretion in asthmatic children. *Pediatr Pulmonol* 1998; **26**:339–43.

87. Prader A, Tanner JM, von Harnack GA. Catch-up growth following illness or starvation. *J Pediatr* 1963;**62**:646–59.

88. Blodgett FM, Burgin L, Iezzoni D, Gribetz D, Talbot NB. Effects of prolonged cortisone therapy on statural growth, skeletal maturation and metabolic status of children. *N Engl J Med* 1965;**254**:636–41.

89. Van Metre TE, Niermann WA, Rosen LJ. Comparison of the growth suppressive effects of cortisone, prednisone and other adrenal cortical hormones. *J Allergy* 1960;**31**:531.

90. Friedman M, Strang LB. Effect of long-term corticosteroids and corticotrophin on the growth of children. *Lancet* 1966;**2**:569–72.

91. Drever JC, Malone DN, Grant IW, Douglas DM, Lutz W. Corticotrophin after corticosteroids in children with asthma and growth retardation. *Br J Dis Chest* 1975;**69**:188–94.

92. Oberger E, Engstrom I, Karlberg J. Long-term treatment with glucocorticoids/ACTH in asthmatic children III Effects on growth and adult height. *Acta Paediatr Scand* 1990;**79**:77–83.

93. Harter JG, Reddy WJ, Thorn GW. Studies on an intermittent corticosteroid dosage regimen. *N Engl J Med* 1963;**269**:591–6.

94. Wolthers OD, Pedersen S. Short term linear growth in asthmatic children during treatment with prednisolone. *Br Med J* 1990;**301**:145–8.

95. Kerrebijn KF, Kroon JD. Effect of height of corticosteroid therapy in asthmatic children. *Arch Dis Child* 1968;**43**:556–61.

96. Brown HM, Storey G. Beclomethasone dipropionate steroid aerosol in treatment of perennial allergic asthma in children. *Br Med J* 1973;**3**:161–4.

97. Godfrey S, König P. Beclomethasone aerosol in childhood asthma. *Arch Dis Child* 1973;**48**:665–70.

98. Kuzemko JA. Growth velocity in children on oral corticosteroids and betamethasone valerate aerosol. *Postgrad Med J* 1974;**50**(Suppl 4):38–40.

99. Godfrey S, Balfour-Lynn L, Tooley M. A three- to five-year follow-up of the use of the aerosol steroid, beclomethasone dipropionate, in childhood asthma. *J Allergy Clin Immunol* 1978;**62**:335–9.

100. Graff-Lonnevig V, Kraepelien S. Long-term treatment with beclomethasone dipropionate aerosol in asthmatic children with special reference to growth. *Allergy* 1979;**34**:57–61.

101. Thomas BC, Stanhope R, Grant DB. Impaired growth in children with asthma during treatment with conventional doses of inhaled corticosteroids. *Acta Paediatr* 1994;**83**:196–9.

102. Littlewood JM, Johnson AW, Edwards PA, Littlewood AE. Growth retardation in asthmatic children treated with inhaled beclomethasone dipropionate. *Lancet* 1988;**i**:115–16.

103. Varsano I, Volovitz B, Malik H, Amir Y. Safety of 1 year of treatment with budesonide in young children with asthma. *J Allergy Clin Immunol* 1990;**85**:914–20.

104. Verini M, Verrotti A, D'Arcangelo A, Misticoni G, Chiarelli F, Morgese G. Long-term therapy in childhood asthma: clinical and auxological effects. *Riv Eur Sci Med Farmacol* 1990;**12**:169–73.

105. Merkus PJFM, Essen-Zandvliet EEM, Duiverman EJ, van Houwelingen HC, Kerrebijn KF, Quanjer PH. Long-term effect of inhaled corticosteroids on growth rate in adolescents with asthma. *Pediatrics* 1993;**91**:1121–6.

106. Agertoft L, Pedersen S. Effects of long-term treatment with an inhaled corticosteroid on growth and pulmonary function in asthmatic children. *Respir Med* 1994;**88**:373–81.

107. Russell G, Ninan TK, Carter PE, Reid IW, Sutherland I. Effects of inhaled corticosteroids on hypothalamo–pituitary–adrenal function and growth in children. *Res Clin Forums* 1989;**11**:77–84.

108. Allen DB, Mullen M, Mullen B. A meta-analysis of the effect of oral and inhaled corticosteroids on growth. *J Allergy Clin Immunol* 1994;**93**:967–76.

109. Wolthers OD, Pedersen S. Growth of asthmatic children during treatment with budesonide: a double blind trial. *Br Med J* 1991;**303**:163–5.

110. Wolthers OD, Pedersen S. Controlled study of linear growth in asthmatic children during treatment with inhaled glucocorticosteroids. *Pediatrics* 1992;**89**:839–42.

111. Bisgaard H. Systemic activity of inhaled topical steroid in toddlers studied by knemometry. *Acta Paediatr* 1993;**82**:1066–71.

112. Heuck C, Wolthers OD, Hansen M, Kollerup G. Short-term growth and collagen turnover in asthmatic adolescents treated with the inhaled glucocorticoid budesonide. *Steroids* 1997;**62**:659–64.

113. Heuck C, Heickendorff L, Wolthers OD. Short-term growth and collagen turnover in asthmatics treated with inhaled formoterol and budesonide. *Eur Respir J* 1999;**14**:42s.

114. Heuck C, Wolthers OD, Kollerup G, Hansen M, Teisner B. Adverse effects of inhaled budesonide (800 micrograms) on growth and collagen turnover in children with asthma: a double-blind comparison of once-daily versus twice-daily administration. *J Pediatr* 1998;**133**:608–12.

115. Reid A, Murphy C, Steen HJ, McGovern V, Shields MD. Linear growth of very young asthmatic children treated with high-dose nebulized budesonide. *Acta Paediatr* 1996;**85**:421–4.

116. Wolthers OD, Pedersen S. Short-term growth during treatment with inhaled fluticasone propionate and beclomethasone dipropionate. *Arch Dis Child* 1993;**68**:673–6.

117. MacKenzie C. Effects of inhaled corticosteroids on growth. *J Allergy Clin Immunol* 1998;**101**:S451–5.

118. Reed CE, Offord KP, Nelson HS, Li JT, Tinkelman DG. Aerosol beclomethasone dipropionate spray compared with theophylline as primary treatment for chronic mild-to-moderate asthma. *J Allergy Clin Immunol* 1998;**101**:14–23.

119. Doull IJ, Freezer NJ, Holgate ST. Growth of prepubertal children with mild asthma treated with inhaled beclomethasone dipropionate. *Am J Respir Crit Care Med* 1995;**151**:1715–19.

120. Simons FER, Dolovich J, Moore DW. A comparison of beclomethasone, salmeterol, and placebo in children with asthma. *New Engl J Med* 1997;**337**:1659–65.

121. Verberne AA, Frost C, Roorda RJ, van der Laag H, Kerrebijn KF. One year treatment with salmeterol compared with beclomethasone in children with asthma. *Am J Respir Crit Care Med* 1997;**156**:688–95.

122. Sharek PJ, Bergman DA. The effect of inhaled steroids on the linear growth of children with asthma: a meta-analysis. *Pediatrics* 2000;**106**:E8.

123. Saha MT, Laippala P, Lenko HL. Clinical observations on catch-up growth in asthmatic children following withdrawal of inhaled glucocorticosteroids. *Pediatr Pulmonol* 1998;**26**:292–4.

124. Agertoft L, Pedersen S. Effect of long-term treatment with inhaled budesonide on adult height in children with asthma. *N Engl J Med* 2000;**343**:1064–9.

125. Silverstein MD, Yunginger JW, Reed CE, Petterson T, Zimmerman D, Li JT, O'Fallon WM. Attained adult height after childhood asthma: effect of glucocorticoid therapy. *J Allergy Clin Immunol* 1997;**99**:466–74.

126. Van Bever HP, Desager KN, Lijssens N, Weyler JJ, Du Caju MV. Does treatment of asthmatic children with inhaled corticosteroids affect their adult height? *Pediatr Pulmonol* 1999;**27**:369–75.

127. Inoue T, Doi S, Takamatsu I, Murayama N, Kameda M, Toyoshima K. Effect of long-term treatment with inhaled beclomethasone dipropionate on growth of asthmatic children. *J Asthma* 1999;**36**:159–64.

128. Larsson L, Norjavaara E, Gerhardsson de Verdier M, Lindmark B. Asthma, steroids and final height. *Am J Respir Crit Care Med* 2000;**161**:A774.

129. Holliday SM, Faulds D, Sorkin EM. Inhaled fluticasone propionate. A review of its pharmacodynamic and pharmacokinetic properties, and therapeutic use in asthma. *Drugs* 1994;**47**:318–31.

130. Barnes NC, Hallett C, Harris TA. Clinical experience with fluticasone propionate in asthma: a meta-analysis of efficacy and systemic activity compared with budesonide and beclomethasone dipropionate at half the microgram dose or less. *Respir Med* 1998;**92**:95–104.

131. Agertoft L, Pedersen S. Short-term knemometry and urine cortisol excretion in children treated with fluticasone propionate and budesonide: a dose response study. *Eur Respir J* 1997;**10**:1507–12.

132. Visser MJ, van AW, Elliott BM, Odink RJ, Brand PL. Short-term growth in asthmatic children using fluticasone propionate. *Chest* 1998;**113**:584–6.

133. Primhak RA, Smith CM, Powell CVE. A comparison of the systemic effects of high dose inhaled steroids in asthmatic children. *Am J Respir Crit Care Med* 1999;**159**:A909.

134. Price JF, Russell G, Hindmarsh PC, Weller P, Heaf DP, Williams J. Growth during one year of treatment with fluticasone propionate or sodium cromoglycate in children with asthma. *Pediatr Pulmonol* 1997;**24**:178–86.

135. Allen DB, Bronsky EA, LaForce CF, Nathan RA, Tinkelman DG, Vandewalker ML, Konig P. Growth in asthmatic children treated with fluticasone propionate. *J Pediatr* 1998;**132**:472–7.

136. Barnes ND, Whitaker K, Gelson W, Barnes JLC. The effect of inhaled dry powder steroids on growth in children with asthma. *Am J Respir Crit Care Med* 1997;**155**:A267.

137. de Benedictis FM, Medley HV, Williams L. Long-term study to compare the safety and efficacy of fluticasone propionate and beclomethasone dipropionate in asthmatic children. *Eur Respir J* 1998;**12**:142.

138. Rao R, Gregson RK, Jones AC, Miles EA, Campbell MJ, Warner JO. Systemic effects of inhaled corticosteroids on growth and bone turnover in childhood asthma: a comparison of fluticasone with beclomethasone. *Eur Respir J* 1999;**13**:87–94.

139. Teper AM, Colon AJ, Cherry HR, Robaldo JF, Kofman CD, Maffet AF, Vidayrreta SM. Effect of fluticasone propionate on asthmatic infants. *Am J Respir Crit Care Med* 1998;**157**:A711.

140. Todd G, Dunlop K, McNaboe J, Ryan MF, Carson D, Shields MD. Growth and adrenal suppression in asthmatic children treated with high-dose fluticasone propionate. *Lancet* 1996;**348**:27–9.

141. Fitzgerald D, Van Asperen P, Mellis C, Honner M, Smith L, Ambler G. Fluticasone propionate 750 micrograms/day versus beclomethasone dipropionate 1500 micrograms/day: comparison of efficacy and adrenal function in paediatric asthma. *Thorax* 1998;**53**:656–61.

142. Doull IJ, Campbell MJ, Holgate ST. Duration of growth suppressive effects of regular inhaled corticosteroids. *Arch Dis Child* 1998;**78**:172–3.

143. Ubhi BS, Brownlee KG. The clinical effect of long term high dose fluticasone propionate on the growth of severe asthmatic children. *Am J Respir Crit Care Med* 1998;**157**:A711.

144. Ferguson AC, Spier S, Manjra A, Versteegh FG, Mark S, Zhang P. Efficacy and safety of high-dose inhaled steroids in children with asthma: a comparison of fluticasone propionate with budesonide. *J Pediatr* 1999;**134**:422–7.

145. Kannisto S, Korppi M, Remes K, Voutilainen R. Adrenal suppression, evaluated by a low dose adrenocorticotropin test, and growth in asthmatic children treated with inhaled steroids. *J Clin Endocrinol Metab* 2000;**85**:652–7.

146. Stempel DA, Blaiss MS, Edwards L, Srebro S. The effect of inhaled corticosteroids (ICS) on growth velocity in children with asthma. *Am J Respir Crit Care Med* 2000;**161**:A774.

147. Price J. The role of inhaled corticosteroids in children with asthma. *Arch Dis Child* 2000;**82**(Suppl 2):ii10–ii14.

148. O'Callaghan C, Barry PW. How to choose delivery devices for asthma. *Arch Dis Child* 2000;**82**:185–7.

149. Leach CL, Davidson PJ, Boudreau RJ. Improved airway targeting with the CFC-free HFA-beclomethasone metered-dose inhaler compared with CFC-beclomethasone. *Eur Respir J* 1998;**12**:1346–53.

150. Lipworth BJ. Clinical pharmacology of corticosteroids in bronchial asthma. *Pharmacol Ther* 1993;**58**:173–209.

151. Gibbs CJ, Coutts II, Lock R, Finnegan OC, White RJ. Premenstrual exacerbation of asthma. *Thorax* 1984;**39**:833–6.

152. Horan JD, Lederman JJ. Possible asthmogenic effect of oral contraceptives. *Can Med Assoc J* 1968;**99**:130–1.

153. Matsuo N, Shimoda T, Matsuse H, Kohno S. A case of menstruation-associated asthma: treatment with oral contraceptives. *Chest* 1999;**116**:252–3.

154. Price J, Kemp, J. The problems of treating adolescent asthma: what are the alternatives to inhaled therapy? *Respir Med* 1999;**93**:677–84.

155. Kravis LP, Kolski GB. Asthma mortality in children: a 16-years experience at Children's Hospital of Philadelphia. *N Engl Reg Allergy Proc* 1986;**7**:442–7.

156. Martin AJ, Campbell DA, Gluyas PA, *et al*. Characteristics of near-fatal asthma in childhood. *Pediatr Pulmonol* 1995;**20**:1–8.

157. Wamboldt FS, Wamboldt MZ, Gavin LA, Roesler TA, Brugman SM. Parental criticism and treatment outcome in adolescents hospitalized for severe, chronic asthma. *J Psychosom Res* 1995;**39**:995–1005.

158. Buston KM, Wood SF. Non-compliance amongst adolescents with asthma: listening to what they tell us about self-management. *Fam Pract* 2000;**17**:134–8.

159. Gibson PG, Henry RL, Vimpani GV, Halliday J. Asthma knowledge, attitudes, and quality of life in adolescents. *Arch Dis Child* 1995;**73**:321–6.

160. Gibson PG, Shah S, Mamoon HA. Peer-led asthma education for adolescents: impact evaluation. *J Adolesc Health* 1998;**22**:66–72.

161. Stocks J, Henschen M, Hoo AF, Costeloe K, Dezateux C. Influence of ethnicity and gender on airway function in preterm infants. *Am J Respir Crit Care Med* 1997;**156**:1855–62.

162. Torday JS, Nielsen HC. The sex difference in fetal lung surfactant production. *Exp Lung Res* 1987;**12**:1–19.

163. Talal N. Sex hormones and immunity. In: IM Roitt, ed. *Encyclopedia of Immunology,* Vol 3. Academic Press, London, 2000.

164. Grossman CJ. Regulation of the immune system by sex steroids. *Endocr Rev* 1984;**5**:435–55.

165. Whitacre CC, Reingold SC, O'Looney PA. A gender gap in autoimmunity. *Science* 1999;**283**:1277–8.

166. Kulig M, Tacke U, Forster J, *et al*. Serum IgE levels during the first 6 years of life. *J Pediatr* 1999;**134**:453–8.

167. Jarvis D, Burney, P. ABC of allergies. The epidemiology of allergic disease. *Br Med J* 1998;**316**:607–10.

168. Olsen NJ, William JK. Gonadal steroids and immunity. *Endocr Rev* 1996;**17**:371–84.

169. Piccinni MP, Giudizi MG, Biagiotti R, *et al*. Progesterone favors the development of human T helper cells producing Th2-type cytokines and promotes both IL-4 production and membrane CD30 expression in established Th1 cell clones. *J Immunol* 1995;**155**:128–33.

170. Prescott SL, Macaubas C, Holt BJ, Smallacombe TB, Loh R, Sly PD, Holt PG. Transplacental priming of the human immune system to environmental allergens: universal skewing of initial T cell responses toward the Th2 cytokine profile. *J Immunol* 1998;**160**:4730–7.

171. Alberts WM. 'Circa menstrual' rhythmicity and asthma. *Chest* 1997;**111**:840–2.

172. De Marco R, Locatelli F, Sunyer J, Burney P. Differences in incidence of reported asthma related to age in men and women. A retrospective analysis of the data of the European Respiratory Health Survey. *Am J Respir Crit Care Med* 2000;**162**:68–74.

173. Venn A, Lewis S, Cooper M, Hill J, Britton J. Questionnaire study of effect of sex and age on the prevalence of wheeze and asthma in adolescence. *Br Med J* 1998;**316**:1945–6.

174. Skobeloff EM, Spivey WH, St Clair SS, Schoffstall JM. The influence of age and sex on asthma admissions. *JAMA* 1992;**268**:3437–40.

175. Wieringa MH, Weyler JJ, Van Bever HP, Nelen VJ, Vermeire PA. Gender differences in respiratory, nasal and skin symptoms: 6–7 versus 13–14-year-old children. *Acta Paediatr* 1999;**88**:147–9.

176. Withers NJ, Low L, Holgate ST, Clough JB. The natural history of respiratory symptoms in a cohort of adolescents. *Am J Respir Crit Care Med* 1998;**158**:352–7.

177. Sears MR. Consequences of long-term inflammation. The natural history of asthma. *Clin Chest Med* 2000;**21**:315–29.

178. Sears MR, Burrows B, Flannery EM, Herbison GP, Holdaway MD. Atopy in childhood. I Gender and allergen related risks for development of hay fever and asthma. *Clin Exp Allergy* 1993;**23**:941–8.

179. Becklake MR, Kauffmann F. Gender differences in airway behaviour over the human life span. *Thorax* 1999;**54**:1119–38.

180. Barbee RA, Halonen M, Kaltenborn W, Lebowitz M, Burrows BA. Longitudinal study of serum IgE in a community cohort: correlations with age, sex, smoking, and atopic status. *J Allergy Clin Immunol* 1987;**79**:919–27.

181. Verity CM, Vanheule B, Carswell F, Hughes AO. Bronchial lability and skin reactivity in siblings of asthmatic children. *Arch Dis Child* 1984; **59**:871–6.

182. Stein RT, Holberg CJ, Morgan WJ, Wright AL, Lombardi E, Taussig L, Martinez FD. Peak flow variability, methacholine responsiveness and atopy as markers for detecting different wheezing phenotypes in childhood. *Thorax* 1997;**52**:946–52.

183. Peat JK, Britton WJ, Salome CM, Woolcock AJ. Bronchial hyperresponsiveness in two populations of Australian schoolchildren. II Relative importance of associated factors. *Clin Allergy* 1987;**17**:283–90.

184. Leynaert B, Bousquet J, Henry C, Liard R, Neukirch F. Is bronchial hyperresponsiveness more frequent in women than in men? A population-based study. *Am J Respir Crit Care Med* 1997;**156**:1413–20.

185. Eliasson O, Scherzer HH. Recurrent respiratory failure in premenstrual asthma. *Conn Med* 1984;**48**:777–8.

186. Pauli BD, Reid RL, Munt PW, Wigle RD, Forkert L. Influence of the menstrual cycle on airway function in asthmatic and normal subjects. *Am Rev Respir Dis* 1989;**140**:358–62.

187. Hanley SP. Asthma variation with menstruation. *Br J Dis Chest* 1981;**75**:306–8.

188. Zimmerman JL, Woodruff PG, Clark S, Camargo CA. Relation between phase of menstrual cycle and emergency department visits for acute asthma. *Am J Respir Crit Care Med* 2000;**162**:512–15.

189. Eliasson O, Scherzer HH, DeGraff AC Jr. Morbidity in asthma in relation to the menstrual cycle. *J Allergy Clin Immunol* 1986;**77**:87–94.

190. Tan KS, McFarlane LC, Lipworth BJ. Loss of normal cyclical beta 2 adrenoceptor regulation and increased premenstrual responsiveness to adenosine monophosphate in stable female asthmatic patients. *Thorax* 1997;**52**:608–11.

191. Tan KS, McFarlane LC, Lipworth BJ. Modulation of airway reactivity and peak flow variability in asthmatics receiving the oral contraceptive pill. *Am J Respir Crit Care Med* 1997;**155**:1273–7.

192. Vellutini M, Viegi G, Parrini D, *et al*. Serum immunoglobulins E are related to menstrual cycle. *Eur J Epidemiol* 1997;**13**:931–5.

193. Kalogeromitros D, Katsarou A, Armenaka M, Rigopoulos D, Zapanti M, Stratigos I. Influence of the menstrual cycle on skin-prick test reactions to histamine, morphine and allergen. *Clin Exp Allergy* 1995;**25**:461–6.

194. Waldblott GL. Estrogenic hormone determination in premenstrual asthma. *J Allergy* 1942; **13**:125–34.

195. Ensom MH. Gender-based differences and menstrual cycle-related changes in specific diseases: implications for pharmacotherapy. *Pharmacotherapy* 2000;**20**:523–39.

196. Troisi RJ, Speizer FE, Willett WC, Trichopoulos D, Rosner B. Menopause, postmenopausal estrogen preparations, and the risk of adult-onset asthma. A prospective cohort study. *Am J Respir Crit Care Med* 1995;**152**:1183–8.

197. Wjst M, Dold S. Is asthma an endocrine disease? *Pediatr Allergy Immunol* 1997;**8**:200–4.

198. Preece MA, Law CM, Davies PS. The growth of children with chronic paediatric disease *Clin Endocrinol Metab* 1986;**15**:453–77.

199. Balfour-Lynn L. Effect of asthma on growth and puberty. *Pediatrician* 1987;**14**:237–41.

200. Ganong WF. *Review of Medical Physiology*, 16th edn. Lange Medical Books, Prentice Hall International, London, 1993.

Asthma in primary care

TRISHA WELLER AND KEVIN JONES

INTRODUCTION

Childhood asthma poses a management challenge, not only to health professionals in hospital centres, but also to those providing medical and healthcare to communities. This chapter examines the organization of services for children with asthma in primary care and takes account of the increasing contribution of nurses. The viewpoint presented unavoidably focuses on the situation in the UK, but parallels are drawn with other countries whenever possible.

Asthma morbidity

In the UK, a recent audit reports that one in seven children have asthma.[1] This condition can be managed effectively within the primary healthcare setting, with specialist referral reserved where there are doubts as to the diagnosis. Evidence from two UK general practices suggested that around 90% of children with asthma had no contact with hospital-based paediatric departments, whether as out- or in-patients, during their years with the illness.[2] Even in the setting of acute asthma attacks, the UK General Practitioners in Asthma Group (GPIAG) national attack audit (1991–92) showed that a similar proportion of acute episodes was managed entirely in the community.[3] However, a large survey of people with asthma undertaken on behalf of the UK National Asthma Campaign (NAC) reported that 19% of children under 5 years experienced asthma symptoms every day, 71% of school-children had taken time off school due to asthma and 13% had had emergency treatment at hospital for asthma during the previous 12 months.[4]

Asthma guidelines

A major advance in asthma care world-wide has been the emergence of consensus statements on the management of the disease. Asthma guidelines in the UK include both adults and children, as well as addressing asthma management in secondary and primary care;[5] the international children's consensus statement was revised in 1998.[6] Most guidelines do not yet include recent therapeutic additions, such as the leukotriene receptor antagonists. Children age 5 years and over are included with adults – a concern because of the potential for the sanctioning of high doses of inhaled corticosteroids in the growing child. Infants and preschool children (under 5) are grouped together, raising similar concerns over the use of inhaled corticosteroids, especially where the diagnosis of asthma in the very young may be in doubt. Revision of these guidelines, taking an evidence-based approach has been completed and are scheduled to be published shortly. In developing countries, the Global Initiative in Asthma (GINA) guidelines[7] may be referred to, but access to appropriate medication is restricted by cost and availability (Chapter 17), restricting their relevance to relatively affluent countries.

ORGANIZATION OF ASTHMA CARE

Because asthma is common, many professionals without specialist training care for children with asthma. It is important that their care is in line with current evidence-based practice and that referral to qualified paediatric pulmonologists should be made if there are problems. A tertiary referral service will need the support of services such as paediatric radiology and lung function laboratories, but these are less widely available. Increasing numbers of paediatricians with a specialist interest in the respiratory field (paediatric pulmonologists) now have an important role in improving secondary care asthma services and developing links with community services.

Direct access to paediatric care is the norm in some countries, such as the United States, but in others distance from appropriate respiratory care or lack of such provision presents a problem. Some UK hospitals operate a direct access scheme for selected difficult or 'brittle' asthma patients with good effect.[8] Rapid access is not available to most children with asthma, but is usually restricted to those with severe disease and those under the care of paediatric pulmonologists. In the UK children with acute asthma are often taken directly to the emergency room of their local hospital, but there is evidence that care delivered there may not be optimal.[9,10] It has been reported that only 50% of those who presented to an emergency room with acute asthma received oral steroids after nebulized bronchodilator therapy and follow-up was generally poor.[11] It is evident that care and communication needs to improve in both primary and secondary care.

Organization of asthma care in general practice

Traditionally, family practice was a reactive service with patients consulting their primary care physicians either in their offices or in their own homes for advice and/or treatment concerning self-perceived health problems. Nurses had minimal involvement within the general practice setting. In 1990, general practice services in the UK changed with the introduction of health promotion clinics, which attracted reimbursement from the National Health Service (NHS).[12] The emphasis switched from illness to health and health promotion is now incorporated within all aspects of healthcare within general practice. Organized care for both asthma and diabetes within a general practice setting also attracts some additional funding. Practice nurses have become increasingly important because of their potential to generate income for practices with health promotion and chronic disease management responsibilities. As a result there has been the escalation in the number of nurses within general practice[13] and an emergence of the practice nurse as a discrete healthcare professional in the UK. This has been a welcome innovation in primary care, but education and training remains essential. There are now some published studies supporting the role of the nurse in asthma management, but there are many nurses in the community who have yet to undertake any formal asthma education.[13a,13b] Even fewer have appropriate paediatric respiratory training and experience.

Asthma care by nurses

Nurse-run asthma clinics have proliferated since their first introduction in 1985 and since formal asthma training programmes were developed for practice nurses.[14,15] Asthma and other respiratory programmes are now run by the UK National Respiratory Training Centre (NRTC), and the asthma course is recognized academically and accredited by several UK universities. Over 11 000 'students' from the UK and Europe have successfully passed the 'gold standard' NRTC Asthma Course module. The role of the nurse in asthma management is defined by Barnes[16] (Figure 16.1) and is appropriate for differing levels of educational expertise and responsibility. The NRTC educational format ensures safe practice and provides a solid foundation for developing additional expertise.

Proactive care of asthma has been shown to improve outcomes in the hospital setting,[17] but scientific studies in UK general practice have been few until recent years. An audit of the effects of a nurse-run asthma clinic reported a reduction in general practitioner consultations, oral steroid courses and acute nebulizations, as well as days lost from work and school, in patients taking prophylactic asthma medication.[18] Results were similar in both adults and children. Increased numbers of patients consulted with the nurse but despite medication changes, prescribing costs were unaffected. This audit demonstrated that using a trained asthma nurse was one way of providing asthma care in general practice. A smaller randomized, controlled study looked at patient self-management in one general practice asthma clinic in London.[19] The clinic patients successfully self-treated episodes of asthma more frequently, but there was no significant difference in reported symptoms, days off or consultations between the groups.

One study reported a reduction in asthma symptoms and fewer asthma attacks but an increase in short courses of oral steroids in those practices where there was a trained asthma nurse. The researchers concluded that there was a case for recommending that all general practices should employ a nurse trained in asthma to improve patient management.[20] An evidence-based approach to care may lessen the likelihood of litigation which is increasing in general practice. Another study using trained asthma nurses, targeted patients with more severe asthma; the nurses were able to make changes to asthma therapy in line with UK guidelines.[21,22]

General practices in south-east London reported no difference in quality of life after an *educational intervention* to improve asthma management.[23] However, only 26% of those taking asthma medications were seen and there was a high turnover of practice nurses, some of whom were inadequately trained. It was unclear from the study how the outcome was assessed and whether there was an emphasis on secondary rather than primary care. There was no mention of how many patients seen in general practice were frequent attenders at emergency departments. Perhaps there was a need for improved hospital discharge policies and better communication with primary care. Madge showed a reduction in the readmission rate from 25% to 8% when she introduced

STRUCTURED ASTHMA CARE AND TRAINING REQUIREMENTS

MINIMUM INVOLVEMENT

ACTIVITIES

1. Compile asthma register
2. Take a structured formal history
3. Take peak flows in a surgery
4. Teach how to use peak flow meter at home, and how to chart a diary card
5. Demonstrate, instruct, and check inhaler technique

SUGGESTED PRELIMINARY TRAINING

- Sit in with clinician/NRTC Asthma Course holder during asthma consultations
- Instruction from NRTC Instructor
- Formal study days set up by Health Commissions/Boards, respiratory pharmaceutical companies etc.

+
EXPERIENCE
↓

MEDIUM INVOLVEMENT

ACTIVITIES 1–5+

6. Carry out diagnostic procedures e.g. reversibility exercise and serial peak flow monitoring
7. Improve asthma education
8. Provide explanatory literature
9. Spot poor control, with referral back to clinician
10. Establish regular follow-up procedure

SUGGESTED INTERMEDIATE TRAINING

- Sit in with clinician/NRTC Asthma Course holder during asthma consultations
- Formal study days and workshops set up by Health Commissions/Boards, respiratory pharmaceutical companies
- Instruction from NRTC Instructor/Trainer

+
EXPERIENCE
↓

IN-DEPTH TRAINING
NRTC Distance Learning Package + NRTC Asthma Course
(input from NRTC Trainer)

+
EXPERIENCE
↓

MAXIMUM INVOLVEMENT/AUTONOMY

ACTIVITIES 1–10+

11. Carry out full assessment and regular follow-up
12. Formulate structured treatment plan in conjunction with clinician + patient

13. Prepare prescription for clinician's signature
14. Give telephone advice/additional appointments where appropriate
15. See patients first in an emergency

NATIONAL
RESPIRATORY
TRAINING
CENTRE

Figure 16.1 *Structured asthma care and training requirements for nurses. Minimum/medium/maximum level of involvement. National Respiratory Training Centre, Warwick, UK, with permission.*

an educational programme for children admitted to hospital with acute asthma.[24] Another study has also shown that structured discharge planning reduces re-admission rates in children.[25]

Ever since Speight first highlighted the problem of *underdiagnosis* of childhood asthma in 1978,[26] this issue has posed one of the most important organizational problems for primary care. Levy and Bell demonstrated in 1984 a median of 16–20 respiratory consultations before a diagnosis of asthma was made in asthmatic children in one general practice with an interest in the disease.[27] There is evidence of improvement[28] and continuing studies by the UK General Practitioners in Asthma Group are documenting further progress.[29]

The widespread use of resources in UK family practice directed towards proactive asthma care without the benefit of rigorous conducted scientific trials, is beginning to be questioned in this day of evidence-based medicine. It is likely that there will be increased research in the future to support the use of asthma-trained nurses in the community. Improving approach to asthma education in secondary care as well as extending asthma training to other nurses within the community, such as public health nurses and school nurses will hopefully prove to be beneficial too.

Many healthcare professionals believe that their acute asthma workload has diminished and that patients are well satisfied with the service offered. The Asthma in Real Life (AIR) study suggested that for doctors and nurses, the focus of asthma care was too heavily biased towards symptoms and not enough towards the patient's wishes. A patient-focused approach may improve motivation with resulting behavioural changes and adherence to therapy.[30] Recent evidence has supported the assumption that new asthma episodes are declining.[31]

General practice (primary care) services are changing with a greater emphasis on nurse-led care and in the future this may lessen the medical model approach to care and control of asthma, with increased emphasis on patient-centred care.

HOSPITAL OR COMMUNITY LIAISON

Children with asthma admitted to hospital with an acute exacerbation may receive an outpatient follow-up appointment after discharge. This may or may not be in a designated asthma clinic, depending on local resources, and a nurse trained in asthma management is not always available. In practice this traditional model is not very effective as only about 10% of asthmatic children enter secondary care at all.[3] Not all patients attending for emergency asthma treatment at hospital receive appropriate asthma management according to guidelines[5] and many receive little or no follow-up in general practice.[8]

A number of possibilities exist to improve this situation. The first of these lies in the concept of 'hospital liaison'. *Hospital liaison* has existed for some time in the care of children with cystic fibrosis, diabetes and malignant diseases where specially trained hospital-based nurses have provided follow-up care to children discharged to the community, either on a short- or long-term basis. This has the advantage of promoting links between hospital staff and families and of building on educational lessons mentioned (but not always recalled) during admission.

The main disadvantage is the exclusion of the primary care team and an over-reliance on the hospital.

Charlton developed the concept of a *nurse-run* clinic within a hospital setting operating on the same lines as a nurse-run clinic within general practice.[32] Essential to the success of the clinic was the cooperation and collaboration of the participating general practitioners. This type of clinic may be much better placed to communicate with practice nurses and general practitioners, conducting home visits where necessary, as well as taking part in educational activities in primary care. An alternative model of care could be for a specialist paediatric respiratory nurse to initially assess and manage new asthma referrals. The child would then return to see the paediatric pulmonologist 4–6 weeks later and any further changes implemented. This model of care may accelerate the return to primary care management and avoid the need for further secondary care appointments.[33]

Simpson showed there is still a need to improve acute asthma care in general practice prior to referral to hospital,[34] but hospital admission rates for children have fallen in recent years, with many children remaining under brief observation rather than being admitted overnight. It has been shown that 70% of children admitted to hospital for acute asthma could be cared for in alternative settings.[35] This is preferable for both the child and the family, as well as reducing costs.

An alternative approach is the employment of asthma liaison nurses within a primary care group for a local population looking specifically at reducing hospital emergency attendance and admission and improving asthma management. Education and training needs of health professionals can be identified and implemented locally. Close liaison with the whole primary care team can result in group protocols for asthma and emergency care and improved communication with the local hospital services. Improved communication locally between the practice nurse, the health visitor and the school nurse should help to improve care for children with asthma at home and at school.

COMMUNITY CARE

Self-management

A key element of asthma management has been the concept of empowering patients to take control of their own disease and learn to vary its treatment according to their own specific impression of need. This has been associated in the past with the recording of peak-flow measurements at home on a daily basis, an onerous and unreliable task. Self-management plans based on only symptoms are just as useful.[36,37] A randomized controlled trial found that peak-flow recording did not add significantly to asthma management when compared with symptom management alone.[38]

Doubling preventer asthma therapy at the first sign of increased symptoms or at the start of a cold is another procedure based on no supporting evidence;[5] in fact there is contrary evidence. Parents need support and feedback to enable them to alter asthma treatment according to symptoms. Not all are happy to take on the responsibility, but some parents will hold a supply of oral prednisolone to be used during episodes of troublesome asthma, following a carefully planned management approach. An Australian study[39] reported that 95% of families did not use any written instructions during an acute asthma attack, and although 44% had been issued with a management plan only 9% of these families used it. There was also a delay in starting reliever medication and seeking help. Increasing the numbers of patients in general practice who have simple and practical self-management plans would be an improvement on the current situation, but is clearly insufficient without parental compliance.

Asthma at school

Children with asthma are very likely to experience symptoms and need treatment while under the care of school staff. Teachers often know little about asthma and its treatment, are worried about having asthmatic children in their care,[40,41] and are also unsure how asthma care at school should be organized.[42] Children with asthma should expect easy access to medication at school. Schools should have an asthma policy with a designated member of staff responsible for their care.[43] Evans reported an increased awareness of asthma in schools as well as increased numbers with asthma policies, but her study still indicated a need for schools to develop policies, for children to be able to have their inhalers easily accessible and for staff to have some training on asthma.[44] Teachers in the UK are allowed to supervise but not administer medication, which presents potential problems for young children.[45] Some areas in the UK have adopted school asthma policies in which a spacer device and short-acting β_2-medication is available at school for use by any child in an emergency situation. However, there are potential problems with this approach since legally, medication must be prescribed for a named individual and a 'generic' device and inhaler for use by whoever needs it is currently unlawful in the UK.

Family physicians and nurses involved with asthma care have an important role in providing specific information to schools. The main liaison between school staff and healthcare professionals in the UK is the school health service normally headed in each district by a community paediatrician. The doctors and nurses working with the service have a major opportunity to recognize under-diagnosed asthma and to initiate the care of children with asthma in school.

School nurses have a valuable role in promoting health to all children. They may be in a position to identify those whose asthma is poorly controlled as a result of non-adherence to treatment, inappropriate or inadequate treatment or where asthma is unrecognized or untreated.[46] In the UK, general practice health records and school nurse records are entirely separate. Improved communication, sharing information and improved referral procedures between general practice and the school nursing service as well as with secondary care must be the way forward. School asthma cards produced by the National Asthma Campaign are a useful way of ensuring that there is documented information about the child's treatment but these records must be updated whenever there is a change in treatment (Figure 16.2).

Children should be encouraged to take part in all school activities. Almost all children with severe asthma are now in mainstream education, whereas in the past some may have attended special schools. Access to inhalers must be unimpeded. Increasing numbers of children attending schools have asthma as well as potentially life-threatening allergies (anaphylaxis). These children may carry adrenaline (epinephrine) injectable pens and it is essential that schools know how and when to administer the injection as well. There are considerable training implications. School nurses have an important role in the training and support of both the child, the parents and the teaching staff.

Teenagers

Teenage asthma presents a challenge and has been shown to be underdiagnosed and under-treated.[47] Compliance with medication may be poor. Adolescence is a time of huge physical and emotional change as well as increasing independence and asthma cannot be treated in isolation from these other issues. Finding out what is important to the teenager is of paramount importance. A drop-in clinic run by a nurse in the community can provide an opportunity to discuss issues such as relationships, smoking, drugs, sexual behaviour and contraception, worries and concerns, as well as asthma. Access to the health professional should be normally at a time when it does not interfere with education. The consultation must be confidential and non-judgmental and the teenager may prefer to be seen without parents.

ASTHMA AUDIT, OUTCOMES AND QUALITY OF LIFE ISSUES

Audit is an integral part of healthcare provision. The information obtained may include the numbers of asthmatic patients on the practice list, the proportion of these reviewed each year and the number of hospital admissions for asthma. To be accurate the information should be prospectively collected and logged on computer. Despite healthcare changes in the UK and different health funding arrangements, there is still a contractual requirement for this information to be supplied by primary care

NATIONAL **ASTHMA** CAMPAIGN
conquering asthma

School asthma card

Child's name
Address

Parent's name
Telephone Home
Work
General Practitioner Name
Telephone
Hospital
Reference number
Telephone
Consultant

This card is for your school. Remember to update it or exchange it for a new one if treatment is changed.

1

Regular (preventer) treatment to be taken in school time

Name and how taken	Dose and when taken

Expiry dates checked

Before exercise

2

Relief treatment when needed

1 For sudden chest tightness, wheeze, breathlessness or cough, give or allow child to take the medication below. After a few minutes the child should feel better and be able to return to normal activity.

Name and how taken	Dose and when taken

Expiry dates checked

Parent's signature

2 If the reliever has no effect after five to ten minutes call the child's doctor or an ambulance.

3 Continue to give the child their reliever medication every few minutes until help arrives.

4 Inform the child's parents.

3

To receive a copy of the National Asthma Campaign School pack (for school staff) or the booklet Asthma at School, please contact the National Asthma Campaign.

National Asthma Campaign
Providence House
Providence Place
London N1 0NT
Telephone 0171 226 2260

National Asthma Campaign Scotland
21 Coates Crescent
Edinburgh EH3 7AF
Telephone 0131 226 2544

Asthma Helpline
0345 01 02 03
Monday to Friday
9am to 7pm

Card checked

Date	Initials

Registered charity number 802364

4

Figure 16.2 *National Asthma Campaign school card.*

practitioners. However, the information is now collected under the clinical governance umbrella which includes audit and is used on a more local basis to determine where health priorities and needs lie.[48] A National Service Framework (NSF) for asthma, which would monitor care against a defined standard seems unlikely.[49,50]

A major need in the assessment of asthma care, whether in the hospital or community sectors, is for widely applicable, validated, sensitive, specific, acceptable and simple *outcome measures*. The absence of a true 'gold standard' for asthma care is a major problem. Inter-instrument variations of peak-flow meters have resulted in potentially unreliable results.[51,52] Re-calibration of some of the portable meters has improved accuracy but poor peak flow technique can render the results unreliable and meaningless. It is important to remember that peak flow readings are used in conjunction with respiratory symptoms and not on their own. Children under the age of 6 or 7 are generally unable to produce reliable, repeatable and meaningful results, common clinical factors are probably more important for the diagnosis of childhood asthma.[53] Spirometry is now used more frequently in primary care, but it is essential to ensure that the operator has had appropriate training in performing the tests, the spirometers have been calibrated and the results interpreted correctly.[54] Intermittent spirometric measurements are far less sensitive than symptoms, as outcome measures for clinical management.

Improved *quality of life* is an important objective for children and their families (Chapter 6e). Where adults are

---

> *In the last week/month*
>
> 1. Have you had difficulty sleeping because of your asthma symptoms (including cough)?
> 2. Have you had your usual asthma symptoms during the day (cough, wheeze, chest tightness or breathlessness)?
> 3. Has your asthma interfered with your usual activities (e.g. sports, work/school etc)?

Figure 16.3 *Questions to determine asthma control.*[49]

concerned with functional ability, children's quality of life depends more on having friends or becoming independent of their parents.[55] During childhood, children change markedly, which French *et al.* acknowledged, by developing a quality of life questionnaire for three different age groups of childhood.[56] Juniper has developed a reliable and validated questionnaire which is specifically for children and is divided into the domains of activity limitation, symptoms and emotional function, matched by a questionnaire for their parents.[57] Quality of life measures are not widely applied either in primary or secondary care, but could be used to identify the real impact of asthma on the child and their family. Specific measures based on the use of simple questions to assess night-time wakening, day-time symptoms and interference with activity in the last week/month, can be used to assess control[49] (Figure 16.3). Although children were not specifically considered in the discussions that led to this report, the outcome measures would be equally applicable to children. Though yet to be validated, these questions are based on earlier, well-researched versions.[58–60]

NEW DEVELOPMENTS

Information technology

Good communication between healthcare workers is paramount in the management of asthmatic children. Admission rates of children to hospital with acute asthma have risen markedly in many countries, but the duration of stay has declined.[61] Children may return home earlier in the course of an attack and therefore may need more prompt attention from their family physician. Traditional discharge notes and full summaries can continue to provide all necessary information, but too often delays prevent their potential being realized. Information, communication and technology (ICT) offers a solution in the long-term. Many programs in use do not 'talk' to each other and hospital outpatient clinics do not have desk-top computers where information can be entered at the time of consultation and then transferred to general practice. The use of a nationally applied software system for collecting data on chronic diseases such as asthma and simplified data entry would provide more accurate and accessible information. Parent held records, either written or on a microchip, may be an alternative approach but this is generally an area which is not yet fully explored.

Asthma developments in primary care

The General Practitioners in Asthma Group (GPIAG) in the UK was established in 1987 to promote good asthma care in general practice and to provide a forum within which interested doctors could discuss such care and present scientific data. The group has made significant contributions to research literature[3,40,62,63] and has its own journal. Similar groups exist in Canada and Australia. Many practice nurses have developed a specific interest in asthma and are often more aware of latest research than their GP colleagues! Allergy is beginning to attract greater interest in primary care too. More nurses are being trained in skin-prick testing to identify allergen sensitivity and are thus able to target specific allergen reduction advice more appropriately. In addition, specific allergy courses have been developed.

The potential of nurses prescribing for chronic disease management such as asthma and diabetes is an exciting prospect.[64]

Safeguards when prescribing for children with asthma may be necessary. Greater involvement of pharmacists, who could spot poor asthma control, provide asthma education and teach and check inhaler technique, is a potential that has not been fully realized. This role may change if pharmacists become able to issue repeat prescriptions.[65]

Considerable investment in asthma research has been made. While much of this will continue to examine the molecular biology of asthma, good studies into the organization and delivery of care for patients with asthma in the community should also emerge from these continuing initiatives.

CONCLUSION

Good asthma care involves an integrated approach from different health professionals and one that is specific for the individual needs of the child. Systems vary between countries and much of the UK picture portrayed in this chapter may be at odds with that found elsewhere – particularly in its emphasis on primary care. However the role of an individual specifically trained in asthma management, could have a wide impact leading to improved asthma care. Asthma is common, chronic and as yet incurable, but it can be controlled with appropriate management and expertise. Children can and should be able to enjoy a childhood where they are unrestricted by asthma symptoms.

REFERENCES

1. National Asthma Campaign. *National Asthma Audit 1999/2000*. Cookham, Berks: Direct Publishing Solutions, 1999.
2. Charlton IH, Bain DJG. The care of children with asthma in general practice: signs of progress? *Br J Gen Pract* 1991;**41**:256.
3. Neville RG, Clark RC, Hoskins G, Smith B, for the General Practitioners in Asthma Group. National asthma attack audit 1991-2. *Br Med J* 1993; **306**:559–62.
4. National Asthma Campaign. *Impact of Asthma Survey Results*. Allen and Hanburys, London, 1996.
5. SIGN/British Thoracic Society Guidelines on Asthma Management. *Thorax* 2002; in press.
6. Warner JO, Naspitz CK. Third International Pediatric Consensus statement on the management of childhood asthma. International Pediatric Asthma Consensus Group. *Pediatr Pulmonol* 1998;**25**:1–17.
7. Global Initiative for Asthma. Global strategy for asthma management and prevention. NIH Publication No. 023659, 2002.
8. Crompton GK, Grant IWB, Bloomfield P. Edinburgh emergency asthma admission service. Report of ten years experience. *Br Med J* 1979; **2**:1199–201.
9. Reed S, Diggle S, Cushley MJ, Sleet RA, Tattersfield AE. Assessment and management of asthma in an accident and emergency department. *Thorax* 1989; **44**:620–6.
10. Chidley KE, Wood-Baker R, Town GI, Sleet RA, Holgate ST. Reassessment of asthma management in an accident and emergency department. *Respir Med* 1991;**85**:373–7.
11. Evans K, Sergeant E, Barnes G, Weller T, Cherry R, Ayres J. Audit of asthma care following hospital attendance and discharge. *Thorax* 1998; **53**(Suppl 4):A77.
12. Health Departments of Great Britain. General Practice in the National Health Service. The 1990 Contract. HMSO, London,1989.
13. Greenfield S, Stilwell B, Drury M. Practice nurses: social and occupational characteristics. *J R Coll Gen Pract* 1987;**37**:341–5.
13a. Jones RDM, Freegard S, Reeves M, Hanney K, Dobbs. The role of the practice nurse in the management of asthma. *Prim Care Resp J* 2001; **10**(4):109–11.
13b. Cave AJ, Wright A, Dorrett J, McErlain M. Evaluation of a nurse-run asthma clinic in general practice. *Prim Care Resp J* 2001;**10**:65–68.
14. Pearson R. The case for asthma clinics in general practice. *Mod Med* 1988;**33**:125–8.
15. Barnes GR. Nurse-run asthma clinics in general practice. *J R Coll Gen Pract* 1985;**35**:447.
16. Barnes GR. The community nurse and childhood asthma. In: *Asthma in Childhood: Symposium chaired by Prof H Simpson, Royal College of Physicians*. Theracom Ltd. Maidenhead, Berks. Clivedon Press Ltd, 1988.
17. Zeiger RS, Heller S, Mellon MH, Wald J, Falkoff R, Schatz M. Facilitated referral to asthma specialist reduces relapses in asthma emergency room visits. *J Allergy Clin Immunol* 1991;**87**:1160–8.
18. Charlton IC, Charlton G, Broomfield J, Mullee MA. Audit of the effect of a nurse run asthma clinic on workload and patient morbidity in a general practice. *Br J Gen Pract* 1991;**41**:227–31.
19. Hayward SA, Jordan M, Golden G, Levy M. A nurse run asthma clinic: assessment of patient self treatment for asthma. *Thorax* 1992;**47**:238P[Abstract].
20. Hoskins G, Neville RG, Smith B, Clark RA. The link between practice nurse training and asthma outcomes. *Br J Commun Nurs* 1999;**5**:222–8.
21. Dickinson J, Hutton S, Atkin A, Jones K. Reducing asthma morbidity in the community: the effect of a nurse-run asthma clinic in an English general practice. *Respir Med* 1997;**91**:634–40.
22. Dickinson J, Hutton S, Atkin A. Implementing the British Thoracic Society's guidelines: the effect of a nurse-run asthma clinic on prescribed treatment in an English general practice. *Respir Med* **92**:264–7.
23. Premaratne UN, Sterne JAC, Marks GB, Webb JR, Azima H, Burney PGJ. Clustered randomised trial of an intervention to improve the management of asthma: Greenwich asthma study. *Br Med J* 1999;**318**:1251–5.
24. Madge P, McColl J, Paton J. Impact of a nurse-led home management training programme in children admitted to hospital with acute asthma: a randomised controlled study. *Thorax* 1997;**25**:223–8.
25. Wesseldine LJ, McCarthy P, Silverman M (1999) Structured discharge procedure for children admitted to hospital with acute asthma: a randomised controlled trial of nursing practice. *Arch Dis Child* **80**:110–14.
26. Speight ANP. Is childhood asthma being underdiagnosed and undertreated? *Br Med J* 1978;**2**:331–2.
27. Levy M, Bell L. General practice audit of asthma in childhood. *Br Med J* 1984;**289**:115–16.
28. Charlton I, Jones KP, Bain J. Delay in diagnosis of childhood asthma and its influence on respiratory consultation rates. *Arch Dis Child* 1991;**66**:633–5.
29. General Practitioners in Asthma Group (GPIAG). Audit of diagnosis of asthma in children. *Thorax* 1993;**48**:451.
30. Price D. The implications of the AIR study. In: B O'Connor, G Barnes, D Pendleton, eds. *Asthma in Real Life: Patient-Centred Management*. Royal Society of Medicine, London, 2000, pp. 13–20.
31. Flemming DM, Sunderland R, Cross KW, Ross AM. Declining incidence of episodes of asthma: a study of

trends in new episodes presenting to general practitioners in the period 1989–98. *Thorax* 2000; **55**:657–61.

32. Charlton I, Antoniou AG, Atkinson J, *et al.* Asthma at the interface: bridging the gap between general practice and a district general hospital. *Arch Dis Child* 1994;**70**:313–18.

33. Silverman M, Dunbar H. Personal Communication, 2000.

34. Simpson AJ, Matusiewicz SP, Brown PH. Emergency pre-hospital management of patients admitted with acute asthma. *Thorax* 2000;**55**:97–101.

35. McConnochie KM, Russo MJ, McBride JT, *et al.* How commonly are children hospitalized for asthma eligible for care in alternative settings. *Arch Ped Adoles Med* 1999;**153**:1:49–55.

36. D'Souza W, Crane J, Burgess C, *et al.* A community trial of a credit card asthma self-management plan. *Eur Respir J* 1995;**7**:1260–5.

37. Uwyyed K, Springer C, Avital A, Bar-Yishay E, Godfrey S. Home recording of PEF in young asthmatics: does it contribute to management? *Eur Respir J* 1996;**9**:872–9.

38. Wensley D, Silverman M. Personal Communication, 2000.

39. Ordonez GA, Phelan PD, Olinsky A, Robertson CF. Preventable factors in hospital admissions for asthma. *Arch Dis Child* 1998;**78**:143–7.

40. Hill RA, Britton JR, Tattersfield AE. Management of asthma in schools. *Arch Dis Child* 1987;**62**:414–15.

41. Storr J, Barrell E, Lenney W. Asthma in primary schools. *Br Med J* 1987;**295**:251–2.

42. Brookes J, Jones K. Schoolteachers' perceptions and knowledge of asthma in primary school-children. *BJGP* 1992;**42**:504–7.

43. National Asthma Campaign. *The Asthma Manifesto*. National Asthma Campaign, London, 1993.

44. Evans KL, Kenkre JE. A study of guidelines for the management of children with asthma in primary schools within Birmingham. *Br J Commun Health Nurs* 1997;**2**(10):479–83.

45. Department for Education and Employment/DOH. *Supporting Children with Medical Needs*. DFEE, London, 1996.

46. Kaur B, Anderson HR, Austin J, Burr M, Harkins LS, Strachan DP, Warner JO. Prevalence of asthma symptoms, diagnosis and treatment in 12–14 year old children across Great Britain (international study of asthma and allergies in childhood, ISAAC UK). *Br Med J* 1998;**316**:118–34.

47. Price J. The transition of management from childhood to adolescence. *Eur Respir Rev* 1997;**7**:19–23.

48. NHS Executive. *The NHS Performance Assessment Framework*. Department of Health, 1999.

49. Royal College of Physicians. *Measuring Clinical Outcome in Asthma*. MG Pearson, Bucknall CE, eds. London, 1999.

50. National Asthma and Respiratory Training Centre. *Respiratory Conditions. Are Health Needs Being Met?* Direct Publishing Solutions, Cookham, 1999.

51. Shapiro SM, Hendler JM, Ogirala RG, Aldrich TK, Shapiro MB. An evaluation of the accuracy of Assess and mini-Wright peak flowmeters. *Chest* 1991; **99**:358–62.

52. Miller MR, Dickinson SA, Higchings DJ. The accuracy of peak flow meters. *Thorax* 1992;**47**:904–9.

53. Werk LN, Steinbach S, Adams WG, Bauchner H. Beliefs about diagnosing asthma in young children. *Pediatrics* 2000;**105**:585–90.

54. British Thoracic Society, Association of Respiratory Technicians and Physiologists. Guidelines for the measurement of respiratory function. *Respir Med* 1994;**88**:165–94.

55. Eiser C. Children's quality of life measures. *Arch Dis Child* 1997;**77**:350–4.

56. French DJ, Christie MJ, West A. Quality of life in childhood asthma: development of the Childhood Asthma Questionnaire. In: M Christie, D French, eds. *Assessment of Quality of Life in Childhood Asthma*. Harwood Academic Publishers, Switzerland, 1994, Ch. 14, pp. 157–80.

57. Juniper EF, Guyatt GH, Feeny DH, Griffith LE, Ferrie PJ. Minimum skills required by children to complete health-related quality of life instruments for asthma: comparison of measurement properties. *Eur Respir J* 1997;**10**:2285–94.

58. Jones KP, Bain DJG, Middleton M, Mullee MA. Correlates of asthma morbidity in primary care. *Br Med J* 1992;**304**:361–4.

59. Jones K, Charlton I, Middleton M, Preece W, Hill A. Targeting asthma care in general practice using a morbidity index. *Br Med J* 1992;**304**:1353–6.

60. Jones PW, Quirk FH, Baveystock CM, Littlejohns P. A self-complete measure of health status for chronic airflow limitation. The St George's Respiratory Questionnaire. *Am Rev Respir Dis* 1992; **145**:1321–7.

61. Mitchell EA. International trends in hospital admission rates for asthma. *Arch Dis Child* 1985;**60**:376–8.

62. Hilton S. An audit of inhaler technique among asthma patients of 34 general practitioners. *Br J Gen Pract* 1990;**40**:505–6.

63. Jones K, General Practitioners in Asthma Group. Impact of an interest on asthma prescribing costs in general practice. *Qual Health Care* 1992;**1**:110–13.

64. Department of Health. *Review of Prescribing, Supply and Administration of Medicines: Final Report*. DOH, London, 1999.

65. Medicines Control Agency. Proposals for supplementary prescribing by nurses and pharmacists and proposed amendments to the prescription only medicine (human use) order 1997. MLX284. Letter. 16 April 2002. MCA, London. www.mca.gov.uk

Sub-Saharan Africa

EZEKIEL M WAFULA

EPIDEMIOLOGY

Definition

Bronchial asthma in children presents as recurrent cough occurring often at night, sometimes accompanied by wheezing. On close review, these children are noted to have other features that are consistent with bronchial asthma. Often, these children are diagnosed to have other respiratory conditions like pneumonia, bronchitis, or wheezy bronchitis. The reluctance to use the term bronchial asthma is partly due to reluctance to stigmatize the child with what is considered a severe disease, and also the mistaken view that the disease is rare or that it affects mainly older children.

Incidence, prevalence, morbidity and mortality

Bronchial asthma is common among children in Sub-Saharan Africa. Children presenting at health facilities tend to have severe forms of the disease, while those with mild disease do not reach such facilities and remain within the home environment. The majority of children with asthma develop clinical features of the disease at a very early age (20% before 6 months, 50% by 1 year, and 70% by 2 years). Consequently, the vast majority of children with bronchial asthma in the Sub-Saharan Africa are aged below 5 years. Most of these children are at home, and not in schools or health facilities where they could easily be accessed and treated.[1]

Most studies on bronchial asthma in Sub-Saharan Africa have been carried out in primary schools, often involving children from the age of 8 years to 12 years. Such studies have revealed varying levels of prevalence that range from <2–10%. The prevalence of bronchial asthma has been rising over the years. However, the prevalence has been shown to be higher among children from urban areas than among those from rural areas and also among those from higher socio-economic status than those from poorer ones.[2–9]

Although bronchial asthma is a significant cause of illness among children, the true magnitude of morbidity and mortality, even at health facilities, is difficult to estimate from the available records since many children presenting with asthma at such facilities are not diagnosed as having asthma.

Risk factors for asthma in the Sub-Saharan Africa

The risk factors that have been identified in the Sub-Saharan Africa include the family history of asthma and eczema, dampness in the household, urban residence, exposure to tobacco smoke, and higher socio-economic status. Race in terms of white or black does not seem to influence the prevalence of asthma.[3,4,10,11]

The house-dust mite, *Dermatophagoides pteronyssinus*, cockroach allergen, feathers, cat allergen and pollen of both grass and flowers have been found to be important allergens. The house-dust mite and the cockroach are prevalent in the Sub-Saharan Africa and their relative contribution to bronchial asthma is likely to be significant.[5,12,13]

Exclusive breast-feeding has been associated with reduction in the prevalence of bronchial asthma while early introduction of cow's milk has been associated with increased prevalence of the disease.[10]

Nonetheless, the prevalence of bronchial asthma in Sub-Saharan Africa has been considered relatively low, presumably because of effect of the large number of infections among children in this region.[13,14] Frequent infections are likely to reduce the prevalence of atopic disease by modulation of the balance of lymphocytes in development and also by the effect of the excessive amounts of IgE produced in response to the parasitic infections. The relationship between intestinal parasitosis, atopy and asthma is complex.[15,16] Many studies of parasite load are confounded by urban/rural differences, the interaction of IgE-dependent mechanisms with parasite clearance or re-infection, and by access to immunization.[17]

One intriguing study of children born in hospital in Tanzania showed a relationship between several prenatal risk factors and wheeze (14% of children) at age 4.[18] Although small in number (3.4% of births), those with malaria parasites in cord blood had an increased risk of wheeze (odds ratio 6.8), while those with high cord IgE had reduced risk (odds ratio 0.24).

CLINICAL FEATURES

Children with bronchial asthma usually present with a history of recurrent cough or wheezing, most of them below 2 years of age. Diagnosis of asthma in such young children is often not made by health workers, who consider it a disease of older children.

There are real difficulties in differentiating between children with bronchial asthma and those with bronchiolitis, although bronchiolitis tends to occur among younger children, peaking at 6 months of age and hardly manifesting after the age of 1 year. On the other hand, asthma is infrequent below the age of 6 months and hardly worth considering below the age of 4 months.

The simple clinical parameters that have been adopted by WHO and UNICEF as reliable diagnostic tools for pneumonia, namely fast breathing and chest in-drawing, have been shown to be effective in identifying pneumonia and severe pneumonia among children.[19] However, a significant number of children classified as having pneumonia have features of bronchial asthma in addition. It is recommended that such children classified as having both pneumonia and bronchial asthma, where asthma is classified on the basis of the presence of a wheeze. The occurrence of pneumonia and asthma together has been noted in a number of children, whose successful treatment has only been achieved by treating both conditions. However, there is no study to date that has been undertaken to examine the possibility of asthma predisposing to pneumonia.

MANAGEMENT

Management of bronchial asthma in children offers special challenges in the Sub-Saharan Africa. These challenges include inadequate health services, the significantly large young population of children with asthma and low socio-economic status.

A large proportion of children with asthma are not appropriately managed because they do not reach the health facilities or the health workers fail to recognize their condition as asthma. This situation has been addressed in a number of countries where asthma has been included as one of the conditions to be managed within the IMCI strategy, where wheezing has been used as a diagnostic sign for asthma and specific guidelines have been given for management of such children. A useful model for asthma management in remote health centres has been described elsewhere.[20]

The significantly large young population of less than 2 years with asthmatic attacks presents special problems in management at the outpatient level. Use of inhalation therapy for bronchial asthma is not feasible for such children, even when spacers are utilized. These children are mainly managed using oral bronchodilators that include sulbutamol and a theophylline, and oral steroids for those who are severely affected, using standard regimens. Those with more severe asthmatic attacks and who get admitted to the hospital receive the standard medication that is described elsewhere in this book.

The low socio-economic status for most populations in the Sub-Saharan Africa limits the use of inhalation therapy even in children who are old enough to cooperate and to use an inhaler because of the high cost of these drugs. However older children and those who can afford are put on inhalation therapy using standard protocols. Necessity is the mother of invention – nowhere more so than in Africa, where old plastic drinks bottles make excellent spacer devices.[21]

The World Health Organization's Integrated Management of Childhood Illness Strategy may fail to distinguish severe asthma from (lower) respiratory tract infection, especially in young children.[19] In an environment where chest radiology is scarce, this leads to the combined need for antibiotic and anti-asthma medication.

Because of the ubiquitous nature of the risk factors for asthma in the Sub-Saharan Africa, and the limited personal resources which are available, preventative strategies are rarely carried out.

REFERENCES

1. Macharia WM, Mirza NM, Wafula EM, Onyango FE, Agwanda RO. Clinical characteristics of childhood asthma as seen at Kenyatta National Hospital. *E Afr Med J* 1990;**67**:837–41.

2. Nganga LW, Odhiambo JA, Omwega MJ, Gicheha EM, Becklake MR, Menzies R, Mohammed N, Macklem PT. Exercise induced bronchospasm: a pilot survey in Nairobi School children. *E Afr Med J* 1997; **74**:694–8.

3. Keeley DJ, Neill P, Gallivan S. Comparison of the prevalence of reversible airway obstruction in rural

and urban Zimbabwean Children. *Thorax* 1991; **46**:549–53.

4. Mohamed N, Nganga L, Odhiambo J, Nyamwaya J, Menzies R. Home environment and asthma in Kenyan School Children: a case control study. *Thorax* 1995; **50**:74–8.

5. Yemaneberhan H, Bekele Z, Venn A, Lewis S, Parry E, Britton J. Prevalence of wheeze and asthma and relation to atopy in urban and rural Ethiopia. *Lancet* 1997;**350**:85–90.

6. Terblanche E, Stewart RI. The prevalence of exercise-induced bronchoconstriction in Cape Town school children. *S Afr Med J* 1990;**78**:744–7.

7. Nganga LW, Odhiambo JA, Mungai MW, Gicheha CM, Nderitu P, Maingi B, Macklem PT, Beclake MR. Prevalence of exercise induced bronchospasm in Kenyan school children: an urban-rural comparison. *Thorax* 1998;**53**:919–26.

8. Van Niekerk CH, Weinberg EG, Shore SC, Heese HV, Van Schalkwyk J. Prevalence of asthma: a comparative study of urban and rural Xhosa children. *Clin Allergy* 1979;**9**:319–4.

9. Addo Tobo EO, Custovic A, Taggart SC, Asafo-Agyei AP, Woodcock A. Exercise induced bronchospasm in Ghana: differences in prevalence between urban and rural school children. *Thorax* 1997;**52**:161–5.

10. Wafula EM, Limbe MS, Onyango FE, Nduati R. Effects of passive smoking and breast feeding on childhood bronchial asthma. *E Afr Med J* 1999;**76**:606–9.

11. Aligne AC, Auinger P, Byrd RS, Weitzman M. Risk factors for pediatric asthma. *Am J Respir Crit Care Med* 2000;**162**:873–7.

12. Awotedu AA, Oyejije CO, Ogunlesi A, Onadeko BO. Skin sensitivity patterns to inhalant allergens in Nigerian asthmatic patients. *E Afr Med J* 1992; **69**:631–5.

13. Shaheen SO, Aaby P, Hall AJ, Barker DJ, Heyes CB, Shiell AW, Goudiaby A. Measles and atopy in Guinea-Bissau. *Lancet* 1996;**347**:1792–6.

14. Cookson WOCM, Moffat MF. Asthma – An epidemic in the absence of infection? *Sci Mag* 1997;**275**:41–2.

15. Scrivener S, Britton J. Immunoglobulin E and allergic disease in Africa. *Clin Exp Allergy* 2000;**30**:304–7.

16. Scrivener S, Yemaneberhan H, Zebenigus M, *et al.* Independent effects of intestinal parasite infection and domestic allergen exposure on risk of wheeze in Ethiopia: a nested case-control study. *Lancet* 2001;**358**:1493–9.

17. Aaby P, Shaheen SO, Heyes CB, Goudiaby A, Hall AJ, Shiell AW, Jensen H, Marchant A. Early BCG vaccination and reduction in atopy in Guinea-Bissau. *Clin Exp Allergy* 2000;**30**:644–50.

18. Sunyer J, Mendendez C, Ventura PJ, Aponte JJ, Schellenberg D, Kahigwa E, Acosta C, Anto JM, Alonso PL. Prenatal risk factors of wheezing at the age of four years in Tanzania. *Thorax* 2001; **56**:290–5.

19. Integrated Management of Childhood Illness Strategy Initiative. *Bull WHO* 1997;**75**:Suppl. 1.

20. Chang AB, Shannon C, O'Neill MC, Tiemann AM, Valery PC, Craig D, Fa'Afoi E, Masters IB. Asthma management in indigenous children of remote community using an indigenous health model. *J Paediatr Child Health* 2000;**36**:249–51.

21. Zar HJ, Brown G, Donson H, Brathwaite N, Mann MD, Weinberg EG. Home-made spacers for bronchodilator therapy in children with acute asthma: a randomised trial. *Lancet* 1999;**354**:979–82.

Indian subcontinent

S NOEL NARAYANAN

INTRODUCTION

Asthma is an important cause of morbidity in children and the prevalence of asthma in different parts of India varies between 4 and 20%.[1] There has been an increase in the incidence and severity of asthma in children in the last two decades, possibly the result of environmental factors and improved diagnosis. It has been suggested that the development of asthma is determined by genetic predisposition, but its severity by environmental factors.[2] A study of Delhi children aged 5–15 years showed that factors associated with the development of asthma were: a positive family history; absence of exclusive breast-feeding; associated atopic disorders; and a past history of bronchiolitis, as in studies elsewhere. An additional finding (confirmed elsewhere in India) was the association with a past history of tuberculosis. The severity of asthma was determined by early onset of symptoms, asthma in grandparents, and smoking of more than 10 cigarettes per day by any family member. Air pollution, overcrowding, and pets were not considered to be significant contributing factors.[3] Children employed in the carpet weaving industry were reported to have significantly lower peak-flow rate than their normal counterparts.[4]

In a tertiary referral centre like Medical College Hospital, Trivandrum, 25% of the children's outpatient attendance was found to be due to asthma. Analysis of data from the Respiratory Clinic during the period of 1996–2000 revealed that 80% of cases of asthma occurred among children aged 1–5 years; 15% of cases were above 5 years; and only 5% of cases occurred in infants below 1 year. A positive family history was obtained in about 45% of cases. The first episode of asthma occurred before 3 years of age in 70% of cases. Thirty per cent of cases were found to be mild episodic, 60% were moderately severe,

and 10% were chronic severe cases. The male:female ratio was about 1.5:1. Asthma also accounted for 14% of hospital admissions, while 30% of cases of respiratory disease admitted to hospital were asthmatic. The annual hospital case fatality rate of children admitted with acute severe asthma was about 0.05%.

TRIGGER FACTORS

The common precipitating factors were upper respiratory tract infections, cold wind, lunar episodes like full moon or new moon days, exercise, oil head-bath, and dust. Parents also mentioned ingestion of 'cold food items' e.g. curd and fruits like bananas and grapes as precipitating factors.

Based on skin-prick tests in our department, 49% of asthma cases showed a positive reaction to multiple allergens. The common allergens detected were cockroach (68%), house-dust mite (44%), cotton dust (28%) and paper dust (38%). Dietary allergens (milk, egg) constituted only 4% of the cases. Total IgE level was above 95th centile for age in 60% of children with a positive skin-prick test. Specific IgE was not done. Passive smoking was often found to be associated with early onset and more severe symptoms of asthma.

In a study from Bombay, it was found that 55% of cases showed positive skin-prick test reaction. The major allergen was dust mite (60%). Significant reactions were also seen with animal epithelium, dust, fungus, and pollen.[5]

In Bangalore city, a report of differential pattern of pollens in ambient air found that 65 types of pollen occurred at 1.5 m, and 75 types at 35 m height; 57 types occurred at both heights. Most common and predominant pollens were *Parthenium*, *Cassurina* and *Eucalyptus*.[6]

Ten per cent of the Indian population is estimated to suffer from pollen allergy.

Episodes of bronchial asthma were increased during the rainy and winter seasons, probably triggered by viral respiratory infections.

Tuberculosis may also occasionally be confused with asthma.[7,8]

MANAGEMENT ISSUES

Traditional medicine

In India therapeutic pluralism exists widely. People seek treatment from various modalities like Allopathy, Ayurveda, Homeopathy, Siddha, and Unani. One curious treatment practised in the indigenous system is the use of a small live fish with an unknown remedy inside its mouth. The patient is instructed to swallow the fish whole and the resulting cure of asthma is believed to be excellent.

In traditional Ayurvedic treatment, medicines used for treatment of asthma are herbal medicines like Dashamoola Kadathrayam, Thamboola Rasayanam, and Kanakasavam. These are mainly used for treatment of chronic cases. Pankaja Kasthoori contains secretions of certain types of deer called Kasthuri, which has a very strong odour and is used along with other herbal compounds for treatment of acute asthma. Certain Unani physicians give concoctions made from Neem oil, Porcupine flesh, camphor, and various heavy metal salts to infants as preventive therapy for asthma. Some physicians also use small doses of arsenic compounds for prevention of asthma.

Western medicine

Evaluation of young children with acute illness in the developing world is undoubtedly facilitated by the Integrated Management of Childhood Illness Programme of WHO/UNICEF.[9] Using these algorithms, however, leads to underdiagnosis of asthma and overdiagnosis of pneumonia in children under 5 years old.[10] They need to be adapted to reflect regional morbidity.

In most hospitals, treatment of chronic cases is based on the severity of asthma. Mild cases are managed with oral β_2-agonists as and when required. Moderately severe cases are often managed with twice-daily sustained release theophylline or inhaled steroids. Sustained release theophylline preparations are preferred over inhaled steroids in chronic asthma as they are cheaper and more acceptable to children. Salbutamol and ipratropium are the drugs commonly used for rescue inhaler therapy. Chronic severe cases are managed with a combination of sustained release theophyllines and inhaled corticosteroids.

Children with a history of life-threatening asthma are given steroids at the beginning of the attack. Oral steroids are seldom used for long-term control. Antibiotics are generally prescribed for acute attacks except in mild cases.

Parents are educated regarding the need for drug compliance and non-pharmacological management, such as avoidance of possible allergens. Increasing emphasis is being given to family therapy and parental involvement.

Organization of care

Acute non-severe asthma is generally managed in the primary healthcare set-up, and severe cases are referred to apex institutions. Nebulization facility is available in the majority of peripheral hospitals. Most centres now resort to nebulization with β_2-agonists along with parenteral theophylline and steroids for treatment of acute cases. Very few cases need ventilatory support and the outcome is usually good. Domiciliary care using home nebulizers and peak-flow monitoring is seldom practised.

REFERENCES

1. The International Study of Asthma and Allergies in Childhood (ISAAC) Steering Committee. Worldwide variation in prevalence of symptoms of asthma, allergic conjunctivitis and atopic eczema. *Lancet* 1998; **351**:1225–32.
2. Arshad SH, Stevens M, Hide DW. The effect of genetic and environmental factors on the prevalence of allergic disorders at the age of 2 years. *Clin Exp Allergy* 1992;**23**:504–11.
3. Ratageri VH, Kabra SK, Dwivedi SN, Seth V. Factors associated with severe asthma. *Indian Pediatr* 2000; **37**:1072–81.
4. Joshi SK, Sharma P, Sharma U, Sitaraman S, Pathak SS. Peak expiratory flow rate of carpet weaving children. *Indian Pediatr* 1996;**33**:105–8.
5. Lahiri K, Boby John KF, Bijur S. IgE level in asthmatic children. *Paediatr Pulmonol* 1996;**8**:30–2.
6. Agasha SN, *et al.* Profile of vertical studies of airborne pollen. *Indian J Allergy Immunol* 1986;**2**:32.
7. Ratageri VH, Kabra SK, Dwivedi SN, Seth V. Factors associated with severe asthma. *Indian Pediatr* 2000; **37**:1072–82.
8. Chugh K. Clinical approach to a patient with cough. *Indian J Pediatr* 2001;**68**:S11–19.
9. Integrated Management of Childhood Illness Strategy Initiative. *Bull WHO* 1997;**75**:Suppl. 1.
10. Shah D, Sachdev HP. Evaluation of the WHO/UNICEF algorithm for integrated management of childhood illness between the age of two months to five years. *Indian Pediatr* 1999;**36**:767–77.

Latin America

ALEJANDRO M TEPER AND CARLOS D KOFMAN

PREVALENCE OF ASTHMA AND ALLERGY

The International Study of Asthma and Allergies in Childhood (ISAAC) which has resulted in an improved understanding of the world-wide variations in the prevalence of reputed asthma and wheezing, has recently reported specifically in the situation in Latin America.[1] The prevalence rates of wheeze in the last 12 months in two age groups (13–14 and 6–7 years) in representative samples of school-children from most regions of the world, were greatest in English speaking countries and Latin America. Regional data from Latin America showed a 16.9% prevalence (range 6.6–27.0) in the older age group and 19.6% (range 8.6–32.1) in the younger group. Countries with the highest incidence (>20%) were Peru, Costa Rica and Brazil. Mexico had the lowest incidence (<10%). Argentina, Chile, Panama, Paraguay and Uruguay showed intermediate rates (10–20%).

No explanation has been found to the differences in prevalence between regions. The global ISAAC study results suggested that the lower prevalence of asthma in some developing areas was primarily accounted for by environmental factors, including poorer hygiene and healthcare that could lead to increased early exposure to infection, which could in turn be protective in the inception of asthma and allergies.[1] However, an analysis of Latin American data shows that wheezing is more prevalent in poorer cities (Lima, San Jose de Costa Rica), than in others with a higher socio-economic level (Buenos Aires, Santiago). In keeping with the observation that air pollution is not a major risk factor for the development of asthma in populations, although it may exacerbate asthma in individuals.[2] In Santiago, Chile, the most polluted city in Latin America,[4] the incidence of asthma in children was <16%. Therefore, other factors are likely to play an important role in the prevalence of asthma in a specific population.

The prevalence of asthma is increasing in the Western world, and also in South America. In Argentina, Salmun et al.[5] in a study conducted 3 years before the ISAAC study, reported a prevalence of wheeze during the last 12 months of 2% and 1% less than the ISAAC figures in the 6 and 12-year-old group, respectively. The same was observed in Chile when comparing epidemiological studies by Medina[6] in 1979 and Moreno[7] in 1992.

Allergic sensitization

In industrialized countries, sensitization to indoor allergens has been invoked in the early inception of asthma. A multinational study of the prevalence of sensitization to mite species in a large asthmatic population conducted in seven Latin American cities with varying climate and geographical characteristics[8–11] showed a high prevalence of sensitization to mite allergens, particularly in tropical regions. Also, in contrast to European studies, high altitude cities, such as Quito, Bogotá and Mexico City, have a high incidence of skin sensitivity to mite allergens, especially *D. pteronyssinus* and *D. farinae,* presumably because of differences in local climatic factors.[9,10]

TREATMENT OF ASTHMA

Cultural, social and economic factors, lack of diagnostic facilities and limited access to healthcare may result in the under-treatment of asthma in Latin America. Sales reports of drugs used in the management of asthma seem to substantiate this hypothesis. Currently, Latin America has a total population of over 500 million people. Based on an estimated 12% prevalence rate, there should be over 60 million asthmatic individuals. If only 30% of them belong to the persistent moderate to severe group (according to the International Consensus Report on Diagnosis and Treatment of Asthma),[11] approximately 18 million asthmatics will require anti-inflammatory treatment for the control of the disease. With regard to inhaled corticosteroids, despite a marked increase in sales during recent years, less than 2 500 000 units/year were prescribed, e.g. only 0.13 units per patient/year, in 1999. In Argentina, Molfino et al. analysed the prescriptions for the treatment of airway diseases between 1983 and 1990.[12–18] Despite improved management of diseases with airflow obstruction, evidenced by a decrease in the use of oral bronchodilators and disodium cromoglycate, and an increase in the use of inhaled bronchodilators and steroids, appropriate treatment of asthma remains insufficient.

It is possible to improve the health of asthmatic children from low income backgrounds by implementing International Guidelines, as a study from urban Brazil has shown.[13]

ASTHMA MORTALITY

Mortality from asthma increased during the 1980s, but in recent years seems to be declining in some countries. However, little is known about trends in mortality in Latin America. In a survey performed a few years ago in 11 countries of the region based on a uniform protocol,[14] the overall death rate was 3.14/100 000. Significant differences were found between countries with the highest death rates in Uruguay and Mexico (5.6/100 000), and the lowest, Paraguay (0.8/100 000) and Colombia (1.4/ 100 000). In South American countries with marked seasonal climatic differences, such as Chile, Uruguay, Paraguay and Argentina, deaths occurred mainly in winter. In most countries, deaths from asthma occurred at home, rather than during hospital admission. The differences found may be due, at least in part, to defective information collected in death certificates. More recently, data on mortality trends in young people in Southern Brazil show a significant increase in asthma-related deaths in the 5–19 year age group (0.04/100 000 in 1970 vs 0.39/100 000 in 1992).[15] Additionally, this increase cannot be ascribed to a shift in labelling from bronchitis to asthma. In some countries, such as Colombia, asthma mortality in all age groups increased from 1979 to 1988, and has since declined.[16] Mean death rates in all the countries considered were similar to those in Great Britain, lower than in Australia, New Zealand, West Germany and Japan, and higher than in the United States and Canada.

DIFFERENTIAL DIAGNOSIS

With regard to the differential diagnosis of asthma in infants and young children, it should be noted that in the southernmost region of South America, Argentina, Chile, Uruguay and South of Brazil, there is a higher incidence than in other parts of the world, of obliterative bronchiolitis among survivors of severe viral infections in early life, particularly by adenovirus. The pathogenic[17] and functional[18] characteristics of post-adenoviral bronchiolitis obliterans in children have been recently described.

SUMMARY

Latin America, due to its geographical, climatic, economic and ethnic differences, has a markedly heterogeneous population that challenges any attempt at global assessment. Moreover, the lack of precise definitions of bronchial asthma and the scarcity of epidemiological studies may result in either an underestimation or an overestimation of its prevalence, although standardization has been attempted world-wide. Asthma is moderating or highly prevalent in most Latin American countries. Poor socio-economic status and limited access to healthcare may be responsible for the frequent under-treatment of asthma. This, in turn, may play a critical role in asthma mortality rates in the region.

REFERENCES

1. Mallol J, Sole D, Innes A, Clayton T, Stein R, Soto-Quiroz S-Q, on behalf of the Latin American ISAAC Collaborators Group. Prevalence of Asthma Symptoms in Latin America: The International Study of Asthma and Allergies in Childhood (ISAAC). *Pediatr Pulmonol* 2000;**30**:439–44.
2. Martinez F. Role of viral infections in the inception of asthma and allergies during childhood: could they be protective? *Thorax* 1994;**49**:1189–91.
3. Schwartz J, Koenig J, Slater D, Larson T. Particulate air pollution and hospital emergency visits for asthma in Seattle. *Am Rev Respir Dis* 1993;**147**:826–31.
4. Salinas M, Vega J. The effect of outdoor air pollution on mortality risk: an ecological study from Santiago, Chile. *World Health Stat Q* 1995; **48**:118–25.
5. Salmun N, Manterola A, Gentile A. Prevalencia del asma en la población escolar argentina. *Medico Interamericano* 1996;**15**:420–5.
6. Medina E, Kaempffer AM. Morbilidad y atención médica en el gran Santiago. *Rev Med Chil* 1979; **107**:155–68.

7. Moreno R, Marambio JA, Donoso H, Sandoval H, Contreras G, Retamal E, Valenzuela P. Crisis obstructivas y antecedentes de asma: encuesta en población general del gran Santiago. *Rev Chil Enf Respir* 1992;**8**:253.

8. Fernandez-Caldas E, Baena-Cagnani CE, Lopez M, *et al.* Cutaneous sensitivity to six mite species in asthmatic patients from five Latin American countries. *J Invest Allergol Clin Immunol* 1993;**3**:245–9.

9. Spieksma F, Spieksma-Boezeman M. High altitude and house dust mites. *Br Med J* 1971;**1**:82–4.

10. Valdivieso R, Estupinan M, Acosta ME. Asthma and its relation with *Dermatophagoides ptereonyssinus* and *Dermatophagoides farinae* in Andean altitudes (Quito, Ecuador). *J Invest Allergol Clin Immunol* 1997;**7**:46–50.

11. National Heart, Lung and Blood Institute. International consensus report on diagnosis and treatment of asthma. *Eur Respir J* 1992;**5**:601–41.

12. Molfino NA, Nannini LJ, Chapman KR, Slutsky AS. Trends in pharmacotherapy for chronic airflow limitations in Argentina: 1983–1990. *Medicina* 1995;**55**:88–90.

13. Cabral A L, *et al.* Are international asthma guidelines effective for low-income Brazilian children with asthma? *Eur Respir J* 1998;**12**:35–40.

14. Neffen H, Baena-Cagnani CE, Malka S, *et al.* Asthma mortality in Latin America. *J Invest Clin Immunol* 1997;**7**:249–53.

15. Chatkin JM, Barreto SM, Fonseca NA, Gutierrez CA, Sears MR. Trends in asthma mortality in young people in southern Brazil. *Ann Allergy Asthma Immunol* 1999;**82**:287.

16. Vergara C, Caraballo L. Asthma mortality in Columbia. *Ann Allergy Asthma Immunol* 1998;**80**:55.

17. Mistchenko A, Diez R, Mariani A, Robaldo J, Maffey A, Bayley Bustamante G. Cytokines in adenoviral disease in children: association of interleukin-6, interleukin-8 and tumor necrosis factor alfa levels with clinical outcome. *J Pediatr* 1994;**124**:714–20.

18. Teper A, Kofman C, Maffey A, Vidaurreta S. Lung function in infants with chronic pulmonary disease after severe adenoviral illness. *J Pediatr* 1999;**134**:730–3.

..

Japan

YOJI IIKURA

INTRODUCTION

The increased prevalence of asthma in children has led to the publication of more extensive treatment and management guidelines world-wide. In Japan, asthma in children is an important health issue, and this article discusses the number of cases and various treatment methods, their effectiveness, and current trends.

PREVALENCE OF ASTHMA IN CHILDREN

In Japan, the number of asthma cases in children has been increasing. This is true not only in large cities, but also in remote islands where levels of industrial pollution are low. An epidemiological study investigating trends within one region, showed an increase in asthma prevalence over the course of 10 years (Table 17d.1). This data clearly indicates a continuous increase in the rates of asthma diagnosis and of reported wheezing in this region.[1]

In another epidemiological study,[2] Hosoi *et al.* investigated asthma in the Kyoto region from June to September 1996, in 17 906 students from 30 elementary and junior high schools, by questionnaire. The completion rate of questionnaires was 90.3%. The results reveal asthma rates of 4.9% in elementary schools and 3.5% in junior high

schools (Table 17d.2), indicating that asthma is as serious a health concern in Japan as in other parts of the world.

TREATMENT OF ASTHMA

Asthma attacks

In Japan, the first guidelines for asthma treatment were published in 1993, and the third revised guidelines in 1998.[3] Treatment options include the initial use of a low-dose of β_2-agonist combined with sodium cromoglycate (SCG) 2 ml administered by a nebulizer for asthma attack. In certain cases, this method has been significantly better in treating asthma attacks than low doses of

Table 17d.1 *Prevalence of asthma in elementary school children in a single region (%)[1]*

Year	Numbers	Asthma	Episodes of wheezing	Total
1971	4893	1.71	1.30	3.01
1981	5272	3.62	4.34	7.96
1991	3876	5.37	5.13	10.50

Table 17d.2 *Prevalence of asthma and wheezing in Kyoto schools (%)[2]*

	Asthma			Wheezing		
	M	F	Total	M	F	Total
Elementary school						
1	4.7	4.1	4.4	8.7	8.5	8.5
2	4.9	3.6	4.3	8.0	7.4	7.7
3	6.2	3.7	4.9	6.1	6.7	6.4
4	6.0	3.1	4.6	7.7	5.0	6.3
5	8.8	3.6	6.1	6.5	4.4	5.5
6	6.4	4.2	5.2	5.4	4.0	4.7
Mean	6.2	3.7	4.9	7.1	6.0	6.5
Junior high						
1	4.2	3.3	3.8	3.0	2.4	2.7
2	3.9	2.5	3.2	2.4	3.0	2.6
3	4.2	2.6	3.4	2.6	2.8	2.7
Mean	4.1	2.8	3.5	2.7	2.7	2.7
Mean	5.6	3.5	4.5	5.9	5.0	5.5

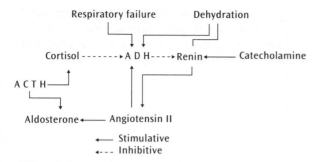

Figure 17d.1 *Interrelationship between anti-diuretic hormone (ADH) and the renin–angiotensin–aldosterone system in acute severe asthma.*[6]

β_2-agonist diluted with saline.[4] Further, long-term use of the SCG solution improves airway responsiveness, evaluated by methacholine inhalation tests. This combination has shown significantly better results than low doses of β_2-agonist combined only with saline. Therefore, the combination of a low dose of β_2-agonist SCG administered by a nebulizer has become the most common method of treatment in Japan.[5] The use of this combination may be a contributory factor to the lower rate of asthma death in children (0.5 per 100 000 cases), compared with that in total population (4.7 per 100 000) in Japan.

In severe asthma attacks, intravenous administration of aminophylline in an early phase is frequently used. This treatment is beneficial for patients suffering from dehydration associated with severe asthma attack and in whom increases in ADH (antidiuretic hormone) are present.[6] The use of β_2-agonists in these patients exacerbates rather than improves their condition (Figure 17d.1).

The standard treatment for patients with severe attacks requiring hospitalization is continuous inhalation of *l*-isoproterenol solution.[7] The author's group used 0.1–0.2 mg *l*-isoproterenol/kg patient weight solution mixed with 500 ml of normal saline, nebulized continuously with 70–100% oxygen. This method was effective in treating severe asthma, only one case requiring intubation for control of severe asthma attacks in 10 years in our hospital.

Long-term treatment of childhood asthma

The characteristic long-term treatment for childhood asthma is the use of oral anti-allergic drugs and theophylline. The efficacy of recently developed leukotriene receptor antagonists has been reported.[8] In the paediatric field, these drugs have been used in Japan. This drug is likely to be widely used for the treatment of asthma in children.

The treatment with theophylline has been associated with 'theophylline related seizure'. In 86 studies which measured the plasma theophylline levels, no seizure was observed in paediatric asthma patients without diseases of the central nervous system (CNS) and whose plasma

theophylline level was below 5 mg/l. Kitabayashi *et al.* reported seizures in five out of 29 children with asthma who also had diseases of the CNS,[9] indicating the need for careful use of theophylline in children.

Recently, a patch-type formulation of tulobuterol, a β_2-agonist, has been developed. This formulation exerts a long-acting effect and the attachment of this patch to the skin at bedtime can control nocturnal asthma attacks.[10]

Currently, inhaled corticosteroid therapy is available for paediatric use in Japan and is widely used even in young children with the Aerochamber. This treatment has resulted in the reduction in the number of children with severe asthma.

Medical payment for long-term hospitalized children with asthma

The medical cost of hospital treatment is covered by the government for children under 18 years with asthma who stay in hospital for more than one month. This system is beneficial for children with severe asthma, enabling them to receive adequate medical care without financial concern. As a result, this system also helped decrease the rate of asthma deaths in children.

REFERENCES

1. Innoue K, Ootani T, Iikura Y, Innui H, Shinagawa Y. Clinical epidemiology of bronchial asthma in children report. *Jpn J Allergol* 1985;**34**:1062.

2. Hosoi S, Asai K, Harasaki T, Furushou K, Mikawa H. An epidemiological study on the prevalence of allergic diseases. *Jpn J Allergol* 1997;**46**:1025–35.

3. Miyamoto A, Makino S, Furusho M. *Japanese Asthma Guideline.* Kyowakikaku, Tokyo, Japan, 1998.

4. Iikura Y, Utida K, Sakamoto Y, Ooto K, Matsumoto T, Tubaki T, Tomikawa M. Inhalation therapy for treatment of asthma. *Allergy Pract* 1996;**16**:26–32.

5. Iikura Y, Fujita K, Youfu S, Tomikawa M. Current topics in allergy treatment. *Jpn J Dev Pharmacol Ther* 1998;**11**:57–62.

6. Iikura Y, Odajima Y, Akasawa A, Nagakura T, Kisida M, Akimoto K. Antidiuretic hormone in acute asthma in children: effects of medical treatment on serum levels and clinical course. *Allergy Pro* 1989;**10**:197–201.

7. Iikura Y, Matumoto T, Otuka T, Obata T, Sakaguchi T, Akasawa A, Koya N. Continuous isoproterenol inhalation therapy in children with severe asthmatic attack. *Int Arch Allergy Immunol* 1997;**113**:370–2.

8. Hamilton A, Failferman I, Stober P, Richard M, O'Byrne P, Pranlukast M. A cysteinyl leukotriene receptor antagonist allergen-induced early and late phase bronchoconstriction and airway

hyperresponsiveness in asthmatic subjects. *J Allergy Clin Immunol* 1998;**102**:177–83.

9. Kitabayashi T, Iikura Y, Akasawa A, *et al*. Study on theophylline related seizures. *Jap J Dev Pharmacol Ther* 1998;**12**:11–15.

10. Iikura Y, Utiyama H, Akimoto K, Ebisawa M, Sakaguchi N, Saito H, Miura K, Onda T. Pharmacokinetics and pharmacodynamics of the tulobuterol patch, HN-078, in children asthma. *Ann Allergy Asthma Immunol* 1995;**74**:147–51.

17e

Hong Kong

K N CHAN

PUBLIC HEALTH ISSUES

Epidemiology

Like many other countries where serial data are available, the prevalence of asthma and allergic disease in Hong Kong has been increasing quite dramatically. Based on an ISAAC study done in the mid-1990s, the prevalence of asthma ever, wheeze ever and current wheeze amongst local school-children was estimated to be 11%, 20% and 12% respectively.[1] This compares with a rate of asthma ever of merely 7–8% in the late 1980s.[2] The cause of the increase remains obscure, but is comparable with the trend recorded in Singapore.[3] Unknown environmental factors are thought to play a major role in the increase.

Given the similar genetic background, there is marked regional variation in disease prevalence. A trend towards a higher prevalence of asthma and allergic disease in the more affluent communities is clearly evident. In a study comparing the rate of asthma and allergic disease in three cities with different levels of affluence in Asia,[4] Hong Kong, being the most westernized, had the highest prevalence of asthma, rhinitis and eczema. The rate was intermediate for those in Kota Kinabalu and lowest in San Bu, considered least affluent. However, the rate of atopy, as determined by skin-prick test to common allergens, was similar for these three places.

On the whole, the prevalence of asthma in the Far East is still low compared with Western developed countries. This does not necessarily mean that Chinese are less susceptible to the development of allergic diseases. The rate of atopy, defined by skin-prick tests to common allergens, is high amongst the Chinese. A study showed that 49% of 12- to 20-year-old Hong Kong Chinese students had one or more positive skin test to common allergens,[5] nearly 90% of whom reacted to house-dust mite and 73% to cockroach. Pollen allergy is uncommon, presumably due to low allergen load in the locality. After emigrating to Australia, where they were exposed to high concentrations of rye grass pollen, up to 60% of the ethnic Chinese migrants acquired sensitization to grass pollen and may develop hay fever. Similarly, the prevalence of asthma increases with length of stay in the new country.

Of other allergic diseases, rhinitis was the commonest, affecting about 50% of the subjects. Eczema was reported in about 15% and hay fever was rare in Hong Kong. Like other series, familial aggregation of allergic diseases is evident. However, a positive parental history is more important in predicting asthma and allergic disease than atopic sensitization.[5]

Environment

House-dust mite, cat and cockroach are ubiquitous indoor allergens in residential homes in Hong Kong. Its hot, humid subtropical climate favours the growth of house-dust mite. Compared with other populations in the Far East, Hong Kong has the highest recorded Der pI levels, although the prevalence of asthma is lower than that of Singapore where the Der pI levels are generally much lower. This implies that the concentration of the allergen is unlikely to be the cause of increasing prevalence of asthma in Hong Kong.

On the other hand, in conjunction with economic growth, there has been tremendous increase in the number of motor vehicles and increase in the average distance travelled by vehicles, particularly diesel-fuelled vehicles in recent years. The pollutants resulting from these diesel engines may enhance the airway response to inhaled allergens in susceptible subjects either directly, or in conjunction with other outdoor pollutants such as NO_2 and O_3.

CLINICAL ISSUES

Clinical diagnosis

The findings in the recent ISAAC study appear to lend support to the suspicion that asthma in Hong Kong is underdiagnosed. There are added difficulties in diagnosing asthma in Hong Kong. There is no word equivalent to 'wheeze' in Cantonese. In addition, Chinese parents often do not recognize or are unwilling to accept their child's symptoms as being due to asthma. On the other hand, they are generally quite willing to accept the more benign-sounding 'sensitive or over-sensitive breathing tubes'. Consequently, there is also some tendency on the part of general practitioners to offer a more acceptable clinical label than a diagnosis of asthma.

Management

The use of traditional Chinese medicine is steeped in the local culture. It is used extensively in Hong Kong. While inhaling vaporized medicines has been an ancient practice, the use of metered-dose inhalers is relatively new and has not been widely accepted. Generally parents still prefer the traditional orally administered medicines to using inhalers.

Methods to improve the take-up of inhaled corticosteroids include the introduction of nurse-based management programs.[6]

REFERENCES

1. Leung R, Wong G, Lau J, Ho A, Chan JKW, Choy D, Douglass C, Lai CKW. Prevalence of asthma and allergy in Hong Kong schoolchildren: an ISAAC study. *Eur Respir J* 1997;**10**:354–60.
2. Ong SG, Liu J, Wong CM, Lam TH, Tam AYC, Daniel L, Hedley AJ. Studies on the respiratory health of primary school children in urban communities of Hong Kong. *Sci Total Environ* 1991;**106**:121–35.
3. Goh DYT, Lee BW, Quek SC, Chew FT, Quek CM. A survey on the prevalence of childhood asthma in Singapore – preliminary findings. *J Singapore Paediat Soc* 1994;**26**:146–52.
4. Leung R, Ho P. Asthma, allergy, and atopy in three South East Asian populations. *Thorax* 1994;**49**:1205–10.
5. Leung R, Jenkins M. Asthma, allergy and atopy in southern Chinese school students. *Clin Exp Allergy* 1994;**24**:353–8.
6. Hui SHL, Leung T-F, Ha G, Wong E, Li AM, Fok T-F. Evaluation of an asthma management program for Chinese children with mild-to-moderate asthma in Hong Kong. *Pedicat Pulmonol* 2002;**32**:22–9.

17f

The Caribbean

JENNIFER M KNIGHT-MADDEN

INTRODUCTION

The Caribbean consists of many islands and two mainland states stretching from Guyana in the South (latitude 10°N) to Bermuda in the North.[1] Islands vary in size, language and culture and also in the ethnic origins of their inhabitants. Whereas in most islands the predominant influence in the gene pool is that of West Africa, Trinidad and Tobago and Guyana have populations that are equally divided between those of East Indian and African descent. All islands have other influences including Chinese, European, Syrian-Lebanese and Indigenous peoples to some extent. In fact, the National Motto of Jamaica is 'Out of many – one people'. This may lead to differences in the genetic predisposition to asthma and atopy among the islands, although this has not yet been demonstrated.

Asthma is acknowledged to be a major problem in the Caribbean. The Caribbean Asthma and Allergy Association was launched in 1997 and through yearly scientific meetings seeks to stimulate asthma and allergy research and to educate health professionals and the general public about asthma. At that time the 'Caribbean Guidelines for Asthma Management and Prevention' was printed and distributed.[2]

EPIDEMIOLOGY

The *prevalence* of asthma reported in the Caribbean varies. Twenty-one per cent of Jamaican school-children were classified as exercise-induced asthmatics using a questionnaire.[3] Asthma was diagnosed by questionnaire in 21% of 1057 Jamaican high school-children, 92.7% of whom reported at least one other manifestation of atopy.[4] Tropical Latin America has also reported high rates such as point and cumulative prevalence rates of 8.8% and 12.2% respectively in Cartegena, a Colombian city on the Caribbean coast.[5] In Barbados, a single hospital provides all accident and emergency care. The average monthly admissions to this A&E department for asthma grew 10-fold from 1970 to 1990 compared with a 10% increase in the island's population. Though little has been published concerning asthma mortality, it is known that the asthma death rate increased in Jamaica from 1980–1989 to over 4 per 100 000 population.[6]

The importance of *allergy*, particularly to house-dust mite and latterly to cockroach has been demonstrated. Skin test reactivity to at least one allergen has been found in 50–81% of asthmatics who were skin tested,[7,8] most commonly to *Dermatophagoides* spp. Sensitivity to house-dust mite allergens correlated with mattress and bedroom dust mite antigen density,[9,10] and was more common in those who lived in more humid concrete houses rather than wooden houses.[8] A recent study in 161 Jamaican adults showed that cockroach sensitivity is next in importance, with mould mix, Bermuda grass, dog and cat being less frequently positive (personal observations).

There are also *climatic* differences which may impact asthma. Those islands to the east are most affected by the influx of Sahara dust as demonstrated in Barbados. Although there is little variation in temperature (24–32°C), the changes of the seasons do affect the incidence of acute episodes of asthma, with the peak being seen during the rainy winter months.[7,11]

The association between *sickle cell disease* and asthma is discussed in Chapter 13a.

TREATMENT

Although many physicians have used the Caribbean guidelines,[2] others do not as evidenced by the continued frequent use of salbutamol (albuterol) as single therapy in many patients, though this is in some ways due to cost constraints. Jamaican popular wisdom suggests that marijuana in various forms may be useful for the treatment of asthma. Cannasol, a product based on marijuana, has been developed and produced in Jamaica.

The cost of the treatment of asthma varies markedly from island to island. In Barbados, the government supplies all asthma therapy free to their citizens. However, in most nations in the region this is not the case and many patients have inadequate care because of the inability to afford medications. Though metered dose inhalers are considered inexpensive, in Jamaica one canister of salbutamol is at least 10% of the minimum weekly wage.

CONCLUSION

Asthma is undoubtedly a significant problem in the Caribbean. In keeping with the recommendations of the study group on the Global Strategy for Asthma Management and Prevention, the Caribbean Asthma and Allergy Association hopes to stimulate more local research so that appropriate strategies can be put into place for improving the management of all those who have this disease in the region.

REFERENCES

1. Monteil MA. Asthma in the English-speaking Caribbean. *West Indian Med J* 1998;**47**:125–8.
2. Picou D *et al. Caribbean Guidelines for Asthma Management and Prevention: A Pocket Guide for Health Care Personnel*. Caribbean Health Research Council.
3. Nichols DJB, Longsworth FG. Prevalence of exercise-induced asthma in school children in Kingston, St Andrew and St Catherine, Jamaica. *West Indian Med J* 1995;**44**:16–19.
4. Lawrence AWW, Segree W. The prevalence of allergic disease in Jamaican adolescents. *West Indian Med J* 1981;**30**:86–9.
5. Caraballo L, Cadivia A, Mendoza J. Prevalence of asthma in a tropical city of Columbia. *Ann Allergy* 1192;**68**:525–9.
6. Scott PW, Mullings RL. Bronchial asthma deaths in Jamaica. *West Indian Med J* 1998;**47**:129–32.
7. Pearson RS. Asthma in Barbados. *Clin Allergy* 1973;**3**:289–97.
8. Barnes KC, Brenner RJ, Helm RM, *et al.* The role of house dust mite and other household pests in the incidence of allergy among Barbadian asthmatics [abstract]. *West Indian Med J* 1992; **41**(Suppl 1):38.
9. Hansen RL, Marx JJ, Twigs JT, *et al.* House dust mite in the West Indies. *Ann Allergy* 1991;**66**:320–3.
10. Pearson RS, Cunnington AM. The importance of house dust mite in sensitivity in Barbadian asthmatics. *Clin Allergy* 1973;**3**:299–306.
11. Deprandine C, Mosley HSL, Roach TR. Weather and bronchial asthma in Barbados; a preliminary investigation [abstract]. *West Indian Med J* 1984;**33**(Suppl 2):24.

Education of children, parents, health professionals and others

JAMES Y PATON

INTRODUCTION

Over the last 30 years, there has been a very large increase in our scientific understanding of childhood asthma. Highly effective pharmacological therapies have been introduced. Yet asthma remains the commonest chronic disease of childhood in developed countries and its prevalence has been increasing, at least until recently.[1] This apparent paradox has led to the conclusion that there is an 'asthma knowledge gap' between clinicians' performance and patients' behaviours.[2,3] Either clinicians are not providing the appropriate care or, if they are, children and their parents are not following the therapeutic recommendations.[4]

EDUCATION IN ASTHMA MANAGEMENT

Why is education important in asthma management?

Since a cure for childhood asthma is not yet possible, the present focus of asthma management is on disease control – controlling symptoms, restoring function and improving quality of life.[5] The main therapeutic route to achieving asthma control has been the long-term use of anti-inflammatory therapy, mainly inhaled corticosteroids, to control chronic airway inflammation. Even in children, inhaled corticosteroids are now the mainstay of preventive treatment.

However, if asthma is to be controlled effectively, parents and children must carry out a number of rather complex tasks. These include using prescribed drugs properly to prevent or control asthma symptoms; being able to identify and, if possible, avoid asthma trigger factors; being able to detect and self-manage most asthma exacerbations; having the necessary interpersonal skills to communicate effectively with healthcare workers and developing the necessary social supports.[3,5] There is an additional layer of complexity because both the asthma and its consequences vary over time. It is children with asthma and their parents who are most aware of these changes. Clinicians are simply not able to give guidance on every contingency or individual circumstance that such families may encounter. Further, children and their families also have information, preferences and beliefs, complementary to the doctor's professional knowledge, which affect the way they behave.

Furthermore children with asthma and their parents have become increasingly interested in being full partners in their own medical care. While all patients must self-manage their asthma to some extent, for example by using relieving medication when necessary, there has been a progressive move towards involving patients more directly in their asthma management.[6] Such self-management or family management[7] requires patients or families to monitor the asthma and adjust the therapy in response to changes in severity, independently of their clinician. However, 'self-management' is not the same as self-treatment. In self-management, the patient provides the individual context and the clinician the general medical backdrop. Both are necessary for effective management and disease control.[8] Ideally, there should be a co-operative, agreed approach to asthma management involving patients, the healthcare team and family members – a process that has been labelled 'guided self-management'. In adults, there is extensive evidence that asthma self-management leads to improved outcomes (reviewed in ref. 9).

Education helps children and their families develop the necessary knowledge, attitudes, beliefs and skills to manage asthma effectively. The importance of education in asthma management has been increasingly recognized, and patient education is now a central component of current asthma guidelines.[5,10] However patients, including children and their parents, are not the sole targets for education about managing asthma. There are many professional groups who have important roles to play in asthma care, and who require education. Indeed, preparing healthcare professionals is turning out to be just as important as preparing the child or the family. If delivering effective asthma care requires a partnership, then all participants must be educated and organized effectively.[11] Indeed, Clark and Gong have suggested that often neither the child and family nor the healthcare professional are adequately prepared for their respective roles in asthma management.[3]

Asthma education and the problem of adherence and concordance

It is self-evident that no treatment regime is likely to be effective unless it is properly followed. Patients must understand how to follow their regimes, and be able and willing to do so. Since the pioneering work of Sackett and Haynes,[12] there has been growing recognition that patients, including asthmatic children and their families, often fail to follow their treatment regime.[13–15] A broad range of evidence suggests that only about a third of patients follow a prescription correctly; one third adhere to the prescription poorly, if at all; and the other third is somewhere in between.[16] Failure to comply is not confined to medication use, but affects all aspects of medical care. For instance, Sackett pointed out that 20–50% of clinic appointments are missed.[12] Changes in behaviour such as stopping smoking or weight reduction are implemented even less

frequently. Unfortunately, clinicians are poor at recognising who is not achieving to the treatment plan, or in predicting which patients will comply.[17] It is also clear that health professionals themselves are not necessarily good at complying.[18]

Theoretical approaches to understanding health behaviours

Given the evidence of poor compliance, it is not surprising that behavioural scientists have tried hard to understand how an individual makes health-related decisions. Initially, scientific efforts were directed to understanding why patients did not comply with therapies. Over time behavioural scientists have expanded the scope of their efforts to include the wider range of activities patients must undertake to manage their health problems effectively. Many theoretical models have been developed, e.g. the health belief model, stages of change theory, self-regulation theory and social learning theory (see Clark and Becker for a brief review[19]). All these theories try to explain the mechanisms that lead to behaviour change.

Self-regulation as a key health behaviour for asthma management

Recently, Clark and colleagues have drawn from both social learning theory[20] and the theory of self-regulation to develop a model of particular application in asthma management[3,19,21] (Figure 18.1). Their model is based on three assumptions. Firstly, several factors predispose a person to manage a disease. Secondly, patient management arises from a conscious use of strategies to manipulate situations to reduce disease impact on daily life. Thirdly, illness management is not an end in itself but merely the means to other ends important to the patient, such as the reduction of symptoms.[3] Families can use self-regulation processes to observe how the disease prevents them achieving their specific goals, to judge what type of action might help the situation, to experiment with behaviours and to draw conclusions or react to the effects of those behaviours. This approach has particular relevance to asthma where there is no definitive formula for optimum

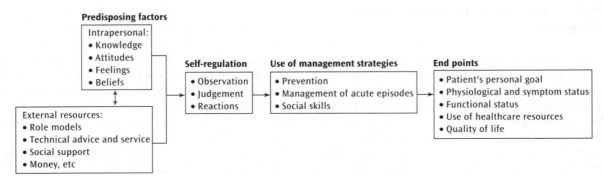

Figure 18.1 *Model of patient management of chronic lung diseases. (From ref. 3.)*

management and where families often have to make decisions about changing treatments on their own without input from health professionals.

The role of behavioural theories in asthma education

These theoretical models of behaviour change generally aim to describe what factors lead to particular health behaviours. Increasingly, such theories have underpinned health educational interventions for asthma. For example, in the self-regulation model, education would have an important role not simply in providing information about the disease but in developing the subject's capacity to observe, to make sensible judgements, to feel confident and recognize good asthma outcomes. These behavioural models often share elements that can be distilled into core principles. Such 'principles of behaviour change and health education' can inform the design and evaluation of any asthma educational programme[2] (Table 18.1). Whatever the merits of any particular theory, a theoretical framework has a number of advantages. Firstly, theoretical insights into the mechanisms that lead to a particular behaviour provide a basis for optimizing that behaviour. Secondly, if an intervention fails, a theoretical framework helps in understanding why failure occurred and how it might be avoided in the future.[3]

Does asthma education work? Evidence for effectiveness

What exactly 'patient education' means is not always clear in published studies. In addition, published asthma education programmes have varied widely in their objectives,

in the content and the educational methods used, in their intensity and duration, and in the educator.[22] Many programmes have aimed to transmit knowledge rather than focusing on behaviours, even though a wide gap often separates knowledge and behaviour. All too frequently, asthma education, whether informal during a consultation or more formal group teaching during a planned session, has been based on an ad hoc set of messages and skills that health professionals believe patients need to know. Unfortunately, these messages have been derived from intuitions, traditions or habits and frequently do not coincide with any theoretical principles (such as listed in Table 18.1) and are then combined with teaching methods that are too didactic. It is hardly surprising that there has been a debate about whether asthma education works.[23]

Nevertheless, since the 1980s a number of well-designed models of asthma education for children and adults have been tested. Clark and Gong have listed well-designed paediatric asthma educational programmes based on relevant behavioural theory that have been evaluated and have been shown to lead to important asthma outcomes such as reduced use of health services.[3] Significant health gains can be made by children with asthma when their primary care physicians are provided with training in asthma care and communication skills.[82] The evidence from adult studies for the effectiveness of differing combination of patient education and self-management has been summarized in a series of Cochrane reviews.[9]

Thus, there is clear evidence that asthma education can be effective in providing patients and families with the understanding, skills and behaviours to allow them to control their asthma effectively. Education can also help patients gain the motivation and confidence to control their illness.[83,84] Education nowadays is recognized as having a central role in changing a patient's behaviour in a way that ultimately leads to more effective asthma

Table 18.1 *Educational principles that should be included in an 'ideal' asthma education programme*[2]

Educational principle	Comment
Educational diagnosis	Involves identification of the causes of the behaviour
Hierarchical approach	States that there is a natural order in the sequence of factors influencing behaviour
Cumulative learning	Experiences must be planned in a sequence that takes into account the patient's past learning and their present learning opportunities
Participation or ownership	Behaviour changes will be greater if the patients have identified their own needs for change and have actively selected a method or approach
Situational specificity	The effectiveness of any educational programme depends on the individual circumstances and characteristics of the patient and the educator ('right audience, right time in right way')
Use of multiple methods	A comprehensive behaviour change programme should employ different methods to take account of patient or situation specific factors
Individualization	Tailoring education allows interventions that are both patient and situation relevant
Relevance	The more relevant the content and methods to the learner's circumstances, the more likely learning and behaviour is to be successful
Feedback	Providing feedback allows the patient to adapt learning and response to his or her own situation or pace
Reinforcement	Behaviour that is rewarded tends to be repeated
Facilitation	An intervention should provide the means to take action or reduce the barriers to action

management. The challenge now is to adapt and implement programmes of proven effectiveness in clinical practice.

PREPARING FOR EFFECTIVE PARTNERSHIPS

Good communication is essential

It is over 30 years since Korsch's classic study documenting the lack of attention paid by paediatricians to parents' fears and concerns about their child's illness and the resulting dissatisfaction with the consultation.[24] Patients clearly valued the doctor being warm and friendly, taking account of their concerns and expectations, providing clear-cut explanations about the diagnosis and cause of the illness and avoiding medical jargon. Significantly, parental satisfaction was not related to the amount of time the doctor spent with patients. Paying attention to initial fears and expectations did not highjack or prolong the consultation, but led to shorter visits. Once urgent concerns had been dealt with, mothers were observed to be more attentive and open to the physician's suggestions. Korsch even described how on occasions the doctor actually wasted time during the consultation by 'ineffective verbalization' – arguing with the parent or needlessly repeating questions that had not been understood. Apart from satisfaction, doctor–patient communication seems to influence other aspects of patients' behaviour such as adherence to treatment, recall and understanding of medical information, disease-coping and quality of life.[25]

Communication between a doctor and a patient has a number of different functions including creating a good personal relationship, exchanging information and making treatment-related plans.[25] A number of behaviours that help clinicians to communicate more effectively have been recognized. They include adopting a congenial demeanour (being friendly and attentive and using humour), showing empathy (through eliciting and acknowledging patient fears and concerns, paraphrasing and reflecting their words and using non-verbal behaviour) and giving encouragement, praise and reassurance.[26] Showing empathy may be particularly important. Good general guidelines for clinician–patient communication exist (Table 18.2) and the resulting benefits for asthma management may be considerable (Figure 18.2). As a result, good communication skills are now accepted as a prerequisite for a satisfactory doctor–patient partnership.[15]

Improving health professionals' communication skills

Unfortunately, for many health professionals these skills do not come naturally. Nor do such skills necessarily improve with experience. Doctors themselves have

reported that their relationships with their patients cause them stress and anxiety due to lack of confidence and competence in communicating.[27]

Fortunately, with training, there is evidence health professionals can improve their communication skills in such a way that patients experience measurably better outcomes.[28,29] One recent randomized trial tested the effect of including specific training in communication skills in an asthma education programme for paediatricians. This intervention included two interactive afternoon seminars based on the self-regulation theory. The educational material included a brief specialist lecture about asthma, a videotape showing effective use of the skills identified in Table 18.2, case studies of troublesome clinical problems, a protocol enabling doctors to assess their own communication skills and a review of key asthma messages and materials to use when teaching. The programme resulted in a significant improvement in the prescribing and communications behaviour of physicians, more favourable patient responses to physicians' actions, patient–physician encounters that were actually of shorter duration and reduced use of health care resources.[30] Training in communication skills is finally becoming more widely available and is now an important component of many undergraduate medical curricula.

Educating health professionals about disease management

Some practical insights from recent research into asthma education have been collated.[31] To be effective, education for healthcare providers had to start with their own input about their perceived needs and preferred teaching methods. Traditional lectures did not alone change behaviour. Effective training of clinicians involved not only developing their asthma management skills, but also providing a supportive environment. Changing only one or two specific aspects of asthma management at a time was more likely to be effective than trying to change everything at once. Involving clinical staff in teaching other clinical staff was effective. Incentives such as CME points or recognition or rewards helped to reinforce active participation. Simplified and convenient prompts and reference materials were helpful as supplementary educational tools. Researchers in New York found that patients were sometimes more comfortable discussing problems and seeking help from non-professional clinical staff, e.g. receptionists or technicians. Training for the entire practice team may then enable non-professional staff to reinforce the health professional's recommendations.

What about improving parents' and children's communication skills?

Whether improving patients' and parents' communications skills through training might also lead to more

Table 18.2 *Good basic communication skills helping physicians to communicate more effectively*

Behaviour category	Specific behaviour	Reason for using
Congenial demeanour	Greet the patient by name. Introduce yourself	Increases patient satisfaction
	Listen attentively e.g. use eye contact, sitting rather than standing, sit at same level, lean forward to attend to discussion. Avoid flustering the patient	Helps establish rapport
	Maintain an interactive conversation e.g. use open-ended questions – 'Tell me about it?'; use simple language; use analogies to teach important concepts	Interactive dialogue produces richer information
	Use appropriate non-verbal encouragement (nodding, smiling)	
	Give verbal praise for things done well	
Reassuring communication	Address any immediate concerns	Increases patient satisfaction and improves understanding
	Elicit parents underlying concerns and worries about their child	Allows family to focus their attention on the information being offered
	Give specific, truthful information that alleviates fears. Check that it is understood	Fear is a distraction; reducing it enables the patient to focus on what the physician is saying, and improves recall
Treatment plan focus	Elicit family's immediate objectives. Reach agreement on a short-term goal that both provider and patient will strive to reach and that both regard as important	Enhances willingness to follow the treatment plan
	Review the physician's long-term therapeutic plan with the patient so the patient knows what to expect over time, when treatment will be modified and criteria for judging success of treatment plan	
	Help patient develop and use criteria for future management decisions e.g. using diary information, guidelines for handling potential problems	
	Provide patients or parents with a written management plan, ideally in their own writing	

effective clinician–patient communication is also under study. The main target for such programmes is usually a parent but children may also benefit. Lewis *et al.* found that brief education during clinic waiting improved the rapport between the physician and the child, encouraging the child to learn more about their condition and to take a more active role in their care.[32]

DESIGNING AND DELIVERING ASTHMA EDUCATIONAL PROGRAMMES

General comments

Because many asthma education programmes have been poorly documented,[22] replicating programmes may be difficult or impossible. A combination of poor design and poor documentation has also made it difficult to identify those components most effective at promoting

changes in behaviour. In the future, there should be a standard description of any educational programme including the theoretical basis, a list of objectives, and a detailed account of what was done.[22]

Core content

From the first generation of asthma education studies, there is reasonable agreement about the essential content of an asthma education programme.[4] The patient with asthma needs to have some understanding of and skills in: (i) Asthma attack prevention; (ii) Asthma attack management; (iii) Communication and interpersonal skills important in the management of asthma.[33,34] *Prevention of an attack* includes the skills and behaviours necessary to recognize early warning signs (including using a peak-flow meter, if appropriate) and to act on these signs to prevent an attack. It also involves identifying and avoiding triggers, understanding about reliever

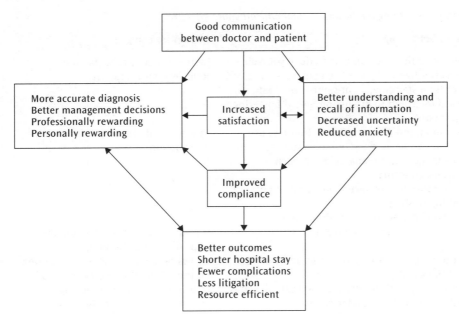

Figure 18.2 *Benefits of the ideal consultation. (From ref. 27.)*

and preventer medications, having proper inhaled device technique and taking prescribed medication correctly and on schedule.[33] *Attack management* comprises resting and staying calm during an attack, taking medications as prescribed and using agreed criteria on when to seek assistance. Finally, the necessary *social skills* include an ability to communicate effectively and to negotiate, as well as skills to manage relationships central to the control of the child's asthma. Thus this educational content covers the knowledge, skills, and behaviours necessary for asthma self-management as well as broader concerns relating to family and environmental influences. A range of suggested topics and useful educational tools addressing these issues can be found in published guidelines.[5] Unanswered questions remain, and further work is needed to refine the essential content and the most effective teaching strategies.[26]

Whom to teach?

CHILD OR PARENT

Parents or carers are usually the main targets of paediatric asthma education. However, this does not mean children should be ignored. Research has suggested that children may be quite able to take part in programmes that develop problem-solving and decision-making skills.[7] Indeed, Lewis and Lewis found that the principal barriers to involving children were firstly, physicians who were reluctant to share power with parents, let alone children, and secondly, some parents whose roles were threatened by increased sharing.[35] A brief video shown to children in the waiting room improved the rapport between the physician and child.[32]

If children are involved in asthma education, then it is important that developmentally appropriate approaches

are used. For 4- to 7-year-old children approaches such as story telling and games can be used. For 8- to 12-year-olds, the emphasis shifts to mastering tasks while for those 13 or older the emphasis should be on social relationships.[7] There may be wider benefits arising from involving children in asthma management education, with one study finding that such children performed better at school performance and achieved higher grades than controls.[36] Recently, peer-led asthma education programmes have proved successful with adolescents.[37]

Another issue is whether children and their parents should be taught together or separately. One common pattern is to separate children and parents for teaching, bringing them together only at the end.[38] This approach may allow the children to report to their parents what they have learned, thus verifying and validating the take-home messages. However, there is surprisingly little detailed advice available.

INDIVIDUALS OR GROUPS?

One issue to consider is whether education is best delivered to patients one at a time, perhaps with a family member present, or in (typically small) groups.[39] As an approach, individual teaching fits more comfortably into a clinic setting. Indeed, every clinical contact may be viewed as providing a 'teachable moment'. Reinforcing behaviour over a number of clinic visits is relatively easy. It is also potentially easier to individualize the education by matching both content and delivery methods to a particular patient's learning style and speed. However, individual educational approaches are likely to be more costly in terms of the educator's time. Group teaching approaches, if successful, may be more cost-effective. Small group education may also provide other benefits such as peer support and group problem solving common problems.

Group approaches may be particularly relevant to children who are used to being taught at school. Organized asthma educational programmes often use group teaching. However, arranging meetings for a group may be difficult, particularly if multiple sessions are planned. A degree of individualization within a group setting is possible through the use of strategies such as worksheets for individual problem solving, or group problem solving of an individual management difficulty.[39]

If a group approach is to be used, there is little guidance about the best group size. In published studies, group size has varied, with between 4 and 10 being common.[38,40] Similarly, there is little information about the most appropriate age composition. There is evidence that children as young as 8 can perform basic self-management practices and by adolescence can handle most self-management tasks.[7] One study included children between 8 and 13 years,[40] but whether mixing older teenagers and younger children is beneficial or otherwise is not clear. Clark et al. found that 8- to 12-year-old children could be taught with children 13 years or older if the educator addressed the needs and interests of the two age groups.[7] Older children may be helpful teaching the younger children.[7]

Reviewing the available evidence, Wilson found that both individual and group education could improve patient outcomes.[39] However, Wilson suggests that it may be most meaningful to recognize that individual and group education may have different roles at different stages in a 'continuum of education' about asthma.[39]

Lesson content, format and duration

The 'ideal' educational programme will include the core asthma messages (outlined above) and will be based on sound health educational principles (Table 18.1). For example, the programme should include an educational diagnosis of the individual patient or group needs, including assessing their past and present experiences; there should be careful sequencing of the educational messages starting with more basic messages before progressing to more complex material; there should be opportunities for later review and feedback to reinforce new behaviours.

A number of sessions over a period of time may be required if significant changes in behaviour are to be achieved. For group programmes, a once-a-week lesson of 45–90 minutes over a number of weeks has been common.[40,41] There are examples of briefer interventions that have also been successful.[42,43] If shorter programmes are used, it may be appropriate to focus on skills that can be adopted rapidly without major changes in daily routine.

Tailoring the content

Often it is neither appropriate nor feasible to arrange a comprehensive programme. An available programme will have to be adapted to a particular local setting. One approach to identifying the most important educational components for a particular setting has been to carry out a local needs assessment. This has been done by interviewing patients, relatives and clinicians;[44] by reviewing critical incidents that resulted in bad asthma outcomes;[45] or through the use of focus groups.[46] The results can then be used to tailor the programme to local needs and circumstances while avoiding wasting time on irrelevant content. For the educators, local adaptation may be a key step in developing local ownership – an important feature for successful implementation.[47]

Just as a programme should be adapted for local circumstances, so an individual educational diagnosis is important in shaping the content to suit an individual's personal goals, needs and learning styles. Children and their parents are usually more interested in issues such as the long-term side effects of drugs or quality of life, rather than objective outcomes such as lung function. Also parents and their children may have different goals. Boys often want to take part in the same physical activities as their peers; parents may be more concerned by nocturnal disturbance. In any programme, it is important to remember that patients are more likely to follow the plan if the goals and objectives are directly relevant to them. The diagnostic approaches used can vary from informal techniques used routinely during a consultation, such as asking about the understanding of medications or checking device technique, to more detailed questionnaires[34] that may be completed while the patient is waiting.

Delivery strategies

BY WHOM?

Asthma education may be delivered by a wide variety of people. In the clinic or ward, it is often a doctor or nurse. In a group setting, studies have also used a behavioural therapist,[40] trained asthma educators or even children themselves.[37] Compared with alternatives, interaction with an 'educator' whether for individuals or groups potentially provides a more stimulating and individualized experience for the subject. However, it is important that the educator engages with the subjects and facilitates their active involvement.[39] Delivering a standard lecture in an identical manner to every patient will be as ineffective as lecturing a larger passive group. There has been increasing recognition of the fact that any member of the clinical team may have opportunities to give asthma education or to reinforce advice. Accordingly, everyone within the healthcare team should be trained to give out consistent messages about asthma management. With the increasing emphasis on partnership between patients and health workers, clinical team members should remember that they can learn from families about the impact of the disease on the child and the family.[34] At present, even the most sophisticated modern technology does not match the flexibility of an individual educator and educational material in the form of interactive CDs, videos, audiotapes and so on is mostly used to supplement verbal massages.

DELIVERY METHODS

The way in which an educational programme is delivered should be developmentally appropriate, acceptable and engaging. Many strategies have been employed including role-play, team games, group discussions, problem-solving worksheets and guided skill acquisition (for example, the educator coaching the child and parent on device technique). Regardless of method, the important point is that the emphasis should be on active learning combined with opportunities for supervised learning, practice of skills and feedback about performance.

WHEN AND WHERE TO TEACH

Asthma education has been carried out in many different settings including hospital wards, emergency rooms, community organizations and schools,[26] but studies comparing their value are not usually available.

Emergency departments and inpatient wards may provide a 'window of opportunity' for asthma education. The available evidence from both paediatric[42] and adult studies (reviewed in ref. 48) is that such interventions can be highly effective with substantial reductions in subsequent healthcare utilization. Patients and families may be particularly receptive to messages about managing asthma during an emergency asthma contact. Constraints of time, and understandable parental distress, mean that any education must be simple and specific. One programme used a simple '1...2...3 Plan' with the plan listing specific steps for taking preventive and relieving medication, steps for responding to warning signs of an attack and encouraging early community follow-up.[31]

Follow-up in primary care offers opportunities for integrating education into routine care and allows review and reinforcement of educational messages. However, general practitioners are often concerned about increases in their workload.[49] The development of asthma nurse clinics may relieve the pressure on busy practitioners. Also, nurses have different consultation styles from doctors, and they may be better able to elicit and respond to patient's fears and concerns.

Schools provide a good opportunity to give asthma education to children. Studies in schools have shown clear benefits from such education in terms of altered health behaviour, reduced asthma symptoms and improved performance.[50,51] An innovative Australian study has described a successful peer-led approach to asthma education for teenagers in schools.[37] Education in the school setting may help to reduce the negative effects of asthma morbidity on school attendance and performance, and

may increase children's confidence in their own ability to control their asthma and lead an active life.[26]

Thus each setting may offer both advantages and limitations that determine what educational goals can actually be achieved.[26] At present, different settings are rarely directly compared, and evidence that one setting is superior to another is usually not available. Ultimately, the best setting may be the one where the individual wants to learn and is most receptive to changing behaviour.[26] Because every setting may offer such opportunities for teaching ('teachable moments'), the view currently is that asthma education should be available at every contact between the child and family and the healthcare system, whatever the setting.

Education to ethnic minority groups

Asthma is a major health problem among disadvantaged children and children from minority groups. They are at particular risk because of language barriers, poverty, lack of access to medical care and culturally-based beliefs about health and illness.[31] Those providing asthma education should be aware of such issues and should be sensitive to attitudes, beliefs, behaviours, reading abilities, language difficulties and ethnic and cultural appropriateness.

DEVELOPING SUPPORTING EDUCATIONAL MATERIALS

Supporting educational materials are an important part of any educational programme. Simple written guidelines or audiovisual materials may enhance a patient's ability to manage asthma successfully. In relation to self-management in adult patients, the inclusion of a written action plan advising on appropriate steps to be taken early in an exacerbation resulted in a greater reduction in admissions to hospital than programmes without a plan.[9]

It is also clear there are huge demands from patients for information to supplement what health professionals tell them. For example, in 1997 the National Asthma Campaign in the UK received 480 000 requests for its information booklets for asthma patients.[26] Satisfying this demand has been called a 'growth industry'[52] and there is growing investment in consumer health information. Despite this the quality of information remains variable, and much is inappropriately targeted and poorly constructed.

Is it the information children and families want?

Health professionals have frequently assumed that they know what information patients need and want. Unfortunately, health professionals are often poor at giving the patients the information they really want. When asked, patients have clear views. They say they want 'life impact information' and information about 'what to do when'. Such information enhances their feeling of control over their lives and is as important to them as the more traditional information about diagnosis and treatment.[53,54]

Similarly, parents report feeling disempowered dealing with acute illness in preschool children because they have difficulty making sense of the illness.[55] Parents feel they are not told how to recognize when illness is severe; when it is appropriate to seek help; and why the doctor has decided on a particular treatment – all information that they would like. Parents want to know about the likely cause of the illness, about any implications of the illness, its treatment and the potential for prevention. Parents have made positive suggestions, for example learning from other parents' experiences dealing with illness would be useful, particularly for inexperienced parents. Although parents suggested information should be free from jargon, they were keen that it should not omit important technical information that would facilitate understanding.[55]

Adult studies echo many of these points. Doctors can significantly underestimate patients' appetite for information.[56] There is also evidence that patients prefer frank rather than reassuring information about drugs and their side effects.[57] Explicit information about side effects does not appear to influence subsequent side effect reporting.[58]

What about the quality of information?

There is currently major concern about the quality of information. Not all available information is of good quality; only a small proportion is based on sound evidence. Concern has particularly arisen because of the variable quality of the information on Internet websites, where the information may be incomplete, badly organized or inaccurate.[59]

In relation to any information, a check on the date of preparation, the sources used, the qualifications of the author and the sponsors of the information may help to give some assessment of the likely accuracy and objectivity. More explicit quality criteria have been developed to evaluate the extent to which material is based on evidence[60] (Table 18.3). Unfortunately, such tools are not yet widely known or used, and few materials satisfy the proposed standards. Tools to rate the reliability of health information on the web are also being developed, but are at a very early stage.[61,62]

Is the information accessible?

If information is to be useful, it has to be accessible. Many adults have poor reading and comprehension skills. For example, it has been estimated that around one quarter

Table 18.3 *Quick reference guide to the DISCERN quality criteria (Discern Handbook)*[60]

A good quality publication about treatment choices will:
- Have explicit aims
- Achieve its aims
- Be relevant to consumers
- Make sources of information explicit
- Make date of information explicit
- Be balance and unbiased
- List additional sources of information
- Refer to areas of uncertainty
- Describe how treatment works
- Describe the benefits of treatment
- Describe the risks of treatment
- Describe what would happen without treatment
- Describe the effects of treatment choices on overall quality of life
- Make it clear there may be more than one possible treatment choice
- Provide support for shared decision making

of the US population have rudimentary reading skills and are functionally illiterate i.e. below 5th grade (approximately 10 years) reading level. Another 25% have marginal reading skills (6–9th grade reading level, 11–14 years). There are similar concerns about readings skills in the UK. Poor reading skills are also associated with poorer health and greater use of health services.[63] Many of the available pamphlets and information sheets about asthma are written at too sophisticated a level, well beyond the reading and comprehension abilities of most of the target population. Patient information material produced for the World Wide Web is, at present, no better.[64]

Unfortunately, parents' self-reported education level does not provide an accurate reflection of their reading level.[65] Structured tests are available to measure patients' reading skills: for example, the Rapid Estimate of Adult Literacy in Medicine (REALM).[66] There are also tests to assess the readability of written materials:[67] for example, the Flesch Reading Ease (FRE)[68] (Table 18.4). Computed readability measures are included in some common word processing programs such as Microsoft Word. Although these measures may be a useful guide, they may not be accurate, particularly in the context of chronic diseases, where patients become familiar with medical jargon.[69]

Is the information delivered in the most appropriate way?

Making sure written information is accessible, particularly to disadvantaged and minority groups, is a key issue. For many low-literacy populations, very simple brochures or comics are more likely to be understood. When written communication is essential, material should be at 5th grade level or lower, and should be supplemented by

Table 18.4 *Flesch Reading Ease Score*[68]

Flesch Reading Ease Scores	Difficulty grading	Example texts	IQ required	% of population who understand
0–30	Very difficult	Scientific journals	126+	4.5
31–50	Difficult	Academic journals	111+	24.0
51–60	Fairly difficult	Quality magazines	104+	40.0
61–70	Standard	Reader's digest	90+	70.0
71–80	Fairly easy	Slick fiction	87+	80.0
81–90	Easy	Pulp fiction	84+	86.0
91–100	Very easy	Comics	81+	90.0

non-written material.[63] Information presented in alternative ways may be necessary: for example, audiotapes or videotape for those with limited reading skills; large print for those with visual impairment people; or Braille for deaf–blind people.[70] Information will often have to be translated into languages other than English. In fact, minority population groups are often particularly poorly catered for, and have to cope with material that is both difficult to read and culturally inappropriate.

Significant changes are occurring in the way information is delivered with the development of the Internet and other electronic formats such as interactive CDs, video discs and touch-screen computers. Computer systems may facilitate tailoring information for the individual.[71] For newer methods, there is frequently little evaluation of the effectiveness or content compared with a well designed more traditional patient leaflet.[52] Whether newer methods of providing information such as the Internet will eventually prove more effective remains to be seen.

Developing good educational materials – some simple guidance

Developing good educational materials requires a systematic approach, including careful assessment of the needs of the target audience, limiting the educational objectives, focusing the content on desired behaviours, presenting the context of the message first, and planning for reader interaction.[72,73] If it is to be understood, written material needs to be prepared carefully with attention to readability, the likely concentration span of the reader and legibility.[74] Such issues may be particularly relevant to children. Simple guidelines to effective writing are available (Table 18.5). Any written material should also be legible; again guidelines are available (Royal National Institute for the Blind's Clear Print Guidelines[75]). Apart from instruments for assessing reading skills and reading levels, other tools for assessing the suitability of written, audiotape or video materials are available.[66]

Ultimately, the best way to assess readability is to ask patients for their opinions.[59] A key step in the preparation of any educational material is, therefore, piloting the material with the target audience to ensure that it is indeed understandable and appropriate.

Table 18.5 *Effective writing for patients*[59]

- Place the most important information first or last
- Write in a conversational style with short words and sentences
- Limit each paragraph to a single message
- Focus on a specific personal experience rather than generalities
- Ensure that the use of words is consistent
- Use headers to alert readers to what is coming
- Cut out irrelevant information
- In general, write in positive sentences
- Use negative sentences when advising patients to avoid actions
- Ask patients to read your draft and to suggest how to improve it

FROM THEORY INTO PRACTICE – INTEGRATING EDUCATIONAL ACTIVITIES INTO CLINICAL CARE

Two broad strategies have been used for integrating asthma education into practice.[26] The core content that all asthmatic patients need will usually be delivered on an individual basis in teaching integrated into normal clinical care. *Teaching self-management skills at clinic visits* has been shown to reduce asthma morbidity and improve quality of life whether attending hospital[76,77] or a nurse-run clinic in the community.[78] Thus all the relevant staff should be appropriately trained and able to deliver education. Even quite brief training may be effective.[30] In many countries, national training centres or training courses are available, and standards for asthma educators and certification examinations are being developed. Certification may be beneficial in ensuring teaching competence and reliable standards of care. Training from a national centre has been shown to be associated with improved clinical outcomes.[79,80] If nothing else, a national programme may help ensure that patients receive consistent, clear and impartial messages about asthma management.

Many patients will want *supplementary education*, which may be effectively provided in a group setting. Children and families can be referred to organized asthma education programmes, usually associated with their particular clinic or hospital. Schools may be another useful setting.[37] However, the time required organizing and attending such programmes means that they will only ever be suitable for relatively few patients. Which approach is best? Wilson has suggested that it may be most meaningful to recognize that individual and group education may have different roles at different stages in a 'continuum of education' about asthma.[39]

Asthma guidelines that include advice about education are now widely available to health professionals and provide another tool to ensure that impartial and consistent messages are given to patients. Unfortunately, adherence to national guidelines is often poor.[18,81] The evidence about how best to implement asthma guidelines is limited but is broadly in line with the evidence from educational interventions in other clinical situations (summarized in ref. 26). While guidelines can change clinician behaviour, there needs to be a clear strategy for implementation. Local adaptation to provide local ownership may be one practical and effective approach. Change is more likely when the guideline is supported by specific educational interventions and when patient-specific reminders are used to prompt clinicians. However, there does not appear to be one strategy for implementation of guidelines that is universally effective. Barriers to change such as pressure of work are commonly identified and need to be addressed – many are reminiscent of issues that have arisen in studies about asthma education for patients.

CONCLUSION

There is increasing recognition that educating patients and their families about asthma management may result in more effective treatment and reduced morbidity. There is little point spending vast sums of money developing sophisticated pharmacological treatments when simple interventions based on currently available information might make a significant difference, if properly implemented. The disparity between 'high technology' skills and 'high touch' skills in asthma management has been emphasized and may explain why asthma morbidity has not improved despite advances in both diagnosis and treatment.[2] Effective asthma education potentially provides a vital bridge between these two positions. A better theoretical understanding of how to persuade patients to change health-related behaviours is resulting in a more rational approach to the development of asthma education programmes. Studies in recent years have made it quite clear that a rigorous research-based approach to asthma education is possible. As a consequence, education programmes can be more appropriately targeted, with a clearer understanding of what will work, when and why. In the long-term, better education is likely to bring substantial benefits to children with asthma and their families.

Acknowledgement   I am grateful to P. Madge for many stimulating discussions about asthma education and for help collating relevant literature.

REFERENCES

1. Anderson HR, Butland BK, Strachan DP. Trends in prevalence and severity of childhood asthma. *Br Med J* 1994;**308**:1600–4.
2. Green LW, Frankish CJ. Theories and principles of health education applied to asthma. *Chest* 1994;**108**:220S–9S.
3. Clark NM, Gong M. Management of chronic disease by practitioners and patients: are we teaching the wrong things? *Br Med J* 2000;**320**:572–5.
4. Clark NM, Bailey WC, Rand C. Advances in prevention and education in lung disease. *Am J Respir Crit Care Med* 1998;**157**:S155–S167.
5. National Asthma Education Program. *Guidelines for the Diagnosis and Management of Asthma*. National Asthma Education Program Expert Panel Report 2. NIH Publication No. 97-4051, 1997. National Institutes of Health, Bethesda, MD.
6. Partridge MR. Self-management in adults with asthma. *Patient Educ Couns* 1997;**32**:S1–S4.
7. Clark NM, Feldman CH, Evans D, *et al*. Managing better: children, parents, and asthma. *Patient Educ Couns* 1986;**8**:27–38.
8. Holman H, Lorig K. Patients as partners in managing chronic disease. *Br Med J* 2000;**320**:527–8.
9. Gibson PG, Coughlan J, Wilson AJ, *et al*. Self-management education and regular practitioner review for adults with asthma (*Cochrane Review*). Issue 4. The Cochrane Library. Update Software, Oxford, 1999.
10. SIGN/BTS Guidelines on Asthma Management. *Thorax* 2002; in press.
11. Sterk PJ, Buist SA, Woolcock AJ, *et al*. The message from the World Asthma Meeting. *Eur Respir J* 1999;**14**:1435–53.
12. Sackett DL, Haynes RB. *Compliance with Therapeutic Regimens*. Baltimore and London: John Hopkins University Press, 1976.
13. Coutts JA, Gibson NA, Paton JY. Measuring compliance with inhaled medication in asthma. *Arch Dis Child* 1992;**67**:332–3.
14. Gibson NA, Ferguson AE, Aitchison TC, Paton JY. Compliance with inhaled asthma medication in preschool children. *Thorax* 1995;**50**:1274–9.
15. Paton J. Compliance or adherence to therapy. In: M Silverman, CP O'Callaghan, eds. *Practical Paediatric Respiratory Medicine*. Arnold, London, 2001.
16. Cochrane GM. Therapeutic compliance in asthma; its magnitude and implications. *Eur Respir J* 1992;**5**:122–4.

17. Gilbert JR, Evans CE, Haynes RB, Tugwell P. Predicting compliance with a regimen of digoxin therapy in family practice. *Can Med Assoc J* 1980;**123**:119–22.

18. Legorreta AP, Christian-Herman J, O'Connor RD, Hasan MM, Evans R, Leung KM. Compliance with national asthma management guidelines and specialty care: a health maintenance organization experience [see comments]. *Arch Intern Med* 1998;**158**: 457–64.

19. Clark NM, Becker MH. Theoretical models and strategies for improving adherence and disease management. In: SA Shumaker, EB Schron, JK Ockene, WL McBee, eds. *Handbook of Health Behavior Change*. Springer Publishing, New York, 1998, pp. 5–31.

20. Bandura A. Social foundations of thought and action: a social cognitive theory. Englewood Cliffs, NJ: Prentice-Hall, 1986.

21. Clark NM, Evans D, Zimmerman BJ, Levison MJ, Mellins RB. Patient and family management of asthma: theory-based techniques for the clinician. *J Asthma* 1994;**31**:427–35.

22. Sudre P, Jacquemet J, Uldry C, Perneger TV. Objectives, methods and content of patient education programmes for adults with asthma: systematic review of studies published between 1979 and 1998. *Thorax* 1999;**54**:681–7.

23. Bernard-Bonnin AC, Stachenko S, Bonin D, Charette C, Rousseau E. Self-management teaching programs and morbidity of pediatric asthma: a meta-analysis. *J Allergy Clin Immunol* 1995;**95**:34–41.

24. Korsch BM, Gozzi EK, Francis V. Gaps in doctor–patient communication. I. Doctor-patient interaction and patient satisfaction. *Pediatrics* 1968;**42**:855–70.

25. Ong LM, de Haes JC, Hoos AM, Lammes FB. Doctor-patient communication: a review of the literature. *Soc Sci Med* 1995;**40**:903–18.

26. Partridge MR, Hill SR. Enhancing care for people with asthma: the role of communication, education, training and self-management. 1998 World Asthma Meeting Education and Delivery of Care Working Group. *Eur Respir J* 2000;**16**:333–48.

27. Fallowfield L. The ideal consultation. *Br J Hosp Med* 1992;**47**:364–7.

28. Stewart MA. Effective physician–patient communication and health outcomes: a review [see comments]. *CMAJ* 1995;**152**:1423–33.

29. Roter DL, Hall JA, Kern DE, Barker LR, Cole KA, Roca RP. Improving physicians' interviewing skills and reducing patients' emotional distress. A randomized clinical trial. *Arch Intern Med* 1995;**155**:1877–84.

30. Clark NM, Gong M, Schork MA, *et al.* Impact of education for physicians on patient outcomes. *Pediatrics* 1998;**101**:831–6.

31. Asthma management in minority children. Practical insights for clinicians, researchers and public health planners. *NIH Publication* No. 96-3675. National Institutes of Health, Bethesda, MD, 1995.

32. Lewis CC, Pantell RH, Sharp L. Increasing patient knowledge, satisfaction, and involvement: randomized trial of a communication intervention. *Pediatrics* 1991;**88**:351–8.

33. Clark NM, Starr Schneidkraut NJ. Management of asthma by patients and families. *Am J Respir Crit Care Med* 1994;**149**:S54–S66.

34. Kohler CL, Davies SL, Bailey WC. How to implement an asthma education program. *Clin Chest Med* 1995;**16**:557–65.

35. Lewis M, Lewis C. Consequences of empowering children to care for themselves. *Pediatrician* 1990; **17**:63–7.

36. Clark NM, Feldman CH, Evans D, Wasilewski Y, Levison MJ. Changes in children's school performance as a result of education for family management of asthma. *J Sch Health* 1984;**54**:143–5.

37. Gibson PG, Shah S, Mamoon HA. Peer-led asthma education for adolescents: impact evaluation. *J Adolesc Health* 1998;**22**:66–72.

38. Lewis CE, Rachelefsky G, Lewis MA, de la SA, Kaplan M. A randomized trial of A.C.T. (asthma care training) for kids. *Pediatrics* 1984;**74**:478–86.

39. Wilson SR. Individual versus group education: Is one better? *Patient Educ Counseling* 1997;**32**:S67–S75.

40. Colland VT. Learning to cope with asthma: a behavioural self-management program for children. *Patient Educ Couns* 1993;**22**:141–52.

41. Ronchetti R, Indinnimeo L, Bonci E, Corrias A, Evans D, Hindi-Alexander M, *et al.* Asthma self-management programmes in a population of Italian children: a multicentric study. Italian Study Group on Asthma Self-Management Programmes. *Eur Respir J* 1997; **10**:1248–53.

42. Madge P, McColl JH, Paton JY. Impact of a nurse-led home-management training programme in children admitted to hospital with acute asthma: a randomised controlled trial. *Thorax* 1997;**52**:223–8.

43. Wesseldine LJ, McCarthy P, Silverman M. Structured discharge procedure for children admitted to hospital with acute asthma: a randomised controlled trial of nursing practice. *Arch Dis Child* 1999;**80**:110–14.

44. Bailey WC, Richards JMJ, Brooks CM, Soong SJ, Windsor RA, Manzella BA. A randomized trial to improve self-management practices of adults with asthma. *Arch Intern Med* 1990;**150**:1664–8.

45. Wilson SR. Patient and physician behavior models related to asthma care. *Med Care* 1993;**31**:MS49–60.

46. Kohler CL, Dolce JJ, Manzella BA, *et al.* Use of focus group methodology to develop an asthma self-management program useful for community-based medical practices. *Health Educ Q* 1993; **20**:421–9.

47. Grimshaw JM, Russell IT. Achieving health gain through clinical guidelines II: Ensuring guidelines

change medical practice. *Qual Health Care* 1994;**3**:45–52.

48. Clark NM, Nothwehr F. Self-management of asthma by adult patients. *Patient Educ Couns* 1997;**32**:S5–S20.

49. Bradley C, Riaz A. Barriers to effective care in inner city general practices. *Eur J Gen Pract* 1998;**4**:65–8.

50. Parcel GS, Nader PR, Tiernan K. A health education program for children with asthma. *J Dev Behav Pediatr* 1980;**1**:128–32.

51. Evans D, Clark NM, Feldman CH, *et al*. A school health education program for children with asthma aged 8–11 years. *Health Educ Q* 1987; **14**:267–79.

52. Meredith P, Emberton M, Wood C. New directions in information for patients. *Br Med J* 1995;**311**:4–5.

53. Dennis KE. Patients' control and the information imperative: clarification and confirmation. *Nursing Res* 1990;**39**:162–6.

54. Clark CR. Creating information messages for health care procedures. *Patient Educ Couns* 1997; **30**:162–6.

55. Kai J. Parents' difficulties and information needs in coping with acute illness in preschool children: a qualitative study. *Br Med J* 1996;**313**:987–90.

56. Doust JA, Morgan TN, Weller BJ, Yuill BJ. Patient desire for information before a total hip replacement operation. *Med J Aust* 1989;**151**:201–3.

57. Morris LA, Kanouse DE. Consumer reactions to the tone of written drug information. *Am J Hosp Pharm* 1981;**38**:667–71.

58. Howland JS, Barker MG, Pie T. Does patient education cause side effects? A controlled trial. *J Fam Pract* 1990;**31**:62–4.

59. Wyatt JC. Information for patients. *J R Soc Med* 2000;**93**:467–71.

60. Charnock D, Shepperd S. DISCERN Online – quality criteria for consumer health information. http://www.discern.org.uk/. 1999.

61. Jadad AR, Gagliardi A. Rating health information on the internet; navigating to knowledge or babel? *JAMA* 1998;**279**:611–14.

62. Kim P, Eng TR, Deering MJ, Maxfield A. Published criteria for evaluating health related web sites: review. *Br Med J* 1999;**318**:647–9.

63. Communicating with patients who have limited literacy skills. Report of the National Work Group on Literacy and Health. *J Fam Pract* 1998; **46**:168–76.

64 Graber MA, Roller CM, Kaeble B. Readability levels of patient education material on the World Wide Web. *J Fam Pract* 1999;**48**:58–61.

65. Davis TC, Mayeaux EJ, Fredrickson D, Bocchini JAJ, Jackson RH, Murphy PW. Reading ability of parents compared with reading level of pediatric patient education materials. *Pediatrics* 1994; **93**:460–8.

66. Doak CC, Doak LG, Rook JH. *Teaching Patients with Low Literacy Skills*, 2nd edn. J.B. Lippincott, Philadelphia, 1996.

67. Spadaro DC, Robinson LA, Smith LT. Assessing readability of patient information materials. *Am J Hosp Pharm* 1980;**37**:215–21.

68. Flesch FR. A new readability yardstick. *J Appl Psychol* 1948;**32**:221–33.

69. Mayberry JF, Mayberry MK. Effective instructions for patients. *J R Coll Physicians Lond* 1996;30:205–8.

70. Raynor DK, Yerassimou N. Medicines information – leaving blind people behind? *Br Med J* 1997; **315**:268.

71. Osman LM, Abdalla MI, Beattie JA, *et al*. Reducing hospital admission through computer supported education for asthma patients. Grampian Asthma Study of Integrated Care (GRASSIC) [see comments]. *Br Med J* 1994;**308**:568–71.

72. Farrell-Miller P, Gentry P. How effective are your patient education materials? Guidelines for developing and evaluating written educational materials. *Diabetes Educ* 1989;**15**:418–22.

73. Doak LG, Doak CC, Meade CD. Strategies to improve cancer education materials. *Oncol Nurs Forum* 1996;**23**:1305–12.

74. Payne S, Large S, Jarrett N, Turner P. Written information given to patients and families by palliative care units: a national survey. *Lancet* 2000;**355**:1792.

75. See it Right Pack. 31-1-2001. London, Royal National Institute for the Blind.

76. Ignacio-Garcia JM, Gonzalez-Santos P. Asthma self-management education program by home monitoring of peak expiratory flow. *Am J Respir Crit Care Med* 1995;**151**:353–9.

77. Lahdensuo A, Haahtela T, Herrala J, *et al*. Randomised comparison of guided self management and traditional treatment of asthma over one year. *Br Med J* 1996;**312**:748–52.

78. Dickinson J, Hutton S, Atkin A. Implementing the British Thoracic Society's guidelines: the effect of a nurse-run asthma clinic on prescribed treatment in an English general practice. *Respir Med* 1998; **92**:264–7.

79. Dickinson J, Hutton S, Atkin A, Jones K. Reducing asthma morbidity in the community: the effect of a targeted nurse-run asthma clinic in an English general practice. *Respir Med* 1997;**91**:634–40.

80. Neville RG, Hoskins G, Smith B, Clark RA. Observations on the structure, process and clinical outcomes of asthma care in general practice [see comments]. *Br J Gen Pract* 1996;**46**:583–7.

81. Lang DM, Sherman MS, Polansky M. Guidelines and realities of asthma management. The Philadelphia story. *Arch Intern Med* 1997;**157**:1193–200.

82. Clark NM, Gong M, Schork MA, Kaciroti N, Evans D, Roloff D, Hurwitz M, Maiman LA, Mellins RB.

Long-term effects of asthma education for physicians on patient satisfaction and use of health services. *Eur Respir J* 2000;**16**:15–21.

83. Feldman CH, Clark NM, Evans D. The role of health education in medical management of asthma.

Some program applications. *Clin Rev Allergy* 1987;**5**:195–205.

84. Parker SR, Mellins RB, Sogn DD. NHLBI workshop summary. Asthma education: a national strategy. *Am Rev Respir Dis* 1989;**140**:848–53.

Appendix: Reference data

ISOBEL M BROOKES

LUNG FUNCTION

Introduction

Interpretation of lung function tests requires knowledge of the expected or reference ('normal') range of values for a particular patient. For this reason reference values are generated to summarize the distribution of lung function indices in different populations. An extensive literature exists concerning reference values in both children and adults, reflecting the fact that no single reference population is appropriate for laboratories throughout the world.

A comprehensive review of lung function testing in children, and reference values from previously published data, can be found in 'Standardization of Lung Function Tests in Paediatrics' prepared by a working group of the European Society for Clinical Respiratory Physiology (SEPCR).[1] Reference values given below for lung function in school-age children are largely taken from a published cross-sectional study of 772 healthy Caucasian United Kingdom school-children over the age range 4–19 years.[2,3]

Sources of variability in lung function measurements

Like all physiological measurements, lung function measurements are subject to variability, both within and between patients, even in the absence of disease. Technical variability results from differences in equipment and procedures. Biological variability exists both within an individual (diurnal and seasonal differences) and between individuals (size, age, race, sex, and environmental factors) and may be the focus of epidemiological or research studies.

The identification of variability due to disease is the focus of clinical measurements. In generating reference values the aim should be to minimize technical variation and account for biological variation. Many regression equations have been formulated which use an independent biological variable such as height to predict the dependent variable, such as FEV_1. The disadvantage of this approach is that a single predicted value is obtained, without any measure of the expected spread of values for a person of that height. Ideally results of lung function test should be reported as a z-score (deviation from the expected value in standard deviations), rather than '% predicted'.

Selection of reference values

It should always be borne in mind that reference values for any index of lung function merely represent data pertaining to a sample of the population. Consideration must therefore be given to the characteristics of the reference population and their relationship to the study population. The reason for performing the test should always be borne in mind, whether it is in screening a healthy population for early signs of disease, or monitoring response to therapy in patients already diagnosed with asthma.

Undue reliance on a test result as conclusive evidence for a particular disease is unwarranted. In addition to the absolute values obtained, the sensitivity and specificity of the test being conducted must be considered (Table A1), along with its repeatability and relevance to the pathophysiology of the disease process under consideration. For clinicians faced with individual patients and their results, the predictive value of a positive or negative test result may be

Table A.1 *Classification of results in relation to true status*

True Status	Test results	
	Positive	**Negative**
Positive	True positive	False negative
Negative	False positive	True negative
Sensitivity:	True positive/(true positive+false negative)	
Specificity:	True negative/(true negative+false positive)	
Predictive value of a positive result:	True positive/(true positive+false positive)	
Predictive value of a negative result:	True negative/(true negative+false negative)	

Table A.2 *Range of mean values for within-subject coefficient of variation (%) for lung function measurements on healthy children during a single test session[4]*

PEF	FEV_1	$FEV_{0.75}$	MEF_{50}
2–6.7	2.7–4.8	5.4	5–12
MEF_{25}	MMEF	VC	FRC_{He}
7.9–11.3	4.6–8.1	2.9–4.0	4.0–7.0

more informative. The prevalence of a disease in the population will have a marked effect on the predictive value of a test, even when the sensitivity and specificity are the same.

In general, claims concerning the *diagnostic sensitivity and specificity* of tests (for bronchial hyperresponsiveness, for example) are wildly exaggerated, because of selection bias in the populations studied. If a test is developed to distinguish severe, atopic, hospital-managed asthma on the one hand, from healthy, symptom-free, non-atopic children, it cannot be expected to provide diagnostic answers in children with borderline symptoms, who fall into the 'grey area' of diagnosis.

The *repeatability* of a test is usually determined by the agreement between duplicate measurements made shortly after each other in healthy subjects. This is obviously important for interpretation of test results and the range of reported percentage coefficients of variation for a number of lung function measurements are given in Table A2.[4] In disease, variability almost always increases.

Selected indices, definitions and reference values for school-children

PEAK EXPIRATORY FLOW (PEF) (1/s)

The maximal flow during a forced expiratory vital capacity manoeuvre commencing from a position of full inspiration.[2]

Sex	Standing height (cm)	Regression equation for predicted mean
M	<162.6	−5.98 + 0.073 Ht
	>162.5	−13.14 + 0.125 Ht
F	<152.6	−6.79 + 0.079 Ht
	>152.5	−3.94 + 0.064 Ht

FORCED EXPIRATORY VOLUME (FEV_t)

The timed forced expiratory volume is the volume of gas exhaled in a specified time (t) from the start of the forced vital capacity manoeuvre. The time interval used conventionally is one second, yielding FEV_1. Healthy children under 6–8 years of age, however, may often exhale a complete vital capacity in less than one second. For this group, $FEV_{0.75}$ is more applicable.

FEV_1 (l)

Sex	Standing height (cm)	Regression equation for predicted mean (Figure A1)[2]
M	<162.6	−2.78 + 0.03425 Ht
	>162.5	−5.108 + 0.0521 Ht
F	<152.6	−2.734 + 0.03316 Ht
	>152.5	−3.680 + 0.04112 Ht

$FEV_{0.75}$ (ml)

Sex	Standing height (cm)	Regression equation for predicted mean[5]
M	100–155	−2297 + 30.0 Ht
F	100–155	−2363 + 30.0 Ht

MAXIMAL EXPIRATORY FLOW AT A SPECIFIED LUNG VOLUME (MEF_X)

The expiratory flow achieved at the designated lung volume during a forced expiratory manoeuvre from full inspiration.

MEF_{50} (l/s) – maximum expiratory flow at 50% of FVC

Sex	Standing height (cm)	Regression equation for predicted mean[2]
M	<162.6	−2.91 + 0.040 Ht
	>162.5	−3.38 + 0.048 Ht
F	<152.6	−3.03 + 0.041 Ht
	>152.5	0.49 + 0.023 Ht

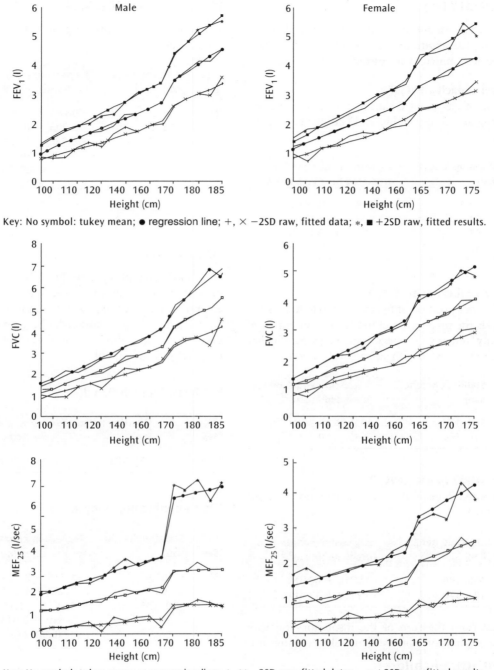

Key: No symbol: tukey mean; ● regression line; +, × −2SD raw, fitted data; *, ■ +2SD raw, fitted results.

Key: No symbol: tukey mean; □ regression line; +, × −2SD raw, fitted data; *, ● +2SD raw, fitted results.

Figure A.1 *Tukey mean (2 SD) results for FEV$_1$, FVC and MEF$_{25}$ related to standing height in males and females together with the fitted mean and SD lines.*

MEF$_{25}$ (l/s) – maximum expiratory flow when 25% of FVC remains to be exhaled

Sex	Standing height (cm)	Regression equation for predicted mean (Figure A1)[2]
M	<162.6	−0.948 + 0.0158 Ht
	>162.5	0.218 + 0.00074 Ht
F	<152.6	−0.807 + 0.015 Ht
	>152.5	−2.12 + 0.027 Ht

Maximal mid expiratory flow (MMEF, FEF$_{25-75\%}$) (l/s)

The mean forced expiratory flow during the middle half of the forced vital capacity (FVC).

Sex	Standing height (cm)	Regression equation for predicted mean[6]
M and F	111–183 cm	−4.38 + 0.05 Ht ± 32.9%

VITAL CAPACITY (VC)

The volume change at the mouth moving from full inspiration to complete expiration (Figure 6b.1, Chapter 6b). This can be determined in any one of the following ways:

Forced vital capacity (FVC) (l)

The volume of gas exhaled during a forced expiration commencing at full inspiration and ending at complete expiration.

Sex	Standing height (cm)	Regression equation for predicted mean (Figure A1)[2]
M	<162.6	$-3.619 + 0.0429\,Ht$
	>162.5	$-7.038 + 0.0678\,Ht$
F	<152.6	$-3.311 + 0.03918\,Ht$
	>152.5	$-3.881 + 0.04512\,Ht$

Inspiratory vital capacity (IVC) (l)

Measured from a position of full expiration to full inspiration. This is the preferred method for measurement of vital capacity in many European centres, giving a higher value than FVC in those with airway obstruction.

Sex	Standing height (cm)	Regression equation for predicted mean[7,8]
M	103–177	$3958 \times 10^{-6}\,Ht^{2.708}$
F	110–162	$1645 \times 10^{-6}\,Ht^{2.86}$

Expiratory vital capacity (EVC) (l)

Measured from full inspiration to full expiration without maximal effort.

Sex	Standing height (cm)	Regression equation for predicted mean[9]
M	100–190	$-5710 + 60\,Ht$
F	105–176	$-4420 + 49\,Ht$

Determined from the sum of the inspiratory capacity (IC) and the expiratory reserve volume (ERV) (Figure 6b.1, Chapter 6b).

Sex	Standing height (cm)	Regression equation for predicted mean[10]
M	110–170	$3722 \times 10^{-6}\,Ht^{2.70}$
F	110–170	$1549 \times 10^{-6}\,Ht^{2.86}$

FEV/FVC

Sex	Regression equation for predicted mean[2]
M	$1 - 0.001\,Ht$ (cm)
F	$1.04 - 0.00098\,Ht$

RESIDUAL VOLUME (RV) (l)

The volume of gas remaining in the lung at the end of a full expiration.

Sex	Standing height (cm)	Regression equation for predicted mean[3]
M	<162.6	$-0.283 + 0.00818\,Ht$
	>162.5	$-3.905 + 0.03095\,Ht$
F	110–175	$610.323 - 20.91427\,Ht$ $+ (0.28586128 \times Ht^2)$ $- (1.94588828 \times 10^{-3} \times H^3)$ $+ (6.594203 \times 10^{-6} \times Ht^4)$ $- (8.8899 \times 10^{-9} \times Ht^5)$

LUNG VOLUME

Functional residual capacity (FRC) is the volume of gas present in the lung and airways at the average end-expiratory level. It is equal to the sum of the expiratory reserve and residual volume. May be determined by a 'gas dilution' method, nitrogen washout, whole body plethysmography or radiography.

FRC by helium dilution (l)

Sex	Standing height (cm)	Regression equation for predicted mean[6]
M and F	111–183	$0.067 \times e^{0.021 \times ht}$

FRC by plethysmography (l)

Sex	Standing height (cm)	Regression equation for predicted mean[3]
M	<162.6	$-1.716 + 0.02394\,Ht$
	>162.5	$-7.036 + 0.05918\,Ht$
F	110–175	$-33.928 + 1.1478 \times Ht - (0.0136745 \times Ht^2) + (6.9822757 \times 10^{-5} \times Ht^3) - (1.2725216 \times 10^{-7} \times Ht^4)$

Total lung capacity (TLC) is the volume of gas in the lung at the end of a full inspiration. Calculated from sum of FRC + IC or the sum of RV + IVC.

Sex	Standing height (cm)	Regression equation for predicted mean[2]
M	<162.6	$-3.828 + 0.04976\,Ht$
F	>162.5	$-10.648 + 0.09586\,Ht$
	110–175	$-234.078 + 7.03067\,Ht - (0.07802979 \times Ht^2) + (3.8100528 \times 10^{-4} \times Ht^3) - (6.859791 \times 10^{-7} \times Ht^4)$

The effects of ethnic origin

Ethnic differences in predicted lung function have been attributed to differences in body proportions. For instance, the ratio of trunk to standing height is smaller in the Afro-Caribbean population than in Caucasians. The use of sitting height related to lung function or the use of the FVC as a surrogate measure of lung size has been advocated as a way of minimizing such apparent differences for predictive purposes.[11] Most of these studies have been carried out in the United States and there are few comparative data available on ethnic variation in lung function in Europe. Significant differences have, however, been noted between European, African and South Asian children studied in the UK, suggesting that separate reference ranges should be developed.[12,13] Both studies demonstrated lower height adjusted values for FEV_1 and FVC in children of South Asian and Afro-Caribbean origin compared with those of European origin. The differences ranged between 8–13%.

The effects of gender and puberty

Gender has a variable effect upon comparative lung function indices between boys and girls, which seems to begin in infancy.[16] This is also the case for measurements of forced expiratory flow made in infancy. Gender is also important at the time of puberty[2] due to the differences in age at which the pubertal growth spurt occurs. The pubertal increase in height precedes the increase in chest dimensions in puberty. The increase in vital capacity in boys may continue after maximal height is achieved.[22] The use of simple regression equations derived from either adult or paediatric patients may be misleading during adolescence. An equation based on developmental rather than chronological age would be ideal, but none is available to date.

Under a height of 152.6 cm no difference was demonstrated between the sexes in the relationship between PEF, MEF_{50} and MEF_{25} and height. Boys, however, had significantly higher values of FEV_1 and FVC (Table A3). For the same height girls had higher values than boys for all spirometric measurements apart from FVC during the

Table A.3 *The mean percentage differences between boys and girls for certain spirometric variables related to standing height[2]*

Height	107.6–152.5 cm	152.5–162.5 cm
Gender	Males greater than females by:	Females greater than males by:
PEF	0	+7.4%
FEV_1	+6%	+7.4%
FVC	+8.5%	0
MEF_{50}	0	+19%
MEF_{25}	0	+36%

period of their pubertal growth spurt over the height range 152.6–162.5 cm but the boys subsequently achieved higher values, the difference increasing thereafter (Table A3, Figure A2).

Infant lung function

Infant lung function measurements are usually carried out under sedation in specialist centres, and in general are much less standardized than those in older more co-operative children. This has made obtaining reference data extremely difficult, although many groups have published 'normative' data which are specific to their population, equipment and precise methodology.

The *rapid thoraco-abdominal compression technique* has been used widely to generate partial forced expiratory manoeuvres and determine maximal flow at functional residual capacity ($V'_{max}FRC$), a measure of peripheral airway function.[14,15]

Recently a multicentre group have collated data on 459 healthy infants measured using similar methods during the first 20 months of life.[16] This is the largest number of healthy infants used to derive reference data for $V'_{max}FRC$.

For the first time sex specific regression equations were recommended, based on length in cm (or age) for predicting $V'_{max}FRC$. (Girls were found to have flows approximately 20% higher than boys during the first 9 months of life.)

For boys:

$$V'_{max}FRC = (4.22 + 0.00210 \times length^2)^2$$

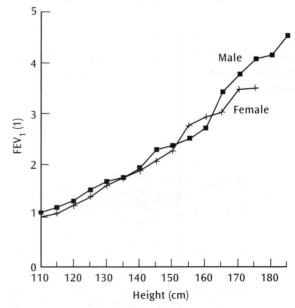

Figure A.2 *Tukey mean results for FEV₁ in males and females. Note the three phases: 107.6–152.6 cm boys have higher values, 152.6–162.5 cm lower values and thereafter higher values again (from ref. 2 with permission).*

For girls:

$$V'_{max}FRC = (-1.23 + 0.0242 \times length)^2$$

Z scores (the number of standard deviations that a value deviates from the mean expected value) were also calculated. These allow the high variability of $V'_{max}FRC$ in healthy infants to be taken into account, when reporting individual results. A range of 0 ± 2 Z scores, can be used as a normal range (see Figure A3).

Preschool children

In recent years there has been increasing interest in measuring lung function in this age group. One technique that has proved popular is *resistance by interruption (Rint)*. Several commercially available systems exist which may not produce comparable data. Two groups have recently published similar reference equations for Rint in healthy preschool children, based on height[17,18] (Figure A4). Each group used a different version of equipment made by the same manufacturer (Micromedical, UK). When using reference data to interpret Rint measurements care must be taken to ensure the equipment, procedure and analysis methods are the same.

NON-INVASIVE MARKERS OF AIRWAY INFLAMMATION

Induced sputum: eosinophils

The analysis of cell counts of induced sputum is a well established research tool in asthma research in adults. Sputum is usually induced by inhalation of hypertonic saline. In healthy controls the dominant cell is the macrophage, in asthma the eosinophil count is raised and increased numbers of desquamated bronchial epithelial cells are seen.[23] Recently published reference data[24,25] comparing healthy children with those with asthma included the following:

	Median eosinophil differential count (interquartile range) (%)
Healthy children	
Newcastle, Australia	
$n = 72$	0.3(0–1.05)
Hammersmith Hospital,	
London $n = 17$	0(0–0)
Children with asthma	
Newcastle, Australia	
$n = 42$	4.3(1.5–14.1)
Controlled asthma	
(*on inhaled corticosteroid*)	2.5(0.75–1.5)
Symptomatic asthma	3.8(2.4–15.1)
Acute exacerbation	8.5(1.5–20.0)
Hammersmith Hospital,	
London $n = 36$	0.02(0–1.3)

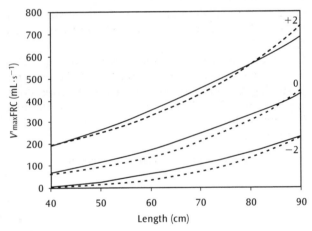

Figure A.3 *Predicted $V'_{max}FRC$ Z scores (0 ± 2 SD) for boys (dashed lines) and girls (solid lines) plotted against length. (From ref. 16.)*

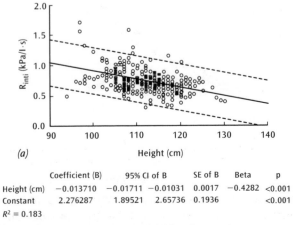

(a)

	Coefficient (B)	95% CI of B		SE of B	Beta	p
Height (cm)	−0.013710	−0.01711	−0.01031	0.0017	−0.4282	<0.001
Constant	2.276287	1.89521	2.65736	0.1936		<0.001

$R^2 = 0.183$

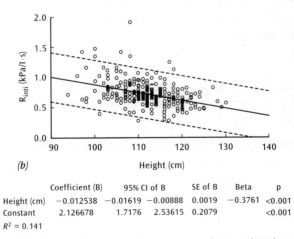

(b)

	Coefficient (B)	95% CI of B		SE of B	Beta	p
Height (cm)	−0.012538	−0.01619	−0.00888	0.0019	−0.3761	<0.001
Constant	2.126678	1.7176	2.53615	0.2079		<0.001

$R^2 = 0.141$

Figure A.4 *Linear regression of (a) inspiratory interrupter resistance (R_{inti}) and (b) expiratory interrupter resistance (R_{inte}) versus height. The solid line indicates the regression line and dashed lines indicate the 95% prediction interval. (From Ref. 18.)*

Both studies showed significantly increased eosinophil differential counts in the sputum of asthmatic children, compared with controls. Atopic children were not excluded from either control group. Only 56% of patients aged 5–15 years tested in the London study were able to produce a satisfactory sample for analysis. When individual eosinophil counts were related to current symptom score or lung function, no relationship could be found.

Exhaled nitric oxide

Exhaled nitric oxide has been demonstrated to be a non-specific marker of inflammation in asthma in adults and children. It is elevated in asthmatics who are not receiving inhaled steroids, during acute exacerbations and after allergen challenge in susceptible individuals.[23] Several methodological options are available for measurement of eNO, and data from each are not comparable.[26]

Recently reference data from healthy children aged 6–15 years were published. The tidal breathing method was used, with nitric oxide levels measured on line using chemilumescence.[27] The authors recommended that each laboratory establishes its own reference values.

REFERENCE DATA FOR SERUM IMMUNOGLOBULINS

Total serum immunoglobulin levels: IgG, IgA and IgE

PRESCHOOL CHILDREN (AGED 6–72 MONTHS)

IgG (g/l)[19]

Square root of mean IgG
$$= 1.16 + 0.2715 \text{ age} - 0.01195 \text{ age}^2 \text{ (mths)}$$
$$SD = 0.45 - 0.00550 \text{ age} + 0.0000945 \text{ age}^2$$

IgA (g/l)[19]

Log mean IgA $= -1.92 + 0.03975 \text{ age}$
$$- 0.0002155 \text{ age}^2 \text{ (mths)}$$

$$SD = 0.658 + 0.0003166 \text{ age} - 0.00002374 \text{ age}^2$$

IgE[20]

Age	Median total serum IgE (U)	95th Centile
Newborn	0.5	5
3 months	3	11
1 year	8	29
5 years	15	52

SCHOOL-CHILDREN

Total serum IgG and IgA[19]

Age (years)	IgG (g/l)	IgA (g/l)
6–9	9.9 (5.4–16.1)	1.3 (0.5–2.4)
9–12	9.9 (5.4–16.1)	1.4 (0.7–2.5)
12–15	9.9 (5.4–16.1)	1.9 (0.8–2.8)

Median ± 95% confidence interval.

Total serum IgE[20]

Age	Total serum IgE (U)	95th Centile
10	18	63
Adult	26	120

IgG Subclasses[21]

PRESCHOOL CHILDREN

Data on three primary subclasses, IgG-1 to IgG-3, from 215 healthy children aged from 6 months to 6 years (Figures A5–7).

IgG-1   Mean IgG-1 $= 3.624 + 0.4428 \text{ age (years)}$
$SD = 2.166 - 0.3797 \text{ age} + 0.06274 \text{ age}^2$

IgG-2   Log mean IgG-2 $= -0.7502 + 0.4377 \text{ age}$
$+ 0.05667 \text{ age}^2$
$SD = 0.541 - 0.09016 \text{ age} + 0.01756 \text{ age}^2$

IgG-3   Log mean IgG-3 $= -1.16$
$SD = 0.4307 - 0.05073 + 0.009497 \text{ age}^2$

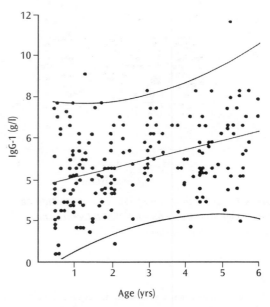

Figure A.5 *Scatter diagram of IgG-1 concentration against age, with age-specific mean and 95% reference range (from ref. 20 with permission).*

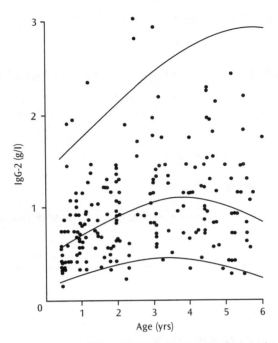

Figure A.6 *Scatter diagram of IgG-2 concentration against age, with age-specific mean and 95% reference range (from ref. 20 with permission).*

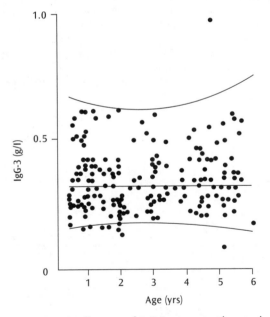

Figure A.7 *Scatter diagram of IgG-3 concentration against age, with age-specific mean and 95% reference range (from ref. 20 with permission).*

IgG-4

Such wide variations were seen in IgG-4 levels in this population that a normal range could not be constructed.

SCHOOL-CHILDREN[20]

Age (years)	IgG-1	IgG-2	IgG-3	IgG-4
10	5.2 (3.6–7.3)	2.6 (1.4–4.5)	0.7 (0.3–1.1)	0.4 (<0.1–1.0)
15	5.4 (3.8–7.7)	2.6 (1.3–4.6)	0.7 (0.2–1.2)	0.4 (<0.1–1.1)

Median (g/l) (5th–95th centile).

REFERENCES

1. European Respiratory Society for Clinical Respiratory Physiology. Report of the working party on standardization of lung function tests in paediatrics. *Eur Respir J* 1989;**2**:117s–265s.
2. Rosenthal M, Bain SH, Cramer D, *et al.* Lung function in white children aged 4 to 19 years. I Spirometry. *Thorax* 1993;**48**:794–802.
3. Rosenthal M, Cramer D, Bain SH, *et al.* Lung function in white children aged 4 to 19 years. II Single breath analysis and plethysmography. *Thorax* 1993;**48**:803–8.
4. Quanjer PH, Stocks J, Polgar G, *et al.* Compilation of reference values for lung function measurements in children. *Eur Respir J* 1989;**2**:184s–261s.
5. Lunn JE. Respiratory measurements of 3556 Sheffield schoolchildren. *Br J Prev Soc Med* 1965;**19**:115–21.
6. Weng TR, Levison H. Standards of pulmonary function in children. *Am Rev Respir Dis* 1969;**99**:879–94.
7. Guerini C, Pistelli G, Paci A, Taddeucci G, Dalle Luche A. Pulmonary volumes in children. I Normal values in males of 6–15 years old. *Bull Eur Physiopathol Respir* 1970;**6**:701–19.
8. Pistelli G, Paci A, Dalle Luche A, Giuntini C. Pulmonary volumes in children. 11 Normal values in female children 6–15 years old. *Bull Eur Physiopathol Respir* 1978;**14**:513–23.
9. Godfrey S, Kamburoff PL, Nairn JL. Spirometry, lung volumes and airway resistance in normal children aged 5 to 18 years. *Br J Dis Chest* 1970;**64**:15–24.
10. Geubelle F, Breny H. Volumes pulmonaires d'enfants sains, ages de 5 a 16 ans. *Le Poumon et le Coeur* 1969;**25**:1051–64.
11. Schwartz J, Katz SA, Fegley RW, Tockman MS. Sex and race differences in the development of lung function. *Am Rev Respir Dis* 1988;**138**:1415–21.
12. Johnston LDA, Bland JM, Anderson HR. Ethnic variation in respiratory morbidity and lung function in childhood. *Thorax* 1987;**42**:542–8.
13. Patrik JM, Patel A. Ethnic differences in the growth of lung function in children: a cross sectional study in Inner City Nottingham. *Ann Hum Biol* 1986; **13**:307–15.

14. Hanrahan JP, Tager LB, Castile RG, *et al*. Pulmonary function measures in healthy infants. Variability and size correction. *Am Rev Respir Dis* 1990;**134**:513–19.

15. Sly PD, Tepper R, Henschen, Gappa M, Stocks J. Tidal forced expirations. ERS/ATS Task Force on Standards for Infant Respiratory Function Testing. European Respiratory Society/American Thoracic Society. *Eur Respir J* 2000;**16**:741–8.

16. Hoo A, Dezateux C, Hanrahan JP, Cole TJ, Tepper RS, Stocks J. Sex-specific prediction equations for $V'_{max}FRC$ in infancy: a multicentre collaborative study. *Am J Respir Crit Care Med* 2002;**165(8)**:1084–92.

17. Merkus PJ, Mijnsbergen JY, Hop WC, de Jongste JC. Interrupter resistance in preschool children: measurement characteristics and reference values. *Am J Respir Crit Care Med* 2001;**163**:1350–5.

18. Lombardi E, Sly PD, Concutelli G, *et al*. Reference values of interrupter respiratory resistance in healthy preschool white children. *Thorax* 2001; **56**:691–5.

19. Isaacs D, Altman DG, Tidmarsh CE, Walman HB, Webster ADB. Serum immunoglobulin concentrations in preschool children measured by laser nephelometry: reference ranges for IgG, IgA, IgM. *J Clin Pathol* 1983;**36**:1193–6.

20. Hinchliffe RF. Reference values. In: JS Lilleyman, LM Hann, eds. *Paediatric Haematology*. Churchill Livingstone, Edinburgh, 1992, pp. 1–22.

21. Bird D, Duffy S, Isaacs D, Webster ADB. Reference ranges for IgG subclasses in preschool children. *Arch Dis Child* 1985;**60**:204–7.

22. Official Statement of the American Thoracic Society. Lung Function testing: selection of reference values and interpretative strategies. *Am Rev Respir Disease* 1991;**144**:1202–18.

23. Gibson PG, Henry RL, Thomas P. Noninvasive assessment of airway inflammation in children: induced sputum, exhaled nitric oxide, and breath condensate. Review 65 refs. *Eur Respir J* 2000; **16**:1008–15.

24. Cai Y, Carty K, Henry RL, Gibson PG. Persistence of sputum eosinophilia in children with controlled asthma when compared with healthy children. *Eur Respir J* 1998;**11**:848–53.

25. Wilson NM, Bridge P, Spanevello A, Silverman M. Induced sputum in children: feasibility, repeatability, and relation of findings to asthma severity. *Thorax* 2000;**55**:768–74.

26. Kissoon N, Duckworth L, Blake K, Murphy S, Silkoff PE. Exhaled nitric oxide measurements in childhood asthma: techniques and interpretation. Review 132 refs. *Pediatr Pulmonol* 1999;**28**:282–96.

27. Baraldi E, Azzolin NM, Cracco A, Zacchello F. Reference values of exhaled nitric oxide for healthy children 6–15 years old. *Pediatr Pulmonol* 1999; **27**:54–8.

Index

References to figures are indicated by 'f' and references to tables are indicated by 't' when they fall on a page not covered by the text reference.